D1398326

OXYGEN TRANSPORT
TO TISSUE XV

ADVANCES IN EXPERIMENTAL MEDICINE AND BIOLOGY

Recent Volumes in this Series

OXYGEN TRANSPORT TO TISSUE XV

Edited by

Peter Vaupel
Rolf Zander

Johannes Gutenberg-Universität
Mainz, Germany

and

Duane F. Bruley

University of Maryland Baltimore County
Baltimore, Maryland

PLENUM PRESS • NEW YORK AND LONDON

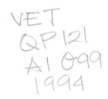

Library of Congress Cataloging-in-Publication Data

Oxygen transport to tissue XV / edited by Peter Vaupel, Rolf Zander,
and Duane F. Bruley.
    p.   cm. -- (Advances in experimental medicine and biology ; v.
345)
  Includes bibliographical references and index.
  "Proceedings of the Twentieth Annual Meeting of the International
Society on Oxygen Transport to Tissue, held August 26-30, 1992, in
Mainz, Germany"--T.p. verso.
  ISBN 0-306-44632-4
  1. Tissue respiration--Congresses. 2. Oxygen--Physiological
transport--Congresses. 3. Tumors--Pathophysiology--Congresses.
I. Vaupel, Peter. II. Zander, R. (Rolf) III. Bruley, Duane F.
IV. International Society on Oxygen Transport to Tissue. Meeting
(20th : 1992 : Mainz, Rhineland-Palatinate, Germany) V. Title:
Oxygen transport to tissue 15. VI. Title: Oxygen transport to
tissue fifteen. VII. Series.
  [DNLM: 1. Oxygen--blood--congresses. 2. Biological Transport-
-congresses. 3. Oxygen Consumption--congresses. W1 AD559 v.345
1993 / QV 312 09786 1993]
QP121.A1099 1993
599'.0113--dc20
DNLM/DLC
for Library of Congress   93-49074
                                            CIP

Proceedings of the twentieth annual meeting of the International Society on Oxygen Transport to Tissue, held August 26–30, 1992, in Mainz, Germany

ISBN 0-306-44632-4

©1994 Plenum Press, New York
A Division of Plenum Publishing Corporation
233 Spring Street, New York, N.Y. 10013

Printed in the United States of America

INTERNATIONAL SOCIETY ON OXYGEN TRANSPORT TO TISSUE
(1992)

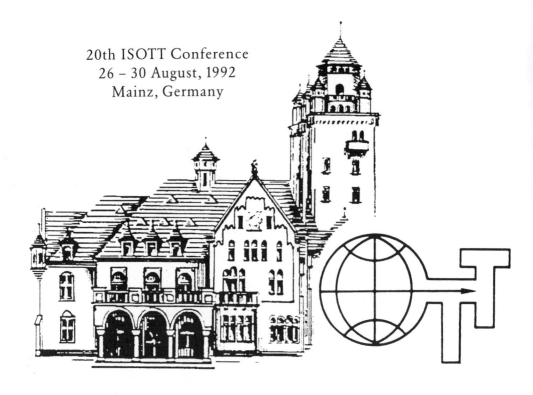

20th ISOTT Conference
26 – 30 August, 1992
Mainz, Germany

ORGANIZING COMMITTEE

Peter Vaupel, President ISOTT
Rolf Zander, Secretary General
Anne Deutschmann-Fleck
Sabine Bua
Debra Kelleher
Winfried Krüger
Anne Mertzlufft
Fritz Mertzlufft
Wolfgang Müller-Klieser
Lieselotte Vaupel
Stefan Walenta

We are most grateful for the financial support for the 1992 ISOTT Conference received from the following:

MAIN SPONSORS

NOVA biomedical
Radiometer Deutschland
Vinzenz von Paul Foundation

SPONSORS

Alliance
Andos
Bayer
Boehringer Ingelheim
Boehringer Mannheim
Braun-Melsungen
Byk-Gulden
Ciba Corning
Corotec
Eppendorf-Netheler-Hinz
Fresenius
Hamamatsu Deutschland
Hoechst
Hoyer
ICI
Immuno
Inner Space
Knoll
M.U.R.
Naglik
Nellcor
Pfrimmer
Schaper & Brümmer
Ulmcke

LIST OF EXHIBITORS

Abbott
Andos
AVL
Baxter
Ciba Corning
Drägerwerk
Eppendorf-Netheler-Hinz
Johnson & Johnson (Critikon)
Lawrenz
Medical Systems
M.U.R.
NOVA biomedical
Oxford Optronics
Physio B.V.
Radiometer Deutschland
Vinzenz von Paul Foundation/Sauter-Sulgen

PREFACE

Seventeen years after the 2nd International Symposium on Oxygen Transport to Tissue, which was held in Mainz in March 1975, the local Organizing Committee and the Board of ISOTT were pleased to host the ISOTT Conference in Mainz on the Rhine again. The venue of the 20th meeting was the prestigious, fully restored Schloss Waldthausen (Waldthausen Castle) which provided a special setting for ISOTT 1992. The beautiful front view of the castle became part of the ISOTT 1992 logo.

The 20th ISOTT Meeting was held in Mainz from August 26th through August 30th, 1992. The Conference attracted 200 active participants from 16 countries. The theme of this meeting emphasized oxygen transport to tumors but as in earlier meetings, essentially all aspects of oxygen transport within the body were covered as demonstrated by the manuscripts comprising this volume of the series "Oxygen Transport to Tissue".

All manuscripts were reviewed. Extensive revisions were made in about 25% and modest revision in about another 30%. Because we had to compromise between the aim of rapid publication on the one hand and the need for thorough review on the other, minor errors in format and some typographical errors were not corrected. Except for some revisions, all of the original camera-ready manuscripts in this volume were prepared by the authors themselves and we greatly appreciate their cooperation. We also wish to acknowledge the skillful, patient and careful work involved in the preparation of this volume by Drs. Debra Bickes-Kelleher and Winfried Krüger. The editors are most grateful to Mrs. Anne Deutschmann-Fleck and Sabine Bua for their assistance in editing the proceedings book. The local Committee also acknowledges the help of all staff members including scientists, technicians and family members without whom the 20th Conference would not have been possible.

We hope that the 1992 ISOTT Conference, like the 2nd International Symposium on Oxygen Transport to Tissue in 1975, is remembered by many members of the ISOTT family. The high scientific standard, the picturesque setting of the venue in the Rhine Valley with its castles and vineyards and the attractive social program provided fond memories both for the participants and their accompanying guests.

The editors congratulate Dr. H. Degens for the honour of being selected as the 1992 Melvin H. Knisely Award Winner for his excellent contributions in the area of research on oxygen transport to tissue.

On behalf of the editors this volume is dedicated to Professor Gerhard Thews as a sign of our sincere gratitude for his outstanding contributions to the world of science in the field of oxygen transport to tissue and on the occassion of his 67th birthday.

For the editors

Peter Vaupel

April, 1993

CONTENTS

SYMPOSIUM DEDICATED TO PROFESSOR THEWS

RESPIRATORY SYSTEM

OXYGEN TRANSPORT IN BLOOD, HYPERBARIC OXYGENATION

ARTIFICIAL OXYGEN CARRIERS IN BLOOD

HEART

OXYGEN SUPPLY TO TUMORS

BRAIN

SKELETAL MUSCLE AND OTHER TISSUES

O_2 CONSUMPTION VS. O_2 SUPPLY

METHODS AND MODELING

SYMPOSIUM DEDICATED TO PROFESSOR THEWS

PROFESSOR DR. DR. GERHARD THEWS: A LIFETIME'S DEDICATION TO RESEARCH ON OXYGEN TRANSPORT TO TISSUE AND ACADEMIC TEACHING

Peter Vaupel, ISOTT President 1992

Institute of Physiology and Pathophysiology
University of Mainz
Duesbergweg 6
D-6500 Mainz, Germany

As President of ISOTT 1992, and on behalf of the ISOTT Executive Committee I wish to dedicate the 20th ISOTT meeting and this volume of Advances in Experimental Medicine and Biology arising from it to Professor Gerhard Thews, as a sign of sincere gratitude for his outstanding contributions to the world of science in the area of oxygen transport to tissues. His innovative and productive work over the last 40 years has been documented in more than 200 scientific papers. These publications are distinguished by their ability to present sophisticated ideas in a simple and precise way. As a result, many of Professor Thews' works are recognized both nationally and internationally as "classics" in the fields of lung and tissue respiration, oxygen transport, and acid-base balance in the blood. The numerous scientific awards which have been presented to Professor Thews further demonstrate the significance of these scientific achievements.

As we gathered in Mainz for the 20th ISOTT meeting, we were all reminded of the important role that Gerhard Thews played as a charter member of the International Committee in the "first hours" of the International Society on Oxygen Transport to Tissue. Gerhard Thews was elected President of this young international society during its 1st International Symposium on Oxygen Transport to Tissue which was held in 1973 in Charleston and Clemson, SC (USA). On taking up this post, he followed in the footsteps of Dr. Melvin H. Knisely, one of the pioneers of microcirculation research, whose spirit is commemorated by the society even today, in the form of the M. Knisely Award for young scientists. Subsequent to his presidency, Gerhard Thews was a member of the ISOTT Executive Committee for many years.

The 2nd International Symposium on Oxygen Transport to Tissue, which was held in Mainz in March 1975 is remembered by many ISOTT members. The high scientific standard and the picturesque setting of this city in the Rhine Valley provided fond memories both for the participants and their accompanying guests.

Oxygen Transport to Tissue XV, Edited by P. Vaupel
et al., Plenum Press, New York, 1994

In the meantime, a new generation of scientists have successfully developed their own careers under the auspices of this "man of the first hour". Many of these scientists have chosen topics related to oxygen transport in living tissues as the focus of their research. As one of these scientists, it was a great honor for me, 17 years after the first meeting in Mainz, to be able to welcome the ISOTT family once again. At the start of this meeting, a special session was held which was also dedicated to Professor Thews. It was therefore fitting for me to present the participants with the following short biography of my mentor and "genius loci".

Gerhard Thews was born in 1926 in Koenigsberg. After finishing his schooling and military service, he and his family became refugees, expelled from their native East Prussia (now a part of Russia). He subsequently studied Physics and Medicine at the University of Kiel. His Physics studies ended in 1954 when he was awarded the title of Doctor of Natural Science, following which he worked as a Research Fellow in the Institute of Physiology at the University of Kiel. During his time in Kiel he qualified as a medical doctor and was awarded the title of Doctor of Medicine in 1957. In 1962 he became Associate Professor of Physiology at the University of Kiel, and only one year later was promoted to Full Professor. In 1963, the offer of a Chair in Physiology came from the University of Mainz. Since then, Gerhard Thews has been Chairman of this Department, despite numerous offers of attractive posts from other Institutions.

Besides receiving a series of scientific awards, his activities as a researcher were honored by his receiving full membership of the Academy of Science and Literature in Mainz. The recognition from this prestigious Academy has had a special meaning in Gerhard Thews' life. He held the post of Vice President from 1977 to 1985, and the post of President from 1985 to 1993.

As most readers of this volume well appreciate, an academic life involves not only research, but also teaching. As a former student of Gerhard Thews, I feel qualified to speak about his abilities in this sphere. His great didactic talents and enthusiasm for academic teaching are reflected in his engagement in student matters and the publication of several widely-used physiology textbooks, which have been translated into several languages. One special characteristic of Gerhard Thews as a University teacher which is remembered and appreciated by a vast number of students, is his pleasant, fair and motivating way of conducting examinations.

He was, and still is, perceived by his colleagues and students as a generous, innovative mentor who always had understanding and respect for them. Due to his broad academic background, Gerhard Thews was prepared to cross the traditional boundaries of physiology and to alert his colleagues to the clinical relevance of many physiological issues. It is therefore not surprising that some of his former assistants today hold leading positions at several hospitals. Two of his former students now hold Chairs in Physiology (J. Grote, University of Bonn) and Tumor Biology and Pathophysiology (P. Vaupel, Harvard Medical School and University of Mainz, respectively).

This short summary of Gerhard Thews' biography, has, I hope, given some insights into the exceptional energy and untiring dedication which distinguish the career of this multi-talented scientist and medical doctor. Those who have had the opportunity of knowing Gerhard Thews more closely have come to appreciate his logical thinking, personal charm and tolerance. Because of his manifold activities and his special personality, it seems inappropriate to say that Professor Gerhard Thews is 66 years old. Instead, it is more apt for us to congratulate him on being 66 years young!

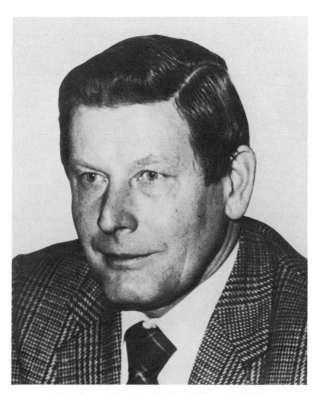

Professor Dr. Dr. Gerhard Thews, 1992

ALVEOLAR-CAPILLARY GAS TRANSFER IN LUNGS:
DEVELOPMENT OF CONCEPTS AND CURRENT STATE

Johannes Piiper

Abteilung Physiologie
Max-Planck-Institut für experimentelle Medizin
Hermann-Rein-Str. 3
D-3400 Göttingen
Germany

Introduction

In the lungs, the alveolar/capillary gas transfer is an intermediate step in gas transport, interposed between ventilation and pulmonary blood flow. A major difficulty in analysing pulmonary gas exchange in terms of ventilation, gas/blood transfer and perfusion is due to the fact that the lung is highly inhomogeneous with respect to these processes and their combination. Moreover, the alveolar-capillary transfer involves diffusion across heterogeneous media and chemical reactions, and in the case of O_2 the binding to hemoglobin.

In the analysis of pulmonary gas exchange, the transfer of O_2 from the alveolar gas phase into blood may be considered as the primary, fundamental process. This process involves diffusion and chemical reaction and the time limits are set by the capillary transit time which is determined by the capillary blood volume and capillary blood flow. The second stage in the analysis of pulmonary gas exchange would be the modeling of the whole lung as a system comprising a large number of unequal pulmonary capillaries, arranged in parallel, with variable perfusion and with variable convective-diffusive transport of oxygen in the airways to the alveolar-capillary barrier.

Gerhard Thews has importantly contributed to our understanding of pulmonary O_2 transfer at both levels: O_2 uptake kinetics by single red blood cells and O_2 transfer in whole lungs with functional inhomogeneities (reviewed by Thews, 1963, 1979). In this report, some of his and his coworkers' methods and results will be briefly evaluated in comparison with corresponding investigations performed by other investigators.

The selection of the cited papers is subjective: no attempt to cover the whole recent pertinent literature will be undertaken. Thus a deplorable omission, due to lack of space, concerns the highly original work of Masaji Mochizuki and his associates, also extending from gas transfer of single red blood cells to that of whole lungs (recently reviewed by Mochizuki, 1991).

I. Oxygen Transfer Kinetics of Red Blood Cells

Most of the recent studies of O_2 and CO transfer of red blood cells (RBC) have been performed using the rapid mixing-stopped flow technique. The method is wrought with the serious problem of diffusion resistance in the stagnant liquid layer surrounding the RBC (Gad-El-Hak et al., 1977; Coin and Olson, 1979; Rice, 1980; Huxley and Kutchai, 1981; Vandegriff and Olson, 1984; Holland et al., 1985; Yamaguchi et al., 1985). Efforts to take into account this stagnant layer effect have been undertaken, but the results are not easily verified (Hook et al., 1988). Also Thews and coworkers have used a modified stopped-flow method (Niesel et al., 1959). A red cell suspension was rapidly mixed into a solution equilibrated at another P_{O_2}, and the subsequent changes in O_2 saturation (S_{O_2}) were measured by an ultrarapid spectral analyzer.

But a new and elegant method devised by Thews was the blood lamella method. The composition of a gas phase surrounding , at both sides, a thin blood lamella in which red cells ideally lay in a unicellular layer, was rapidly changed and the subsequent reequilibration of hemoglobin O_2 saturation (S_{O_2}) was measured by spectrophotometry as rate of change of S_{O_2} (Thews, 1959; Thews, 1961; Frech et al., 1968).

This procedure matches the conditions in the lungs much better than the rapid-mixing technique since the equilibration occurs with a constant (gas phase) P_{O_2}. Indeed, a good agreement with alveolar-to-end-capillary P_{O_2} difference as measured in hypoxia in man was reported (Thews, 1979). However, the resulting pulmonary capillary transit times, 0.2 to 0.3 sec, were shorter than the generally accepted values around 0.7 sec resulting from analysis of CO uptake (Roughton and Forster, 1957).

In recent years, Heidelberger and Reeves (1990a, 1990b) have developed a technique which, in principle, resembles the blood lamella technique of Thews. They succeeded in producing a unicellular layer of blood between two sheets of highly gas-permeable Gore-Tex membrane (an open mesh of Teflon fibrils, 78% porosity). Dual-wavelength measurements of S_{O_2} were done after a step change in P_{O_2}. The kinetics, as characterized by values of half-time, were much faster, and the effective specific O_2 conductances (θ_{O_2}) were much higher than those obtained by the rapid mixing and stopped-flow techniques, even after attempted corrections for the stagnant layer effects. The authors attributed the difference mainly to an essential reduction of the boundary-layer error in the unicellular thin layer method. Even more striking was the result that the calculated θ_{O_2} varied largely with S_{O_2} and equilibration time, thus generally calling into question the usefulness of the index θ_{O_2}.

In my laboratory in Göttingen, RBC O_2 uptake and release kinetics were studied using the rapid-mixing stopped-flow technique (Holland et al., 1985). Various checks and corrections were applied in order to eliminate the stagnant layer effect (Yamaguchi et al., 1985; Hook et al., 1988). Indeed, a θ_{O_2} of 3.9 ml / (min·Torr·ml blood) was obtained for human blood, a value higher than the values previously obtained by rapid-mixing techniques, but considerably below the range resulting from the measurements by Heidelberger and Reeves (1990b).

According to the Roughton-Forster (1957) equation applied to O_2 transfer,

$$1/D_{L_{O_2}} = 1/D_{M_{O_2}} + 1/(\theta_{O_2} \cdot V_c)$$

a higher θ_{O_2}, with same pulmonary O_2 diffusing capacity ($D_{L_{O_2}}$) and pulmonary capillary volume (V_c), leads to a smaller D_M, meaning that a larger part of the resistance to alveolar-capillary diffusion of O_2 is to be located outside the capillary blood, i.e. in the tissue barrier ("membrane"), in gas phase ("stratification") or has to be attributed to various functional inhomogeneities (see below).

A sensitivity analysis of the model derived from experimental data revealed that the diffusivity of O_2 was the main factor limiting red blood cell O_2 transfer, diffusion of hemoglobin and reaction of hemoglobin with O_2 being of lesser influence (Hook et al., 1988). A similar conclusion was drawn from measurements of O_2 kinetics at varied temperatures (37°, 27°, 17°C). The measured rates had same temperature coefficients as diffusion coefficients of O_2 (and hemoglobin) and were much less than those of O_2-

hemoglobin reactions (Yamaguchi et al., 1987). Of course, this behavior would have been expected if the kinetics had been essentially limited by extracellular diffusion of O_2 (stagnant layer).

II. Gas Exchange in Functionally Inhomogeneous Lungs

Thews and coworkers (Thews and Vogel, 1968; Vogel and Thews, 1968; Vogel et al., 1968; Schmidt and Schnabel, 1970; Thews, Schmidt and Schnabel, 1971; Schmidt et al., 1972; Thews and Schmidt, 1976) have elaborated a technique, based on step-wise changes of inspired gas composition, to detect and quantify the unequal distribution of alveolar ventilation ($\dot{V}A$), pulmonary diffusing capacity (DL) and pulmonary blood flow ($\dot{Q}$) in normal humans and in pulmonary patients. The pulmonary wash-in/wash-out kinetics of CO_2, O_2 and Ar was measured following a step change of inspired gases (O_2 from 12% to 21%; CO_2 from 0% to 5%; Ar from 10% to 0%). According to modeling, the wash-in/wash-out kinetics of the three test gases was expected to be determined by the following parameters: (1) Ar, by $\dot{V}A/VA$ (VA, alveolar lung volume); (2) CO_2, by $\dot{V}A/VA$ and $\dot{V}A/\dot{Q}$; (3) O_2, by $\dot{V}A/VA$, $\dot{V}A/\dot{Q}$, and $DL/\dot{Q}$.

In most cases, a model comprising two compartments with different $\dot{V}A/VA$. $\dot{V}A/\dot{Q}$, and $DL/\dot{Q}$, and a shunt, was sufficient for explaining the measured data. From the obtained ventilation/diffusion/perfusion patterns in normal persons and in patients with restrictive and obstructive lung diseases the alveolar-arterial P_{O_2} differences (AaD_{O_2}) were calculated, and subdivided into components due to shunt, $\dot{V}A/\dot{Q}$ distribution, and diffusion limitation (including finite DL and its distribution).

In recent years, Vidal Melo et al. (1990) have elaborated a modeling approach that is similar to that of Thews and associates as it is based on a two-compartment lung, with different $\dot{V}A/\dot{Q}$ but same and finite $DL/\dot{Q}$, and shunt. Arterial and end-expired gases and DL_{CO} (steady state) were used for calculations. For diffusion-limited O_2 transfer, Bohr integration was performed for each compartment. It was shown that in chronic obstructive lung disease the relative role of diffusion limitation increased with severity of the disease.

The multiple inert gas elimination method (MIGET), now in use in many clinical laboratories, is a powerful tool for quantitative determination of the $\dot{V}A/\dot{Q}$ inhomogeneity in lungs (Wagner et al., 1974; West, 1977a,b). The difference between the arterial P_{O_2} predicted from the $\dot{V}A/\dot{Q}$ inequality derived from MIGET, assuming no diffusion limitation, and the measured arterial P_{O_2} was attributed to diffusion limitation. This P_{O_2} difference was found to increase in exercise in hypoxia (Torre-Bueno et al., 1985), but also at very high levels of O_2 uptake in normoxia (Hammond et al., 1986).

The effects of $DL/\dot{Q}$ variance and of combinations of $\dot{V}A/\dot{Q}$ and $DL/\dot{Q}$ variances has been investigated in a number of papers, both in theory and in application to experimental data (Piiper, 1961a,b; Piiper et al., 1961; Chinet et al., 1971; Geiser et al., 1983; Hammond and Hempleman, 1987; Hempleman and Gray, 1988; Gray, 1991). Chinet et al. (1971) were among the first to demonstrate that not only the extent of $\dot{V}A/\dot{Q}$ and $DL/\dot{Q}$ variances, but also their reciprocal correlation is important in determining the effects on gas exchange. They showed that in a lung with $\dot{V}A/\dot{Q}$ inequality the effects on gas exchange were different when DL was distributed in such a manner that DL/VA was constant from those observed with constant $DL/\dot{Q}$.

In recent years, a group in Tokyo (Yamaguchi et al., 1991), has attempted to measure both the $\dot{V}A/\dot{Q}$ and $DL/\dot{Q}$ distributions and their correlation. $\dot{V}A/\dot{Q}$ was measured by MIGET, whereas DL and $DL/\dot{Q}$ distribution was derived from simultaneously determined steady-state DL for CO, and arterial P_{O_2} and P_{CO_2}. The results were plotted as distribution of $\dot{Q}$ in a $\dot{V}A/\dot{Q}$ - $DL/\dot{Q}$ field, as suggested many years ago (Piiper, 1961b).

III. Pulmonary Diffusing Capacity for Oxygen

The overall pulmonary diffusing capacity is an important physiological index.

Moreover, it can be compared to morphometric measurements of effective alveolar and capillary surface area and air/blood barrier thickness (Weibel, 1973; Gehr et al., 1978).

One approach to arrive at D_L of a functionally inhomogeneous lung is to determine the inhomogeneities as accurately as possible and take them into account (as discussed above in connection with MIGET). The alternative approach is to create conditions in which the inhomogeneity effects are reduced in such a manner that they can be disregarded. This can be achieved by vigorous rebreathing of a hypoxic-hypercapnic gas mixture, leading to a large reduction of inspired-alveolar partial pressure differences as well as of alveolar partial pressure differences between lung areas with different $\dot{V}_A/\dot{Q}$ or $D_L/\dot{Q}$. From the subsequent equilibration kinetics of alveolar gas with mixed venous blood, recorded by mass spectrometry, the diffusing capacity D_L can be obtained (Adaro et al., 1973; Cerretelli et al., 1974; Veicsteinas et al., 1976; Piiper et al., 1978; Meyer et al., 1981).

In simultaneous determinations of $D_{L_{O_2}}$ and $D_{L_{CO}}$ in man in hypoxia at rest and running on a treadmill, the ratio $D_{L_{O_2}}/D_{L_{CO}}$ averaged 1.2, which is close to the Krogh's diffusion coefficient ratio for tissue (Meyer et al., 1981). This result suggested that the conductance derived from the measurements was really diffusive, i.e. a diffusing capacity, not essentially contanimated by other effects, in particular not by chemical reaction of hemoglobin (which is much slower for CO).

Nitric oxide (NO) has recently attracted much interest as it is considered to be the physiological endothelial relaxing factor. As test gas for alveolar-capillary diffusion, its important characteristics are its high affinity for hemoglobin (even higher than of CO) and its fast combination rate with hemoglobin (very much faster than of CO). In anesthetized dogs the ratio of simultaneously determined $D_{L_{NO}}/D_{L_{CO}}$ in hypoxia averaged 3.3, whereas the Krogh diffusion constant ratio was estimated at 1.9 (Meyer et al., 1990). Although other explanations cannot be excluded, this result points to a strong reaction limitation of pulmonary CO uptake in hypoxia. This result conduces us to reinterpret the ratio $D_{L_{O_2}}/D_{L_{CO}}$. Assuming that also here CO uptake is in part reaction-limited, "true" $D_{L_{CO}}$ must be higher than the measured value and the "corrected" ratio $D_{L_{O_2}}/D_{L_{CO}}$ falls below the Krogh diffusion constant ratio. This means that $D_{L_{O_2}}$ may have been underestimated. An explanation for an underestimation of $D_{L_{O_2}}$ may be $D_L/\dot{Q}$ inhomogeneity whose effects are not expected to be reduced by rebreathing., because $D_L/\dot{Q}$ inequality effects would be present in a lung with homogeneous alveolar gas (Piiper, 1992).

The importance of the $D_L/\dot{Q}$ ratio and its variance for alveolar-capillary O_2 transfer follows from the fact that gas equilibration in pulmonary blood in simple models is determined by the ratio $D_{L_{O_2}}/(\dot{Q} \cdot \beta_{O_2})$ where β_{O_2} designates the slope of blood O_2 dissociation curve (Piiper and Scheid, 1981, 1983). Also this aspect has been explicitly recognized by Thews (1961).

Conclusions and Outlook

In spite of continuous research efforts, to which Gerhard Thews and his associates have importantly contributed, the various mechanisms of pulmonary O_2 transfer have not yet been satisfactorily elucidated. In some cases, new results obtained with improved methods have called basic concepts into question. The following areas and aspects may deserve particular attention.

(1) The measurements of red blood cell O_2 kinetics as obtained on stationary thin blood lamellae need verification and extension.

(2) Diffusion limitation effects observed in hypoxia and in heavy exercise should be verified and quantified in terms of $D_{L_{O_2}}$ and its unequal distribution.

(3) The relationships between D_L values for various gases, in particular for O_2 and CO, need a systematic analysis at all levels (from single red blood cells to whole lungs).

(4) The limiting role of mixing of inspired with resident gas in normal and diseased lungs (not covered in this report) is still rather controversial, but deserves attention particularly in diseased lungs.

Summary

Progress in research on pulmonary gas exchange, with special reference to the contribution of Gerhard Thews and associates, is reviewed. In particular, the following aspects are considered.

(1) *Oxygen transfer kinetics of red blood cells.* Recent measurements, particularly on red blood cells in thin blood films, yield more rapid equilibration kinetics than previously recorded. A reevaluation of the roles of diffusion and chemical reaction in alveolar O_2 uptake may become necessary.

(2) *Gas exchange in functionally inhomogeneous lungs.* Besides the classical ventilation/perfusion ($\dot{V}A/\dot{Q}$) inequality, a variation of the diffusing capacity-to-perfusion ratio ($DL/\dot{Q}$) appears to be of importance. The combination of $\dot{V}A/\dot{Q}$ and $DL/\dot{Q}$ inequalities may lead to a better understanding of alveolar gas exchange, particularly in diseased lungs.

(3) *Pulmonary diffusing capacity (DL) for oxygen.* The rebreathing technique, which strongly reduces the effects of inequal $\dot{V}A/\dot{Q}$ distribution effects, appears to be particularly suited for measurement of overall alveolar-capillary diffusion. But neither the factors determining DL, obtained by rebreathing or other methods, nor the relationships between DL for various gases are yet fully understood.

References

Adaro, F., Scheid, P., Teichmann J., and Piiper, J., 1973, A rebreathing method for estimating pulmonary D_{O_2}: theory and measurements in dog lungs, *Respir. Physiol.* 18:43-63.

Cerretelli, P., Veicsteinas, A., Teichmann, J., Magnussen, H., and Piiper, J., 1974, Estimation by a rebreathing method of pulmonary O_2 diffusing capacity in man, *J. Appl. Physiol.* 56:553-563.

Chinet, A., Micheli, J.L., and Haab, P., 1971, Imhomogeneity effects on O_2 and CO pulmonary diffusing capacity estimates by steady-state methods. Theory, *Respir. Physiol.* 13:1-22.

Coin, J.T., and Olson, J.S., 1979, The rate of oxygen uptake by human red blood cells, *Biol. Chem.* 254:1178-1190.

Frech, W.-E., Schultenhinrichs, D., Vogel, H.R., und Thews, G., 1968, Modelluntersuchungen zum Austausch der Atemgase. I. Die O_2-Aufnahmezeit des Erythrocyten unter den Bedingungen des Lungencapillarblutes, *Pflügers Arch. ges. Physiol.* 301:292-301.

Gad-El-Hak, M., Morton, J.B., and Kutchai, H., 1977, Turbulent flow of red cells in dilute suspensions. Effect on kinetics of O_2 uptake. *Biophys. J.*18:289-300.

Gehr, P., Bachofen, M., and Weibel, E.R., 1978, The normal human lung: ultrastructure and morphometric estimation of diffusion capacity. *Respir. Physiol.* 32:121-140.

Geiser, J., Schibli, H., and Haab, P., 1983, Simultaneous O_2 and CO diffusing capacity estimates from assumed lognormal $\dot{V}A$, $\dot{Q}$ and DL distributions, *Respir. Physiol.* 52:53-67.

Gray, A.T., 1991, The effects of $\dot{V}A/\dot{Q}$ and $D/\dot{V}A$ inequalities on pulmonary oxygen diffusing capacity estimates, *Respir. Physiol.* 84:287-293.

Hammond, M.D., Gale, G.E., Kapitan, K.S., Ries, A., and Wagner, P.D., 1986, Pulmonary gas exchange in humans during exercise at sea level, *J. Appl. Physiol.* 60:1590-1598.

Hammond, M.D., and Hempleman, S.C., 1987, Oxygen diffusing capacity estimates derived from measured $\dot{V}A/\dot{Q}$ distributions in man, *Respir. Physiol.* 69:129-147.

Heidelberger, E., and Reeves, R.B., 1990a, O_2 transfer kinetics in a whole blood unicellular thin layer, *J. Appl. Physiol.* 68:1854-1864.

Heidelberger, E., and Reeves, R.B., 1990b, Factors affecting whole blood O_2 transfer kinetics: implications for $\theta(O_2)$, *J. Appl. Physiol.* 68:1865-1874.

Hempleman, S.C., and Gray, A.T., 1988, Estimating steady-state DL_{O_2} with nonlinear dissociation curves and $\dot{V}A/\dot{Q}$ inequality, *Respir. Physiol.* 73:279-288.

Holland, R.A.B., Shibata, H., Scheid, P., and Piiper, J., 1985, Kinetics of O_2 uptake and release by red cells in stopped-flow apparatus: effects of unstirred layer, *Respir. Physiol.* 59:71-91.

Hook, C., Yamaguchi, K., Scheid, P., and Piiper, J., 1988, Oxygen transfer of red blood cells: experimental data and model analysis, *Respir. Physiol.* 72:65-82.

Huxley, V.H., and Kutchai, H., 1981, The effect of the red cell membrane and a diffusion boundary layer on the rate of oxygen uptake by human erythrocytes, *J. Physiol. (London)* 316: 75-88.

Meyer, M., Scheid, P., Riepl. G., Wagner, H.J., and Piiper J., 1981, Pulmonary diffusing capacities for O_2 and CO measured by a rebreathing technique, *J. Appl. Physiol.* 51:1643-1650.

Meyer, M., Schuster, K.D., Schulz, H., Mohr, M., and Piiper, J., 1990, Pulmonary diffusing capacities for nitric oxide and carbon monoxide determined by rebreathing in dogs, *J. Appl. Physiol.* 68:2344-2357.

Mochizuki, M., 1991, "Blood Gas Exchange Kinetics", Nishimaruyama Hospital, Sapporo.

Niesel, W., Thews, G., und Lübbers, D.W., 1959, Die Messung des zeitlichen Verlaufs der O_2-Aufsättigung und -Entsättigung menschlicher Erythrocyten mit dem Kurzzeit-Spektralanalysator, *Pflügers Arch. ges. Physiol.* 268:296-307.

Piiper, J., 1961a, Unequal distribution of pulmonary diffusing capacity and the alveolar-arterial P_{O_2} differences: theory, *J. Appl. Physiol.* 16:493-498.

Piiper, J., 1961b, Variations of ventilation and diffusing capacity to perfusion determining the alveolar-arterial O_2 difference: theory, *J. Appl. Physiol.* 16:507-510.

Piiper, J., 1992, Diffusion-perfusion inhomogeneity and alveolar-arterial O_2 diffusion limitation: theory, *Respir. Physiol.* 87:349-356.

Piiper, J., Haab, P., and Rahn, H., 1961, Unequal distribution of pulmonary diffusing capacity in the anesthetized dog, *J. Appl. Physiol.* 16:499-506.

Piiper, J., Meyer, M., and Scheid, P., 1978, Pulmonary diffusing capacity for O_2 and CO at rest and during exercise, *Bull. Eur. Physiopathol. Respir.* 15:145-150.

Piiper, J., and Scheid, P., 1981, Model for capillary-alveolar equilibration with special reference to O_2 uptake in hypoxia, *Respir. Physiol.* 46:193-208.

Piiper, J., and Scheid, P., 1983, Comparison of diffusion and perfusion limitations in alveolar gas exchange, *Respir. Physiol.* 51:287-290.

Rice, S.A., 1980, Hydrodynamics and diffusion consideration of rapid-mix experiments with red blood cells, *Biophys. J.* 29:65-78.

Roughton, F.J.W., and Forster, R.E., 1957, Relative importance of diffusion and chemical reaction rates in determining rate of exchange of gases in the human lung, with special reference to true diffusing capacity of pulmonary membrane and volume of blood in the lung capillaries, *J. Appl. Physiol.* 11:291-302.

Schmidt, W., und Schnabel, K.H., 1970, Methodische Verbesserungen des Verfahrens der Verteilungsanalyse von Ventilation, Perfusion und O_2-Diffusionskapazität der Lunge, *Respiration* 27:15-23.

Schmidt, W., Thews, G., and Schnabel, K.H., 1972, Results of distribution analysis of ventilation, perfusion, and O_2 diffusing capacity in the human lung. Investigations in healthy subjects and in patients with obstructive lung disease, *Respiration* 29:1-16.

Thews, G., 1959, Untersuchung der Sauerstoffaufnahme und -abgabe sehr dünner Blutlamellen, *Pflügers Arch. ges. Physiol.* 268:308-317.

Thews, G., 1961, Die Sauerstoffdiffusion in den Lungencapillaren, *in:* "Physiologie und Pathologie des Gasaustausches in der Lunge" (Bad Oeynhausener Gespräche IV), H. Bartels, and E. Witzleb, eds., Springer, Berlin, Göttingen, Heidelberg, pp. 1-19.

Thews, G., 1963, Die theoretischen Grundlagen der Sauerstoffaufnahme in der Lunge. *Ergebn. Physiol.* 53:42-107.

Thews, G., 1979, Der Einfluss von Ventilation, Diffusion und Distribution auf den pulmonalen Gasaustausch. Analyse der Lungenfunktion unter physiologischen und pathologischen Bedingungen. Funktionsanalyse biologischer Systeme 7. Akademie der Wissenschaften und der Literatur, Mainz/Steinkopf Wiesbaden, pp. 1-126.

Thews, G., and Schmidt, W., 1976, Partitioning of the alveolar-arterial O_2 pressure difference under normal, hypoxic and hyperoxic conditions. *Respiration* 33:245-255.

Thews, G., Schmidt, W., and Schnabel, K.H., (1971), Analysis of distribution inhomogeneities of ventilation, perfusion, and O_2 diffusing capacity in the human lung. *Respiration* 28:197-215.

Thews, G., und Vogel, H.R., (1968), Die Verteilungsanalyse von Ventilation, Perfusion und O_2-Diffusionskapazität in der Lunge durch Konzentrationswechsel dreier Inspirationsgase. I. Theorie. *Pflügers Arch. ges. Physiol.* 303:195-205.

Torre-Bueno, J.R., Wagner, P.D., Saltzman, H.A., Gale, G.E., and Moon, R.E., 1985, Diffusion limitation in normal humans during exercise at sea level and simulated altitude, *J. Appl. Physiol.* 58:989-995.

Vandegriff, K.D., and Olson, J.S., 1984, Morphological and physiological factors affecting oxygen uptake and release by red blood cells, *J. Biol. Chem.* 259: 12619-12627.

Veicsteinas, A., Magnussen, H., Meyer, M., and Cerretelli, P., 1976, Pulmonary O_2 diffusing capacity at exercise by a modified rebreathing method, *Eur. J. Appl. Physiol.* 35:79-88.

Vidal Melo, M.F., Caprihan, A., Luft, U.C., and Loeppky, J.A., 1990, Distribution of ventilation and diffusion with perfusion in a two-compartment model of gas exchange, *in:* "Oxygen Transport to Tissue XIII," (Advances in Experimental Medicine and Biology, Vol. 277), Piiper, J., Goldstick, T.K., and Meyer, M., eds., Plenum Press, New York and London, pp. 653-664.

Vogel, H.R., and Thews, G., 1968, Die Verteilungsanalyse von Ventilation, Perfusion und O_2-Diffusionskapazität in der Lunge durch Konzentrationswechsel dreier Inspirationsgase. II. Durchführung des Verfahrens, *Pflügers Arch.* 303:206-217.

Vogel, H.R., Thews, G., Schulz, V., and Mengden, H.J., 1968, Die Verteilungsanalyse von Ventilation, Perfusion und O_2-Diffusionskapazität in der Lunge durch Konzentrationswechsel dreier Inspirationsgase. III. Untersuchung von Jugendlichen, älteren Personen und Schwangeren, *Pflügers Arch.* 303:218-229.

Wagner, P.D., Saltzman, H.A., and West, J.B., 1974, Measurement of continuous distributions of ventilation-perfusion ratios: theory, *J. Appl. Physiol.* 36:588-599.

Weibel, E.R., 1973, Morphological basis of alveolar gas exchange, *Physiol. Rev.* 53:419-495.

West, J.B., 1977a, "Ventilation/Blood Flow and Gas Exchange," 3rd ed., Blackwell, Oxford.

West, J.B., 1977b, State of the art: ventilation-perfusion relationships, *Am. Rev. Respir. Dis.* 116:919-943.

Yamaguchi, K., Glahn, J., Scheid, P., and Piiper, J., 1987, Oxygen transfer conductance of human red blood cells at varied pH and temperature, *Respir. Physiol.* 67:209-223.

Yamaguchi, K., Kawai, A., Mori, M., Asano, K., Takasugi, T., Umeda, A., Kawashiro, T., and Yokoyama, T., 1991, Distribution of ventilation and diffusing capacity to perfusion in the lung, *Respir. Physiol.* 86:171-187.

Yamaguchi, K., Nguyen-Phu, D., Scheid, P., and Piiper, J., 1985, Kinetics of O_2 uptake and release by human red blood cells studied by a stopped-flow technique, *J. Appl. Physiol.* 58:1215-1224.

O_2 TRANSPORT IN SKELETAL MUSCLE: DEVELOPMENT OF CONCEPTS AND CURRENT STATE

K. Groebe

Institut für Physiologie und Pathophysiologie
Johannes Gutenberg-Universität Mainz
Saarstr. 21, D-6500 Mainz, Germany

When comparing oxygen consumption rates $(\dot{V}_{O_2})$ of various organs — as shown in Fig. 1 — skeletal muscle is exceptional in two respects: Its consumption rate attains the second largest absolute value of all organs and may vary between rest $(0.2\ ml\,O_2{\cdot}100\ g^{-1}{\cdot}min^{-1})$ and maximum performance $(16\ ml\,O_2{\cdot}100\ g^{-1}{\cdot}min^{-1}$ for electrical stimulation) by a factor of 80, thus covering a range that is by far larger than in any other tissue. In order to understand muscle O_2 transport one has to identify transport mechanisms and evaluate their importance towards bringing about the observed high O_2 fluxes and allowing for their enormous variability.

Muscle oxygen transport involves four subprocesses that interact in supplying oxygen from arterial blood to the O_2 consumers, the mitochondria: *(i)* Convective O_2 transport in blood, *(ii)* O_2 release from blood vessels, *(iii)* free O_2, and *(iv)* myoglobin-facilitated O_2 diffusion from vessel wall to mitochondria. In addition, understanding O_2 transport is complicated by *(v)* heterogeneities in microvascular geometries and blood flows.

SOME FORMER WORK ON O_2 TRANSPORT IN MUSCLE

A first part of this article shall review some of the work that has been directed towards elucidating mechanisms important for muscle O_2 transport. The first and best known approach by August Krogh [8,9] describes P_{O_2} drops in a circular tissue cylinder surrounding an individual capillary for a given P_{O_2} at the capillary wall. Krogh showed that tissue O_2 transport in muscle at rest and in post-contraction hyperemia can be explained by diffusion of free oxygen directed radially away from the capillary. The Krogh model has been refined and extended by the work of Thews [11,12,13,14] and other researchers to also include others of the mentioned mechanisms as red blood cell (RBC) O_2 unloading along the capillary or P_{O_2} drop inside the capillary, moreover, time dependence of P_{O_2} profiles due to changes in O_2 delivery or demand, O_2 diffusion parallel to the capillary direction (longitudinal diffusion), and tissue cylinders of cross-sectional shapes other than circular. Applying such improved models, steady state and transient P_{O_2} distributions in an entire capillary domain as well as time dependence of O_2 consumption during dynamic work could be calculated. Fig. 2 demonstrates the effects of longitudinal diffusion in heavily working muscle by means of P_{O_2} distributions along the capillary direction, calculated from a more recent model. It shows P_{O_2} profiles within the capillary (upper traces), at the capillary-fiber interface (middle traces), and at the outer rim of the supplied tissue volume (lower traces). Solid curves are with, dahed curves are without longitudinal diffusion. Obviously, longitudinal diffusion introduces

Oxygen Transport to Tissue XV, Edited by P. Vaupel
et al., Plenum Press, New York, 1994

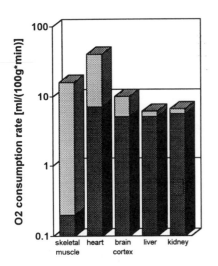

Figure 1. O_2 consumption rates of various organs. Lightly shaded portions of columns represent variability. Note logarithmic scaling of the ordinate.

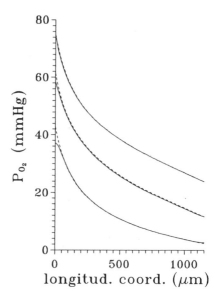

longitud. coord. (μm)

Figure 2. Effect of longitudinal diffusion in heavily working skeletal muscle. Shown are modelled P_{O_2} distributions along the capillary direction within the capillary (upper traces), at the capillary-fiber interface (middle traces), and at the outer rim of the supplied tissue volume (lower traces). Solid curves are with, dashed curves without longitudinal diffusion.

but small changes in tissue P_{O_2}, the largest ones amounting to 2–4 $mm\,Hg$. This observation agrees well with results by THEWS [11,12] who in 1953 had predicted effects of 2–3 $mm\,Hg$ and by that explained the differences in critical venous P_{O_2}s of the brain found experimentally for the cases of hypoxic versus ischemic hypoxia. As a further model application, THEWS [13] calculated the change in average muscle tissue O_2 concentration following step changes in O_2 consumption rate. These calculated time courses of O_2 concentration may, in turn, be used to determine highly resolved time courses of O_2 consumption rate by fitting them to measured P_{O_2} time courses.

In view of the many studies mentioned, it came as a big surprise when HONIG and co-workers [5] presented measured P_{O_2} distributions in cross sections of working dog gracilis muscles which were largely different from the ones predicted before and one of which is shown in Fig. 3. The numbers state Mb-O_2 saturation and — in parentheses — P_{O_2}. Fairly independent of performance, muscle P_{O_2} was extremely uniform at low levels of no more than a few $mm\,Hg$. These profiles could only be understood if resistance to O_2 diffusion in and next to capillaries compared to resistance in the rest of the tissue was much larger than assumed in most former model studies. Explanations of larger capillary resistance may be offered by the following observations: *(i)* The capillary surface is maximally effective in O_2 exchange only at sites at which RBCs are located (see [4]). *(ii)* The RBCs from which the oxygen emerges are surrounded by a plasma sleeve, the capillary endothelium, and the interstitial space which together form a layer not containing the O_2 carrier myoglobin (carrier-free region, CFR) and therefore exhibiting a higher resistance (see [6]). *(iii)* The carrier myoglobin is very little

Another breakthrough in understanding red muscle O_2 transport was the introduction of myoglobin-facilitated O_2 diffusion in muscle fibers (see WITTENBERG, [16]), the outstanding importance of which has been documented in a vast number of publications. In a heavily working muscle fiber, for example, presence of myoglobin (Mb) may reduce the P_{O_2} drop between sarcolemma and fiber center, necessary to drive the required O_2 flux by 40 % [1]. For a recent review on Mb-facilitated O_2 diffusion see, *e.g.*, KREUZER and HOOFD [7].

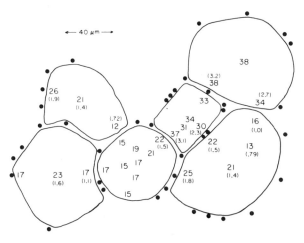

Figure 3. Cross section through muscle fibers and capillaries (●) in maximally working dog gracilis muscle. Measured Mb-O_2 saturations and — in parentheses — corresponding P_{O_2}s are shown for various measurement sites. From [5].

functional at the high P_{O_2} values prevailing next to capillaries which adds another layer of larger resistance surrounding the capillary (region deficient of functional carrier or carrier-deficient region, CDR). In addition to considerable peri-capillary resistance, O_2 flux density (*i.e.* diffusive O_2 flux divided by cross-sectional area occupied by the flux) is largest there also, together resulting in steep P_{O_2} drops in and next to the capillary.

In order to test for the correctness of the measured low muscle fiber P_{O_2} values, one may calculate the times required by RBCs to unload their oxygen for different values of tissue P_{O_2} and compare them to hemodynamic estimates of red cell capillary transit times. HONIG et al. [5] showed that even for a tissue P_{O_2} of $0\,mm\,Hg$, O_2 unloading times calculated for the case of maximum performance (see Tab. 1, left) are substantially longer than estimated transit times (median 84 ms, inter-quartile range 59–111 ms) furnishing strong evidence against the assumption of negligible intra- and peri-capillary resistance. THEWS calculated time courses of RBC O_2 release for dynamic work on the bicycle ergometer at maximum performance and found unloading times that confirmed HONIG et al.'s conclusions on the one hand but were much closer to estimated capillary transit times on the other (Tab. 1, right). Furthermore, THEWS determined O_2 diffusing capacities of the human leg musculature that are roughly two thirds of lung diffusing capacity at moderate work.

Directly comparing modelled P_{O_2} distributions to measured ones is a more straightforward way of checking both measurements and theoretical concepts that are thought to explain experimental findings. Fig. 4 shows cumulative P_{O_2} frequency distributions in heavily working

Table 1. O_2 unloading times for RBCs of 4 μm diameter, for saturation ranges and CFR thicknesses as given in table, and for a P_{O_2} of $0\,mm\,Hg$ at the outer rim of the CFR as calculated by HONIG et al. [5] and THEWS [15]. In the rightmost column, estimates of diffusing capacity of the human leg musculature are quoted from [15]. All unloading times are substantially longer than transit times estimated in [5]: Median transit time is 84 ms and inter-quartile range is 59–111 ms.

HONIG et al. [5]				THEWS [15]				
saturation change		O_2 unloading time for CFR thickness		saturation change		O_2 unloading time for CFR thickness		O_2 diffusing capacity
in	out	1 μm	2 μm	in	out	1 μm	2 μm	$\frac{ml\,O_2}{min \cdot mm\,Hg}$
85 %	40 %	327 ms	481 ms	85 %	40 %	118 ms	143 ms	31
85 %	30 %	451 ms	657 ms	85 %	26.5 %	189 ms	229 ms	47

dog gracilis muscle which have been measured (solid, from [2]) or calculated by means of the below model (dashed) and which are almost congruent. This indicates that modelled P_{O_2} distributions are indeed in good agreement with measurements if the above mentioned effects — which increase peri-capillary resistance to O_2 diffusion relative to tissue resistance — are accounted for.

The above modelling results implicitly assume homogeneous muscle geometry and perfusion. However, heterogeneities in capillary blood flow greatly complicate understanding of muscle O_2 transport. It has been shown by POPEL et al. [10] that such heterogeneities may have marked effects on muscle P_{O_2} distributions depending on their magnitude and relation to geometric heterogeneities. Inhomogeneity might be of particular importance in resting muscle: Median fiber P_{O_2} has been measured by HONIG and GAYESKI to be about 30–50 $mm\,Hg$ below venous outflow P_{O_2} (HONIG, personal communication), whereas models assuming homogeneous flow would predict a few $mm\,Hg$ for this difference at the most. This finding may be explained by pronounced inter-regional flow heterogeneities which are characterized by periodic switching between states of flow and flow stop, brought about by rhythmic arteriolar activity.

ANALYSIS OF THE SYSTEM OF DIFFUSIVE O₂ TRANSPORT IN MUSCLE

In the remainder of this paper, diffusive oxygen transport in myoglobin containing muscle will be analyzed somewhat more systematically. To this end, P_{O_2} distributions in the tissue surrounding a capillary are calculated for various muscle performances, covering the range experimentally found in electrically stimulated dog gracilis muscles. Geometry of the mathematical model used for this purpose is diagrammed in Fig. 5. The model considers red blood cell O_2 unloading along the capillary, the particulate nature of blood, free and hemoglobin-facilitated O_2 diffusion and hemoglobin-O_2 reaction kinetics within red cells, a region devoid of an O_2 carrier surrounding red cells, and myoglobin-facilitated O_2 diffusion in the tissue.

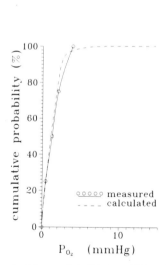

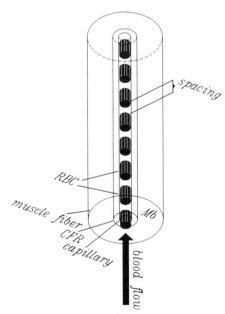

Figure 4. Measured (solid, from [2]) and calculated (dashed) cumulative P_{O_2} frequency distributions in heavily working dog gracilis muscle.

Figure 5. Schematic drawing of model geometry. Large cylinder: Capillary domain supplied by central capillary. RBC: Red blood cells within the capillary, separated by plasma-filled gaps ("spacing"). Mb: Oxygen carrier myoglobin, present in muscle fibers. CFR: Carrier-free region separating erythrocytes and muscle fiber.

Table 2. Data specific to the five stimulation frequencies studied.

stimulation frequency	1	2	4	6	8	Hz
O_2 consumption rate, $\dot{V}_{O_2}$	3	6	11	13	15	$\frac{ml\,O_2}{100g\cdot min}$
blood flow rate	26	40.5	68.5	84	119	$\frac{ml}{100\,g\cdot min}$
venous Hb-O_2 saturation	0.45	0.30	0.25	0.275	0.40	
functional capillary density	800	950	1000	950	650	mm^{-2}
RBC spacing	1.25	1	0.75	0.6	0.5	RBC lengths
organ-venous blood pH	7.37	7.31	7.26	7.24	7.20	
Hill coefficient of Hb	3.02	3.19	3.34	3.41	3.95	
half saturation P_{O_2} of Hb	29.0	30.2	31.2	31.6	34.0	$mm\,Hg$

Further details of the model are going to be published elsewhere. In this presentation only the situation near the venous capillary ending will be discussed because this is the most critical region for O_2 supply and the effects to be described are most pronounced there. General input data have been chosen as specified in [3]. Input data specific to the the five performances considered (see Tab. 2) correspond to electrical stimulation rates of 1, 2, 4, 6, and 8 Hz, and are taken from measurements by HONIG and GAYESKI (HONIG, personal communication).

Fig. 6 shows calculated radial P_{O_2} profiles near the venous capillary ending for the five performances considered. Three regions are delineated by vertical lines: The red blood cell (RBC, in which only average P_{O_2} is displayed), the carrier-free region (CFR), and the muscle fiber (*fiber*). The profiles for twitch rates of 1 and 2 Hz resemble results from classical Krogh models without facilitated diffusion. At higher O_2 consumption rates, however, profiles exhibit steep peri-capillary P_{O_2} drops and but shallow P_{O_2} gradients further into the fiber.

These observations are due to the fact that facilitation of O_2 diffusion by Mb is P_{O_2} dependent: Facilitation is proportional to the slope of the myoglobin oxygen dissociation curve (ODC) at the actual P_{O_2}. This is illustrated in Fig. 7 which shows Mb-O_2 saturation S and

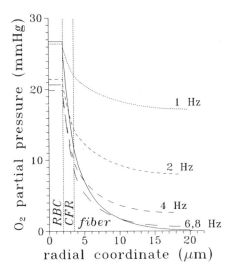

Figure 6. Radial P_{O_2} profiles near the venous capillary ending for stimulation rates of 1–8 Hz. Red blood cell (RBC), carrier-free region (CFR), and muscle fiber (*fiber*) are delineated by vertical dotted lines.

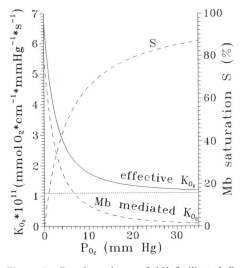

Figure 7. P_{O_2} dependence of Mb facilitated O_2 diffusion. Dashed curves: Mb oxygen dissociation curve S, and Mb-mediated O_2 diffusion conductivity K_{O_2}. Solid curve: Effective O_2 diffusion conductivity. Dotted line: free O_2 conductivity.

Mb-mediated O_2 diffusion conductivity K_{O_2} (dashed curves) as functions of P_{O_2}. Facilitated conductivity is six times free O_2 conductivity (dotted line) at $P_{O_2} = 0\,mm\,Hg$ and becomes negligible at high P_{O_2}s. Effective O_2 diffusion conductivity or effective "Krogh's diffusion constant" (solid curve) is the sum of free O_2 conductivity and Mb mediated conductivity.

P_{O_2} dependence of effective conductivity has two important consequences:

1. O_2 transport is maximally enhanced, and fiber P_{O_2} drops are most efficiently reduced as aerobic capacity is approached since this causes fiber P_{O_2} to fall to low values.

2. Due to the small gradients necessary within the fiber, P_{O_2} at the interface between CFR and muscle cell can be set to low values even at the highest O_2 fluxes. This promotes RBC O_2 unloading in that it allows for the large peri-capillary P_{O_2} gradients necessary to drive the oxygen out of the blood vessel.

In the above, it has been mentioned that in the CFR O_2 conductivity is lowest — since no O_2 carrier is present — and O_2 flux density is highest, both together resulting in the steepest P_{O_2} gradients to achieve the required flux. On the other hand, the CFR is thin and despite its adverse material properties it would be of very little effect on P_{O_2} drop (which is the integral of P_{O_2} gradient over distance) if it were only thin enough. Therefore, in order to evaluate its relevance one needs to employ a more integral measure of its importance for O_2 transport. One such measure could simply be the P_{O_2} drop across the CFR, but in order to cancel the obvious dependencies of this measure on O_2 consumption rate and capillary density, one rather employs O_2 flux per unit volume of tissue divided by the P_{O_2} drop, which is a volume-related lumped conductance or diffusing capacity.

Fig. 8 shows the P_{O_2} drops across CFR and muscle fiber, $\Delta P_{O_2 CFR}$ ($\triangle$, solid) and $\Delta P_{O_2 M}$ ($\triangle$, dashed), respectively, as functions of stimulation rate. Moreover, volume-related diffusing capacities of entire capillary domain, C_{tot} ($\bullet$, dotted), of CFR, C_{CFR} ($\bullet$, solid), and of fiber, C_M ($\bullet$, dashed), computed according to the above definition are displayed. Between 1 and 6 Hz, $\Delta P_{O_2 M}$ is kept remarkably stable in spite of a 4.3-fold increase in $\dot{V}_{O_2}$. Accordingly, C_M increases by a factor of 2.8 which is brought about by the fall in fiber P_{O_2} improving Mb-mediated conductivity as discussed before. Capillary recruitment — which is known to occur with higher performance — explains another part of this rise in conductance.

Despite the small dimensions of the CFR, P_{O_2} drop across the CFR, $\Delta P_{O_2 CFR}$, is of same magnitude or larger than P_{O_2} drop across the fiber, $\Delta P_{O_2 M}$. This is due to the unfavourable geometry and to lack of an O_2 carrier in the CFR, and is reflected by the fact that at high performance fiber conductance, C_M, becomes much larger than CFR conductance, C_{CFR}, even though muscle fiber radius is an order of magnitude larger than CFR thickness. In other words, in the CFR not only P_{O_2} gradients are steepest but also the transport resistance offered by the CFR may contribute over 60 % of total transport resistance, although the CFR accounts for no more than 10–15 % of total diffusion path length. This observation indicates that *the bottleneck of diffusional O_2 transport is the CFR*.

As the radial P_{O_2} profiles in Fig. 6 show, minimum cell P_{O_2} at a stimulation rate of 4 Hz is only 2 $mm\,Hg$, and the muscle's diffusional transport capacity appears to be almost exhausted even though it is working far from its aerobic capacity. This is even more surprising because at maximum $\dot{V}_{O_2}$ capillary derecruitment occurs which has the maladaptive effect that functional capillary density fcd — i.e. the number of capillaries open to red cells per mm^2 of cross-sectional area in sections perpendicular to the capillary direction — is only two thirds the one at 4 Hz. Thus, at maximal $\dot{V}_{O_2}$ capillary domains are by 50 % larger and functional capillaries supply more than twice the transcapillary O_2 flux. Doubling of transcapillary O_2 flux has to be achieved by a small increase in driving force since tissue P_{O_2} cannot fall by more than 2 $mm\,Hg$. This suggests the existence of some enormous reserve in transport capacity which is utilized at increasing performance.

The maximum diffusive oxygen flux per unit volume of tissue that can be supported in a given physiological situation may be calculated as follows: O_2 conductance per unit length (u.l.) of a supply unit — i.e. capillary domain — times number of supply units per (u.l.)^2 of muscle cross section — i.e. functional capillary density fcd — times capillary P_{O_2}. Since

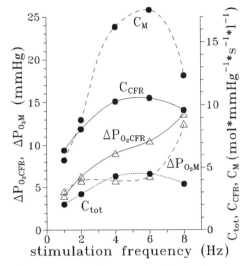

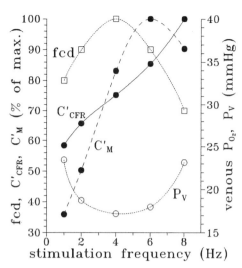

Figure 8. P_{O_2} drops across CFR and muscle fiber (ΔP_{O_2CFR}: $\triangle$, solid and ΔP_{O_2M}: $\triangle$, dashed), and volume-related diffusing capacities of entire capillary domain, CFR, and muscle fiber (C_{tot}: $\bullet$, dotted. C_{CFR}: $\bullet$, dashed. C_M: $\bullet$, solid) as functions of stimulation rate.

Figure 9. Functional capillary density (fcd: $\square$, dotted), diffusing capacities of CFR and fiber in individual capillary domains (C'_{CFR}: $\bullet$, solid; C'_M: $\bullet$, dashed) — all graphed as % of their maximal values —, and capillary venous P_{O_2} (P_V: $\bigcirc$, dotted) as functions of stimulation rate.

in a capillary domain CFR and muscle fiber are arranged in series, their diffusive resistances are additive and supply unit O_2 conductance is $\left(C'_{CFR}{}^{-1} + C'_M{}^{-1}\right)^{-1}$. In this expression conductances relating to a capillary domain rather than to a tissue volume are marked by a prime. All four quantities C'_{CFR}, C'_M, fcd, and capillary P_{O_2} (in particular P_{O_2} at the venous capillary ending, P_V) change with performance as displayed in Fig. 9, and thus represent mechanisms for adapting O_2 transport capacity to consumption rate:

1. The most obvious mechanism is a decrease in O_2 extraction measured by HONIG et al. [5] and the acid-induced shift in the Hb ODC which together increase venous P_{O_2}, P_V ($\bigcirc$, dotted). It effects an additional 6.7 $mm\,Hg$ of driving force (compared to 4 Hz) at sites where capillary P_{O_2} is lowest. This moderate gain in driving force is traded in at the cost of an excessive increase in blood flow rate, so capillary transit times become short enough to maintain high venous O_2 saturation and P_{O_2}. According to this interpretation, the observed convective O_2 shunt would not be indicative of deteriorating control of blood flow distribution or the like, but would represent the ultimate adaptive response to extreme rises in O_2 demand.

2. The second and most important contribution towards the reserve in O_2 transport capacity is the increase in muscle fiber O_2 conductivity with decreasing local P_{O_2} which entails an increase in diffusing capacity C'_M with performance ($\bullet$, dashed).

3. Intra-capillary red cell spacings tend to become smaller at high perfusion rates thus increasing effective O_2 exchange area and O_2 conductance of the CFR, C'_{CFR} ($\bullet$, solid).

4. Finally, capillary density fcd changes with performance ($\square$, dotted), inducing roughly proportional changes in O_2 conductance per volume of tissue. Following an initial increase in fcd, at 6 and 8 Hz capillary derecruitment occurs — which may be an effect of the special conditions in electrically stimulated muscles and may not be present during physiological work.

CONCLUSION

In red muscle there is a large reserve in O_2 transport capacity which is recruited with increasing O_2 demand. The characteristic P_{O_2} dependence of Mb-facilitated O_2 diffusion makes up for the largest part of the reserve. Other contributions are made by the convective O_2 shunt at maximum stimulation rate and by changes in functional capillary density and intra-capillary red cell spacing with performance. Comparison of O_2 diffusing capacities in carrier-free region and muscle fiber indicates that the bottleneck of diffusional O_2 transport is the carrier-free region.

REFERENCES

[1] W.J. Federspiel, A model study of intracellular oxygen gradients in a myoglobin-containing skeletal muscle fiber, *Biophys.J.* 49:857–868 (1986)

[2] T.E.J. Gayeski, C.R. Honig, Intracellular P_{O_2} in long axis of individual fibers in working dog gracilis muscle, *Am.J.Physiol.* 254:H1179–H1186 (1988)

[3] K. Groebe, A versatile model of steady state O_2 supply to tissue. Application to skeletal muscle, *Biophys.J.* 57:485–498 (1990)

[4] J.D. Hellums, The resistance to oxygen transport in the capillaries relative to that in the surrounding tissue, *Microvasc.Res.* 13:131–136 (1977)

[5] C.R. Honig, T.E.J. Gayeski, W. Federspiel, A. Clark, P. Clark, Muscle O_2 gradients from hemoglobin to cytochrome: new concepts, new complexities, *Adv.Exp.Med.Biol.* 169:23–38 (1984)

[6] C.R. Honig, T.E.J. Gayeski, K. Groebe, Myoglobin and oxygen Gradients, pp. 1489–1496 **in:** "The Lung, Scientific Foundations", R.G. Crystal, J.B. West et al. (eds.), Raven, New York, 1990

[7] F. Kreuzer, L. Hoofd, Facilitated diffusion of oxygen and carbon dioxide, pp. 89–111 **in:** "Handbook of Physiology, Sect. 3: The Respiratory System, Vol. IV: Gas Exchange", L.E. Fahri, S.M. Tenney, eds., American Physiological Society, Bethesda, 1987

[8] A. Krogh, The number and distribution of capillaries in muscles with calculations of the oxygen pressure head necessary for supplying the tissue, *J.Physiol.(London)* 52:409–415 (1918–1919 A)

[9] A. Krogh, The supply of oxygen to the tissues and the regulation of the capillary circulation, *J.Physiol.(London)* 52:457–474 (1918–1919 A)

[10] A.S. Popel, C.K. Charny, A.S. Dvinsky, Effect of heterogeneous oxygen delivery on the oxygen distribution in skeletal muscle, *Math.Biosci.* 81:91–113 (1986)

[11] G. Thews, Über die mathematische Behandlung physiologischer Diffusionsprozesse in zylinderförmigen Objekten, *Acta Biotheoretica* 10:105–137 (1953)

[12] G. Thews, Die Sauerstoffdiffusion im Gehirn, *Pflügers Arch.* 271:197–226 (1960)

[13] G. Thews, Theoretische Grundlagen für die Bestimmung der Verbrauchsfunktion des kontraktionsabhängig atmenden Muskels, *Pflügers Arch.* 273:367–379 (1961)

[14] G. Thews, Die Sauerstoffdrücke im Herzmuskelgewebe, *Pflügers Arch.* 276:166–181 (1962)

[15] G. Thews, Oxygen supply to the dynamically working skeletal muscle, pp. 63–75 **in:** "Funktionsanalyse biologischer Systeme, Bd. 16", M. Meyer, N. Heisler (eds.), Akademie der Wissenschaften und der Literatur, G. Fischer, Stuttgart, 1986

[16] J.B. Wittenberg, Myoglobin-facilitated oxygen diffusion: Role of myoglobin in oxygen entry into muscle, *Physiol.Rev.* 50:559–636 (1970)

CURRENT STATE OF METHODOLOGY ON HEMOGLOBIN OXIMETRY IN TISSUES

Britton Chance

University of Pennsylvania
Department of Biochemistry and Biophysics
Johnson Research Foundation
Philadelphia, PA 19104-6089 USA

INTRODUCTION

It is a great pleasure to honor Dr. Thews. I am going to talk about two aspects of his works, the optical method and the diffusion process. In the 1870's, Tyndall devised the dual wavelength spectrophotometric method using a single light source and spectrometer with a differential galvanometer (Fig. 1).

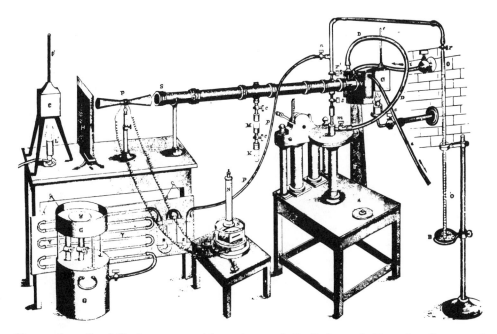

Figure 1. Tyndall Apparatus: Absorption and Radiation of Heat by Gases and Vapors (1).

In the 1930's, Glen Millikan made a dual wavelength spectrophotometer, identified as a "metabolic microscope". He made the important observation that the deoxygenation of hemoglobin and myoglobin in the cat soleus muscle was

Oxygen Transport to Tissue XV, Edited by P. Vaupel
et al., Plenum Press, New York, 1994

as great in contraction as it was in ischemia. While he attributed this to what was then called muscle hemoglobin, we now find that he probably observed hemoglobin. He also devised a very sensitive dual wavelength spectrophotometer for oximetry in the ear that was the forerunner of pulse oximetry. He recognized the problem of light scattering and its wavelength dependence with green and red light (Fig. 2). In a footnote of his 1949 paper he observed that the near-infrared would be better than green and red light as indeed Kramer had found that the deep red light was much better for penetrating tissue[*].

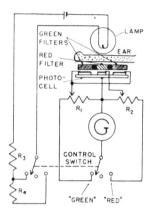

Figure 2. Circuit diagram for multiple scale oximeter to be used with the galvanometer scale: $R_1=R_2$=critical damping resistance of the galvanometer. R_3 and R_4 control the lamp brightness. They should be adjusted to fulfill the following two conditions: 1. The lamp must be bright enough on "red" to maintain the ear in a fully flushed state (normal lamp voltage: 5.3). 2. The lamp must be bright enough on "green" to give full scale deflection with "standard A" filter (normal lamp voltage: 7.7) (2).

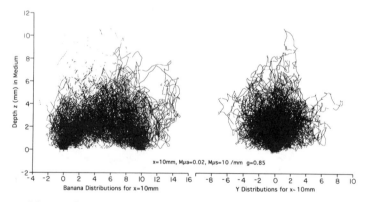

Figure 3a. Monte Carlo simulation of photon migration in scatterer/absorber (simulating human breast) (3).

---

[*] "It has been shown by independent research of the Coleman Electric Company that the most effective crossover wave-length of this filter-ear-photo-cell combination is not in the green, as the author had supposed, but in the near infra-red. The blood thickness of the ear is sufficient to block the green light almost completely. This discovery does not affect the principle of operation, as the "green" color is defined by its property of being equally absorbed by the two pigments; it was, however, importaning a serious weakness in the early standardization procedure, and in indif remedying the difficulty" from (2).

The diffusion of heat and light, particularly the diffusion of continuous light into tissue as modeled by Monte Carlo looks like "tousled hair", but this is indeed a probability distribution shown laterally and End-on (Fig. 3a). The light penetrates the tissue at depth roughly half that of the modeling separation between input and output. It has been a problem of spectrophotometry of the 60s and 80s as to just how long this pathlength ($<L>$) was and how it varied in different human subjects (Fig. 3b).

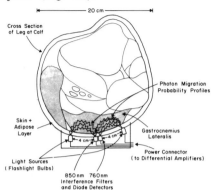

Figure 3b. Illustration of "Run-Man" monitoring Hb and Mb leg muscle.

Assuming a constancy of $<L>$, a very simple apparatus has been devised to study the human gastrocnemius by migrating photons from continuous light sources taking into account that the light is highly scattered. Silicon diode detectors and interference filters are used to measure the deoxygenation of hemoglobin and the hemoglobin concentration. The device is quite small (about the size of a cigar box).

Multiple units permit a comparison of the muscles of the quadriceps, the *vastus medialis*, the *lateralis*, and the *rectus femoris*, during bicycle exercise (Fig. 4a). During a ramp exercise (Fig. 4b), there is progressive deoxygenation and the decrease over and above that due to exercise levels of 250 watts occasioned by cuff ischemia is negligible when the *laterals* and the *medialis* are measured. The *femoris*, which is less activated by exercise, shows a further change on cuff ischemia (5). These results suggest that the oxygen extraction from hemoglobin can approach completeness at high exercise levels [in contrast to the previous talk (see Groebe, this volume)]. The mitochondria are a very good system for oxygen extraction from the tissue and indeed appears to create a steep O_2 gradient, as found surely in heart (5). The display of Fig. 4b does not show how much myoglobin contributed to the absorbance changes.

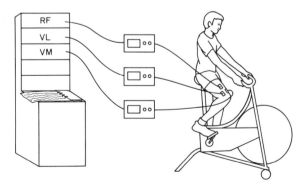

Figure 4a. Continuous wave measurement of hemoglobin and myoglobin deoxygenation at 760-800 nm in bicycle ergometry (4).

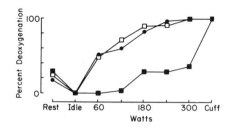

Figure 4b. Time course of deoxygenation of hemoglobin and myoglobin in the *vastus lateralis* (squares), *vastus medialis* (filled circles) and *rectus femoris* (squares). Characteristic idling causes oxygenation while work at 60 to 300 W causes the deoxygenation in all muscles but to a significantly greater extent in the *vastus* than in the *femoris* muscles. Cuff ischemia while exercising shows no change in the *vastus* and a large change in the *femoris*, indicative of the relative oxygen supply/demand characteristic at these workloads evoked by bicycle exercise.

^{1}H NMR permits the measurement of deoxymyoglobin specifically, the proximal histidine proton in paramagnetically shifted by the deoxy form. Myoglobin is measured over 10 times more sensitively than hemoglobin in solution and to a greater extent when Hb is in red blood cells (6). We have been able to combine optical and ^{1}H NMR studies in the NMR magnet by making a non-magnetic optical probe with fiber optic coupling for measuring simultaneously the optical and ^{1}H NMR responses to plantar flexion of the dog gastrocnemius in electrical stimulation (Fig. 5). There is a continuous deoxygenation of hemoglobin to the 40% desaturation level [calibrated in separate studies by cuff hypoxia]. The myoglobin is deoxygenated to a resting value of 100% oxygenated myoglobin when hypoxia is introduced. This corresponds to tissue PO_2 of < 5 torr. Thus, the myoglobin is deoxygenated when the hemoglobin is over 76% deoxygenated for the dog muscle. Thus the combination of optical spectroscopy and proton NMR spectroscopy affords a direct approach to the previously unsolved problem of the relationship of hemoglobin and myoglobin deoxygenation in exercising skeletal muscle.

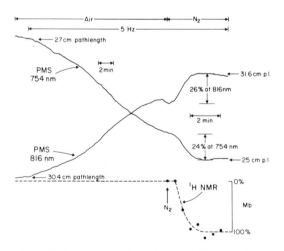

Figure 5. Correlation of time resolved optical (PMS) and ^{1}H NMR of Hb + Mb kinetics in dog gastocnemius muscle.

My second tribute to Thews is his contribution to diffusion theory. Lord Rayleigh established the equations for the random walk 1919 (Fig. 6a). However, Thews pointed out the connectivity between the physical chemical diffusion problem, the heat flow problem, and electricity. We have recently added the next chapter in, i.e., that photons diffuse in tissues, and have made

THE

LONDON, EDINBURGH, and DUBLIN

PHILOSOPHICAL MAGAZINE

AND

JOURNAL OF SCIENCE.

[SIXTH SERIES.]

APRIL 1919.

XXXI. *On the Problem of Random Vibrations, and of Random Flights in one, two, or three Dimensions. By* Lord RAYLEIGH, *O.M., F.R.S.*

Figure 6a. Title Page of Lord Rayleigh derivations of equations for random walk in 1, 2 and 3 dimensions (7).

the connectivity between flux and fluence, concentration and storage, diffusional conductivity, and photon diffusion coefficients (Table I). The heat flow equations and the chemical equations model the flow of light in highly scattering medium. Thus, the basic equations for random walk and for thermal diffusion can be linked together in the novel study of photon diffusion in tissue.

The time resolved flow of photons into a scattering medium can be modeled by a Monte Carlo simulation (see Fig. 3).

Table 1

Analogue relations between diffusion, heat conduction, electricity, and optics photon diffusion that result from the analogous differential equations, which with the aid of electrical computer methods can be referred to for the solution of diffusion or heat conduction problems. (After THEWS, 1963)

Physical-Chemical Diffusion	Heat Conduction	Electricity	Optics Photon Diffusion
Chemical Flux	Heat flux	Current	Photon Flux/Fluence
Concentration (N)	Temperature	Potential	Photon Storage
Solubility	Specific heat	Specific capacitance	—
Diffusional conductivity K	Heat conductivity	Conductance	Photon diffusion coefficient
—	—	Impedance	—

Methods of Measurement

The two approaches to the experimental study of photon diffusion in tissues are depicted in Figure 7a where on the left a pulse of 150 picoseconds impinges upon the tissue and the ensuing evolution of a migration pattern occurs over the next 10 nanoseconds as indicated in the left hand side. The pattern of photon migration is banana-shaped due to the fact that photons that attempt to travel between source and detector along the service of the model at any moment have a 50% chance of escaping into the atmosphere and never returning to the model (8). Those that travel deeply within the model will be absorbed and not reach the detector. The second method, frequency resolved spectroscopy, depends upon a time delay between the phase delay of a sinusoid of high frequency, which modulates the light source and is received with shifted phase at the detector.

The time evolution of photon migration (Figs. 7a,b) for a light pulse input gives the light progression of the diffusive wave deeper into the scatter with time.

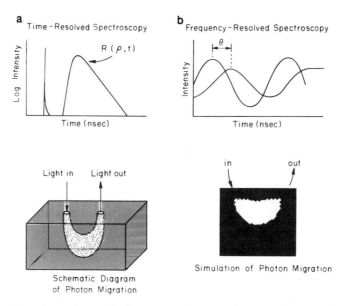

Figure 7. Examples of two basic approaches to photon diffusion in tissue (left, time resolved spectroscopy; right, frequency resolved spectroscopy).

Diffusive Waves in Scattering Medium in Frequency Resolved Spectroscopy

In frequency resolved spectroscopy using a rapidly oscillating light, the mean pathlength is fixed and the diffusion wave of photons gives a fixed phase shift into the tissue (10). A simple phase meter is used to demonstrate diffusive waves in a scattering medium (Fig. 8a).

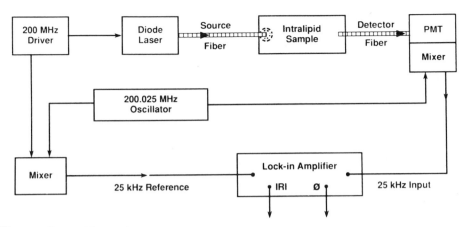

Figure 8a. Illustrating the technology for measuring photon diffusive waves in a scattering medium (intralipid sample).

The phase contours(10) are measured at various distances of the detector from the source, and thus a progressive phase shift of 20-80° are shown. One wavelength of 360o phase shift corresponds to 11 cm for 360° (Fig. 8b). The graph shows the phase shift to be linear with the distance and to reach 360° at 11.5 cm. The exponential attenuation is linear in log coordinates. Thus, a wave front propagates in the diffusive medium at a velocity small compared to the velocity of light. The photons themselves are diffusing randomly, but the diffusive waves maintain phase over one wavelength. This is a new kind of lightwave in scattering medium, which can be used to study the properties of tissue since it is very responsive to heterogeneity of absorption or scattering factor.

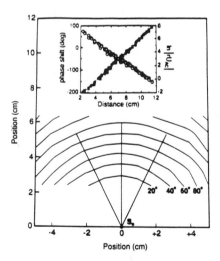

Figure 8b. Illustrating the wavefronts of increasing phase shift generated by a 200 MHz light source in a 0.5% intralipid sample. The inset plots the phase delay as a function of distance. Take note the 360° is achieved at 11.5 cm wavelength while the exponential attenuation occurs over the 12 cm of measurement.

Experimental Verification

A particular application of this technique is to localize small objects in tumors (Fig. 9a). We have employed the obvious alternative of coding the light beams of the photon diffusion wave, by in-phase and anti-phase coding so that two light sources here are at phase zero at 200 MHz, while two are coded at 180°. Thus, one region of migration is distinguished from the other by the phase of the diffusive wave. One can further explore the sensitivity to an absorber placed between the transmitter and receiver. In the near field, therefore, coherence is maintained.

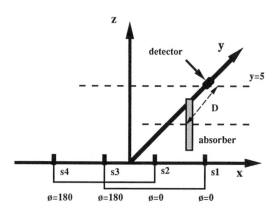

Figure 9a. Four element array configuration showing the moving detector to detect the amplitude null in the phase transition and the movable absorber to illustrate the sensitivity of detector of the localized absorber.

If we traverse the detector from the region where the phase is zero, to where the phase is 180°, we observe a sharp amplitude node of the halfwidth of 1 cm (Figs 9b). We can easily detect a 1 mm movement. Phase shift gives a position measure which is relatively independent of the distance away from the source (Fig. 9c). The phase shift is zero to the left of the center and to 180° on the right. Thus we have now magnified our detectability tremendously because of the very sharp phase transition appropriate to localization of a small object in tumors. As stated in the abstract, an 0.8 millimeter object is detected very sensitively.

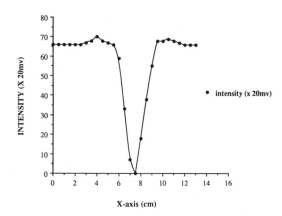

Figure 9b. Illustration of amplitude null for an four element array indicated in Figure 9a. The detector is scanned along the x-axis as indicated in Figure 9a.

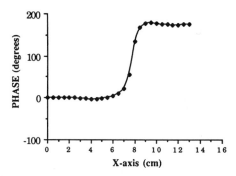

Figure 9c. Illustration of an experimentally determined phase transition by scanning the detector across the null line when two of the transmitters are phase 0 and two of the transmitters are phase 180. The slope of the transition is approximately 20°/mm movement of the detector but the sensitivity is probably limited by the size of the detecting fiber (8 mm).

A 5 millimeter rod (Fig 10), 1 cm long is placed in the optical field and translated through the phase transition shift causing a phase perturbation which is very large for a black rod, from -60 to +50°, 110° of phase shift. With an absorber (cardiogreen) at 3.5 milligram/ml we find 1.2° phase shift per millimeter with this rather dilute sample, in the nanomolar region, near the level of sensitivity of Positron Emission Tomography.

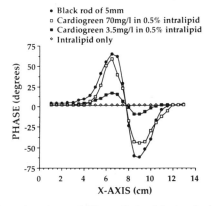

Figure 10. Illustrating the detectability of 4 objects (solid circle, black rod of 5 mm diameter; open square, cardiogreen at 70 mg/liter in 0.5% intralipid; solid square, cardiogreen at 3.5 mg/liter in 0.5 intralipid; open diamonds, intralipid only).

SUMMARY

Photon migration provides sensitive tissue oximetry in which the optical pathlength is known. Phase array gives the precise location of a sub-nanomolar amount of hidden absorber in highly scattering medium.

ACKNOWLEDGMENTS

This work was supported in part by NIH Grants NS-27346 and HL-44125

REFERENCES

1. J. Tyndall. "Contributions to Molecular Physics in the Domain of Radiant Heat," Appleton & Co., New York, 1873.
2. G.A. Millikan. *Experiments on muscle haemoglobin*, Proc. Roy. Soc. London B. 123:218-244 (1937).
3. Feng, S. person. commun.
4. Chance, B., Dait, M.T., Chang, C., Hamaoka, T. and Hagerman, F. (1991) Non-invasive Evaluation of Deoxygenation during Intense Exercise and Recovery of Oxygenation of Hemoglobin and Myoglobin in the Quadriceps Muscles of Elite Competitive Rowers. Am. J. Physiol. 262:C766-C775.
5. Chance, B., (1989) Metabolic Heterogeneities in Rapidly Metabolizing Tissues. J. Applied Cardiology 4:207-221.
6. Wang, Z.; Wang, D.-J.; Noyszewski, E.A.; Bogdan, A.R.; Haselgrove, J.C.; Zimmerman, R.A.; Leigh, J.S: (1992) *SMRM Eleventh Annual Scientific Meeting*, August 8-14, Berlin, Germany, p. 2712.
7. Lord Rayleigh, *Phil. Mag.* **37**, 321; 1919.
8. Sevick, E.M. and Chance, B. (1991) Quantitation of Time-and Frequency-Resolved Optical Spectra for the Determination of Tissue Oxygenation. Anal. Biochem. 195: 330-351.
9. Cui, W., Kumar, C. and Chance. B. (1991) Experimental study of migration depth for the photons measured at sample surface In: Proceedings of Time-Resolved Spectroscopy and Imaging of Tissues, SPIE (B. Chance, ed) SPIE, Bellingham, WA, pages 1431:180-191.
10. O'Leary, M.A., Boas, D.A., Chance, B. and Yodh, A.G. (1992) Refraction of Diffuse Photon Density Waves. Phys. Rev. 69:2658-2661.

MODELING OXYGEN TRANSPORT: DEVELOPMENT OF METHODS AND CURRENT STATE

Duane F. Bruley

University of Maryland Baltimore County, College of Engineering
5401 Wilkens Avenue, Baltimore, Maryland 21228

INTRODUCTION

It is a privilege and a pleasure to be a participant in a symposium in honor of Professor Gehard Thews. This is a special occasion for me because my professional career is closely tied to Professor Thews and his early work in mathematical modeling oxygen transport in the microcirculation of tissue.

In the spring of 1962 I had the good fortune of meeting one of the pioneers in the study of microcirculation at the Medical College of South Carolina in Charleston, South Carolina. The encounter was by chance since a colleague (Dr. William Barlage) and I had just about completed our one and one-half day visit to the Medical College when Dr. Melvin H. Knisely, then Head of the Anatomy Department, stopped and asked where we were from and what our interests were. When we told him we were chemical engineering Professor's from Clemson University, he invited us to lunch. At lunch he learned that I had just completed my Ph.D. and my dissertation included the simulation of the Thermal dynamics of a wetted-wall column (time dependent-coupled partial differential equations in cylindrical coordinates) on a digital computer. He immediately asked if I would be interested in modeling and simulating oxygen transport in the microcirculation of nervous tissue. Being turned on by the idea he said he would furnish me a publication that he felt was leading the field with the request that I evaluate the work and discern whether or not we could collaborate and even further enhance the calculations. The publication was **"Oxygen Diffusion In the Brain A Contribution to the Question of the Oxygen Supply of the Organs,"** Pflugers Archives, 271:197-226, 1960 by DR. GEHARD THEWS. After translating the article and reviewing the work I was extremely interested and impressed. I then told Dr. Knisely that I would like to work on the project and that I thought we could make a contribution by extending Dr. Thews analytical solutions to computer simulations so we could investigate system non-linearities, such as the oxygen dissociation curve. With that commitment I studied the physiology (being a traditional chemical engineer all of my past experience was with non-living systems) of the microcirculation for about one year and then derived an initial set of coupled partial differential equations describing the Krogh capillary-tissue system. The set of PDE's was then solved by standard techniques for normal and many pathological cases.

From that initial encounter with Dr. Melvin H. Knisely and the review of Dr. Gehard Thews paper, I have been involved with experimental and theoretical work related to oxygen transport in the microcirculation. Dr. Haim Bicher joined our team in 1968 to contribute to the experimental side of our studies. In 1971, I invited Dr. Bicher to join me in sponsoring a symposium on oxygen transport to tissue. As a result of our effort to develop the meeting we organized and founded ISOTT in 1973 at the Charleston-Clemson meeting selecting Dr. Knisely as the honorary first meeting president. Therefore, I am very pleased to be part of this symposium in honor of Dr. Gehard Thews, particularly at an ISOTT meeting.

Oxygen Transport to Tissue XV, Edited by P. Vaupel
et al., Plenum Press, New York, 1994

Partial Historical Developments

August Krogh (1, 2, 3) was the first researcher to apply a mathematical analysis to the relation of capillary distribution and tissue oxygen supply. He felt that the effectiveness of oxygen delivery to the tissues was strongly dependent on the distribution of capillaries and the permeabilities of capillary walls and tissue.

Krogh was also the first to experimentally measure oxygen diffusion through tissue and to report an effective diffusivity. Most significantly, he concluded that the capillaries were distributed with such regularity in some cases that tissue oxygenation could be adequately represented by a single capillary surrounded by an annular volume element of tissue. Krogh determined the average dimensions of this representative model and then collaborated with the Danish mathematician Erlang to mathematically describe the oxygen transport in tissue.

Despite its overt simplicity, the Krogh tissue cylinder has been used by many as the basis for oxygen transport studies (4).

A.V. Hill (5) derived equations describing the transport of oxygen, lactic acid, and carbon dioxide in several geometric configurations of tissue. His work is important to the theoretical understanding of gas diffusion in living tissue and was organized in a four part paper.

Opitz and Schneider (6) were among the first to conduct combined theoretical and experimental investigations on oxygen supply in brain tissue. In their theoretical work, Opitz and Schneider modified the steady state equations describing oxygen transport in the Krogh tissue cylinder to include axial diffusion. These were used to study oxygen delivery at the cellular level. From this work they concluded that an oxygen excess existed in the healthy brain, and that axial diffusion contributed to the oxygen supply to the tissue at the venous end of the capillary.

F. J. W. Roughton (7) applied Bessel function solutions to the steady and unsteady state diffusion of oxygen into the Krogh cylinder. He applied Krogh's assumptions and obtained solutions of oxygen tension as a function of time and radial distance at a given axial position. These simulations included diffusion of oxygen without reaction, with zero order kinetics and with first order kinetics.

Seymor S. Kety (8) reviewed previous work on the Krogh model and derived an equation giving the average oxyhemoglobin saturation over a capillary cross-section. This average was linear along the capillary and assumed homogeneous tissue oxygen consumption and negligible axial diffusion. Kety indicated the neglect of axial diffusion may have introduced considerable error.

GEHARD THEWS (9) published the article, referred to earlier in this manuscript, in 1960 summarizing his work in oxygen transport to the tissues. He was apparently the first to consider oxygen gradients in the capillary. Dr. Thews maintained the significance of an oxygen tension gradient across the capillary to the radial oxygen transport. Considering a homogeneous distribution of capillaries unlikely, he employed an alternate method for determining tissues radius. The consumption of oxygen was treated as by Opitz and Schneider, with the same metabolic rate for gray matter being employed. However, new diffusion coefficients were measured and presented. Dr. Thews mitigated the nonlinear effects by simulating the venous end of the capillary and assuming a stationary, nonflow arrangement.

Dr. Thews chief concern was the lethal corner oxygen tension. He employed his technique to calculate the oxygen tension at the wall, and applied Krogh's equation to calculate the tension at the lethal corner. He concluded that there was not an oxygen excess in the brain.

D. F. Bruley, M. H. Knisely, D. D. Reneau and T. A. McCracken published two papers (10, 11) which present and numerically solve equations (as derived by Bruley) describing the transport and reaction of oxygen in the capillary and gray matter of the brain. The numerical solutions employed the Krogh tissue cylinder geometrical model, homogeneous metabolic activity, radial and axial diffusion, and the nonlinearity of the oxyhemoglobin saturation curve.

The first work simulated the steady state distribution of oxygen tension in the capillary and tissue. Axial diffusion in blood and tissue was neglected in the first version to study the effects of flat and parabolic blood velocity profiles in the capillary. The effect of arterial carbon dioxide tension on the venous oxygen partial pressure was also investigated.

The second study included axial diffusion and was compared to the first particularly for the cases of arterial and venous hypoxia. The results led to the conclusion that axial diffusion did little to modify oxygen delivery at the venous end. Later calculations by McCracken, Bruley, and Knisely (12) showed that axial diffusion was in fact important to the difference between arterial and venous hypoxia. In venous hypoxia, only the venous end suffers oxygen difficiency. In arterial hypoxia, the oxygen tension is low at the entrance to the capillary as well. (It is hypothesized that the tissue withstands venous hypoxia better because supplementary oxygen can diffuse from the tissue at the arterial end of the capillary.)

The second paper also considered the simulation of transient oxygen tension profiles in blood and tissue. This method included both radial and axial diffusion, constant tissue metabolic rate, and a term to account for oxygen release from the erythrocyte. The system was forced with step changes in oxygen tension applied to steady state arterial hypoxia. The results were presented graphically and showed not only the expected pure diffusion axially in the tissue, but also in the capillary.

T. A. McCracken, D. F. Bruley, and M. H. Knisely (16) collaborated on the development of a distributed parameter model describing the simultaneous transport of oxygen, carbon dioxide and glucose for both capillaries and tissue in the human brain. The model was solved for steady state cases to give the interactions of the three components.

Over the years, mathematical modeling has not been limited to the Krogh cylinder geometry. Metzger (13), Grunewald (14), and Hutten, Thews, and Vaupel (15) have conducted simulations of oxygen transport with a variety of geometric configurations. Grunewald compared the experimental results with those of mathematical models for asymmetric, concurrent, and countercurrent flow. Hutten, Thews, and Vaupel constructed a transistor-resistor analog to a capillary-tissue array. Herman Metzger worked with alternate geometries, and introduced work on both countercurrent models and a three dimensional mesh system. The first (13) allowed for inhomogeneous blood flow and was used to analyze concurrent and countercurrent flow systems for normoxia and arterial hypoxia in brain tissue. The latter paper (17) dealt with the three dimensional modeling of a mesh of orthogonal capillaries in brain tissue. The model incorporated inhomogeneous blood flow and was used to evaluate the influence of several important physiological parameters upon the oxygen tension frequency distribution pattern.

D. F. Bruley, D. D. Reneau, H. I. Bicher and M. H. Knisely devised a lumped parameter model for the erythrocyte, plasma, and tissue (18). This model gave a venous oxygen tension which correlated with that of distributed parameter models. It was noted that the lumped parameter model provided space averaged values, whereas the determination of point values, such as lethal corner oxygen tension, required a distributed parameter model. In these simulations, however, the emphasis was on the AUTOREGULATORY effect produced by low oxygen tension in the brain tissue.

An experimental program was conducted to measure tissue and blood oxygen tension in anesthetized, curarized cats. Oxygen deficiency at the arteriole end produced tissue anoxia. However, autoregulatory mechanisms appear to delay the onset of anoxia for a longer time than if solely diffusion and convection effects were at play. Experimental and theoretical results indicated two possible autoregulatory effects: first flow changes occur, and second, the tissue metabolism is reduced, apparently by Michaelis-Menten kinetics.

Another model was derived to simulate the dynamic relationship of oxygen levels, entering the lungs and the response of the cerebral cortex oxygen tension. This model provided a convenient and useful method for elucidating such physiological phenomena as the transport of anabolites and metabolites in the capillary tissue system and the effect of superimposed autoregulation. Results indicated that autoregulation based upon oxygen tension levels did have a protective function in the survival of single neurons during hypoxia. The concept of OXYGEN SENSITIVE AUTOREGULATION resulted from this work.

J. E. Fletcher (19) employed a Krogh cylinder model to study the effects of nonequilibrium kinetics and the shift of the Hb-O_2 saturation curve on the steady state oxygen tension profiles in tissue. The simulation included axial diffusion in the tissue and an equation governing the kinetics of O_2 release from the hemoglobin.

D. F. Bruley, L. F. Groome, D. H. Hunt, H. I. Bicher, and M. H. Knisely (20) devised a pseudo-steady state model of oxygen transport to tissue. A Krogh cylinder geometry was employed, finite differenced and solved on a hybrid computer. Results from previous dynamic solutions the pseudo steady state approach to be valid, for small time constant systems with relatively slow changing inputs (this is true in the microcirculation due to the filtering effect in the lungs and vascular systems and the "1" second time constant of the Krogh capillary tissue configuration).

L.F. Groome, D.F. Bruley and M.H. Knisely (28) used a stochastic approach to simulate tissue oxygenation from single erythrocytes. The results when several erythrocytes were used compared well with deterministic models solved by finite difference calculus.

T. Ono and H. Tazawa (21) conducted microphotmetric studies with Masaji Mochizuki (22) on the reaction of oxygen and carbon monoxide with red cells. A mathematical analysis of the oxygen transport mechanism coupled with the experimental velocity data was used to determine a mass transfer coefficient for the red cell wall.

D. F. Bruley, D. D. Reneau, H. I. Bicher, and N. H. Knisely developed and tested mathematical simulations of nonequilibrium erythrocyte deoxygenation (18). Both steady state and dynamic models were presented and incorporated a first order expression for the release kinetics of oxyghemoglobin. The steady state model employed a distributed parameter system with the Krogh cylinder geometry, and was solved digitally by the method of lines.

R.S. Artique, D.F. Bruley and C.W. Williford - developed a steady state mathematical model of oxygen and carbon dioxide transport at the capillary level to test the effect of the experimentally determined red blood cell mass transfer coefficient on tissue oxygen delivery, (23,24). The model includes axial convection and diffusion in the capillary and radial diffusion in a metabolically homogeneous tissue.

Many other investigators have made important contributions to the understanding of oxygen transport in the microcirculation via mathematical modeling. Some of these investigators include, D. Lübbers, K. Groebe, A.S. Popel, Y.Kislykov, N. Busch, M.Halberg, D. Hellums, D. Wodick, L. Hoofd, Z. Turek and many others to numerous to mention with limited space. The computers and methodologies being used today allow much more sophisticated approaches over the purely analytical approaches and the early computer solution techniques. This historical paper will now elaborate on a particular computer scheme that began development in 1962 and is now evolving as a competitive strategy for doing large scale computations of transport phenomena on relatively small computers.

The mathematical models and computer simulations for mass transfer in biological systems have been difficult to develop because of the complexity of biological systems and the lack of suitable and efficient computational techniques to solve the resulting equations. Especially, the heterogeneity of biological systems is very difficult to deal with by conventional numerical techniques. While traditional stochastic or probabilistic methods might handle the heterogeneous systems, they consume a tremendous amount of computation time.

The Bruley-Williford-Kang (B-W-K) Technique (26, 27) evolved out of the W-B method (25) and is a novel and promising technique for solving mass or heat transport problems because of its ability to calculate three dimensional, time dependent solutions in heterogeneous, convection, diffusion and reaction systems. This technique solves explicitly by using the mean distance calculated from the transient probability density function (pdf) during a short discrete time. This method is faster than other stochastic/probabilistic techniques since it uses the mean distance of the movement of molecules between two adjacent grid points in the system instead of performing actual random walks and is capable of dealing with heterogeneities because each grid point can use different probability density functions in the the three dimensions.

The B-W-K Technique is, in a sense, a combination of probabilistic and numerical methods capitalizing on advantages of both methods. Some of these are as follows:

1. There are no differential equations to deal with. Only the mean distance of a density function representing the system between two grid points is computed.
2. The calculations involved in this technique are simple.

3. The computation time, compared to other probabilistic or stochastic methods, is much less because the mean distance of the molecular movement is used instead of performing random walk calculations.
4. Three dimensional, time dependent, diffusion (conduction), convection, and reaction problems can be solved by this technique.
5. This technique is capable of dealing with heterogeneous problems if the heterogeneity can be discretized in grids.

UNDERLYING THEORIES OF B-W-K

I. Green's Function and Probability Density Function

One of the advantages of using the Green's Function is that the general solution of the non-homogeneous mass or heat transfer problems can be expressed by the functions satisfying homogeneous boundary conditions. However, generally it is not easy to obtain the Green's Function except in a few cases and even in cases where the Green's Function solution can be obtained, the calculation of the solution is not simple. Therefore, in the B-W-K technique, the system is discretized in space, and the space between two nodal points is assumed to be part of a homogeneous system for a very small discretized time step except for the grids at the boundaries.

When there is diffusion, convection, and reaction (in this particular case, the zeroth order reaction rate) with no boundary (e.g., $-\infty < x, y, z < +\infty$), mass transfer in the system can be expressed as follows;

$$\frac{\partial C}{\partial t} = D_x \frac{\partial^2 C}{\partial x^2} + D_y \frac{\partial^2 C}{\partial y^2} + D_z \frac{\partial^2 C}{\partial z^2} - v_x \frac{\partial C}{\partial x} - v_y \frac{\partial C}{\partial y} - v_z \frac{\partial C}{\partial z} + R_x \tag{1}$$

where,

C: Concentration
D: Diffusion coefficient
R_X: Reaction rate (in this particular case, Rx is the zeroth order reaction rate)
t: Time at the solution point
v: Convective velocity

subscript x,y,z: x,y, and z direction, respectively.

When the initial condition, C', at a spatial point, x', y', and z' is given at time of t' as a point source, the solution, C_s at the point, x.y. and z at time, t, is:

$$C_s(x,y,z,t) = \int \int_{-\infty}^{\infty} \int C'(x', y', z', t')(\frac{\varepsilon_x \varepsilon_y \varepsilon_z}{\pi^3})^{\frac{1}{2}} \text{Exp} [-\varepsilon_x (x - x' - v_x t)^2$$
$$- \varepsilon_y (y - y' - v_y t)^2 - \varepsilon_z (z - z' - v_z t)^2 \, dx' \, dy' \, dz' + \int_{t'}^{t} R_x \, dt' \tag{2}$$

where ε is $\dfrac{1}{(4D\,t)}$

After rearranging, equation (2) can be written as follows:

$$C_s(x,y\,z,t) = \int_{-\infty}^{\infty} (\frac{\varepsilon_x}{\pi})^{\frac{1}{2}} \text{Exp} [-\varepsilon_x (z - z' - v_z t)^2 \, dz' \int_{-\infty}^{\infty} (\frac{\varepsilon_y}{\pi})^{\frac{1}{2}} \text{Exp} [-\varepsilon_y (y - y' - v_y t)^2 \, dy'$$
$$\int_{-\infty}^{\infty} (\frac{\varepsilon_z}{\pi})^{\frac{1}{2}} \text{Exp} [-\varepsilon_z (x - x - v_x t)^2] \, dx' \, C'(x', y', z', t') + \int_{t'}^{t} R_x \, dt' \tag{3}$$

In the case that only one dimension is considered, this equation becomes,

$$C_{1s}(x,t) = (\frac{\varepsilon_x}{\pi})^{\frac{1}{2}} \int_{-\infty}^{+\infty} C_1(x',t') \, \text{Exp}[-\varepsilon_x(x - x' - v_x t)^2] \, dx' + \int_{t'}^{t} R_x \, dt' \tag{4}$$

where C_{1s} is the solution for one dimensional problem and C_1 is the concentration of one dimensional problem at the time $t=t'$ and the position $x=x'$.

To compute the concentration at the position $x = 0.0$ at the next time step, for the initial condition $x = x'$, $t' = 0.0$, equation (4) may be written as:

$$C_{1s}(0,\Delta t) = (\frac{\varepsilon_x}{\pi})^{\frac{1}{2}} \int_{-\infty}^{+\infty} C_1(x',0) \, \text{Exp}[-\varepsilon_x(-x' - v_x \Delta t)^2 \, dx' + R_x \Delta t$$

where $\Delta t = t - t'$ and ε_x becomes $\dfrac{1}{(4 D \Delta t)}$. $\tag{5}$

Equation (5) means that the next time step concentration at a grid point (i.e. after one time step size) is the effect of the sum of two terms. One term is given by the mass transport by diffusion and convection between two grid points,

$$G_v(x', \Delta t) = (\frac{\varepsilon_x}{\pi})^{\frac{1}{2}} \, \text{Exp}[-\varepsilon_x(-x' - v_x \Delta t)^2], \tag{6}$$

where G_v is the Green's density function for the system of diffusion and convection without any boundary. The other term of equation (5) is from the reaction which occurs between two grid points during the time step size, Δt. This second term can be treated separately from the first term.

Equation (6) is also analogous to the Gaussian density function when the term,

$(\frac{\varepsilon_x}{\pi})^{1/2} \, \text{Exp}[-\varepsilon_x(x' + v_x \Delta t)^2]$, is changed to $(2\varepsilon_x)^{1/2}(2\pi)^{-1/2} \, \text{Exp}[\frac{-\varepsilon_x(x' + v_x \Delta t)^2}{2} 2]$.

Then Equation (5) becomes

$$G_v(x') = \sqrt{\frac{2\varepsilon_x}{2\pi}} \, \text{Exp}[\frac{-[\sqrt{2\varepsilon_x}(-x' - v_x \Delta t)]^2}{2}]. \tag{7}$$

Equation (7) is exactly the same as the Gaussian density function,

$$\Phi(x', \sigma^2) = (\frac{1}{\sqrt{2\pi}\,\sigma}) \, \text{Exp}[\frac{-(x' - \mu)^2}{2\sigma^2}] \tag{8}$$

where the terms, $-v_x \Delta t$ and $\dfrac{1}{\sqrt{2}\,\varepsilon_x}$, are replaced by μ and σ (mean and standard deviation of the normal density function).

Equation (7) is the transient density function between two nodal points for a single time step, Δt.

II.   Mean Value Theorem

One of the assumptions of the B-W-K Technique is the "Linear Interpolation' of the solution values between two nodal points. Therefore, the solutions for one time step ahead are calculated using the linearized current solutions and the transient density function between two spatial grid points, while other probabilistic or stochastic techniques perform the actual random walks, thus consuming a tremendous amount of computation time.

When a function, $\eta(x)$, is a real valued function of a real variable defined for all real numbers, the expectation of the function, $E[\eta(x)]$, can be calculated as follows.

$$E[\eta(x)] = \int_a^b \eta(x) f(x)\, dx \tag{9}$$

where $f(x)$ is the probability density function and $\int_a^b f(x)\, dx = 1$.

The second mean value theorem says that if the functions $\eta(x)$ and $f(x)$ are continuous on the interval $[a,b]$, then, there is a number, λ, in the open interval (a,b) such that

$$\int_a^b \eta(x) f(x)\, dx = \eta(\lambda) \int_a^b f(x)\, dx \tag{10}$$

Let us suppose that the $\eta(x)$ is a linear function, $\eta(x) = Ax+B$, where A and B are constants and $f(x)$ is a probability desnity function (i.e. $f(x) \geq 0$, $\int_a^b f(x) = 1$ and $f(x)$ is continuous).

In the B-W-K Technique the density function $f(x)$ is a transient density function between t and t+Δt as well as a function of the spatial variable, x. In other words, each value of the function, $\eta(x)$, at the position, x, has probability density value of $D(x,\Delta t)$ to affect to the solution point, X_S, after the time interval, Δt. For the computation of a solution by this method, only one side of the transient density function from the solution point, X_S, is dealt with at a time, i.e. either $[-\infty, X_S]$ or $[X_S, \infty]$. Therefore, the density function at each side has to be re-normalized (i.e. divide by the term, $[\int_a^b D(x)\, dx]$ to obtain the mean value. Then, the density function, $f(x)$ becomes

$[\dfrac{D(x)}{\int_a^b D(x)\, dx]}]$ and the mean value (or the expectation of function, $E[\eta(x)]$ is

$$E[\eta(x)] = \frac{\int_a^b \eta(x) D(x,\Delta t)\, dx}{\int_a^b D(x, \Delta t)\, dx} \tag{a}$$

$$= \frac{\int_a^b (Ax + B) D(x,\Delta t)\, dx}{\int_a^b D(x, \Delta t)\, dx} \tag{b}$$

$$= \frac{A\int_a^b x\, D(x,\Delta t)\, dx}{\int_a^b D(x,\Delta t)\, dx} + \frac{\int_a^b B\, D(x,\Delta t)\, dx}{\int_a^b D(x,\Delta t)\, dx} \qquad (c) \qquad\qquad (11)$$

The value for a is $-\infty$ (or Xs) and b is Xs (or ∞) and the computation of mean values can be mathematically expressed as the following equation.

$$\eta(\lambda) = A\,\lambda + B \qquad\qquad (12)$$

The value, λ, is analogous to the center of mass and $\dfrac{D(x,\Delta t)\, dx}{\int_a^b D(x,\Delta t)\, dx}$, as the mass elements between two nodal points. When the functional values between two grid points are linear, the mean value between two grid points is the functional value at the mean distance of the density function between two points.

III.   Markov Property

In the B-W-K Technique, for the computation of the solution from the time step, $(t+\Delta t)$, to the time step, $(t+2\Delta t)$, the Markov Property was applied. The Markov Property assumes that if a particle moves from one state to another state, there is a certain set of transient probabilities regardless of what state it has been in before. Once the new time solutions are computed at the time, $(t+\Delta t)$, by the method described in the section B, the solutions at $(t+\Delta t)$ are used as the a prior time solutions for the computation of solution at $(t+2\Delta t)$ which is one more time step ahead.

Summary

Many investigators have contributed to the quantitative understanding of oxygen transport to tissue. Computers continue to improve in speed and architecture thus allowing more sophisticated modeling approaches to be employed. This paper highlights the development of a unique computational strategy, the B-W-K method, that was developed to handle large simulations on small computers. It has proven to be very effective for the solution of large-scale problems in oxygen transport to tissue.

References

1.   Krogh, August. "The Rate of Diffusion of Gases Through Animal Tissues with Some Remarks on the Coefficient of Invasion," Jour. Physiol. 52:391-408. 1918-1919.

2.   Krogh, August. "The Number and Distribution of Capillaries in Muscles with Calculations of the Oxygen Pressure Head Necessary for Supplying the Tissue," Jour. Physiol. 52:409-415. 1918-1919.

3.   Krogh, August. "The Supply of Oxygen to the Tissues and the Regulations of the Capillary Circulation," Jour. Physiol. 52:457-474 1918-1919.

4.   Krogh, August. The Anatomy and Physiology of Capillaries, Yale University Press, New Havenm, Conn., led. 1922.

5.   Hill, A.V. "The Diffusion of Oxygen and Lactic Acid Through Tissues," Proc. Roy. Soc. B 104:39-96, 1928.

6.   Opitz, Erich and Max Schneider. "The Oxygen Supply of the Brain and the Mechanism of Deficiency Effects," <u>Ergebnisse der Physiologie, biologische Chemie.</u>

7.   Roughton, F.J. W. "Diffusion and Chemical Reaction Velocity as Joint Factors in Determining the Rate Uptake of Oxygen and Carbon Monoxide by the Red Corpuscles," <u>Proc. Roy. Soc.</u> B 111:1-36, 1932.

8.   Kety, Seymour S. "Determinants of Tissue Oxygen Tension," Ped. Proc. 16:666-670. 1957.

9.   Thews, Gehard. "Oxygen Diffusion in the Brain. A Contribution to the Question of the Oxygen Supply of the Organs,"Pflugers Archiv. 271:197-226, 1960.

10.   McCracken, T.A., Bruley, D.F., Reneau, D.D., Bicher, H.I. and M.H. Knisely. "Systems Analysis of Transport Processes in Human Brain; O_2, CO_2, Glucose," 1st Pacific Chemical Engineering Congress, Kyoto, Japan, October, 1972.

11.   Reneau, D.D., D.F. Bruley, M.H. Knisely. "Digital Simulation of Transient Oxygen Transport in Capillary - Tissue Systems "Cerebral Gray Matter"," Amer. Inst. Chem. Eng. J. Vol. 15:916-925, 1969.

12.   McCracken, T.A., Bruley, D.F. and M.H. Knisely. "A Systems Analysis for the Transport of Oxygen and the Simultaneous Transport of Oxygen, Carbon Dioxide, and Glucose in the Capillaries and Tissue of the Human Brain," Unpublished Ph.D. Dissertation, Clemson University, Clemson, South Carolina, 1971.

13.   Metzger, H. "PO_2 Histogram of Three Dimensional Systems with Homogeneous and Inhomogeneous Microcirculation, a Digital Computer Study," Oxygen Transport in Tissue Workshop, Dortmund, Germany, July, 1971.

14.   Grunewald, W. "Method of Comparison of Calculated and Measured Oxygen Distribution," Oxygen Transport in Tissue Workshop. Dortmund, Germany, July, 1971.

15.   Hutten, H., G. Thews, and P. Vaupel. "Some Special Problems Concerning the Oxygen Supply to Tissue, as Studies by an Analog Computer," Oxygen Transport in Tissue Workshop, Dortmund, Germany, July, 1971.

16.   McCracken, T.A., Bruley, D.F. and M.H. Knisely. "A Systems Analysis for the Transport of Oxygen and the Simultaneous Transport of Oxygen, Carbon Dioxide and Glucose in the Capillaries and Tissue of the Human Brain," Chemical Engineering Department Report, Clemson University, Clemson, S.C.

17.   Metzger, H. "Advances in Experimental Medicine and Biology," Vol. 37 A & B, Plenum Press, N.Y., 1973.

18.   Bruley, D.F., D.D. Reneau, H.I. Bicher and M.H. Knisely. "Theoretical Studies of Brain Tissue Oxygenation Considering the Deoxygenation Rate of the Red Cell," VIIth Conf. of the Europ. Soc. for Proc. of Microcirc., Aberdeen, Scotland, Bibl. anat., <u>11</u>, 507 (Karger, Basel 1973).

19.   Fletcher, J.E. "Advances in Experimental Medicine and Biology", Plenum Press, New York, 1975.

20.   Bruley, D.F., L. Groome, D.H. Hunt, H.I. Bicher, and M.H. Knisely, "Predicting Oxygen Supply to Brain Tissue Using a Pseudo Dynamic

Model Simulation Technique," presented at the Eighth European Conference in Microcirculation, Le Touquet, France, June, 1974.

21. Ono, Tsukasa, and Hiroshi Tazawa. "Microphotometric Methods for Measuring the Oxygenation and Deoxygenation Rate in a Single Red Blood Cell," Japanese J. of Physiol. 25, 93-107, 1975.

22. Mochizuki, Masaji. "On the Velocity of Oxygen Dissociation of Human Hemoglobin and Red Cell," Japanese J. of Physiol., Vol. 16, No. 6, Dec. 15, 1966.

23. Artigue, R., D.F. Bruley, D. Von Rosenberg, M. Mochizuki. "The Effect of the Red Blood Cell Deoxygenation Rate on Oxygen Delivery to Tissue," 9th Europ. Conf. Microcirculation, Antwerp 1976. Bibl. anat., No. 15, pp. 405-508 (Karger, Basel 1977).

24. Artigue, R. S., D. F. Bruley and C. Williford. "Oxygen and Carbon Dioxide Transport in Human Brain: Effect of the Mass Transfer Coefficient of the Red Blood Cell," Rose-Hulman Institute of Technology, Terre Haute, IN, and Tulane University, New Orleans, LA. Unpublished at this printing.

25. Williford, C., D. Bruley and R. Artique. "Probabilistic Modelling of Oxygen Transport on Brain Tissue," Neuro Research 2, 153-170 (1974).

26. Kang, K., D. Bruley and H. Bicher. "A Computer Simulation of Simultaneous Heat and Oxygen Transport During Three Dimensional Tumor Hyperthermia", Oxygen Transport to Tissue X, Advances in Experimental Medicine and Biology, Plenum Press, Vol. 222, 747-756 (1988).

27. Kang, K. and D. Bruley. "A Simulation of Three Dimensional Oxygen Transport In Brain Tissue with A Single Neuron-Single Capillary System by the Williford-Bruley Technique," Oxygen Transport to Tissue - VI, Advances in Experimental Medicine and Biology, Plenum Press, Vol. 180, 887-899 (1984).

28. Groome, L.J., Bruley, D.F. and M.H. Knisely, "A Stochastic Model for the Transport of Oxygen to the Brain", Oxygen Transport to Tissue - II; Advances in Experimental Medicine and Biology, Plenum Publishing Corporation 75, pp. 267-277, 1976.

RESPIRATORY SYSTEM

OPTIMAL PRE-OXYGENATION: THE NASORAL-SYSTEM

Fritz Mertzlufft,[1] and Rolf Zander[2]

[1] Clinic of Anaesthesiology and Intensive Care Medicine
Saarland-University Medical School at Homburg
D-6650 Homburg-Saar, Germany
[2] Institute of Physiology and Pathophysiology
Johannes Gutenberg-University at Mainz
D-6500 Mainz, Germany

INTRODUCTION

The human body's intra- and extrapulmonary O_2 reserves, i.e. the oxygen stores of the functional residual capacity (FRC) and the blood, will be rapidly depleted during any kind of respiratory arrest (apnea). Application of oxygen prior to iatrogenic apnea (e.g. for endotracheal intubation procedures), therefore, commonly is discussed [e.g. Miller, 1990] as the proposed measure designed to achieve an increase in the human body's oxygen stores sufficient to avoid hypoxemia. This prophylactic application of oxygen simply has become to be termed "pre-oxygenation", regardless of the amount of increase in the O_2 stores actually achieved. A myriad of different techniques and procedures are practically used, although only few information has been provided by textbooks referring to this so-called "pre-oxygenation" [e.g. Atkinson et al., 1986; Larsen, 1989; Miller, 1990].

However, the true goal behind any "pre-oxygenation" procedure is to achieve a total intrapulmonary replacement of the existing gas mixture, nitrogen in particular, by pure oxygen in order to really improve patient's safety. This total intrapulmonary oxygen enrichment, in contrast to simple oxygen application maneuvers (i.e. pre-oxygenation), has become to be termed »optimal pre-oxygenation« [Zander and Mertzlufft, 1992; Mertzlufft and Zander, 1992].

As the result of such optimal pre-oxygenation (i.e. total nitrogen washout), the alveolar pO_2 (pAO_2) theoretically should increase to 673 mmHg at standard conditions, i.e. barometric pressure (pB) 760 mmHg, alveolar carbon dioxide partial pressure ($pACO_2$) 40 mmHg, and 47 mmHg water vapour pressure (pH_2O). This pAO_2 of 673 mmHg corresponds to 88.6% alveolar O_2 concentration and, based on a FRC of 3,000 mL, represents an intrapulmonary oxygen reservoir of 2,650 mL O_2 within the FRC, thus providing about 10 minutes of maximum safety concerning O_2 supply for patients at rest (O_2 consumption $\approx$ 250 mL/min).

Oxygen Transport to Tissue XV, Edited by P. Vaupel
et al., Plenum Press, New York, 1994

Unfortunately, total intrapulmonary oxygen enrichment, and hence nitrogen washout, can hardly be achieved in clinical practice due to the specific problems of the systems available [Berthoud et al., 1983; Mertzlufft and Zander,1992; Sandersen, 1972]: Assessment of how much denitrogenation is needed, i.e. the oxygen stores can be filled, includes minute volume in relation to the size of the FRC, FIO_2, and all mishaps of rebreathing. Since these limitations are widely accepted, literature necessarily reflects the ongoing attempts to provide clinicians with an oxygenation system allowing for optimal pre-oxygenation in every-day-practice [e.g. Ooi et al., 1992].

In this context it appears meaningful to consider the recently introduced NasOral-System [Mertzlufft and Zander, 1992] as beeing a promising contribution to such unsolved practical demands. Described as a simple oxygen applicator, the NasOral-System provides unidirectional (i.e.nasal-to-oral) flow of pure oxygen.

The present study, therefore, was designed to investigate the capability of the NasOral-System for optimal pre-oxygenation in a clinical routine setting.

METHODS

With written informed consent and following institutional approval, 20 patients (according to the ASA classification II and III) scheduled for neurosurgical treatment participated. With the exception of their neurosurgical illness, none of them suffered from any additional disease, particularly not from respiratory or cardiac disorders.

Premedication consisted of Lormetazepam 1 mg the evening before and two hours prior to the operation and induction of anesthesia.

Before discharge of the patient from the ward to the operation theatre the following set up was initiated: (1) both the blood gas analyzer (STAT Profile 5, NOVA biomedical, Waltham, USA) and the respiratory gas analyzer (AGM 1304, Brüel & Kjaer, Copenhagen, Denmark) were calibrated according to the actual barometric pressure (depending on actual climate and height above sea level), (2) the attempted inspired O_2 partial pressure (pIO_2; mmHg) was calculated for the FIO_2 of 1.0 as required for optimal pre-oxygenation at BTPS conditions (pB - 47 mmHg pH_2O), (3) the thread of the oxygen nut and liner union of the anesthetic circle system (providing piped medical oxygen delivered by liquid oxygen plants) was connected to the respiratory gas analyzer for comparison of the resulting measured pIO_2 (BTPS) with the calculated value, (4) the thread of the oxygen unit was connected in sealing-tight manner with the NasOral-System (fig. 1) which was flushed for 1 min with pure oxygen using a flow rate of 6 L/min, and then the respiratory gas analyzer (AGM 1304) and a mechanical spirometer (Volumeter 3000, Dräger) were connected to the oral gas outlet of the NasOral-System.

After arrival of the patient in the anesthesia induction room monitoring, instrumentation, and optimal pre-oxygenation were performed subsequently as usual: (1) Electrocardiogramm (PM 8014, Dräger), blood pressure (Dinamap 8100, J & J Critikon), and pulse oxymetry (OxyShuttle; J & J Critikon); (2) local anesthesia (2 mL Mepivacain 1%) and peripheral-venous (Venflon 2, 17G, Viggo) and radial artery cannulation (Insyte-W 2, 20G, Becton Dickinson); (3) fluid administration (1,000 mL of cristalloids, Schiwa); (4) optimal pre-oxygenation (NasOral-System) (fig. 1).

The NasOral-System was placed by the Anesthesia Nurse Assistent whereas optimal pre-oxygenation was performed by the patient himself using individual O_2 flow rates (4 -

8 L/min), regulated on demand with the help of the nurse staff.

The alveolar oxygen and carbon dioxide partial pressures (pAO_2, $pACO_2$; mmHg) during the total O_2 enrichment procedure were recorded endexpiratory (oral gas outlet of the NasOral-System, i.e $peEO_2$, $peECO_2$; mmHg) and continuously (exhalation-to-exhalation analysis) by means of photoacoustic-infrared technique using the AGM 1304 side-stream capnometer (Brüel & Kjaer) with proven accuracy [Zander and Mertzlufft, 1992] and registered with a Videoprinter (UP-850, Sony).
Simultaneously, the minute ventilation volumes were obtained by means of the Dräger spirometer (connected to the oral gas outlet of the NasOral-System). The oxygen and carbon dioxide partial pressures for arterial blood (paO_2, $paCO_2$; mmHg) were determined simultaneously at the end of the total O_2 enrichment, i.e. after total N_2 washout (i.e. pAO_2 = pIO_2 - $pACO_2$). Blood samples were obtained from the indwelling permanent arterial line by 2 mL plastic syringes. Measurements were double estimations with the NOVA blood gas analyzer.

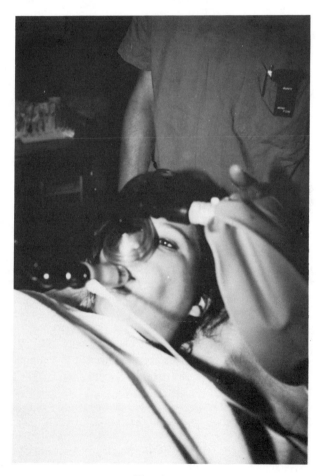

Fig. 1

The NasOral-System in operation: Nasal oxygen inflow via mask and reservoir bag, oral gas outlet comprizing one way valve and side-stream capnometer connection (according to Mertzlufft and Zander, 1992).

RESULTS

A total of 20 patients was investigated, 12 males and 8 females of various height, weight and age. The mean body height was 171.1 ± 9 cm, mean body weight was 65.8 ± 12 kg. The average life age was 36.2 ± 14 years. The minute volume for all patients was found to be 8.7 ± 2.2 L/min on average.

The mean barometric pressure (pB) during the course of the study was 734.9 ± 4.9 mmHg.

The results obtained ar summarized by table 1.

Table 1. Optimal pre-oxygenation by means of total O_2 enrichment of the FRC using the NasOral-System. 20 patients, O_2 flow 4 - 8 L/min on demand, minute volume 8.7 ± 2.2 L/min. Inspiratory and alveolar partial pressures (BTPS) obtained by side-stream capnometry, measured arterial partial pressures obtained by blood gas analysis.

PARTIAL PRESSURES [mmHg]			
pB	734.9	±	4.9
pIO_2 calculated (STPD)	735.0		
pIO_2 calculated (BTPS)	688.0		
pIO_2 measured (BTPS)	689.5	±	5.5
$pACO_2$ measured (peECO$_2$)	32.0	±	6.7
pAO_2 calculated (BTPS)	656.0		
pAO_2 measured (peEO$_2$)	658.0	±	8.7
paO_2 measured	625.0	±	9.8
$paCO_2$ measured	34.0	±	6.5

The time needed to achieve an oxygen enrichment of only 98% by using the NasOral-System was 50.9 ± 7.8 seconds, whereas the time needed to optimally fill the intrapulmonary O_2 store with 100% oxygen was 3.2 ± 0.3 min.

CONCLUSIONS

Among jeopardizing events due to unsuspected problems related to the intubation procedure are hypoxemia and hypercapnia. Respiratory deteriorations and inadequate measures of prevention and/or surveillance still are reported as the major causes for anesthesia related deaths [Larsen, 1989]. From these, particularly hypoxemia could easily be ruled out if the single oxygen store of the human body that routinely allows for therapeutic maneuvers, i.e. the intrapulmonary oxygen store of the functional residual capacity

(FRC), is only rigorously used for optimal oxygen enrichment before initiating apnea (e.g. for induction of anesthesia and endotracheal intubation). Moreover, the procedure of optimal pre-oxygenation, i.e. total oxygen enrichment of the FRC, must be considered the single measure to safely avoid the most common risk of hypoxemia. The term pre-oxygenation as commonly used for such a procedure is rather incorrectly and confusing and should be abandoned in order to avoid any mismanagement, since it only describes just some kind of oxygen application instead of the true goal, i.e. total intrapulmonary oxygen enrichment.

As shown by the results obtained with the present study (cf. table 1), within only a few seconds the intrapulmonary O_2 store increases to about 2,650 mL O_2, indeed, if the oxygenation system applied provides the gas mixture within the functional residual capacity (ca. 3,000 mL) being replaced by pure oxygen, i.e. if nitrogen can be washed out almost completely.

Thus, the oxygen applicator used for this study, i.e. the NasOral-System as introduced recently (fig. 1), has been proved to be a well-suitable and easy-to-use tool for performing optimal pre-oxygenation or, even more correct, total intrapulmonary O_2 enrichment by nitrogen washout (cf. table 1). It is an essential feature of this NasOral-System that, the oxygen supply takes place solely via the nose (nasal inflow route) whereas oxygen overflow and exhalation pass through the mouth (oral outflow route) which is prevented from drawing in ambient air by the one-way valve, i.e. that gas flow is allowed following a "nas-oral" route only. An additional benefit has been comprized by it's ease of operation, i.e. the obvious independency of any potential user's skills: The patients themselves took care for their individual nitrogen washout, and hence total intrapulmonary O_2 enrichment, without any complaint or cease of function. Moreover, neither anxiety (as occuring with contemporary systems) or increased salivation (as expected due to the oral part of the NasOral-System) nor any other event (that potentially may be obstaculous to optimal pre-oxygenation) could be observed with that new oxygen applicator. Concerning the time consuming obligatory pre-induction management of monitoring, instrumentation and pre-oxygenation, it appeared to be a further major benefit of the NasOral-System that, instead of only pre-oxygenation, optimal pre-oxygenation could be performed simultaneously rather than subsequently.

Furthermore, despite the heterogeneity of the morphometric and respiratory data of the 20 patients investigated, N_2 washout was achieved within a considerable and clinically relevant short time period ($\approx$ < 1 min for 98% oxygen enrichment) and with most economic low oxygen flow rates ($\approx$ 4 L/min). The respective alveolar pO_2 values as obtained end-expiratory by side-stream capnometry (table 1), accurately represent the expected (predominated) values. Even the arterial pO_2 as obtained by blood samples taken with plastic syringes gives indirect evidence for the appropriate function of the NasOral-System. Both values, alveolar and arterial pO_2, on secondary consideration seem to indicate that, the concept of increasing alveolar-to-arterial pO_2 difference ($AaDO_2$; mmHg) with increasing inspired O_2 fraction (FIO_2) [e.g. Falke, 1991] may be mainly influenced by the techniques of measurement. With respect to this it appears necessary to re-evaluate this concept and, however, to put it to discussion again. On the other hand, it also became rather obvious, that the relationship between alveolar and arterial pCO_2 ($AaDCO_2$; mmHg) as described by serious investigators [Nunn, 1987; Whitesell et al., 1981] regularly occurs under clinical conditions rather than being a theoretical (or clinically irrelevant) and unmeasurable variable for routine settings.

From the results found with this investigation we feel encouraged to summarize that, with respect to the safety margins (maintained O_2 supply for approx. 10 min due to the achieved optimal pAO_2) and to considerations of economic working conditions (instrumentation, connection of monitors and optimal pre-oxygenation can be performed simultaneously), the used oxygen applicator appears to be superior to any other oxygenation system actually available. If a patient is still connected to the NasOral-System (with or without the one-way valve in situ) following such optimal pre-oxygenation, however, the gas now taken up by mass-movement can only be O_2: After a 10 min period of apnea the pAO_2 then decreases from 673 to 556 mmHg only (still providing an O_2 reserve of 73.2%) [Zander and Mertzlufft, 1992]; this so-called apneic oxygenation has already been demonstrated [e.g. Nunn, 1987].

Therefore, optimal pre-oxygenation prior to apnea plus supply with pure O_2 during apnea will provide adequate O_2 supply with very high security, if required for at least 30 minutes.

We finally conclude that, the oxygen applicator "NasOral-System" has the potential to develop the standard procedure for oxygenating a patient.

REFERENCES

Atkinson, R.S., Rushman, G.B., Lee, J.A., 1986, "Synopsis der Anästhesie", 2nd ed., G. Fischer Verlag, New York.

Berthoud, M., Read, D.H., Norman, J., 1983, Pre-oxygenation - how long? Anaesthesia. 38:96.

Falke, K.J., 1991, Therapeutic thresholds for acute changes in arterial O_2 partial pressure, in: "The Oxygen Status of Arterial Blood", R. Zander and F. Mertzlufft, eds., Karger, Basel, p. 64.

Larsen, R., 1989, "Anaesthesie", Urban & Schwarzenberg, 3rd ed., München, pp. 131.

Mertzlufft, F., Zander, R., 1992, A new device for the oxygenation of patients: the «NasOral-System», Adv Exp Med Biol, Oxygen Transport to Tissue XIV. (in press).

Mertzlufft, F., Zander, R., 1992, A new oxygenation device: The NasOral-System, Abstracts 10th World Congress of Anaesthesiologists. A:493.

Miller, R.D., 1990, "Anesthesia", 3rd ed., Churchill Livingstone, New York.

Nunn, J.F., 1987, "Applied Respiratory Physiology", 3rd ed., Butterworths, London, p. 224.

Ooi, R., Pattison, J., Joshi, P., Feldman, S., Soni, N., 1992, Preoxygenation: An alternative technique, Anesth Analg. 74:S224.

Sandersen, R.G., 1972, "The Cardiac Patient", W.B. Saunders, Philadelphia.

Whitesell, L., Asiddao, C., Gollmann, D., Jablonski, J., 1981, Relationship between arterial and peak expired carbon dioxide pressure during anesthesia and factors influencing the difference, Anesth Analg. 60:508.

Zander, R., Mertzlufft, F., 1992, Clinical use of oxygen stores: pre-oxygenation and apneic oxygenation, Adv Exp Med Biol, Oxygen Transport to Tissue XIV. (in press).

Zander, R., Mertzlufft, F., 1992, Assessing the precision of capnometers, AINS Anästhesiol Intensivmed Notfallmed Schmerzther. 27:42.

EFFECTS OF PROGRESSIVE INTRATRACHEAL ADMINISTRATION OF PERFLUBRON DURING CONVENTIONAL GAS VENTILATION IN ANESTHETIZED DOGS WITH OLEIC ACID LUNG INJURY

Scott E. Curtis and Julie T. Peek

Department of Pediatrics, University of Alabama at Birmingham
Birmingham, Al 35294-0005, U.S.A.

INTRODUCTION

The respiratory distress syndrome of prematurity (RDS) is due to immaturity of alveolar type II cells which fail to produce adequate surfactant. The resultant increase in alveolar surface tension leads to both alveolar flooding and alveolar collapse, decreased compliance, and increased shunt with hypoxemia. Exogenous replacement of surfactant has reduced morbidity and mortality from RDS, though the most premature infants often fail to respond. Another possible therapy for RDS is liquid breathing (LB). Introduced by Kylstra et al. (1962), LB refers to a ventilatory mode in which the lungs are filled with a liquid perfluorocarbon (PFC) or hyperbarically oxygenated saline to functional residual capacity (FRC) followed by tidal ventilation with additional liquid. Using PFC's with surface tensions of $\approx$ 15 dynes/cm, Shaffer et al. (1983a, 1983b) showed markedly improved arterial oxygenation during LB compared to gas ventilation in surfactant-deficient, very premature lambs. Interestingly, even after drainage of PFC from the lungs of these lambs, persistent improvements in FRC, compliance, and gas exchange were seen, suggesting that residual PFC coating the alveoli improved alveolar surface tension.

In the adult respiratory distress syndrome (ARDS), pulmonary capillary injury leads to alveolar flooding with serum that inactivates surfactant (Petty et al., 1977). Deficient surfactant production due to injury of type II cells has also been postulated to occur in ARDS. Extrapolating from the success of surfactant therapy in RDS, such therapy is being investigated in animal and human trials of ARDS but with mixed results (Holm and Matalon, 1989; Zelter et al., 1990; Lachman, 1989). Success may be limited by poor distribution of surfactant within injured lungs (Jobe et al., 1984). This may be improved with larger surfactant doses (Gilliard et al., 1990), though the safety and efficacy of larger doses has not been shown. It is logical to ask whether another low surface tension material such as PFC could yield superior gas exchange in ARDS, as it has in animal models of RDS. A new substance, perfluorooctylbromide (perflubron, PFB) has excellent spreadability (o/w +2.7 dyne/cm), low surface tension (18 dyne/cm), and high O_2

solubility (50 vol% at 25°C). We hypothesized that intratracheal administration of PFB could improve lung mechanics and oxygenation in acute lung injury. In particular, we wished to see if any benefit would occur with simple bolus installation of PFB into the lungs without resorting to the more technically difficult traditional LB technique. Unlike surfactant, the high solubility of PFB for O_2 and CO_2 should not mitigate against intratracheal dosing as large as FRC. This was recently demonstrated by Fuhrman et al. (1991) who noted no change in PaO_2 or $PaCO_2$ in healthy pigs in going from conventional gas ventilation to gas ventilation with a full FRC dose of PFC. We tested our hypothesis in a canine model of severe acute lung injury induced by oleic acid. PFB was administered in six doses, each dose equal to one-sixth of FRC, so that the lungs were eventually filled to FRC with PFB. For comparison, another group of dogs were identically injured and ventilated but received no PFB.

METHODS

We studied 16 adult dogs of either sex with a mean±SD weight of 18.1±2.6 kg. All dogs were anesthetized with 30 mg/kg of IV pentobarbital, intubated, and restrained in the supine position. Anesthesia was supplemented periodically if a strong toe pinch elicited a change in heart rate or blood pressure. Muscle relaxation was achieved with a bolus IM injection of succinylcholine followed by a continuous drip. Ventilation was begun with FiO_2 of 1.0, positive end-expiratory pressure of 6 cm H_2O, rate of 20 bpm, I:E ratio of 1:1, and tidal volume adjusted to a $PaCO_2$ of 35 to 45 Torr. We placed silastic catheters in the left external jugular vein (EJV) and carotid artery and floated a 7.5 Fr Swan-Ganz catheter into the pulmonary artery (PA) via the right EJV, for blood sampling and measurement of mean arterial pressure, mean pulmonary artery pressure (MPAP) and pulmonary capillary wedge pressure (PCWP). Core temperature was monitored with the PA catheter and kept near 37°C using warming lamps. Blood gas tensions were measured and corrected to the animal's temperature. Hemoglobin and O_2 concentrations were measured and total O_2 content calculated to include dissolved O_2. Cardiac output (CO) was determined by the thermodilution technique using 5 ml injections of iced saline. Systemic O_2 delivery and uptake (DO_2 and VO_2) were determined from CO and arterial and mixed venous O_2 contents. Pulmonary vascular resistance (PVR) was calculated as the quantity MPAP minus PCWP divided by cardiac index (CI, CO/dog weight) and reported as PRU·kg. Lactate concentrations were immediately measured from drawn arterial blood. Blood volume was measured four times during each study using Evans Blue dye. Mean and peak airway pressure were recorded from the ventilator display and static respiratory system compliance (Crs) determined with the interrupter technique (Sly et al., 1987).

After the preparation was complete and all monitored values were stable, data collection began (time zero). Oleic acid (0.15 ml/kg) was then infused over 20 min. via the left EJV. Measurements were repeated at 30, 60, and 90 min. At 90 min. animals were randomized to either a control group or a PFB group (n=8 each). Both groups continued to receive gas ventilation at the initial settings until 270 min. with data collected every 20 min. In the PFB group, a dose (10 ml/kg) of PFB estimated to be one-sixth of FRC was instilled into the lungs after data collection at min. 90, 120, 140, 160, and 180. After data collection at min. 200, enough additional PFB was instilled to produce a meniscus in the ET tube parallel to the anterior surface of the dog's chest. The PFB was instilled via a side-port in the ET tube while ventilation continued and the dog was tilted in different body positions. After data sampling at min. 240, PFB was removed from the lung by putting the dog head down and suctioning the airway. In both groups,

a 10 ml/kg bolus of Dextran 70 was given IV anytime CI decreased to < 90 ml·min⁻¹·kg⁻¹.
Sodium bicarbonate (7.5%) was given as needed to keep arterial HCO_3 > 20 meq/dl.

The data from the 16 dogs prior to randomization (time 0-90 min.) were treated as
one group and analyzed by repeated measures ANOVA. After minute 120, statistically
significant differences within a group versus time and significant between group
differences were detected by ANOVA with correction for multiple comparisons done
using the conservative Duncan's multiple range test.

RESULTS

Gas exchange

Data are presented as means±SE unless otherwise stated. PaO_2 decreased
dramatically with oleic acid infusion, from 499±13 Torr to 127±22 Torr by min. 90
(Fig.1). After that, PaO_2 continued to decrease in control dogs and was in the low 50's
for the remainder of the study. In contrast, PaO_2 in PFB treated dogs was significantly
higher by the third dose (108±26 Torr vs. 55±3 Torr). The difference between groups
increased further with subsequent doses, peaking with the 6th dose (198±46 Torr vs. 51±3
Torr). Total PFB instilled to achieve FRC was 61±7 ml/kg (mean±SD). With removal
of PFB (mean±SD retrieved 29±5 ml/kg) PaO_2 decreased and was not significantly
different from controls (77±9 Torr vs. 53±3 Torr). $PaCO_2$ increased significantly with
lung injury (39±2 Torr at min. 0 to 45±3 Torr at min. 90) but did not change after min.
120. The only significant between group difference occurred at min. 270 (after PFB
removal) when $PaCO_2$ was lower in PFB dogs (44±2 Torr vs. 50±2 Torr) at the same
effective tidal volume (16±1 ml/kg). Arterial HCO_3 levels were well maintained in both
groups. On average, 0.6 meq/kg of exogenous $NaHCO_3$ was required to keep serum
HCO_3 levels greater than 20 meq/l, with no between group differences.

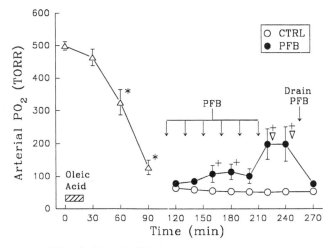

Figure 1. Data are mean±SE. * significantly different from time 0, + significantly different from controls
at same time, ▽ significantly different from time 120.

Lung mechanics

Static respiratory system compliance (Crs) decreased significantly from baseline to min. 90 (1.46 ± 0.06 ml·cmH$_2$O^{-1}·kg^{-1} to 1.13 ± 0.07 ml·cmH$_2$O^{-1}·kg^{-1}) (Fig.2). In controls, Crs continued to decrease and reached a nadir of 0.93 ml·cmH$_2$O^{-1}·kg^{-1}. Crs in PFB dogs was significantly higher than controls after the first 4 PFB doses, but declined to match controls with further lung filling. With PFB removal there was a marked increase in Crs (1.52 ± 0.15 ml·cmH$_2$O^{-1}·kg^{-1}) so that it was again significantly higher than in controls. Mean airway pressure (mPaw) increased significantly after oleic acid infusion in all dogs (9.1 ± 0.5 to 10.7 ± 2.3 cmH$_2$O). mPaw was lower in PFB dogs after the first 2 doses of PFB, but increased with subsequent doses so that mPaw was higher in PFB dogs after the 5th and 6th doses. With PFB removal mPaw again was significantly lower in PFB dogs.

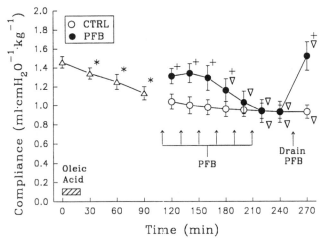

Figure 2. Data are mean$\pm$SE. * significantly different from min. 0, + significantly different from controls at same time, ▽ significantly different from min. 120.

Hemodynamics

Cardiac index decreased immediately with oleic acid infusion, from 170 ± 13 ml·min^{-1}·kg^{-1} to 107 ± 9 ml·min^{-1}·kg^{-1} by min. 30. It did not change significantly thereafter and remained above 100 ml·min^{-1}·kg^{-1} in both groups. An average total of 23.8 ± 3.1 ml/kg of Dextran 70 was required to maintain this CI, with no between group differences. Initially, changes in DO$_2$ paralleled CI, but DO$_2$ was significantly higher in PFB dogs than controls for the last 5 measurements (Fig.3). VO$_2$ did not differ from baseline at any time in either group, averaging 6.75 ± 0.12 ml·min^{-1}·kg^{-1}. Still, arterial lactate rose significantly from 1.7 ± 0.3 mmoles/l at baseline to 2.5 ± 0.5 mmoles/l at min. 90, but did not change after that or differ between groups. PVR also increased significantly with oleate infusion (0.74 ± 0.05 PRU·kg at baseline to 1.02 ± 0.07 PRU·kg at min. 90). Although PVR did not change significantly in either group after min. 120, it was lower in PFB dogs in 4 of the last 8 measurements. Blood volume was well maintained in both groups throughout the study, with an average value of 88 ± 2 ml/kg. Mean arterial pressure decreased immediately with oleate infusion, from 118 ± 5 Torr to 87 ± 4 Torr but soon rebounded and remained > 100 Torr for the rest of the study. Despite some obvious pulmonary hemorrhage in all dogs, Hct did not change significantly over the course of the study and averaged 40±1%. HR decreased significantly during the oleic acid infusion (from 151±6 bpm to 118±5 bpm) and averaged 121±2 bpm thereafter in the two groups.

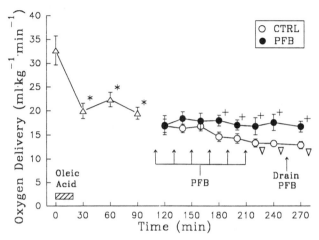

Figure 3. Data are mean±SE. * significantly different from min. 0, + significantly different from controls at same time, ▽ significanlty different from min. 120.

DISCUSSION

The adult respiratory distress syndrome (ARDS) is responsible for roughly 75,000 adult and pediatric deaths per year in the U.S. (Shale, 1987). In addition, survivors often exhibit residual lung dysfunction. The initial lung injury in ARDS is reversible, but the therapy used to maintain adequate arterial oxygenation, high FiO_2 and airway pressures, adds significant iatrogenic injury to the primary process. Efforts to interrupt the inflammatory process have failed to improve survival (Bone et al., 1987). Alternative ventilatory strategies such as high-frequency ventilation have also not altered outcome (Holzapfel et al., 1987). Extensive work demonstrating surfactant dysfunction in ARDS has prompted trials of replacement therapy (Lachman, 1989; Richman et al., 1989), and early results are encouraging. Because ARDS involves surfactant inactivation and not just deficiency, larger volumes may be needed than in RDS, and there may be limitations to the amount of surfactant that can be instilled. Perfluorocarbons are low surface tension materials (10 to 20 dyne/cm) that have been shown to improve lung mechanics in animal models of RDS (Shaffer et al., 1983b) and in one human trial (Greenspan et al., 1990). When the lungs are completely filled with PFC, lung recoil is greatly reduced (Kylstra and Schoenfish, 1972). There are, however, no PFC's that are approved for clinical use in liquid breathing. Perflubron, a pharmaceutical grade PFC, is a highly purified substance with excellent physical properties: low surface tension, high spreadability, short retention time, and high O_2 and CO_2 solubility. This study tested the hypothesis that intratracheal administration of PFB could improve lung mechanics and gas exchange in ARDS-type injury, and sought to determine the optimal dose.

We tested this use of PFB in a severe model of lung injury that produces a large amount of alveolar flooding. Oleic acid (OA) is a naturally occurring substance released into the circulation with long bone fractures and pancreatitis, two events often followed by ARDS. Infusion of OA into the pulmonary circulation results in direct damage of pulmonary capillary endothelial cells, followed by leakage of plasma and red blood cells into lung alveoli and interstitium (Motohiro et al., 1986). This causes decreased lung compliance, decreased FRC, increased shunt, and increased VD/VT. Though the mechanism is unknown, it also leads to decreased contractility and heart rate. With doses of 0.15 ml/kg, pulmonary dysfunction is usually maximum by 90 min. after infusion. Our animals demonstrated typical findings, with markedly decreased PaO_2 and Crs and increased $PaCO_2$, mPaw, and PVR. Also, CO, MAP, and HR decreased acutely with OA, necessitating volume resuscitation. This is a rather severe emulation of the lung findings early in ARDS, and one could argue that ARDS patients may show a more dramatic response than OA treated animals to any tested therapy. For example, despite using a lower dose of OA (0.037 ml/kg) than in this study, Zelter et al. (1990) were unable to show any benefit with an aerosolized surfactant in sheep.

Nevertheless, in this study PaO_2 appeared to improve after the first PFB dose, with statistical significance occurring by the third dose. This is in spite of the fact that alveolar PO_2 must be lower in PFB dogs due to the presence of PFB vapor (10.4 Torr). Crs was significantly higher than in controls after the very first dose of PFB suggesting that it may have improved alveolar surface tension. Although we have not solved the dilemma of how to measure FRC in a partially fluid-filled lung (the gas *and* liquid compartments), the increased oxygenation implies that lung recruitment and improved V/Q relations did occur. Of interest is the large improvement in oxygenation that occurred after the 6th PFB dose, as instilled volume finally equalled FRC, while static Crs *decreased* in PFB dogs from the 4th dose on. The decrease in Crs as the lungs approached filling may have represented over-distension: our total instilled dose of 61 ± 7 ml/kg can not be interpreted as an FRC of 61 ± 7 ml/kg, since some PFB was probably lost via evaporation. Still, resting volume of excised dog lungs filled with PFC was 50 ml/kg (Kylstra and Schoenfish, 1972) and, in vivo, the additional outward recoil of the chest wall should increase FRC slightly further. Thus, end-inspiration in PFB dogs was probably occurring near total lung capacity (70 to 80 ml/kg) and the flat portion of the pressure-volume curve. This may have obscured any improvement in alveolar surface tension and explain the late decrease in Crs in PFB dogs as the lungs filled. Still, it is important to note that at its highest, mPaw was only 3 cmH_2O greater in PFB dogs than in controls.

The doubling of PaO_2 with dose 6 of PFB indicates a sudden improvement of V/Q matching. Studies in saline-filled (West et al., 1965) and in PFC-filled lungs (Lowe and Shaffer, 1986) have shown a redistribution of pulmonary blood flow, away from posterior lung towards the anterior, due to the hydrostatic effects of the fluid. It is likely then that a significant portion of pulmonary blood flow in our partially PFB filled lungs went to anterior lung segments. The sudden improvement in PaO_2 with the addition of only slightly more PFB at dose six might be explained by a recruitment of anterior lung segments that were previously perfused but poorly ventilated. Lung recruitment is probably more important for gas exchange than the net effect upon compliance.

Paradoxically, PFB removal (50% of instilled dose) resulted in normalization of Crs but a loss of the previous improvement in PaO_2, implying increased V/Q mismatch. Perfusion may have resumed a more normal basal distribution, while ventilation occurred in the now more compliant PFB coated anterior segments. The mass effects of PFB, which is nearly twice the density of water, may act to keep alveoli open, displace edema fluid, and redistribute blood flow. These effects may be more important to its efficacy than a simple lowering of surface tension.

Hemodynamics were well maintained throughout the study in PFB dogs, even when lungs were filled to FRC. Early studies using traditional liquid breathing demonstrated decreases of CO of about 40% with subsequent lactic acidosis (Lowe et al., 1979). This was presumed due to moderate increases in PVR and right ventricular afterload (Lowe and Shaffer, 1986) as well as effects of the heavy, PFC-filled lung on venous return and cardiac compliance. However, it has since been shown that mean alveolar pressure is not excessive during LB (Curtis et al., 1990) and that maintenance of intravascular volume prevents any decrease in CO (Curtis et al., 1991). Adverse cardiopulmonary interactions should be even less in the partially liquid-filled lung than in full liquid breathing. Blood volume was normal in both our groups throughout this study, and PFB dogs required no more blood volume supplements than control dogs. In actual practice, a therapy that improves PaO_2 and DO_2 would allow downward adjustment of FiO_2 and mPaw, to reduce resultant O_2 toxicity and barotrauma, a major goal of such therapy.

Hemorrhagic foam was noted in the ET tube of most dogs, particularly in PFB treated dogs. No dogs were suctioned (except for PFB drainage at min. 240) because PFB would have been removed and the progressive dosing protocol disrupted. Traditional tidal liquid breathing with removal of this edema fluid may prove more efficacious than our method of partial liquid breathing. Following canine lung injury by sucrose installation, significantly more edema fluid was removed during one hour of full liquid breathing than in control dogs whose airways were simply suctioned (Calderwood et al., 1973). After PFC drainage, PaO_2 was significantly higher than in controls. Richman et al. (1990) also were able to show significant improvement in PaO_2 following lung lavage with PFC in cat lungs injured with both oleic acid and saline washout. Saline lavage has been used to treat various lung diseases, but acutely worsens lung function due to surfactant washout (Rogers et al., 1972; Kylstra et al., 1971). Also, one lung must be simultaneously gas ventilated to maintain gas exchange, which is not physically possible in small patients.

A significant unknown in this study was the distribution of PFB within the lungs. We slowly poured each dose through a side port in the ET tube while positive pressure ventilation continued. Each dose was divided into thirds, given with the dog supine, left side down, and right side down. It is not known whether aerosolization of the PFB would provide better dispersion, and whether this would translate into improved mechanics and gas exchange. The density of PFB is 1.9 gm/ml, so it is also possible that with time, some PFB in superior lung segments drains to inferior lung segments. Studies of PFB dispersion are needed, including methods of administration and the effects of rotating the subject after administration.

In summary, a severe restrictive defect characterized by decreased Crs and PaO_2 was produced in anesthetized dogs undergoing conventional gas ventilation. Partial filling of the lungs with PFB resulted in significant increases in oxygenation and Crs with no impairment in CO_2 elimination. The procedure was well tolerated with no adverse hemodynamic consequences. Questions of how to best administer PFB, how to measure FRC during PLV, and the possible benefits of a true lung lavage with PFB remain to be answered.

ACKNOWLEDGEMENT

This study was funded by the Children's Hospital of Alabama Research Foundation. SEC is supported in part by an American Lung Association Trudeau Research Scholar Award. PFB was generously supplied by Alliance Pharmaceutical Corp., San Diego, Ca. We thank Siemens-Elema, ventilator division, for the loan of equipment. We also acknowledge the expert technical assistance of Glenda Clyde and W. Edward Bradley.

REFERENCES

Bone, R.C., Fisher, C.J., Clemmer, T.P., et al., 1987, A controlled clinical trial of high dose methylprednisolone in the treatment of severe sepsis and septic shock, *N. Engl. J. Med.* 317:653.

Calderwood, H.W., Modell, J.H., Ruiz, B.C., et al., 1973, Pulmonary lavage with liquid fluorocarbon in a model of pulmonary edema, *Anesthesiology* 38:141.

Curtis, S.E., Howland, D.F., and Furhman, B.P., 1990, Airway and alveolar pressures during liquid (fluorocarbon) breathing, *J. Appl. Physiol.* 68:2322.

Curtis, S.E., Fuhrman, B.P., Motoyama, E.K., et al., 1991, Cardiac output during liquid breathing in newborn piglets, *Crit. Care Med.* 19:225.

Fuhrman, B.P., Paczan, P.R., and DeFrancisis, M., 1991, Perfluorocarbon associated gas exchange, *Crit. Care Med.* 19:712.

Gilliard, N., Richman, P.M., Merritt, T.A., and Spragg, R.G., 1990, Effect of volume and dose on the pulmonary distribution of exogenous surfactant administered to normal rabbits or to rabbits with oleic acid lung injury, *Am. Rev. Resp. Dis.* 141:743.

Greenspan, J.S., Wolfson, M.R., Rubenstein, D., and Shaffer, T.H., 1990, Liquid ventilation of human preterm neonates, *J. Pediatr.* 117:106.

Holm, B.A., and Matalon, S., 1989, Role of pulmonary surfactant in the development and treatment of adult respiratory distress syndrome, *Anesth. Analg.* 69:805.

Holzapfel, L., Perrin, R.F., Gaussorgues, P., and Giudicelli, D.P., 1987, Comparison of high frequency jet ventilation in adults with respiratory distress syndrome, *Intens. Care Med.* 13:100.

Jobe, A., Ikegami, M., Jacobs, H., and Jones, S., 1984, Surfactant and pulmonary blood flow distributions following treatment of premature lambs with natural surfactant, *J. Clin. Invest.* 73:848.

Kylstra, J.A., Tissing, M.O., and Maen, A., 1962, Of mice as fish, *Trans. Amer. Soc. Artif. Intern. Organs* 8:378.

Kylstra, J.A., Rausch, D.C., Hall, K.D., and Spock, A., 1971, Volume-controlled lung lavage in the treatment of asthma, bronchiectasis and mucoviscidosis, *Am. Rev. Resp. Dis.* 103:651.

Kylstra, J.A. and Schoenfish, W.H., 1972, Alveolar surface tension in fluorocarbon-filled lungs, *J. Appl. Physiol.* 33:32.

Lachman, B., 1989, Animal models and clinical pilot studies of surfactant replacement in adult respiratory distress syndrome, *Eur. Respir. J.* 2:98S.

Lowe, C.A., Tuma, R.F., Sivieri, E.M., and Shaffer, T.H., 1979, Liquid ventilation: Cardiovascular adjustments with secondary hyperlactatemia and acidosis, *J. Appl. Physiol.* 47:1051.

Lowe, C.A., and Shaffer, T.H., 1986, Pulmonary vascular resistance in the fluorocarbon-filled lung, *J. Appl. Physiol.* 60:154.

Motohiro, A., Furukawa, T., Yasumato, K., and Inokuchi, K., 1986, Mechanisms involved in acute lung edema induced in dogs by oleic acid, *Eur. Surg. Res.* 18:50.

Petty, T.L., Reiss, O.K., Paul, G.W., et al., 1977, Characteristics of pulmonary surfactant in adult respiratory distress syndrome associated with trauma and shock, *Am. Rev. Respir. Dis.* 115:531.

Richman, P.S., Spragg, R.G., Merritt, T.A., and Curstedt, T., 1989, The adult respirtory distress syndrome: first trials with surfactant replacement, *Eur. Respir. J.* 2:109S.

Richman, P.S., Wolfson, M.R., Shaffer, T.H., and Kelsen, S.G., 1990, Lung lavage with oxygenated fluorocarbon improves gas exchange and lung compliance in cats with acute lung injury, *Am. Rev. Respir. Dis.* 141:A773.

Rogers, R.M., Braunstein, M.S., and Shuman, J.F., 1972, Role of bronchopulmonary lavage in the treatment of respiratory failure: a review, *Chest* 62:95.

Shaffer, T.H., Tran, N., Bhutani, V.K., and Sivieri, E.M., 1983a, Cardiopulmonary function in very preterm lambs during liquid ventilation, *Pediatr. Res.* 17:680.

Shaffer, T.H, Douglas, P.R., Lowe, C.A., and Bhutani, V.K., 1983b, The effects of liquid ventilation on cardiopulmonary function in preterm lambs, *Pediat. Res.* 17:303.

Shale, D.J., 1987, The adult respiratory distress syndrome-20 years on, *Thorax* 42:641.

Sly, P.D., Bates, J.H.T., and Milic-Emili, J., 1987, Measurement of respiratory mechanics using the Siemens Servo Ventilator 900c, *Pediatr. Pulm.* 3:400.

West, J.B., Dollery, C.T., Matthews, C.M.E., and Zardini, P., 1965, Distribution of blood flow and ventilation in saline-filled lung, *J. Appl. Physiol.* 20:1107.

Zelter, M., Escudier, J., Hoeffel, J.M., and Murray, J.F., 1990, Effects of aerosolized artificial surfactant on repeated oleic acid injury in sheep, *Am. Rev. Respir. Dis.* 141:1014.

ROLES OF ANTIOXIDANT ENZYMES IN ERYTHROCYTES ON HYPOXIC PULMONARY VASOCONSTRICTION

Kazuhiro Yamaguchi, Koichiro Asano, Tomoaki Takasugi, Akira Kawai, Masaaki Mori, Akira Umeda, Takeo Kawashiro and Tetsuro Yokoyama

Department of Medicine School of Medicine, Keio University Tokyo 160, Japan

INTRODUCTION

Hypoxic pulmonary vasoconstriction (HPV) is of importance in regulating the distribution of blood flow in the lung, thus allowing the lung to maintain a pertinent matching between ventilation and blood flow. Recently, several authors (cf. Archer et al, 1989b) have reported that endogenous products of reactive O_2 species (ROS) in the lung are the important factor for initiating HPV.

Excessive ROS has been known as the substantial substances in the pathogenesis of acute lung injuries, all of which are similarly characterized by hyporesponsiveness (i.e. vascular paresis) of the pulmonary microcirculation to some vasoactive stimuli, especially to alveolar hypoxia (Archer et al., 1989a). The vascular paresis for alveolar hypoxia is important factor for worsening the accumulation of edema fluid in the lung (Yamaguchi et al., 1991). Hydrogen peroxide (H_2O_2) and/or hydroxyl radical have been recognized to induce significant endothelial damage associated with alveolar flooding, but superoxide seems to be less effective for oxidant-induced lung injury (Heffner and Repine, 1989). On the other hand, superoxide may be important to alter the pulmonary vascular reactivity to various stimuli including alveolar hypoxia under oxidative stress (Archer et al., 1989a).

Although importance of vascular smooth muscle and endothelium on HPV have been studied in details (cf. Gurtner and Wolin, 1991), rheological components affecting HPV have received only a little attention. Red blood cells (RBCs) contribute to blood viscosity and, therefore, vascular resistance. McMurtry et al. (1978) have elucidated the increase and prolongation of the reactivity of rat pulmonary vasculature to hypoxia by addition of RBCs to plasma. Since RBCs are rich in enzymes protecting oxidation, it has been well known that RBCs augment lung antioxidant capacity and play a role in preventing oxidant-induced pulmonary edema

Oxygen Transport to Tissue XV, Edited by P. Vaupel
et al., Plenum Press, New York, 1994

(Heffner and repine, 1989). In such a way, importance of RBCs in pulmonary circulation for protecting pulmonary edema has been recognized, however, their possible roles for altering pulmonary vascular reactivity under a condition with or without oxidative stress has not been fully studied.

The present study was undertaken to systematically know whether or not antioxidant enzymes in RBCs such as superoxide dismutase (SOD), catalase (CAT) and glutathione peroxidase (GSH-Px) would play a significant role for modulating physiological HPV as well as for restoring HPV under a condition with a considerable amount of ROS.

METHODS

Isolated Perfused Lungs

Japanese male rabbits weighing 2.0 - 3.0 kg received 1000 U/kg heparin through the ear vein and were anesthetized with pentobarbital sodium (25 mg/kg). Subsequently, a sternotomy was performed and the chest was open widely. The animal was killed by rapid exsanguination using a 15G polyethylene catheter inserted into the left ventricle. The pulmonary artery was cannulated with a 18G rigid polyethylene tube and the catheter in the left ventricle was advanced to the left atrium. The isolated lungs were perfused in a recirculating manner at 70 ml/min with a modified Krebs-Henseleit buffer, 3% albumin to maintain isooncotic pressure and 20 uM indomethacin to inhibit cyclooxygenase activity. pH of the perfusate was kept at 7.4 by using a gas mixture containing 5% CO_2 as an inspired gas. Pressures were continuously monitored in the pulmonary artery and the trachea.

Preparation of RBCs

Blood collected from the rabbits was used to assess the effects of antioxidant enzymes in RBCs on HPV under both conditions with and without exogenous oxidant stress. The fresh blood was centrifuged (3000 rpm) at 4°C for 15 min. The plasma and buffy coat were discarded, and the packed RBCs were added into cold phosphate-buffered saline (PBS). RBC suspensions thus prepared were then incubated with either 50 mM N,N-diethyldithiocarbamate (DDC: SOD inhibitor) (Michiels and Remacle, 1988), 0.1 mM 4,4'-diisothiocyano-2,2' disulfonic acid stilbene (DIDS: anion channel blocker) (Lynch and Fridovich, 1978), 30 mM 3-amino-1,2,4-triazole (AMT: CAT inhibitor) (Michiels and Remacle, 1988), or 0.2 mM mercaptosuccinate (MS: GSH-Px inactivator) (Michiels and Remacle, 1988). If necessary, RBC suspension in PBS was treated with both AMT and MS to inhibit H_2O_2 scavengers in RBCs concurrently. Since irreversible inhibition of CAT only occurs when the enzyme is in the form of compound I, treatment of RBCs by AMT was performed in the presence of 0.4 mM H_2O_2 (Burke and Wolin, 1987). The incubation was done at 37°C and RBCs treated with agents were washed three times with cold PBS to remove any agent remaining.

Protocol 1

After the stabilization period (20 min) of mean pulmonary arterial pressure (Ppa) in the isolated lung, inspired gas was changed from 21% O_2

(normoxic ventilation) to 3% O_2 (hypoxic ventilation) for 10 min keeping CO_2 concentration in the inspired gas at 5%. When the plateau of Ppa during hypoxic ventilation was attained, normoxic ventilation was begun again for 10 min. Such a cycle was repeated three times and the averaged Ppa difference between normoxic and hypoxic ventilation was used as a measure of pulmonary vascular responsiveness to alveolar hypoxia (HPV). After these measurements, the second cycles comprised of three hypoxic challenges, as well, were performed under the different experimental condition from the first cycles. Using this protocol, following experiments were done; (1) comparison between HPV during perfusion simply with the buffer and HPV in the perfusate containing control RBCs (not treated by inhibitors of antioxidant enzymes but incubated only by PBS), (2) comparison between HPV in the perfusate with control RBCs and HPV during perfusion with the solution containing either DDC-, DIDS-, AMT-, or MS-treated RBCs, (3) to elucidate, directly, the importance of antioxidant mechanisms in vascular lumen for modulating HPV, effects of SOD (75 U/ml) and CAT (1000 U/ml) added to the perfusate without RBCs were also examined. When RBC suspension was used, hematocrit of the perfusate was adjusted to 7% in all measurements.

Protocol 2

To analyze possible roles of antioxidant enzymes in RBCs for modulating HPV under exogenous oxidative stress, xanthine (X) and xanthine oxidase (XO) were administered to the reservoir for intravascular genesis of reactive O_2 metabolites. Essential schedule on experiments was the same as the protocol 1. After the necessary period for stabilization of pulmonary hemodynamics, xanthine was added to the perfusate to achieve the final concentration at 100 µM, and the first cycles of measurements (three hypoxic ventilation) were made at a given experimental condition. At the end of the first cycles, xanthine oxidase (10 mU/ml) was added to the perfusate and the second cycles of measurements (three hypoxic ventilation) were performed. After completion of each experiment, the lung was excised and its wet-to-dry weight ratio (W/D) was determined. Based on this protocol, following measurements were made before and after the addition of X/XO in the perfusate; (1) HPV in the perfusate with or without control RBCs, (2) HPV in the presence of either DDC- or DIDS-treated RBCs, (3) HPV in the presence of RBCs treated with AMT, MS or both, (4) concerning HPV in the perfusate containing DDC-treated RBCs, additional observations were made by the administration of either SOD (75 U/ml), CAT (1000 U/ml) or desferrioxamine (DF: 1.5 mg/ml, iron chelator) to the reservoir. Hematocrit of the perfusate containing RBCs was adjusted to 7% in each measurement.

RESULTS

HPV without exogenous oxidative stress

HPV obtained from the perfusion containing control RBCs was significantly greater than that without RBCs.

Inhibition of SOD in RBCs by DDC did not attenuate HPV appreciably as compared to that obtained from the presence of control RBCs. Similarly, impediment in permeation of superoxide through RBC membrane by treatment with DIDS did not influence the magnitude of HPV.

Presence of RBCs treated with either CAT inhibitor, AMT, or GSH-Px inhibitor, MS, did not exert any significant influence on HPV.

Addition of either SOD or CAT to the perfusate (without RBCs) did not enhance HPV.

HPV with exogenous oxidative stress

Exogenous ROS generated by X and XO distinctly attenuated HPV during the perfusion with the buffer alone, while the addition of control RBCs to the perfusate did preserve HPV.

Treatment of RBCs with either DDC or DIDS was unable to preserve HPV after adding X and XO to the reservoir (Figure 1). Diminishing HPV by X and XO during the perfusion with DDC-treated RBCs was restored by the administration of either SOD or DF to the perfusate, whereas the addition of CAT failed to do so (Figure 2).

AMT- or MS-treated RBCs did not attenuate HPV under oxidative stress. Simultaneous treatment of RBCs with AMT and MS did not alter HPV before and after the imposition of oxidative stress, as well.

Lung W/D ratios in the presence of X and XO were not different from those obtained in the absence of X and XO irrespective of the agents used for inhibiting antioxidant enzymes in RBCs.

DISCUSSION

Critique of the method

The crucial point of this study is that chemical inhibitor of one antioxidant enzyme has influence on other antioxidant enzymes (Michiels and Remacle, 1988). For inhibition of SOD in RBCs, we used DDC which was a copper-chelating agent removing copper from the active site of SOD. DDC at 50 mM, the concentration used in the present study, was shown to inhibit SOD in human fibroblasts completely but it also significantly restrained other antioxidants including CAT, GSH-Px and GSH (Michiels and Remacle, 1988). Therefore, the effects of DDC-treated RBCs on pulmonary hemodynamics are complicated and might be considered as a consequence of suppressing nearly whole antioxidant mechanisms in RBCs.

DIDS, a family of sulfonated stilbenes which binds irreversibly to band 3 of the RBC membrane, is known to restrain the exchange of anions across the RBC membrane powerfully and specifically (Lynch and Fridovich, 1978).

AMT is an irreversible inhibitor of CAT in the form of compound I (Burke and Wolin, 1987). More than 90% inhibition of CAT by AMT was observed at the concentration over 10 mM without any effect on SOD or GSH-Px activity in human fibroblasts (Michiels and Remacle, 1988). AMT also reacts irreversibly with several heme peroxidases, however with the exception of cyclooxygenase, little evidence exists for the involvement of heme peroxidases in the regulation of vascular tone (Burke-Wolin and Wolin, 1989). Cyclooxygenase activity was actually inhibited by indomethacin in all measurements of the present study (see methods).

Among mercaptocarboxylic acids which were shown to inhibit GSH-Px, the key enzyme in the GSH redox cycle, mercaptosuccinate (MS) appears to be the most potent (Michiels and Remacle, 1988).

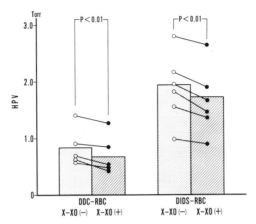

Figure 1. HPV during perfusion with DDC- or DIDS-RBC under oxidative stress (see text for further details).

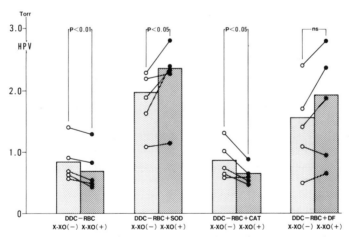

Figure 2. Effects of SOD, CAT and DF on HPV in the perfusate with DDC-RBCs under oxidative stress (see text for further explanation).

HPV without exogenous oxidative stress

The significant roles of redox state in the lung tissue, especially in the vasculature for governing pulmonary vascular tone, have been suggested by several authors (cf. Archer et al., 1989b: Burke-Wolin and Wolin, 1989). Although RBCs contain abundant antioxidant enzymes and may act as sinks in the pulmonary microcirculation for extinguishing ROS, the potential effects of antioxidants in RBCs on pulmonary vascular reactivity to various stimuli have not been fully evaluated. Using isolated rat lungs, McMurtry et al. (1978) found that the addition of RBCs to plasma prolonged the period of pulmonary vascular responsiveness to hypoxia and concluded that RBCs prevented accumulation of an inhibitor or released a factor which enhanced HPV. More recently, Archer et al. (1989b) reported the very fascinating results showing that the isolated rat lung produced superoxide anion as the main physiological ROS, which decreased in proportion to the degree of alveolar hypoxia and radical levels fell during hypoxia before the onset of pulmonary vasoconstriction. Joining the findings of McMurtry et al. (1978) and Archer et al. (1989b), it is possible to conjecture that antioxidant enzymes in RBCs can act as a modulator for HPV even in a physiological condition. Therefore, we attempted, in this study, to clarify a potential role of antioxidant enzymes in RBCs for modulating HPV. However, experimental results exhibited that any procedure suppressing antioxidant mechanisms within RBCs did not alter HPV significantly. Further, addition of either SOD or CAT to the perfusate failed to augment HPV.

This study demonstrated that, although the presence of RBCs in the perfusate significantly enhanced the pressor responses of the pulmonary microcirculation to alveolar hypoxia, these responses were not mediated by antioxidant enzymes in RBCs under a physiological condition.

HPV with exogenous oxidative stress

Although beneficial effects of RBCs on preventing ROS-induced pulmonary edema by supplying their intracellular antioxidants to the pulmonary microcirculation has been confirmed by several authors (cf. Heffner and Repine, 1989), important roles of antioxidants in RBCs in modulating pulmonary vascular tone as well as reactivity under oxidative stress have not been systematically investigated.

To know whether or not antioxidant enzymes in RBCs would be of importance for preserving pulmonary vascular reactivity to hypoxia, we measured HPV before and after the addition of X and XO to the perfusate containing RBCs which were previously incubated with inacivators of SOD, CAT or GSH-Px. It is very difficult to evaluate the pulmonary vascular reactivity under oxidative stress because an excessive quantity of ROS may induce a considerable accumulation of edema fluid in the alveolar space and interstitium, leading to a mechanical compression accompanied by a increasing outflow pressure of the pulmonary microcirculation. The compressed microvessels may fail to react on a variety of stimuli including alveolar hypoxia. In addition, the hypoxic gas may not reach the flooded alveoli and the alveolar PO_2 may not be altered in these regions, resulting in no significant response to lowering an inspired O_2 concentration even in the case that vascular reactivity to O_2 is maintained. Therefore, it is essentially important to analyze the problem of vascular reactivity under a condition without an overt pulmonary edema.

To avoid a significant accumulation of edema fluid, we applied a relatively small amount of XO, i.e. 10 mU/ml. In fact, lung W/D ratios after administrating X and XO in the perfusate did not differ from those obtained without X and XO.

The present study demonstrated that ROS generated by X and XO considerably diminished reactivity of the pulmonary vascular bed to hypoxia. These hemodynamic effects of X and XO were achieved without the development of overt pulmonary edema. Addition of control RBCs (not treated with any reagent) to the perfusate successfully restored the pulmonary vascular responsiveness to hypoxia, indicating that antioxidants within RBCs were importantly working so as to protect attenuated HPV under oxidative stress.

DDC-treated RBCs could not restore HPV after the administration of XO (Figure 1), resulting in that superoxide and its scavengers in RBCs would play significant roles in promoting and avoiding ROS-induced vascular paresis for HPV, respectively. However, interpretation of the results on DDC-treated RBCs should be cautious. As described above, DDC may not be a specific inhibitor for SOD and has a distinct influence on both CAT and GSH-redox cycle (Michiels and Remacle, 1988). Thus, we can not conclude simply that attenuated HPV observed during the perfusion with DDC-treated RBCs is caused by the restraint of SOD in RBCs. To know a relative contribution of the scavengers of superoxide and H_2O_2 in RBCs to preserving HPV, we further investigated the effects of exogenous SOD, CAT and DF on HPV in the perfusate containing DDC-treated RBCS. Addition of SOD to the perfusate did restore the attenuated HPV caused by X and XO whereas exogenous CAT did not (Figure 2), leading to the conclusion that the observed effects of DDC would be principally explicable from its inhibitory action on SOD in RBCs. Administration of DF to the perfusate also protect a loss of pulmonary vascular reactivity to hypoxia under oxidative stress (Figure 2). DF is traditionally thought to act as an low-molecular-weight iron chelator entering the cells and eliminating hydroxyl radicals which are mainly yielded from the interaction of H_2O_2 with intracellular iron (Habar-Weiss reaction) (Archer et al., 1989a). Thereby, restoration of HPV by the addition of DF in DDC experiments seemingly indicates the importance of hydroxyl radicals to alter intrinsic vascular reactivity to hypoxia. However, this finding is highly inconsistent with the results on the addition of CAT exogenously to the perfusate with DDC-treated RBCs (Figure 2). If hydroxyl radicals significantly affect the vascular reactivity, exogenous CAT should also improve HPV in the suspension of DDC-treated RBCs because CAT removes intravascular H_2O_2 which passes through the cells constituting the pulmonary vascular walls and contributes to the formation of hydroxyl radicals. It was proposed that DF might impair XO by inhibiting two iron-sulfur centers which were crucial to XO activity (Archer et al., 1989a), leading to the possibility that the presence of DF significantly reduced the genesis of ROS in itself. In addition, DF may scavenge superoxide by a mechanism which appears to be distinct from its effects on iron chelator (Sinaceur et al., 1984). We are convinced that beneficial effects of DF observed in our study are explicable from its effects on XO activity and/or superoxide but not from the inhibition of hydroxyl radical formation.

DIDS-treated RBCs failed to restore HPV in the presence of X and XO (Figure 1), again indicating the importance of superoxide to cause vascular paresis for hypoxia under oxidative stress. Our experimental results are likely to be qualitatively consistent with Archer et al.(1989a) who exhibited that exogenously produced superoxide by X and XO was a main cause for a loss of reactivity to alveolar hypoxia in the isolated rat lung without a significant pulmonary edema.

Inhibition of either CAT (by AMT) or GSH-Px (by MS) in RBCs did not attenuate HPV under oxidative stress. In addition, simultaneous inhibition of CAT and GSH-Px in RBCs also failed to reduce the magnitude of HPV after the administration of X and XO, suggesting that H_2O_2 scavenging mechanisms in RBCs were not essential for preserving HPV under oxidative stress.

In conclusion, (1) RBCs in the pulmonary vascular lumen enhance the pressure response to alveolar hypoxia under a physiological condition, i.e. without an excessive oxidant stress. These effects of RBCs are not mediated by antioxidant enzymes in RBCs. (2) The presence of RBCs in the microcirculation is essentially important to preserve hypoxic pulmonary vasoconstriction under oxidative stress. This phenomenon is shown to be mainly mediated by superoxide dismutase within RBCs, but neither by catalase nor by glutathione redox cycle.

REFERENCES

Archer, S.L., Peterson, D., Nelson, D.P., DeMaster, E.G., Kelly, B., Eaton, J.W., and Weir, E.K., 1989a, Oxygen radicals and antioxidant enzymes alter pulmonary vascular reactivity in the rat lung, J. Appl. Physiol. 66:102-111.

Archer, S.L., Nelson, D.P., and Weir, E.K.,1989b, Simultaneous measurement of O_2 radical and pulmonary vascular ractivity in rat lung, J. Appl. Physiol. 67:1903-1911.

Burke, T.M., and Wolin, M.S., 1987, Hydrogen peroxide elicits pulmonary arterial relaxation and guanylate cyclase activation, Am. J. Physiol. 252:H721-H732.

Burke-Wolin, T., and Wolin, M.S., 1989, H_2O_2 and cGMP may function as an O_2 sensor in the pulmonary artery, J. Appl. Physiol. 66:167-170.

Gurtner, G.M., and Wolin, T.B., 1991, Interactions of oxidant stress and vascular reactivity, Am. J. Physiol. 260:L207-L211.

Heffner, J.E., and Repine, J.E., 1989, Pulmonary strategies of antioxidant defense, Am. Rev. Respir. Dis. 140:531-554.

Lynch, R.E., and Fridovich, I., 1978, Permeation of the erythrocyte stroma by superoxide radical, J. Biol. Chem. 253:4697-4699.

McMurtry, I.F., Hookway, B.W., and Roos, S.D., 1978, Red blood cells but not platlets prolong vascular reactivity of isolated rat lungs, Am. J. Physiol. 234:H186-H191.

Michiels, C., and Remacle, J., 1988, Use of the inhibition of enzymatic antioxidant systems in order to evaluate their physiological importance, Eur. J. Biochem. 177:435-441.

Sinaceur, J., Ribiere, C., Nordmann, J., and Nordmann, R, 1984, Desferrioxamine: a scavenger of superoxide radicals ?, Biochem. Pharmacol. 33:1693-1694.

Yamaguchi, K., Mori, M., Kawai, A., Asano, K., Takasugi, T., Umeda, A., Yokoyama, T., 1991, Impairment of gas exchange in acute lung injury, Jap. J. Thorac. Dis. 29:133-144.

ROLES OF HYPOXIA AND BLOOD FLOW IN MODULATING $\dot{V}_A/\dot{Q}$ HETEROGENEITY IN THE LUNGS

Michael P. Hlastala[1,2] and Karen B. Domino[3]

[1]Department of Physiology and Biophysics
[2]Department of Medicine
[3]Department of Anesthesiology
University of Washington
Seattle, WA 98195, USA

INTRODUCTION

The distribution of ventilation to perfusion ratio ($\dot{V}_A/\dot{Q}$) within the lungs is heterogeneous due to the influence of gravity as well as local factors. $\dot{V}_A/\dot{Q}$ heterogeneity is critical in determining the efficiency of O_2 transfer by the lungs. In recent years, data have been accumulated revealing a minimal role of gravity, with respect to both ventilation and perfusion. Other factors such as vascular resistance, airway resistance, lung compliance, hypoxic vasoconstriction, hypercapnic bronchodilation, etc., dominate. This report presents an accumulation of several experiments[1,2,3,4] designed to assess the role of hypoxia and blood flow in regulating local $\dot{V}_A/\dot{Q}$ ratio.

METHODS

Mongrel dogs of either sex (23 - 28 kg) were anesthetized with pentobarbital sodium (30 mg/kg iv, supplemented with 25-50 mg hourly), had their trachea intubated, and were ventilated with a tidal volume of 15 ml/kg. Respiratory rate was adjusted to maintain arterial PCO_2 between 30 and 35 Torr, and diaphragmatic paralysis was secured with succinylcholine (100 mg im, supplemented with 20-40 mg iv hourly).

Oxygen Transport to Tissue XV, Edited by P. Vaupel
et al., Plenum Press, New York, 1994

An isolated left lower lobe preparation[1] was used which allows separate and simultaneous determinations of $\dot{V}_A/\dot{Q}$ distributions in the LLL and in the right lung using the multiple inert gas elimination technique. Carotid and pulmonary arterial catheters were placed via peripheral cutdown. Bilateral thoracotomies were performed. To facilitate isolation of the left lower lobe (LLL) pulmonary venous circulation, the left upper lobe was surgically resected. The LLL pulmonary vein was cannulated retrograde via the left atrial appendage. Because the LLL pulmonary vein has two to four contributory branches, the catheter was positioned in the main trunk of the lobar vein just proximal to its junction with the left atrium. The sampling line was positioned midstream within the lumen of a 1-cm-long 5-mm-ID 9-mm-OD rigid tube. Previous work has demonstrated that a mixed sample of pulmonary venous blood is obtained from the LLL pulmonary venous catheter.

LLL pulmonary blood flow ($\dot{Q}_{LLL}$) was measured by an electromagnetic flow probe placed around the left main pulmonary artery. The flow probe was precalibrated *in situ*. Adjustable vascular snares were placed around the right pulmonary artery and left pulmonary artery distal to the flow probe. LLL pulmonary arterial pressure (Ppa$_{LLL}$) was measured by a catheter inserted into the left pulmonary artery distal to the flow probe and vascular snare. Both thoracotomies were covered with plastic to conserve heat and moisture. $\dot{Q}_T$ was obtained in triplicate by the thermodilution method with the use of iced 5% dextrose in water.

With the animal supine, a bronchial divider was placed through a tracheostomy to allow separate ventilation of the LLL and right lung (RL). The RL was ventilated with an $F_IO_2 = 0.5$ at a tidal volume of 9 ml/kg. The LLL was ventilated with a relatively greater volume per lung mass to permit constant alveolar CO_2 when LLL perfusion was increased. CO_2 was not added when $\dot{Q}_{LLL}$ was increased. Five centimeters of water PEEP was administered to compensate for the absence of distending transpulmonary pressure with the chest open. Tidal volume of LLL and RL was measured by spirometer and minute ventilations of LLL and RL were calculated. After completions of the surgical preparation, heparin (7500 U iv followed by 500 U iv hourly) was administered.

In some animals the effect of acute oleic acid pulmonary edema on the response to LLL alveolar hypoxia was studied. In these animals, gas exchange of the LLL was studied before injury and 1 h following intravenous injection of 0.05 ml/kg of oleic acid into the right atrium over 10 min (post-injury). During administration of oleic acid, the electromagnetic flow probe was removed and the RL and LLL were ventilated with 100% O_2. The respiratory rate was increased after injury to maintain constant $PaCO_2$. Immediately after administration of oleic acid, ventilation of the LLL with the hypoxic gas was resumed. After 1 h of hypoxia, hemodynamic, blood gas, and inert gas measurements were obtained. After 2 h of hypoxic ventilation, the animals were killed with an overdose of sodium thiopental and the right lower lobe (RLL) and LLL were quickly removed, weighted, and prepared for gravimetric analysis. Blood-free wet weight-to-dry weight ratios were obtained using the cyanomethemoglobin method to estimate blood content.

MIGET measurements, performed by the use of standard method, were adapted to assess gas exchange of the LLL. Briefly, a dilute solution of six inert gases (sulfur hexafluoride, ethane, cyclopropane, halothane, diethyl ether and acetone) dissolved in 5% dextrose was infused into a peripheral vein for at least 30 min before the first MIGET samples were drawn. Inert gas partial pressures were measured in blood simultaneously collected from the main pulmonary artery (P_v) and the LLL pulmonary vein (P_{lpv}) and in mixed expired gas from the LLL. Duplicate samples were obtained at each study phase. Exhaled gas specimens were maintained at >40°C before analysis to avoid condensation and loss of highly soluble gases.

The concentrations of inert gases in the gas samples were measured on a gas chromatogaph (Varian 3300) equipped with a flame ionization detector and an electron capture detector. The gas extraction method of Wagner et al[12] was used to determine the concentration of inert gases in the blood samples. $\dot{V}_A/\dot{Q}$ heterogeneity was assessed by changes in the perfusion and ventilation distributions predicted by the 50-compartment model and by heterogeneity indices [(a-A)D area or $DISP_{R*}$] derived from retention and excretion data. Inert gas shunt ($\dot{Q}_s/\dot{Q}_T$), inert gas dead space (V_D/V_T), mean $\dot{V}_A/\dot{Q}$ ratio of the perfusion (mean $\dot{V}_A/\dot{Q}$ of $\dot{Q}$) and ventilation (mean $\dot{V}_A/\dot{Q}$ of $\dot{V}$) distributions. Log standard deviations of the perfusion (log $SD_{\dot{Q}}$) and ventilation (log $SD_{\dot{V}}$) distributions were calculated from the 50-compartment distribution.

RESULTS

In the hypoxic LLL experiments, the general cardiopulmonary status, including temperature (37.5 ± 0.5°C), heart rate, systemic arterial pressure, Ppcw, $\dot{Q}_T$, arterial PO_2, arterial PCO_2, mixed venous PO_2, and Hb did not change throughout the experiment. $\dot{Q}_{LLL}$ (lpv) obtained by inert gases correlated highly with $\dot{Q}_{LLL}$ obtained by the electromagnetic flow probe [$\dot{Q}_{LLL}$ (lpv) = 0.982 ($\dot{Q}_{LLL}$ flow probe) + 0.03, r=0.90, p<0.001]. Hypoxic ventilation of the LLL resulted in a decrease in $\dot{Q}_{LLL}$ and an increase $\dot{Q}_{RL}$. $\dot{Q}_{LLL}/\dot{Q}_T$ decreased from 24 ± 2 to 11 ± 2 % with LLL hypoxia. P_{pa} increased and P_aO_2, P_vO_2 and $P_{lpv}O_2$ were significantly reduced with LLL hypoxia. Hypoxic ventilation of the LLL resulted in an increase in $\dot{V}_A/\dot{Q}$ heterogeneity as indicated by an increase in DISP$_{R*}$ from 5.52 ± 0.93 during hyperoxia to 7.72 ± 0.89 during hypoxia (P<0.05).

In the altered flow, normoxic LLL experiments, the circulatory parameters did not change throughout the experiment. $\dot{Q}_{LLL}$ during baseline was 919 ± 48 ml/min and P_{pa} was 18.3 ± 1.5 Torr. Gas exchange of the LLL demonstrated a mean $\dot{V}_A/\dot{Q}$ ratio of the perfusion distribution of 1.00 ± 0.09 and a mean $\dot{V}_A/\dot{Q}$ ratio of the ventilation distribution of 4.71 ± 0.66. $\dot{Q}_s/\dot{Q}_T$ was low (0.7 ± 0.2%), and perfusion of low $\dot{V}_A/\dot{Q}$ units was not present under baseline conditions. Partially occluding the right pulmonary artery increased $\dot{Q}_{LLL}$ to 1358 ± 93 ml/min, main P_{pa} to 25.2 ± 2.0 Torr, $P_{pa}LLL$ to 22.1 ± 2.6 Torr, and P_{lpv} to 12.8 ± 1.6 Torr without affecting other hemodynamics. With a 50% increase in $\dot{Q}_{LLL}$, gas exchange in the LLL deteriorated as shown by an increase by 23% in DISP$_{R*}$. Further increases in $\dot{Q}_{LLL}$ caused by increasing cardiac output with an arterial-venous fistula resulted in a further increase in $\dot{Q}_{LLL}$ by 100% and 200% resulting in an increase in heterogeneity index by 42% and 54%, respectively. Partial occlusion of the LLL pulmonary artery reduced $\dot{Q}_{LLL}$ to 50% normal and increased DISP$_{R*}$ by 13%.

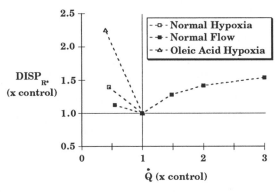

Figure 1. $\dot{V}_A/\dot{Q}$ Heterogeneity index (DISP$_{R*}$) vs. LLL perfusion. Hypoxia induced changes in normal lungs is indicated by open square. Normoxic changes in perfusion in normal lungs is indicated by closed squares. Hypoxia induced changes in oleic acid injured lungs is indicated by open triangles.

In the oleic acid injured dog lungs, hypoxic ventilation of the LLL resulted in a greater decrease in $\dot{Q}_{LLL}$ to 291 ± 48 ml/min from 715 ± 93 ml/min during hyperoxia. Hypoxic ventilation of the LLL resulted in very large increase in $\dot{V}_A/\dot{Q}$ heterogeneity as indicated by an increase in $DISP_{R*}$ from 5.39 ± 0.63 during hyperoxia to 12.05 ± 1.97 during hypoxia (P<0.05).

DISCUSSION

We chose our experimental preparation to alter pulmonary blood flow in vivo without the complicating influences of drug effects; increases in sympathetic tone; and changes in systemic hemodynamics, P_vO_2, acid-base status, lung volume, minute ventilation and alveolar PO_2 and PCO_2. The surgical preparation was hemodynamically stable, edema of the LLL did not occur, and gas exchange was unchanged between pre- and post-baseline controls. The preparation is more physiological than an *in situ* lobe preparation (Ohlsson et al, 1989), as the circulation to the LLL was never interrupted and the LLL was perfused with normal mixed venous blood at physiological flow rates. Tidal volume, respiratory rate and lung volume did not change, which may occur when PEEP or exercise is used to alter pulmonary blood flow. Because changes in alveolar CO_2 composition may affect $\dot{V}_A/\dot{Q}$ heterogeneity[11], the LLL was relatively hyperventilated compared with its mass and inspired CO_2 was added to maintain a constant LLL alveolar PCO_2, indicated by a lack of change in $P_{lpv}CO_2$.

Increases in hypoxic lobe $\dot{V}_A/\dot{Q}$ heterogeneity are partially due to HPV-induced decreases in hypoxic lobe blood flow. LLL hypoxia resulted in a 54% diversion of pulmonary blood flow to the hyperoxic RL and a 15% increase in P_{pa}. Previous studies have examined gas exchange when pulmonary blood flow was reduced by decreasing perfusion rate[9], hemorrhage[6,10] and positive end expiratory pressure[5,7]. Increases in $\dot{V}_A/\dot{Q}$ heterogeneity with hemorrhage and PEEP have been attributed to interregional lung differences by creating additional zone 1 regions. However, we do not believe that regional HPV creates additional zone 1 regions, since P_{pa} increased with hypoxia.

The magnitude of the change observed with changes in $\dot{Q}_{LLL}$ was smaller than those obtained with a similar degree of flow reduction induced by HPV or *in situ* perfusion rate. The findings suggest that hypoxia has a role in altering $\dot{V}_A/\dot{Q}$ heterogeneity that is independent of the reduction in perfusion.

In oleic acid-injured lungs, alveolar hypoxia resulted in greater $\dot{V}_A/\dot{Q}$ mismatch because of the addition of a heterogeneous HPV response between normal and injured lung regions. The percentage of perfusion of normal $\dot{V}_A/\dot{Q}$ units and absolute blood flow to normal $\dot{V}_A/\dot{Q}$ units in the LLL were both decreased in the LLL. In contrast shunt-like vessels exhibited an attenuated vasoconstrictor response to hypoxic ventilation. The percentage of perfusion of shunt and low $\dot{V}_A/\dot{Q}$ units was markedly greater in the HPV group, suggesting that these shunt-like vessels exhibited a reduced response to alveolar hypoxia. The heterogeneous response to LLL hypoxia therefore contributed to the increase in $\dot{V}_A/\dot{Q}$ heterogeneity with hypoxic gas ventilation in oleic acid pulmonary edema compared with normal lungs.

REFERENCES

1. K.B. Domino, M.P. Hlastala, B.L. Eisenstein, and F.W. Cheney, Effect of regional alveolar hypoxia on gas exchange in dogs. *J. Appl. Physiol.* 67:730 (1989).

2. K.B. Domino, B.L. Eisenstein, F.W. Cheney, and M.P. Hlastala, Pulmonary blood flow and ventilation-perfusion heterogeneity. *J. Appl. Physiol.* 71:252 (1991).

3. K.B., Domino, F.W. Cheney, B.L. Eisenstein, and M.P. Hlastala, Effect of regional alveolar hypoxia on gas exchange in pulmonary edema. *Am. Rev. Respir. Dis.* 145:340 (1992a).

4. K.B., Domino, B.L. Eisenstein, Y.M. Lu, T. Tran, and M.P. Hlastala, Lobar $\dot{V}_A/\dot{Q}$ heterogeneity is increased by increased lobar pulmonary blood flow (Abstract). *FASEB J.* 6:A1477 (1992b).

5. R. Dueck, P.D. Wagner, and J.B. West, Effects of positive end-expiratory pressure on gas exchange in dogs with normal and edematous lungs. *Anesthesiol.* 47:359 (1977).

6. J.B. Fortune, R.W. Mazzone, and P.D. Wagner, Ventilation-perfusion relationships during hemorrhagic hypotension and reinfusion in the dog. *J. Appl. Physiol.* 54:1071 (1983).

7. G. Hedenstierna, F.C. White, R. Mazzone, and P.D. Wagner, Redistribution of pulmonary blood flow in the dog with PEEP ventilation. *J. Appl. Physiol.* 46:278 (1979).

8. M.P. Hlastala, Multiple inert gas elimination technique. *J. Appl. Physiol.* 56:1 (1984).

9. J. Ohlsson, M. Middaugh, and M.P. Hlastala, Reduction in lung perfusion increases $\dot{V}_A/\dot{Q}$ heterogeneity. *J. Appl. Physiol.* 66:2423 (1989).

10. N.B. Robinson, E.Y. Chi, and H.T. Robertson, Ventilation-perfusion relationships after hemorrhage and resuscitation: an inert gas analysis. *J. Appl. Physiol.* 54:1131 (1983).

11. E.R. Swenson, H.T. Robertson, M.E. Middaugh, and M.P. Hlastala, Inspiration of CO_2 improves ventilation-perfusion matching in the dog (Abstract). *FASEB J.* 2:924 (1988).

12. P.D. Wagner, H.A. Saltzman, and J.B. West, Measurement of continuous distributions of ventilation-perfusion ratios: theory. *J. Appl. Physiol.* 36:588 (1974).

13. P.D. Wagner, P.F. Naumann, and R.B. Laravuso, Simultaneous measurement of eight foreign gases in blood by gas chromatography. *J. Appl. Physiol.* 36:600 (1974).

EFFECTS OF 5-HYDROXYTRYPTAMINE INHIBITION ON GAS EXCHANGE AND PULMONARY HEMODYNAMICS IN ACUTE CANINE PULMONARY EMBOLISM

A. Kawai, A. Umeda, M. Mori, T. Takasugi,
K. Yamaguchi, and T. Kawashiro

Department of Medicine, Keio University
School of Medicine, Tokyo, 160 Japan

INTRODUCTION

5-Hydroxytryptamine (Serotonin; 5-HT), a potent vasoconstrictor of pulmonary arteries, has been reported to play an important role in cardiopulmonary dysfunction that accompanies pulmonary embolization (Huval et al.,1983). The quantitative effects of 5-HT on gas exchange efficiency, however, have not been systematically investigated in pulmonary embolism. Using a new type of selective serotonin receptor antagonist, we examined the distribution of ventilation-perfusion (V_A/Q) ratios and pulmonary hemodynamics to clarify the effects of serotonin on gas exchange in acute canine pulmonary embolism.

MATERIALS AND METHODS

Fourteen healthy mongrel dogs weighing between 10 and 15 kg were studied. Each was anesthetized with pentobarbital sodium (25 mg/kg iv) and paralyzed with pancuronium bromide (0.2 mg/kg iv). Their lungs were mechanically ventilated with room air in supine position. The tidal volume was 10 ml/kg and the respiratory rate was adjusted between 20 and 30 /min. Polyethylene catheters were placed in the internal jugular vein and the femoral vein and artery. A thermal dilution Swan-Ganz catheter was positioned in the pulmonary artery and cardiac output as well as pulmonary arterial pressure were measured (Model RMP-6008, Nihon Kohden, Tokyo). A specially made 5 F thermodilution-impedance catheter (Model HE-2900, Elecath Inc., NJ) was positioned in the abdominal aorta through the femoral artery. Using the thermal-saline double indicator dilution method (Ishibe et al., 1987), we measured extra-vascular lung water volume with a lung water computer

Oxygen Transport to Tissue XV, Edited by P. Vaupel
et al., Plenum Press, New York, 1994

(Model MTV-1100K, Nihon Kohden, Tokyo). Normal saline containing six inert gases, including SF_6, ethane, cyclopropane, halothane, diethyl ether and acetone, was infused at a rate of 2.0 ml/min for 40 minutes through the femoral vein. Under a steady state, we collected expired gas and arterial and mixed venous blood samples to measure the concentrations of the indicator gases with a gaschromatograph (Model GC-163 Hitachi Ltd.).

After these control measurements were obtained, glass-beads (diameter 0.1mm), 0.4-0.6 g/kg, were given intravenously via the internal jugular vein until mean pulmonary arterial pressure (PAP) reached between double and triple the baseline. Thirty minutes later we again collected the expired gas and the arterial and mixed venous blood samples under a steady state.

One half of the animals were randomly assigned to a treatment group (DV(+) group) and the others were assigned to a control group(DV(-) group). The DV(+) group received a bolus injection of 0.1 mg/kg of DV-7028 (a new type of selective $5-HT_2$ receptor antagonist) when PAP reached maximum and was followed by the continuous infusion at a rate of 1 mg/kg/hr.

Gas exchange was assessed by alveolar-arterial Po_2 gradient (AaDo$_2$), the continuous $\dot{V}_A/\dot{Q}$ distributions, retention of SF_6 (R_{SF6}) and 1- excretion of acetone (1-$E_{acetone}$). We used the multiple inert gas elimination technique reported by Wagner et al. (1974) to determine the continuous $\dot{V}_A/\dot{Q}$ distributions. We calculated R_{SF6} and 1-$E_{acetone}$ by the following equations.

$$R_{SF6} = Pa_{SF6} / Pv_{SF6}$$

$$1-E_{acetone} = 1- P_{Eacetone} / P_{Vacetone}$$

Pa_{SF6} is the arterial partial pressure of SF6; Pv_{SF6} is the mixed venous partial pressure of SF6; $P_{Eacetone}$ is the mixed expired gas partial pressure of acetone; $P_{Vacetone}$ is the mixed venous partial pressure of acetone.

All data in the table and text are presented as the mean $\pm$ standard deviation. Statistical ananlysis was performed using Wilcoxon's rank sum test for the paired data and Student's t-test for the non-paired data. We accepted $p < 0.05$ as statistically significant.

RESULTS

Changes of gas exchange, hemodynamic variables, airway pressure, hematological parameters and arterial blood serotonin 30 minutes after glass-bead embolization are shown in Table 1. After embolization Pao$_2$ decreased in both groups and AaDo$_2$ increased only in the DV(-) group. Shunt and dead space also increased in some cases of both groups but showed no statistical significance. Mean pulmonary arterial pressure (PAP), pulmonary vascular resistance (PVR) and airway pressure (P_{AIRWAY}) increased significantly in both groups.

Extra-vascular lung water volume index (ETVI) increased only in the DV(-) group. Paco$_2$ and cardiac output (C.O.) in both groups and ETVI in the DV(+) group did not change. Arterial blood serotonin and platelet counts declined in both groups after pulmonary embolization. The counts of white blood cell (WBC) and red blood cell(RBC) did not change. Compared to the DV(-) group after embolization, the increase of AaDo2, PAP

Table 1. Changes of gas exchange, pulmonary circulation, airway pressure, hematological parameters and blood serotonin after embolization

	DV (-) group		DV (+) group	
	Pre-Embolization	Post-Embolization	Pre-Embolization	Post-Embolization
Pa$_{O_2}$ (Torr)	93.6 ± 10.3	59.9 ± 5.9 **	91.0 ± 7.9	59.1 ± 16.4 **
Pa$_{CO_2}$ (Torr)	31.9 ± 5.4	31.1 ± 8.5	32.7 ± 7.7	42.6 ± 11.3
AaD$_{O_2}$ (Torr)▲	19.2 ± 16.5	53.9 ± 14.6*	22.7 ± 11.3	38.1±20.9
Shunt (%)	1.1 ± 1.5	4.0 ± 5.0	1.8 ± 1.9	3.9±2.2
Dead space (%)	16.4 ± 13.6	25.0 ± 14.2	22.0 ± 28.2	25.8 ± 12.5
PAP (mm Hg)▲	14.6 ± 4..0	37.3 ± 4.3 **	17.2 ± 3.3	29.1 ± 3.3 *
PVR ▲ (dyne·sec·cm^{-5})	273 ± 91	928 ± 187 **	292 ± 95	676 ± 190 *
C.O. (L/min)	3.33 ± 1.4	2.94 ± 0.78	3.31 ± 1.35	2.87 ± 0.84
ETVI (ml/kg)	11.3 ± 3.5	14.5 ± 8.2 *	9.3 ± 2.9	10.1 ± 1.8
P$_{AIRWAY}$ (mm Hg)	2.07 ± 0.53	2.63 ± 0.30 *	2.04 ± 0.45	2.42 ± 0.41 *
5-HT (ng/ml)	265 ± 108	206 ± 84 *	121 ± 52	100 ± 57 *
Platelet(x10^3/μl)	16.3 ± 6.1	11.9 ±5.7 *	13.8 ± 4.1	11.1 ± 3.1 *
WBC(x10^3/μl)	4.4 ± 2.6	5.7 ± 4.3	6.9 ± 2.1	8.7 ± 2.0
RBC(x10^4/μl)	686 ± 64	693 ± 57	641 ± 85	592 ± 64

*P< 0.05 ** P< 0.01 from previous column.   ▲P<0.05 comparing DV(-) group with DV(+) group. AaD$_{O_2}$: Alveolar arterial P$_{O_2}$ gradient; PAP: Mean pulmonary arterial pressure; PVR: Pulmonary vascular resistance;   C.O.: Cardiac output; ETVI: Extra-vascular lung water volume index; P$_{AIRWAY}$: Airway pressure; 5-HT: arterial blood serotonin concentration.

and PVR in the DV(+) group was significantly inhibited by DV-7028.

The course of PAP in both groups after embolization is shown in Fig. 2. PAP immediately reached a maximum value then gradually decreased. The PAP of the DV(+) group was significantly lower than that of the DV(-) group within 60 minutes after embolization.

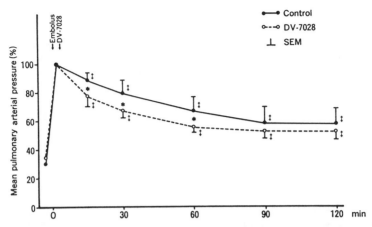

Fig. 1 The course of mean pulmonary arterial pressure (PAP) in both groups after embolization. Closed circle designates the mean value of the DV(-) group and open circle means the mean value of the DV(+) group. Each value was represented as a percentage of the maximum PAP.

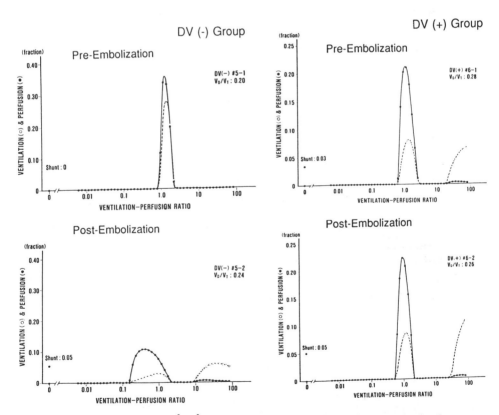

Fig. 2 The continuous $\dot{V}_A/\dot{Q}$ distributions obtained from typical cases of the DV(-) group (left) and the DV(+) group (right). The distributions of Pre-embolization is represented above and those of Post-embolization is below.

The continuous $\dot{V}_A/\dot{Q}$ distributions obtained from typical cases of both groups are revealed in Fig. 2. In all cases of the DV(-) group, glass-bead embolization made the distribution of $\dot{V}_A/\dot{Q}$ apparently worse with development of lung units with low or high $\dot{V}_A/\dot{Q}$ ratios (Fig. 2, left). In four of seven cases of the DV(+) group (Fig. 2, right), however, glass-bead embolization did not deteriorate the distribution of $\dot{V}_A/\dot{Q}$.

AaDo$_2$ 30 minutes after embolization of both groups are shown in Fig. 3. AaDo$_2$ of the DV(+) group was significantly lower than that of the DV(-) group. DV-7028 inhibited the increase in AaDo$_2$ after embolization. Effects of DV-7028 for R_{SF6} in all cases are represented in Fig. 4. R_{SF6} significantly increased after embolization in the DV(-) group. But in the DV(+) group R_{SF6} did not change. DV-7028 inhibited the increase in R_{SF6}. Effects of DV-7028 for 1-$E_{acetone}$ in all cases are represented in Fig. 5. 1-$E_{acetone}$ did not change after embolization in both groups.

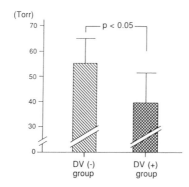

Fig. 3 Effect of DV-7028 for AaDo$_2$ after pulmonary embolization.

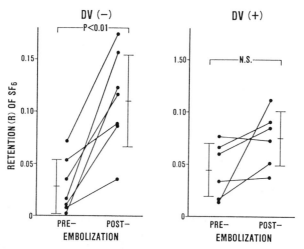

Fig. 4 Effects of DV-7028 for R_{SF6} in all cases.

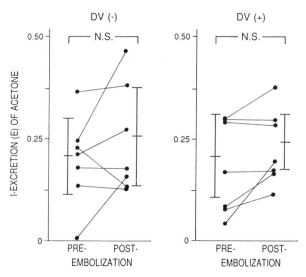

Fig. 5 Effects of DV-7028 for 1-E$_{acetone}$ in all cases.

DISCUSSION

Release of Vasoactive Agents from Circulating Platelets in Pulmonary Embolization. Pulmonary embolization causes profound alternations in cardiopulmonary hemodynamics, gas exchange and lung extra-vascular water accumulation, which can be attributed to the release of some vasoactive agents. A substantial component of the hemodynamic effects are mediated by platelet-derived vasoactive agent, such as thromboxane A$_2$ (Utsonomiya et al., 1982) and serotonin (Levy and Simmons, 1971; Hyland J.W.et al., 1963). To investigate the role of serotonin in pulmonary embolism, we used DV-7028 which inhibits 5-HT$_2$ receptor selectively (Morishima, 1991). In the present study, glass-bead embolization caused the reduction of circulating platelet numbers and arterial blood serotonin. A precipitous decline in circulating platelets was reported early in experimental pulmonary embolization(Thomas and Gurewich, 1966). These platelets layered on the exposed surfaces of the emboli and were activated (Thomas et al., 1966). Our results suggest that fresh clots formed around the glass-bead emboli which might have led to platelet activation and serotonin release.

Changes of Pulmonary Hemodynamics Following Pulmonary Embolization. After embolization PAP and PVR increased significantly. The PAP and PVR of the DV(+) group was significantly lower than those of the DV(-) group within 60 minutes after embolization. These results are almost the same as those reported using a relatively selective serotonin receptor antagonist, ketanserin (Huval et al, 1983). The results from our study shows that serotonin was a component that increased PAP and PVR after pulmonary embolization and its effects were apparent within 60 minutes.

Gas Exchange Impairment in Pulmonary Embolization. Pulmonary embolization causes severe gas exchange impairment and hypoxia. The responsible mechanism has been attributed to shunt (Caldini,P., 1965; Cheney,F., 1973) and ventilation-perfusion mismatching (Dantzker,D.R., 1978). Using two different-sized glass-beads, Delcroix(1990) reported that only small bead (0.1 mm diameter) embolization generated a shunt and both bead sizes deteriorate the distribution of $\dot{V}_A/\dot{Q}$ ratios. Therefore we used the small-sized beads to investigate the mechanism of gas exchange impairment in pulmonary embolization.

The Effects of Serotonin on Gas Exchange Following Pulmonary Embolization. There have been several studies which investigated the effects of serotonin on gas exchange. Huval et al.(1983) found a decrease of shunt fraction using ketanserin after embolization. Thompson et al.(1986) reported that serotonin is responsible for the fall in Pao_2 following pulmonary embolization. We assessed gas exchange systematically by $AaDo_2$, the continuous $\dot{V}_A/\dot{Q}$ distributions, R_{SF6} and $1-E_{acetone}$. The continuous $\dot{V}_A/\dot{Q}$ distributions had never been investigated for the effects of serotonin in pulmonary embolization.

Serotonin inhibition by DV-7028 substantially attenuated the increase in $AaDo_2$ after pulmonary embolization. Shunt and dead space were not significantly changed by DV-7028. Because neither shunt nor dead space could account for the attenuation of the increase in $AaDo_2$ after embolization, changes of the distribution of $\dot{V}_A/\dot{Q}$ might be the main cause. Without DV-7028, glass-bead embolization made the distribution of $\dot{V}_A/\dot{Q}$ apparently worse. With DV-7028, the embolization did not deteriorate the distribution of $\dot{V}_A/\dot{Q}$ in 4 of 7 cases. As it is difficult to know the amount of changes of $\dot{V}_A/\dot{Q}$ distribution, we introduced R_{SF6} and $1-E_{acetone}$. Changes of R_{SF6} indicate changes of low $\dot{V}_A/\dot{Q}$ lung units and shunt. Changes of $1-E_{acetone}$ indicate changes of high $\dot{V}_A/\dot{Q}$ lung units and dead space. In the present study, serotonin inhibition by DV-7028 led to inhibition of the increase of R_{SF6} after embolization, which meant inhibition in the increase of low $\dot{V}_A/\dot{Q}$ lung units and shunt. Thus it seems reasonable to conclude that serotonin deteriorates gas exchange in pulmonary embolization due to the increase of low $\dot{V}_A/\dot{Q}$ lung unit and shunt.

There are some possibile reasons why serotonin increased low $\dot{V}_A/\dot{Q}$ lung unit and shunt. One possible reason is that serotonin increases extravascular lung water in alveoli, which induces low $\dot{V}_A/\dot{Q}$ lung units and shunt. Serotonin inhibition blocked the increase in extravascular lung water index after embolization in our study (Table 1). Another possible reason is that serotonin causes constriction of peripheral bronchioles as shown by Colebatch(1966). Airway pressure increased after embolization, but serotonin inhibition did not change the result (Table 1). The very peripheral site of broncho-constriction, however, may account for the difficulty in demonstrating the change of airway pressure.

CONCLUSION

Serotonin deteriorates gas exchange due to the increase of low $\dot{V}_A/\dot{Q}$ lung units and shunt in acute canine pulmonary embolism.

REFERENCES

Caldini, P., 1965, Pulmonary hemodynamics and arterial oxygen saturation in pulmonary emboli, J.Appl.Physiol. 20: 184-190.

Cheney, F., Paulin, J., and Ferene, B.S., 1973, Effect of pulmonary microembolism on arteriovenous shunt flow, J.Thorac.Cardiovasc.Surg. 4: 473-477.

Colebatch, H.J.H., Olsen, C.R.,and Nadel, J.A.,1966, Effect of histamine, serotonin and acetylcholine on the peripheral airway, J.Appl.Physiol. 21: 217-226.

Huval, W.V., Mathieson, M.A., Stemp, L.I., Dunham, B.M., Jones, A.G., Shepro, D., and Hechtman, H.B., 1983, Therapeutic benefits of 5-hydroxytyptamine inhibition following pulmonary embolism, Ann.Surg.197:220-225.

Hyland, J.W., Piemme T.E., and Alexander S., 1963, Behavior of pulmonary hypertension produced by serotonin and emboli, Am. J. Physiol. 205: 591-597.

Ishibe, Y.,.Suekane, K., Nakamura,M., Izumi,T., Umeda,T., Sagawa,Y., Satoh, K., and Oh, M., 1987, Measurement of lung water with double indicator dilution method using heat and sodium ions in dogs, Jap.Anesth.J.Rev. 2:5-7.

Levy S.E., Simmons, D.H., 1971, Serotonin pulmonary hypertension and airway constriction in the anesthetized dog, Pro. Sci. Exp.Biol.Med. 138:365-368.

Morishima, Y., Tanaka, T., Watanabe, K., Igarashi, T., Yasuoka,M., and Shibano,T.,1991, Prevention by DV-7028, a selective $5-HT_2$ receptor antagonist, of the formation coronary thrombi in dogs, Cardiovasc.Resear. 25: 727-730.

Thomas, D.P.,and Gurewich, V., 1966, Role of platelets in sudden death induced by experimental pulmonary emboli, Circulation 22: 207-209.

Thomas, D.P., Gurewich, V., and Ashford T.P., 1966, Platelet adherence to thromboembolism, N. Engl. J. Med. 274: 952-958.

Thompson, J.A., Millen, J.E., Glauser, F.L., and Hess, M.L., 1986, Role of $5-HT_2$ receptor inhibition in pulmonary embolism, Circulatory Shock 20:299-309.

Utsonomiya, T., Krausz, M.M., Levine, L., Shepro, D., and Hechtman, H.B., 1982, Thromboxane mediation of cardiopulmonary effects of embolism, J. Clin. Invest. 70:361-368.

Wagner, P.D., Saltzman,H.A., and West, J.B., 1974, Measurement of continuous distribution of ventilation-perfusion ratios: Theory, J.Appl.Physiol. 36:588-599.

SURFACTANT REPLACEMENT THERAPY IN ANIMAL MODELS OF RESPIRATORY FAILURE DUE TO VIRAL INFECTION

A. van 't Veen, K.L. So and B. Lachmann

Dept. of Anaesthesiology
Erasmus University Rotterdam
The Netherlands

INTRODUCTION

Several studies have shown that during the development of respiratory failure in the adult respiratory distress syndrome (ARDS), the pulmonary surfactant system is disturbed[1-5]. One of the current promising therapeutic approaches in ARDS is, therefore, re-establishment of the functional integrity of the damaged surfactant system by intratracheal instillation of surfactant. The first clinical trials[6,7] and results from experimental studies on ARDS have shown that exogenous surfactant application can restore lung function in ARDS (for review see references 8 and 9). Due to the great variance in etiology of ARDS it is, however, a necessity to investigate surfactant replacement therapy in different models of respiratory failure. Therefore, we studied the effect of surfactant substitution in two animal models of severe respiratory failure due to viral pneumonia.

In the first model, mice were infected with influenza A virus resulting in a lethal pneumonia. Infection with influenza A virus causes severe damage to the alveolar capillary membrane and can lead to pulmonary edema, hemorrhage and death from respiratory failure and shock[10,11]. In this model, the effect of surfactant replacement on lung mechanics was studied. Thorax-lung compliance (C_{tl}) was measured and postmortem lung volume at 5 cm H_2O (V_5) positive end-expiratory pressure (PEEP). It is not possible to measure functional residual capacity (FRC) in small laboratory

Oxygen Transport to Tissue XV, Edited by P. Vaupel
et al., Plenum Press, New York, 1994

animals effectively, however, it is possible to measure postmortem lung volumes with a method based on Archimedes principle. It is speculated that the V_5 is the cumulative outcome of postmortem lung volume at end-expiration (approximating FRC), the added lung volume, resulting from 5 cm H_2O PEEP and the amount of fluid in the alveoli. V_5 is likely to give a valuable impression of pulmonary stability of the surfactant system. Additionally, changes in surface tensions of bronchoalveolar lavage (BAL) fluid during infection was measured.

In the second model, rats were infected with Sendai virus resulting in a pneumonia with acute respiratory failure closely resembling ARDS[12]. In this model it was possible to investigate the effect of surfactant substitution on arterial blood gas tensions.

METHODS AND MATERIALS

Animals

All experiments were approved by the institutional committee on animal care according to the rules on animal welfare of the European Committee. Male Swiss-bred mice n = 80 (SPF, 20-25 g) and male Sprague-Dawley rats n=41 (180-200 g, SPF) supplied by Harlan/CPB, Zeist, The Netherlands, were used. Animals were housed under conventional conditions; food and water were given ad libitum. Infected animals were housed under the same conditions, under filtered bonnets, in a separate facility.

Virus preparation and infection procedure

Influenza A virus (A/PR8/34, H1N1) was passed once in 10-day embryonated chicken eggs. The allantoid fluid was clarified by centrifugation, diluted once in sucrose and then stored at -70°C. The hemagglutination (HA) titer of this stock solution was 1:400. For a lethal infection, mice were exposed once for 30 min to an aerosol of live influenza A virus by placing them in an aerosol chamber through which an 8-fold dilution of the stock solution was nebulized.

Sendai virus (Myxovirus parainfluenza type 1) was propagated in 11-day embryonated chicken eggs. The stock solution, similarly prepared as with influenza A virus, had a HA titer of 1 : 3000. For inoculation animals were placed for 90 min in an aerosol chamber in which a one-fold dilution of the stock solution was nebulized.

Preparation of animals for ventilation and/or lung mechanics measurement

Animals, both mice and rats, were anesthetized by intraperitoneal injection of 60 mg/kg pentobarbital (Nembutal®; Algin BV, Maassluis, The Netherlands) and tracheotomized using a metal cannula as tracheal tube. Paralyzation was achieved by intramuscular injection of pancuronium bromide, 0.1 mg/kg (Pavulon®; Organon Technika, Boxtel, The Netherlands). Additionally in rats, the carotid artery was canalized for drawing arterial blood samples for measuring blood gas tensions.

Bronchoalveolar lavage and surface tension measurement

BAL was performed three times in mice with a volume of 1 ml sterile saline preheated to 38°C. BAL cells were removed from the lavage fluid by centrifugation (800 x g, 10 min, 4°C). Surface activity in BAL fluid was measured with a modified Wilhelmy balance by applying 400 μl of BAL fluid onto a 71.3 cm^3 trough. For measurement of minimal surface tensions the area was compressed to 20% of the initial value.

Lung mechanics in influenza A model

Mice were randomly divided into ten groups (n = 8 per group). Two groups were not infected and served as controls, eight groups were infected. On days 1, 3 and 5 after infection, thorax-lung compliance (C_{tl}), lung volume at 5 cm H_2O (V_5) and the ratio wet/dry lung weight (ratio$_{w/d}$) were measured and in three other infected groups BAL was performed. On day five after infection these parameters, except BAL, were studied in two additional groups: one was treated with surfactant and one was sham-treated with the vehicle for surfactant (VFS = 1:2 mixture H_2O and saline). From these two groups the lungs were prepared for histologic examination.

C_{tl} **measurement.** Anesthetized and tracheotomized mice were placed in a multichambered body plethysmograph[13] and connected to a ventilator system for pressure-controlled ventilation. Initial ventilatory settings: 30 pulses/min (30 bf), inspiration/expiration (I/E) ratio 1:2 , peak pressure (P_{peak}) 25 cm H_2O (25/0) and F_{IO2} = 1. After 10 min C_{tl} was recorded at a breath frequency of 10/min. For calculation of compliance per kilogram body weight ($C_{tl/kg}$), the bodyweight (BW) registered on the day of infection was used.

V_5 **measurement.** After registration of C_{tl}, animals were euthanized with an overdose of pentobarbital. The thorax was excised, carefully leaving the diaphragm intact and leaving the intratracheal cannula in place. These excised lungs were reexpanded with 0.5 ml of air to reopen atelectic areas induced by the surgical procedure. Next, the lungs were left to collapse for 10 min against a positive pressure of 5 cm H_2O 100% nitrogen. Afterwards the trachea was bound and the cannula removed, maintaining the positive pressure in the lungs. First the total weight (W) of the thorax was measured, followed by the measurement of the thorax weight immersed in saline at a preset depth to measure upward force (F) caused by displacement of a volume of saline equal to the volume of the thorax. V_5 was calculated by the following formula (for details see reference 14):

$$V_5 = 0.99 * F - 0.94 * W$$

For the correction for BW (V_5/kg), the BW registered on the day of infection was used.

Ratio$_{w/d}$. Dry lung weight was obtained after drying the excised lungs in a conventional microwave oven at 250 W for 1 h[15].

Surfactant/VFS installation. After measurement of C_{tl} a PEEP of 4-5 cm H_2O was added, keeping the remaining ventilatory settings unchanged. Next 0.15 ml of a natural bovine surfactant (200 mg/kg BW dissolved in 1:2 mixture of H_2O and saline), extracted in basically the same manner as described by others[16], or 0.15 ml of the VFS was instilled into the lungs. Ten minutes later C_{tl} was registered again; hereafter V_5 was measured as described above.

Arterial blood gas tension measurement in Sendai virus model

Thirty-six hours after infection of the rats, seven animals were prepared for ventilation and measurement of arterial blood gases. The remaining animals were prepared 48 hours after infection.

The ventilator was set in a pressure-controlled mode, 35 b/min, P_{peak} 15/0, I/E ratio of 1:2 and 100% oxygen (F_{IO2} = 1). To assess the severity of respiratory failure, blood gas tensions were measured at increased ventilatory airway pressures. P_{peak} was first increased to 20/0 then to 25/4 adding a PEEP of 4 cm H_2O. After each ventilatory change 15 min was allowed for stabilization before a 0.3 ml blood sample was drawn from the carotid artery for blood gas tension measurements.

Treatment with surfactant or VFS was performed only in animals with an arterial oxygen tension (PaO_2) below 150 mm Hg ventilated at 15/0 and in which increased ventilatory airway pressures (25/4) did not increase PaO_2 above 175 mm Hg. Twenty-two animals met these preset criteria at 48 hours after infection and were randomly divided into three groups. Nine animals received 1.5 ml of surfactant (200 mg/kg BW) intratracheally, seven animals received 1.5 ml VFS intratracheally and six animals received no treatment whatsoever except for continuation of the same ventilatory support that was used in the treated animals (25/4). After treatment ventilatory settings remained unchanged and blood gas tensions were monitored for 2 hours.

Histologic examination

In both models the lungs were prepared and excised for histologic examination. In mice, the thorax was opened and a cannula inserted into the right ventricle. A pressure of 5 cm H_2O in the lungs was maintained while the lungs were perfused with formalin (4%) via the right ventricle. In rats, the chest of each animal was opened at the end of the experiment and a cannula was inserted into the pulmonary artery and an inflation pressure of 20 cm H_2O was maintained. After this procedure the lungs were removed and kept in a 10% formalin solution for at least 48 hours. Paraffin sections were stained with hematoxylin-eosin and examined microscopically.

Statistical analysis and presentation of the data

Statistical analysis of data was performed using the Mann-Whitney U test for analysis of intergroup differences or Wilcoxon's test for analysis of intragroup differences. Statistical significance was accepted at $p \leq 0.05$ (two-tailed). All data are expressed as mean ± SD.

RESULTS

Lung mechanics and surface tensions

Both minimal and maximal surface tension of BAL fluid were significantly increased on the fifth day after infection with influenza A virus compared to noninfected control values (table 1). C_{tl}/kg and V_5/kg in mice were significantly decreased on the third and the fifth day after infection (table 1). Furthermore ratio$_{w/d}$ was significantly increased on the third and fifth day after infection in animals (table 1).

Surfactant instillation on the fifth day significantly increased C_{tl}/kg in these animals, whereas VFS instillation did not significantly improve C_{tl}/kg (table 2). To take into account the effect of the instilled amount of fluid into the lungs 0.15 ml should be subtracted from control values to correct for the reduction of V_5 by the volume of the instilled dose (assuming no absorption of fluid has taken place). Table 2 shows the corrected values for $V_{5/kg}$.

Table 1. Changes in lung mechanics and surfactant system during influenza A pneumonia

days after infection	controls	1	3	5
$R_{w/d}$	4.28	4.21	4.83[*]	5.34[*]
	(0.51)	(0.22)	(0.28)	(0.78)
V_5/kg (ml/kg)	20.8	20.0	14.1[*]	9.5[*]
	(2.5)	(2.1)	(2.1)	(3.3)
C_{tl}/kg	0.57	0.56	0.46[*]	0.41[*]
(ml/kg/cm H_2O)	(0.08)	(0.06)	(0.06)	(0.14)
maximal surface tension (dynes/cm)	58.3	58.5	55.5	63.9[*]
	(3.7)	(4.2)	(6.6)	(1.7)
minimal surface tension (dynes/cm)	22.5	21.6	21.1	32.2[*]
	(1.7)	(1.4)	(3.3)	(2.1)

Changes in ratio$_{w/d}$, lung volume at 5 cm H_2O PEEP (V_5/kg), thorax-lung compliance (C_{tl}) of control mice and mice infected with a lethal dose of influenza A virus. Mean (SD), n=8/group. * = p ≤ 0.05 Mann-Whitney U test.(Partly reprinted with permission from ref.14)

Table 2. Effect of exogenous surfactant instillation on lung mechanics during influenza A pneumonia

	surfactant group		VFS group	
	before	after	before	after
C_{tl} (ml/kg/H_2O)	0.34	0.52 *	0.35	0.32
	(0.15)	(0.28)	(0.14)	(0.15)
	healthy corrected	untreated	surfactant	VFS
V_5/kg (ml/kg)	14.7	9.5	14.0*#	4.3
	(2.2)	(3.3)	(2.3)	(1.9)

Influence of surfactant or VFS instillation on thorax-lung compliance (C_{tl}/kg) and postmortem lung volume at 5 cm H_2O PEEP on the fifth day after infection with lethal dose influenza A virus. C_{tl}/kg at 25 cm H_2O before and 10 min after instillation of 0.15 ml surfactant or VFS. Mean (SD), n=8/group. * = p ≤ 0.05 Wilcoxin test compared to values before treatment. V_5/kg at 5 cm H_2O, after instillation of surfactant or VFS. * = p ≤ 0.05 compared to solvent treated group, # = p ≤ 0.05 compared to untreated animals at the fifth day after infection. Mann-Whitney U test. (Reprinted with permission from ref. 14)

Evaluation of the effect of surfactant instillation (table 2) shows that surfactant almost completely restored V_5/kg (from 9.5 ± 3.3 ml/kg in untreated animals on the fifth day after infection to 14.0 ± 2.3 ml/kg in surfactant treated animals). VFS significantly reduced V_5/kg.

Arterial blood gas tensions

At 36 h after infection, animals already showed severe signs of respiratory insufficiency. Increasing the ventilatory airway pressure from 15/0 to 25/4, however, almost completely restored arterial blood gas tensions to normal values: PaO_2 from 152.2 ± 18.7 to 456.5 ± 65.6 mm Hg, PCO_2 from 65.3 ± 19.2 to 46.8 ± 8.2 mm Hg. Criteria for treatment of surfactant or VFS were not met.

Twelve hours later, six animals had died spontaneously and another five animals died during ventilation with 15/0. After this higher airway pressures were applied immediately after tracheotomy. PO_2 values, however, remained low; 101.8 ± 20.7 at 20/0 (n=22) and 123.7 ± 34.1 at 25/4 (n=22). These animals were then randomly assigned to three groups. Before treatment there existed no significant differences in PaO_2, PCO_2, arterial pH and arterial HCO_3^- concentrations between these groups (table 3)

Within five minutes after surfactant instillation, PaO_2 significantly increased and remained significantly higher during the entire observation period than in the saline treated and untreated groups (Fig. 1).

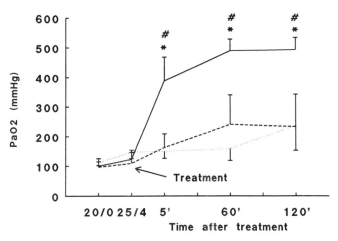

Figure 1. PaO_2 values (mean $\pm$ SD) 48 hours after infection with Sendai virus, during artificial ventilation and after treatment with surfactant (solid line, n = 9), saline (broken line, n = 7), respiratory support only (dotted line, n = 6). * P $\leq$ 0.05, surfactant treated animals versus saline treated and untreated controls. # P $\leq$ 0.05, surfactant versus pretreatment values at the same ventilator settings. Mann-Whitney U test. (Reprinted with permission from: Anesth Analg 1991;72:589).

As a result of the ventilation, PaO_2 increased slightly, though not significantly, in the saline treated and untreated groups.

In the surfactant treated group and in both control groups, PCO_2 decreased and pH concurrently increased during the 2 hour ventilation period with no significant difference between these three groups. Only in the surfactant group did, PCO_2 values reach physiological values (table 3).

Table 3. $PaCO_2$ and pH values

	Before		After treatment		
	20/0	25/4	5 min	60 min	120 min
$PaCO_2$ (mm HG)					
surfactant	105.8	95.1	61.9	46.9#	42.6#
	(57.0)	(43.6)	(14.9)	(8.2)	(8.3)
VFS	74.5	76.7	68.1	49.2#	54.6
	(21.0)	(17.6)	(21.2)	(12.7)	(15.9)
untreated	122.9	97.6	80.4	63.7#	55.9#
	(27.1)	(23.2)	(11.3)	(5.3)	(7.3)
pH					
surfactant	7.13	7.12	7.22#	7.33#	7.33#
	(0.18)	(0.16)	(0.09)	(0.06)	(0.11)
VFS	7.22	7.19	7.22	7.32#	7.31#
	(0.11)	(0.11)	(0.14)	(0.08)	(0.09)
untreated	7.03	7.09	7.13	7.23#	7.29#
	(0.05)	(0.07)	(0.04)	(0.03)	(0.03)

Values are expressed as mean (SD) and were taken 48 hours after a lethal dose of Sendai virus, during artificial ventilation and after treatment with surfactant, VFS or respiratory support only. Animals were ventilated in a pressure controlled mode, at a rate of 35/min, I/E ratio 1:2 and 100% O_2. Different settings were applied, treatment with surfactant or VFS was done at 25/4 ventilatory pressures and ventilatory pressures were kept unchanged during the entire observation period.

# $p < 0.05$ compared with pretreatment valeus at the same ventilator settings (25/4). (Reprinted with permission from: Anesth. Analg.72:589(1991)).

Histologic examination

Histologic examination of mouse lungs five days after infection with influenza A virus showed severe atelectasis and alveolar filling with leucocyte-rich exudate.

Histologic examination of rat lungs infected with Sendai virus showed swelling of the alveolar walls and alveolar edema containing inflammatory cells. Swelling of bronchial epithelial cells and atelectic areas were present. In both models, lungs treated with surfactant showed a clear improvement of lung aeration compared with VFS treated lungs or untreated lungs.

DISCUSSION

An intact surfactant system is indispensable for the maintenance of proper lung function and, therefore, any type of surfactant deficiency whether primary or secondary will contribute to the development of severe pulmonary pathology. Malfunction of the pulmonary surfactant system leads to decreased lung distensibility, collapse of alveoli and small airways[17,18]. This results in atelectasis, enlargement of the right to left shunt, hypoxemia and acidosis[19,20]. Furthermore the surfactant system, through stabilization of the fluid balance in the lung, plays an important role in the prevention of pulmonary edema[21-23].

During the development of respiratory failure, we found in both models a loss of lung function. In the influenza A model pulmonary edema, in this study reflected by increased ratio$_{w/d}$, was associated with decreased pulmonary compliance, decreased V_5, and decreased surfactant activity in BAL fluid. Studies on lung function with the Sendai model showed a decrease in C_{tl} during the course of infection[12] and a severe impairment of gas exchange, as confirmed by the results of the present study. The necessity to use PEEP for restoring gas exchange at 36 h after infection and so preventing alveolar collapse indicates the presence of surfactant deficiency.

From this study it cannot be concluded at which stage during the infection impairment of surfactant function significantly contributes to changes in pulmonary mechanics. Increased surface tension in BAL fluid on the fifth day after infection with influenza A virus, clearly indicates decreased surfactant function. This can be caused by loss or by inhibition of surfactant. The fact that on the third day, in vitro surface tensions of BAL fluid were not changed, despite changes in lung mechanics, does not necessarily mean that impairment of surfactant function was not present in vivo.

The loss of pulmonary function and development of respiratory failure as observed in this study can be explained by an impairment of the surfactant system. Severe viral pneumonia may cause destruction of type I cells which results in the disruption of the integrity of the alveolar-capillary membrane causing the development of permeability edema[24-26]. Edema constituents like albumin, fibrinogen and other plasma components are potent inhibitors of the surfactant system[27-31]. A deficit of surfactant itself may result from destruction of the surfactant producing type II cells by the inflammatory reaction to virus or by virus replication itself[26]. Because the surfactant system is essential for the prevention of pulmonary edema, a vicious circle may develop where inhibition of the surfactant function by edema components accelerates the formation of pulmonary edema and the development of respiratory failure.

Surfactant substitution on the fifth day after lethal infection with influenza A virus restored C_{tl}/kg of infected animals almost to normal, from 60% of noninfected control values before substitution to 91% after surfactant substitution. Postmortem V_5 of infected animals was also almost restored to normal after substitution of surfactant; postmortem $V_{5/kg}$ of the surfactant treated group was 95% of volume-corrected noninfected control values, whereas $V_{5/kg}$ in the VFS-treated group was only 29% of volume-corrected noninfected control values. Introduction of PEEP initially could restore gas exchange during a lethal infection with Sendai virus. In a later stage of the disease, however, a higher P_{peak} with PEEP had no significant effect because the opening pressure of the lungs is increased. Intratracheal instillation of surfactant reduces the opening pressure, prevents alveolar collapse and combined with ventilatory support, restores gas exchange to almost normal.

Findings in this study indicate that reduced arterial oxygenation, pulmonary compliance and V_5 caused by loss of surfactant function during viral pneumonia can almost completely be restored by surfactant replacement therapy, which is an indirect proof for a shortage of surfactant during viral pneumonia. On the basis of earlier observations and these findings we conclude that surfactant replacement therapy seems a promising approach for the treatment of respiratory failure during severe viral pneumonia.

REFERENCES

1. M. Hallmann, R. Spragg, J.H. Harrel, K.M. Moser and L. Gluck, Evidence of lung surfactant abnormality in respiratory failure, *J. Clin. Invest.* 70:673(1982)
2. W. Seeger, U. Pison and R. Buchhorn, Alterations in alveolar surfactant following severe multiple trauma, *in*: "Basic research on lung surfactant," P. Von Wichert, ed., Prog. Respir. Dis., Basel (1990)
3. P. Von Wichert, P.V. Kohl, Decreased dipalmitoyl lecithin content found in lung specimens from patients with so-called shock-lung, *Intensive Care Med.* 3:27(1977)
4. T.L. Petty, G.W. Silvers, G.W. Paul and R.E. Stanford, Abnormalities in lung elastic properties and surfactant function in adult respiratory distress syndrome,*Chest.* 75:571(1979)
5. B. Lachmann and E. Danzmann, Adult respiratory distress syndrome,*in*: "Pulmonary surfactant," B. Robertson, ed.,Elsevier, Amsterdam(1984)
6. B. Lachmann, The role of pulmonary surfactant in the pathogenesis and therapy of ARDS,*in*: "Update in intensive care and emergency medicine," J.L. Vincent,ed.,Springer-verslag, Berlin(1987)
7. P.S. Richman, R.G. Spragg, B. Robertson, T.A. Merrit and T. Curstedt, The adult respiratory distress

syndrome: first trials with surfactant replacement, *Eur. Respir. J.* 2:109S(1989)

8. B.A. Holm and S. Matalon, Role of pulmonary surfactant in the development and treatment of adult respiratory distress syndrome, *Anesth. Analg.* 69:805(1989)

9. B. Lachmann, Surfactant replacement, *Appl. Cardiopulm. Physiol.* 3:3(1989)

10. H. Herzog, H. Staub and R. Richterich, Ga-analytical studies in severe pneumonia. Observations during the 1957 influenza epidemic, *Lancet.* i:593(1959)

11. D.B. Louria, H.L. Blumenfeld, J.T. Ellis, E.D. Kilbourn and D.E. Rogers, Studies on influenza in the pandemic of 1957-58. II Pulmonary complications of influenza, *J. Clin. Invest.* 38:213(1959)

12. G.J. van Daal, E.P. Eijking, K.L. So and B. Lachmann, Acute respiratory failure during pneumonia induced by Sendai virus, *Adv. Exp. Med. Biol. (in press)*

13. B. Lachmann, P. Berggren, T. Curstedt, G. Grossmann and B. Robertson, Combined effects of surfactant substitution and prolongation of inspiratory phase in artificially ventilated premature newborn rabbits, *Pediatr. Res.* 16:921(1982)

14. G.J. van Daal, J.A.H. Bos, E.P. Eijking, D. Gommers E. Hannappel and B. Lachmann, Surfactant replacement therapy improves pulmonary mechanics in end-stage influenza A pneumonia in mice, *Am. Rev. Respir. Dis.* 145:859(1992)

15. B.T. Peterson, J.A. Brooks and A.G. Zack, Use of microwave oven for determination of postmortem water volume of lungs, *J. Appl. Physiol.* 49:34(1982)

16. I.L. Metcalfe, G. Enhorning, F. Possmayer, Pulmonary surfactant-associated proteins: their role in the expression of surface activity, *J. Appl. Physiol.* 49:34(1980)

17. J.A. Clements, Function of the alveolar lining, *Am. Rev. Respir. Dis.* 115:S67(1977)

18. J. Goerke, Lung surfactant, *Biochem. Biophys. Acta.* 344:241(1974)

19. B.A. Holm, S. Matalon and R.H. Notter, Pulmonary surfactant effects and replacements in oxygen toxicity and other ARDS-type lung injuries, *in*: "Surfactant replacement therapy in neonatal and adult respiratory distress syndrome," B. Lachmann, ed. Springer-Verlag, Berlin Heidelberg(1988)

20. B. Lachmann, Surfactant replacement therapy in neonatal and respiratory distress syndrome, *in*: "Surfactant replacement therapy in neonatal and adult respiratory distress syndrome," B. Lachmann, ed. Springer-Verlag, Berlin Heidelberg(1988)

21. J.A. Clements, Pulmonary edema and permeability of alveolar membranes, *Arch. Environ. Health.* 104(1961)

22. R.K. Albert, S. Lakshminarayan, J. Hildebrandt, W. Kirk, and J. Butler, Increased surface tension favors pulmonary edema formation in anesthetized dogs' lungs, *J. Clin. Invest.* 63:1015(1979)

23. G.F. Nieman and C.E. Bredenberg, Pulmonary edema induced by high alveolar surface tension, *Prog. Respir. Res.* 18:204(1984)

24. C. Sweet and H. Smith, Pathogenicity of influenza virus, *Microbiol. Rev.* 44:303(1980)

25. D.G. Brownstein, Sendai virus infection, lung, mouse and rat, *in*: "Monographs on pathology of laboratory animals," T.C. Jones, ed., International Life Sciences Institute, Washington D.C.(1985)

26. S.F. Stinson, D.P. Ryan, M.S. Hertweck, J.D. Hardy, S.Y. Hwang-Kow and CG Loosli, Epithelial and surfactant changes in influenza pulmonary lesions, *Arch. Pathol. Lab. Med.* 100:147(1976)

27. F.B. Taylor and M.E. Abrams, Effects of surface active lipoprotein on clotting and fibrinolysis and of fibrinogen on surface tension of surface active lipoprotein, *Am. J. Med.* 40:346(1966)

28. M. Ikegami, A. Jobe, H. Jacobs and R. Lam, A protein from airways of premature lambs that inhibits surfactant function, *J. Appl. Physiol.* 57:1134(1984)

29. B.A. Holm, R.H. Notter and J.N. Finkelstein, Surface property changes from interactions of albumine with natural lung surfactant and extracted lung lipids, *Chem. Phys. Lipids.* 38:287(1985)

30. W. Seeger, G. Stohr, H.R. Wolf and H. Neuhof, Alteration of surfactant function due to protein

leakage: special interaction with fibrin monomer, *J. Appl. Physiol. 58:326(1985)*

31. B.A. Holm, G.E. Enhorning and R.H. Notter, A biophysical mechanism by which plasma proteins inhibit surfactant activity, *Chem. Phys. Lipids.* 49:49(1988)

EFFECTS OF DIFFERENT MODES OF VENTILATION ON OXYGENATION AND INTRACRANIAL PRESSURE OF PIGS WITH SURFACTANT DEPLETED LUNGS

J. Kesecioglu,[1,2] T. Denkel,[2] F. Esen,[2] L. Telci,[2] K. Akpir,[2] W. Erdmann,[1] and B. Lachmann[1]

[1]Department of Anesthesiology, Erasmus University Hospital
Dijkzigt, Rotterdam, The Netherlands
[2]Department of Anesthesiology, University of Istanbul, Faculty of
Medicine, Istanbul, Turkey

INTRODUCTION

In cases where the diseased state of the patient is caused or further complicated by a brain injury, conflict can arise between the conceptions of providing adequate gas exchange and the simultaneous need of brain protection against a possible increase of intracranial pressure (ICP) due to the ventilatory modes used.

The effect of positive end-expiratory pressure (PEEP) on ICP has been reported by various investigators, without any consensus being reached[1-10]. While the application of PEEP resulted in increases in ICP in some studies[1,2], other researches failed to demonstrate an increase of this parameter with a clinical consequence[3]. Because of this reason volume controlled ventilation (VCV) with PEEP, pressure regulated volume controlled ventilation (PRVCV) with an inspiratory/expiratory (I/E) ratio of 4:1 and low frequency positive pressure ventilation with extracorporeal CO_2 removal (LFPPV-$ECCO_2R$) were compared in normovolemic pigs in supine posture, with surfactant depleted lungs. The aim being to achieve similar $PaCO_2$ tensions the changes produced in ICP were investigated.

METHODS

Six male pigs, 41.2 ± 2.7 kg were premedicated with midazolam (0.5 mg/kg) intramuscularly. Anesthesia was induced with thiopentone (2-4 mg/kg), given through a 20 G cannula placed into an ear vein. Tracheostomy was performed and a portex tube with an internal diameter of 7 mm was inserted. The tube was fixed to the trachea with stitches and the cuff was inflated to avoid air leakage. Lungs were ventilated with a Servo 900C (Siemens-Elema, Solna, Sweden) ventilator thereafter. Anesthesia was maintained by infusion of midazolam (0.2 mg/kg/min) and fentanyl (2 μg/kg/min). Pancuronium bromide (0.08 mg/kg/min) infusion was administered after a bolus of 0.2 mg/kg for muscle relaxation.

Oxygen Transport to Tissue XV, Edited by P. Vaupel
et al., Plenum Press, New York, 1994

A 7F three lumen catheter for adequate fluid replacement to avoid hypovolemia and a 7F thermodilution catheter for hemodynamic monitoring were inserted to the surgically exposed right and left internal jugular veins respectively. The needle and the Seldinger guide wire provided with the system were used for insertion and the ligature of the vessels was avoided in order not to obstruct venous flow.

Two 20F cannula were inserted to the right and left femoral veins for the administration of extracorporeal circulation. Femoral artery was cannulated for blood sampling and invasive blood pressure monitoring. An 18F urine catheter was placed into the bladder by cystostomy to monitor urine output.

ICP was monitored by a 22G catheter introduced to the ventricule through a twist drill hole, 2 cm lateral to the midline and 1 cm posterior to the coronary suture. ICP and cardiac output (CO) measurements were made on a Horizon 2000 (Mennen Medical, Rehovot, Israel) monitor.

Arterial blood gases were determined by ABL 300 and OSM Hemoximeter (Radiometer, Copenhagen, Denmark). Total static lung compliance (TSLC) and best-PEEP were measured with the Compli 80 System (Kontron, Milan, Italy). In this system, the pressure-volume curve was determined by using a stepwise inflation of the lungs (100 ml per step), starting at atmospheric pressure and continuing to a total volume of 10 ml/kg inflation. TSLC was computed as the ratio between the volume from the inflation limb of the pressure-volume and the corresponding pressure difference. Best-PEEP was computed as the minimal pressure at which the slope of the pressure-volume curve became linear. Internal PEEP [PEEPi = static PEEP (PEEPs) + auto-PEEP] of PRVCV modes were displayed by the ventilator by pressing the end-expiratory hold button. Centrifugal pump (Biomedicus, Minneapolis, U.S.A.) and membrane lungs (SciMed, Minneapolis, U.S.A.) were used for $ECCO_2R$. The membrane lungs were each ventilated with 10 L of humidified O_2.

After completing baseline measurements pigs were subjected to lung lavage; 50 ml/kg of warm saline solution was used to establish a model of ARDS. $PaO_2 < 100$ mm Hg at CM 2 was accepted as ARDS.

Randomly applied modes of ventilation were as follows:

CM 1: VCV with a preset PEEPs 4 cm H_2O, V_t 10-15 ml/kg, frequency (f) 12 breaths/min and I/E ratio 1:2 (25% I, 10% pause).

CM 2: Same as CM 1. After lung lavage.

Mode (M) 1: VCV with measured best-PEEP, V_t 10-15 ml/kg, f 12 breaths/min and I/E ratio 1:2 (25% I, 10% pause).

M 2: PRVCV with PEEPs 4 cm H_2O, PIP adjusted to get a V_t 10-15 ml/kg, f 12 breaths/min and I/E ratio 4:1 (80% I).

M 3: LFPPV with measured best-PEEP, V_t 5 ml/kg, f 5 breaths/min and I/E ratio 1:2 (25% I, 10% pause) 1-2 L/min O_2, given through a catheter (ID 1 mm), inserted through the tracheal tube and advanced to the level of the carina; $ECCO_2R$ with a pump speed of 20-30% of the CO measured during CM2 and two membrane lungs with a surface area of 3.5 m² each.

FiO_2 was 1 in all modes. Measurements were made 60 min after changing the ventilatory mode. The ventilation modes were adjusted to get similar $PaCO_2$ and PaO_2 above 350 mm Hg. ARDS was reconfirmed when switching from one mode to the other by CM. Lung lavage was repeated when PaO_2 was $\geq$ 100 mmHg. Pigs which became hemodynamically unstable at any time during the course of the study were excluded.

Data were compared among the groups by two way analysis of variance (ANOVA test). All data are expressed as mean ± SD. Student's t-test was used for pairwise comparison. Significance was considered at P < 0.01.

RESULTS

The arterial blood gas values as PaO_2 and $PaCO_2$ are shown in Figures 1 and 2. Higher PaO_2 values were obtained with the application of M3. $PaCO_2$ values were kept similar in all modes of both groups.

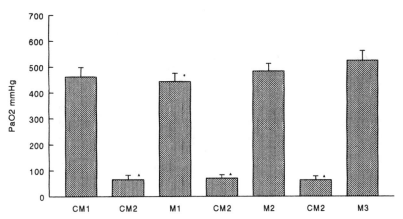

Figure 1. PaO_2 data of the trial modes. ▲ different from CM1, M1, M2 and M3; * different from M3.

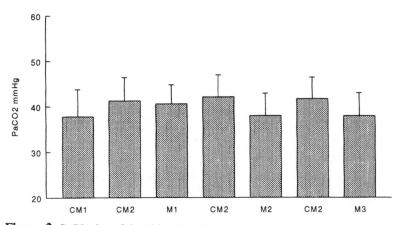

Figure 2. $PaCO_2$ data of the trial modes. No differences were found between the groups.

Changes in ICP and CO during the application of each mode along with the baseline measurements in both groups are shown in Figure 3. No significant change of ICP and CO was observed with the treatment modes compared to the control mode after lung lavage. No differences were observed between the effects of M1, M2 and M3 on ICP and CO in both groups.

Data on PEEPi and TSLC are depicted in Table 1. No difference was observed between the PEEPi levels in M1, M2 and M3. TSLC was decreased significantly after the application of lung lavage.

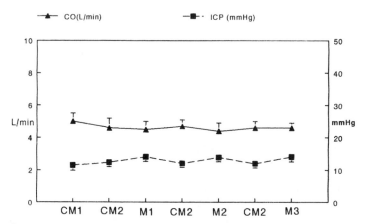

Figure 3. ICP and CO data of the trial models. No differences were found between the groups.

Table 1. TSLC and PEEPi values measured during the administration of trial modes of ventilation (mean ± SD)

	TSLC (ml/cm H_2O)	PEEPi (cm H_2O)
CM1	44.9±4.6[a]	4[b]
CM2	21.5±3.9[b]	4[b]
M1	33.1±2.6	12.9±1.7
CM2	22 ±3.4[b]	4[b]
M2	33 ±2.5	13.6±1.4
CM2	21.8±3.7[b]	4[b]
M3	35.1±2.1	14.3±1.3

TSLC= total static lung compliance; PEEPi= internal-PEEP; values shown in CM1, CM2, M1 and M3 are static-PEEP and in M2 is static-PEEP + auto-PEEP.
a= different from CM2,M1, M2 and M3
b= different from M1, M2 and M3

DISCUSSION

The aim of ventilatory therapy in ARDS is to provide oxygenation and opening of the recruitable alveoli. A critical pressure has to be applied to the alveoli in order to achieve these goals. A meticulous selection of ventilatory mode and pressures are essential to avoid complications such as barotrauma, hemodynamic depression or increased ICP[11]. On the other hand serious depression of circulation or increase in ICP should not be expected as long as the applied pressure is precisely adjusted to balance the surface tension and preventing its transmission to the vascular bed[12].

In this study best-PEEP measurements allowed us to apply the right amount of end expiratory pressure to provide adequate gas exchange and avoid an elevation of ICP.

The results of this study show that PRVCV and LFPPV-ECCO$_2$R yielded higher PaO$_2$ values compared to VCV with PEEP. Minimal changes in ICP and CO were observed after lung lavage suggesting the existence of a protective mechanism of the ARDS in this model. This protection was probably due to a significant decrease in TSLC due to the surfactant depletion caused by lung lavage.

PRVCV and LFPPV-ECCO$_2$R proved to be superior modes compared to VCV with PEEP since in addition to the lack of their negative effect on ICP and hemodynamics they provided better oxygenation, suggesting their safe use in ARDS patients with elevated ICP and deteriorated surfactant system.

ACKNOWLEGDMENTS

We thank Sharida Santoe for typing the manuscript and Laraine Visser-Isles for English language editing.

REFERENCES

1. D.D. Doblar, T.V. Santiago, A.U. Kahn, and N.H. Edelman, The effect of positive end-expiratory pressure ventilation (PEEP) on cerebral blood flow and cerebrospinal fluid pressure in goats, *Anesthesiology* 55:244-250 (1981).
2. K.J. Burchiel, T.D. Steege, and A.R. Wyler, Intracranial pressure change in brain-injured patients requiring positive end-expiratory pressure ventilation, *Neurosurgery* 8:443-449 (1981).
3. E.A.M. Frost, Effects of positive end-expiratory pressure of intracranial pressure and compliance in brain-injured patients, *J Neurosurg* 47:195-200 (1977).
4. J.M. Luce, J.S. Huseby, W. Kirk, and J. Butler. Mechanism by which positive end-expiratory pressure increased cerebrospinal fluid pressure in dogs, *J Appl Physiol* 52:231-235 (1982).
5. S.J. Aidinis, J. Lafferty, and H.M. Shapiro, Intracranial responses to PEEP, *Anesthesiology* 45:275-285 (1976).
6. M.L.J. Apuzzo, M.H. Weiss, V. Petersons, R. Baldwin Small, T. Kurze, and J.S. Heiden, Effect of positive end expiratory pressure ventilation on intracranial pressure in man, *J Neurosury* 46:277-232 (1976).
7. J.S. Huseby, E.G. Pavlin, and J. Butler, Effect of positive end-expiratory pressure on intracranial pressure in dogs, *J Appl Physiol* 44:25-27 (1978).
8. S. Lodrini, M. Montolivo, F. Pluchino, and V. Borroni, Positive end-expiratory

pressure in supine and sitting positions: Its effects on intrathoracic and intracranial pressures, *Neurosurgery* 24:873-877 (1989).

9. K.R. Cooper, P.A. Boswell, and S.C. Choi, Safe use of PEEP in patients with severe head injury, *J Neurosurg* 63:552-555 (1985).

10. J.M. Hurst, T.G. Saul, C.B. DeHaven, and R. Branson, Use of high frequency Jet ventilation during mechanical hyperventilation to reduce intracranial pressure in patients with multiple organ system injury, *Neurosurgery* 4:530-435 (1984).

11. B. Lachmann, E. Danzmann, B. Haendly, and B. Jonson, Ventilator settings and gas exchange in respiratory distress syndrome, *in*: Applied Physiology in Clinical Respiratory Care, O. Prakash, ed., Martinus Nijhoff Publishers, The Hague (1982).

12. B. Lachmann, B. Jonson, M. Lindroth, and B. Robertson, Modes of artificial ventilation in severe respiratory distress syndrome, *Critical Care Medicine* 10:724-732 (1982).

EFFECTS OF HYPERTONIC SALINE ON THE PULMONARY GAS EXCHANGE

L. Hannemann, W. Schaffartzik, A. Meier-Hellmann, K. Reinhart

Department of Anesthesiology and Surgical Intensive Care Medicine
Steglitz Medical Center, Free University of Berlin
Hindenburgdamm 30, D-1000 Berlin 45, Germany

INTRODUCTION

Hypertonic saline solution (HSS) increases cardiac output (Q_T) in animals as well as in patients with hypovolemic shock. It has been observed on several occasions that elevations of Q_T resulted in a concomitant increase of venous admixture (Q_{VA}/Q_T) and/or intrapulmonary shunt (Q_S/Q_T).[1,2,3] However, Constable et al.[4] showed in endotoxemic calves that HSS had no effect on Q_{VA}/Q_T despite an increase of Q_T. It was the purpose of this study to examine the effect of HSS on Q_{VA}/Q_T in humans with hyperdynamic septic shock.

MATERIAL AND METHODS

PATIENTS

Twenty-one patients with septic shock requiring ventilatory support and pulmonary artery catheterization were studied after having obtained informed consent and approval by our local ethic committee. All patients had clinical and laboratory parameters which fulfilled the widely accepted criteria of sepsis.[5] All patients were deeply anesthetized by continuous infusions of fentanyl (maximal dosage: 0.24 mg/hr) and dehydrobenzperidol (maximal dosage: 3.0 mg/hr). Mechanical ventilation was

Oxygen Transport to Tissue XV, Edited by P. Vaupel
et al., Plenum Press, New York, 1994

accomplished with a volume-cycled respirator (Siemens Servo 900 B) at tidal volumes of 12 to 15 ml per kilogram of body weight, an inspiratory/ expiratory ratio of 1:2, a positive end-expiratory pressure as clinically indicated (up to 12 cm H_2O), and a constant F_IO_2. These parameters were kept constant during the study period. All patients were studied within 24 to 36 hours after the diagnosis of septic shock was confirmed.

DETERMINATION OF HEMODYNAMIC AND OXYGEN TRANSPORT RELATED VARIABLES

In all patients, pulmonary and radial arterial catheters had been placed for hemodynamic monitoring (Swan-Ganz catheters: Edwards Laboratories LA, USA; transducers 5265 039: Viggo-Spectramed, Bilthoven, electronically derived means, with reference to the midaxillary line; cardiac output [thermodilution at temperatures between 6 and 12^0 C]: SAT II cardiac output computer, Edwards Laboratories LA, USA). Arterial pressure, pulmonary artery pressure, pulmonary capillary wedge pressure (PCWP), and Q_T were determined immediately before simultaneously withdrawl of arterial and mixed venous blood. The blood samples were used for measurement of the blood gas status, pH (ABL 2, Radiometer, Copenhagen), and hemoglobin concentration (Hemoximeter Osm 3, Radiometer, Copenhagen). Blood gases were corrected for blood temperature measured in the pulmonary artery. Oxygen concentration and venous admixture were calculated using the standard equation.

HEMODYNAMIC STABILIZATION

Prior to baseline measurements (BSL) patients were hemodynamically stabilized by adequate volume loading until there was no further increase in Q_T. All patients required additional inotropic support. If dobutamine in a dosage of up to 16 g kg^{-1} min^{-1} was insufficient to achieve a mean arterial blood pressure (MAP) about 70 mm Hg, norepinephrine was added, "titrated" as low as possible, to obtain the desired MAP.

Measurements were taken after the patients had been hemodynamically stable for at least 30 min. Patients with change in body temperature $> \pm 0.5^0$ C were withdrawn from the study. After baseline measurements 2-4 ml kg^{-1} body weight 7.5% NaCl (2400 mosmol/l) in 6% hydroxyethyl starch were infused within 15 min via a central venous line. Measurements including a hemodynamic profile with calculation of oxygen transport related variables were repeated immediately at the end of the infusion (0 min), and 30, 60, and 90 minutes thereafter.

Data are reported as means ± SEM. Comparisons between BSL and the subsequent measurements were done by Wilcoxon test and significance (*) was accepted at p < 0.05.

RESULTS

All patients received dobutamine (range 2.9 to 16.6 g kg^{-1} min^{-1}, mean 11.5 ± 3.8 g kg^{-1} min^{-1}), and twelve of them norepinephrine (0.10 to 1.40 g kg^{-1} min^{-1}, mean 0.76 ± 0.68 g kg^{-1} min^{-1}).

Q_T increased significantly by 35% (p<0.05) immediately after the infusion was completed, and PCWP by 64% (p<0.05). Arterial oxygen tension remained unchanged (0 min) and decreased by only 8% 30 min after the end of HSS infusion, whereas venous admixture increased 26% (p<0.05). The most marked changes in hemodynamics and O_2 transport were observed immediately at the end of the infusion (Table 1). Heart rate, systolic, mean, and diastolic arterial blood pressures remained unchanged. Results are summarized in table 1.

Table 1. Cardiac Output (Q_T), Venous Admixture (Q_{VA}/Q_T), Arterial Partial Pressure of O_2 (PaO_2), Mean Pulmonary Artery Pressure (PAPM) and Pulmonary Capillary Wedge Pressure (PCWP) before, at the end of HSS-Infusion and 30, 60 and 90 min thereafter.

	Before HSS BSL	After HSS 0 min	After HSS 30 min	After HSS 60 min	After HSS 90 min
Q_T [L/min]	7.8 ± 0.4	10.5 ± 0.5*	9.2 ± 0.4*	9.0 ± 0.5*	8.5 ± 0.4*
Q_{VA}/Q_T [%]	11.3 ± 1.7	14.2 ± 2.0*	13.2 ± 1.7*	12.8 ± 1.6*	12.6 ± 2.0*
PaO_2 [mm Hg]	126.8 ± 6.0	123.1 ± 6.0	113.2 ± 5.3*	119.0 ± 5.3	123.8 ± 5.3
PAPM [mm Hg]	29 ± 1	36 ± 1*	33 ± 1*	30 ± 1	30.9 ± 1.2*
PCWP [mm Hg]	14 ± 3	23 ± 1*	18 ± 1*	17 ± 1*	16 ± 1*

* = p < 0.05 compared with baseline measurement.

DISCUSSION

Q_T increased by about 35% and Q_{VA}/Q_T by about 25% after the infusion of HSS (0 min). This (Q_{VA}/Q_T)/Q_T- relationship can be seen whether Q_{VA}/Q_T or Q_S/Q_T are measured by classical methods based on arterial and mixed venous O_2

levels as in our study or by O_2-independent methods such as the multiple inert gas elimination technique.[1,3] Furthermore, this phenomenon can be seen regardless of whether Q_T is altered by pharmcological means such as HSS or mechanical means such as arteriovenous fistulas.[3]

Despite the increase of Q_{VA}/Q_T arterial (a) PO_2 did not change (0 min). It is possible that HSS improved the blood flow in the pulmonary capillaries. This hypothesis is supported by the observation of Rocha-e-Silva et al.[5] who reported an improvement of pulmonary microcirculation in patients with hemorrhagic shock treated with HSS. This improvement could have overcome the effect of increasing Q_T on the $(Q_{VA}/Q_T)/Q_T$- relationship resulting in a nearly unchanged PaO_2. Of course, we cannot discern from our data between candidate mechanisms, e.g. whether this was due to an improved homogeneity of the distribution of ventilation/ perfusion-ratios, changes in alveolar-capillary diffusion properties of O_2 or other mechanisms.

It is also possible that the fall of PaO_2 (30 minutes after the infusion was completed) was induced by an extravasation of fluid into the interstitial tissue with rising mean pulmonary artery pressure and PCWP. This could have led to a thickening of the blood gas barrier and could have interfered with O_2 diffusion as well as with the distribution of ventilation/ perfusion-ratios.

However, the underlying mechanisms of how rising cardiac output increases venous admixture or intrapulmonary shunt remains unclear and await further investigation.

REFERENCES

1. P.H. Breen, P.T. Schumacker, G. Hedenstierna, J. Ali, P.D. Wagner, L.D.H. Wood. How does increased cardiac output increase shunt in pulmonary edema? J Appl Physiol 53:1273-1280 (1982)

2. J.D. Michenfelder, W.S. Fowler, R.A. Theye. CO2 levels and pulmonary shunting in anesthetized man. J Appl Physiol 21:1471-1476 (1966)

3. P.D. Wagner, W. Schaffartzik, R. Prediletto, D.R. Knight. Relationship among cardiac output, shunt, and inspired O2 concentration. J Appl Physiol 71:2191-2197 (1991)

4. P.D. Constable, L.M. Schmall, W.W. Muir, G.F. Hoffsis. Respiratory, renal, hematologic, and serum biochemical effects of hypertonic saline solution in endotoxemic calves. Am J Vet Res 52:990-998 (1991)

5. R.C. Bone, C.J. Fisher, T.P. Clemmer, G.J. Slotman, C.A. Metz, R.A. Balk, J.N. Sheagren. A controlled clinical trial of high dose methylprednisolone in the treatment of severe sepsis and septic shock. N Engl J Med 317:653-58 (1987)

6. M. Rocha E Silva, E.A. Negraes, A.M. Soares, V. Pontieri, L. Loppnow. Hypertonic resuscitation from severe hemorrhagic shock; pattern of regional circulation. Circ Shock 19:165-175 (1986)

DIFFUSION AND PERFUSION LIMITATIONS IN PATIENTS SUFFERING FIBROSING LUNG DISEASE

H. Kobayashi, P. Scheid*, and T. Tomita

Department of Medicine, Kitasato University, Kanagawa 228
Japan
*Institut für Physiologie, Ruhr-Universität Bochum, 4630
Bochum, F.R.G.

INTRODUCTION

Using a simple alveolar model, Piiper and Scheid (1981, 1983) evaluated the limitations imposed by diffusion (Ldiff) and perfusion (Lperf). Their approach enabled one to quantitatively estimate the limitations in gas transport with respect to diffusion and perfusion, and has been applied to several aspects of gas transport (Piiper and Scheid, 1975).

The estimation of the limitations is of a particular interest for the patients with decreased pulmonary diffusing capacity, *e.g.*, fibrosing lung disease (FLD). Evaluation of alveolar gas transport using Ldiff and Lperf has not yet been applied to FLD patients at normoxia, since the original calculations done by Piiper and Scheid (1981, 1983) were based on a linear O_2 equilibrium curve (OEC). The assumption of a linear OEC in Ldiff and Lperf calculation is not applicable to the case of high metabolic rate or decreased diffusing capacity at normoxia (Kobayashi *et al.*, 1991).

Using a physiological OEC, we calculated the Ldiff and Lperf in patients with a diffusing capacity of about one-third normal and compared the results with the limitations in healthy subjects. We chose a simple homogeneous alveolar model to evaluate the specific effect of diffusion impairment on diffusional and perfusional oxygen transport, excluding the effect of regional functional inhomogeneity.

MODEL AND CALCULATIONS

A simple homogeneous lung model was used, consisting of an air space with constant alveolar P_{O_2}, P_A, of 100 Torr and capillary perfusion rate, $\dot{Q}$, separated by a barrier with diffusing capacity, D.

Limitation indicates a fractional increase of gas transfer that would occur if pulmonary conductance (diffusing capacity for Ldiff, and perfusion rate for Lperf) was raised to infinite values (fig. 1). We used an alinear OEC (Kelman, 1966), Pa_{CO_2} being at 40 Torr, pH at 7.40, body temperature at 37 °C, O_2 capacity of blood at 9 mmol/L.

Ldiff and Lperf were calculated according to eqs. (7) and (8) of Kobayashi *et al.* (1991), as

$$Ldiff = (C_A - Ca)/(C_A - C\bar{v}) \tag{1}$$

$$Lperf = 1-(\dot{Q}/D) \cdot (Ca-C\bar{v})/(P_A-P\bar{v}) \tag{2},$$

where C_A is the oxygen concentration of blood in equilibrium with alveolar gas; Ca: oxygen concentration of arterial blood; $C\bar{v}$: oxygen concentration of mixed venous blood. Alveolar oxygen partial pressure, P_A, was fixed at 100 Torr as a normoxic condition.

Given a set of P_A (=100 Torr), $\dot{M}/\dot{Q}$ (=Ca-$C\bar{v}$), and $D/\dot{Q}$, and applying the alinear OEC, the arterial and venous blood composition (Pa, Ca, $P\bar{v}$, and $C\bar{v}$) can be calculated (Kobayshi *et al.*, 1991), and Ldiff and Lperf were obtained according to eqs. (1) and (2). Ldiff and Lperf were thus calculated for ranges of the ratios $\dot{M}/\dot{Q}$ (0.5 to 5,0 mmol·L^{-1}) and $D/\dot{Q}$ (0.05 to 0.5 mmol·Torr^{-1}·L^{-1}).

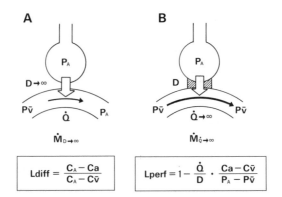

Figure 1. A:Diffusion limitation. Under the maximal oxygen transport rate with infinite diffusing capacity, $Pa = P_A$. $\dot{M}max$ and Ldiff can thus be calculated. B:Perfusion limitation. Under the maximal oxygen transport rate with infinite perfusion rate, $Pa = P\bar{v}$. $\dot{M}max$ and Lperf can thus be calculated.

The assumed values were (Table 1): for healthy subjects at rest, $\dot{M}$ = 10 mmol·min^{-1}, D = 1.5 mmol·Torr^{-1}·min^{-1}, and $\dot{Q}$ = 5 L·min^{-1}, while on 60 Watt exercise, $\dot{M}$ = 30 mmol·min^{-1}, D = 2.0 mmol·Torr^{-1}·min^{-1}, and $\dot{Q}$ = 10 L·min^{-1}. For FLD patients at rest $\dot{M}$ = 10 mmol·min^{-1}, D = 0.5 mmol·Torr^{-1}·min^{-1}, and $\dot{Q}$ = 5 L·min^{-1}, while on 60 Watt exercise $\dot{M}$ = 40 mmol·min^{-1}, D = 0.5 mmol·Torr^{-1}·min^{-1}, and $\dot{Q}$ = 10 L·min^{-1} based on the report by Hughes *et al.* (1991).

Table 1. Data set in this study. $\dot{M}$:oxygen consumption rate, $\dot{Q}$: perfusion rate, D: diffusing capacity.

		Healthy subjects		Patients with FLD	
		at rest	on exercise	at rest	on exercise
$\dot{M}$	$mmol \cdot min^{-1}$	10	30	10	40
D	$mmol \cdot Torr^{-1} \cdot min^{-1}$	1.5	2.0	0.5	0.5
$\dot{Q}$	$L \cdot min^{-1}$	5	10	5	10
$\dot{M}/\dot{Q}$	$mmol \cdot L^{-1}$	2.0	3.0	2.0	4.0
$D/\dot{Q}$	$mmol \cdot Torr^{-1} \cdot L^{-1}$	0.3	0.2	0.1	0.05

Ldiff and Lperf were also obtained with respect to $D/(\dot{Q}ß)$, where ß is the capacitance coefficient for oxygen in the blood, *i.e.*,

$$ß = (Ca - C\bar{v})/(Pa - P\bar{v}) \tag{3}.$$

RESULTS OF CALCULATIONS

Fig.2 shows the dependence of Ldiff on $D/\dot{Q}$ and $\dot{M}/\dot{Q}$ at a fixed P_A of 100 Torr.

Ldiff became significant only in the case with a lower $D/\dot{Q}$ (less than 0.05 $mmol \cdot Torr^{-1} \cdot min^{-1}$) and a higher $\dot{M}/\dot{Q}$ (more than 2.5 mmol/L). In healthy subjects, Ldiff was close to zero both at rest and during mild exercise. In the FLD patients, Ldiff was close to zero at rest, but rose to 0.50 during mild exercise (table 2).

Fig.3 shows the dependence of Lperf on $D/\dot{Q}$ and $\dot{M}/\dot{Q}$ at a fixed P_A of 100 Torr.

Lperf decreased gradually as $D/\dot{Q}$ decreased, but was rather insensitive to $\dot{M}/\dot{Q}$ changes. In healthy subjects, Lperf was 0.89 at rest, and was decreased to 0.77 on exercise, Lperf being larger than Ldiff both at rest and on exercise. In the FLD patients, Lperf was 0.66 at rest and was decreased to 0.10 on the 60 Watt exercise, Ldiff being larger than Lperf on exercise (table 2).

Table 2. Ldiff and Lperf in healthy subjects and FLD patients at rest and on exercise.

	Healthy subjects		Patients with FLD	
	at rest	on exercise	at rest	on exercise
Ldiff	0.00	0.00	0.00	0.50
Lperf	0.89	0.77	0.66	0.10

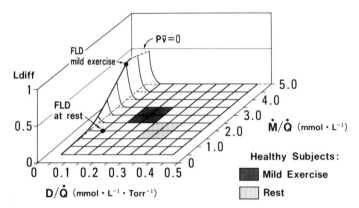

Figure 2. Diffusion limitation with respect to D/Q̇ and Ṁ/Q̇. The limitation values for the healthy subjects at rest and on mild (60 Watt) exercise are shown in the middle of the dotted and shaded area (normal ranges). The limitation is calculated where Pv̄ is larger than 0.

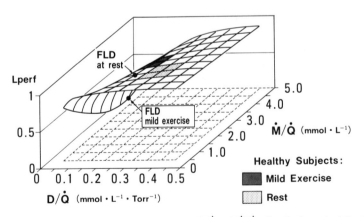

Figure 3. Perfusion limitation with respect to D/Q̇ and Ṁ/Q̇. See the legend of fig. 2.

Fig. 4 also shows Ldiff and Lperf vs. $D/(\dot{Q}ß)$. Since Ldiff and Lperf values at any given $D/(\dot{Q}ß)$ was only slightly dependent on $\dot{M}/\dot{Q}$, Ldiff and Lperf were shown on the same curve with a $\dot{M}/\dot{Q}$ of 2 mmol·L^{-1}. Ldiff and Lperf based on a linear OEC are also shown. Lperf with the alinear OEC was similar to Lperf with the linear OEC, but Ldiff with the alinear OEC was smaller than the Ldiff with the linear OEC at a given $D/(\dot{Q}ß)$. At a lower $D/(\dot{Q}ß)$, there exist turns both for Ldiff and Lperf curves and thus exist two values for a given $D/(\dot{Q}ß)$. The turn occurs when $P\bar{v}$ is about 10 Torr, and the curves start when $P\bar{v} = 0$. The Limitation curves between the starting point and the turn do not, therefore, exist physiologically.

In the healthy subjects, Ldiff remained zero on exercise, Lperf decreasing slightly. In the FLD patients, Ldiff increased considerably to 0.50 on exercise, while Lperf decreased down to 0.10.

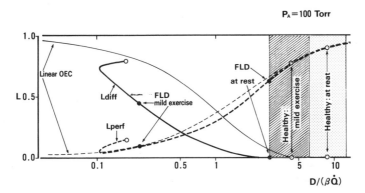

Figure 4. Ldiff and Lperf with respect to $D/(\dot{Q}ß)$. Ldiff with the alinear OEC deviates down from the Ldiff with the linear OEC, while Lperf is only slightly different from each other. On 60 Watt exercise in the FLD patients, Lperf decreased and Ldiff increased considerably.

DISCUSSION

Critique of Methods

In this study we neglected the finite reaction velocity between oxygen and hemoglobin, changes in pH and P_{CO_2} in the blood during the passage through the pulmonary circulation, and functional heterogeneity with shunt in the lungs. We rather used a simple alveolar model, excluding other factors which might influence the oxygen transport in the lungs. This approach enabled us to investigate the specific effect of diffusion impairment on alveolar gas transport with respect to diffusion and perfusion, excluding other factors.

The heterogeneity with shunt in the lungs, should further deteriorate the oxygen transport in real lungs of FLD patients (Wagner *et al.*, 1976; Jernudd-Wilhelmsson *et al.*, 1986; Hempleman and Hughes, 1991; Yamaguchi *et al.*, 1992).

Limitations in Gas Transport in the Healthy Subjects and the FLD Patients

In healthy subjects, Ldiff was close to zero both at rest and on mild exercise of 60 Watt. The amount of the diffusional oxygen transport in the lung can thus be considered to be almost the same as in the case with the lung having infinite diffusing capacity. The diffusing capacity is thus large enough for the oxygen transport in healthy subjects, and the perfusion is the predominant limiting factor for oxygen transport. This has also been shown by others (see Kobayashi *et al.*, 1991).

It can be intuitively understood that, since arterial blood is almost fully saturated both at rest and on exercise, cardiac output is the determinant factor to carry oxygen to the tissue in healthy subjects.

In the FLD patients with reduced diffusing capacity, Ldiff was still zero at rest. The cardiac output was thus the determinant factor, and has been reported to be kept at the value of healthy subjects (Hughes *et al.*, 1991) in spite of the increased resistance of pulmonary vessels. In a case with heterogeneous lungs, the Pa value and thus Ca would be lower, and the perfusion rate would be more important for the oxygen transport to the tissue.

During 60 Watt exercise, Ldiff became the predominant factor and Lperf decreased accordingly. The perfusion rate can be considered to be high enough for oxygen transport, and any further increase in the cardiac output would not contribute much to the oxygen transport to the tissue. The infinite cardiac output would add only 10% increase in oxygen transport.

The arterial hypoxemia reflects a decreased diffusing capacity (fig. 1A) and/or a higher perfusion rate (fig. 1B). Arterial hypoxemia induced by diffusion impairment reduces the oxygen transport to the tissue, but the arterial hypoxemia induced by a higher perfusion rate would not necessarily result in a decreased oxygen transport. To evaluate the oxygen transport, particularly the convective oxygen transport, to the tissue, it is apparent that, not only the Pa or Ca, but also the perfusion rate should be taken into account.

It should be noted that eq. (1) is the same formula as the physiological shunt equation. In the real lung, diffusion limitation is not separable from physiological shunt. Eqs. (1) and (2) should not be applied to the real lungs with heterogeneity and shunt without reservations.

CONCLUSION

In healthy subjects, diffusion limitation is negligible both at rest and during 60 Watt exercise, perfusion being the major factor that limits alveolar O_2 uptake. In patients with FLD, diffusion likewise does not limit O_2 uptake at rest. During exercise, however, diffusion becomes the main limiting factor, while perfusion is less important. Thus, for patients suffering FLD increasing pulmonary perfusion is not expected to substantially improve alveolar O_2 uptake.

References

Agusti, A.G.N., Roca, J., Rodriguez-Roisin, R., Gea, J., Xaubet, A., and Wagner, P.P., 1987, Role of O_2 diffusion limitation in idiopathic pulmonary fibrosis, *Am. Rev. Repir. Dis.*, 135: A307.

Hempleman, S.C., and Hughes, J.M.B., 1991, Estimating exercise DL_{O2} and diffusion limitation in patients with interstitial fibrosis, *Respir. Physiol.*, 83: 167-178.

Hughes, J.M.B., Lockwood, D.N.A., Jones, H.A., and Clark, R.J., 1991, $DL_{CO}/\dot{Q}$ and diffusion limitation at rest and on exercise in patients with interstitial fibrosis, *Respir. physiol.*, 83, 155-166.

Jernudd-Wilhelmsson, Y., Hörnblad, Y., and Hedenstierna, G., 1986, Ventilation-perfusion relationships in interstitial lung disease, *Eur. J. Respir. Dis.*, 68:39-49.

Kelman, G.R., 1966, Digital computer subroutine for the conversion of oxygen tension into saturation, *J. Appl. Physiol.*, 21:1375-1376.

Kobayashi, H., Pelster, B., Piiper, J., and Scheid.,P., 1991, Diffusion and perfusion limitation in alveolar O_2 exchange: shape of the blood O_2 equilibrium curve, *Respir. Physiol.*, 83:23-34.

Piiper, J., and Scheid, P., 1975, Gas transport efficacy of gills, lungs and skin: theory and experimental data. *Respir. Physiol.*, 23:209-221.

Piiper, J., and Scheid, P., 1981, Model for capillary-alveolar equilibration with special reference to O_2 uptake in hypoxia, *Respir. Physiol.*, 46:193-208.

Piiper, J., and Scheid, P., 1983, Comparison of diffusion and perfusion limitations in alveolar gas exchange, *Respir. Physiol.*, 51:287-290.

Wagner, P.D., Dantzker, D.R., Dereck, R., de Polo, J.L., Wasserman, K., and West, J., 1976, Distribution of ventilation-perfusion ratios in patients with interstitial lung disease, *Chest*, 69, Suppl. 2:256.

Yamaguchi,K.,Kawai,A.,Mori,M.,Asano,K.,Takasugi,T.,Umeda,A.,Kawashiro,T.,and Yokoyama,T., 1991, Distribution of ventilation and of diffusing capacity to perfusion in the lung, *Respir. Physiol.*, 86:171-187.

REGULATION OF BLOOD FLOW IN PULMONARY MICROCIRCULATION BY VASOACTIVE ARACHIDONIC ACID METABOLITES - ANALYSIS IN ACUTE LUNG INJURY

Kazuhiro Yamaguchi, Masaaki Mori, Akira Kawai, Koichiro Asano, Tomoaki Takasugi, Akira Umeda, Takeo Kawashiro and Tetsuro Yokoyama

Department of Medicine, School of Medicine, Keio University Tokyo 160, Japan

INTRODUCTION

In order to assess the physiological abnormalities and the pathogenesis of adult respiratory distress syndrome (ARDS), especially that associated with pulmonary fat embolism, acute lung injury caused by monounsaturated nonsterified fat oleic acid (cis-9-octadecenoic acid) has been widely used in animal experiments. This lung injury results in an extensive, multifocal, and heterogeneously distributed lung damage with alveolar flooding, interstitial edema and microatelectasis. The ability to reduce the perfusion entering into damaged and edematous areas is essentially important in preserving blood oxygenation in ARDS.

In normal lungs, hypoxic pulmonary vasoconstriction (HPV) has been commonly accepted as the essential factor to govern the distribution of pulmonary perfusion and to serve for maintaining gas exchange, as pulmonary blood flow from hypoxic region is directed to better oxygenated areas of the lung (Fishman, 1976). If HPV is deteriorated at hypoxic regions, gas exchange efficiency would be lowered because of a relative increase in blood flow to the hypoxic areas.

Eicosanoids have been implicated as mediators of a variety of afflictions to the lungs. Cyclooxygenase and lipoxygenase products of arachidonic acid appear in high concentrations in lung lymph and blood after infusion of either oleic acid or endotoxin (Olanoff et al., 1984; Ball et al., 1989; Chang et al., 1989). These arachidonic acid metabolites, which are vasoactive and expected to be elaborated mainly in injured areas, may modulate HPV.

The present study was undertaken to test the hypothesis that HPV would be significantly altered especially in diseased areas of acute lung injury induced by administrating oleic acid. Additionally, possible roles of locally accumulating vasoactive arachidonate metabolites in modifying the vascular reactivity to hypoxic spell were also examined.

Oxygen Transport to Tissue XV, Edited by P. Vaupel
et al., Plenum Press, New York, 1994

MATERIALS AND METHODS

Fifty mongrel dogs of either sex weighing 10-15 kg were anesthetized with a slow injection of pentobarbital sodium (25 mg/kg), placed in a supine position and had their trachea intubated. Ventilation was maintained with a tidal volume of 10-15 ml/kg without positive end-expiratory pressure. Respiratory rate was adjusted to maintain arterial PCO_2 ($PaCO_2$) between 30 and 40 Torr, and diaphragmatic paralysis was secured with pancuronium bromide (4 mg iv, repeated as necessary). The temperature of the animal at the aortic arch was kept at 37-38°C with a thermostatically regulated heating pad. A 5-Fr catheter with thermistor and conductivity electrodes in close proximity (HE-2900, Electro-Catheter Corp., Rahway, NJ) was passed through the femoral artery to the arch of the aorta, and was used to quantitate the extravascular lung water (ETVI) in terms of a standard double-indicator-dilution technique (Nobel and Severinghaus, 1972). A 7-Fr double-lumen Swan-Ganz catheter was placed just inside the main pulmonary artery to measure cardiac output (Q_T) and pulmonary arterial pressures. Q_T was obtained by the method of thermodilution injecting 5 ml of 3% saline kept at zero degree. This injectate simultaneously allowed us to estimate the amount of ETVI using heat as a diffusible indicator and sodium ion as a nondiffusible indicator, respectively (Nobel and Severinghaus, 1972). The validity of ETVI determined with the double-indicator-dilution technique was confirmed by comparing it with the value obtained from the direct method proposed by Pearce et al. (1965). ETVI was expressed in an unit of ml/kg (body weight). Minute ventilation and respiratory frequency were monitored by means of a pneumotachograph of Fleisch with a differential pressure transducer. PO_2, PCO_2 and pH in blood samples were analyzed with electrodes.

The animal was given an injection of oleic acid at a dose of 0.08 ml/kg into the femoral vein. Since a quasi steady state concerning hemodynamics and arterial blood gases was established nearly 90 min after oleic acid injection, necessary measurements were performed between 90 and 180 min after the administration of oleic acid.

To examine the fractional blood flow entering into the damaged areas of the lung, exceedingly low soluble gas, sulfur hexafluoride (SF_6), dissolved in a normal saline was intravenously infused at a constant rate for at least 30 min. After a steady state was attained, the samples of both arterial and mixed venous blood were simultaneously taken and the expired gas was collected. The concentrations of SF_6 in the samples were measured with a gas chromatograph (model 163, Hitachi Ltd., Tokyo) equipped with an electron capture detector. Blood-gas partition coefficient for SF_6 was determined for each animal by applying the extraction method of Wagner et al. (1974). After correcting for experimental error, retention (R) of SF_6, defined as a quotient between the partial pressure of the indicator gas in arterial blood and that in mixed venous blood (Wagner et al., 1974), was calculated. In theory, R value is indicative of fractional shunt flow (Q_S/Q_T) which is mainly caused by the blood flow passing through the injured areas with alveolar flooding and collapse (Yamaguchi, et al., 1991).

After the stable lung injury was achieved, i.e. 90 min following oleic acid injection, base-line values of Q_S/Q_T and ETVI were measured while allowing the animal to breathe the gas mixture containing O_2 concentration (FIO_2) at 0.21. Thereafter, observations were repeated 40 min after either change of FIO_2 from 0.21 to 0.6 or administration of the following agents. (1) normal saline, (2) indomethacin (5 mg/kg); a noble cyclooxygenase inhibitor, (3) OKY-046 (100 µg/kg/min); thromboxane A_2 (TXA_2) synthase inhibitor, (4) sysnthetic prostacyclin (PGI_2: 0.1 µg/kg/min), (5) AA-861 (30 µg/kg/min; 5-lipoxygenase inhibitor, and (6) synthetic leukotriene D_4 (LTD_4: 10 ng/kg/min). The efficacy and selectivity of the agents as described above were confirmed by measuring the arterial concentrations of thromboxane B_2 (TXB_2), 6-keto-prostaglandin F1a (PGF) and leukotriene B_4 (LTB_4) by radioimmunoassay. Since sulfidopeptide leukotrienes (LTs) have been known to act as important stimuli for cyclooxygenase metabolism (Coggeshall et al., 1988), the experiments focused on elucidating the effects of LTs on Q_S/Q_T and ETVI, i.e. either AA-861 or LTD_4 infusion, were performed simultaneously inhibiting cyclooxygenase by indomethacin, thus allowing us to judge simple effects of LTs on pulmonary microcirculation in injured lungs.

RESULTS

Administration of oleic acid caused a noticeable hypoxemia with a significant increase in pulmonary vascular resistance (PVR), Q_S/Q_T and ETVI, accompanied by a considerable accumulation of TXB_2, PGF and LTB_4 in the arterial blood.

Hyperoxic gas breathing (FIO_2: 0.6) significantly decreased PVR, Q_S/Q_T and hourly gain of ETVI as compared with those obtained during normoxic gas breathing (FIO_2: 0.21). Alteration of FIO_2 from 0.21 to 0.6 increased mixed venous PO_2 (PvO_2) from 33 to 45 Torr without any change of Q_T.

Administration of indomethacin decreased the arterial concentration of TXB_2 and PGF but did not change that of LTB_4. The pressor response in the pulmonary circulation after indomethacin infusion was markedly augmented, i.e. PVR increased by 50% with little change of Q_T. Indomethacin produced a significant reduction of both Q_S/Q_T and hourly gain of ETVI as compared to those obtained from the injured animals treated with normal saline in place of indomethacin infusion (control group) (Figures 1 and 2).

Inhibition of TXA_2 synthesis by OKY-046 yielded a sufficient decline in TXB_2 but an obvious increase of PGF in the arterial blood, resulting in no significant change of Q_T and PVR but leading to an augmentation of Q_S/Q_T (Figure 1). Although hourly gain of ETVI obtained under a condition of OKY-046 administration was inclined to increase as compared with that of control group, there was no statistical difference between them (Figure 2).

Synthetic PGI_2 infusion decreased PVR without any change of Q_T and enhanced Q_S/Q_T (Figure 1). Hourly gain of ETVI during PGI_2 infusion was not significantly different from that of control group (Figure 2).

AA-861 successfully suppressed the leukotriene biosynthesis but did not yield any significant change of both Q_T and PVR. AA-861, however, augmented Q_S/Q_T (Figure 1). Hourly gain of ETVI estimated during AA-861 administration was much larger than that observed for the animals treated with indomethacin (Figure 2).

LTD_4 infusion in injured animals pretreated with indomethacin enhanced PVR without any alteration of Q_T. Although LTD_4 administration appreciably diminished Q_S/Q_T, hourly gain of ETVI was found to increase

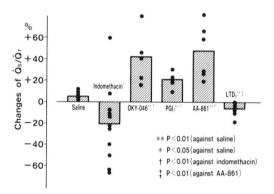

Figure 1. Changes of shunt flow by various agents in oleic-acid-lung injury (see text for further details).

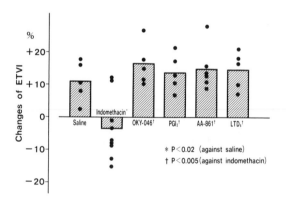

Figure 2. Changes of ETVI by various agents in oleic-acid-lung injury (see text for explanation).

considerably as compared to that obtained for the animals treated with indomethacin alone (Figures 1 and 2).

DISCUSSION

Pulmonary fat embolism is a frequent clinical complication following major trauma, particularly that involving long-bone fracture (Sherr et al., 1974). This often causes ARDS within 24-72 hours after traumatic event (Sherr et al., 1974). Fat emboli appear to consist largely of triglycerates, which is hydrolyzed to fatty acids by pulmonary lipases (Sherr et al., 1974). Experimental study (Sherr et al., 1974) showed that oleic acid comprised about 50% of the total fatty acids present in pulmonary emboli subjected to long-bone trauma, indicating that oleic acid might be one of the major substances to induce ARDS associated with pulmonary fat embolism. Thus, the model of lung injury produced by injection of oleic acid may be useful to study the pathophysiological abnormalities accompanied with ARDS induced by fat emboli.

Intravenous administration of oleic acid causes a leakage of protein-rich fluid into the interstitium and alveoli. The injury is multifocal and tends to favor peripheral sites while sparing normal parenchyma. Pulmonary edema may be the result of oleic-acid-induced free radicals assaulting the microvascular endothelium, because the increased permeability can be attenuated by antioxidant pretreatment (Townsley et al., 1985).

The distribution of pulmonary blood flow is predominantly determined by the resistance of arterioles, which is regulated by the local vascular tone sensitive to alveolar and mixed venous O_2 tension (Fishman 1976). In normal lungs, hypoxic and hyperoxic regions elicit vasoconstriction (HPV) and vasodilation, respectively, shifting the blood flow from hypoxic areas to better oxygenated areas, thus maintaining gas exchange efficiency as a whole. If tissue damage distorts HPV, vascular beds in hypoxic areas fail to be contracted, leading to a relative increase of perfusion in injured and edematous areas of the lung. This causes the augmentation of Q_S/Q_T and worsens the gas exchange efficiency.

When animals were ventilated with a hyperoxic gas mixture (FIO_2: 0.6), lungs damaged by oleic acid yielded a significant increase of PvO_2 followed by a decrease in PVR, Q_S/Q_T and ETVI without an appreciable change in Q_T. If the vascular reactivity to O_2 is preserved at any area in diseased lungs, relative change of microvascular diameter induced by varying PO_2 should be potentially greater in the hypoxic areas, i.e. in the injured areas. If so, hyperoxic gas breathing which increases alveolar PO_2 at any region in the lung as well as mixed venous PO_2 should dilate microvessels in injured regions more effectively, thus shifting the blood flow from relatively normal to injured regions. This is sharply contrary to the observed experimental results, indicating that vascular reactivity to O_2 in injured areas is likely to be distinctly impaired. These results also indicate that, at a higher FIO_2, there appears to be a nonuniform reduction in the vascular tone of pulmonary microvessels and a sizable shift in perfusion from diseased areas to those preserved from tissue damage, leading to a considerable diminution in Q_S/Q_T, which may reduce the amount of accumulation of extravascular lung water in injured areas.

Several authors (Olanoff et al., 1984; Ball et al., 1989) have reported that considerable increase of thromboxane, prostaglandins as well as leukotrienes is seen both in bronchoalveolar lavage fluid and in plasma after oleic acid injection, the trend being qualitatively similar to the results obtained in the present study. The products derived from arachidonic acid are potent mediators either constricting or dilating smooth muscles of airway tracts and of vascular trees (Coggeshall et al., 1988). Among them, PGI_2, one of the cyclooxygenase products, is a noble vasodilator and its local accumulation may cope with the vasoconstriction initiated by hypoxia in injured areas of the lung treated with oleic acid (Schulman et al., 1988; Yamaguchi et al., 1991), thus yielding a paralysis of vascular response to O_2. Abolition of PGI_2 biosynthesis by the administration of indomethacin caused a significant increase of PVR with a concomitant decline in both Q_S/Q_T and hourly gain of ETVI (Figures 1 and 2). The findings may support the idea that reduction of vasodilator prostaglandins such as PGI_2 restores local hypoxic pressor response and diminishes blood flow to the injured areas, resulting in reducing the rate of edema formation. The importance of PGI_2 attenuating responsiveness of the pulmonary microvessels to O_2 was also confirmed by OKY-046 administration which augmented the production of PGI_2 as measured by PGF in the blood and by synthetic PGI_2 infusion, both of which significantly increased Q_S/Q_T and tended to worsen the edema formation (Figures 1 and 2).

Restraint on cyclooxygenase pathway also attenuates the production of TXA_2, which is accepted as one of the important mediators for alterations in lung mechanics such as resistance to airflow in injured lungs (Coggeshall et al., 1988). Moreover, TXA_2 is known as the mediator acting mainly to constrict postcapillary venules in the pulmonary microcirculation (Kadowitz and Hyman, 1984) and thus reduces blood flow into injured areas but increases edema formation (Yoshimura et al., 1989; Hellewell et al., 1991). Therefore, if TXA_2 is important in regulating blood flow in lungs damaged by oleic acid, inhibition of TXA_2 generation by either indomethacin or OKY-046 should enhance Q_S/Q_T but diminish ETVI. This is highly inconsistent with the experimental results obtained from indomethacin or OKY-046 administration, indicating that TXA_2 is not essential factor for modulation of pulmonary blood flow in the diseased microcirculation at least in oleic-acid-lung injury (Figures 1 and 2).

Although Inhibition of cyclooxygenase activity has been reported to divert arachidonic acid into the lipoxygenase pathway (Morris et al., 1980), the present study failed to show such an effect as far as genesis of LTB_4 was considered.

Importance of sulfidopeptide LTs such as LTC_4, D_4, E_4 was assessed either by inhibiting 5-lipoxygenase with AA-861 or by administrating LTD_4. LTs have been reported to constrict the precapillary arterioles and the postcapillary venules, both of which are attributed in part to the secondary generation of TXA_2 from the pulmonary vascular tissue (Ohtaka et al., 1987). To avoid the possible effects mediated by TXA_2 in a series of experiments on AA-861 and LTD_4 infusion, the animal was pretreated with indomethacin, thus allowing us to know simple effects of LTs on pulmonary microvasculature. AA-861 caused the increase of Q_S/Q_T and worsened the edema formation, while LTD_4 infusion reduced Q_S/Q_T significantly but enhanced the edema formation (Figures 1 and 2). These findings may indicate that LTs per se restore the pressure response to O_2 of the arterioles and reduce the blood flow into the injured areas but they augment the edema formation either by constricting the postcapillary venules or by increasing permeability.

In conclusion, local regulation of blood flow by vasoconstriction and vasodilation responding to O_2 is considerably attenuated in the injured areas induced by oleic acid administration, leading to the augmented edema formation. This is mainly caused by the local accumulation of vasodilator prostaglandin, PGI_2. Vasoconstrictive leukotrienes effectively copes with the vasodilator effects of PGI_2 and diminishes blood flow entering into injured area but does not reduce the edema formation. On the other hand, TXA_2 seems to be of minor importance for modulating blood flow and edema formation at least in acute lung injury induced by oleic acid.

REFERENCES

Ball, H.A., Cook, J.A., Spicer, K.M., Wise, W.C., and Halushka, P.V., 1989, Essential fatty acid-deficient rats are resistant to oleic acid-induced pulmonary injury, J. Appl. Physiol., 67:811-816.

Chang, S., Westcott, J.Y., Pickett, W.C., Murphy, R.C., and Volkel, N.F., 1989, Endotoxin-induced lung injury in rats: role of eicosanoids, J. Appl. Physiol., 66:2407-2418.

Coggeshall, J.W., Christman, B.W., Lefferts, P.L., Serafin, W.E., Blair, I.A., Butterfield, M.J., and Snapper, J.R., 1988, Effects of inhibition of 5-lipoxygenase metabolism of arachidonic acid on response to endotoxemia in sheep, J. Appl. Physiol., 65:1351-1359.

Fishman, A.P., 1976, Hypoxia and pulmonary circulation, Cir. Res., 38:221-231.

Hellewell, P.G., Henson, P.T., Downey, G.R., and Worthen, S., 1991, Control of local blood flow in pulmonary inflammation: role for neutrophils, PAF, and thromboxane, J. Appl. Physiol., 70:1184-1193.

Kadowitz, P.J., and Hyman, A.L., 1984, Analysis of responses of leukotriene D_4 in the pulmonary vascular bed, Cir. Res., 55:707-717.

Morris, H.R., Piper, P.J., Taylor, G.W., and Tippins, J.R., 1980, The role of arachidonate lipoxygenase in the release of SRS-A from guinea pig chopped lung, Prostaglandins 19:371-383.

Nobel, W.H., and Severinghaus, J.W., 1972, Thermal and conductivity dilution curves for rapid quantitation of pulmonary edema, J. Appl. Physiol., 32:770-775.

Ohtaka, H., Tsang, J.Y., Foster, A., Hogg, J.C., and Schellenberg, R.R., 1987, Comparative effects of leukotrienes on porcine pulmonary circulation in vitro and in vivo, J. Appl. Physiol., 63:582-588.

Olanoff, L.S., Reines, H.D., Spicer, K.M., and Halushka, P.V., 1984, Effects of oleic acid on pulmonary capillary leak and thromboxanes, J. Surg. Res., 36:597-605.

Pearce, M.L., Yamashita, J., Beazell, J., 1965, Measurement of pulmonary edema, Cir. Res., 16:482-488.

Sherr, S., Montemurno, R., and Raffer, P., 1974, Lipids of recovered pulmonary fat emboli following trauma, J. Trauma, 14:242-246.

Schulman, L.L., Lennon, P.F., Ratner, S.J., and Enson, Y., 1988, Meclofenamate enhances blood oxygenation in acute oleic acid lung injury, J. Appl. Physiol., 64:710-718.

Tounsley, M.I., Taylor, G.E., Korthuis, R.J., and Taylor, A.E., 1985, Promethazine or DPPD pretreatment attenuates oleic acid-induced injury in isolated canine lungs, J. Appl. Physiol., 59:39-46.

Wagner, P.D., Saltzmann, H.A., and West, J.B., 1974, Measurement of continuous distributions of ventilation-perfusion ratios: theory, J. Appl. Physiol., 36:588-599.

Yamaguchi, K., Mori, M., Kawai, A., Asano, K., Takasugi, T., Umeda, A., and Yokoyama, T., 1991, Impairment of gas exchange in acute lung injury, Jap. J. Thorac. Dis. 29:134-144.

Yoshimura, K., Tod, M., Pier, K.G., and Rubin, L.J., 1989, Role of venoconstriction in thromboxane-induced pulmonary hypertension and edema in lambs, J. Appl. Physiol., 66:929-935.

PULMONARY VAGAL AFFERENTS VERSUS CENTRAL CHEMOSENSITIVITY IN THE VENTILATORY RESPONSE TO HYPOXIA AND LACTIC ACIDOSIS

H. Kalhoff[2], H. Kiwull-Schöne[1], and P. Kiwull[1]

[1]Department of Physiology, Ruhr-University
 D-4630 Bochum, Germany
[2]Pediatric Clinic, D-4600 Dortmund, Germany

INTRODUCTION

After peripheral chemodenervation, hypoxia is generally expected to cause ventilatory depression, but also tachypnea has been observed[1]. The latter response appeared to depend on the integrity of the vagus nerves[2]. Furthermore, according to the "Reaction Theory"[3], hypoxia-induced systemic lactic acidosis should increase pulmonary ventilation via central chemosensitivity, provided the extracellular fluid (ECF) pH in the brainstem is thereby reduced. However, hypoxia-induced systemic lactic acidosis failed to stimulate ventilation in peripherally chemodenervated cats in spite of a pronounced fall in ECF-pH[4].

Disfunction of central chemosensitive control together with impaired or immature peripheral afferent input could help to explain the prolonged apnoeic periods in prematures and small infants[5], thereby probably increasing the risk for "sudden infant death syndrome" (SIDS). In the present animal-model, the carotid chemoreflexes were eliminated and reversible differential cold-blockade of the vagus nerves was performed to quantify the minor role of central chemosensitivity and the functional significance of myelinated pulmonary vagal afferents in ventilatory control during hypoxia and post-hypoxic adaptation.

METHODS

The experiments were performed in 10 spontaneously breathing rabbits weighing 3.0 ±0.2 kg, anaesthetized by an initial dose of 56.0 ±2.1 mg/kg pentobarbital sodium i.v., followed by continuous infusion of 9.2 ±0.4 mg/kg/h. The tracheotomized animals were usually breathing oxygen-enriched air from an open system. The carotid sinus nerves were cut. Both cervical vagus nerves were exposed for a distance of 10-12 cm along the neck and were put without tensile load on thermodes through which alcohol of selected alternating temperatures between 38° and 0°C was circulated[6].

Oxygen Transport to Tissue XV, Edited by P. Vaupel
et al., Plenum Press, New York, 1994

The animals underwent alternating 5 min-periods of either severe hypoxia (mean $PaO_2=3.9 \pm 0.08$ kPa) or normoxia (mean $PaO_2=13.5 \pm 0.3$ kPa). The vagus nerves were left intact or cold-blocked either completely to 0-2°C or partially to 6-8°C, in the latter range of nerve temperature myelinated fibre conductivity being selectively impaired[6, 7, 8]. Each vagal blockade was followed by a control period with intact vagus nerves. Tidal volume (V_T) and inspiratory/expiratory durations (T_I, T_E) were continuously measured by pneumotachography to calculate total cycle duration ($T_T = T_I + T_E$) and minute ventilation ($\dot{V} = 60 \cdot V_T/T_T$). Gas partial pressures (PaO_2, $PaCO_2$), standard bicarbonate concentration ($HCO_3^- st$) and pH (pHa) were determined from arterial blood samples. Differences of group means $\pm SEM$ were regarded as being significant for $P_D \leq 0.05$ (paired t-test).

RESULTS

Effects of repeated Hypoxic Periods on Pulmonary Ventilation, arterial PCO_2 and pH

During the course of the experiments (Fig. 1), repeated periods of hypoxia caused a progressive metabolic acidosis, with a reduction of $HCO_3^- st$ from 20.6 ± 1.1 to 14.3 ± 1.1 mM and a fall in pHa by up to 0.170 units. This considerable overall decrease in pHa during the course of experiments was entirely due to metabolic acidosis, since the

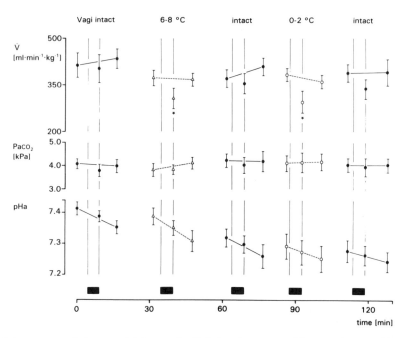

Fig. 1 Pulmonary ventilation, arterial PCO_2 and pH during the course of the experiments with repeated periods of hypoxia (black bars). The vagus nerves were reversibly cold-blocked either partially (6-8°) or completely (0-2°C). Mean values $\pm SEM$ in 8 carotid chemodenervated rabbits. No overall ventilatory reaction to progressive metabolic acidosis, hypoxic depression only during vagal blockade.
* Significant difference compared to normoxic control before hypoxia, $P_D \leq 0.05$ (paired t-test)

PaCO$_2$ did not change significantly (from 4.08 $\pm$0.21 to 4.04 $\pm$0.31 kPa). Likewise, comparing start and end of experiments each under normoxic control conditions, there were significant changes neither in pulmonary ventilation (from 413.7 $\pm$38.8 to 391.8 $\pm$41.5 ml·min^{-1}·kg^{-1}) nor in tidal volume (from 7.8 $\pm$0.7 to 7.4 $\pm$0.7 ml·kg^{-1}), hence respiratory control being rather independent of the progressively developing metabolic acidosis throughout about 2 hours. However, ventilatory reactions both during hypoxia and normoxic recovery were significantly modified by pulmonary vagal afferents.

Contribution of Pulmonary Vagal Afferents to Pulmonary Ventilation and Breathing Pattern during Hypoxia and Post-hypoxic Adaptation

In order to separate possible influences of pulmonary vagal afferents and systemic time-dependent effects, ventilatory variables, blood-gases and acid-base data were averaged for the repeated intermittent periods with intact vagus nerves and compared to those during partial or total vagal blockade (Table 1, Figs. 2 and 3).

During the periods of hypoxia, a significant ventilatory depression did only occur when the vagus nerves were either blocked completely or when at least the myelinated afferent fibre portion was selectively blocked (Table 1). Analysis of the volume- and time-pattern of breathing (Fig. 2) showed that this ventilatory depression during hypoxia was

Table 1. Respiratory data and arterial acid-base status under different conditions of oxygenation and vagal afferent input

Variable	Vagi intact			Vagi 6-8 °C			Vagi 0-2°C		
FIO$_2$	0.27	0.07	0.27	0.27	0.07	0.27	0.27	0.07	0.27
$\dot{V}$ [ml·kg^{-1}·min^{-1}]	392.0 $\pm$18.4	367.2 $\pm$21.8	412.8* $\pm$19.0	372.8 $\pm$24.9	307.2* $\pm$32.5	367.6 $\pm$20.7	383.9 $\pm$20.9	296.8* $\pm$35.0	361.7* $\pm$22.1
VT [ml·kg^{-1}]	7.7 $\pm$0.4	7.0* $\pm$0.3	7.8 $\pm$0.4	9.2 $\pm$0.9	8.5 $\pm$0.7	9.8* $\pm$1.0	9.7 $\pm$1.0	8.8 $\pm$0.7	8.9 $\pm$0.7
TI [s]	0.46 $\pm$0.02	0.42* $\pm$0.02	0.45 $\pm$0.01	0.60 $\pm$0.03	0.58 $\pm$0.03	0.61 $\pm$0.03	0.59 $\pm$0.03	0.56 $\pm$0.03	0.57 $\pm$0.02
TE [s]	0.74 $\pm$0.03	0.82 $\pm$0.07	0.71 $\pm$0.03	0.89 $\pm$0.08	1.22* $\pm$0.16	0.99* $\pm$0.10	0.92 $\pm$0.08	1.33* $\pm$0.16	0.90 $\pm$0.07
PaO$_2$ [kPa]	14.30 $\pm$0.61	3.88* $\pm$0.10	12.95* $\pm$0.49	14.40 $\pm$0.93	3.79* $\pm$0.38	12.25* $\pm$0.85	14.09 $\pm$0.97	3.84* $\pm$0.20	12.36* $\pm$0.81
PaCO$_2$ [kPa]	4.13 $\pm$0.15	3.93* $\pm$0.19	4.08 $\pm$ 0.19	3.81 $\pm$0.29	3.83 $\pm$0.21	4.12 $\pm$0.25	4.12 $\pm$0.35	4.15 $\pm$0.42	4.18 $\pm$0.35
HCO$_3^-$st [mM]	17.9 $\pm$0.8	15.6* $\pm$0.6	15.8* $\pm$0.6	18.8 $\pm$1.0	16.6* $\pm$0.9	16.6* $\pm$1.1	16.1 $\pm$1.2	14.4* $\pm$0.9	14.8* $\pm$1.2
pHa	7.334 $\pm$0.019	7.316* $\pm$0.018	7.287* $\pm$0.020	7.387 $\pm$0.027	7.350* $\pm$0.024	7.308* $\pm$0.034	7.292 $\pm$0.040	7.273 $\pm$0.039	7.252* $\pm$0.042

Volume- and time components of pulmonary ventilation (N=10), blood-gases and acid-base values (N=8) under steady state conditions before hypoxia, at the end of 5 min hypoxia and after 5 min of post-hypoxic recovery. Means $\pm$SEM in carotid chemodenervated rabbits, with either intact or cold-blocked vagus nerves.

* Significant difference compared to normoxic control before hypoxia, P$_D$$\leq$0.05 (paired t-test)

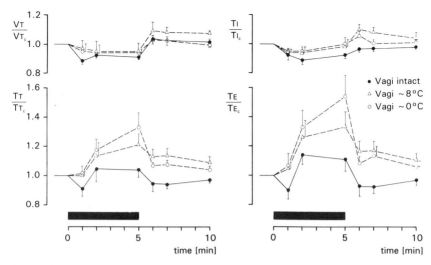

Fig. 2 Volume- and time components of pulmonary ventilation during hypoxia (black bars) and post-hypoxic recovery. Means ±SEM of relative changes against normoxic control in 10 carotid chemo-denervated rabbits. Contribution of pulmonary vagal afferents.

caused by respiratory frequency rather than by tidal volume. The pronounced prolongation of respiratory cycle duration was mainly caused by rises in T_E up to 33.7 ±10.1% or 54.0 ±14.3% during partial and total vagal blockade, respectively ($P_D \leq 0.01$). With intact vagus nerves, the small but significant reduction of V_T was not worsened by respiratory frequency, there being significant rises in neither T_T nor T_E.

During the post-hypoxic recovery periods, a transient rise in ventilatory drive (up to 13.3 ±5.7% in the first minute, $P_D \leq 0.05$) could only be discerned when the pulmonary vagal reflexes were left intact. This drive was due to both rise in mean inspiratory flow (V_T/T_I) up to 6.7 ±2.8% and shift of the breathing pattern (T_I/T_E) in favour of inspiration by up to 12.2 ±5.7%, as calculated from the primary data of Fig. 2.

Analysis of Ventilatory Reactions to Hypoxia-induced Metabolic Acidosis compared to CO_2-induced Respiratory Acidosis

In order to analyze the ventilatory reactions to hypoxia-induced metabolic lact-acidosis, pulmonary ventilation under post-hypoxic normoxic conditions was compared to pre-hypoxic control, and the resulting changes in $\dot{V}$ were plotted against changes in pHa (Fig. 3). With intact pulmonary vagal afferents, there was a transient rise in ventilation above the control level with a maximum after one minute of normoxic recovery following hypoxia. After five minutes, $\dot{V}$ was only increased by about 22 ml· min⁻¹·kg⁻¹ in spite of a pHa decrease of about 0.06 units, corresponding to less than 10% of the ventilatory sensitivity to the same change in pHa following CO_2-inhalation (previous data, unpublished). Moreover, this relatively small and transient ventilatory drive was entirely dependent on the integrity of myelinated vagal afferent fibres. Their influence became even more pronounced, when isocapnic conditions were considered by correcting the small concomitant deviations in Pa_{CO_2} (Fig. 3, right-hand diagram). With both partially and completely abolished pulmonary vagal reflexes, ventilation in response to post-hypoxic metabolic acidosis was rather diminished than enhanced, thus bearing a striking contrast to respiratory acidosis under the same conditions.

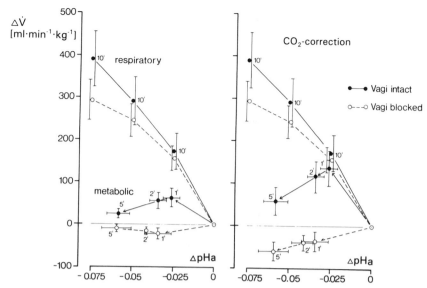

Fig. 3 Ventilatory responses to changes in arterial pH due to hypoxia-induced metabolic acidosis compared to CO_2-induced respiratory acidosis and contribution of pulmonary vagal afferents.

Metabolic acidosis: Means $\pm$SEM of absolute post-hypoxic changes against pre-hypoxic control in 10 carotid chemodenervated rabbits with either intact or cold-blocked (to 8° or 0°C) vagus nerves.

Small changes in $PaCO_2$ caused by $\Delta\dot{V}$ were corrected to isocapnic contol conditions (right-hand diagram)

Respiratory acidosis: Means $\pm$SEM of ventilatory responses to CO_2-inhalation taken from previous measurements in carotid chemodenervated rabbits with either intact (N=12) or cut (N=11) vagus nerves.

DISCUSSION

The two main findings presented here are (1) the complete insignificance of an even pronounced metabolic acidosis as central ventilatory chemoreflex drive and (2) the significant role of pulmonary vagal afferents for control of breathing during hypoxia and post-hypoxic adaptation.

In discrepancy to the unique function between brainstem ECF-pH and ventilation postulated by Loeschcke[3], a complete lack of ventilatory reaction to hypoxia-induced brainstem lactic acidosis has also been observed in cats[4, 9, 10], although the sensitivity of ventilation against CO_2-induced changes in ECF-pH remained invariably high[4, 10]. Therefore, brainstem ECF-pH as the adequate stimulus for central chemoreception was tentatively replaced by the intra/extracellular H^+-gradient[4, 9], which would explain the central hypoxic ventilatory depression and lack of post-hypoxic ventilatory drive by intracellular lactic acid accumulation[11]. However, the H^+-gradient hypothesis cannot explain the likewise small or even lacking respiratory effects of exogenous metabolic brainstem acidosis due to acid infusion described in cats[12, 13, 14] and rabbits[10], respectively. Thus, at the moment, there is no unifying theory to explain the striking differences in central chemosensitivity to metabolic versus respiratory acidosis.

Inferentially for the present experiments, endogenous lactic acidosis cannot be expected to sustain a ventilatory drive during hypoxia or post-hypoxic adaptation in peripherally chemodenervated animals. The small and transient post-hypoxic respiratory drive observed with intact vagus nerves may be attributed to a CO_2-release by the Haldane effect on switching from hypoxia to normoxia (Table 1) rather than to metabolic acidosis. Interestingly, this "respiratory drive" can only be discerned, when myelinated pulmonary vagal afferent input is intact to prevent any ventilatory depression during the foregoing hypoxic period.

In general, the ventilatory response to systemic hypoxia in peripherally chemo-denervated rabbits, apparently lacking any additional central chemosensitive drive by concomitant metabolic acidosis, is still controversial. In earlier experiments, we were able to observe both, tachypnea and ventilatory depression, depending on whether the vagus nerves were left intact or cold-blocked[2, 8]. Tachypneic hyperventilation is thereby funda-mentally different from chemoreflexogenic drive generation in terms of mean inspiratory flow rate (VT/TI). Accordingly, the present results have shown that there was no rise in VT/TI during hypoxia. This lack of a "true" chemoreflex drive in rabbits with cut carotid sinus nerves but intact vagus nerves does support earlier notions in the literature that in this species aortic chemoreflexes neither mediated by the vagus nerves nor by the depressor nerves are of any functional importance[15].

More detailed experiments in rabbits have shown that cooling the vagus nerves to temperatures of 6-8°C selectively blocked myelinated fibres' conductivity, leaving C-fibres still active to a considerable extent, whereas nerve-cooling to 0-2°C completely blocked any fibre activity[6,7,8]. Since in the present study, effects of partial and total vagal blockade on breathing pattern were statistically indistinguishable, the most probable candidates of pulmonary vagal afferents to prevent the central hypoxic depression and to sustain the small transient ventilatory drive during post-hypoxic adaptation seem to be among the myelinated fibre portion.

A-fibre afferents from slowly adapting pulmonary stretch receptors (SARs) are known to to mediate the Hering-Breuer inflation reflex (HBIR) switching off inspiration and promoting expiration, thereby decreasing the TI/TE-ratio. B-fibre afferents from rapidly adapting receptors (RARs) were assumed to sustain the pulmonary deflation reflex by promoting inspiration and shortening expiration, thereby increasing the TI/TE-ratio[6, 8].

Although A- and B-fibre activity cannot be separated completely by differential vagal cooling[6, 8], the functional significance of the vagus nerves during systemic hypoxia most likely refers to the lung deflation reflex or myelinated B-fibre afferents. In fact, during moderate hypoxia, tachypneic hyperventilation was accompanied by a considerable shift of the central respiratory rhythm towards inspiration[8]. Thereby the predominant inhibition of inspiratory neurons by both the HBIR and systemic hypoxia was effectively counteracted. Due to more severe hypoxia in the present study, the characteristic type of breathing pattern with an increased TI/TE-ratio and concomitant hyperventilation did persist but for one minute. However, the overall balance in favour of inspiration pre-vented ventilatory depression at least throughout the entire hypoxic period.

Recent data in the literature support the presented view that vagal myelinated fibres are important for hypoxic breathing and post-hypoxic recovery. As nerve myelination is not yet completed at birth, maturation of respiratory responses to hypoxia in new-born rabbits has been reported, whereby, interestingly, the threshold for the HBIR was lower in younger animals[16]. This points to a lack of the counteracting deflation reflex and thus to a possible immaturity of pulmonary vagal B-fibres. Moreover, in newborn guinea pigs, there was direct evidence for a functional immaturity of these vagal afferent fibres normally mediating histamine-induced bronchoconstrictions[17]. Likewise, a decreased number of small myelinated fibres in the vagus nerve in SIDS victims compared with age-matched controls has been found[18]. These reports and the present data suggest, that maturation of myelinated vagal afferents plays an important role in the respiratory defence reactions during and after periods of hypoxic apnea in situations with insufficient periph-eral and central chemoreflex function.

Acknowledgement

We would like to thank Ms S. Adler and Ms C. Bräuer for their excellent help with the drawings and the fotographs.

REFERENCES

1. M.J. Miller and S.M. Tenney, Hypoxia-induced tachypnea in carotid deafferented cats, *Respir. Physiol.* 23:31 (1975)
2. H. Kiwull-Schöne and P. Kiwull, The role of the vagus nerves in the ventilatory response to lowered PaO$_2$ with intact and eliminated carotid chemoreflexes, *Pflügers Arch.* 381:1 (1979)
3. H.H. Loeschcke, Central chemosensitivity and the reaction theory, *J. Physiol.(Lond.)* 322:1 (1982)
4. H. Kiwull-Schöne and P. Kiwull, Hypoxic modulation of central chemosensitivity, in:"Central Neurone Environment and the Control Systems of Breathing and Circulation", M.E. Schläfke, H.P. Koepchen, and W.R. See, eds., Springer, Berlin-Heidelberg-New York (1983)
5. D.P. Southall, Role of apnea in the sudden infant death syndrome: a personal view, *Pediatrics* 81: 73-84 (1988)
6. H. Kalhoff, Die Bedeutung pulmonaler Afferenzen im N. vagus für die Atmung nach Ausschaltung der peripheren Chemoreflexe, Thesis, Faculty of Medicine, Ruhr-University Bochum (1988)
7. H. Kalhoff, H. Kiwull-Schöne und P. Kiwull, Leitungscharakteristik pulmonaler Afferenzen des N. vagus bei differentieller Kälteblockade, *Atemw.-Lungenkrkh.* 13:368 (1987)
8. H. Kalhoff, H. Kiwull-Schöne, and P. Kiwull, Pulmonary vagal afferents involved in the hypoxic breathing without arterial chemoreflexes, in: "Arterial Chemoreception", C. Eyzaguirre, S.J. Fidone, R.S. Fitzgerald, S. Lahiri, and D.M. McDonald, eds., Springer, New York (1990)
9. F.D. Xu, M.J. Spellman Jr., M. Sato, J.E. Baumgartner, S.F. Ciricillo, and J.W. Severinghaus,Anomalous hypoxic acidification of medullary ventral surface, *J. Appl. Physiol.* 71:2211 (1991)
10. H. Kiwull-Schöne and P. Kiwull, Hypoxia and the "reaction theory" of central respiratory chemosensitivity, in: "Oxygen Transport to Tissue XIII", M. McCabe, D. Maguire and T.K. Goldstick, eds., Plenum Press, New York (1992)
11. J.A. Neubauer, A. Simone, and N.H. Edelman, Role of brain lactic acidosis in hypoxic depression of respiration, *J. Appl. Physiol.* 65:1324 (1988)
12. F.L. Eldridge, J.P. Kiley, and D.E. Millhorn, Respiratory responses to medullary hydrogen ion changes in cats: Different effects of respiratory and metabolic acidoses, *J. Physiol. (Lond.)* 358:285 (1985)
13. H. Shams, Differential effects of CO$_2$ and H$^+$ as central stimuli of respiration in the cat, *J. Appl. Physiol.* 58:357 (1985)
14. L.J. Teppema, P.W.J.A. Barts, H.Th. Folgering, and J.A.M. Evers, Effects of respiratory and (isocapnic) metabolic arterial acid-base disturbances on medullary extracellular fluid pH and ventilation in cats, *Respir. Physiol.* 53:379 (1983)
15. B.E. Gernandt, A study of the respiratory reflexes elicited from the aortic and carotid bodies, *Acta Physiol. Scand.* 11, Suppl.35:1 (1946)
16. K.M. Wangsnes and B.J. Koos, Maturation of respiratory responses to graded hypoxia in rabbits, *Biol. Neonate* 59:219 (1991)
17. C. Clerici, A.Harf, C. Gaultier, and F. Roudot, Cholinergic component of histamine-induced bronchoconstriction in newborn guinea pigs, *J. Appl. Physiol.* 66:2145 (1989)
18. P.N. Sachis, D.L. Armstrong, L.E. Becker, and A.Ch. Bryan, The vagus nerve and sudden infant death syndrome: A morphometric study, *J. Pediatrics* 98:278 (1981)

MICROVASCULAR PO$_2$ REGULATION AND CHEMORECEPTION

IN THE CAT CAROTID BODY

S. Lahiri, D. F. Wilson*, R. Iturriaga and W. L. Rumsey[#]

Departments of Physiology, and Biochemistry and Biophysics*
University of Pennsylvania School of Medicine, Philadelphia
PA 19104 and Bristol-Myers Squibb Pharmaceutical Institute[#]
New Brunswick, NJ 08903, USA.

INTRODUCTION

Regulation of carotid body microcirculation and microvascular PO$_2$ is in itself of great physiological interest, and understanding their roles in the integrated cellular and sensory functions is critical. Now that a sensitive optical method, based on quenching of phosphorescence of lumiphors is available (Vanderkooi et al., 1987; Wilson et al., 1988), we investigated the effects of arterial PCO$_2$ and PO$_2$ changes on the cat carotid body microvascular PO$_2$ (CBM PO$_2$) simultaneously with the chemosensory activity <u>in vivo</u>. The working hypothesis was that PCO$_2$-pH changes do not change CBM PO$_2$ but affects the sensory discharge directly.

METHODS

Cats of either sex were anesthetized with sodium pentobarbitone (30-40 mg/kg, initially) and carotid bodies were exposed. The carotid sinus nerve and other nerve supplies to the carotid body areas were cut. A few chemosensory afferents were isolated and their activities were recorded as described previously (Lahiri and Delaney), 1975). The cats were paralyzed and artificially ventilated through a tracheal canula. The femoral arteries were cannulated for blood pressure and blood sampling and a vein to administer drugs and saline. The inspired gas was made continuously from the gas tanks of compressed air, O$_2$, N$_2$ and CO$_2$, and was adjusted to obtain the desired end-tidal PO$_2$ and PCO$_2$ which were continuously monitored with the Beckman analyzers.

Quenching of phorescence of the probe, Pd complex of tetra-(4-carboxyphenyl) porphine (20 mg/kg, bound to serum albumin in solution), by oxygen was the basis

Oxygen Transport to Tissue XV, Edited by P. Vaupel
et al., Plenum Press, New York, 1994

of microvascular PO_2 measurement. The illuminating light for the epifluorescence attachment was a 45 watt Xenon lamp with flash duration less than 5 μsec. The delay time after the flash was 20, 40, 80, 160, 300, 600 and 2,500 μsec. The images were taken with Xybion intensified CCD camera. The mean excitation wavelength was 537 nm and emission 630 nm. The image was magnified with a Wild Makroscope, placed 5-7 cm above the carotid body. The images were digitized and processed with a computer and recorded with a video recorder. A data analysis software system (Pawlowski and Wilson, licensed to Medical Systems Corporation) was used to calculate phosphorescence lifetime for each pixel location of the image. For details of the methods, see Rumsey et al. (1988) and Wilson et al. (1988).

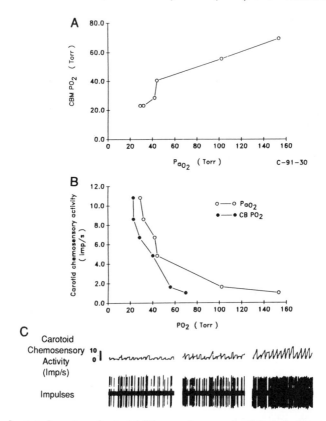

Fig. 1. Steady-state lowering of arterial PO_2 on microvascular PO_2 and chemosensory discharge of cat carotid body in vivo. A. CBM PO_2 fell as PaO_2 was lowered, the fall being greater at PaO_2 lower than 60 Torr, paralleling PaO_2 more closely. B. Chemosensory discharge in relation to PO_2. The response became steeper as the fall of PaO_2 reduced the CBM PO_2 below 50 Torr. Thereafter, the arterial-CBM PO_2 gradient was about 10 Torr, and the sensory response was increasinly intense. Thus, there was a CBM PO_2 threshold of about 50 Torr to the chemosensory response. C. Carotid chemosensory impulses at 3 levels of PO_2.

RESULTS

The oxygen pressure images of the carotid body did not show any significant heterogeneity. Neither was there any spontaneous shift of the relative oxygen pressures in the carotid body from one part to another at any PaO_2, such as would occur if there were local alterations in blood flow.

Effects of lowering arterial PO$_2$ on CBM PO$_2$. Fig. 1 shows an example of the effects of steady state levels of arterial PO$_2$ on CBM PO$_2$ and carotid chemosensory discharge. CBM PO$_2$ fell linearly from about 72 Torr to 40 Torr as PaO$_2$ was lowered from 155 Torr to about 50 Torr, and thereafter fell more steeply (Fig. 1A). Thus, in the high range of arterial PO$_2$, the oxygen pressure difference between arterial and CBM PO$_2$ was large but this narrowed in the lower range of arterial PO$_2$, - a result consistent with the shape of the O$_2$ equilibrium curve of blood assuming the tissues were extracting the same amount of O$_2$ for a smaller arterio-venous O$_2$ difference.

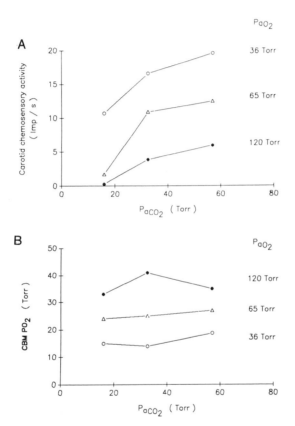

Fig. 2. Effects of steady state hypocapnia and hypercapnia on carotid chemosensory activity (A) and microvascular PO$_2$ (B). A. Increasing PaCO$_2$ increased carotid chemosensory activities at any PaO$_2$, and decreasing PaO$_2$ further stimulated the activity, the effect being greater at higher PaCO$_2$. B. PaCO$_2$ changes did not alter CB (microvascular) PO$_2$ at any PaO$_2$. Decreasing PaO$_2$ however decreased the microvascular PO$_2$.

Effects of arterial PCO$_2$ and pH on CBM PO$_2$. Fig. 2 shows an example of the responses of the carotid chemosensory discharge and CBM PO$_2$ to steady-state hypocapnia and hypercapnia. The sensory discharge increased with the increasing PaCO$_2$ at a constant PaO$_2$, and the effects of CO$_2$ -H$^+$ was augmented by hypoxia. However, the CBM PO$_2$ at a given PaO$_2$ did not change with the changes of PaCO$_2$; lowering of PaO$_2$ reduced CBM PO$_2$, as seen in Fig. 1.

DISCUSSION

At normal PaO_2 of 100 Torr, CBM PO_2 was about 50 Torr. With further lowering of PaO_2, CBM PO_2 decreased more sharply, narrowing the arterial-CBM PO_2 difference. The constitutive chemosensory discharge rate increased sharply at about CBM PO_2 of 50 Torr. Arterial PCO_2 changes at a constant PaO_2 did not show any significant effect on CBM PO_2.

The cellular PO_2 would have to be lower than CBM PO_2. Thus, the CBM PO_2 in the cat carotid body in vivo, measured by the new optical method is more consistent with the values reported by Acker and his colleagues (see Acker, 1989 for review) than those by Whalen and Nair (1983). Whalen and Nair (1983) reported a relatively high CB tissue PO_2 particularly during normoxia. Their data suggested that oxygen extraction per unit volume of blood flow was small, either due to high tissue blood flow or to low O_2 consumption, or a combination of both. Our present CBM PO_2 data indicated a significant amount of O_2 extraction which could still be compatible with a high tissue blood flow and a relatively large O_2 consumption. Carotid body is particularly well known for its extensive microvasculature (DeCastro and Rubio, 1968), and microsphere (9-15 μm) studies recorded high tissue blood flow (Barnett et al., 1988). Unfortunately, the rate of O_2 consumption by the carotid body is still a controversial issue (see Acker, 1989). Our microvascular PO_2 data clearly indicated a substantial O_2 extraction, and a lowering of tissue PO_2 with hypoxia in the range which could influence the metabolic state (Wilson et al., 1988). This is consistent with the hypothesis that O_2 chemoreception in the carotid body is mediated, at least in part, by a shift in the metabolic energy production (Anichkov and Belenkii, 1963; Mulligan et al., 1981). A decrease in the energy state could change ATPase dependent ion balance and Ca^{2+} mobilization which, in turn, activate neurotransmitter release and increase the sensory discharge.

Using three types of metabolic inhibitors (antimycin A, for electron transport, FCCP, as protonophore and dissipation of energy, and oligomycin for blockade of ATP synthesis) we previously showed (Mulligan et al. 1981) that O_2 chemoreception can be blocked specifically without attenuating CO_2 chemosensory response, evidence supporting the metabolic hypothesis of O_2 chemoreception. Biscoe and Duchen (1990) and Duchen and Biscoe (1992 a,b) made parallel findings in the glomus cell responses with respect to intracellular Ca^{2+} and mitochondrial membrane potential. However, Gonzalez and colleagues (Obeso et al, 1989) opposed the metabolic hypothesis on the ground that dinitrophenol, an uncoupler of oxidative phosphorylation, did not decrease carotid body ATP concentration but caused release of dopamine. There are several problems with this line of reasoning: [ATP] alone particularly measured in the whole carotid body may be insensitive to changes in the chemoreceptor cells. Also, the phosphate potential [ATP]/[ATP]/[P_I] must be decreased by a large amount to decrease the [ATP] (Wilson et al., 1979). As for DNP effect, one must note that it is a weak acid that can increase intracellular acidity; it is a protonophore which drives equilibrates [H^+] across the plasma membrane; and it uncouples oxidative phosphorylation, raising O_2 consumption and heat production and decreasing phosphate potential. Thus, intracellular acidification could have produced the most effect.

Gonzalez prefers the view that hypoxia depolarizes glomus cells, permitting Ca^{2+} entry and neurotransmitter release (1992). But it is not clear whether the glomus cells are indeed depolarized by hypoxia. Biscoe and his colleagues believe that hypoxia hyperpolarizes glomus cell membrane (Biscoe and Duchen, 1990) but depolarizes its mitochondrial membrane (Duchen and Biscoe 1992a,b. Calcium appears to be involved in chemosensory activity but there remains a considerable uncertainty about its role. In the hands of Duchen and Biscoe (1992b) and Sato et al. (1991) hypoxia consistently resulted in $[Ca^{2+}]_i$ increase whereas Donnelly and Kholwadwala (1992) reported that hypoxia resulted in a decrease in $[Ca^{2+}]_i$. Most studies have indicated that extracellular Ca^{2+} concentration is important but it may not be critical under all conditions (Delpiano and Acker 1989; Shirahata and Fitzgerald, 1991; Iturriage et al., 1992a). Thus, it is premature to discuss further how Ca^{2+} mobilization is linked to hypoxia.

On the basis of their observations that chromaffin cells, unlike glomus, manifested autofluorescence and $[Ca^{2+}]_i$ responses only to very low PO_2, below 5 Torr, Duchen and Biscoe (1992a,b) shared the view of Mills and Jobsis (1972) that a specialized cytochrome oxidase with low affinity for oxygen acted as the O_2 receptor. Metabolic inhibitors, however, would not make a distinction between the two cytochrome oxidase, and it is not clear how Duchen and Biscoe (1992a,b) made the distinction. However, a distinction can be made by using CO, the affinity of which for the heme pigments is likely to vary because of their differential affinity for O_2. Recently, we used CO to test the hypothesis that not just cytochrome oxidase but also other heme pigment(s) may be involved in the initiation of O_2 chemoreception (unpublished observations). We confirmed the brief report that high PCO stimulates carotid chemosensory discharge and that this stimulation is reversed by light (Joels and Neil, 1962). We anticipate that action spectra studies will unambiguously identify photosensitive CO compound involved in O_2 chemoreception (sensory discharge, neurotransmitter release, Ca^{2+} mobilization, etc.). Our preliminary measurements of the photochemical action spectrum indicates that the major component is the mitochonrdrial cytochrome c oxidase. Convergence of metabolism, and membrane initiated responses are an essential part of the metabolic hypothesis of chemoreception. In several instances, ATP generated by metabolism controls membrane events (e.g., Miller, 1990) and in others, for example in taste receptor cells, membrane receptors (Kinnamon and Cummings, 1992) initiate the cellular responses.

Alterations in $PaCO_2$ -H^+ changed the chemosensory discharge without changing the CBM PO_2. Furthermore, the sensory response showed PCO_2 -PO_2 stimulus interaction (e.g., Lahiri and Delany, 1975) without any similar interaction in the CBM PO_2. Accordingly, the effect of CO_2 -H^+ was not mediated through CBM PO_2, even though the Bohr effect of CO_2 -H^+ significantly changed O_2 content of the arterial blood. This lack of effect of O_2 content is consistent with the effects of moderate anemia and carboxyhemoglobinemia and hypotension (see Lahiri et al, 1983, for review) at a given arterial PO_2. The observation that the hypoxic chemoreception is not mediated by intracellular acidosis (Iturriaga et al., 1992) is relevatnt in the context.

It is primarily PO_2 which determined CBM PO_2. The lack of PCO_2 -pH effect on CBM PO_2 despite its effect on the chemosensory discharge (hence oxygen utilization) and on O_2 transport, indicated that CB microcirculation was not regulated by CO_2 -H^+. Thus, measurements of microvascular PO_2 in vivo have provided an important tool for the study of microcirculation of the carotid body and resolved the issue of its tissue PO_2, as it relates to the metabolic mechanisms of O_2 chemoreception.

ACKNOWLEDGEMENTS

We owe thanks to Anil Mokashi for his help with the experiments and to Suzanne Hyndman for her secretarial assistance. The work was supported by the grant HL-43413.

REFERENCES

Acker, H., 1989, PO_2 Chemoreception in arterial chemoreceptors, <u>Annu. Review Physiol.</u> 51:835-844.

Anichkov, S. V., and Belinkii, M. L., 1963, Pharmacology of the Carotid Body Chemoreceptors, Pergamon Press, New York.

Barnett, S., Mulligan, E., Wagerle, L., C., and Lahiri, S., 1988, Measurement of carotid body blood flow in the cat using radioactive microspheres, <u>J. Appl. Physiol.</u> 65:2484.

Biscoe, T. J., and Duchen, M. R., 1990, The cellular basis of transduction in carotid body chemoreceptors, <u>Am. J. Physiol.</u> 258:271.

DeCastro, F., and Rubio, M., 1968, The anatomy and innervation of the blood vessels of the carotid body and the role of chemoreceptive reactions in the autoregulation of the blood flow, in: <u>Arterial Chemoreceptors</u>, R. W. Torrance, ed., Blackwell, Oxford.

Delpiano, M., and Acker, H., 1989, Hypoxic and hypercapnic responses of $[Ca^{2+}]_o$ and $[K^+]_o$ in the cat carotid body in vitro, <u>Brain Res.</u> 482:235.

Donnelly and Kholwadwala, K., 1992, Hypoxia decreases intracellular calcium in adult rat carotid body glomus cells, <u>J. Neurophysiol.</u> 67:1543.

Duchen, M. R. and Biscoe, T. J., 1992a, Mitochondrial function in type I cells isolated from rabbit arterial chemoreceptors, <u>J. Physiol. Lond.</u> 450:13.

Duchen, M. R. and Biscoe, T. J., 1992b, Relative mitochondrial membrane potential and $[Ca^{2+}]_i$ in type I cells isolated from the rabbit carotid body, <u>J. Physiol. Lond.</u> 450:33.

Gonzalez, C., Almaraz, L., Obeso, A., and Riqual, R., 1992, Oxygen and acid chemoreception in the carotid body chemoreceptors, TINS 15:146.

Iturriaga, R., and Lahiri, S., 1992a, Effects of verapamil and external calcium removal on carotid chemoreception <u>in vitro</u>, <u>FASEB J.</u> 6:A1171.

Iturriaga, R., Rumsey, W. L., Lahiri, S., Spergel, D., and Wilson, D. F., 1992a, Intracellular pH and oxygen chemoreception in the cat carotid body *in vitro*, <u>J. Appl. Physiol.</u> 72:2259.

Joels, N., and Neil, E., 1962, The action of high tensions of carbon monoxide on the carotid chemoreceptors, <u>Arch. Int. Pharmacodyn.</u> 138:528.

Kinnamon, S. C., and Cummings, T. A., 1992, Chemosensory transduction mechanisms in taste, <u>Annu. Rev. Physiol.</u> 54:715.

Lahiri, S. and Delaney, R. G., 1975, Stimulus interaction in the responses of carotid body chemoreceptor single afferent fibres, <u>Respir. Physiol.</u> 24:249.

Lahiri, S., Smatresk, N. J., and Mulligan, E., 1983, Responses of peripheral chemoreceptors to natural stimula, in: <u>Physiology of the Peripheral Arterial Chemoreceptors</u>, H. Acker and R. G. O'Regan, eds., Elsevier, Amsterdam, pp. 221.

Miller, D., 1990, Glucose-regulation of potassium channels are sweet news for neurobiologists, TINS. 13:197.

Mills, E., and Jobsis, F. F., 1972, Mitochondrial respiratory chain of carotid body and chemoreceptor response to changes in oxygen tension, <u>J. Neurophysiol.</u> 35:405.

Mulligan, E., Lahiri, S., and Storey, B., 1981, Carotid body O_2 chemoreception and mitochondrial oxidative phosphorylation, <u>J. Appl. Physiol.</u> 51:438.

Obeseo, A., Almaraj, L., and Gonzalez, C., 1989, Effects of cyanide and uncouplers on chemoreceptor activity and ATP content of the cat carotid body, <u>Brain Res.</u> 481:250.

Sato, M., Ikeda, K., Yoshizaki, K., and Koyano, H., 1991, Response of cytosolic calcium to anoxia and cyanide in cultured glomus cells of newborn rabbit carotid body, <u>Brain Res.</u> 551:527.

Shirahata, M., and Fitzgerald, R. S., 1991, Dependency of hypoxic chemotransduction in cat carotid body on voltage-gated calcium channels, <u>J. Appl. Physiol.</u> 71: 1062.

Rumsey, W., Vanderkooi, J., and Wilson, D. F., 1988, Imaging of phosphorescence: a novel method for measuring the distribution of oxygen in perfused tissue, <u>Science</u> 241, 1649-1651.

Vanderkooi, J. M., Maniara, G., Green, T. J., and Wilson, D. F., 1987, An optical method for measuring dioxygen concentration based on quenching of phosphorescence, <u>J. Biol. Chem.</u> 262, 5476.

Whalen, W. J., and Nair, P., 1983, Oxidative metabolism and tissue PO_2 of the carotid body, in: Physiology of the Peripheral Arterial Chemoreceptors, H. Acker and R. G. O'Regan, eds., Elsevier, New York.

Wilson, D. F., Owen, C. S., and Erecinska, M., 1979, Quantitative dependence of mitochondrial oxidative phosphorylation on oxygen concentration, <u>Arch. Biochem. Biophys.</u> 195:494.

Wilson, D. F., Rumsey, W. L., Green, T. J., and Vanderkooi, J. M., 1988, The oxygen dependence of mitochondrial oxidative phosphorylation measured by a new optical method for measuring oxygen concentration, <u>J. Biol. Chem.</u> 263:2712.

OXYGEN TRANSPORT IN BLOOD, HYPERBARIC OXYGENATION

HEMOGLOBIN OXYGEN AFFINITY AND ACID-BASE STATUS IN BLOOD OF CHRONIC HEMODIALYSIS PATIENTS

M. Wehler, J. Grote, and H. U. Klehr*

Physiologisches Institut, *Medizinische Klinik der Universität Bonn
5300 Bonn, FRG

INTRODUCTION

It has been demonstrated that in critically ill patients less dialysis-induced morbidity and hemodynamic instability occured with bicarbonate-dialysis compared to acetate-dialysis (Graefe et al., 1978; Scribner, 1979; Vincent et al., 1982). However, the advantages of using bicarbonate dialysate in stable outpatient chronic dialysis patients has been the subject of debate (Man et al., 1982; Mehta et al., 1983; Hakim et al, 1985). The recent introduction of a new bicarbonate dialysate preparation that can be used in central delivery systems makes bicarbonate-dialysis affordable in outpatient dialysis centers. Since previous studies on the influence of hemodialysis on the blood oxygen dissociation curve (ODC) showed contradictory results (Cannella et al., 1982; Soliani et al., 1990), we investigated the oxygen affinity and the acid-base status of blood under the conditions of acetate- and bicarbonate-hemodialysis in stable chronic dialysis patients.

METHODS

Ten chronic stable outpatient dialysis patients (5 female, 5 male, mean age 59 ± 14.3 years) with chronic renal failure participated in the study and informed consent was obtained. They had no current symptoms of fluid overload or cardio-respiratory diseases. The dialysis program consisted of 4 hour sessions three times weekly. During the course of the study acetate-dialysis was changed to bicarbonate-dialysis, so the influence of each dialysate could be examined at one and the same patient. Arterial blood samples drawn anaerobically in heparinized syringes before and immediately after hemodialysis were used to determine the ODC at $PCO2 = 40mmHg$ and $T = 37°C$, the pH-logPCO$_2$-equilibration curves at (SO$_2$ = 100 and 0 %), the respiratory gas tensions, the acid-base status and the concentrations of 2,3-DPG, hemoglobin and electrolytes. Blood samples were kept in icewater and analysed within the next two hours. Micro-bloodsamples were equilibrated with gas mixtures of known oxygen and carbondioxide content (BMS2, Radiometer, Copenhagen) and the functional- and fractional oxygen saturation were measured (OSM3 Hemoximeter, Radiometer, Copenhagen). Simultaneously the pH-log PCO_2-equilibration curve was determined in oxygenated and in deoxygenated blood by the Astrup micromethod (Siggaard-Andersen, 1974). Using the derived data the ODC for a constant pH of 7.4 was calculated. The concentrations of Hb, COHb and MetHb were measured by the OSM3 Oximeter while the 2,3-DPG concentration was enzymatically assayed (Boehringer, Mannheim). For determination of arterial PO_2, PCO_2 and pH capillary blood samples were analysed (AVL Gas Check, Typ 939, AVL Biomedical Instruments, Graz, Austria).

RESULTS AND DISCUSSION

All patients on acetate-dialysis showed before hemodialysis a minor non-respiratory acidosis with a mean arterial pH of 7.3. During dialysis plasma pH returned to 7.4 due to an increase in mean BE from -6.6 to -2.8 mmol/l. The fluid loss caused a rise in hemoglobin concentration of about 15 %. The 2,3-DPG concentration was found to be significantly elevated to 5.44 mmol/l RBC before hemodialysis (Table 1). The accompanying blood ODCs measured at constant PCO_2 of 40 mmHg were shifted to the left (Figure 1). After normalisation for pH 7.4 using the simultaneously determined pH-logPCO_2-equilibration curves given in figure 2 the derived standard ODCs showed a significant increase in O_2-affinity with a mean half saturation pressure of the standard ODC ($P_{50, 7.4}$) of 24 and 24.6 mmHg for the blood samples taken before and after acetate-hemodialysis. The mean standard ODC determined after dialysis can be found in figure 3.

Table 1. Arterial pH and concentrations of Hb, 2,3-DPG and BE in blood of 10 chronic hemodialysis patients before and after acetate- (AcHD) and bicarbonate-hemodialysis (BiHD). Given are mean values ± SD.

Dialysis	Hb (g/dl)	2,3-DPG (mmol/l RBC)	pHa	BE (mmol/l)
before AcHD	10.9 ±1.9	5.44 ±0.30	7.33 ±0.05	-6.6 ±2.6
after AcHD	12.3 ±1.8	5.39 ±0.29	7.40 ±0.04	-2.8 ±1.8
before BiHD	10.6 ±0.9	5.52 ±0.27	7.37 ±0.05	-3.8 ±2.6
after BiHD	11.7 ±1.2	5.45 ±0.31	7.46 ±0.02	+2.9 ±1.2

After changing from acetate- to bicarbonate-dialysis therapy the patients showed before dialysis a mild non-respiratory acidosis with a mean BE of -3.8 mmol/l, having completed the dialysis a mean BE of +2.9 mmol/l was found as given in table 1. The 2,3-DPG concentration was elevated to 5.5 mmol/l RBC. As during acetate-dialysis the blood O_2-affinity was increased. Standardization of the O_2-dissociation curves determined before hemodialysis resulted in slightly leftshifted curves with a mean $P_{50, 7.4}$ of 25 mmHg (Figure 3). Bicarbonate-dialysis induced a small decrease in O_2-affinity with a mean $P_{50, 7.4}$ of 26 mmHg. Table 2 summarizes the mean values of the standard ODCs measured before and after acetate- as well as bicarbonate-hemodialysis.

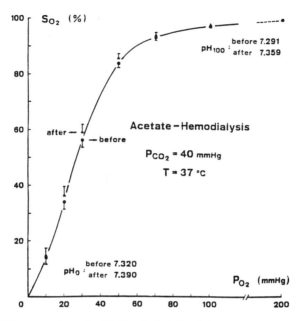

Fig. 1. O_2-dissociation curve determined in blood of 10 chronic hemodialysis patients before and after acetate-hemodialysis. Given are mean values ± SD.

Table 2. Mean values ± SD of the standard O_2-dissociation curves determined before and after acetate- (AcHD) and bicarbonate-hemodialysis (BiHD).

SO_2 (%)	control	PO_2 (mmHg) before AcHD	after AcHD	before BiHD	after BiHD
10	10.3	7.7 ±1.2	7.7 ±1.3	8.7 ±1.5	9.5 ±1.5
20	15.4	12.6 ±1.4	12.8 ±1.4	13.5 ±1.8	14.4 ±1.7
30	19.2	16.5 ±1.5	16.9 ±1.4	17.5 ±1.9	18.3 ±1.9
40	22.8	20.2 ±1.6	20.7 ±1.5	21.1 ±2.0	22.1 ±2.0
50	26.6	24.0 ±1.6	24.6 ±1.6	25.0 ±2.2	25.9 ±2.1
60	31.2	28.4 ±1.7	29.1 ±1.7	29.3 ±2.3	30.3 ±2.3
70	36.9	33.9 ±1.7	34.8 ±1.8	34.7 ±2.4	35.7 ±2.4
80	44.5	41.8 ±1.9	42.9 ±2.1	42.6 ±2.6	43.6 ±2.7
90	57.8	57.1 ±2.2	58.6 ±2.8	57.8 ±3.1	58.9 ±3.3

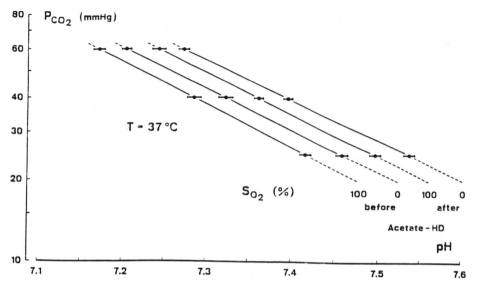

Fig. 2. pH-logPCO₂-equilibration curves determined in blood of 10 chronic hemodialysis patients before and after acetate-hemodialysis. Given are mean values $\pm$ SD.

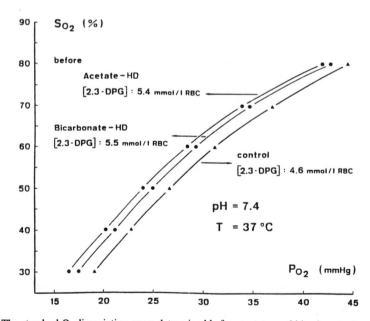

Fig. 3. The standard O₂-dissociation curve determined before acetate- and bicarbonate- hemodialysis. For comparison, the O₂-dissociation curve of controls is given. Given are mean values $\pm$ SD.

As shown in figure 4 in spite of significantly elevated 2,3-DPG concentrations the blood O_2-affinity of both compared groups was increased before as well as after hemodialysis. The changes were less pronounced in bicarbonate-hemodialysis patients. During hemodialysis the $P_{50, 7.4}$ increased without reaching normal levels. The leftshift of the ODC in hemodialysis patients can yet not be explained. Among the factors influencing the O_2-affinity the plasma chloride concentration and the HbCO fraction were within normal range. The observed increase in the 2,3-DPG concentration of the erythrocytes should result in a decrease of hemoglobin O_2-affinity. According to Edwards and Rigas, 1967 and Schmidt et al., 1987 a shift of the ODC to the left has to be expected with increasing red blood cell age. Since the anemic patients were treated with recombinant human erythropoetin the red blood cell age of the investigated blood samples, however, has to be expected below normal.

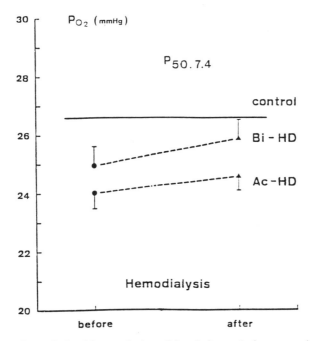

Fig. 4. P_{50} values calculated for standard conditions before and after acetate (Ac-HD) and bicarbonate-hemodialysis (Bi-HD). Given are mean values ± SEM.

CONCLUSIONS

Blood of chronic dialysis patients shows in spite of significantly elevated 2,3-DPG concentrations a pronounced increase in hemoglobin O_2-affinity. Since the O_2-affinity remains increased after acetate- or bicarbonate-hemodialysis a lasting impairment of O_2 transfer from blood to tissue has to be expected.

REFERENCES

Cannella, G., V. Maccagnola, B. Guiliani, R. Maiorca, E. Draghin (1982): The oxyhemoglobin dissociation curve during acetate and bicarbonate dialysis. *Nephron* 32: 378.

Edwards, M. J., D. A. Rigas (1967): Electrolyte labile increase of oxygen affinity during in vivo aging of hemoglobin. *J Clin Invest* 46: 1579 - 1588.

Graefe, U., J. Milutinovich, W. C. Follette, J. E. Vizzo, A. L. Babb, B. H. Scribner (1978): Less dialysis-induced morbidity and vascular instability with bicarbonate in dialysate. *Ann Intern Med* 88: 332 - 336.

Hakim, R. M., M. A. Pontzer, D. Tilton, J. M. Lazarus, M. N. Gottlieb (1985): Effects of acetate and bicarbonate dialysate in stable chronic dialysis patients. *Kidney Int* 28: 535 - 540.

Man, N. K., G. Fournier, P. Thireau, J. L. Gaillard, J. L. Funck-Brentano (1982): The effect of bicarbonate containing dialysate on chronic hemodialysis patients: A comparative study. *Artif Organs* 6: 421 - 428.

Mehta, B. R., D. Fischer, M. Ahmed, T. D. Dubose (1983): Effects of acetate and bicarbonate hemodialysis on cardiac function in chronic dialysis patients. *Kidney Int* 24: 240 - 245.

Schmidt, W., D. Böning, K. M. Braumann (1987): Red cell age effects on metabolism and oxygen affinity in humans. *Respir Physiol* 68: 215 - 225.

Scribner, B. H. (1979):Substitution of bicarbonate for acetate in the dialysate for care of a critically ill patient. *Dial Trans* 6: 26.

Soliani, F., T. Lusenti, V. Franco, G. Lindner, V. Davoli, A. Parisoli, M. Brini, P. P. Borgatti (1990): Intradialytic variations in hemoglobin affinity for oxygen during bicarbonate dialysis and hemodiafiltration. *Int J Artif Org* 13: 321-322.

Vincent, J. L., J. L. Vanherweghem, J. P. Degaute, J. Berre, P. Dufaye, R. J. Kahn (1982): Acetate-induced myocardial depression during hemodialysis for acute renal failure. *Kidney Int* 22: 653 - 657.

THE EFFECT OF INCREASED BLOOD CARBON MONOXIDE LEVELS
ON THE HEMOGLOBIN OXYGEN AFFINITY DURING PREGNANCY

J. Grote, P. Dall, K. Oltmanns, and W. Stolp*

Physiologisches Institut der Universität Bonn
*Johanniter-Krankenhaus, 5300 Bonn, FRG

INTRODUCTION

Since tobacco smoke contains 1.5-4.5 % carbon monoxide cigarette smoking induces a rise in the blood CO-hemoglobin concentration with a subsequent decrease in the O_2-capacity and a simultaneous increase in the hemoglobin O_2-affinity. Both effects cause a restriction of respiratory gas exchange. Aim of the present study was to investigate the influence of tobacco smoking during pregnancy on the O_2-affinity and the CO_2-binding of maternal blood. Using the derived results, a model describing the blood O_2-dissociation curve for the conditions of increased concentrations of CO-hemoglobin and of 2,3-DPG was developed. In addition, maternal to fetal oxygen transfer at elevated CO-hemoglobin fractions in maternal blood was analysed.

METHODS

In venous blood samples taken from 17 smoking (A) and 9 non-smoking (B) pregnant women (3rd. trimester) the O_2-dissociation curve (ODC) was determined at $PCO_2 = 40$ mmHg and T = 37°C. In the majority of cases (A, B) micro-bloodsamples were equilibrated with gas mixtures of known oxygen and carbondioxide content (BMS2, Radiometer, Copenhagen) and the functional- and fractional oxygen saturation were measured (OSM3 Hemoximeter, Radiometer, Copenhagen). In some cases (B) a modified method for continuous ODC recording according to Niesel and Thews (1961) was applied. Simultaneously the pH-log PCO_2-equilibration curve was determined in oxygenated and in deoxygenated blood by the Astrup micromethod (Siggaard-Andersen, 1974). Using the derived data the ODC for a constant pH of 7.4 was calculated.
The concentrations of Hb, COHb and MetHb were measured by an OSM3 Hemoximeter (Radiometer, Copenhagen) while the 2,3-DPG concentration was enzymatically assayed

Oxygen Transport to Tissue XV, Edited by P. Vaupel
et al., Plenum Press, New York, 1994

(Boehringer, Mannheim). For determination of arterial PO_2, PCO_2 and pH capillary blood samples were analysed (ABL 330, Radiometer, Copenhagen). All measurements were completed within 2 hours after the blood samples were taken.

RESULTS AND DISCUSSION

The oxygen dissociation curves determined in blood of smoking pregnant women showed in spite of significantly elevated 2,3-DPG concentrations an increased O_2-affinity as summarized in Tab.1. The mean P_{50} calculated for standard conditions was found to be 24.4 mmHg in blood samples with CO-hemoglobin fractions between 2 and 4 % (A I) and 23.2 mmHg in samples with CO-hemoglobin fractions below 4 % (A II). Both oxygen tensions were significantly below the comparable value of 26.7 mmHg found in non-pregnant, non-smoking young women at a mean 2,3-DPG concentration of 4.6 mmol/l RBC (Grote, 1986).

Tab.1 Concentrations of Hb, COHb and 2,3-DPG as well as P_{50} and n_{50} (pH $=7.4$) in blood of smoking (A) and non-smoking (B) pregnant women. Given are mean values $\pm$ SD. (A I $= 9$, A II $= 8$, B $= 9$)

	COHb (% Hb)	Hb (g/dl)	2,3-DPG (mmol/l RBC)	$P_{50,7.4}$ (mmHg)	n_{50}
A I	2.7 $\pm$ 0.6	13.1 $\pm$ 1.6	5.6 $\pm$ 0.5	24.4 $\pm$ 0.7	2.28
A II	5.7 $\pm$ 1.7	12.1 $\pm$ 1.2	5.7 $\pm$ 0.8	23.2 $\pm$ 0.6	2.26
B	< 1	11.6 $\pm$ 0.3	5.8 $\pm$ 0.6	28.8 $\pm$ 1.2	2.86

Besides the leftshift all O_2-dissociation curves of blood containing CO-hemoglobin in concentrations above normal levels were characterized by a decrease in slope. The mean Hill coefficients at half-saturation (n_{50}) were 2.28 in group A I and 2.26 in group A II, respectively. For standard conditions in human whole blood n_{50} values between 2.5 and 2.7 are commonly accepted to be normal (Severinghaus, 1979; Reeves, 1980; Braumann et al., 1982; Grote, 1986). The mean ODC determined for constant pH of 7.4 in blood samples of smoking pregnant women with a mean CO-hemoglobin fraction of 5.7 % and a mean 2,3-DPG concentration of 5.7 mmol/l RBC (A II) is given in Fig. 1.

To describe the clearance of carbon monoxide the half-live period of the CO-hemoglobin concentration after heavy smoking was determined in 5 male volunteers. The observed mean value was 3.8 hours. For comparison, Zander (1986) calculated a half-live period of 8.3 hours using data measured 12 and 18 hours following CO load due to cigarette smoking.

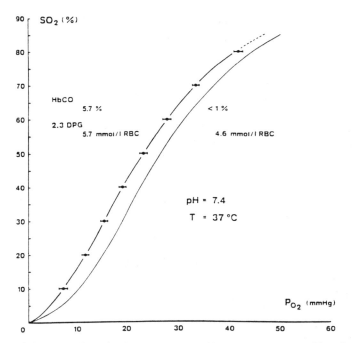

Fig. 1. O₂-dissociation curve determined in blood of 8 smoking pregnant women with an increased mean COHb level of 5.7 % (A II). Given are mean values ± SD.

For comparison, the blood O₂-dissociation curve of non-smoking, non-pregnant women is given.

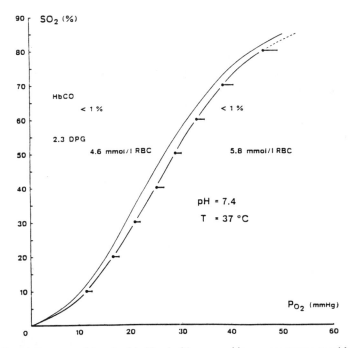

Fig. 2. O₂-dissociation curve determined in blood of 9 non-smoking pregnant women with normal COHb levels (B). Given are mean values ± SD.

For comparison, the blood O₂-dissociation curve of non-smoking, non-pregnant women is given.

The blood samples of the non-smoking pregnant women (B) with CO-hemoglobin fractions below 1 % showed increased 2,3-DPG concentrations comparable to those observed in the blood of smoking pregnant women but in contrast they exhibited a marked decrease in O_2-affinity (Fig. 2). The mean P_{50} of 28.8 mmHg calculated for standard conditions was significantly greater than the normal value as well as the mean values determined in the groups A I and A II (Tab. 1). The Hill coefficient was found to be above normal range, the mean n_{50} value was 2.86. For standard conditions Lucius et al. (1970) determined a mean P_{50} of 27.8 mmHg in blood samples taken between the 10th to 40th week of gestation while Bauer et al. (1969) observed a mean half-saturation tension of 30.5 mmHg approx. 2 hours before delivery.

Based on conceptions of Haldane (1912/13) and Forster (1970) the observed influence of increased concentrations of CO-hemoglobin and of 2,3-DPG on the blood oxygen dissociation curve can be described according to Adair (1925) by the equation :

$$Hb_{O2} + Hb_{CO} = \frac{A_1 \cdot x + 2 A_2 \cdot x^2 + 3 A_3 \cdot x^3 + 4 A_4 \cdot x^4}{4 (1 + A_1 \cdot x + A_2 \cdot x^2 + A_3 \cdot x^3 + A_4 \cdot x^4)}$$

with $x = (P_{O2} + M \cdot P_{CO}) \, 10^{c \cdot DPG}$.

$M \cdot P_{CO}$ - the P_{O2} equivalent of P_{CO} - was found to be 4.04 mmHg in group A I and 7.02 mmHg in group A II. Taking into account a normal 2,3-DPG concentration of 4.6 mmol/l RBC a mean value of -0.025 was calculated for c. The accompanying dissociation curve for HbO_2 + HbCO as a function of PO_2 + M PCO for the investigated blood samples of smoking women with high CO-hemoglobin fractions (A II) is given in Fig. 3.

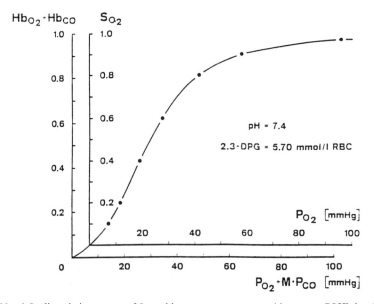

Fig. 3. Blood O_2-dissociation curve of 8 smoking pregnant women with a mean COHb level of 5.7 % (A II) plotted according to Forster (1970).

148

The P_{50} values calculated according to Forster (1970) for different CO-hemoglobin levels but normal 2,3-DPG concentrations are in good agreement with the oxygen tensions determined at half-saturation in blood samples with comparable CO-hemoglobin fractions corrected for a 2,3-DPG concentration of 4.6 mmol/l RBC. Calculations based on a model described by Collier (1976) resulted in P_{50} values systematically 1-3 mmHg above the determined data (Fig. 4).

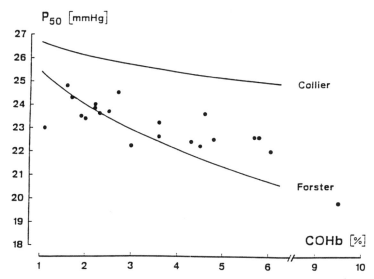

Fig. 4. Effects of COHb concentration on $P_{50, 7.4}$.

Dots represent determined P_{50} values corrected for normal 2,3-DPG concentrations.

For comparison, the P_{50} - COHb relationship calculated according to Collier and Forster is given.

The derived O_2-dissociation curves and acid-base data were used to analyse the effect of increased CO-hemoglobin levels in maternal blood on the respiratory gas exchange in the placenta. Considering the mean values for the respiratory gas tensions and the pH as observed in group A II of PO_2 = 97 mmHg, PCO_2 = 32 mmHg, pH = 7.454, a maternal placental blood flow of 450 ml/min and a fetal oxygen uptake of 24 ml/min (Longo, 1987) an oxygen tension of 30 mmHg was calculated for the blood in the uterine vein. This value is about 8 mmHg below the normal mean PO_2 in blood of the uterine vein. The results indicate the presence of hypoxia in fetal blood caused by the changes in O_2-affinity and O_2-capacity of maternal blood due to increased CO-hemoglobin levels after heavy smoking. Comparable calculations based on the oxygen dissociation curve observed in blood samples of non-smoking pregnant women resulted in a normal PO_2 of 37 mmHg in the uterine vein.

CONCLUSIONS

The CO binding to hemoglobin in the blood of smoking pregnant women induces in spite of significantly elevated 2,3-DPG concentrations a pronounced left-shift of the O_2-dissociation curve. The increase in O_2-affinity and the decrease in O_2-capacity of maternal blood with CO-hemoglobin fractions above normal cause an impairment of respiratory gas exchange in the placenta which may lead to arterial hypoxia of the fetus under conditions of high CO-hemoglobin concentrations.

REFERENCES

Adair, G. S. (1925): The hemoglobin system. VI. The oxygen dissociation curve of hemoglobin. *J. Biol. Chem.* 63, 529-545.

Bauer, Ch., M. Ludwig, I. Ludwig, and H. Bartels (1969): Factors governing the oxygen affinity of human adult and fetal blood. *Respir. Physiol.* 7, 271-277.

Braumann, K.-M., D. Böning, and F. Trost (1982): Bohr effect and slope of the oxygen dissociation curve after physical training. *J. Appl. Physiol.* 52, 1524-1529.

Forster, R.E. (1970): Carbon monoxide and the partial pressure of oxygen in tissue. Ann. NY Acad. Sci. 174: 233-241.

Grote, J. (1986): Oxygen affinity and erythrocyte 2,3-diphosphoglycerate in blood during anemia of pregnancy. *In:* Funktionsanalyse biologischer Systeme 16:33-39.

Haldane, J.B.S. (1912/13): The dissociation of oxyhaemoglobin in human blood during partial CO poisoning. *J. Physiol.*, London 45: XXII-XXIV.

Hlastala, M.P., H.P. McKenna, R.L. Franada, and J.C. Detter (1976): Influence of carbon monoxide on hemoglobin-oxygen binding. *J. Appl. Physiol.* 41, 893-899.

Lucius, H., H. Gahlenbeck, H.-O. Kleine, H. Fabel, and H. Bartels (1970): Respiratory functions, buffer system, and electrolyte concentrations of blood during human pregnancy. *Respir. Physiol.* 9, 311-317.

Niesel, W., und G. Thews (1961): Ein neues Verfahren zur schnellen und genauen Aufnahme der Sauerstoffbindungskurve des Blutes und konzentrierter Hämoproteinlösungen. *Pflügers Arch.* 273, 380-395.

Okada, Y., I. Tyuma, Y. Ueda, and T. Sugimoto (1976): Effect of carbon monoxide on equilibrium between oxygen and hemoglobin. *Am. J. Physiol.* 230, 471-475.

Reeves, R.B. (1980): A rapid micro method for obtaining oxygen equilibrium curves on whole blood. *Respir. Physiol.* 42, 299-315.

Severinghaus, J.W. (1979): Simple, accurate equations for human blood O_2 dissociation computation. *J. Appl. Physiol.* 46, 599-602.

Zander, R. (1986): COHb-Konzentrationen im Blut bei Rauchern und Nichtrauchern. *In*: Der Sauerstoff-Status des arteriellen Blutes, Zander, R., Mertzlufft, F.O. (eds.), pp. 183 - 186, Basel: Karger.

Zwart, A., G. Kwant, B. Oeseburg, and W.G. Zijlstra (1984): Human whole-blood oxygen affinity: effect of carbon monoxide. *J. Appl. Physiol.* 57, 14-20.

MODELING BLOOD GAS EQUILIBRIA OF HUMAN BLOOD

Jacob P. Zock

Department of Medical Physiology
University of Groningen
Bloemsingel 10, 9712 KZ Groningen, The Netherlands

INTRODUCTION

Although not always recognized as such, mathematical models of blood gas and acid-base equilibria are widely used, mostly in blood gas apparatus, to calculate the values of quantities that are not measured, such as base excess, standard base excess, oxygen saturation or 2,3-DPG concentration [1, 2].

Already in the early days the complexity of blood gas and acid-base equilibria led to the implementation in a mathematical model: L.J.Henderson published in his book "Blood" a large number of nomograms for calculating values of the various blood gas quantities [3]. Many algorithms for the calculation of blood gas and acid-base quantities under clinical circumstances have been published (e.g. [4, 5, 6, 7, 8]). Even until fairly recently they were published in the form of nomograms [7]. Computers have made the use of nomograms obsolete and allow complex calculations to be done [1]. Mathematical models can be made more elaborate and complex. Nowadays, algorithms concerning blood gas equilibria and acid-base state are build-in applications in blood gas analyzing apparatus [2]. The algorithms are often based on empirical relations and a consistent representation of the underlying mechanisms is not the primary objective.

In the model described below basic physico-chemical relations are used as much as possible. The development of the model began with calculations concerning the acid-base equilibria in plasma and blood when temperature is changed [13, 14]. Blood is considered as a two compartment system. The two compartments, plasma and erythrocyte content, are separated by a membrane which is selectively permeable for a number of substances. The model consists of the equations of equilibria in plasma and in the erythrocyte solution and of the coupling between the two solutions across the membrane. Constraints are further imposed by physico-chemical properties such as osmotic equilibrium and electroneutrality.

A model of blood gas equilibria should show that delivery of oxygen from the blood enhances the uptake of carbon dioxide and H^+ ions, and that binding of oxygen in the lungs promotes the delivery of carbon dioxide. This behavior is caused by the special properties of the hemoglobin molecule. Equations which model the hemoglobin molecule should represent these properties in a consistent way.

In the first versions of the model the properties of hemoglobin regarding oxygen binding, proton buffering, carbon dioxide binding and the influence of the latter two on oxygen binding were modelled separately [14]. Interactions between them were described in additional, empirical equations. Influence of 2,3-DPG was not accounted for at all.

On the basis of Wyman's theory of the interactions in complex molecules [9, 11] and the two state model of hemoglobin, a mathematical description of the molecule was developed in which the important binding properties and their interactions were represented [10]. In fact, the binding of oxygen, protons, carbon dioxide and 2,3-DPG to hemoglobin and their mutual influences can be implemented as a single mathematical function: Wyman's binding potential function. In our implementation the binding potential function is partitioned into a set of equations which form the core of the mathematical model of blood [10]. This representation has the required properties without the need of additional equations. Hemoglobin strongly reacts with carbon monoxide in competition with oxygen. The binding potential function can be made to represent this properties of hemoglobin concerning the binding of carbon monoxide as well [12].

It has to be understood that the representation in a model means a great reduction of the complexity of the hemoglobin molecule. Groups chosen to represent the influence of CO_2, H^+ and 2,3-DPG on oxygen affinity — the so called bohr groups — offer a reasonable approximation for purposes of reproducing binding curves, but should not be taken to necessarily properly describe the actual groups responsible for this effect.

Comparison of experimental curves with oxygen saturation curves of blood calculated with the model shows that the binding of oxygen in blood, including the influences of pH, pCO_2 and 2,3-DPG on it, is well represented by this model.

MODEL

As far as blood gas transport is concerned a fairly simple picture of blood can be used. Blood consists of erythrocytes dispersed in plasma. Plasma is a solution of proteins and electrolytes in water. The erythrocytes contain a solution of hemoglobin and electrolytes in water. In the model the red cells are taken together into one compartment. Blood thus consists of two homogeneous compartments: plasma and red cells (Fig. 1). A number of substances can exchange across the erythrocyte membrane: O_2, CO_2, water, Cl^-, HCO_3^-, and H^+. This couples the equilibria inside the erythrocytes to those in plasma.

Red cells are for a substantial part filled with hemoglobin. Hemoglobin cannot normally leave the red cells, nor can plasma proteins enter them. Therefore, electrical charges on these proteins are fixed to their compartments. Ions that can freely pass the membranes are distributed according to a Gibbs-Donnan equilibrium. Ions that practically satisfy this requirement are Cl^-, HCO_3^-, H^+.

The net negative charge of plasma protein depends on pH in plasma. Plasma pH results from two equilibria: proton release from the CO_2/HCO_3^- equilibrium and proton binding to protein buffers. The net negative charge of hemoglobin depends on

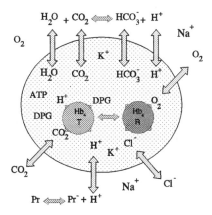

Figure 1. Blood as a two compartment system with equilibria considered.

pH inside the erythrocytes and on substances that are bound to hemoglobin. These are, besides oxygen and protons, carbon dioxide and 2,3-DPG. By consequence, the Gibbs-Donnan distribution changes when there are changes *e.g.* in pH or in pO_2 or pCO_2.

Water can freely pass the cell membrane. A redistribution is reflected in a change in hematocrit. Such changes follow from redistribution of electric charges where charges on proteins are replaced by charges on free HCO_3^- ions. Furthermore, substances that do not pass the red cell membrane — like plasma proteins, hemoglobin, ATP and 2,3-DPG — also determine the distribution of water between the red cells and plasma.

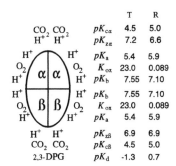

Figure 2. Equilibrium constants used in the two state model of hemoglobin

Hemoglobin binds oxygen and the other ligands in a reversible reaction. Binding changes the distribution between the different structures of the molecule and this causes changes in the average affinities for all ligands. Various theories exist on the mechanisms of these changes. In the model a two state representation — T and R — was used. Changes in the overall affinity of a certain ligand are here caused by a change in the partition over the two states.

Carbon dioxide is involved in more equilibria than oxygen. The major part of carbon dioxide is present as bicarbonate ions which are distributed between blood plasma and the intracellular compartment of the red cells. Bicarbonate ions formed in the red cell pass the cell membrane either in exchange for a chloride ion or together with a proton. In this way bicarbonate and chloride are distributed in a Gibbs-Donnan equilibrium. The protons coming free are bound to plasma proteins and to hemoglobin. In the latter case this binding diminishes the affinity of hemoglobin for oxygen. Protons, too, are supposed to be distributed between plasma and red cell content according to the Gibbs-Donnan equilibrium. The influence of carbon dioxide on oxygen binding is largely exerted by the concomitant change in pH.

Carbon dioxide is also bound directly to amino groups on the globin protein as carbamino groups. Just like protons and 2,3-DPG, carbon dioxide bound to hemoglobin diminishes the affinity of hemoglobin for oxygen.

A small part of carbon dioxide is present as dissolved carbon dioxide. The very small amount of carbonic acid is proportional to the concentration of dissolved gas. In calculations it is usually included in this fraction by using a proportionally larger value for the solubility coefficient of carbon dioxide.

Three sets of relations can be considered: those describing the equilibria in plasma, those in erythrocyte content and those describing the equilibria across the membrane. Values of the constants in the equations determine the characteristics of the model. A subset of the equations and initial values of a number of quantities fix the standard state of the model. Examples are given in table 1.

Table 1. Composition supposed at start

Quantity	Value	Unit
Plasma sodium concentration	145	mmol/L
Plasma protein concentration	70	g/L
Blood Hb concentration	150	g/L
Cell Hb concentration	330	g/L
2,3-DPG amount	$0.92 \cdot tHb_4$	mmol

The kations Na^+ and K^+ are supposed to be contained in their compartments and are the only kations considered. Furthermore, the amounts of plasma protein, hemoglobin, chloride, ATP, 2,3-DPG and water are all determined at the start of the calculations assuming a standard state with plasma pH of 7.4, cell pH of 7.192, pO_2 of 14 kPa, pCO_2 of 5.33 kPa at a temperature of 310 K.

CALCULATIONS

The model was implemented as a PASCAL computer program and consisted of a number of nested loops. Calculation starts with an initial guess of red cell pH. Then the Gibbs-Donnan ratio, and thus red cell pH, and the concomitant water distribution is calculated in the plasma–cell loop.

The innermost loop calculates 2,3-DPG bound to hemoglobin at that cell pH, pO_2, and pCO_2. It is entered with each new value of intracellular pH. After the water distribution and the Gibbs-Donnan ratio are calculated, a new plasma pH results because plasma concentrations have changed. The initial pH and that calculated are

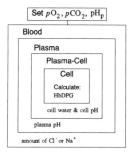

Figure 3. Nesting of loops to calculate Cl^- for a combination of pO_2, pCO_2, and pH.

compared. If they differ less than the set error level the loop is left, otherwise the loop is repeated with a new pH value. In the outermost loop the calculated pH is compared with the requested value. After comparison the amount of Cl^- or Na^+ is adjusted to shift pH in the desired direction. The calculation stops if the requested pH is approximated within the chosen precision.

RESULTS AND DISCUSSION

The model can be used to calculate various graphical and numerical relations between blood gas and acid-base quantities. Figure 4 shows the oxygen saturation curves calculated for human blood with normal, low, and high concentrations of 2,3-DPG present. Also shown in the figure are curves drawn through points of which the values are taken from the literature. The curves for normal 2,3-DPG concentration almost coincide. An enlarged part of it is shown in the right hand panel. Measured values were taken from [5]: center line, [15]: dashed line, and [16]: dotted line. The

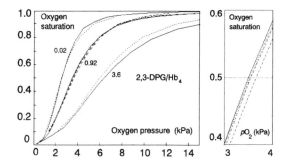

Figure 4. Effects of 2,3-DPG/Hb$_4$ ratio on oxygen saturation curve.

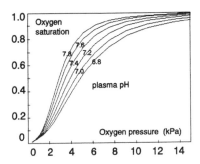

Figure 5. Effects of plasma pH at $pCO_2=5.33$ kPa on oxygen saturation curve.

values for high and low 2,3-DPG were also measured by Zwart. Solid lines were plotted through calculated points.

Figure 4 shows that the calculated curves for a normal 2,3-DPG/Hb_4 ratio agree well with experimental curves. For the lower ratio the calculated curves also agree well with those determined by Zwart, but for the high ratio there is a difference between the calculated and the measured curves [16]. This difference might be caused by the way kations are dealt with in the model. They are thought to be confined to their compartment. In reality there is a continuous leakage of them opposed by pumping through the membrane. This may lead to different osmotic behavior and a different Gibbs-Donnan distribution. Different pH values and 2,3-DPG binding may result, giving the difference between the curves. Apart from the high 2,3-DPG/Hb_4 ratio the influence of 2,3-DPG oxygen binding in human blood is well represented by the model. Oxygen saturation curves of blood at some values of plasma pH and constant pCO_2 of 5.33 kPa are shown in figure 5. The show the H^+ bohr effect in whole blood. Similar

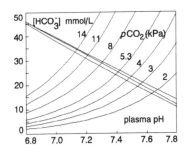

Figure 6. CO_2 bufferlines at three values of pO_2.

pictures are easily calculated for the case that pH is kept constant and pCO_2 is the parameter.

Changes in blood gases go along with changes in acid-base state. The latter may be represented in a HCO_3^--pH diagram. Figure 6 shows three CO_2 bufferlines, each one calculated at a fixed value of pO_2. The uppermost curve is that at $pO_2=14$ kPa, the lowest curve that at $pO_2=0.035$ kPa and the curve in between at $pO_2=3.5$ kPa. The last one is steeper because oxygen saturation of hemoglobin, and thus saturation and the amount of H^+ bound, strongly depends on pH.

The model is characterized by many constants and relations. They have been chosen to be as representative as possible. Especially those of hemoglobin are difficult to verify. In part, this is caused by the fact that the molecule is strongly simplified. Experimental values of constants had sometimes to be changed slightly to get agreement between calculated and experimental curves. The value of L_0, which determines the partition between the T and the R state of hemoglobin when not liganded is chosen in the range of experimental values [17, 18], *i.e.* $\ln L_0 = 9.5$. The oxygen affinity of the T state is about the one found for blood [18], that of the R state is higher, so that the ratio between them is higher than reported. The ratio between the 2,3-DPG affinities, 100, is at the high end of the range of experimental values 25–100.

Overall, the model gives a good approximation of the properties of blood at the temperature of 310 K. Temperature dependencies of a number of parameters are lacking. This makes that the model cannot calculate the behavior at temperatures other than normal body temperature.

ACKNOWLEDGEMENT

This work was supported by the Groningen Centre for Biomedical Technology (BMTC) as part of the CAD project.

REFERENCES

1. O. Siggaard-Andersen and M. Siggaard-Andersen, The oxygen status algorithm: a computer program for calculating and displaying pH and blood gas data, *Scand. J. Clin. Lab. Invest. 50, Suppl.* 203: 29-45 (1990).
2. O. Siggaard-Andersen, P.D. Wimberley, N. Fogh-Andersen and I.H. Gothgen, Measured and derived quantities with modern pH and blood gas equipment: calculation algorithms with 54 equations, *Scand. J. Clin. Lab. Invest., Suppl.* 189: 7-15 (1988).
3. L.J. Henderson, "Blood: A Study in General Physiology," Yale University Press, New Haven (Conn.) (1928).
4. R.B. Singer and A.B. Hastings, An improved clinical method for the estimation of disturbances of the acid-base balance of human blood, *Medicine* 27: 223-42 (1948).
5. J.W. Severinghaus, Blood gas calculator, *J. Appl. Physiol.* 21: 1108-16 (1966).
6. L.J. Thomas Jr., Algorithms for selected blood acid-base and blood gas calculations, *J. Appl. Physiol.* 33: 154-8 (1972).
7. P. Rispens, J.R. Brunsting, J.P. Zock and W.G. Zijlstra, A modified Singer-Hastings nomogram, *J. Appl. Physiol.* 34, 377-82 (1973).

8. R.G. Ryall and C.J. Story, Equilibrium model of the oxygen association curve of normal human erythrocytes under standardized conditions, *Clin. Chem.* 29: 1819-22 (1983).

9. J. Wyman, The binding potential, a neglected linkage concept, *J. Molec. Biol.* 11: 631-44 (1965).

10. J.P. Zock, Mathematical model of the physiological properties of human hemoglobin, *Proc. Kon. Ned. Akad. Wet.* C90: 493-508 (1987).

11. J. Wyman and S.J. Gill, "Binding and Linkage," University Science Books, Mill Valley (1990).

12. J.P. Zock, Carbon monoxide binding in a model of hemoglobin differs between the T and the R conformation, *in*: J. Piiper, T.K. Goldstick and M. Meyer(eds), "Oxygen Transport to Tissue XII," Plenum Press, New York (1990).

13. P. Rispens, "Significance of Plasma Bicarbonate for the Evaluation of H^+ Homeostasis," Thesis, Groningen (1970).

14. J.P. Zock, "CO_2 and O_2 Equilibria in Human Blood and Interstitial Fluid," Thesis, Groningen (1985).

15. G. Arthurson, L. Garby, M. Robert and B. Zaar, The oxygen dissociation curve of normal human blood with special reference to the influence of physiological effector ligands, *Scand. J. Clin. Lab. Invest.* 34: 9-13 (1974).

16. A. Zwart, "Spectral and Functional Properties of Haemoglobin in Human Whole Blood," Thesis, Groningen (1983).

17. L. Garby and J. Meldon, "The Respiratory Functions of Blood," Plenum Press, New York (1977).

18. T. Groth, L. Garby and C.H. de Verdier, Estimation of parameters in a multi-affinity-state model for haemoglobin from oxygen binding data in whole blood and in concentrated haemoglobin solutions, *J. Molec. Biol.* 121: 507-22 (1978).

HIGH COOPERATIVITY OF HEMOGLOBIN-OXYGEN BINDING IN EMBRYONIC RABBIT BLOOD

Robert A. B. Holland and Susan J. Calvert

School of Physiology & Pharmacology
University of New South Wales
Kensington, Sydney, NSW 2033
Australia

INTRODUCTION

This paper reports experiments that examine whether the functional unit of hemoglobin in the blood of mammalian embryos is the tetramer. This has generally been assumed to be the case in all mammalian blood - adult, fetal and embryonic, although measurements on blood from other classes of vertebrates have indicated that the functional unit may contain more than four subunits.

Much of the evidence is based on the Hill plots of the oxygen equilibrium curves (OECs). In an OEC, the percentage saturation is found as a function of oxygen tension under specified conditions, and the normal mammalian OEC has the well known sigmoid shape. The points of this curve may be plotted according to the logarithmic form of the Hill equation,

$$\log \{Y/(1-Y)\} = n_H \log PO_2 - n_H \log P_{50} \tag{1}$$

where Y is fractional saturation, P_{50} is the oxygen tension at half-saturation, and n_H (Hill "n") is the slope of the plot. The value of n_H indicates how many subunits of hemoglobin appear to be oxygenating or deoxygenating together and it is therefore known as an index of interaction or cooperativity. Examples of Hill plots are in the results section of this paper (Fig. 2). In normal mammalian blood the Hill plot is linear or nearly linear between about 20% and 85% saturation, the value of n_H being in the range 2.6 to 3.3 in this middle region, and less at higher or lower saturations. The failure to find n_H values greater

Oxygen Transport to Tissue XV, Edited by P. Vaupel
et al., Plenum Press, New York, 1994

than 4 has indicated that in normal mammalian blood there are never more than 4 subunits oxygenating or deoxygenating together, and therefore that the functional unit is likely to be the tetramer.

However, over recent years, studies of blood of marsupials at an early stage of development have shown that, before birth and in the first few days after birth, the OEC climbs steeply above about 50% saturation. Their Hill plots showed a marked bend at about 50% saturation, the value of n_H in the upper part of the plot being significantly greater than 4; and in some cases over 6. These findings were made in the Tammar Wallaby, *Macropus eugenii* (Holland et al., 1988; Tibben et al., 1991; Calvert et al., 1992); and in two other species from different families: the Common Brushtail Possum, *Trichosurus vulpecula* (Holland et al., 1991) and the very small Fat-tailed Dunnart, *Sminthopsis crassicaudata* (Holland, Calvert, Hope and Chesson, unpublished observations, 1992). Since marsupial blood is at the embryonic stage till several days after birth (nucleated red cells and multiple hemoglobins), it appeared worthwhile to look for a similar feature in the blood of embryos of eutherian (placental) mammals.

For the experiments reported here, we chose the rabbit. This species has been studied in the late embryonic and fetal stage by Jelkmann and Bauer (1977) and also it has no fetal hemoglobin; as in the marsupials there is a direct changeover from embryonic to adult type hemoglobins.

METHODS

We studied blood from 25 embryonic rabbits of the New Zealand White strain. Of these, 10 came from 2 mothers 13 days after fertilization; and 15 came from 3 mothers, 14 days after fertilization.

After pregnancy had been confirmed by palpation, the mothers were anaesthetized with intramuscular xylazine hydrochloride (Rompun), 10 mgm/kg body weight; and ketamine hydrochloride, 70 mg/kg. Supplementary doses were administered every half-hour. The embryos were dissected out and blood taken from the umbilical vessels of individual embryos. After the blood sample had been taken from the last embryo, the mother was painlessly killed by an overdose of anaesthetic and a bilateral pneumothorax.

In general the methods were as described by Holland et al. (1988). The embryonic blood was placed on ice and the OEC of the whole blood was determined within four hours of the blood being taken. In addition OECs were determined on the blood of four of the mothers. The OEC determinations were done by a thin-film method using a modified HEM-O-SCAN. In this the blood (as little as 1 μlitre) is held between two gas-permeable membranes and, after calibration, the gas surrounding it is changed from 0% oxygen to 30% oxygen. During oxygenation the PO_2 in the gas surrounding the blood film was read by an oxygen electrode, and the oxygen saturation of the blood in the film was read by spectrophotometry, using a beam-splitter, interference filters at 559 and 577 nm, and two photodiodes. The OEC so obtained is recorded on an X-Y plotter. In our modified procedure we introduced the oxygenating gas in pulses so that we obtained a number of discrete points on the OEC rather than a continuous curve. In all the OEC determinations described here, the Pco_2 was 42 mm Hg and the temperature was 37°C.

The P_{50} of each OEC was read from the curve and a Hill plot made of the entire curve using equation 1. The value of n_H, the index of co-operativity, was calculated for each interval using this equation, and the values at "low saturation" and "high saturation" compared. For low saturation n_H we took the n_H value at the 25% saturation point; for high saturation n_H we took the value at the 75% saturation point.

The blood of each adult and embryonic rabbit was examined microscopically after it had been stained with Wright's stain. Also, cell lysate was examined for hemoglobin types by isoelectric focusing on polyacrylamide ampholine gels, stained with benzidine.

RESULTS

Blood was obtained from 25 embryos. Fifteen were 14 days from fertilization, four coming from each of two mothers, and seven from the third. Ten were 13 days from fertilization, five being from each of two mothers. In addition, blood from four of the mothers was studied.

Table 1. Characteristics of Oxygen-Hemoglobin Equilibrium Curves in Rabbits, Embryonic and Adult; 37°C, $P_{CO2} = 42$ mm Hg.

Gest. Age[1] (days)	Number of mothers	Number of embryos	P_{50} mm Hg	n_H low	n_H high
13	2	10	28.7	2.17 (0.07)[2]	5.72 (0.15)[2]
14	3	15	27.6	2.09 (0.07)[2]	5.17 (0.16)[2]
Adult	4		32.4	3.2	

[1] Gest. Age = Gestational Age.
[2] The figures in brackets represent one S.E. of the mean of the relevant n_H values.

Typical OECs of adult and embryonic rabbit blood are shown in Figure 1 and their Hill plots are in Figure 2. The results are summarized in Table 1. The P_{50} of the embryonic rabbits was a little less than that of the mothers. All samples of embryonic blood showed a Hill plot bent upwards at about 50% saturation. In all but one embryo, the high saturation n_H was greater than 4 and in some it was higher than 6. The highest value of low saturation n_H was 2.53.

By the "t" test, the mean high saturation n_H was greater than 4 in both the 13 day and in the 14 day embryos ($P < 0.001$). The mean high saturation n_H was higher for the 13 day than for the 14 day embryos ($0.02 < P < 0.05$).

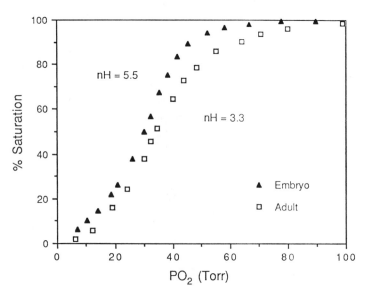

Figure 1. Oxygen equilibrium curves of blood from an adult rabbit, and a rabbit embryo 14 days after fertilization. Curves were determined at 37°C and Pco_2 = 42 mmHg.

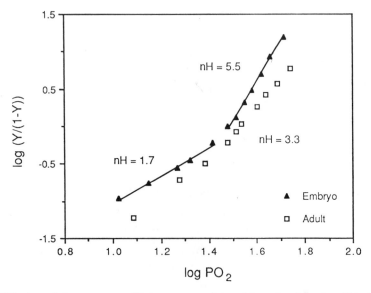

Figure 2. Hill plots of the oxygen equilibrium curves of the adult and embryonic rabbit (14 days after fertilization). The plots are from the curves shown in Figure 1.

One concern when a steeply climbing OEC is found is that it could be an artefact caused by progressive depletion of a co-factor such as 2,3-diphosphoglycerate (2,3-DPG) during the determination of the curve. Because 2,3-DPG shifts the OEC to the right, its progressive depletion would cause a shifting of the upper points of the curve to the left; thus producing an appearance of a steeply climbing curve. The possibility of this artefact was excluded by doing repeat OECs in 13 of the embryonic samples. These were completed about half an hour after the first curve. If there had been a significant systematic shift of points to the left, the P_{50} of the second curve would have been substantially lower than that of the first. The P_{50} of the repeat curves was 0.4 mm Hg lower than that of the corresponding final curves (S.E. = 0.23 mmHg), a very small change, so it was concluded that high n_H values found were genuine, and were not an artefact caused by co-factor depletion.

The adult Hill plots appeared straight in the middle and a single n_H was determined for each of the adults, the mean value being 3.2.

All embryonic blood had more than one hemoglobin present and one of the components appeared similar to adult rabbit hemoglobin. Our stained gels had a high background and it was not possible to distinguish clearly different embryonic hemoglobin types.

Microscopic examination of blood smears from each embryo showed that the great majority of the red cells were of the embryonic type, being large and nucleated. In one sample, up to 40% of the red cells were non-nucleated. In two other smears, up to 20% of the red cells were non-nucleated, and in the others, non-nucleated cells were 10% or less. Some of the non-nucleated cells may have been embryonic cells that had lost their nuclei; some may have been maternal red cells contaminating the sample. We do not consider that the presence of small numbers of maternal cells invalidate our finding of a high n_H value - their effect on the value found for n_H is to make it lower than n_H for uncontaminated blood.

DISCUSSION

The results clearly show a high degree of interaction between subunits of embryonic hemoglobin. The high values of n_H show that more than four subunits of hemoglobin oxygenate or deoxygenate together. This can be achieved either by the functional unit of hemoglobin having more than four subunits, or by there being positive interaction between adjacent hemoglobin subunits. In either case, the functional unit, at least in the higher saturations, is not the tetramer, but contains a larger number of subunits. It should be noted that this high n_H was not found in adult red cells, but only in those of embryonic type with embryonic hemoglobin.

The number of subunits in a functional unit cannot be calculated from the value of n_H found in cells containing a mixture of hemoglobins. Holland et al. (1988) showed in a model that with the upper part of the OEC reflecting the oxygenation of a component whose n_H value was 8, the value of n_H found in this upper region was only 5.21. This was because the higher affinity component was still being oxygenated to some extent in the upper part of the OEC. Also Gill et al. (1978) found that for part of the OEC, human sickle cell hemoglobin, known to aggregate into long chains in the deoxy form, had a maximum n_H value of 5-6. Therefore while we are confident that the embryonic hemoglobin functional unit is larger than a tetramer, we cannot say what it is, or put an upper limit on its size.

This is the first demonstration of an n_H value greater than 4 in any normal eutherian blood and in this respect the rabbit embryonic blood is similar to that of marsupials (see introduction). The physiological advantage of the steeply climbing OEC (manifested by the high n_H value) is that it enables oxygen exchange by the embryonic blood in the placenta or tissues to take place with minimal change in oxygen tension. However, we do not know the oxygen tensions in the placenta or embryonic tissues, so we cannot be more specific about this advantage.

Embryonic rabbit hemoglobin contains six components (Steinheider et al., 1975; Jelkmann and Bauer, 1978). However we have not done OECs on individual components so we cannot say which components give rise to the high n_H value, and we cannot give a chemical explanation for this phenomenon.

Lower values of n_H have been reported in embryonic red cells of other mammals. Wells and Brittain (1983) in very early sheep embryos, found OECs of a hyperbolic shape with n_H below 1.3. The same authors (Wells and Brittain, 1981) working with mouse embryonic blood separated the OEC into two parts: a lower saturation part that was hyperbolic and without co-operativity, and an upper part with co-operativity. However, in this upper part, the highest value found for n_H in any of their embryos was 3.5 It is therefore not possible to say how widespread in mammals is the high n_H in embryonic blood.

In contrast to our previous findings in embryonic type marsupial blood, the P_{50} of the embryonic rabbit blood is a little lower than that of the mother, that is to say the embryonic OEC is left-shifted when compared to that of the mother. Our values for P_{50} in the 13 and 14 day embryos (28.7 and 27.6 mm Hg respectively) were close to those reported by Jelkmann and Bauer (1977) for 14 day embryos (29 mm Hg). It has not yet been possible to study embryos earlier than 13 days from conception so we do not know whether the relative positions of the maternal and embryonic OECs are reversed at the earliest stages.

SUMMARY

In rabbit embryos, 13 or 14 days after conception, the oxygen equilibrium curve climbs steeply above about 50% saturation. The value of the Hill coefficient (n_H) in the upper part of the curve is significantly greater than 4, indicating aggregation of tetramers or interaction between adjacent tetramers. This is the first time this has been described in blood of a normal eutherian (placental) mammal.

ACKNOWLEDGEMENTS

We thank the staff at the Animal Breeding and Holding Unit of the University of New South Wales for the supply of time-mated rabbits.

The work reported here was supported by the Australian Research Council.

REFERENCES

Calvert, S.J., Holland, R.A.B., and Hinds, L.A., 1992, Blood oxygen carriage and change in hemoglobins during embryonic development of a marsupial, the Tammar Wallaby (*Macropus eugenii*), *Respir. Physiol.*, in Press.

Gill, S.J., Skold, R., Fall, L., Schaeffer, T., Spokane, R., and Wyman, J., 1978, Aggregation effects on oxygen binding of sickle cell hemoglobin, *Science* 201:362-363.

Holland, R.A.B., Calvert, S.J., and Gemmell, R.T., 1991, Oxygen carriage in blood of neonatals and adults of the Brushtail Possum (*Trichosurus vulpecula*, Marsupiala, Phalangeridae), *Proc. Aust. Physiol. Pharmacol. Soc.* 22:117P.

Holland, R.A.B., Rimes, A.F., Comis, A., and Tyndale-Biscoe, C.H., 1988, Oxygen carriage and carbonic anhydrase activity in the blood of a marsupial, the Tammar Wallaby (*Macropus eugenii*), during early development, *Respir. Physiol.* 73:69-86.

Jelkmann, W., and Bauer, C., 1977, Oxygen affinity and phosphate compounds of red blood cells during intrauterine development of rabbits, *Pflügers Arch.* 372:149-156.

Jelkmann, W., and Bauer, C., 1978, Embryonic hemoglobins: dependency of functional characteristics on tetramer composition, *Pflügers Arch.* 377:75-80.

Steinheider, G., Melderis, H., and Ostertag, W., 1975, Embryonic ϵ chains of mice and rabbits, *Nature* 257:714-716.

Tibben, E.A., Holland, R.A.B., and Tyndale-Biscoe, C.H., 1991, Blood oxygen carriage in the marsupial, tammar wallaby, at prenatal and neonatal stages, *Respir. Physiol.* 84:93-104.

Wells, R.M.G., and Brittain, T., 1981, Transition to cooperative oxygen-binding by embryonic haemoglobin in mice, *J. Exp. Biol.* 40:351-355.

Wells, R.M.G., and Brittain, T., 1983, Non-cooperative oxygen binding in the erythocytes of pre-implanted sheep embryos, *Comp. Biochem. Physiol.* 76A:387-388.

MATHEMATICAL SIMULATION OF GAS TRANSPORT AND ACID/BASE REGULATION BY BLOOD FLOWING IN MICROVESSELS -- THE Cl⁻/HCO₃⁻ EXCHANGE ACROSS THE RED CELL MEMBRANE

N.S. Huang[1], J.D. Hellums[2] and J.S. Olson[3]

[1,2]Cox Laboratory for Biomedical Engineering
[3] Department of Biochemistry and Cell Biology
Rice University
Houston, TX 77251-1892

INTRODUCTION

Prior workers have often treated the exchange of HCO_3^- and Cl^- by use of phenomenological permeability coefficients[1-4]. However, discrepancies of several orders of magnitude between the Cl^- permeability as measured by isotope exchange and by net (or conductive) flow with direct electrical measurements practically ruled out the possibility that anions as such diffuse across the membrane[5]. Those data and other experimental evidence suggest that the exchange mechanism is carrier-mediated; the carrier is capable of one-for one exchange of anions, but does not permit the net flow of anions across the membrane. As a result, the permeability values are only "effective" and must be interpreted accordingly. Therefore, in this work, we studied a mediated-transport system. Most of the experimental evidence on the exchange kinetics point toward the single-site "ping-pong" mechanism with obligatory exchange[5-11]. The general features of the ping-pong mechanism are illustrated in Figure 1. In the ping-pong mechanism, the anions take turns crossing the membrane rather than switching place simultaneously; and the protein has two structurally distinct states, an inward-facing state and an outward-facing state. Thus, it is an alternating site transporter possessing a single transport site which is alternatively exposed to the opposite sides of the membrane. This site can only cross the membrane when it is occupied by a substrate anion; it then undergoes a conformational change to face the opposite side of the membrane and releases the transported ion. The transported site can now bind another (or the same) anion and return to the original membrane face, release the anion to complete a cycle of anion exchange.

---

[1] N. S. Huang is now with Exxon Production Research Co., Houston, Texas.
[2] Author for correspondence.
This work was supported by the NIH under grant R01 HL 19824.

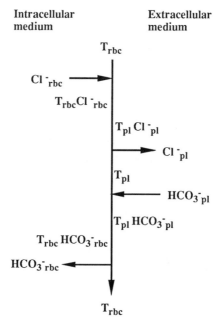

Intracellular medium

Extracellular medium

T_{rbc}

Cl^-_{rbc} →

$T_{rbc}Cl^-_{rbc}$

$T_{pl}Cl^-_{pl}$

→ Cl^-_{pl}

T_{pl}

← $HCO_3^-_{pl}$

$T_{pl}HCO_3^-_{pl}$

$T_{rbc}HCO_3^-_{rbc}$

$HCO_3^-_{rbc}$ ←

T_{rbc}

Figure 1. Diagram of a ping-pong mechanism for anion transport. Shown here is the exchange of an intracellular Cl^- for an extracellular HCO_3^-.

SIMPLIFICATION OF THE PING-PONG MECHANISM

The scheme illustrated in Figure 2 was proposed by Frohlich and Gunn [9]. They attempted to use the minimal number of reaction steps and different kinetic states of the anion transporter that are necessary to describe the one-for-one exchange of the anions. They decomposed the exchange process into three steps: (1) binding of the anion to the transport molecule at one surface of the membrane, (2) translocation of the anion across the membrane, and (3) dissociation of the anion from the transport molecule at the opposite surface.

Detailed mathematical description of the exchange kinetics at this level would be cumbersome. Falke and co-workers [7, 12] utilized $^{35}Cl^-$ nuclear magnetic resonance (NMR) and $^{37}Cl^-$ NMR to set lower limits on the rates of chloride binding and dissociation at the saturated inward- and outward-facing transport sites. Their data showed that Cl^- binding and dissociation at the saturated sites are not rate-limiting, indicating that translocation of bound Cl^- across the membrane is the slowest step in the overall transport cycle. If the translocation step is also relatively slower than the HCO_3^- dissociation step, one can then simplify the kinetic analysis by letting the translocation step be rate limiting or alternatively by letting the association and dissociation reactions be at equilibrium. In addition, the principle of microscopic reversibility for a passive system requires that for the hexagonal scheme of Figure 2: $k_1k_2k_{-3}k_4k_{-5}k_{-6} = k_{-1}k_{-2}k_3k_{-4}k_5k_6$ which in turn becomes: $K_1K_2K_4/K_3K_5K_6=1$, where the $K_i = k_i/k_{-i}$.

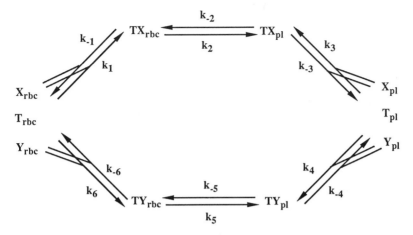

Figure 2. Description of the catalytic cycle of anion exchange according to the ping-pong scheme.

where

T_{rbc} and T_{pl} are the unloaded forms of the transporter in which a single anion binding/transport site is accessible to only intra- or extracellular anions, respectively,

TX_{rbc}, TX_{pl}, TY_{rbc} and TY_{pl} denote the complexes of the transporter with the anions X (Cl^-) and Y (HCO_3^-).

k_1, k_3, k_4 and k_6 are the association rate constants.

k_{-1}, k_{-3}, k_{-4} and k_{-6} are the dissociation rate constants.

k_2 and k_5 are the outward translocation rate constants.

k_{-2} and k_{-5} are the inward translocation rate constants.

For a first order approximation of the anion exchange, additional assumptions are introduced to further simplify the expression for the flux.

(1)   The translocation step is assumed to be the rate limiting step.

(2) k_{trans}, the translocation rate constant, is assumed to be independent of the type of bound anions as well as independent of the direction of the translocation. Therefore, $k_{trans}=k_2=k_{-2}=k_5=k_{-5}$.

(3)   Equilibrium association constants (K_As) for Cl^- and HCO_3^- are assumed to be the same in both membrane compartments (i.e., facing-inward and facing-outward) as suggested by Lemon[17]. Therefore, $K_A=K_1=K_3=K_4=K_6$.

(4)   Both k_{trans} and K_A are assumed to be independent of pH based on reports by several prior works [13-16].

Upon introducing assumptions (1) - (4), a simplified flux expression was developed. It is mathematically more tractable and contains only two kinetic parameters, k_{trans} and K_A.

$$Flux_{HCO3} = T_{tot}\, k_{trans}\, K_A \left([Cl^-]_{rbc}\, [HCO_3^-]_{pl} - [Cl^-]_{pl}\, [HCO_3^-]_{rbc} \right) \Big/$$
$$\left\{ [Cl^-]_{rbc} + [Cl^-]_{pl} + [HCO_3^-]_{rbc} + [HCO_3^-]_{pl} + 2\, K_A \left([Cl^-]_{rbc}\, [Cl^-]_{pl} + \right.\right.$$
$$\left.\left. [HCO_3^-]_{rbc}\, [HCO_3^-]_{pl} + [Cl^-]_{rbc}\, [HCO_3^-]_{pl} + [Cl^-]_{pl}\, [HCO_3^-]_{rbc} \right) \right\} \quad (1)$$

Equation (1) predicts that there is a net influx of HCO_3^- into RBCs or a net efflux of Cl^- entering the extracellular medium as long as

$$\frac{[HCO_3^-]_{pl}}{[HCO_3^-]_{rbc}} > \frac{[Cl^-]_{pl}}{[Cl^-]_{rbc}} \qquad (2)$$

Cabantchik[5] pointed out that for thermodynamic reasons even in the carrier model in which no electrical driving force is considered and in which ions are assumed to carry no current across the membrane, one would predict the same relationship between the equilibrium distribution ratio of the various ions. Therefore Equation (1) is consistent with the Donnan-type distribution of ions (Equation (2)) which is approached at equilibrium when the net flux must be zero.

METHODS OF VALIDATION OF THE SIMPLIFIED PING-PONG MODEL

The transmembrane movements of the Cl^- can be monitored without serious complications, but movements of HCO_3^- must take into account the following equilibria: $CO_2 + H_2O \Leftrightarrow H_2CO_3 \Leftrightarrow H^+ + HCO_3^-$. Two methods of overcoming this difficulty are discussed below.

When an intracellular Cl^- exchanges for an extracellular HCO_3^-, subsequent operation of Jacobs-Stewart Cycle (Figure 3) leads to production of one extracellular H^+ and the absorption of one intracellular H^+. In principle, it is therefore possible to measure Cl^-/HCO_3^- exchange by following changes in extracellular pH, provided that the anion exchange is the rate-limiting step in the cycle and that the pH measuring technique has a sufficiently fast response. In human red blood cells under normal circumstances steps 2 and 3, as illustrated in Figure 3, are very much faster than anion exchange (step 1) because intracellular hydration of CO_2 is catalyzed by carbonic anhydrase and the physical diffusion of CO_2 cross the membrane is rapid. The rate of hydration of extracellular H_2CO_3 is much slower. This difficulty can be overcome by adding carbonic anhydrase to the extracellular medium in a concentration sufficient to leave Cl^-/HCO_3^- exchange as the rate-limiting step in the cycle. The rate of change in pH which reflects the operation of Jacobs-Stewart cycle, can then be taken as a measure of the rate of Cl^-/HCO_3^- exchange. This method was used by Chow et al. [1], Obaid and Crandall [13] and Lemon [17].

An alternative approach to measurement of the anion exchange is one in which the Jacobs-Stewart cycle is prevented by inhibiting the catalyzed hydration of CO_2 by carbonic anhydrase. When this is done, rates of CO_2 transport become very slow compared with rates of anion exchange and isotopically labeled HCO_3^- can be used to monitor HCO_3^- movement. The carbonic anhydrase activity is effectively eliminated by using resealed red cell ghosts in which the enzyme is replaced by an inhibitor of carbonic anhydrase. In this method, Cl^--containing cells are placed in a Cl^--free medium that contains $H^{14}CO_3^-$ ion, and the influx of radioactivity is a good measure of HCO_3^- transport [18]. Other experiments in the presence of carbonic anhydrase inhibitor have measured Cl^- concentration to follow the exchange (Illsley and Verkman's [19]; Klocke[3]).

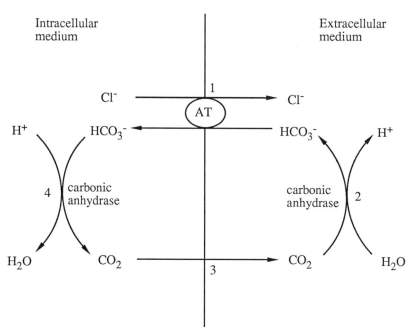

Figure 3. Operation of the Jacobs-Stewart cycle and rapid acidification of the extracellular medium by Cl^-/HCO_3^- exchange after addition of packed RBCs to a Cl^--free media which contains carbonic anhydrase enzyme.

The goal is to characterize k_{trans} and K_A by utilizing available experimental data in the literature. The numerical procedure is initiated by input of the experimental measurements, immediately followed by the usage of a natural cubic spline to smooth the raw data and generate $[C_i]_{exp}$, where C_i denotes all the species that are involved in a particular system. The next step is to supply the inlet or initial conditions and guesses for k_{trans} and K_A. The transient material balance differential equations are then solved with a numerical method; and k_{trans} and K_A are then searched for by a nonlinear least squares fitting method. The nonlinear least squares fitting method searches for the values of both parameters that best fit the experimental data $\{[C_i]_{exp}\}$. In other words, one seeks the values of k_{trans} and K_A which minimize an objective function (A mean square deviation between the calculated and experimental concentrations.). Details of all aspects of the procedure are given by Huang[20].

COMPARISON OF THE SIMULATION RESULTS WITH EXPERIMENTAL DATA

Numerical simulations with iterative determination of the "optimum" values of the two parameters k_{trans} and K_A were carried out for the experiments by each group of investigators discussed above. In addition, the numerical simulations were carried out by use of the passive electrodiffusion model and the "optimum" values of the phenomenological permeabilities, P_{Cl} and P_{HCO3}, were determined. In a number of cases, the simulations were also carried out using values of P_{Cl} and P_{HCO3} from the literature. The methods, conditions and results are given in detail by Huang[21]. Typical simulation results for one case are given in Figure 4.

Figure 4 shows the comparison of the calculations obtained by both models and Illsley and Verkman's [19] red cell ghost chloride/HCO_3 exchange results. Figure 4 illustrates the decrease in intracellular Cl^- concentration following mixture of Cl^--containing ghosts with bicarbonate buffer. The solid line represents the computed $[Cl^-]_{rbc}$ versus time calculated using the simplified ping-pong model with k_{trans}=4.5x10^4 sec^{-1}, K_A=200 M^{-1} (optimum values). The dashed lines in the right-hand-side panel are the computational results generated using the phenomenological permeability coefficients. The results are shown for different values of permeability coefficients, using the set P_{HCO3}=1.1x10^{-3} and P_{Cl} =1.1x10^{-4} cm/sec which represents typical values reported in the literature for anion transport at 37 °C, and the set P_{HCO3} =1.58x10^{-3} and P_{Cl}=4.6x10^{-4} cm/sec which represents the best-fitted values obtained in this study. As can be seen the agreement between the experimental data and the computational results generated by simplified ping-pong model is slightly better than that calculated by the electrodiffusion model. However, the electrodiffusion model can be made to represent the data by choice of permeabilities. The best-fitted kinetic parameters used for both the simplified ping-pong and electrodiffusion simulations for various experimental systems are listed in Table 1.

Permeability coefficients for the best-fitted electrodiffusion for various experimental systems are also listed in Table 1. As illustrated in Figure 4, the usage of permeabilities which are reported in the literature gives predictions that are sometimes in poor agreement with the observed rate of transport. As another illustration, the best-fitted result for Weith's system is achieved using permeabilities which are an order of magnitude higher than the reported literature values. Permeabilities can be found to fit any one set of data adequately. However, there is a wide variation of permeability coefficients reported both in the literature and in this study, because the concentrations of Cl^- and HCO_3^- were varied experimentally over a wide range.

Table 1. Kinetic parameters obtained for Cl^-/HCO_3^- exchange across the RBC membrane from analyzing different workers' experimental data using Equation (4).

	k_{trans} (sec^{-1})	K_A (M^{-1})	P_{HCO3} (cm/sec)	P_{Cl} (cm/sec)
Exchange at 0 °C				
Weith [18]	504	390	3.02x10^{-5}	1.35x10^{-5}
Exchange at 25 °C				
Lemon [17]	1.1x10^4	200	3.16x10^{-4}	3.16x10^{-4}
Exchange at 37 °C				
Klocke [3]	4-6x10^4	200	1.10x10^{-3}	1.10x10^{-4}
Illsley and Verkman [19]	4.5x10^4	200	1.58x10^{-3}	4.60x10^{-4}

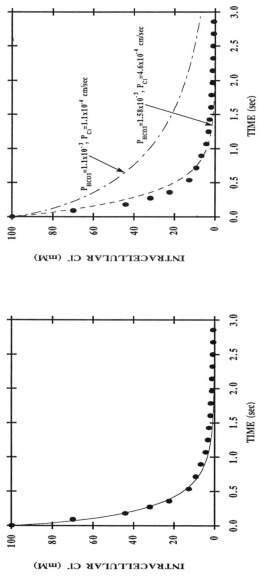

Figure 4. Change in intracellular Cl⁻ concentration following mixture of Cl⁻-loaded RBCs with a Cl⁻-free, HCO₃⁻-containing buffer at 37°C. Illsley and Verkman's experimental results (Illsley and Verkman, 1987) are represented as filled circles. The left panel gives the comparison of simulation result generated using simplified ping-pong model with the experimental data. The theoretical line (———) is calculated with k_{trans} = 4.5x10⁴ sec⁻¹ and K_A = 200 M⁻¹. The right panel gives the comparison of simulation result generated using the constant field electrodiffusion with phenomenological permeability coefficients with the experimental data. The theoretical curve (- - - -) is calculated assuming P_{HCO3}=1.58x10⁻³ and P_{Cl}=4.60x10⁻⁴ cm/sec; (— · —), P_{HCO_3} =1.10x10⁻³ and P_{Cl} =1.10x10⁻⁴ cm/sec.

CONCLUSION

Compared to the electrodiffusion model, the simplified ping-pong model is both on a more satisfactory theoretical basis, and consistently provides better agreement with the available experimental data. Therefore, the conclusion of present work is that simplified ping-pong model has substantial advantages in the mathematical simulation of anion exchange. The ping-pong transporter is suitable for incorporation into a comprehensive model for simulation of gas transport and pH regulation in the microcirculation.

REFERENCES

1. E.I. Chow, E.D. Crandall, and R.E. Forster, Kinetics of bicarbonate-chloride exchange across the human red blood cell membrane. *J. Gen. Physiol.* 68:633 (1976).
2. E.D. Crandall, R.A. Klocke, and R.E. Forster, Hydroxyl ion movements across the human erythrocyte membrane, *J. Gen Physiol* 57:664 (1971).
3. R.A. Klocke, Rate of bicarbonate-chloride exchange in human red cells at 37^0C, *J. Appl. Physiol.* 40:707 (1976).
4. E.P. Salathe, R. Fayad, and S.W. Schaffer, Mathematical analysis of carbon dioxide transport by blood, *Math. Biosci.* 57:109 (1981).
5. Z.I. Cabantchik, P.A. Knauf, and A. Rothstein, The anion transport system of the red blood cell: The role of membrane protein evaluated by the use of probes, *Biochim. Biophys. Acta* 515:239 (1978).
6. A.G. Lowe and A. Lamber, Chloride-bicarbonate exchange and related transport processes, *Biochim. Biophys. Acta* 694:353 (1983).
7. J.J. Falke and S.I. Chan, Evidence that anion transport by band 3 proceeds via a ping-pong mechanism involving a single transport site, *J. Biol. Chem.* 260:2537 (1985).
8. M.L. Jennings, Kinetics and mechanism of anion transport in red blood cells, *Ann. Rev. Physiol.* 47:519 (1985).
9. O. Frohlich and R.B. Gunn, Erythrocyte anion transport: The kinetics of a single-site obligatory exchange system, *Biochim. Biophys. Acta* 864:169 (1986).
10. H. Passow, Molecular aspects of band 3 protein-mediated anion transport across the red blood cell membrane, *Rev. Physiol. Biochem. Pharmacol.* 103:63 (1986).
11. M.L. Jennings, Structure and function of the red blood cell anion transport protein, *Ann. Rev. Biophys. Chem.* 18:397 (1989).
12. J.J. Falke, J.J. Kanes, and S.I. Chan, The kinetic equation for the chloride transport cycle of band 3, *J. Biol. Chem.* 260:9545 (1985).
13. A.L. Obaid and E.D. Crandall, HCO_3^-/Cl^- exchange across the human erythrocyte membrane: Effects of pH and temperature, *J. Membr. Biol.* 50:23 (1979).
14. J.O. Weith, J. Brahm, and J. Funder, Transport and interactions of anions and proteins in the red blood cell membrane, *Ann. N.Y. Acad. Sci* 341:394 (1980).
15. J.O. Weith and P.J. Bjerrum, Titration of transport and modifier sites in the red cell anion transport system, *J. Gen. Physiol.* 79:253 (1982).
16. J.O. Weith, O.S. Andersen, J. Brahm, P.J. Bjerrum, and C.L. Borders, Chloride-bicarbonate exchange in the red cells: Physiology of transport and chemical modification of binding sites, *Phil. Trans. R. Soc. Lond.* 299:383 (1982).
17. D.D. Lemon, Oxygen and carbon dioxide exchange by human hemoglobin and erythrocytes, Ph.D. Thesis, Rice University (1989).
18. J.O. Weith, Bicarbonate exchange through the human red cell membrane determined with [^{14}C] bicarbonate, *J. Physiol.* 294:521 (1979).
19. N.P. Illsley and A.S. Verkman, Membrane chloride transport measured using a chloride-sensitive probe, *Biochemistry* 26:1215 (1987).
20. N.A. Huang, Mathematical simulation of gas transport and acid/base regulation by blood flowing in microvessels, Ph.D. thesis, Rice University (1991).

RED BLOOD CELL VELOCITY IN NAILFOLD CAPILLARIES

DURING HYPERBARIC OXYGENATION

A.J. van der Kleij[1], H. Vink[2], Ch. P. Henny[3],
D.J. Bakker[1], J.A.E Spaan[2]

[1] Departments of Surgery & Hyperbaric Medicine
[2] Departments of Medical Physics & Informatics
[3] Department of Anaesthesiology & Intensive Care
University of Amsterdam & Academic Medical Center
Meibergdreef 9, 1105 AZ Amsterdam,   The Netherlands

INTRODUCTION

Problem wounds are wounds that fail to heal after standard treatment e. g. surgical necrotic tissue debridement, absces drainage, vascular reconstruction etc. Since problem wounds are characterised by hypoxia, hyperbaric oxygen therapy (HBO) is used for treatment, especially in patients with peripheral arterial occlusive disease (Visona et al. 1989). Several authors (Bird and Telfer, 1965; Reich et al., 1970, Hammerlund et al., 1988) have studied the effects of normobaric and hyperbaric oxygen breathing on forearm blood flow in healthy persons and reported a reduction in blood flow apparently counteracting the benefit of hyperoxygenation. On the other hand during hyperoxygenation transcutaneous PO_2 values of over 900 mm Hg have been reported (Dooley and Mehm, 1990, Mathieu et al.,1990) indicating high concentrations of available molecular oxygen in the dermal microcirculation. Intravital capillary microscopy of the nailfold provides information about capillary nutritional blood flow in patients with compromised skin oxygenation (Jacobs et al. 1992). It is not known in what way HBO affects skin capillary nutritional blood flow and how intravital nailfold microscopy can assess the state of hyperoxygenation. The aim of this study was to evaluate the influence of HBO on microcirculatory skin blood flow in healthy volunteers by means of intravital microscopy.

MATERIAL AND METHODS

Measurements were performed in a Multi-Place (93 m³) hyperbaric chamber. Intravital video microscopy (objective: ULWD MSpal 20, NA = 0.40, Olympus) was

Oxygen Transport to Tissue XV, Edited by P. Vaupel
et al., Plenum Press, New York, 1994

used to visualise red blood cell movements in capillaries of healthy volunteers (N=7, age: 22-31 years, male:female ratio = 3:4). As it has been reported (Houben et al., 1992) that day-time variations in micro- and macrocirculatory parameters occur. Therefore each experiment was performed in the early afternoon. Each volunteer was sitting in an upright position with the investigated hand in pronation under the microscope. A drop of glycerin was applied to the skin of the distal phalanx to optimize microscopical visualisation.Subsequently one nailfold capillary of the fourth finger of the left hand was concentrated upon. The optical image was directed to a CCD-camera (model MX1, HCS), mounted on the microscope and directly displayed on a televison monitor (4LC4050, Philips). The final magnification on the monitor screen was 1000 x. Each dimension was calibrated in reference to a stage micrometer (100 X 0.01 = 1mm., Olympus).

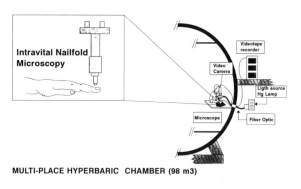

RED BLOOD CELL VELOCITY DURING HYPEROXYGENATION

MULTI-PLACE HYPERBARIC CHAMBER (98 m3)

Department of Hyperbaric Medicine
A M C, AMSTERDAM

Figure 1. Schematic representation of experimental set up. Light source and video recording were placed outside the hyperbaric chamber.

To determine red blood cell velocities (Vrbc) images were recorded on videotape (VTR) for off-line analysis (TV model V6650, Philips) by the frame to frame method. Ambient temperature was registered with a mercury thermometer placed on the examination table, skin temperature of the hand was continuously recorded using an attachable surface temperature-probe (HP, 21078 A). Transcutaneous PO_2 electrodes (heated to 45 °C, TINA™, Radiometer) were applied on the dorsum of the hand (4th metatarsal). Brachial systolic and diastolic blood pressures were measured on the contralateral upperarm. Arterial oxygen saturation and pulse rate were continuously monitored by means of a pulse oximeter (Nellcor, N-180). When $TcPO_2$ was stable each volunteer received 8 liters/min humified (Rendall, aquapack) oxygen by nose-mouth mask (Hudson one, no. 1007). After the trancutaneous partial oxygen pressure had reached a plateau, the ambient pressure was increased from 1 atmosphere (1 ATA) to 3 ATA in approximately 30 minutes. This hyperbaric oxygenation state was maintained for one hour. During this period Vrbc measurements were performed at 5 (T-5), 20 (=T-20), 40 (=T-40) and 60 (=T-60) minutes after reaching 3 ATA (see figure). Subsequently the ambient pressure was reduced back to 1 ATA and the last Vrbc was measured without additional oxygen after the TcPO$_2$ had restabilised (T-120, see figure). All parameters were registered at the same time intervals.

RESULTS

We observed a wide range in ambient temperatures in the time period between changing from normobaric to hyperbaric conditions. As alterations in ambient and skin temperature highly influence mean capillary blood cell velocity (P. Gasser, 1991), we considered the period after the hyperoxygenation state (T-120) as the control period. During hyperbaric conditions ambient temperature remained constant at 27.9 $\pm$ 0.3 °C and the skin temperature at 33.3 $\pm$ 0.6 °C. The results of the microcirculatory parameters are summarized in Table 1. Vrbc showed a continuous increase during the hyperbaric oxygenation state (see figure 2). During control conditions (T=120 minutes), 0.43 $\pm$ 0.12 mm. sec^{-1} (mean $\pm$ sem), Vrbc was significantly (* = P < 0.05) lower compared to Vrbc at the end of hyperbaric oxygenation . Vrbc at T=60 was 0.62 $\pm$ 0.16 (mean $\pm$ sem). TcpO$_2$ values were all significantly increased during the hyperbaric oxygenation state. The temperature of the hand (T$_h$) was significantly decreased during this period.

Table 1. Mean $\pm$ standard error of the mean of microcirculatory parameters, transcutaneous pO$_2$ (TcpO$_2$, mmHg), red blood cell velocity (Vrbc, mm"sec^{-1}), temperature of the hand (T$_h$, °C) and ambient temperature (T$_a$, °C). * means significantly different (P < 0.05) from control (T-120).

	TcpO$_2$	Vrbc	T$_h$	T$_a$
T-5	609.6 $\pm$ 55.7*	411.57 $\pm$ 71.59	32.8 $\pm$ 0.6*	27.5 $\pm$ 0.5
T-20	696.3 $\pm$ 65.5*	416.21 $\pm$ 103.26	32.9 $\pm$ 0.6*	28.0 $\pm$ 0.3
T-40	633.6 $\pm$ 55.9*	565.08 $\pm$ 114.34*	33.3 $\pm$ 0.7*	28.2 $\pm$ 0.2
T-60	683.3 $\pm$ 66.4*	622.94 $\pm$ 156.67*	33.2 $\pm$ 0.6*	28.0 $\pm$ 0.2
T-120	98.1 $\pm$ 8.0	432.39 $\pm$ 120.07	34.4 $\pm$ 0.2	28.0 $\pm$ 0.5

The results of the macrocirculatory parameters are summarized in Table 2. Pulse rate was significantly decreased during hyperoxygenation states (T-20, T-40, T-60) compared to control conditions, whereas no significant changes in mean systolic- and diastolic blood pressure were observed during the same period.

Table 2. Mean $\pm$ Standard error of the mean of macrocirculatory parameters, heart rate (Hr, sec^{-1}), systolic blood pressure (Syst. BP, mm Hg) and diastolic bloodpressure (Diast BP, mm Hg). * means significantly different (P < 0.05) from control (T-120).

	Hr	Syst. BP.	Diast BP.
T-5	75.3 $\pm$ 2.9	127 $\pm$ 5.5	89 $\pm$ 5.4
T-20	67.4 $\pm$ 3.3 *	124 $\pm$ 5.2	85 $\pm$ 5.5
T-40	69.6 $\pm$ 3.0 *	126 $\pm$ 4.5	86 $\pm$ 4.3
T-60	66.6 $\pm$ 2.6 *	124 $\pm$ 4.6	89 $\pm$ 3.6
T-120	74.3 $\pm$ 4.5	126 $\pm$ 7.3	87 $\pm$ 4.8

DISCUSSION

In animals as well as in man hyperoxygenation is associated with blood flow reduction and redistribution (Ackerman and Brinkley, 1966, Muhvich et al., 1992), (Bird and Telfer, 1968; Kenmure et al, 1972; Hansen and Madsen, 1973; Hammerlund et al., 1988; Dooley and Mehm, 1990). While breathing oxygen by mask with an efficacy of 90% and using venous occlusion plethysmography with a Whitney mercury-in-rubber strain gauge at 2 ATA, Bird and Telfer (1966) reported a forearm blood flow reduction of 18.9 % and a calculated oxygen content increase of 18%. These results suggest an unchanged "available oxygen" for (hypoxic) tissue. Consequently the authors hypothesized the existence of a homeostatic mechanism, which under hyperbaric oxigen conditions prevents the high arterial content of available molecular oxygen to reach the tissues. The plethysmographical method is a macrocirculatory parameter, which provides

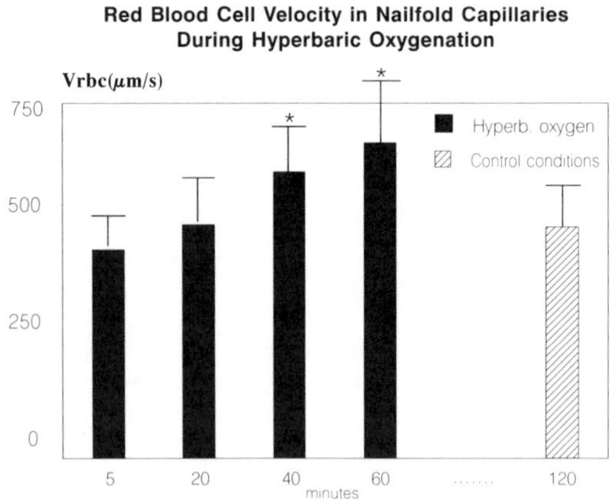

Red Blood Cell Velocity in Nailfold Capillaries During Hyperbaric Oxygenation

Figure 2. Continuous increase of Vrbc during hyperbaric conditions(T-5, T-20, T-40, T60). At T-40 and T-60 Vrbc was significantly increased compared to control conditions, T-120)

limited information about actual functional conditions in the microcirculation. Recently this relative poor correlation between macro and microcirculation has been discussed by Gaehtgens (1992), who emphasized that more knowledge about the relation between variation of total blood flow and microcirculatory network heterogeneity may give a better insight into the discrepancy between these two different types of circulation.

Several indirect and direct methods have been developed, to assess the functional state of the microcirculation. Transcutaneous partial oxygen tension ($TcpO_2$) measurement, as described by Huch et al.(1975), is an indirect method to assess the nutritional skin microcirculation. This method is widely used as assessment method for the severity of peripheral vascular occlusive disease, to select the level of amputation in cases of critical limb ischemia, to monitor tissue viabilty of skin flaps, or after vascular reconstructive procedures (Wyss et al., 1984, Urk van and Feenstra, 1988, Mathieu et al.,1990). Our $TcpO_2$ results coincide with the results reported by other authors (Wyss et al. 1984, Mathieu et al., 1990, Muhvich et al., 1992).

Laser Doppler flowmetry (LDF), another indirect method, was used by Hammerlund et al. (1988) to evaluate the effects of oxygen breathing under hyperbaric conditions. These authors reported a decrease in flow induced by hyperbaric oxygenation. Since most of the LDF signal ($> 80\%$) is dominated by nonnutritional, thermo-regulatory, shunt vessels of the skin (Bollinger and Fagrell, 1990), the findings of Hammerlund et al. indicate a decrease in nonnutritional shunt vessel flow and not a decrease in flow of the nutritional capillaries. The exposure time to hyperoxygenation however was 8 minutes whereas in our study the total exposure time was 60 minutes. In our study the onset of a significant change of Vrbc in nutritional capillaries occurred after a longer exposure to hyperoxygenation (20 minutes), indicating that a longer period of hyperbaric oxygenation may be necessary to be able to find changes within the nutritional capillary network.

During hyperbaric oxygenation the temperature of the hand was significantly decreased compared to control conditions (T-120). This may indicate a reduction in flow within the thermoregulatory capillaries. Since we observed a concurrent increase in Vrbc this may be explained by a flow redistribution form the thermoregulatory capillaries to the nutritional network.

In our opinion it may not be concluded that (hypoxic) tissue can not benefit of hyperbaric oxygenation, since Vrbc increases in the nutritional capillaries which is accompanied by increased TcpO$_2$ values .

CONCLUSIONS

The present study has shown that, in healthy volunteers, during hyperbaric oxygenation, red blood cell velocities in nutritional skin capillaries increased and was accompanied by a significant increase in transcutaneous partial oxygen tension and a significant decrease in the temperature of the hand. It is hypothesized that a redistribution of blood flow between thermoregulatory and nutritional capillaries occurs during hyperbaric oxygenation. Further studies should be performed to investigate whether an increase in red blood cell velocity in the nutritional capillaries during hyperbaric oxygenation will also occur in ischemic tissue .

SUMMARY

Microcirculatory hemodynamics of the skin during hyperbaric oxygenation were assessed by determination of nailfold capillary red blood cell velocity (Vrbc) . Under hyperbaric conditions a continuous increase in Vrbc was found. Control values, 0.43 ± 0.12 mm. sec^{-1} (mean $\pm$ sem), were significantly ($P < 0.05$) lower compared with Vrbc at the end of hyperbaric oxygenation (0.62 ± 0.16 mm. sec^{-1}).

REFERENCES

Ackerman N.B. and Brinkley F.B., 1966, Oxygen tension in normal and ischemic tissues during hyperbaric therapy. *JAMA*. Vol 198, no 12, 1280-1283.

Bird A.D., Telfer A.B.M., 1965, Effect of hyperbaric oxygen on limb circulation. *Lancet*. 1:355-356, 1965.

Bollinger A., Fagrell B., 1990, Clinical Capillaroscopy. A Guide to its Use in Clinical Research and Practice. Publisher Hogrefe & Huber, Toronto, Lewiston NY, Bern, Göttingen, Stuttgart.

Dooley, J.W., Mehm, W.J., 1990, Noninvasive assessment of the vasoconstrictive effects of hyperoxygenation. *Journal of Hyperbaric Medicine.* Vol. 4, No. 4, 177-187.

Gaehtgens P., 1992, Why networks? *Int. J. Microcirc: Clin Exp* 11: 123-132.

Gasser P., 1991, Video-nailfold-microscopy and local cold test: Morphological and hemodynamic correlates in 124 healthy subjects. *Vasa.* Band 20, Heft 3. 244-251.

Hammerlund C., Castenfors J., Svedman P., 1988, Dermal vascular response to hyperoxia in healthy volunteers. In: Hyperbaric Medicine Proceedings on the 2nd Swiss symposium on Hyperbaric Medicine September. p. 55-59. ISBN: 3-908 229-01-4.

Hansen M., Madsen J., 1973, Estimation of relative changes in resting muscle blood flow by ^{133}Xe washout: The effect of oxygen. *Scand. J. clin. Lab. Invest.* 31, 133-139.

Houben A.J.H.M., Schaper N.C., Slaaf D.W., Nieuwenhuijzen Kruseman A.C., 1992, Day time variations in peripheral micro and macrocirculation in man. *Int. J. Microcirculation.* Clin. Exp. Vol 11, Suppl I, S 59.

Jacobs M.J.H.M., Ubbink D.Th., Kitslaar P.J.E.H.M., Tordoir J.H.M., Slaaf D.W., Reneman R.S., 1992, Assessment of the microcirculation provides additional information in critical limb ischemia. *Eur. J. Vasc. Surg.* 6, 135-141.

Kenmure A.C.F., Murdoch W.R., Hutton I., Cameron A. J. V., 1972, Hemodynamic effects of oxygen at 1 and 2 Ata pressure in healthy subjects. *J. Appl. Physiol.* Vol. 32: 2, 223-226.

Mathieu, D., Wattel, F., Bouachour, G., Billard, V., Defoin J.F., 1990, Post-traumatic limb ischemia: Prediction of final outcome by transcutaneous oxygen measurement in hyperbaric oxygen. *J. Trauma.* 30:307-314, 1990.

Muhvich K.H., Piano M.R., Myers R.A.M., Ferguson J.L., Maszella L., 1992, Hyperbaric oxygenation decreases blood flows in normal and septic rats. *Undersea Biomedical Research.* Vol. 19, No.1, 31-40.

Reich T., Tuckman J., Naftchi N.E., Jacobson J.H., 1970, Effect of normo- and hyperbaric oxygenation on resting and postexercise calf blood flow. *J. Appl. Physiol.* 28(3): 275-278.

Urk van H., Feenstra W.A., What can transcutaneous oxygen measurements tell us?, in:"Limb Salvage and Amputation for Vascular Disease, " R. M. Greenhalg, C. W. Jamieson, A. N. Nicolaides, ed., W. B. Saunders Company, Philadelphia, London, Toronto, Montreal, Sidney, Tokyo, 1988.

Visona A., Lusiani L., Rusca F., Barboero D., Ursini F., Pagnan A. Therapeutic, Hemodynamic, And Metabolic effects of hyperbaric oxygenation in peripheral vascular disease. *Angiology.* November, 994-1000, 1989.

Wyss C.R., Matsen III F.A., Simmons C.W., Burgess E.M. Transcutaneous oxygen tension measurements on limbs of diabetic and nondiabetic patients with peripheral vascular disease. *Surgery.* 95, 339-345, 1984.

IMPROVEMENT OF WOUND HEALING IN CHRONIC ULCERS BY HYPERBARIC OXYGENATION AND BY WATERFILTERED ULTRARED A INDUCED LOCALIZED HYPERTHERMIA

Gerd Hoffmann

Sportsmedical Institute Frankfurt/Main
of the Johann Wolfgang Goethe University
Otto-Fleck-Schneise 10, D-W 6000 Frankfurt/Main 71
Federal Republic of Germany

BASICS OF HYPERBARIC OXYGENATION AND WATERFILTERED ULTRARED A INDUCED LOCALIZED HYPERTHERMIA IN DERMATOLOGY

Hyperbaric oxygenation (*HBO*, the intermittent inhalation of pure oxygen with partial pressures higher than normal atmospheric pressure at sea level, nowadays preferably performed in multiplace chambers by breathing pure oxygen through a face mask) can be used to improve healing of problem wounds, like chronic skin ulcers, necrotizing infections, thermal burns, soft tissue radionecrosis and skin grafts (reviews: Fischer et al., 1988; Jain, 1990; Buslau and Hoffmann, 1992).

A decreased oxygen partial pressure in the compromised tissue (hypoxia) is characteristic for wounds. HBO gives benefit to wound healing by increasing oxygen partial pressure in the blood and thereby facilitating oxygen diffusion to the wound tissue (multiplied oxygen partial pressure gradient overwhelms even diffusion difficulties): the increased oxygen partial pressure and raised oxygen amount in the problem tissue improves repair processes, collagen synthesis, neovascularization, epithelialization, phagocyte function and has antimicrobial effects (directly on bacteria and via improved phagocytosis) and reduces oedema by the vasoconstrictive effect of oxygen (Irvin et al., 1966; Winter and Perrins, 1969; Hunt and Pai, 1972; Kivisaari et al., 1975; Hohn, 1977; Knighton et al., 1981; Knighton et al., 1984; Kühne et al., 1985; Fischer et al., 1988; Elstner, 1990; Jain, 1990; Oriani et al., 1990b; Niinikoski et al., 1991; Buslau and Hoffmann, 1992).

These basic pathophysiological principles are as well true to the main subject of interest, the treatment of nonhealing wounds, especially ulcers of different origins, like arterial insufficiency, venous stasis, diabetes, decubitus, or pyoderma gangrenosum:

In most cases chronic ischemic condition is a main underlying factor and therefore HBO has beneficial effects, either as an adjunctive or even as one of the main parts of a therapeutical regimen (Fischer, 1975; Olejniczak, 1975; Hart and Strauss, 1979; Kizer et al., 1982; Heng et al., 1984; Sakakibara, 1987; Yagi, 1987; Yagi, 1990).

Healing or improvement in patients with ulcers, caused by arterial insufficiency, was achieved in the majority of treated patients (Perrins and Barr, 1986; Wattel et al., 1990; Yagi, 1990). Adjunctive HBO is as well successful in venous stasis ulcers (Bass, 1970; Perrins and Barr, 1986; Buslau and Hoffmann, 1992) and in decubital ulcers.

Wound healing improvement in ulcers due to diabetes mellitus is well described (Davis et al., 1988; Cianci et al., 1990; Unger and Lucca, 1990): healing could be achieved in more than 85% (Mathieu and Wattel, 1990), and foot or leg amputations could be avoided e.g. in 95% (compared to 67% without adjunctive HBO) (Oriani et al., 1990a).

Even ulcers, caused by pyoderma gangrenosum, can be treated by HBO up to complete healing (Barr et al., 1972; Thomas et al., 1974; Weyrick et al., 1978; Barr and Perrins, 1987; Buslau and Hoffmann, 1992). Although the pathophysiology of pyoderma gangrenosum is not yet completely understood, it is interpreted as an immunologic process (Göring and Raith, 1989) with reactive vascular changes or an intense vasculitis, causing ischemic ulcers: HBO seems to have effect by improving oxygen partial pressure and suppressing immune responses (Saito et al., 1991; Buslau and Hoffmann, 1992).

HBO has been proven both in healthy persons and in patients to increase oxygen partial pressure in blood and in oxygen consuming tissue (e.g. muscle or skin) (Böhmer, 1990; Hoffmann, 1990; Hoffmann et al., 1990; Böhmer, 1991a).

Localized hyperthermia induced by waterfiltered ultrared A (URA) radiation is a different approach to improve wound healing in chronic ulcers:

Heat acts by two ways: increasing tissue temperature speeds up all metabolic reactions unspecifically, which is especially desired in all regenerative processes including wound healing. In addition heat application is a stimulus to which the human body reacts depending from kind, intensity, duration, and region (local or systemic). In the special situation of chronic ulcers including their infection problems, a contact free method of heat application is most desirable. Ultrared A radiation has good qualities with sufficient depth of penetration: even in the case of relatively superficial absorption of the ultrared A radiation heat transfer by the blood stream and heat conduction lead to a therapeutically usable heat field of deeper tissue regions (Hecht and Schuhmann, 1990; Bickes-Kelleher and Vaupel, 1991; Schaefer et al., 1991; Vaupel et al., 1991).

A speciality of the used ultrared A hyperthermia projector ("Ultrarot A Hyperthermie Projektor 450 W") is, that the radiation is waterfiltered, by this way mostly excluding especially these frequencies or wave lengths, which usually interact with water molecules in the superior layers of the skin and by this cause discomfort. As water is the problematic resonance system in the skin, water is the ideal filter system (Rzeznik and Wangorsch, 1986; Rzeznik and Wangorsch, 1988; Staudt and Ippen, 1989; Braun, 1991; Hoffmann, 1992). Beside the exclusion of ultrared B and C and the border wave length between ultrared A and B (above approx. 1350 nm) as well additional critical wave lengths of 940 and 1130 nm are excluded (Vaupel et al., 1991). The used ultrared A hyperthermia projector overwhelms the necessity of running water as cooling and filtering system. The new ultrared projector stands at the end of a development, which started with the first use of waterfiltered radiation for light and heat therapy in humans at the end of the 19th century. Waterfiltered ultrared A induced hyperthermia causes a remarkable increase in tissue oxygen partial pressure (e.g. measured in muscles) during and even some minutes after administering of ultrared A radiation (Böhmer, 1991b), which is interpreted as increase of microcirculation with post effects greater than with fango.

Ultrared radiation has already been used successfully in the treatment of chronic venous ulcers (Mester and Mester, 1987; Braverman et al., 1988; Sugrue et al., 1990;

Hoffmann, 1992), although others (Staudt and Ippen, 1989) reported no beneficial effects. Even the induction of immunological reactions by ultrared radiation was discussed concerning healing improvement in dermatology (Junaid, 1986).

Common to both methods - HBO and waterfiltered ultrared A induced localized hyperthermia - is, that they do not need any direct mechanical contact to the wound area of the ulcers, by this avoiding additional infection problems. If used correctly and regarding indications and contraindications, both methods are save (concerning HBO: Braun, 1988; Buslau and Hoffmann, 1992; concerning waterfiltered ultrared A induced localized hyperthermia: Staudt and Ippen, 1989; Hoffmann, 1992).

OWN EXPERIENCES

Methods

Patients with mostly chronic leg ulcers (e.g. due to venous insufficiency, arthrogenic reasons, diabetes or pyoderma gangrenosum), already dermatologically treated without success over long periods (up to several years) including all resources of a university dermatologic department, underwent *hyperbaric oxygenation* (45 minutes under full pressure of 1,5 ATA, 5 treatments per week) and / or *localized hyperthermia, induced by a waterfiltered ultrared A radiation* ("Ultrarot-Hyperthermie-Projektor 450 W", Max-Braun-Stiftung, Frankfurt/Main) (starting with 15 minutes, increasing up to 45 minutes per day, 5-7 treatments per week, 275 mW/cm^2 at the wound, 30 cm distance between light projector and wound). Due to the small number of patients available for treatment (including inhomogeneous basic illnesses), the documentation was done casuistically, including photodocumentation.

Results

Improvement of wound healing - from partial effects up to complete wound healing - could be reached by hyperbaric oxygenation and / or waterfiltered ultrared A induced localized hyperthermia.

Both methods were felt to be comfortable: even the direct radiation of wounds by the waterfiltered ultrared A did not cause any pain or discomfort (Hoffmann, 1992).

Example 1. 60 year old female patient, normal weight, without diabetes mellitus or hypertension, borderline cholesterol concentration, no other known risk factors, palpable pedal pulses. In the age of 31 years (1961) fracture of the left lower leg with consecutive Sudeck's atrophy. One year later (1962) first occurrence of a lower leg ulceration. Later on recurring ulcerations, even after a skin transplantation. Since 1988 continuously existing ulceration, mostly without pain: chronic ulcer of the left distal lower leg, phlebologically proofed insufficiency of the vena saphena parva. With conservative treatment (dermatologic local therapy, including silver folium, silver salt chelate gel of phosphorus acid mono-(2-amino-aethyl-)ester, compression etc.) even during a phase of hospitalization, hardly any improvement of the local situation was achieved: In August 1990 a large ulcer with a dimension of approx. 15-20 cm by 8 cm and a depth of 10-15 mm was present.

At that time starting with hyperbaric oxygenation (HBO) as an adjunct. Initially fast diminution of the ulcer: after 15 HBO sessions the ulcer area was decreased to half size with only 2 mm depth. Advantageous change from gram negative to gram positive bacteria. After 40 HBO treatments only three residual ulcers were left. Further wound healing was

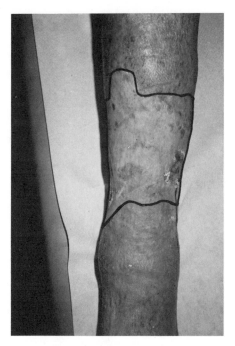

Figure 1. Marked area:
ulcer area before HBO treatment

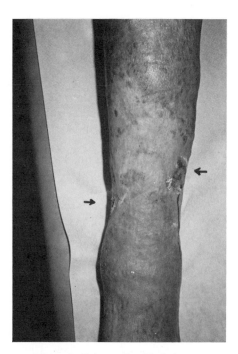

Figure 2. Only small residual ulcers
after 125 HBO treatments

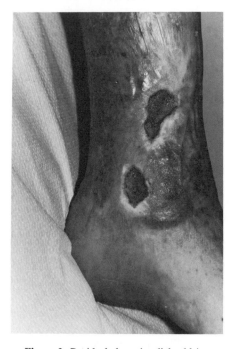

Figure 3. Residual ulcers (medial ankle)
after 175 HBO treatments,
before waterfiltered ultrared A induced
localized hyperthermia

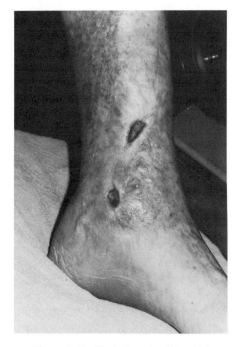

Figure 4. Residual ulcers (medial ankle)
after 175 HBO treatments,
after 65 waterfiltered ultrared A induced
localized hyperthermias

Figures 1 to 4. 60 year old female with chronic ulcer of the left lower leg, chronic venous insufficiency.
(cf. example 1 of text)

more difficult, but successful: After 125 HBO treatments (April 1991) proximal medial long narrow shaped ulcer with a width of only approx. 3 mm, point ulcer at the medial ankle, and lateral ulcer of 2,7 cm by 1,5 cm.

The difference between before HBO and after 125 HBO treatments is striking: the marked area in figure 1 shows the ulcer area before treatment (still recognizable by a lighter skin colour), figure 2 demonstrates the location of the small residual ulcers.

The next four month with additional 50 HBO treatments revealed stagnation with small increases of the area of the three residual ulcers: After one year treatment with a total of 175 HBO sessions the proximal medial ulcer was roundish up to 2 cm diameter, the ulcer at the medial ankle roundish up to 1,5 cm diameter (both shown in figure 3) and the lateral one up to 4 cm diameter.

The stagnation was successfully overcome by waterfiltered ultrared A induced localized hyperthermia, administered five times a week between September and December 1991, even without continuation of HBO. Wound healing improvement with a decreasing area after 13 weeks is documented in figure 4 (Hoffmann, 1992).

Example 2.   A second patient with the use of both methods, HBO and waterfiltered ultrared A induced localized hyperthermia, was a 63 year old slim female (Buslau and Hoffmann, 1992; Hoffmann, 1992). In the age of 23 years (1950) poliomyelitis with consecutive remaining lesions: decreased muscle mass of the left lower leg, stiffness of the left ankle joint, gait disturbance. 1982 fracture of the left femur. Since April 1986 continuously existing lower leg ulcer: arthrogenic (stiffness of the ankle joint, lack of muscle pump function to the veins) with additional toxic compound as side effect of a self administered local therapy. In October 1990 widespread circumferential very painful lower leg ulcer with infection and desolate smeared wound ground and a length of 21 cm.

Within two weeks of HBO treatment (11 sessions) improvement of wound healing with fresh granulation tissue (Buslau and Hoffmann, 1992). After additional skin transplant with unplanned pausing of HBO and thyroid gland problems (including operation) deterioration. Till August 1991 (within 10 month) approx. 150 HBO treatments were given with the effect, that a very serious period with the expected problem of amputation could be overcome and that the usual deterioration in the summer months could be avoided, although wound area kept constant.

Since end of August 1991 up to now (August 1992) waterfiltered ultrared A induced localized hyperthermia was used, resulting in improvement of wound ground (showing better capillarization, freshness and better tendencies towards epithelialization) and in keeping the circumferential ulcer free of infections and avoiding deterioration, although a striking decrease of wound area was not achieved. With the exception of one month, HBO treatment could be stopped (to avoid side effects of very high numbers of HBO sessions).

Example 3.   56 year old female patient with an insulin-dependent diabetes mellitus. More than half a year existing ulcer of the plantar area of the left foot (shown in figure 5). Good improvement within 16 days by 10 HBO treatments (figure 6).

Example 4.   64 year old female patient with chronic venous insufficiency of the left leg (Vena saphena magna and parva), since one year ulcer at the left medial ankle. The improvement of the ulcer by 30 HBO treatments and a few waterfiltered ultrared A induced localized hyperthermias with decreasing area of the ulcer and normalization of the initially highly inflammatory dark red skin towards nearly normal colour is shown in figures 7 (before HBO), 8 (after 3 weeks with 15 HBO treatments), and 9 (after a total of 6 weeks with 30 HBO treatments).

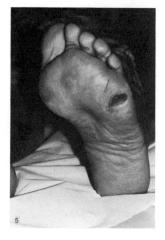 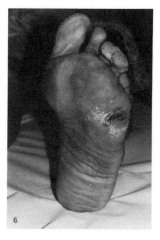

Figures 5 and 6. 56 year old female with chronic plantar ulcer, insulin-dependent diabetes mellitus. Before (fig. 5) and after (fig. 6) 10 hyperbaric oxygenations within 16 days. (cf. example 3 of text)

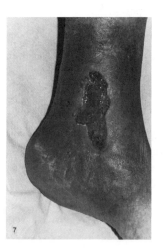 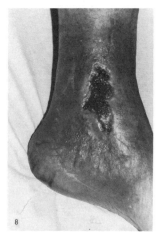 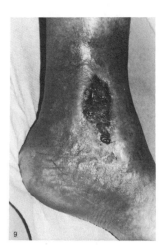

Figures 7, 8, 9. 64 year old female with chronic ulcer at the left medial ankle, chronic venous insufficiency. Before (fig. 7), after 15 (fig. 8), and after 30 (fig. 9) hyperbaric oxygenations.
(cf. example 4 of text)

Example 5. 59 year old overweight male patient. 1 1/2 years existing painful ulcerations of large and increasing size of both dorsal lower legs, suppurating very much, fibrinously covered, marked tissue loss: pyoderma gangrenosum. Parallel to cortisone therapy, HBO and waterfiltered ultrared A induced localized hyperthermia were used, resulting in fresh granulation especially with marked decrease of the initially deep step at the wound borders and with gain of substance (Hoffmann, 1992). Therapy was broken off by the interference of a bleeding gastric ulcer caused by cortisone and analgesics.

Example 6. 37 year old female patient with Crohn's disease (regional ileitis). Since one year recurring lower leg ulceration, evaluated as pyoderma gangrenosum, resistant to immunosuppressive therapy. The combination of 10 HBO treatments with a short period of systemic cortisone therapy resulted in a complete healing of the ulcer within a few weeks, reaching a stable situation (Buslau and Hoffmann, 1992).

Conclusion

Oxygen partial pressure is often diminished in problem wounds or ulcers. HBO is able to increase markedly oxygen partial pressure in tissue, even in problem wounds, and to give by this the basis for a proper wound healing. Ultrared A induced localized hyperthermia increases regional blood flow, oxygen partial pressure and metabolism: this improves wound healing, probably depending from radiation intensity, which can explain the discrepancy to the above quoted negative findings (Staudt and Ippen, 1989), using higher intensities ($500 \, mW/cm^2$).

ACKNOWLEDGMENTS

I want to express my most sincere gratitude for having the chance to use a HBO multiplace chamber and a waterfiltered ultrared A projector to the Vinzenz von Paul Foundation, Basel/Switzerland, and the Max Braun Foundation, Frankfurt/Main, and especially to Dr. med. h.c. Erwin Braun, to whom this work is dedicated.

REFERENCES

Barr, P.O., Enfors, W., Eriksson, G., 1972, Hyperbaric oxygen therapy in dermatology, Br.J.Dermatol.86:631.
Barr, P.O., Perrins, D.J.D., 1987, Prolonged use of hyperbaric oxygen (HBO) in undulant ulcers of the leg, in: Proceeding of the 8th International Congress on Hyperbaric Medicine 1984, Best Publishing Company.
Bass, B.H., 1970, The treatment of varicose leg ulcers by hyperbaric oxygenation, Postgrad. Med. J. 46:407.
Bickes-Kelleher, D.K., Vaupel, P., 1991, Messungen der Temperaturverteilung in einem Agar-Phantom bei Infrarot-A-Bestrahlung und Verwendung einer Wasserkuvette. Abstract for the "12th Conference of the European Society for Hyperthermic Oncology" in Bergen/Norway, June 26-29, 1991.
Böhmer, D., 1990, Influence of hyperbaric oxygenation on muscle pO2, lecture at the "Concilium Hyperbaricum" in Nagoya/Japan, April 13, 1990.
Böhmer, D., 1991a, Der Einfluß der hyperbaren Sauerstoffatmung auf den pO2 des Muskels, in: Sport und Medizin - Pro und Contra, 32. Deutscher Sportärztekongreß vom 18.-21. Oktober 1990 in München, P. Bernett, D. Jeschke, eds., Zuckschwerdt, München.
Böhmer, D., 1991b, Erste Ergebnisse mit dem Ultrarot-Hyperthermie-Projektor 450 W bezüglich intramuskulärem Temperatur- und Sauerstoffpartialdruck-Verlauf im Vergleich zu einer Fangoanwendung, November 19, 1991, Frankfurt/Main.
Braun, E., 1988, Hyperbaric chambers and ancillary equipment: safety, complications and contraindications, in: Handbook of Hyperbaric Oxygen Therapy, B. Fischer, K.K. Jain, E. Braun, S. Lehrl, eds., Springer, Berlin.
Braun, W., and coworkers, 1991, Physik und Technik, in: Ultrarot-Hyperthermie-Projektor 450 W mit maxshydrocuvette, Max Braun Foundation, Frankfurt/Main.
Braverman, B., McCarthy, R.J., Ivankovich, A.D., Tool, K., Overfeld, M., Bapna, M.S., 1988, Evaluation of helium/neon and infrared laser irradiation on wound healing in rabbits, in: ICALEO'87, Proceedings of the Conference on Laser Research in Medicine, San Diego, USA, November 9-11, 1987.
Buslau, M., Hoffmann, G., 1992, Hyperbaric oxygen therapy in the treatment of skin diseases, in: Oxidative Stress in Dermatology, J. Fuchs, L. Packer, eds., Marcel Dekker, New York, in press.
Cianci, P., Petrone, G., Drager, S., Lueders, H., Lee, H., Shapiro, R., 1990, Salvage of the difficult wound/ potential amputation in the diabetic patient, in: Hyperbaric Medicine, Proceedings of the Joint Meeting, held in Basel, on September 22-24, 1988, D. Bakker, J. Schmutz, eds., Foundation for Hyperbaric Medicine, Basel.
Davis, J.C., Buckley, C.J., Barr, P., 1988, Compromised soft tissue wounds: correction of wound hypoxia, in: Problem Wounds - The Role of Oxygen, J.C. Davis, T.K. Hunt, eds., Elsevier, New York.
Elstner, E.F., 1990, Der Sauerstoff, BI-Wissenschaftsverlag, Mannheim.
Fischer, B., Jain, K.K., Braun, E., Lehrl, S., 1988, Handbook of Hyperbaric Oxygen Therapy, Springer, Berlin
Fischer, B.H., 1975, Treatment of ulcers on the legs with hyperbaric oxygen. J. Dermatol. Surg. Onc. 1:45.
Göring, H.D., Raith, L., 1989, Immundermatologie, Ueberreuther, Wien.
Hart, G.B., Strauss, M.B., 1979, Responses of ischaemic ulcerative conditions to OHP, in: Hyperbaric Medicine, G. Smith, ed., Aberdeen University Press, Aberdeen.
Hecht, H.C., Schuhmann, E., 1990, Die Infrarot-A-Strahlung, ein therapeutisches Mittel mit Tiefenwirkung, lecture at the "6. Treffpunkt Medizintechnik", November 15, 1990, Berlin.
Heng, M.C.Y., Pilgrim, J.P., Beck, F.W.J., 1984, A simplified hyperbaric oxygen technique for leg ulcers. Arch. Dermatol. 120:640.

Hoffmann, G., 1990, Experiences with hyperbaric oxygenation in the Sportsmedical Institute Frankfurt/Main, lecture at the "Concilium Hyperbaricum" in Nagoya/Japan, April 13, 1990.

Hoffmann, G., 1992, Grundlagen und Anwendungen des Ultrarot-Hyperthermie-Projektors 450 W aus internistischer und sportmedizinischer Sicht, Frankfurt/Main, 1992.

Hoffmann, G., Böhmer, D., Ambrus, C., Zimmer, P., 1990, Working capacity and changes of blood variables during exercise tests before and after hyperbaric oxygenation. Undersea Biomed. Res. 17(suppl.):62.

Hohn, D., 1977, Leucocyte phagocytic function and dysfunction. Surg. Gynecol. Obstet. 144:99.

Hunt, T.K., Pai, M.P., 1972, The effect of varying ambient oxygen tensions on wound metabolism and collagen synthesis. Surg. Gynecol. Obstet. 135:561.

Irvin, T.T., Norman, J.N., Suwanagul, A., Smith, G., 1966, Hyperbaric oxygen in the treatment of infections by aerobic microorganisms, Lancet 1966:392.

Jain, K.K., 1990, Textbook of Hyperbaric Medicine, Hogrefe and Huber, Toronto.

Junaid, A.J., 1986, Treatment of cutaneous leishmaniasis with infrared heat, Int. J. Dermatol. 25:470.

Kivisaari, J., Vihersaari, T., Renvall, S., Niinikowski, J., 1975, Energy metabolism of experimental wounds at various oxygen environments, Ann. Surg. 181:823.

Kizer, K.W., Kramm, J., Dobbs, L., 1982, Hyperbaric oxygen therapy of refractory skin ulcers, in: Proceeding of the VIIth Annual Conference on Clinical Applications of HBO, Anaheim, California.

Knighton, D.R., Halliday, B., Hunt, T.K., 1984, Oxygen as an antibiotic, the effect of inspired oxygen on infection, Arch. Surg. 121:199.

Knighton, J., Silver, A., Hunt, T.K., 1981, Regulation of wound-healing angiogenesis - effect of oxygen gradients and inspired oxygen concentration, Surgery 90:262.

Kühne, H.H., Ullmann, U, Kühne, F.W., 1985, New aspects on the pathophysiology of wound infection and wound healing - the problem of lowered oxygen pressure in the tissue, Infection 13:52.

Mathieu, D., Wattel, F., 1990, Hyperbaric oxygen in the treatment of the diabetic foot, Undersea Biomed. Res. 17(suppl.):160.

Mester, A., Mester, A.F., 1987, Data for laser biostimulation in wound-healing, in: Laser Optoelectronics in Medicine, vol. 2, Springer, Berlin.

Niinikoski, J., Gottrup, F., Hunt, T.K., 1991, The role of oxygen in wound repair, H. Janssen, R. Rooman, J.I.S. Robertson, eds., Wrightson Biomedical Publishing, Petersfield.

Olejniczak, S., 1975, Employment of low hyperbaric therapy in management of leg ulcers, Mich. Med. 74:1067

Oriani, G., Mazza, D., Sacchi, C., Faglia, E., Favales, F., Mazzola, E., Mastropasqua, A., Pizzi, G.L., 1990a, Hyperbaric oxygen therapy in treatment of diabetic gangrene, Undersea Biomed. Res. 17(suppl.):160.

Oriani, G., Pedesini, G., Nicolosi, M., Meazza, D., Sacchi, C., 1990b, Complicated peripheral wounds and hyperbaric oxygen therapy, in: Hyperbaric Medicine, Proceedings of the Joint Meeting, held in Basel, on September 22-24, 1988, D. Bakker, J. Schmutz, eds., Foundation for Hyperbaric Medicine, Basel.

Perrins, J.D., Barr, P.O., 1986, Hyperbaric oxygenation and wound healing, in: Proceedings of the 1st Swiss Symposium on Hyperbaric Medicine, J. Schmutz, ed., Foundation for Hyperbaric Medicine, Basel.

Rzeznik, J., Wangorsch, G., 1986, Physikalische Grundlagen der IR-A-Hyperthermie, geriatrics pregeriatrics rehabilitation 2: no. 73.

Rzeznik, J., Wangorsch, G., 1988, Physikalische Grundlagen der lokalen Hyperthermie, Geriatrie Rehabil. 1:35

Saito, K., Tanaka, Y., Ota, T., Eto, S., Yamashita, U., 1991, Suppressive effect of hyperbaric oxygenation on immune responses of normal and autoimmune mice. Clin. Exp. Immunol. 86:322.

Sakakibara, K., Takahashi, H., Kobayashi, S., 1987, The role of hyperbaric oxygen in the salvage of ischemic limbs from inevitable amputation in chronic peripheral vascular disease with particular reference to those having had unsuccessful surgery, in: Proceedings of the 8th International Congress on Hyperbaric Medicine, 1984, Best Publishing Company.

Schaefer, C., Kelleher, D.K., Vaupel, P., 1991, Tumor energy status and metabolic changes upon localized hyperthermia using water-filtered infrared-A-radiation, Strahlentherapie Onkologie 167:354.

Staudt, R., Ippen, H., 1989, Erfahrungen mit einem neuartigen Infra-Rot-Strahler - eine Entwicklung des Erwin Braun Institutes, Basel, Geriatrie Rehabilitation 2:71.

Sugrue, M.E., Carolan, J., Leen, E.J., Feeley, T.M., Moore, D.J., Shanik, G.D., 1990, The use of infrared laser therapy in the treatment of venous ulceration, Ann. Vasc. Surg. 4:179.

Thomas, C.Y., Crouch, J.A., Guastello, J., 1974, Hyperbaric oxygen therapy for pyoderma gangrenosum, Arch. Dermatol. 110:445.

Unger, H.D., Lucca, M., 1990, The role of hyperbaric oxygen therapy in the treatment of diabetic foot ulcers and refractory osteomyelitis, Clin. Podiatr. Med. Surg. 7:483.

Vaupel, P., Stohrer, M., Groebe, K., Rzeznik, J., 1991, Localized hyperthermia in superficial tumors using waterfiltered infrared-A-radiation: evaluation of temperature distribution and tissue oxygenation in subcutaneous rat tumors, Strahlentherapie Onkologie 167:353.

Wattel, F., Mathieu, G., Coget, J.M., Billard, V., 1990, Hyperbaric oxygen therapy in chronic vascular wound management, Angiology 59.

Weyrick, W.J., Mader, J.T., Butler, E., Hulet, W.H., 1978, Hyperbaric oxygen treatment of pyoderma gangrenosum, Arch. Dermatol. 114:1232.

Winter, G.D., Perrins, D.J.D., 1969, Effects of hyperbaric oxygen therapy on epidermal regeneration, in: H. Wada, T. Iwa, eds., William and Wilkins, Baltimore.

Yagi, H., 1987, On the hyperbaric oxygen therapy for severe infected granulation wounds (ulcers) of upper and lower extremities, Jpn. J. Hyperbaric Med. 22:27.

Yagi, H., Okadome, K., Fukuda, A., Funahashi, S., Sugimachi, K., 1990, Therapy for problem wounds of ischemic limb with hyperbaric oxygen, in: EUBS 1990 Proceedings, W. Sterk, L. Geeraedts, eds., Foundation for Hyperbaric Medicine, Amsterdam.

LIPID PEROXIDE-RELATED HEMODILUTION DURING REPETITIVE HYPERBARIC OXYGENATION

Monika Brichta[1], Lutz Hock[2], Jürgen Plöse[2], Hermann Kappus[3], Ralph Beneke[1], and Claus Behn[1*]

[1] Institute of Sports Medicine, UKS
[2] Institute of Hyperbaric and Diving Medicine , OHH
[3] Department of Dermatology, UKRV
   Free University Berlin
   D-W1000 Berlin 33
   Germany

INTRODUCTION

Tissue oxygen tension can be elevated under controlled conditions by simultaneously increasing the O_2 concentration of inspired air and the ambient pressure (Jamieson and Van Den Brank,1963). Increasing tissue oxygen tension by hyperbaric oxygenation (HBO) reduces organ blood flow (Muhvich et al.,1992; Bergö and Tyssebotn,1992) as well as some forms of edema (Nylander et al.,1985; Yamaguchi et al.,1990; Gehrs et al.,1991). An acutely reversible decrease of blood hemoglobin concentration by HBO (Bergö and Tyssebotn, 1992) further suggests hyperoxia affecting body fluid distribution.

Increasing tissue oxygen tension augments oxygen radical production (Freeman and Crapo,1981; Freeman et al.,1982). HBO leads to oxidative damage by producing reactive O_2 intermediates (Jamieson et al., 1986; Thom and Marquis,1987; Yusa et al.,1987; Zhang and Piantadosi,1991). Lipid peroxidation seems to be an immediate cause of tissue damage (Hiramitsu et al.,1976; Torbati et al.,1991; Monstrey et al.,1991). Lipid peroxides also lead to vasoconstriction (Simon et al.,1990). HBO-induced vasoconstriction is prevented by antioxidants (Jacobson et al.,1992).

Brief episodes of lipid peroxidation can lead to persistent changes in cell function (Flohe et al.,1978; Kappus,1985). Moreover, lipid peroxidation reaction products may diffuse away from the production site, leading to further damage at distant sites (Benedetti et al., 1979). Lipid peroxidation products and/or effects may, therefore, accumulate when, as under clinical conditions, HBO is repetitively applied. Renal blood flow remains depressed in rats

---

* On leave to Department of Physiology and Biophysics, University of Chile, POB 70005, Santiago 7, Chile, where correspondence should be addressed

for at least 20 min after an acute HBO exposure (100% O_2, 202.6 kPa) of similar duration (Muhvich et al.,1992). Blood flow also remains reduced in some cerebral regions after HBO (Bergö and Tyssebotn,1992). Thus, it is not unlikely that repetitive HBO leads to sustained vasoconstriction implying corresponding changes in capillary filtration equilibrium. Red blood cell count (RBC), blood hemoglobin concentration (Hb), hematocrit (Hct) and plasma protein concentration (TPC) were, therefore, measured in HBO-exposed volunteers to search for shifts in extracellular fluid distribution. Lipid peroxidation was estimated by measuring plasma thiobarbituric acid-reactive substances (TBARS) in plasma as well as urine chemiluminescence (CHL). Oxidative stress resulting from HBO was further investigated by administering high doses of the antioxidant vitamins C and E.

METHODS

Ten healthy male volunteers (30±6 years) were exposed for one hour daily to 240 kPa ambient pressure while breathing 100% O_2. For HBO application up to four volunteers entered a Starmed 2000/5,5 hyperbaric chamber (Haux, Karlsbad-Ittersbach) which was air pressurized within two min to 240 kPa. The volunteers were then provided with 100% oxygen supplied from external flasks via tight-fitting oronasal masks. Expired air was conducted through a valve to the outside of the chamber. After one hour, the chamber was decompressed within two min down to atmospheric pressure, and the O_2 administration terminated. During HBO application the contact with the volunteers was maintained by phone and video. Temperature and total pressure, as well as O_2 and CO_2 concentrations inside the chamber were continuously monitored. After completing a five-day series of HBO exposure (series A), the volunteers were supplemented for 18 days with vitamin C and E in oral doses of 3g/die, respectively. During the final four days of antioxidant vitamin supplementation, HBO was applied again as above (series B), the subjects acting as their own controls.

Blood (antecubital vein puncture) and urine samples were collected immediately before and after each HBO application. Heparinized blood was used for the determination of RBC, Hb and Hct by standard methods (Coulter Counter Electronics, Krefeld). In serum obtained from untreated blood samples, TPC and bilirubin (Br) concentration were assayed by the Biuret and the diazonium method, respectively, using an Hitachi Boehringer Mannheim 704 Automatic Analyzer. Plasma haptoglobin concentration (Hp) was determined by using NOR-Partigen-Immunodiffusion plates (Behringwerke, Marburg). Plasma separated by centrifugation of EDTA treated blood (3000 rpm, 10 min) was stored at -80° C for later asssessment of lipid peroxidation by measuring TBARS in thawed samples with a Shimadzu RF 540 spectrofluorimeter (Yagi, 1976), the results being expressed in malondialdehyde (MDA) equivalents.

Degradation of lipid peroxidation products is accompanied by light emission (Boveris et al.,1980). Lipid peroxide levels in urine were, therefore, estimated by measurement of CHL according to Lissi (personal communication). Immediately after being collected, urine samples were gassed with N_2 for 2 min and stored at $^-$80°C until further processing. Prior to measurement the urine was thawed, titrated to pH 6 and diluted with aqua dest. to an extinction of 0.2. The titrated and diluted urine was subjected to photon counting for light emission in a Biolumat 9500 chemiluminometer (Berthold, Wildbad), the results being standardized for creatinin concentration (Boehringer Mannheim). Results from samples obtained immediately before and after each HBO application were averaged to yield individual values. Data are reported as means±SE. For analysis of differences Student's paired t test was applied. Statistical significance was defined as $p < 0.05$.

RESULTS

Repetitive HBO reduces RBC, Hb, Hct and TPC. This effect is abolished if a vitamin supplement is given. Hp and Br are not affected by HBO (Table 1).

MDA, on the other hand, is increased by HBO, if supplemental vitamins are not given. Supplemental vitamin intake also prevents the HBO-induced MDA increase. CHL is reduced in the presence as compared to the absence of supplemental vitamins (p<0.05). In the latter case, however, CHL decreases in the course of repetitive HBO application (Table 1).

Table 1. Hematological and lipid peroxidation parameters in volunteers subjected to repetitive HBO (100% O_2, 240 kPa, 1 h/die) without (A) and with (B) a supplement of either 3g/die vitamin C and E. Mean values ± SE (n=10).

Series	A		B	
Days	1	5	1	4
RBC (T/l)	4.86 ± 0.11	4.66 ± 0.11[a]	4.75 ± 0.12	4.68 ± 0.11
Hb (g/l)	149 ± 3	143 ± 2 [a]	144 ± 2	143 ± 2
Hct (%)	45.3 ± 0.8	43.4 ± 0.6 [a]	43.9 ± 0.6	43.8 ± 0.8
TPC (g/l)	75.8 ± 0.8	72.0 ± 0.9 [a]	74.7 ± 0.9	73.6 ± 0.8
Hp (g/l)	1.42 ± 0.20	1.47 ± 0.21	1.53 ± 0.21	1.37 ± 0.19
Br (mg/l)	6.7 ± 0.8	6.8 ± 0.7	6.0 ± 0.8	7.3 ± 0.8
MDA (µmol/l)	6.6 ± 0.3	12.4 ± 1.3[a]	6.1 ± 0.4	5.4 ± 0.3
CHL (RU/mg cr)	42.8 ± 5.4	28.9 ± 2.1[b]	24.5 ± 1.7	23.7 ± 0.8

RBC, red blood cell count; Hb, blood hemoglobin concentration; Hct, hematocrit; TPC, total plasma protein concentration; Hp, plasma haptoglobin concentration; Br, serum bilirubin concentration; MDA, plasma malondialdehyde concentration; CHL, urine chemiluminescence; RU, relative units; cr, creatinine.
[a] Significantly different from day 1 value of the same series (p<0.001).
[b] id. (p<0.01).

The evolution of RBC count and MDA during HBO application with and without supplemental vitamin intake is shown in Fig.1. In the absence of supplemental vitamins, RBC and MDA appear to be interrelated (Fig. 2).

DISCUSSION

Repetitive HBO is shown in the present study to induce hemodilution, which occurs together with an increase in lipid peroxidation, both effects apparently being prevented by high doses of antioxidant vitamins. HBO may lead to extracellular fluid redistribution, and/or to body fluid retention, via lipid peroxide mediated vascular effects.

Evidence for HBO-induced hemodilution is provided by the decrease of RBC, Hb, Hct and TPC occurring in the absence of vitamin supplementation (Table 1). HBO is known to reduce RBC survival (Landaw et al.,1979) and Hct (Buxton, et al., 1964; Pilgramm et al.,1986) as well as to increase Br (Pilgramm et al.,1986). Hp and Br, however, did not change during HBO application in the present study (Table 1). It is possible that some hemolysis occured, but was not detected. Even if increased by HBO, hemolysis does not

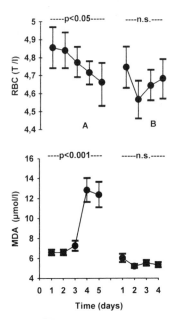

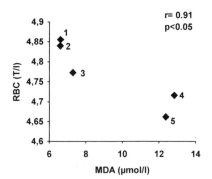

Fig. 1. Red blood cell count (RBC) and plasma malondialdehyde concentration (MDA) during repetitive HBO (100% O_2, 240 kPa, 1h/die). Series A without and B with vitamin C and E supplementation (3g/die, respectively). Means ± SE (n=10).

Fig. 2. Relationship between red blood cell count (RBC) and plasma malondialdehyde concentration (MDA) during repetitive HBO (100% O_2, 240 kPa, 1h/die). The points represent mean values obtained in 10 volunteers subjected to HBO for five days without vitamin supplement. The markers of the points indicate the day of HBO application.

seem to constitute the sole cause of the observed RBC reduction. The fact that HBO-induced RBC reduction occurs in the absence of significant changes in hemolysis and individual cell volume and is accompanied by a decrease in TPC (Table 1) suggests its major cause being hemodilution.

HBO-induced hemodilution has been shown in the present study to be prevented by a supplement of antioxidant vitamins (Table 1). MDA, an indicator of lipid peroxidation, increases when RBC decreases as a consequence of HBO (Fig. 1). MDA appears, moreover, to be linearly related to RBC (Fig. 2). Lipid peroxidation seems, therefore, to be involved in HBO-induced hemodilution.

A single 90 min HBO (200 kPa) application does not have measurable effects on MDA (Grim et al.,1989). In the present study we observed an increase in MDA beginning at day 4 if no supplemental vitamins were given (Fig.1). Lipid peroxidation tends to self perpetuate (Kappus,1985). Lipid peroxides may, therefore, accumulate, particularly, if HBO is repetitively applied. In the absence of supplemental antioxidant vitamins, elimination of lipid peroxides may then be exceeded by their production. Elimination may, moreover, be decreased by reduction of renal excretion. CHL appears to be elevated during series A with respect to series B ($p<0.05$) corresponding with the absence and presence of antioxidant vitamins, respectively (Table 1). The decrease of CHL during series A (Table 1) could be the result of retention of lipid peroxides by the kidney. Renal blood flow reduction by HBO (Muhvich et al.,1992) could, thus, be involved in lipid peroxide as well as in fluid retention.

Oxidatively modified LDLs have been shown by Simon et al. (1990) to induce vasoconstriction by impairment of normal endothelial vasodilator function. The oxidant lipid peroxide *tert*-butyl hydroperoxide (Gurtner et al.,1985) increases thromboxane synthesis, this effect being inhibited by vitamin E. An increase of thromboxane synthesis seems to be a major cause of HBO-induced vasoconstriction (Jacobson et al.,1992).

In summary, HBO may lead to extracellular fluid redistribution and/or body fluid retention, possibly by lipid peroxide-mediated vasoconstriction.

Acknowledgments

We thank Dr. M. Artuc from the Deparment of Dermatology, UKRV, Free University Berlin (FUB) and Professor E. Lissi, Department of Chemistry, University of Santiago (Chile), for advice on MDA determination and CHL measurement, respectively. We are grateful to Mrs. Jutta Nadol and Mrs. Evelyne Rütz (Institute of Sports Medicine) as well as to Ms. Manuela Lücke and Mr. K. Petruschke (Institute of Hyperbaric and Diving Medicine) for valuable technical help. Thank also to Dr. E. Schwartz (Faculty of Biology, FUB) for critical reading the paper.

REFERENCES

Benedetti, A., Casini, A.F., Ferrali, M.,and Comporti, M., 1979, Effects of difusible products of peroxidation of rat liver microsomal lipids, *Biochemical J.* 180:303.

Bergö, G.W. and Tyssebotn, I. ,1992, Cerebral blood flow distribution during exposure to 5 bar oxygen in awake rats, *Undersea Biomed. Res.* 19:339.

Boveris, A., Cadenas, E., Reiter, R., Filipkowski, M., Nakase, Y. and Chance, B., 1989, Organ chemiluminescence: noninvassive assay for oxidative radical reactions, *Proc. Natl. Acad. Sci.* 77:347-351.

Buxton, J.T. et al. ,1964, Haematocrit changes under hyperbaric oxygen, *Ann. Surg.* 30: 18.

Flohe, L., Nieback, G., and Reiber, H., 1978, Zur Wirkung von Divicin in menschlichen Erythrozyten, *Zeitschr. Klin. Chem. Klin. Biochem.* 9:431.

Freeman, B.A.,and Crapo, J.D., 1981, Hyperoxia increases oxygen radical production in rat lungs and lung mitochondria, *J. Biol. Chem.* 256:10986.

Freeman, B.A., Topolosky,M.,K., and Crapo, J.D. ,1982, Hyperoxia increases oxygen radical production in rat lung homogenates, *Arch. Biochem. Biophys.* 216:477.

Gehrs, K. Tiedeman, J., Moon, R.E., Shelton, D.L.,and Buesser , P.J.,1991, Hyperbaric oxygen therapy (HBO) for diabetic macular edema, *Undersea Biomed. Res.* 18(S):20.

Grim, P.S., Nahum, A., Gottlieb,, L., Wilbert, C., Hawe, E., and Sznajder, J. ,1989, Lack of measurable oxidative stress during HBO therapy in burn patients, *Undersea Biomed. Res.* 16(S):22.

Hiramitsu, T. , Hasegawa, Y., Hirata, K. et al. ,1976, Formation of lipoperoxide in the retina of rabbit exposed to high concentration of oxygen, *Experientia* 32: 622.

Jacobson, J.M. , Michael, J.R., Meyers, R.A., Bradley, M.B., Sciuto, A.M. and Gurtner, G.H. ,1992, Hyperbaric oxygen toxicity: role of thromboxane. *J. Appl. Physiol.* 72:416.

Jamieson, D. and Van Den Brank, H.A.S. ,1963, Measurement of oxygen tensions in cerebral tissues of rats exposed to high pressure of oxygen, *J. Appl. Physiol.* 18:869.

Jamieson, D., Chance, B., Cadenas, E. and Boveris, A., 1986, The relation of free radical production to hyperoxia. *Ann. Rev. Physiol.* 48:703.

Kappus, H., 1985, Lipid peroxidation: mechanisms, analysis, enzymology and biological relevance, *in*:"Oxidative Stress", H.Sies, ed., Acad. Press Inc., London.

Landaw , S.A., Leon, H.A.,and Winchell, H.S. ,1979, Effects of hyperoxia on red blood cell survival in the normal rat. *Aerospace Med.* 41:48.

Monstrey, S.M., Mullick, P., Narayanan, K. Liang, M. and Ramasastry, S.S. ,1991, Free radical cytotoxicity and hyperbaric oxygen (HBO) therapy.,*Undersea Biomed. Res.* 18(S):41.

Muhvich, K.H., Piano, M.R., Myers, R.A.M., Ferguson, J.L. and Marzella , L.,1992, Hyperbaric oxygenation decreases blood flows in normal and septic rats, *Undersea Biomed. Res.* 19:31.

Nylander, G., Lewis, D., Nordström, H.,and Larsson, J., 1985, Reduction of postischemic edema with hyperbaric oxygen, *Plast. Reconstr. Surg.* 76:596.

Pilgramm, M., Roth, M.,and Fischer, B., 1987, The change in rheological parameters of the blood under hyperbaric oxygen therapy in inner ear patients, *in*: "Proc. 1st Swiss Symp. Hyperbaric Med.", J. Schmutz, ed., Found. Hyperbaric Med., Basel.

Simon, B.C., Cunningham, L.D. and Cohen, R.A. ,1990, Oxidized low density lipoproteins cause contraction and inhibit endothelium-dependent relaxation in the pig coronary artery. *J. Clin. Invest.* 86: 75.

Thom S.R.,and Marquis, R.E. ,1987, Free radical reactions and the inhibitory and lethal actions of high-pressure gases, *Undersea Biomed. Res.* 14:485.

Torbati, D., Church, D.F., Keller, J.M. and Pryor , W.A., 1991, Organs lipid peroxidation in conscious rats exposed to hyperbaric oxygenation (HBO),*Undersea Biomed Res.* 18(S):37.

Yagi, K. ,1976, A simple fluorometric assay for lipidperoxide in blood plasma , *Biochem. Med.* 15: 212.

Yamaguchi, K.T., Taira, M.T., Stewart, R.J., Roshdieh, B.B., Mason, S.W., Dabbasi, N.I.,and Naito, M.S., 1990, Thermal and inhalation injury:effects of fluid administration and hyperbaric oxygen, *J. Hyperbaric Med.* 5:103.

Yusa T., Beckmann, J.S., Crapo, J.D., and Freeman, B.A., 1987, Hyperoxia increases H_2O_2 production by brain in vivo, *J. Appl. Physiol.* 63:353.

Zhang, J. and Piantadosi, C.A., 1991, Prevention of H_2O_2 generation by monoamine oxidase protects against CNS O_2 toxicity , *Undersea Biomed. Res.* 18(S):28.

ARTIFICIAL OXYGEN CARRIERS IN BLOOD

OXYGEN DELIVERY AUGMENTATION BY LOW-DOSE PERFLUOROCHEMICAL EMULSION DURING PROFOUND NORMOVOLEMIC HEMODILUTION

Peter E. Keipert,[1] N. Simon Faithfull,[1] JoAnn D. Bradley,[1] Diane Y. Hazard,[1] James Hogan,[2] Matteo S. Levisetti,[2] and Richard M. Peters[2]

[1] Alliance Pharmaceutical Corp., 3040 Science Park Road, San Diego, CA and [2] Department of Surgery, University of California, San Diego, CA

INTRODUCTION

Perfluorochemical (PFC) liquids are inert compounds with high solubility for all gases. Physiological oxygen and carbon dioxide transport was first demonstrated in 1966 by the survival of mice subjected to liquid breathing by being completely submerged in an oxygenated liquid PFC.[1] PFCs are insoluble in water, and for the past 25 years significant efforts have been directed towards the development of biocompatible PFC emulsions for use as intravenous oxygen carriers.[2] The first product developed was *Fluosol®* (Green Cross Corp., Japan),[3] which was recently approved by the FDA for use as an oxygen carrier in high-risk patients undergoing percutaneous transluminal coronary balloon angioplasty (PTCA) procedures.[4] Major disadvantages of *Fluosol* include its low concentration of PFC (20% w/v) and the necessity for frozen storage (due to the inherent instability of the emulsion).

In 1986 second-generation perfluorochemical emulsions were developed which were both stable at room temperature and highly concentrated.[5] One of these emulsions, known as *Oxygent™ HT* (made by Alliance Pharmaceutical Corp., San Diego, CA), contains 90% w/v perflubron (perfluorooctylbromide; $C_8F_{17}Br$; PFOB). This product is being developed as a temporary oxygen carrier for use in surgical procedures which employ autologous blood transfusion techniques, including both predonation and intraoperative acute normovolemic hemodilution (ANH).[6] Predonation involves the collection of several units of a patient's blood during the six weeks leading up to surgery. ANH is a procedure whereby blood is withdrawn immediately prior to surgery and simultaneously replaced with either a crystalloid or colloid plasma volume expander.[7]

The present study was performed to evaluate the oxygen delivery capability of a low dose of *Oxygent HT* during profound normovolemic hemodilution in dogs.

METHODS

The physical and chemical properties of *Oxygent HT* are listed in Table I. The final emulsion contains 90% w/v perflubron (equivalent to about 47% vol/vol since the density of perflubron is 1.92 g/mL), is buffered, has physiological osmolality, is terminally sterilized, and is pyrogen free.

Oxygen Transport to Tissue XV, Edited by P. Vaupel
et al., Plenum Press, New York, 1994

Table I. Physical and chemical properties of *Oxygent™ HT*.

Perflubron concentration	(% w/v)	90 ± 4.5
Egg yolk phospholipid	(%w/v)	4.0 ± 0.4
Mean particle size	(μm)	0.25 ± 0.5
Osmolality	(mOsm/kg)	300 ± 50
pH		7.2 ± 0.3
Oxygen solubility	(vol%)	~25 ± 1
CO_2 solubility	(vol%)	~100

Data shown are Means ± Standard Deviation

Mongrel dogs were anesthetized with isoflurane and mechanically ventilated to maintain normocapnia. Catheters were placed in the femoral arteries and vein for arterial pressure monitoring and intravenous infusions. An Oxymetrix Swan-Ganz catheter was advanced into the pulmonary artery from the jugular vein. Blood pressures and EKG were recorded using a Hewlett Packard (Model 7700) polygraph recording system. Cardiac output (measured by thermodilution), mean systemic and pulmonary artery pressures, heart rate, end tidal CO_2, and mixed venous oxygen saturation were monitored. Arterial and mixed venous blood samples were collected for measurement of hematocrit (Hct), blood gases, and total oxygen content (LexO$_2$Con).

A flow-chart describing the acute hemodilution protocol is shown below in Figure 1. Just prior to hemodilution, all dogs received an intravenous bolus of epinephrine (12.5 μg/kg) to contract the spleen and release sequestered red blood cells. Dogs were initially subjected to normovolemic hemodilution to a Hct of 25%, by replacing the blood that was removed with 3 times the volume of Ringer's-lactate. The volume of blood to be removed was calculated from the formula:[6]

$$\text{Blood volume to remove} = \text{Total blood volume} \times \frac{[\text{Hct (initial)} - \text{Hct (final)}]}{\text{Hct (average)}}$$

The animals were then ventilated with 100% oxygen. To mimic additional surgical blood loss while maintaining normovolemia, the dogs were bled to a target hemodilution Hct of 10%. Shed blood was replaced with 1.5 volumes of autologous dog plasma supplemented with 5% human serum albumin in Ringers-lactate solution. The animals were randomly assigned to two groups; the first group of 5 dogs (body weight [BW] of 20 ± 2 kg) were injected intravenously with 3.3 mL/kg of *Oxygent HT* (equivalent to 3.0 g perflubron/kg), while the second group of 4 control dogs (18 ± 1 kg) received 3.3 mL/kg Ringers-lactate solution. All dogs were then monitored for an additional 3 hours post-injection.

The arterial and mixed venous oxygen saturations were calculated from the Kelman computer subroutine for conversion of oxygen tension into saturation.[8] Oxygen content in plasma was calculated according to Henry's Law based on the solubility coefficient of oxygen in plasma and the blood PO$_2$ levels. The contribution of PFC-carried oxygen was calculated from total oxygen contents and agreed closely with the theoretical values calculated from the known oxygen solubility of perflubron.

Results throughout this paper are expressed as Means ± SEM (standard errors of the mean) unless otherwise noted. Statistics performed included either paired or unpaired Student t-tests and analyses of variance. The null hypothesis was rejected at a p value of < 0.05.

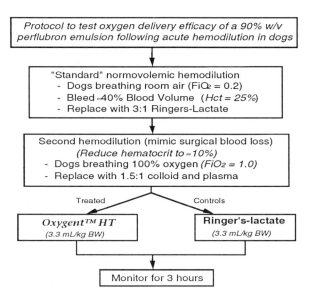

Figure 1. Schematic outline of the acute hemodilution protocol used to evaluate the oxygen delivery capability of a low dose (3.3 mL/kg BW) of *Oxygent HT* (90% w/v perflubron emulsion) administered following a profound reduction in Hct.

RESULTS

From determination of perflubron levels in blood (measured by gas chromatography following quantitative organic phase extraction from blood), the intravascular half-life for *Oxygent HT* was estimated to be approximately 5-6 hours for the dose used. The Hct levels in these mongrel dogs were low initially (<40%), due to the animals' ability to sequester red blood cells in the spleen. After contraction of the spleen by a bolus injection of epinephrine, the Hct levels increased significantly to $48 \pm 2\%$. By the end of the second hemodilution procedure, the final Hct level achieved was $12 \pm 2\%$.

Cardiac output, shown in Figure 2, rose significantly in all the dogs during and after hemodilution. While the mean levels of cardiac output were higher in the treated animals, this difference did not reach statistical significance in the small size sample being compared. The higher cardiac outputs in the treated group were due to a rise in both heart rate and stroke volume. The rise is heart rate contributed more to the difference in cardiac output than the increased stroke volume. The hemodilution and the increased cardiac output did not result in any significant differences, within or between the two groups, in pulmonary capillary wedge pressure or in mean systolic blood pressure. As a result, the calculated rate pressure product (RPP = heart rate x systolic pressure) was significantly higher in the *Oxygent HT* treated dogs.

Dogs receiving *Oxygent HT* had higher oxygen contents in both mixed venous and arterial blood. The combination of increased cardiac output with an increased oxygen carrying capacity of the blood in the *Oxygent HT* group, resulted in higher total oxygen delivery (475 ± 75 mL/min) compared to controls (320 ± 50). The arterial PO_2 levels during ventilation with 100% oxygen were 400 to 450 mmHg and were not really affected by injection of *Oxygent HT*. However, as shown in Figure 3, in the *Oxygent HT* treated dogs, mixed venous PO_2 levels (PvO_2, a reflection of mean tissue oxygenation) and consequently the mixed venous oxyhemoglobin saturation were significantly higher at all of the sampling times during the 3 hour monitoring phase than in the control dogs. The gradual decrease over time in PvO_2 (see Fig. 3) is most likely due to the rate of removal of *Oxygent HT* from the blood and correlated with the previously described plasma half-life of 5-6 hours for this dose in dogs.

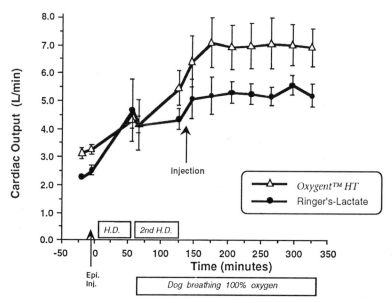

Figure 2. Cardiac output in anesthetized dogs during and following acute normovolemic hemodilution. A bolus of intravenous epinephrine (Epi) was use to contract the spleen to release sequestered red cells. Injection time for the *Oxygent HT* (n = 5) or the Ringer's-lactate (n = 4) following hemodilution (HD) is indicated by the arrow. Data shown are Means ± SEM.

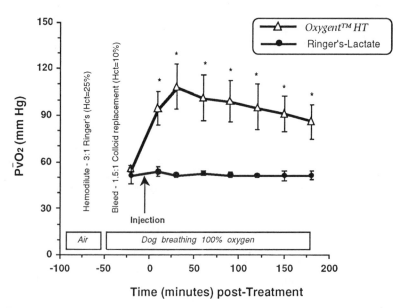

Figure 3. Mixed venous PO_2 levels in anesthetized dogs during and following acute normovolemic hemodilution. Injection time for the *Oxygent HT* (n = 5) or Ringer's-lactate (n = 4) is indicated by the arrow. *Indicates a significant difference between the two groups. Data shown are Means ± SEM.

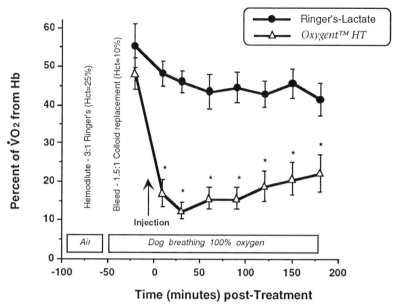

Figure 4. Percentage of the total oxygen consumption (VO₂) contributed by oxygen carried only by hemoglobin (Hb) in anesthetized dogs during and following acute normovolemic hemodilution. Injection time for the *Oxygent HT* (n = 5) or the Ringer's-lactate (n = 4) is indicated by the arrow. *Indicates a significant difference between the two groups. Data shown are Means ± SEM.

Total oxygen consumption (VO₂) following profound hemodilution was not affected by the subsequent infusion of *Oxygent HT* and was maintained at similar levels (110 ± 20 mL/min) in both the treated and control groups throughout the 3 hour monitoring period. The perflubron-dissolved oxygen alone delivered 8-10% of the total oxygen delivery, and, because of the high oxygen extraction coefficient for perflubron, accounted for 25-30% of VO₂. The percent of VO₂ contributed by only the Hb-carried oxygen is shown in Figure 4, and was significantly lower in the *Oxygent HT* treated dogs (15 ± 3%) compared to control dogs (46 ± 4%). The gradual increase observed in the percent of total VO₂ coming from Hb-carried oxygen in the *Oxygent HT* treated animals, resulted from the gradual clearance of emulsion particles from the circulation (plasma half-life ~ 5-6 hours).

DISCUSSION

The total amount of autologous blood feasible to collect using acute normovolemic hemodilution (with or without prior predonation) for harvesting blood, to replace blood lost during surgery, is limited by the degree of anemia tolerated by the patient. If red blood cells lost during surgery could in part be replaced by the use of an oxygen carrier with a limited half-life in the blood, then the need for autologous blood transfusion could be delayed and the autologous blood might not be wasted during periods of acute intraoperative blood loss. The result would be an extension of the potential for preoperative harvesting of blood to replace blood loss, and may permit even more aggressive intraoperative use of autologous blood techniques.[9] During surgery, the use of a PFC-based oxygen carrier would be effective in augmenting oxygen delivery. Because venous oxygen tension remains high in the presence of PFCs, a persistently larger oxygen gradient will exist between the blood and the tissues, thereby facilitating diffusion of oxygen to the tissues.[10] This could serve to further decrease the likelihood of the need for homologous blood transfusions in many surgical procedures.

The results from this study indicated that, in treated dogs in which the Hct has been reduced to 12% by hemodilution, a clinically safe dose of *Oxygent HT* can significantly increase the mean total oxygen delivery by 40%. The increased total oxygen delivery was due to a combination of 30% higher cardiac output and a 10% higher arterial oxygen content in the *Oxygent HT* treated dogs. The higher cardiac output in the treated dogs was mainly the result of the increased heart rate, although stroke volume was somewhat increased as well. There were no differences between the two groups in systemic blood pressure or in pulmonary capillary wedge pressure. The rate pressure product (RPP) is thought to reflect myocardial oxygen consumption and is often used as an index for the onset of ischemia in exercising cardiac patients, or as a guide to myocardial oxygen consumption during cardiac surgery.[11] It is known that to raise the cardiac output by raising heart rate increases oxygen demand of the myocardium more than an equivalent increase in the stroke volume. As a result, the higher cardiac output in the treated animals, with the same preload and afterload, required more work of the myocardium, and therefore yielded a significantly greater RPP.

It is interesting to speculate as to the reasons for this observation. The mean Hct level in these dogs was above the critical Hct of 10% at which oxygen consumption would begin to fall during hemodilution while respiring air.[12] The fact that the dogs were breathing 100% oxygen and had mean PaO_2 values greater than 400 mm Hg would serve to increase the total myocardial oxygen supply and thereby lower the critical Hct at which cardiac output response to hemodilution would begin to fail. In a separate investigation working with an isolated perfused Langendorf heart preparation, Biro and coworkers also noticed that the myocardium appeared to be able to perform more work than would be expected, presumably by extracting more of the dissolved oxygen from a perfusate containing PFC emulsion.[13] This reflects the oxygen diffusion facilitation effect of PFCs,[10] which is due primarily to the elevated oxygen gradient created between the PFC-containing blood compartment and the tissues.

Because PFCs carry significant oxygen at elevated PO_2 levels, and since PFCs have a linear dissociation curve, the utilization of oxygen (i.e., VO_2) will come preferentially from the PFC-dissolved oxygen which is more readily available than oxygen bound to Hb in the red blood cells. The difference between the two groups post-injection, in the percent of total VO_2 coming from Hb-carried oxygen (see Fig. 4), indicated that the perflubron-dissolved oxygen was utilized preferentially before the oxygen carried by hemoglobin. This therefore leaves the Hb-bound oxygen as a safety reserve of oxygen, and represents a margin of safety during hemodilution or acute blood loss that can be provided by perflubron-carried oxygen.

Figure 5 compares the sigmoid shape of the oxyhemoglobin dissociation curve to the linear dissociation curves of *Oxygent HT*, *Fluosol* and plasma. Above a PaO_2 of 100 mmHg Hb is fully saturated, meaning that at elevated PO_2 levels, no additional oxygen can be carried bound to Hb and no oxygen will be released from Hb. Any increases in the PaO_2 will only add to the blood, a small additional amount of oxygen dissolved in the plasma. Since *Fluosol* and *Oxygent HT* have linear dissociation curves, any increase in PaO_2 will increase the amount of oxygen dissolved in the PFC emulsion carried in the blood. The low concentration of PFCs in *Fluosol* (11% by volume) makes the increase in total oxygen carried small. In contrast, *Oxygent HT* (47% by volume) contains more than 4 times the PFC and therefore carries at least 4 times more oxygen.

PFC emulsions have a very high oxygen extraction coefficient when the animals are breathing gases with high concentrations of oxygen. This means that between a PaO_2 of 400 mmHg and a PvO_2 of 100 mmHg, the *Oxygent HT* will give up almost all of its oxygen prior to any bound oxygen being released from hemoglobin. Thus, *Oxygent HT* provides a method for increasing the amount of oxygen carried in blood when the PaO_2 is raised above 90-100 mmHg. By serving as the first dispenser of oxygen to tissues it protects the oxyhemoglobin saturation level. This explains why perflubron-dissolved oxygen could account for a higher percentage (25% to 30%) of oxygen consumption than it was actually contributing to the total oxygen delivery (8-10%). It is reasonable to conclude that the greater increase in the cardiac output seen in the *Oxygent HT* animals might be due to the provision of more oxygen to the myocardium to support a greater increase in the high oxygen demand of a higher heart rate.

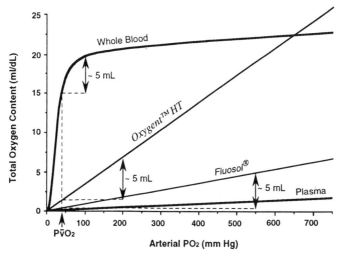

Figure 5. Total oxygen carrying capacity of *Oxygent HT* (90% w/v perflubron emulsion) compared to whole blood, *Fluosol* (a 20% w/v PFC emulsion), and plasma. The arterial PO_2 required to deliver 5 vol.% oxygen is indicated by the arrows. Note that the solubility of oxygen in PFCs obeys Henry's law and depends only on the PO_2 present in the blood.

The potential clinical implications of this study may be viewed in the context of being able to provide a margin of safety for a patient whose blood has been hemodiluted. This may occur following ANH, or following surgical blood loss and restoration of normovolemia by administration of suitable volumes of crystalloid or colloid plasma expanders. From the results of this study it appears reasonable to assume that administration of *Oxygent HT* will cause an increase in PvO_2 and spare oxygen delivery from hemoglobin. The degree to which these changes will occur will depend on a number of interrelated factors. There is always some degree of increase in cardiac output as Hb concentration (and hence blood viscosity) is lowered. The greater the cardiac output response, the greater the PvO_2 and hemoglobin sparing will be in the presence of PFCs. The magnitude of this effect will be increased when oxygen consumption is low and will be directly proportional to the arterial PO_2 levels.

Infused *Oxygent HT* will be lost when there is blood loss, and when it is cleared from the circulation as emulsion particles are taken up by the macrophages of the reticuloendothelial system. Additional loss will occur with time as the perflubron gets excreted from the body via expiration through the lungs. Calculations reveal that a clinical dose of *Oxygent HT* will have an effect equivalent to raising the Hct by 5-10%, and should allow a lower Hct to be used as a trigger for reinfusion of preoperatively collected blood. When bleeding is controlled, the anemia could then be corrected with a smaller total amount of red blood cells. This more aggressive use of autologous blood collection would in turn allow for a reduction in the need for additional homologous blood transfusion.[9]

In conclusion, this study has demonstrated that by adding to blood a PFC emulsion which can increase the amount of oxygen dissolved in the plasma compartment without increasing blood viscosity (as results from red cell infusion) nor affecting control of cardiac output response to a decrease in Hct, *Oxygent HT* can provide substantial augmentation of oxygen delivery to tissues. In contrast, acellular crosslinked Hb solutions being developed for use as blood substitutes[14] have been shown to cause vasoconstriction, presumably due to binding of the endothelium-derived relaxing factor, nitric oxide, to the Hb. As a result, it has been demonstrated that following hemodilution with Hb solutions the cardiac output does not increase.[15] In addition, the perflubron-dissolved oxygen carried by the *Oxygent HT* emulsion will transfer more readily to tissues, compared to oxygen which is bound to either crosslinked Hb molecules in solution or Hb inside of the red blood cells. This implies that when a PFC-based oxygen carrier is used, the hemoglobin-bound oxygen inside the circulating red blood cells will be held in reserve and would therefore still be available to deliver this oxygen under conditions of severe blood loss and anemia.

REFERENCES

1. L.C. Clark and R. Gollan, Survival of mammals breathing organic liquids equilibrated with oxygen at atmospheric pressure, *Science* 152:179 (1966).

2. R.P. Geyer, PFC as blood substitutes - An overview, *in*: "Advances In Blood Substitute Research," R.B. Bolin, R.P. Geyer, G.J. Nemo, eds., Alan R. Liss, New York: 157 (1983).

3. R. Naito and K. Yokoyama, "Perfluorochemical Blood Substitutes," Technical Information Series No. 5., Green Cross Corp, Osaka, Japan (1978).

4. *Fluosol®*. Summary Basis of Approval, Reference number OB-NDA 86-0909. December 26, 1989.

5. J.G. Riess, Fluorocarbon-based in vivo oxygen transport and delivery systems, *Vox Sanguinis* 61:225 (1991).

6. P.E. Keipert, N.S. Faithfull, R.M. Peters, Enhancement of oxygen delivery by a perfluorochemical emulsion following acute hemodilution in dogs, *FASEB J.* 6:A1350 (1992).

7. L. Stehling and H.L. Zauder, Acute normovolemic hemodilution, *Transfusion* 31:857 (1991).

8. G.R. Kelman, Digital computer subroutine for the conversion of oxygen tension into saturation, *J. Appl. Physiol.* 21:1375 (1966).

9. T.F. Zuck and P.M. Carey, Autologous transfusion practice, *Vox Sanguinis* 58:234 (1990).

10. N.S. Faithfull, Oxygen delivery from fluorocarbon emulsions - aspects of convective and diffusive transport, *Biomat., Artif. Cells, Immob. Biotech.* 20: 797 (1992).

11. J.A. Kaplan, Hemodynamic Monitoring, *in*: "Cardiac Anesthesia", J.A. Kaplan. ed, Grune and Stratton, New York, San Francisco, London (1979).

12. S.M. Cain, Oxygen delivery and uptake in dogs during anemic and hypoxic hypoxia, *J. Appl. Physiol.* 42:228 (1979).

13. G.P. Biro, M. Masika, B. Korecky, Oxygen delivery and performance in the isolated, perfused rat heart: comparison of perfusion with aqueous and perfluorocarbon-containing media. *Adv. Exp. Biol. Med.* 248:509 (1989).

14. P.E. Keipert, Properties of chemically crosslinked hemoglobin solutions designed as temporary oxygen carriers. *in:* "Oxygen Transport to Tissues XIV," W. Erdmann, D.F. Bruley, eds., Plenum Press, New York: 453 (1992).

15. G. Lenz, H. Junger, R. van den Ende, B. Brotman, A.M. Prince, Hemodynamic effects after partial exchange transfusion with pyridoxylated polyhemoglobin in chimpanzees, *Biomat. Artif. Cells Immob. Biotech.* 19:709 (1991).

DIVINYL SULFONE CROSS-LINKED HYPERPOLYMERIC HUMAN HAEMOGLOBIN AS AN ARTIFICIAL OXYGEN CARRIER IN ANAESTHETIZED SPONTANEOUSLY BREATHING RATS

Harald Pötzschke[*], Stefan Guth[*], and Wolfgang K.R. Barnikol

Institut für Physiologie und Pathophysiologie
Johannes Gutenberg-Universität
Saarstraße 21, D-6500 Mainz
BR Deutschland

INTRODUCTION

Hyperpolymeric haemoglobin in concentrations necessary to transport oxygen in organism to a significant extent exhibits a negligible oncotic pressure as compared to that of plasma. This property makes hyperpolymeric haemoglobins suitable for development of an artificial oxygen transporting blood additive. With such an additive - in contrast to an oxygen transporting plasma expander - combating a chronic oxygen deficit of tissue (brain, heart, kidney, extremities or in case of anaemia) is possible. Using in these cases an isoncotic oxygen carrying plasma expander instead of an additive would be even more detrimental because of fluid load to heart, at least in case of heart injury. Chronic oxygen deficit is more frequent than acute one, e.g. sudden blood loss. But also a blood loss may be compensated with the aid of an artificial oxygen carrying blood additive in simultaneously applying a plasma expander. Advantage of this procedure is, that the doctor has the possibility to adjust the application of additive and expander to the individual case.

The nature itself gives models for an artificial oxygen transporting (hyponcotic) blood additive: In vertebrates the oxygen transporting system (red blood cells) has an oncotic pressure of about 10^{-8} mbar; in primitive animals (earthworm, snail) this pressure is about 0.4 mbar (soluble huge oxygen transporting proteins: Erythrocruorin and haemocya-

---

[*] This publication contains parts of their theses.
This investigation was supported by the "Bundesminister für Forschung und Technologie (BMFT)", grant-No.: 0702573.

nine with molecular weights 3.4 and 8.3 x 10^6 g/mol, resp. As a consequence both, the oxygen binding capacity and the oncotic pressure and therewith the volume distribution of body fluids - may be governed independently in organism, the first by erythropoietin, the second by liver and kidneys: both systems are decoupled.

We are developing an artificial oxygen carrying blood additive by imitating the "model" of primitive animals. Soluble and stable hyperpolymer haemoglobin are obtainable by crosslinking natural haemoglobins in very high concentration[1,2,3,4], preferring a one-step-reaction to avoid formation of oxidized haemoglobin. There are strong indications, that haemoglobins in high concentration form paracristalline associates[5,6,7], which are fixated covalently by the crosslinkers.

With the following investigations we wanted to demonstrate that preparation of hyperpolymer haemoglobins, exhibiting a sufficiently low viscosity together with a low oncotic pressure, is possible, and that those polymers are tolerated when being applied in organism, and that they are able to transport oxygen to tissues. For this purpose we performed stepwise isovolemic exchanges of blood in rats[8] with suitable solutions under assessment of relevant parameters, using human haemoglobin polymers produced with divinyl sulfone as a crosslinker[9].

MATERIALS, METHODS, AND PROCEDURES

Rat RINGER solution (RaRi) contains 143 mM NaCl, 5 mM KCl, 0.45 mM $CaCl_2$; haemoglobin (Hb) contents (GHb) were measured with the haemiglobin cyanide method; fractions with a CO-Oximeter (INSTRUMENTATION LABORATORY/Lexington (MA)/USA); oxygen pressures of half saturation of haemoglobin ($p_{50}O_2$), mean HILL's indices ($\bar{n}_{50}$: $0.4 < sO_2 < 0.6$; sO_2 = saturation of Hb with oxygen) both at pH 7.4, pCO_2 = 40 Torr, temperature (t) = 37 °C, and BOHR's Coeffizients (b^{pH} = $\partial lg\ p_{50}O_2 / \partial\ pH$, b^{CO_2} = $\partial lg\ p_{50}O_2 / \partial lg\ pCO_2$) were measured with the photometric thin layer method of BARNIKOL[10]. Kinematic viscosities (ν) were measured with micro UBBELOHDE viscometers (SCHOTT/Mainz/D) at 37 °C, oncotic (colloid osmotic) pressures (π_{onk}) with a membrane-osmometer (KNAUER/Bad Homburg/D). The number average molecular weights ($\bar{M}n$) of polymers were calculated from oncotic pressure measurements. Weight average molecular weights ($\bar{M}_w^{GPC}$) were calculated with datas of molecular weight distribution from gel permeation chromatography (GPC) on Sephacryl S-400 HR gels (PHARMACIA/Freiburg/D)[4,11,12,13] using native proteins as calibration substances.

Preparation of haemoglobin hyperpolymers: Pr I (Pr II) is preparation No. I (No. II) used for exchange experiments V I (V IIa and V IIb). All preparations were done at 4 °C. Human erythrocytes from fresh, heparinized blood were separated from the plasma by centrifugation (2000 g, 10 min). Packed washed erythrocytes (haematocrit (HKT) ca. 0.985) were prepared by repeated washing with 0.15 M $NaHCO_3$ solution. Packed erythrocytes were desoxygenated for 24 h with nitrogen. Per mmol haemoglobin ($\alpha_2\beta_2$) 18 mmol of Vinyl sulfone (Divinyl sulfone) were added. The reaction time was 48 h. For haemolysis 2.1 l water per mmol Hb were added, and after 2 h 300 mmol D-Lysine to neutralize free vinyl-groups. After 3 days soluted polymers were separated from non-soluble material by centrifugation, followed by a filtration of the supernatant through a 0,2 μm filter. Then we removed non-desired solutes, adjusted a desired ionic milieu (removed low polymeric haemoglobin molecules in Pr II) and concentrated the polymers by ultrafiltration (MINISETTE-UF-system, with OMEGA filter cassettes of nominal molecular weight limit 30 kD (Pr I) or 300 kD (Pr II): FILTRON/Karlstein/D) against at least ten times the volume of RaRi solution.

Blood exchange experiments - experimental design: Three male Sprague-Dawley rats weighting 325 g (2) and 425 g were used. The rats were anaesthetized with pentobarbital sodium given intraperitoneally using 4 mg per 100 g body weight (mK). We placed heparinized PE-catheters in both femoral arteries, in one femoral vein and in the right atrium via the right external jugular vein. Into the trachea we inserted a short tube for connecting the animal to a two-way breathing gas micro valve (own development). The spontaneously breathing animals could inspire air or different gas mixtures. The expired gas flow was detected with a FLEISCH pneumotachograph (with pressure detector: GANSHORN ELECTRONIC/Munnerstadt/D; signal damping: model 193: EG&G PARC/Princeton (NJ)/USA)) giving the ventilation (Vt). After drying the mixed expired gas passed an oxygen detector (Clark-electrode, E5647; PHM 72 MK2 Digital Acid-Base Analyzer: RADIOMETER/Copenhagen/DK) for measuring oxygen partial pressure, after calibration.

The rats lay on a heated table of 38 °C to maintain body temperature (tK), controlled by a rectal thermometer. We performed the isovolemic blood exchange via two femoral vessels. Withdrawal (arterie) and infusion (vein) were done simultaneously by coupling of two equal syringes, which were fixed in opposite direction at one perfusor syringe drive (Perfusor VI: BRAUN/Melsungen/D). To the withdrawn blood we added heparin (25 IE/5 ml blood) to prevent clotting. Mean arterial pressure ($\overline{p}_a$BL) and heart rate (fHA) were measured via the second femoral arterie with a pressure transducer (P21D; SP 1400-amplifier: GOULD-STATHAM Div./Oxynard (Cal)/USA). This catheter was also used to withdraw samples for measuring arterial oxygen content (G_aO_2) with a Lex-O_2-Con (LEXINGTON INSTRUMENTS/Waltham (MA)/USA), the acid base status (pH_a, p_aO_2, p_aCO_2) with a blood gas analyzer (BGM 1312: INSTRUMENTATION LABORATORIES/ Lexington (MA)/USA), haematocrit (HKT) by the micro haematocrit method and haemoglobin content (GHb). Analogous mixed-venous samples were taken from the catheter in the jugular vein.

Protocoll of experiments: First all quantities mentioned above were measured. Then we pre-exchanged the rat blood with bovine serum albumin solution (56 g/ l) in RaRi to a haematocrit of approximately 0.3 - 0.2 to reach the same haemoglobin content in the rat blood as in the polyhaemoglobin solution. Exchanges with polyhaemoglobin solution followed stepwise, each time 5 ml in 5 minutes. A period of 25 minutes ensued, in which, after restitution (constance of blood pressure, ventilation, heart frequency) we again determined all quantities. With continuing reduction of haematocrit we increased the inspiratory oxygen fraction ($F_I O_2$) to provide a high oxygen saturation of polyhaemoglobin in the lung capillaries.

Calculations: With the aid of the initial values of haematocrit (HKT_0) and haemoglobin content (GHb_0) of blood we calculated the actual rat haemoglobin content as:

$$G^{RHb}Hb = HKT \cdot GHb_0/HKT_0 \tag{1}$$

and the actual polyhaemoglobin content as:

$$G^{PHb}Hb = GHb - G^{RHb}Hb \tag{2}$$

The measured oxygen content is the sum of the concentration of dissolved oxygen ($c^{BL}O_2$) and the contents of oxygen bound to the two haemoglobin species:

$$GO_2 = c^{BL}O_2 + G^{RHb}O_2 + G^{PHb}O_2. \tag{3}$$

The oxygen concentration was calculated using a practical average oxygen solubility coefficient of blood ($\alpha^{BL}O_2 = 0.0034$ ml O_2 STPD/(Torr·dl):

$$c^{BL}O_2 = \alpha^{BL}O_2 \cdot pO_2 \tag{4}$$

The oxygen content of oxygen bound to rat haemoglobin was calculated:

$$G^{RHb}O_2 = G^{RHb}Hb \cdot HFZ \cdot s^{RHb}O_2 \tag{5}$$

where HFZ is HÜFNER's number (practical value = 1.36 ml O_2 STPD/g Hb) and saturation of rat haemoglobin ($s^{RHb}O_2$) was calculated using pO_2 and a mean standard oxygen binding curve of rat whole blood, corrected for the actual acid base parameters.

The content of oxygen bound by polyhaemoglobin ($G^{PHb}O_2$) was calculated:

$$G^{PHb}O_2 = GO_2 - (c^{BL}O_2 + G^{RHb}O_2) \tag{6}$$

The validity of this kind of analysis was verified in blood exchange experiments with albumin solutions alone.
The oxygen uptake ($\dot{V}O_2$ = netto oxygen transport rate) was calculated as:

$$\dot{V}O_2 = Vt \cdot (F_I O_2 - F_E O_2), \tag{7}$$

where $F_I O_2$ ($F_E O_2$) is the oxygen fraction of inspired (expired) gas.
Cardiac output (HZV) was calculated using FICK's equation:

$$HZV = \dot{V}O_2 / avDO_2 \qquad (8)$$

where $avDO_2$ is the arterio-venous difference of oxygen contents.
The partial netto oxygen transport rates ($\dot{V}O_2^X$) are the product of HZV and the partial arterio-mixed venous differences of oxygen contents ($avDO_2^X$):

$$\dot{V}O_2^X = HZV \cdot avDO_2^X \qquad (x = BL, RHb, PHb) \qquad (9)$$

Specific netto oxygen transport rates ($(\dot{V}O_2)_{sp}$) are netto oxygen transport rate over body weight:

$$(\dot{V}O_2)_{sp} = \dot{V}O_2 / mK \qquad (10)$$

RESULTS

Properties of haemoglobin hyperpolymer solutions (in vitro-characterisation): Table 1 summerizes the most important properties of the two prepared solutions (Pr I and Pr II) used for the exchange experiments. In fig. 1 colloid osmotic pressure and kinematic viscosity of the second preparation (Pr II) as a function of polyhaemoglobin-concentration are shown. In the range of concentration reached in the animals (see below) the colloid osmotic pressure is very small as compared with that of plasma (about 2.5 kPa); the kinematic viscosity does not exceed the value of normal rat blood (4-5 cSt).

In vivo characteristic of oxygen transport in the animals: Figure 2 gives the results of the animal experiments in summarized form; especially it shows the raising part of the specific oxygen uptake assessed by

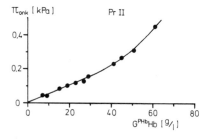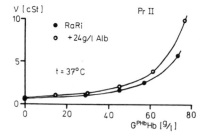

Fig. 1. Colloid osmotic pressure (π_{onk}) and kinematic viscosity (ν) of the second preparation (PrII) versus content of haemoglobin hyperpolymers ($G^{PHb}Hb$): ● in RaRi, ○ in RaRi with 24 g/l bovine serum albumine (Alb).

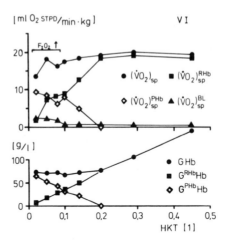

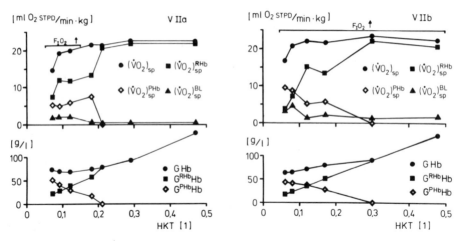

Fig. 2. Data from three animal experiments: V I, V IIa and V IIb. Upper diagrams: total $((\dot{V}O_2)_{sp})$ and partial $((\dot{V}O_2)^x_{sp})$ specific netto oxygen transport rates of the oxygen transporting systems involved (x) versus haematocrit (HKT). The oxygen transport systems are: RHb: rat haemoglobin, PHb: haemoglobin hyperpolymers, BL: the physically dissolved oxygen. F_IO_2 together with the bar indicates those measurements done with increased inspiratory fraction of oxygen. Lower diagramms: The contents (in blood fluid) of rat haemoglobin (G^{RHb}Hb), of polyhaemoglobin (G^{PHb}Hb), and of the sum of both (GHb) dependent on haematocrit (HKT).

Table 1. Left part: properties of haemoglobin hyperpolymers; right part: properties of special solutions used for blood exchange. $P_{50}O_2$: oxygen partial pressure at half saturation of haemoglobin, $\bar{n}_{50}$: mean HILL's index; $\bar{M}_n$: number average molecular weight; $\bar{M}_n^{GPC}$: weight average molecular weight; $G^{PHb}Hb$: content of haemoglobin polymers; cAlb: concentration of bovine serum albumine; π_{onk}: colloid osmotic pressure; ν: kinematic viscosity; Osm: osmolarity; FHb^{III}: fraction of methaemoglobin.

	$P_{50}O_2$ [Torr]	$\bar{n}_{50}$ [1]	$\bar{M}_n$ [$10^6 \cdot g/mol$]	$\bar{M}_w^{GPC}$	$c^{PHb}Hb$ [g/l]	cAlb [g/l]	π_{onk} [kPa]	ν [cSt]	FHb^{III} [1]	Osm [mosm/l]
Pr I	52	1.1	—	9.41	80	0	2.5	3	0.08	300
Pr IIa Pr IIb	24	0.8	0.54	4.67	70	24	2.4	7	0.09	300

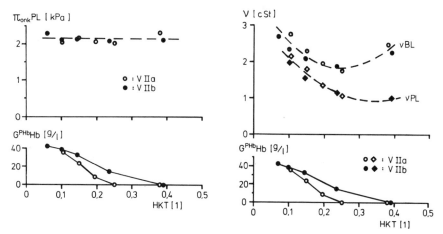

Fig. 3. Upper parts: colloid osmotic pressure of the plasma fluid ($\pi_{onk}PL$) and kinematic viscosity of whole blood (νBL) and the plasma fluid (νPL) versus the haematocrit (HKT) of the blood fluid drawn from the animals in each step of exchange experiments (V IIa and V IIb); lower parts: corresponding contents of polyhaemoglobin ($G^{PHb}Hb$).

the polyhaemoglobin dependent on haematocrit, which means raising degree of blood exchange and polyhaemoglobin blood content, as shown in the lower part of the three diagrams. The relative specific oxygen uptake at the lowest haematocrit achieved were 69% in V I (HKT 0.02), 36% in V IIa (HKT = 0.07) and 57% in V IIb (HKT = 0.06).

Ex vivo measurement of physico-chemical properties of "blood": In fig. 3 the results of physico-chemical ex vivo measurements are shown. These measurements where made in experiments V IIa and V IIb. The oncotic pressure of blood fluid, which was drawn in 5 ml-portions in each step of exchange, remained constant throughout the exchange procedure (see figure 3). The kinematic viscosities of both, blood and plasma exhibit a minimum between hematocrit 0.25 and 0.4, and raised up with increasing content of polyhaemoglobin, but they did not exceed 3 cSt, which is definitely lower than the values of normal rat whole blood (ca. 4.5 cSt).

DISCUSSION

Tab. 1 indicates the possibility of producing hyperpolymer haemoglobins with different oxygen affinities ($P_{50}O_2$). We found that this is achieved by variation of the condition of the crosslinking reaction. So, oxygen affinity may be adjusted to need. To do this the degree of oxygenation of the haemoglobin to be crosslinked is of great importance. In all cases we observed a decrease of cooperativity as assessed by the n_{50}-value. It would be very desirable to keep cooperativity high or even to increase it with crosslinking.

Our results make evident that it is possible to produce hyperpolymers in suitable concentration with such a low viscosity and with such a low oncotic pressure, that they can transport oxygen to tissues at a sufficient scale as an blood additive. But fig. 2 shows also that there is a limitation at about 70 g/l in that both, the viscosity and the oncotic pressure, increase exponentially; this would not be tolerated by organism. On the other side tab. 1 show the enormous nonuniformity of the hyperpolymers - compare the values of $\overline{M}_n$ and $\overline{M}_w$ GPC. According to EINSTEIN's law of viscosity[3] uniform spheric hyperpolymers would have a viscosity independent from molecular weight. So, uniform hyperpolymers would be very desirable, like the natural hyperpolymer oxygen carriers: erythrocruorin and haemocyanine.

The ability of our synthetized hyperpolymers to transport oxygen to tissue also shows that the uptake and release of the oxygen molecule in the lung and in the capillaries, resp. is roughly quick enough. But the kinetics of the reaction may retard the oxygen transitions. To exclude this the kinetics of oxygen with the hyperpolymer haemoglobins should be investigated.

SUMMARY

The production of hyperpolymer haemoglobins, exhibiting sufficiently low colloid osmotic pressure and sufficiently low viscosity is possible, even in concentrations, and therewith oxygen transport capacity, high enough to supply an organism adequatly with oxygen. Such hyperpolymers, when infused, are tolerated by anaesthetized rats in acute blood exchange experiments. Ex vivo determinations of plasma colloid osmotic pressure and both, plasma and whole blood kinematic viscosity during blood exchange showed, that corresponding properties found in vivo were refound within the animal. Furthermore we could show that hyperpolymers produced from desoxygenated human haemoglobin with divinyl sulfone as a crosslinker take part in tissue supply of oxygen to a substantial degree (about 50%) without and with increased inspiratory oxygen fraction, demonstrating the principal ability of hyperpolymers to transport oxygen in blood and to deliver it to tissues.

REFERENCES

1. W.K.R. Barnikol and O. Burkhard, Highly polymerized human haemoglobin for oxygen carrying blood substitute, Adv. Exp. Med. Biol. 215:129 (1987).
2. W.K.R. Barnikol and O. Burkhard, Huge compact soluble molecules: a new old concept to develop an oxygen carrying blood substitute, Biomat., Art. Cells, Artif. Organs 16:639 (1988).
3. W.K.R. Barnikol and O. Burkhard, Low viscosity of densely and highly polymerized human hemoglobin in aqueous solution - the problem of stability, Adv. Exp. Med. Biol. 248: 335 (1989).
4. H. Pötzschke and W.K.R. Barnikol, A new type of artificial oxygen carrier: soluble hyperpolymeric haemoglobin with negligible oncotic pressure - production of stable hyperpolymers from human blood with glutaraldehyde as cross-linker, Biomat., Artif. Cells, Immob. Biotech., in press.
5. O. Burkhard and W.K.R. Barnikol, Die Konzentrationsabhängigkeit molekularspezifischer physikalisch-chemischer und biologischer Eigenschaften des humanen Hämoglobins als Beweis für intertetramere Wechselwirkungen, Funkt. Biol. Med. 2:185 (1983).
6. E. Friederichs, et al., Zum Einfluß von 2,3-Diphosphoglyzerat und Kalzium-Ionen auf die Löslichkeit desoxygenierten Human-Hämoglobins, in: "Hämorheologie und Hämatologie", W. Tillmann, A.M. Ehrly, ed., Verlag Münchener Wissenschaftliche Publikationen, München (1986).
7. I.L. Cameron and G.D. Fullerton, A model to explain the osmotic pressure behavior of hemoglobin and serum albumin, Biochem. Cell Biol. 68:894 (1990).
8. St. Guth and W.K.R. Barnikol, Respiration-stimulus caused by acute anemia in air breathing narcotisized rats, Pfluegers Arch. 418:R 112 (1991).
9. K.C. Morris et al., US Patent 4,061,736, Dec. 6, 1977.
10. W.K.R. Barnikol, W. Döhring, and W. Wahler, Eine verbesserte Modifikation der Mikromethode nach NIESEL und THEWS (1961) zur Messung von O_2-Hb-Bindungskurven in Vollblut und konzentrierten Hb-Lösungen, Respiration 36:86 (1978).
11. W.K.R. Barnikol, O. Burkhard, and H. Pötzschke, Das Erythrocruorin des Regenwurms (Lubricus terrestris) als Eichsubstanz in der Gelchromatographie, J. Chromatogr. 497:231 (1989).
12. W.K.R. Barnikol and H. Pötzschke, Bestimmung des Ausschlußvolumens in der Gel-Chromatographie mit Hilfe fixierter menschlicher Thrombozyten, Biol. Chem. Hoppe-Seyler 371:757 (1990).
13. W.K.R. Barnikol and H. Pötzschke, Das Hämocyanin der Weinbergschnecke (Helix pomatia) als Eichsubstanz in der Gel-Permeations-Chromatographie, Biol. Chem. Hoppe-Seyler 372:629 (1991).

MAGNETOMETRIC MEASUREMENTS OF MACROPHAGE ACTIVITY IN THE LIVER AFTER ADMINISTRATION OF DIFFERENT PERFLUOROCHEMICALS

M.B. Koester and J. Lutz

Physiologisches Institut der Universitaet Wuerzburg
Roentgenring 9, D-W 8700 Wuerzburg, Germany

INTRODUCTION

Ferromagnetic particles, phagocytosed by macrophages of the liver, can be sensed magnetometrically after application of a strong external magnetic field.[1-5] Immediately after the end of magnetization, a loss of alignment of the phagocytosed particles begins, called magnetic relaxation,[6,7] which can be measured by means of a sensitive magnetic probe. The velocity of this disalignment depends on phagosomal motion within the cells and thus is an indirect measure of phagocytic activity.[7-10] Artificial oxygen carriers like perfluorochemicals are taken up by the same cell type within the reticuloendothelial system (RES).[11-14] However, large differences seem to exist between several generations of these blood substitutes and diagnostic agents. The first generation, represented by Fluosol[R]-DA (FSD),[15-17] offered the disadvantage of needing a frozen state to be conserved, a low concentration of the effective emulsion and a prolonged retention within tissues. These handicaps seem widely overcome by second generation fluorochemical emulsions based on perfluoroctylbromide (PFOB,[18,19] perflubron, Oxygent[TM] HT). The above mentioned method was therefore applied to test differences between both types of oxygen carriers concerning their effects on cells of the RES. Since the measurements are non-invasive, longitudinal studies in the same animals of a group can be undertaken after different time periods following administration of the substances.

Oxygen Transport to Tissue XV, Edited by P. Vaupel
et al., Plenum Press, New York, 1994

METHODS

A detailed description of the applied magnetic method was given in a previous paper[5]. Briefly, it includes the following steps: Male Wistar rats were injected iv. (penile vein) with 5 mg/kg b.wt. of γ-Fe_2O_3 particles. Later on the animals were slightly anesthetized with 30 mg/kg b.wt of pentobarbital and magnetized in a magnetic field of 0.26 Tesla (2600 Gauss) for 30 s. Immediately thereafter the animals were put into a magnetically shielded chamber. The depilated skin area above the right lower costal angle was brought in close contact to a double FOERSTER probe (Magnetoscop 1.068, Inst. Dr. Foerster, Reutlingen, FRG) in a gradiometer mode of field detection. From the curves of declining magnetism different parameters were calculated following the equation

$$y = y_o * e^{-k * t} + C$$

y = total magnetic field strength at time t, y_o = "dynamic" field strength; k = relaxation constant, C = "static" or "stable" field strength.

The ratio $y_o/(y_o+C)$, the relation of dynamic to static magnetic field strength during the alignment of magnetic particles, was used as indicator of mobility within cellular structures, independent of small variations of the total magnetic field strength and more sensitive than k, as described in an earlier article.[5]
FSD (Green Cross Corp.,Osaka, Japan) as well as PFOB in form of Oxygent™ HT (90% w/v PFOB emulsion, Alliance Pharmaceutical Corp., San Diego, CA) were given i.v. in comparable doses of either 1 or 3 g/kg b.wt. to four groups of rats; a fifth group served as control. Longitudinal studies of the magnetic relaxation were performed in controls and test groups on the days following, up to the 32th day after injection in geometric increasing time periods. Statistically a $p < .05$ was considered to indicate significance.

RESULTS

After administration of 1 g FSD/kg b. wt., the magnetic relaxation was significantly depressed until the 24 th day after injection (Fig.1). In contrast, after 1 g Oxygent™ TH/kg b. wt., the magnetic relaxation was depressed only until the second day following the injection of this artificial oxygen carrier (Fig.2).
After administration of 3 g FSD/kg b. wt., the magnetic relaxation was significantly depressed until 32 days after injection, with a certain restitution in this time. In clear contrast, the magnetic relaxation was restored after administration of 3 g Oxygent™ HT)/kg b.wt. at 16 days, although a statistically significant depression could be seen before this date (Fig.3).

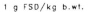

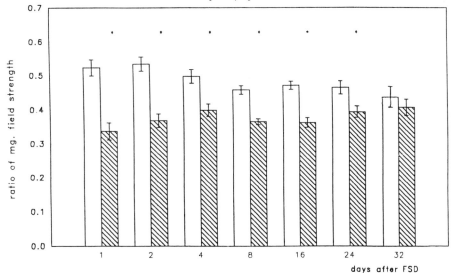

Fig.1. Longitudinal magnetometric studies in two groups of rats. One group served as control (white bars), the other had received 1 g/kg b.wt. of Fluosol^R-DA. Asterisks mark statistically significant differences, which persisted until the 24th day after Fluosol^R-DA administration. Error bars depict the standard error of the mean.

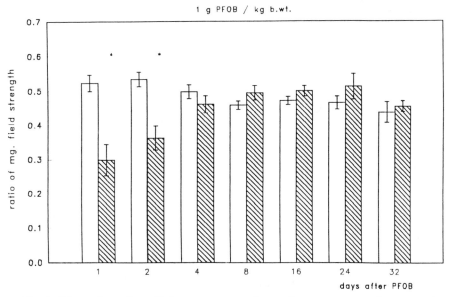

Fig.2. The ratio $y_o/(y_o + C)$ in two groups of rats. One group served as control (white bars), the other had received 1 g/kg b.wt. of PFOB (Oxygent^{TM} TH). Statistically significant differences occurred only during the first two days after administration of PFOB.

DISCUSSION

The need for artificial oxygen carriers ("blood substitutes") is widely recognized today. However, the first generation of PFCs showed (besides its problems with stability) very long dwell times in organs like liver and spleen[11,16].

Although various emulsions had been prepared, only FSD was manufactured in a mercantile style. Besides a transitory preparation of 35 % (w/v), which was withdrawn,

3 g PFOB/kg b.wt.

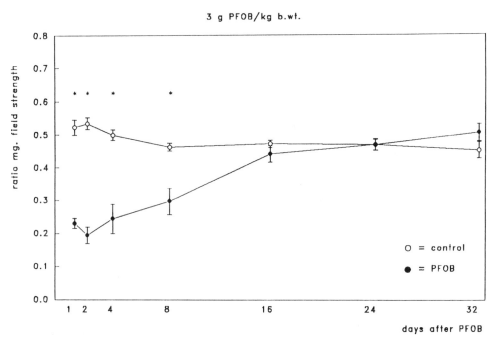

Fig.3. Longitudinal magnetometric studies with the ratio $y_o/(y_o + C)$ in two groups of rats. One group served as control (open circles), the other had received 3 g/kg b.wt. of PFOB (Oxygent[TM] HT). Statistically differences occurred during 8 days after administration of PFOB.

the normal concentration was 20 % (w/v), that means on a volume/volume base it amounted to about 11% v/v.

Among the products of the second generation, PFOB has gained increasing importance. With this substance emulsions were prepared in concentrations of 100% (w/v) and more,[18] equal to about 52 % (v/v). It is this volume relationship which is responsible for the high oxygen capacity (ca. 20 ml O_2/dl/atm). We used a 90% (w/v) preparation of PFOB at the same weight bases (1 and 3 g/kg b.wt.) as FSD and compared their influence on the RES of the liver. Results obtained with the magnetometric method were more sensitive compared with those of the carbon clearance,[20] and the studies presented here were performed each time on the same animal, without the need to kill serial groups. Certain differences may be attributed to the fact that the clearance of carbon is caused by the entire RES, whereas the magnetometric method measures the contribution of the RES especially within the liver.

The results demonstrate that the utilized PFOB (Oxygent™ HT) causes a smaller extent and a shorter time period of inactivation of RES phagocytic activity, most likely attributable to its shorter RES half-life within the RES. It thereby preserves better the functionality of the RES for host defense[14] and detoxification of endotoxins.[21]

ABSTRACT

The activity of liver macrophages was evaluated using a magnetometric method after administration of different perfluorochemicals. Following treatment with perfluoroctylbromide a significant shorter time period of diminished macrophage activity was found compared with a mixture of perfluorodecalin and perfluorotripropylamine. Results obtained with the magnetometric method on liver macrophages were more sensitive compared with those of colloidal carbon clearance of total body RES.

REFERENCES

1. Gehr P, Brain JD, Bloom SB, Valberg PA (1983): Magnetic particles in the liver: a probe for intracellular movement. Nature 302, 336-338

2. Gehr P, Brain JD, Bloom SB (1984): Noninvasive studies of Kupffer cells in situ by magnetometry. J. Leukocyte Biol. 35, 19-30

3. Weinstock SB, Brain JD, Keller-McGandy CE, Taylor KR et al. (1986): Measurement of phagosomal motion by non-invasive magnetometry in Kupffer cells of rats treated with perfluorochemicals. In: Cells of the Hepatic Sinusoid Vol.1 (Ed. A Kirn, DL Knook and E Wisse) Acad. Press NY p. 51-52

4. Weinstock SB, Brain JD (1988): Comparison of particle clearance and macrophage phagosomal motion in liver and lungs of rats. J. Appl. Physiol. 65, 1811-1820

5. Lutz J, Augustin AJ, Schwegler JS, Milz J (1992): Magnetometric studies on the reticuloendothelial system of the liver after administration of different lipid emulsions. Life Sciences 50, 1503-1510

6. Cohen D (1973): Ferromagnetic contamination in the lungs and other organs of the human body. Science 180, 745-748

7. Brain JD, Bloom SB, Valberg PA, Gehr P (1984): Correlation between the behavior of magnetic iron oxide particles in the lung of rabbits and phagocytosis. Exp. Lung Res. 6, 115-131

8. Valberg PA (1984): Magnetometry of ingested particles in pulmonary macrophages. Science 224, 513-516

9. Valberg PA, Albertini, DF (1985): Cytoplasmic motions, rheology, and structure probed by a novel magnetic particle method. J Cell Biol. 101, 130-140

10. Gehr P, Brain JD, Nemoto I, Bloom SB (1983): Behavior of magnetic particles in hamster lungs: estimates of clearance and cytoplasmic motility. J. Appl. Physiol. 55, 1196-1202

11. Lutz J, Metzenauer P (1980): Effects of potential blood substitutes (perfluorochemicals) on rat liver and spleen. Pflueg. Arch. (Europ. J. Physiol.) 387, 175-181

12. Fujita T, Suzuki C, Ogawa R (1983): Effect of Fluosol-DA on the reticulo-endothelial system function in surgical patients. Prog. Clin. Biol. Res. 122, 265-272

13. Castro O, Nesbitt E, Lyles D (1984): Effect of a perfluorocarbon emulsion (Fluosol-DA) on reticuloendothelial system clearance function. Am. J. Hematol 16, 15-21

14. Lutz J (1985): Effect of perfluorochemicals on host defense, especially on the reticuloendothelial system. Int. Anesthesiol. Clinics 23, 63-93

15. Naito R, Yokoyama K (1978): Perfluorochemical blood substitutes Fluosol-43, Fluosol-DA 20% and 35%. Technical Information No 5, Green Cross Corp., Osaka

16. Yokoyama K, Yamanouchi K, Ohyanagi H, Mitsuno T (1978): Fate of perfluorochemicals in animals after intravenous injection or hemodilution with their emulsions. Chem. Pharm. Bull. 26, 956-966

17. Naito R (1980): Synthetic blood, what is it? And what will be its effect on the blood/plasma system? Plasma Forum/Amer.Blood Resources Ass. 1980, 154-171

18. Long DM, Long DC, Mattrey RF, Long RA, Burgan AR, Herrick WC, Shellhamer DF (1988): An overview of perfluoroctylbromide - application as a synthetic oxygen carrier and imaging agent for x-ray, ultrasound and nuclear magnetic resonance. Biomat. Art. Cells Art. Organs 16, 411-420

19. Faithfull NS (1992): Oxygen delivery from fluorocarbon emulsions - Aspects of convective and diffusive transport. Biomat. Art Cells Immob. Biotech. 20, 797-804

20. Jäger LJE, Lutz J (1993) Phagocytosis of colloidal carbon after administration of artificial oxygen carriers of first and second generation. Advances in Exp. Med. & Biol. (This volume, in press)

21. Lutz J, Barthel U, Metzenauer P (1982) Variation in toxicity of Escherichia coli endotoxin after treatment with perfluorinated blood substitutes in mice. Circ. Shock 9, 99-106

PHAGOCYTOSIS OF COLLOIDAL CARBON AFTER ADMINISTRATION OF PERFLUOROCHEMICALS OF FIRST AND SECOND GENERATION

L.J.E. Jäger and J. Lutz

Physiologisches Institut der Universitaet Wuerzburg,
Roentgenring 9, D-W 8700 Wuerzburg, Germany

INTRODUCTION

Artificial oxygen carriers of the perfluorochemical type are marked by their high capacity for carrying dissolved oxygen[1-3]. After circulating in the blood stream they are removed from the circulation and stored for a certain time period chiefly by cells of the reticulo-endothelial system (RES).[4-7] To indirectly assess the duration of this storage, the elimination of colloidal carbon particles from the blood stream can be used as an indicator of the residual phagocytic activity of these cells.[4,8-10]
For this reason the colloid carbon clearance was determined after administrating the same doses of two types of perfluorochemical emulsions (PFC): one of the first generation (Fluosol[R]-DA, FSD), a mixture of 7 parts of perfluorodecalin and 3 parts of perfluorotripropylamine in 2.5% Pluronic F68,[11-13] and one of the second generation: Oxygent™ HT, an emulsion made of perfluorooctylbromide (PFOB, perflubron) in egg lecithin.[14,15]

METHODS

Male rats of the Wistar strain were used throughout the experiments. They were housed in groups of four in macrolon cages, kept on standard diet and had unrestricted access to water. Several groups, each consisting of 4 animals and randomly chosen, received 3 g/kg b. wt. of one of either perfluorochemical emulsions intravenously, while an additional group served as control. Fluosol[R]-DA is a product of Green Cross Corp., Osaka, Japan; Oxygent™ HT is a product of Alliance Pharmaceutical Corp.,

Oxygen Transport to Tissue XV, Edited by P. Vaupel
et al., Plenum Press, New York, 1994

San Diego, CA. The colloidal carbon used was a commercial preparation of India ink (type 17, Pelikan, G. Wagner, Hannover, FRG) that was centrifuged and 1/10 diluted in saline; the given dose was 0.2 ml/100 g b.wt. Three to 24 hours and 2 - 8 days after the administration of PFC, the carbon clearance was determined from spectrophotometric measurements of diluted blood samples at $\lambda = 695$ nm for the first 12 min after carbon injection.

The clearance of the administered carbon was expressed by the elimination con-

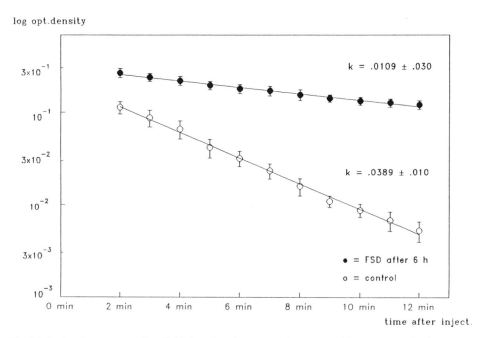

Fig.1 Elimination curves of colloidal carbon in a control group and in a group of animals that had received 3 g Fluosol[R]-DA/kg b.wt. 6 hours before blood analysis. Each group consisted of 4 animals.

stant k according to the equation $k = (\ln c_1 - \ln c_2)/(t_2 - t_1)$, where c_1 and c_2 are concentrations at time t_1 and t_2. Calculation was done by approximating the true regression line using the least-squares trend line for logarithmic values of c.

If a difference between mean k values was established, each of the groups was compared with the control group using the unpaired t test, considering significant results giving p values < 0.05. Error bars in the figures depict the standard error of the mean (SEM).

RESULTS

Two elimination curves of colloidal carbon, expressed as the optical density at $\lambda = 695$ nm and measured for 12 min are depicted in Fig.1. With a logarithmic scale, the curves show a linear decrease and can be calculated according to the method of least squares. From such curves the calculations for the results of the following groups were done.

A depression of the colloidal carbon clearance was noted after both PFCs for the first 3 - 24 hours. Thereafter, however, large differences between the two types were observed. On the second day after FSD, k was still depressed below 60 % (Fig.2); after Oxygent™ HT, it had regained 84.5% of control values (Fig.3). After four days the difference was still impressive: FSD values were less than 65% of controls, whereas those in Oxygent™ HT treated animals were not significantly different from controls (102.5 $\pm$ 3.2 %). It took 8 days for the FSD treated animals to reach carbon clearance values in the range of the controls.

DISCUSSION

PFOB emulsions have distinguished themselves by being capable of carrying greater oxygen quantities than FSD.[2,3,14] Thus according to the difference of concentrations, PFOB emulsions dissolve about 4.5 times the amount of oxygen compared to FSD, whereas the coefficients of solubility, expressed for the pure substance, do not differ markedly.[2,3] Our studies were performed to discriminate between these two PFCs according to their effects on RES activity. The differences observed are probably attributable to the shorter half-life of PFOB in the RES, relative to that of PFCs in FSD. Among the constituents of FSD, perfluorotripropylamine was found to accumulate with time in liver and spleen with half-lives of 53.6 and 72.2 days, respectively.[4] (Pure perfluortripropylamine emulsions seem to have still longer dwell times in these organs[16], while t/2 of FSD in the circulation amounts to about 10-30 hours[12,17]). Measurements of the dwell time especially in cells of the RES are difficult to obtain, so we have used another method of determination of their functionality by means of a magnetometric method.[18,19] By this procedure the response of macrophages in the liver can be evaluated,[20-22] and still longer periods of diminished activity were found, although nearly in the same ratio between FSD and PFOB.

The results presented here reveal that, following equivalent PFC doses, PFOB causes a lesser degree of RES suppression which persists for significantly shorter time periods than after FSD. Thus they offer a distinct advantage of PFOB over FSD during times when the RES is being called upon for life saving tasks like host defense against bacterial invasion[7] and endotoxin neutralization.[23]

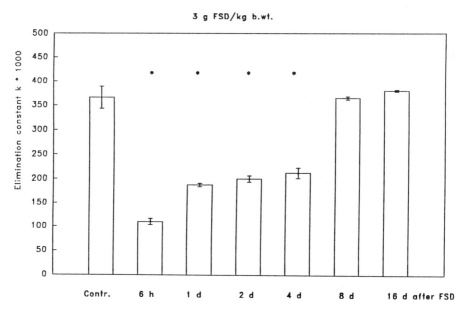

Fig.2 Bar diagram with the result of longitudinal studies after administration of 3 g Fluosol[R]-DA/kg b.wt. in six groups of rats and a control group. Each group consisted of 4 animals.

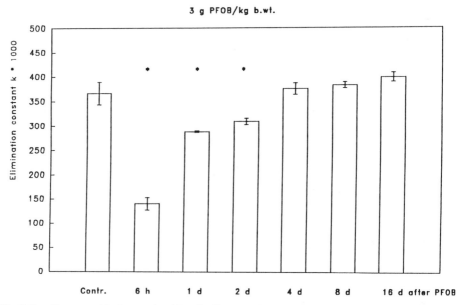

Fig.3 Bar diagram with the result of longitudinal studies after administration of 3 g PFOB (Oxygent[TM] HT)/kg b.wt. in six groups of rats and a control group. Each group consisted of 4 animals.

ABSTRACT

By means of colloidal carbon clearance loading of cells of the reticulo-endothelial system (RES) in rats was estimated after administration of perfluorochemicals. Perfluoroctylbromid revealed a significant lower depression of RES function than an equally dosed (g/kg b.wt.) mixture of perfluorodecalin and perfluorotripropylamine. Compared with a magnetometrical measurement of liver macrophage activity, shorter periods of cell loading was determined.

REFERENCES

1. Geyer RP (1975): Review of perfluorochemical-type blood substitutes. Proceedings of the Xth Int. Congress for Nutrition, Kyoto 1975, 3-19

2. Riess JG, Le Blanc M (1982): Solubility and transport phenomena in perfluorochemicals relevant to blood substitution and other biomedical applications. Pure & Appl. Chem. 54, 2383-2406

3. Long DM, Long DC, Mattrey RF, Long RA, Burgan AR, Herrick WC, Shellhamer DF (1988): An overview of perfluoroctylbromide - application as a synthetic oxygen carrier and imaging agent for x-ray, ultrasound and nuclear magnetic resonance. Biomat. Art. Cells Art. Organs 16, 411-420

4. Lutz J, Metzenauer P (1980): Effects of potential blood substitutes (perfluorochemicals) on rat liver and spleen. Pflueg. Arch. (Europ. J. Physiol.) 387, 175-181

5. Fujita T, Suzuki C, Ogawa R (1983): Effect of Fluosol-DA on the reticulo-endothelial system function in surgical patients. Prog. Clin. Biol. Res. 122, 265-272

6. Castro O, Nesbitt E, Lyles D (1984): Effect of a perfluorocarbon emulsion (Fluosol-DA) on reticuloendothelial system clearance function. Am. J. Hematol 16, 15-21

7. Lutz J (1985): Effect of perfluorochemicals on host defense, especially on the reticuloendothelial system. Int. Anesthesiol. Clinics 23, 63-93

8. Biozzi G, Benacerraf B, Halpern BN (1953): Quantitative study of the granulopectic activity of the reticulo-endothelial system. Br. J. Pathol. 34, 441-457

9. Biozzi G, Stiffel C (1965): The physiopathology of the reticulo-endothelial cells of the liver and spleen. In: Progress in Liver Diseases Vol.2. (Eds. Poper H, Schaffner F) Grune & Stratton, New York, p.166-191

10. Altura BM (1974): Hemorrhagic shock and reticuloendothelial system phagocytic function in pathogen-free animals. Circ. Shock 1, 295-300

11. Naito R, Yokoyama K (1978): Perfluorochemical blood substitutes Fluosol-43, Fluosol-DA 20% and 35%. Technical Information No 5, Green Cross Corp., Osaka, 1-177

12. Yokoyama K, Yamanouchi K, Ohyanagi H, Mitsuno T (1978): Fate of perfluorochemicals in animals after intravenous injection or hemodilution with their emulsions. Chem. Pharm. Bull. 26, 956-966

13. Naito R (1980): Synthetic blood, what is it? And what will be its effect on the blood/plasma system? Plasma Forum / Amer. Blood Resources Ass. 1980, 154-171

14. Faithfull NS (1992): Oxygen delivery from fluorocarbon emulsions - aspects of convective and diffusive transport. Biomat. Art. Cells Immob. Biotech. 20, 797-804

15. Flaim SF, Hazard DR, Hogan J, Peters RM (1991): Characterization and mechanism of side-effects of oxygent™ HT (highly concentrated fluorocarbon emulsion) in swine. Biomat. Art. Cells Immob. Biotech. 19, 383

16. Meyer KL, Carvlin MJ, Mukherji B, Sloviter H, Joseph PM (1992): Fluorinated blood substitute retention in the rat measured by fluorine-19 magnetic resonance imaging. Investig. Radiology 8, 620-627

17. Lutz J, Stark M (1987): Half life and changes in the composition of a perfluorochemical emulsion within the vascular system of rats. Europ. J. Physiol. 410, 181-184

18. Gehr P, Brain JD, Bloom SB, Valberg PA (1983): Magnetic particles in the liver: a probe for intracellular movement. Nature 302, 336-338

19. Gehr P, Brain JD, Bloom SB (1984): Noninvasive studies of Kupffer cells in situ by magnetometry. J. Leukocyte Biol. 35, 19-30

20. Weinstock SB, Brain JD (1988): Comparison of particle clearance and macrophage phagosomal motion in liver and lungs of rats. J. Appl. Physiol. 65, 1811-1820

21. Lutz J, Augustin AJ, Schwegler JS, Milz J (1992): Magnetometric studies on the reticuloendothelial system of the liver after administration of different lipid emulsions. Life Sciences 50, 1503-1510

22. Koester MB, Lutz J (1993) Magnetometric measurements of macrophage activity in the liver after administration of artificial oxygen carriers. Advances in Exp. Med. & Biol. (This volume, in press)

23. Lutz J, Barthel U, Metzenauer P (1982): Variation in toxicity of Escherichia coli endotoxin after treatment with perfluorinated blood substitutes in mice. Circ. Shock 9, 99-106

NOVEL FLUOROCARBON-BASED INJECTABLE OXYGEN-CARRYING FORMULATIONS WITH LONG-TERM ROOM-TEMPERATURE STORAGE STABILITY

J.G. Riess[1], C. Cornelus[1], R. Follana[2], M. P. Krafft[1], A. M. Mahé[2], M. Postel[1] and L. Zarif[1]

1 Unité de Chimie Moléculaire, associée au CNRS. Université de Nice-Sophia Antipolis, Faculté des Sciences. 06108 Nice Cedex, France.
2 Centre Départemental de Transfusion Sanguine, Avenue du Dr M. Donat, 06700 St Laurent du Var, France.

INTRODUCTION

The stability of the first generation of injectable fluorocarbon-based oxygen-carriers, exemplified by *Fluosol®* (Green Cross Corp., Osaka, Japan ; licensed for Percutaneous Transluminal Coronary Angioplasty), is insufficient for convenient general use. It needs to be shipped in the frozen state, thawed and reconstituted prior to use ; it must then be used within 8 hours.

A second generation of products (*Oxygent*™, Alliance Pharmaceutical Corp., San Diego, USA ; presently in clinical trials), in addition to being considerably more concentrated and consequently more efficacious, is also much more stable. It is ready for use and can be stored for over one year at 5-10°C, and for several months at room temperature [1,2]. Further efforts are being devoted to developing still more stable emulsions which would meet the requirements imposed by field use [3].

This paper focuses on the implementation of a novel stabilization concept based on the use of mixed linear fluorocarbon/hydrocarbon amphiphiles playing the role of molecular dowels, and on the development of novel fluorocarbon emulsion formulations with long-term shelf-stability. Preliminary biological tests affirm the inertness of the dowels themselves. Their excretion was monitored by ^{19}F NMR. The efficacy and in-vivo tolerance of an emulsion stabilized by a molecular dowel were evaluated in rats and mice.

MIXED FLUOROCARBON / HYDROCARBON AMPHIPHILES AS MOLECULAR DOWELS FOR STABILIZING FLUOROCARBON EMULSIONS

The Dowel Concept

A new approach to emulsion stabilization utilizing linear mixed fluorocarbon-hydrocarbon amphiphiles to improve the cohesion between the surfactant film (egg yolk phospholipid, EYP) and the fluorocarbon phase has recently been proposed [4]. The hydrocarbon extremity of the mixed molecule was expected to display good affinity for the fatty acid chain zone of the phospholipid membrane, while the fluorinated extremity was expected to penetrate the fluorocarbon phase, thus achieving improved adherence of the phospholipid coating to the fluorocarbon droplet. Such compounds thus play the role of a dowel, at the molecular level, between the fluorocarbon phase and the EYP membrane (Fig 1)

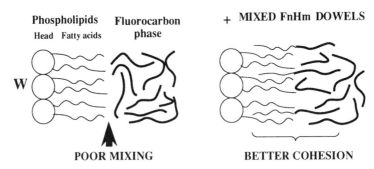

Figure 1. The dowel concept.

These expectations were borne out, and remarkable stabilization effects have indeed been obtained by using this concept [3,4]. Thus, for example, with one mole of the dowel molecule C_8F_{17}-CH=CH-C_8H_{17} (F8H8E ; 2.85% w/v) per mole of egg yolk phospholipids (4% w/v), little or no detectable increase in average particle size has been observed in a concentrated emulsion of perfluorooctyl bromide ($C_8F_{17}Br$ or perflubron ; 90% w/v) after 9 months of storage at 40°C, after an initial equilibration period of *ca* 10 days. During the same period of time, the droplet size of the reference emulsion prepared in the same conditions but without the dowel molecule has doubled (from 0.25 μm to 0.49 μm) when stored at only 25°C.

Biological Tolerance of the Dowels

The dowels are devoid of any reactive functional group and were therefore expected to be chemically and biologically rather inert.

No effect has been observed indeed on the survival and growth of mice after intraperitoneal administration of 30 g of the dowel molecules per Kg body weight (limit of the protocol). Such a dose represents *ca* 600 times the amount of dowel that would be administrated i.v. in a clinically relevant dose (3 g of fluorocarbon per Kg body weight) of the

Table 1 . Preliminary biological results on the neat molecular dowels

DOWEL	Cells Cultures growth / viability [a]	i.p. Injections in mice DOSE	survival ratio
F6H10E	125 / 76	28 g/kg	10 / 10
F8H8E	69/87	30 g/kg	9 / 10
F6H10	70/89	30 g/kg	10 / 10
F8H10	81 / 81	—	—

a   Expressed as percentages with respect to controls

emulsion described below. Incubation for 4 days of the molecular dowels with Namalva lymphoblastoid cell cultures [6] did not affect their growth and viability (Table 1).

Biodistribution, Retention Time in Organs, Metabolism and Excretion

The best candidate fluorocarbons for intravascular oxygen delivery consist of well-defined and pure linear fluorocarbons derived from tetrafluoroethylene which have acceptable organ retention times [1]. Among these, perflubron stands out for its exceptionnally low organ-retention time and for the stability of its EYP-based emulsions ; both of these features are due to the more lipophilic character induced by the terminal bromine atom [5]. Fluorocarbons are excreted by exhalation, without being metabolized, after initial transcient uptake by the reticuloendothelial system (RES) [7].

To study the biodistribution, possible metabolism and excretion rate of a typical example, the mixed fluorocarbon/hydrocarbon dowel $C_6F_{13}CH=CHC_{10}H_{21}$ (F6H10E), was formulated as a 25% (w/v) emulsion with 6% (w/v) egg-yolk phospholipids. The emulsion was prepared by microfluidization and sterilized under standard conditions (121°C, 15 min, 15 psi). Its pH and osmolarity were measured as 7.06 and 265 mOsm respectively. It was injected into anesthesized, catheterized OFA female rats, 10 weeks old, at a 14.4 ml/kg body weight dose (*i.e.* 3.6 g/Kg bw dose of dowel) through the right jugular vein at a rate of 1mL/min. The rats behaved normally after the injection and none of the 33 animals died prior to the programmed sacrifice date.

Quantitative determination of the fluorinated compounds in the main organs of the RES was performed using Fourier transform ^{19}F NMR (188.3 MHz   Bruker AC 200 spectrometer ; CF_3CH_2OH as an internal standard). The animals were sacrificed at regular intervals : 2, 4, 8, 24 and 48 hours, 4, 10, 15 and 21 days, 1, 2.5, 3 and 4 months) and their organs were analysed after homogeneisation using an Ultra-Turrax mixer [8]. ^{19}F NMR is expected to detect all exogenous perfluoroalkylated molecules present, including possible metabolites.

After 4 months F6H10E was still the only fluorinated compound detected in all the spectra recorded, indicating that the F6H10E dowel is not metabolized. Figure 2 illustrates this point by comparing the ^{19}F NMR spectra measured on the emulsion, and on the homogenized rat liver 15 days after its administration.

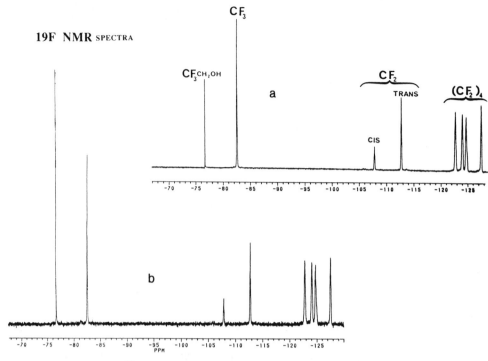

Figure 2 . Typical ^{19}F NMR spectra of F6H10E a) in a F6H10E/EYP emulsion (25/6% w/v) prior to administration, b) in homogenized rat liver 15 days after its administration.

One day after the injection, the dowel distribution is 70% in the liver, 20% in the spleen, 4% in the lungs, 2% in the kidneys and 2% in the blood (Fig 3). Its concentration appears to reach a maximum after one day in the liver (70% of the injected dose) and then decreases. The half retention time of the dowel in the liver is estimated to be 25 ± 5 days. In the spleen maximum accumulation is found after 7 days (25 % of the injected dose).

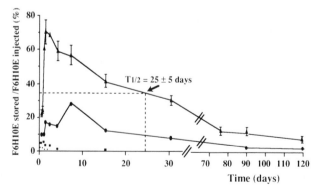

Figure 3 . Evolution of the concentration of F6H10E vs time in liver (▲), spleen (●), lungs (■), kidneys (•).

In the lungs, the dowel content appears to decrease rapidly and becomes undetectable after 3 weeks. In the kidneys the percentage is always very low : it decreases from *ca* 2% of the total injected dose two hours after injection and reaches the sensitivity limit of the method (10^{-4}M, i.e. 0.02% of the initial dose) after 4 days.

PREPARATION OF A DOWEL-STABILIZED PERFLUBRON STEM-EMULSION

Formulation and Preparation

Formulation has a determinant impact on the emulsion's characteristics and properties [9]. A high concentration of fluorocarbon is desirable to assure high oxygen transport efficacy [1,10,11]. An optimal balance was sought between ingredient concentrations, efficacy, fluidity and stability. The average particle size depends to some extend on the fluorocarbon/phospholipid ratio, but an excess of EYP has been shown to be detrimental to emulsion stability [12]. Finally, since fluorocarbon emulsions are thermodynamically unstable systems, their characteristics depend also on the conditions of preparations [13].

Table 2 . New, stable, concentrated (90% w/v) fluorocarbon emulsions with molecular dowels

Perfluorooctyl bromide	90 g (47 mL)	
Egg yolk phospholipids	2.0 g	*equimolar*
F6H10 *Dowel* $C_6F_{13}C_{10}H_{21}$	1.4 g	
NaH$_2$PO$_4$. H$_2$O	0.052 g	
Na$_2$HPO$_4$. 7 H$_2$O	0.355 g	
d-α tocopherol	0.002 g	
Na$_2$Ca EDTA	0.02 g	
NaCl	0.25 g	
water for injection	q.s. ad 100 mL	

Formulation optimization research led to a composition consisting of 90% w/v perflubron , 2% w/v EYP, an *equimolecular* amount of the mixed compound $C_6F_{13}C_{10}H_{21}$ (F6H10), d-α tocopherol as an anti-oxydant, EDTA as a metal chelator, both to protect EYP again oxydation, a phosphate buffer and sodium chloride (Table 2). It is noteworthy that the use of the dowel molecule allows a reduction of the amount of EYP required, without increase in particle size. Such a reduction is desirable as it lowers the amount of hydrolysis products which can form upon storage, allowing for an extention of the expiration date.

Perflubron (Hoescht) and the dowel molecule F6H10 (synthesized in this Laboratory, 98% purity assessed by GC) were detoxified [6] and filtered on a 0.22 μm millipore membrane prior to use. The same batch of injectable grade EYP (Asahi), stored at -20°C, has been used throughout this study. All the ingredients were tested as to their biological acceptance separately before use, perflubron (neat), F6H10 (neat), EYP (20% dispersion) by i.p. injection in mice (10/10 survival).

Among the different procedures applicable to emulsifying fluorocarbons, microfluidization, a mechanical impinging jet homogenizing method, was chosen for its consistency [14].

The emulsions (1L size-batches) were prepared by dispersing the phospholipids with an Ultra-Turrax mixer (8000 rpm) for 3 min at 20°C, dispersing the dowel molecule in this EYP dispersion for 1 min, then adding the perflubron in 10 min under Ultra-Turrax mixing at 8000 rpm. This coarse premix was mixed vigorously for 1 min at 24000 rpm and 20°C. The final emulsion was obtained by cycling the premix 10 times through the Microfluidizer (model 110T) at a pressure of 12000 psi, while the temperature was maintained between 20° and 30°C. All these operations were performed under thorough exclusion of oxygen using argon. The emulsions were then bottled in 50 mL vials (head-space *ca* 8%, Teflon lined stoppers) and heat-sterilized under standard conditions (121°C, 15 min, 15 psi) immediately after preparation.

This intravascular oxygen-carrying emulsion (IVO$_2$), formulated as indicated in table 2, is calculated to dissolve 25 vol % of oxygen when equilibrated with oxygen under atmospheric pressure.

Particle Size Characteristics ; Stability

The above emulsions have been characterized after preparation, after sterilization and during accelerated ageing at 40°C. The freshly sterilized emulsion's pH and osmolarity of a typical batch were measured to be 6.9 and 288 mOsm. Its viscosity coefficient was 17 cp (20.2 cp at 0.73 s^{-1}; Rheo LV8). After one month at 40°C, the viscosity coefficient had decreased to 15 cp and remained unchanged after 3 months at this temperature; the pH was then 6.8.

Figure 4 illustrates the particle size data (±5%), measured by photosedimentation (Horiba Capa-700), of a dowel-based emulsion, compared to those of a reference emulsion prepared in the same conditions without dowel. It shows that the average particle sizes and size distributions of the dowel-based emulsion and of the reference emulsion were similar after preparation and sterilization. This was no longer true after storage at 40°C. A remarkable stabilization effect was then observed with the dowel.

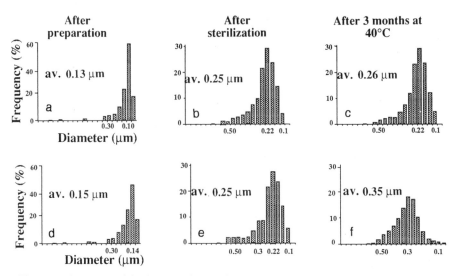

Figure 4 . Average particle sizes and size distributions of a perflubron/EYP/F6H10 (90/2/1.4 % w/v) emulsion (a-c) and of a reference perflubron/EYP (90/2 % w/v) emulsion (d-f).

Thus, after 3 months at 40°C, the dowel-containing emulsion still had essentially the same average particle size and particle size distribution. On the other hand, under the same conditions and over the same period of time, the average droplet size of the reference emulsion had increased from 0.25 to 0.35 μm and displayed a much broader distribution of sizes (Fig. 4f). Such extended particle size stability is obviously of great value in any experiment where particle size can influence the results.

EFFICACY AND IN-VIVO TOLERANCE

Exchange Perfusion of the Conscious Rat

Close-to-total isovolemic exchange perfusion of the conscious rat [15] was performed with the new dowel-stabilized emulsion. For this purpose, the emulsion was diluted to 50% w/v in perflubron, with appropriate solutions of human albumin and salts, allowing for the adjustment of the oncotic pressure, osmolarity (298 mOsm) and pH (7.15).

The animals (SPF OFA Sprague Dawley rats of about 200g) were implanted with a double lumen catheter in the right atrium through the right jugular vein. During the exchange perfusion they were conscious and unrestricted and were breathing an oxygen enriched atmosphere ($FiO_2 = 0.6$). They showed no sign of distress or concern while their hematocrit was reduced to 3-4% by perfusion with ca 2.5 times their blood volume. The oxygen enriched atmosphere was kept for five days, then lowered progressively over the next two days. The survival ratio after a 10 day observation period was 73% (n = 15). This result indicates that this formulation is efficacious in delivering oxygen *in vivo*.

In Vivo Tolerance in Mice

Intravenous injections were also performed in mice with large doses of the 90% w/v concentrated stem emulsion to ascertain its *in vivo* biological tolerance. Ten OF1 male mice (*ca* 20g) received a 52 ml/kg bw dose by infusion via the tail vein (0.7 mL/min). This dose was well tolerated and all the animals survived the one month observation period.

CONCLUSIONS

A new injectable fluorocarbon formulation has been devised which incorporates a molecular dowel to improve the cohesion between the fluorocarbon phase and the phospholipid surfactant film. This results in considerable emulsion stabilization. The new formulation is also characterized by a reduced amount of phospholipid.

The dowel-stabilized emulsion displays long-term shelf stability, was tolerated in mice at doses of at least 52 ml/kg body weight and demonstrated efficacy in a close-to-total exchange perfusion in a rat model.

Preliminary biological assessment indicates that the dowel molecules themselves are biologically inert and tolerated at at least 30g/kg body weight i.p. in mice. No metabolism was found and the half-residence time in the liver of rats, after massive *i.v.* injection in emulsion form (3.6g/kg body weight), was of *ca* 25 days for a typical product, $C_6F_{13}CH=CHC_{10}H_{21}$. The absence of metabolism is particularly favorable to their use as emulsion stabilizers rather than fluorinated surfactants, (although their effectiveness has been demonstrated[1-3]), as it should greatly simplify the pharmacologic and toxicologic studies.

ACKNOWLEDGMENTS   We wish to thank the Centre National de la Recherche Scientifique, the Lions Club and "Applications et Transferts de Technologies Avancées" for their support.

REFERENCES

1. J. G. Riess, *Vox Sanguinis*, 61:225 (1991).
2. J. G. Riess, *Biomat., Art. Cells, Immob. Biotech.*, 20:183 (1992) .
3. J. G. Riess, M. Postel, *Biomat., Art. Cells, Immob. Biotech.*, 20:819 (1992).
4. J. G. Riess, L. Sole violan, M. Postel, *J. Disp. Sci. and Technol.*, 13:349 (1992).
5. J. G. Riess, *Curr. Surg.*, 45:365 (1988).
6. M. Le Blanc, J. G. Riess, D. Poggi, R. Follana, *Pharm. Res.*, 195 (1988).
7. a) R. P. Geyer, *New Engl. J. Med.* 289:1077-1082 (1973). b) J. G. Riess, *Art. Org.* 8:44-56 (1984). c) Y. Tsuda, K. Yamanouchi, H. Okamoto, K. Yokoyama, C. Heldebrant, *J. Pharmacobio. Dyn.*, 13:165 (1990).
8. L. Zarif, M. Postel, B. Septe, J.G. Riess, A.M. Mahe and R. Follana, *J. Pharm. Res.* XXX (1993).
9. T. J. Pelura, C. S. Johnson, T. E. Tarara, *Biomat., Art. Cells, Immob. Biotech.*, 20:845 (1992).
10. N. S. Faithfull, in *"Blood Substitutes. Preparation, physiology and medical applications"*, Horwood, Chichester, 130 (1988).
11. G. P. Biro, P. Blais, *Crit. Rev. Oncol. Hematol.*, 6:311 (1987).
12. M. P. Krafft, J. G. Rolland, J. G. Riess, *J. Phys. Chem.*, 95:5673 (1991).
13. J. G. Riess, M. P. Krafft, in *"Oxygen Transport to Tissues XIV"* W. Erdmann, D. F. Bruley (eds), Plenum Publ. Corp. New York, vol 317, 465 (1992).
14. E. Mayhew, R. Lazo, W. J. Wail, J. King, A. M. Creen, *Biochim. Biophys. Acta*, 775:169 (1984).
15. T. H. Goodin, W. P. Clarke, K. Taylor, R. Eccles, R. P. Geyer, L. E. McCoy, *Am. J. Physiol.*, 245 (Heart Circul. Physiol. 14) :H 519 (1983).

RESUSCITATION OF DOGS FROM ENDOTOXIC SHOCK BY CONTINUOUS DEXTRAN INFUSION WITH AND WITHOUT PERFLUBRON ADDED

S. M. Cain[1], S. E. Curtis[2], B. Vallet[1], and W. E. Bradley[1]

[1]Departments of Physiology and Biophysics and [2]Pediatrics
University of Alabama at Birmingham, Birmingham, Alabama 35294-0005, U.S.A.

INTRODUCTION

In the anesthetized dog infused with endotoxin, cardiac output falls and a hypodynamic shock state ensues (Cain and Curtis, 1992). If supportive therapy, boluses of donor red cells and dextran, is given then this can be converted to the hyperdynamic and hypermetabolic condition so often observed in human sepsis with adequate volume resuscitation (Cain and Curtis, 1991). Other evidence from experimental animals indicated that endotoxin infusion caused arterial conductance increases and venous constriction with consequent pooling in capillary beds of muscle (Bond et al., 1992) and the splanchnic bed (Abel and Beck, 1992). The decrease in venous return to the heart was one of the reasons that volume treatment was necessary to reverse the shock state. Other consequences of the powerful cytokines liberated by endotoxin infusions can be capillary plugging and endothelial damage so that microcirculatory function and peripheral oxygenation are adversely affected (Cain, 1986). As a result, even with adequate or elevated levels of cardiac output, the potential for severe tissue hypoxia in peripheral organ systems has been postulated to be very high as O_2 consumption becomes markedly flow-dependent (Rackow and Astiz, 1991).

For the choice of volume expanders, dextran-70 has been shown to be superior to others such as Ringer's acetate (Modig, 1988). Aside from other arguments about the relative advantages of colloids over crystalloids, dextran was shown to have better rheological effects by virtue of its reported reductions in granulocyte and platelet adhesiveness and aggregation after induction of septic shock (Modig, 1988). Another aspect of extensive volume treatment with a colloidal expander such as dextran is the resultant hemodilution. By increasing blood fluidity, hemodilution itself may be beneficial to tissue oxygenation. Tissue PO_2 in various organ systems has been shown to increase as hematocrits were lowered in nonseptic anesthetized dogs to 25% (Messmer et al., 1973).

Yet another factor in hemodilution is the increase in plasma space between red cells. This may offer an increased resistance to the movement of O_2 from red cell interior to outside the capillary wall and thereby hinder tissue oxygenation (Homer, et al., 1981; Gutierrez, 1986). Because the increased resistance is related to the low solubility for O_2 in the plasma phase, increasing O_2 solubility would be expected to increase O_2 transfer to tissue if that is a significant factor. We had seen in an earlier experiment that resuscitation by dextran alone in endotoxic dogs was apparently very efficacious even though hematocrit fell to 20% over the course of treatment (Cain and Curtis, 1992).

Oxygen Transport to Tissue XV, Edited by P. Vaupel
et al., Plenum Press, New York, 1994

Our question in the present experiments was whether any improvement in O_2 delivery and utilization could be noted if small amounts of perflubron, a brominated perfluorocarbon, were added to the dextran solution to increase O_2 solubility in the plasma phase but without any increase in inspired O_2 fraction.

METHODS

Anesthetized (30 mg/kg pentobarbital sodium iv) and paralyzed (30 mg succinylcholine chloride im + 0.1 mg/min iv) dogs (n = 18) were pump-ventilated with air. Catheters were placed in carotid and pulmonary arteries and in the right femoral vein. Venous outflows from the left hindlimb muscles and from a segment of ileum were isolated as previously described (Stork et al., 1989). Flow from both regions was returned via a reservoir that drained into the right femoral vein. Both areas were autoperfused and innervated. Regional blood flows were measured every 15 min at the time that arterial and venous blood was sampled. Regional O_2 delivery and uptake were calculated from the results. Whole body O_2 uptake (VO_2) was calculated from the analyses and measurement of expired gas volume. Cardiac output was calculated from VO_2 and arteriovenous O_2 content difference. Arterial and regional venous blood lactate concentrations were measured by electrode (YSI Model 23). Lactate flux across muscle or gut was calculated as the venous-arterial difference in concentration times the blood flow. Gut intramural pH was calculated as described by Fiddian-Green et al. (1986) using arterial bicarbonate concentration and the PCO_2 measured in a tonometric balloon placed in the gut segment adjacent to the segment that was vascularly isolated.

When all preparations were complete and the animal was stable with respect to blood pressure, cardiac output, and whole body VO_2, the experimental protocol was begun. We took one set of samples and measurements before beginning infusion of endotoxin (Difco *E. coli* lipopolysaccharide, LPS) at the rate of 33.3 µg/kg·min for 60 min (total dose of 2 mg/kg). To this point, all animals were treated the same. At the end of the LPS infusion period, dextran infusion at the rate of 0.5 ml/kg·min was begun. In half the experiments, perflubron was added to the infusate so that the animals received a total amount of 10 ml/kg over the 2-hr period of volume resuscitation. This was the PFB group. In the other 9 experiments, the animals received the same amount of carrier emulsion with the dextran infusate to serve as the control or comparison group (VEH group). At the end of the experiment and after the animals were euthanized by bleeding, the amounts of perfused muscle and gut were excised and weighed. All regional values are reported per kg of either muscle or gut.

Results were analyzed by repeated measures ANOVA and significant differences were identified by Duncan's multiple range test with significance accepted at $p < 0.05$.

RESULTS

Because neither treatment nor responses differed through the end of the LPS infusion, the data have been pooled for all animals up to that point. During LPS infusion, VO_2 did not change significantly in whole body (Fig. 1) or limb muscle (Fig. 2) but did decrease significantly in the gut segment (Fig. 3). O_2 delivery decreased in the whole body and both organ systems, primarily as a result of decreased flow. Increased O_2 extraction compensated for this to maintain VO_2 but was unable to do so in the gut. Tonometric results (Fig. 4) indicated that the gut wall had become significantly more acid by that time. Vascular resistance fell in the whole body but did not change significantly in the two organ systems. Arterial lactate concentration increased but the flux across the organ systems showed little change with LPS infusion.

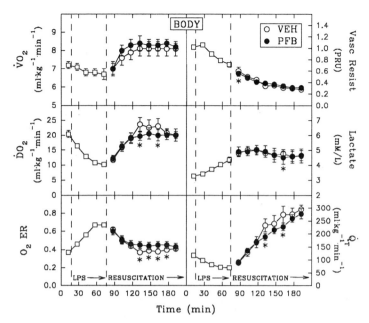

Figure 1. Whole body values (mean±SE) for O₂ uptake (VO₂), O₂ delivery (DO₂), O₂ extraction ratio (O₂ER), vascular resistance, arterial lactate concentration, and cardiac output (Q_T). Asterisks denote p<0.05; filled circles are the PFB group; unfilled circles are the VEH group.

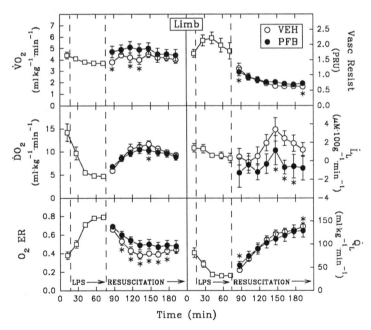

Figure 2. Limb values (mean±SE) for O₂ uptake (VO₂), O₂ delivery (DO₂), O₂ extraction ratio (O₂ER), vascular resistance, lactate flux (L_L), and blood flow (Q_L). Asterisks denote p<0.05; filled circles are PFB group; unfilled circles are VEH group.

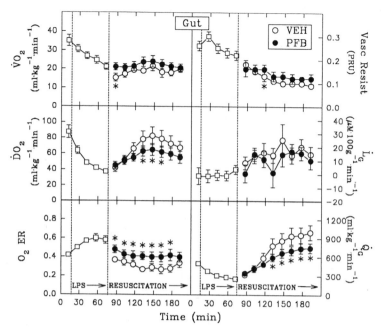

Figure 3. Gut values (mean±SE) for O_2 uptake (VO_2), O_2 delivery (DO_2), O_2 extraction ratio (O_2ER), vascular resistance, lactate flux (L_G), and blood flow (Q_G). Asterisks denote $p<0.05$; filled circles are PFB group; unfilled circles are VEH group.

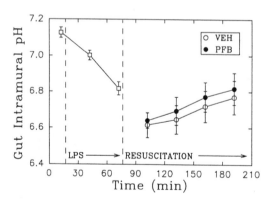

Figure 4. Values for gut intramural pH (mean±SE). Filled circles are PFB group; unfilled circles are VEH group.

One hour after beginning volume resuscitation (a total of 30 ml/kg to that time), cardiac output and both regional blood flows were significantly increased as was O_2 delivery. VO_2 in whole body and in muscle increased significantly by that time but gut VO_2 remained depressed. Consistent with that, gut intramural pH failed to increase significantly. Hematocrit, which started at 40%, had fallen to 25% with one hour of progressive hemodilution but the decrease in arterial O_2 content was more than compensated by the increase in blood flow everywhere.

During the second hour of resuscitation, few further changes were noted in any variable except cardiac output and regional blood flows which continued to show an upward trend. With continuing hemodilution, hematocrits fell to a final value of 20±2% in the PFB group and to 17±1% in the VEH group (p>0.05). O_2 delivery tended to decline but VO_2 remained stable in the whole body and both regions during the last hour of dextran infusion.

The addition of perflubron (PFB) to the infusate had the general effects of raising O_2 extraction while lowering cardiac output or blood flow. This was particularly noticed in the gut but higher O_2 extraction in the limb was also associated with a lesser efflux of lactate. Except for a few time points, however, no significant differences were noted in whole body or regional VO_2. It should be noted that even by the end of the experiment, very little PFB was actually present in the blood. The fluocrit at that time was less than 3%. This made no measurable difference in arterial O_2 content since the animals were ventilated with room air. The asterisks in the figures denoted a significant difference (p < 0.05) between measurements at the same time in the two treatment groups.

DISCUSSION

In earlier experiments, we found that approximately 60 ml/kg of intravenous fluid was necessary to keep mean systemic arterial pressure above 80 mmHg and to maintain cardiac output near or above control levels in dogs given endotoxin intravenously, either as a bolus or as a slow infusion (Bredle and Cain, 1991; Cain and Curtis, 1991a; Curtis and Cain, 1992). In those studies, bolus mixtures of donor red blood cells and dextran were used to keep hematocrit near 40%. Evidence has been cited for capillary pooling as a result of endotoxin treatment (Bond et al., 1992; Abel and Beck, 1992) and the usual picture of endotoxic shock and a hypodynamic circulatory state will result if resuscitative measures, such as volume treatment, is not undertaken. If such a state is allowed to develop, then the consequences of ischemia, capillary plugging, and microvascular injury, particularly upon reperfusion, are likely events (Cain, 1986; Cain, 1991).

In yet another set of experiments, a different resuscitative measure was taken to overcome some of these ischemic sequelae (Cain and Curtis, 1992). Instead of using donor red cells and attempting to maintain hematocrit, we used a continuous dextran infusion of 0.5 ml/kg·min for 2 h after allowing an endotoxic shock state to develop fully. The experimental protocol was exactly the same as that used in these experiments and, indeed, served as the model. Another group was not given any treatment following endotoxin. The treated group showed results entirely consistent with those reported here. Whole body O_2 delivery began to rise very soon after dextran infusion was begun and VO_2 rose to be significantly greater than in the untreated group. Of particular interest was the fact that gut VO_2 still tended to decrease in spite of adequate O_2 delivery to the gut. Nevertheless, it was still higher than in the untreated group, in which 4 out of 6 animals were at or near total cardiovascular collapse by the end of the protocol. An additional piece of information in the current study was the gut intramural pH which affirmed the failure of the gut to maintain energetic status even in the face of supercritical O_2 delivery (Fink, 1991). Resuscitation with an acellular colloid appeared to be very efficacious in the earlier experiments as it was in the present ones, although somewhat less effective in the gut. A question we wished to answer was whether the resultant hemodilution was a positive or negative factor.

Tissues apparently maintain tissue oxygenation and even increase tissue PO_2 with hemodilution down to and below hematocrits of 25% (Messmer, 1973). There are several reasons for this. Hematocrit does not decrease in the microcirculation as much as it does in the systemic circulation and, with the increase in red cell velocity, there is less diffusional shunting in the microcirculation (Kuo and Pittman, 1988; Mirhashemi et al., 1987). There may also be a more homogeneous distribution of red cells within the microcirculation (Pries et al., 1992). These and other considerations have led to hemodilution as a recommended therapeutic procedure in any ischemic condition in which cardiac function is not a problem (Messmer, 1988). Dextran, the diluent in the present experiments, reduces granulocyte and platelet adhesion to endothelial surfaces after endotoxic shock, properties which may have offered additional advantages (Modig, 1988). The possible drawback to intentional hemodilution is that it also increases the median spacing of red cells within a tissue capillary. The added plasma distance between cells may offer an impediment to the equilibration of PO_2 between red cell and plasma phases (Homer, et al., 1981; Gutierrez, 1986; Federspiel and Sarelius, 1984).

Homer et al. (1981) suggested that an increase in O_2 solubility of the plasma would help to overcome its diffusional impediment. They based this on theoretical calculations that predicted a variable PO_2 difference between red cells and plasma, depending on various assumptions. One calculation showed a gradient of 12 mmHg at hematocrit of 20%. They believed that this was a very significant factor based on results of Moss et al. (1976) who showed that for the same reduction of total O_2 capacity by hemodilution, no increase in cardiac output occurred if half the hemoglobin was present in solution in the plasma phase. Homer et al. (1981) actually suggested the use of flurocarbon blood substitutes as a way of testing their theory that capillary PO_2 was a regulatory factor for cardiac output.

Faithfull and Cain (1988) showed that hemodilution with Fluosol did lower critical O_2 delivery to the limb muscles of dogs compared with dextran. However, a subsequent trial with perflubron failed to replicate those results (Cain et al., 1992). The suggested reason was that Fluosol had caused severe microcirculatory disturbance whereas perflubron did not. The authors concluded that in a normal microcirculation, low plasma solubility for O_2 offers no measurable barrier to tissue O_2 extraction. This was a major factor for the rationale of the current study. We reasoned that the microcirculatory disruption attributed to endotoxin and its consequences would amplify any diffusional barrier posed by low O_2 solubility in the plasma. That was the reason for adding perflubron to the diluent used for volume resuscitation. Based on our results, we must conclude that even in endotoxin treated animals, an increase in plasma O_2 solubility had only a small effect on O_2 transfer to tissues. The reason, we believe, is that the red cell to plasma PO_2 gradient is always very small and not an important factor. The effect of plasma hemoglobin that led Homer et al. (1981) to believe that the PO_2 gradient was important may have resulted from a totally different cause. As Biro et al. (1992) recently showed, plasma hemoglobin increased peripheral resistance, probably by its inhibition of EDRF, and did not enhance critical O_2 delivery to canine limb. We suggest that the increase in resistance affected cardiac output in the experiments of Moss et al. (1976) and that any alteration in capillary plasma PO_2 was of minimal importance. Interestingly, a noticeable trend in our PFB group was toward lower cardiac output and regional blood flows, particularly in the gut.

In conclusion, volume therapy of endotoxic shock with acellular colloid solution was very effective in spite of, or possibly because of, the resultant hemodilution. Perfluorocarbon addition made only little improvement on that effectiveness because any effects of a PO_2 gradient between red cell and plasma were probably negligible. Conversely, use of larger concentrations of perflubron may be of benefit by raising the O_2 concentration in capillaries while still preserving the other postulated rheological benefits of hemodilution when microcirculatory function has been disturbed.

ACKNOWLEDGEMENT

Funds for these studies were provided by NIH Grant #HL 26927 and by Alliance Pharmaceutical Corp. who also furnished the perflubron and carrier vehicle. B. Vallet received fellowship grants from the Ministère des Affaires Etrangères (Bourse Lavoisier), the Société de Réanimation de Langue Française (Bourse Nedey), and the Société Française d'Anesthésie-Réanimation.

REFERENCES

Abel, F.L. and Beck, R.R., 1992, Portal venous compliance in canine endotoxin shock, *Circ. Shock* (in press).

Biro, G.P., Anderson, P.J., Curtis, S.E., and Cain, S.M., 1991, Stroma-free hemoglobin: Its presence does not improve oxygen supply to the resting hindlimb vascular bed of anesthetized dogs, *Can. J. Physiol. Pharmacol.* 69:1656.

Bond, R.F., Krech, L.H., and Hershey, J.C., 1992, Effect of ibuprofen upon denervated skeletal muscle resistance and compliance vessels during endotoxemia, *Circ. Shock* 37:145.

Bredle, D.L. and Cain, S.M., 1991, Systemic and muscle O_2 uptake/delivery after dopexamine infusion in endotoxic dogs, *Crit. Care Med.* 19:198.

Cain, S.M., 1986, Assessment of tissue oxygenation, *Crit. Care Clin.* 2:537.

Cain, S.M., 1991, Physiological and pathological oxygen supply dependency, *in*: "Update in Intensive Care and Emergency Medicine 12; Tissue Oxygen Utilization," Gutierrez, G. and Vincent, J.L., eds., Springer-Verlag, Berlin.

Cain, S.M. and Curtis, S.E., 1991, Experimental models of pathologic oxygen supply dependency, *Crit. Care Med.* 19:603.

Cain, S.M. and Curtis, S.E., 1991a, Systemic and regional oxygen uptake and delivery and lactate flux in endotoxic dogs infused with dopexamine, *Crit. Care Med.* 19:1552.

Cain, S.M. and Curtis, S.E., 1992, Systemic and regional oxygen uptake and lactate flux in endotoxic dogs resuscitated with dextran and dopexamine or dextran alone, *Circ. Shock* (in press).

Cain, S.M., Curtis, S.E., and Bradley, W.E., 1992, Facilitation of oxygen transfer by perflubron in hemodiluted dogs, *Adv. Exp. Med. Biol.* (in press).

Curtis, S.E. and Cain, S.M., 1992, Regional and systemic oxygen delivery/uptake relations and lactate flux in hyperdynamic, endotoxin-treated dogs, *Am. Rev. Respir. Dis.* 145:348.

Faithfull, N.S. and Cain, S.M., 1988, Critical levels of O_2 extraction following hemodilution with dextran or Fluosol-DA, *J. Crit. Care* 3:14.

Federspiel, W.J. and I. H. Sarelius, 1984, An examination of the contribution of red cell spacing to the uniformity of oxygen flux at the capillary wall, *Microvasc. Res.* 27:273.

Fiddian-Green, R.G., Amelin, P.M., Hermann, J.B., Arous, E., Cutler, B.S., Schiedler, M., Wheeler, B., and Baker, S., 1986, Prediction of the development of sigmoid ischemia on the day of aortic operations. Indirect measurements of intramural pH in the colon, *Arch. Surg.* 121:654.

Fink, M.P., 1991, Gastrointestinal mucosal injury in experimental models of shock, trauma, and sepsis, *Crit. Care Med.* 19:627.

Gutierrez, G., 1986, The rate of oxygen release and its effect on capillary PO_2 tension: a mathematical analysis, *Resp. Physiol.* 63:79.

Homer, L.D., Weathersby, P.K., and Kiesow, L.A., 1981, Oxygen gradients between red blood cells in the microcirculation, *Microvasc. Res.* 22:308.

Kuo, L and Pittman, R.N., 1988, Effect of hemodilution on oxygen transport in arteriolar networks of hamster striated muscle, *Am. J. Physiol.* 254:H331.

Messmer, K., 1988, Hemodilution - possibilities and safety aspects, *Acta Anaesthesiol. Scand.* 32: Suppl. (89):49.

Messmer, K., Sunder-Plassmann, L., Jesch, F., Gornandt, L., Sinagowitz, E., and Kessler, M., 1973, Oxygen supply to the tissues during limited normovolemic hemodilution, *Res. Exp. Med.* 159:152.

Mirhashemi, S., Ertefai, S., Messmer, K., and Intaglietta, M., 1987, Model analysis of the enhancement of tissue oxygenation by hemodilution due to increased microvascular flow velocity, *Microvasc. Res.* 34,:290.

Modig, J., 1988, Comparison of effects of dextran-70 and Ringer's acetate on pulmonary function, hemodynamics, and survival in experimental septic shock, *Crit. Care Med.* 16:266.

Moss, G.S., Dewoskin, R., Rosen, A.L., Levine, H., and Palani, C.K., 1976, Transport of oxygen and carbon dioxide by hemoglobin-saline solution in the red-cell-free primate, *Surg. Gynecol. Obstet.* 142:357.

Pries, A.R., Fritzsche, A., Ley, K., and Gaehtgens, P., 1992, Redistribution of red blood cell flow in microcirculatory networks by hemodilution, *Circ. Res.* 70:1113.

Rackow, E.C. and Astiz, M.E., 1991, Pathophysiology and treatment of septic shock, *JAMA* 266:548.

Stork, R.L., Dodd, S.L., Chapler, C.K., and Cain, S.M., 1989, Regional hemodynamic responses to hypoxia and hypermetabolism in polycythemic dogs, *J. Appl. Physiol.* 67:96.

HEART

CAPILLARY FLOW DIRECTION
IN THE ISOLATED PERFUSED RAT HEART

Nicholas Cicutti and Karel Rakusan

Department of Physiology
Faculty of Medicine, University of Ottawa,
Ottawa, Ontario, Canada, K1H 8M5

INTRODUCTION

Despite the importance of delineating a specific microvascular flow pattern adapted to the functioning of the heart, this objective has proven particulary difficult in view of the intrinsic contractile nature of cardiac activity. In this context, the direction of blood flow in neighboring coronary capillaries i.e., concurrent vs countercurrent flow has been regarded as potentially significant with respect to tissue oxygenation (Diemer, 1965; Lubbers, 1976). Capillary flow direction, in vivo, has been characterized in normal adult rat myocardium utilizing the colored microsphere technique (Reeves and Rakusan, 1988) and more recently, with respect to regional differences in normal hearts and hearts subjected to pressure overload hypertrophy (Cicutti and Rakusan, 1992).

The objective of the present investigation was firstly to determine whether the isolated perfused heart according to Langendorff was a suitable model for the determination of capillary flow vectors using our colored microsphere technique. To validate the model, results obtained from our in vivo method were used as standards for comparison with those obtained in the present study.

The Langendorff heart offers a comparative ease of preparation and certain technical advantages next to an in vivo model. The ability to precisely control experimental parameters and maintain stable mechanical function over extended periods is superior to that possible under in vivo conditions. For the purposes of the present study, the infusion of microspheres via the ascending aorta into the coronary vasculature is technically less difficult compared to in vivo infusion into the left atrium, and requires only approximately 5-6% of the total number of microspheres needed in vivo. This approach becomes particularly advantageous in the case of smaller hearts in younger animals. In contrast, in vivo infusion of microspheres in the smaller, developing heart presents formidable technical challenges.

It is recognized that the capillary network in the developing heart exhibits systematic differences in capillary geometry relative to the adult heart (Batra and Rakusan, 1992). Therefore, using the Langendorff model, we were interested in characterizing capillary flow vectors in the developing heart relative to the adult heart, in order to determine if the reported changes in the capillary net with growth are reflected by similar changes in capillary flow direction.

METHODS

Animal Preparation

To investigate regional capillary flow direction in rat myocardium an isolated perfused "Langendorff" model was utilized for the sequential infusion of differently colored microsphere suspensions. Sprague-Dawley rats 6-7 week old (n=10), as well as 3-week old (n=34) were anesthetized with sodium pentobarbital (0.1ml/100g body weight). A midline laparotomy was performed with the inferior vena cava isolated. Heparin (0.1ml/100 g body weight) was then injected and allowed to circulate for one minute. Subsequently, the abdominal aorta and inferior vena cava were severed to bleed the animal. Once breathing had ceased, the heart was exposed and loosely packed with crushed ice to arrest it. The aorta was then isolated with a small incision made below the branch of the right carotid artery. A stainless steel canula primed with saline (containing 0.5 mM $CaCl_2$) was inserted into the aorta with 4/0 silk suture tightened around the aorta and cannula. The heart was quickly excised with the cannula attached to a Langendorff perfusion apparatus. Hearts were perfused at a constant presssure 80 cm of H_2O in adult and 65 cm of H_2O in 3-week old hearts respectively. These levels were chosen to reflect the in vivo difference in arterial blood presure in both age groups. The Krebs-Henseleit bicarbonate perfusate contained (mmol·1^{-1}) : NaCl 118.0; KCl 4.7; $CaCl_2$ 2.5; $MgSO_4$ 1.2; $NaHCO_3$ 25.0; KH_2PO_4 1.2; glucose 7.0; sodium pyruvate 2.0, and mannitol 1.1; pH 7.4. The perfusate was equilibrated with 95% O_2-5% CO_2 and warmed to 37°C in a water-jacketed column.

A compliant balloon-tipped catheter was placed in the left ventricle (deflated) and held in place by the mitral valve. A small known volume of water was added to the balloon in order to produce an end-diastolic pressure of approximately 6 mmHg. The peripheral end of the catheter was attached to a transducer (Statham Db 23) and recorder (Grass Model 7) to monitor left ventricular developed pressure, and dP/dt continuously. The hearts were electrically stimulated at a constant rate of 300 beats/minute using small, silver spiral electrodes connected to the base of the right ventricle. Coronary flow rate (effluent from the right ventricle) was measured using a graduated cylinder.

Colored microsphere procedure

Non-radioactive red and blue microspheres with diameters of 10 ± 0.23 μm were purchased from E-Z Trac, Los Angeles, CA. Prior to injection, the microspheres were suspended at a concentration of 6 x 10^6/ml^{-1} in saline containing .01% Tween solution, and lightly agitated in a vortex mixer for one minute. Microsphere aggregates were not observed during microscopic examination of the suspension. Thereafter, differently colored 2 ml microsphere aliquots, each containing approximately 60 x10^4 red or blue microspheres were infused sequentially into the ascending aorta (retrograde perfusion through the coronary vasculature) at constant and identical rates of 0.2 ml/min for 10 minutes (adult) or 3 minutes (3-week) via a Sage Instruments Model 355 syringe pump. A timed 5-minute interval elapsed between injections. After all injections were concluded, the hearts were weighed, dissected, and the samples quick frozen for cryotomic preparation of 40 μm longitudinal sections from midmyocardial and subendocardial regions.

The rationale behind the use of the colored microsphere technique for the characterization of capillary flow direction has previously been described (see Cicutti and Rakusan, 1992). The sequential infusion of two differently colored microsphere suspensions results in the formation of three distinct aggregation patterns within the coronary microcirculation.

(1) Single sphere.
(2) Aggregates of one color only.
(3) Aggregates containing more than one injected color.

According to aggregation patterns, a "flow vector" was established based on the sequence of microsphere colors entrapped within each capillary (Figure 1). Detailed micro-

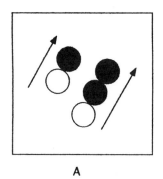 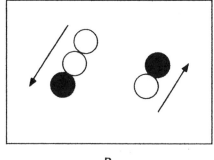

A   B

Figure 1. Schematic representation of capillary flow vectors in myocardium based on sequence of microspheres colors trapped in coronary capillaries; arrows indicate flow direction. (**A**) concurrent flow illustrated between adjacent capillaries. (**B**) example of countercurrent flow depicted.

scopic examination of flow vectors obtained from neighboring capillaries enabled the characterization of regional capillary flow direction.

RESULTS

A comparison of regional myocardial flow vector observations from our earlier in vivo study and the present isolated heart experiments in adult and 3-week old hearts hearts according to capillary ranking is summarized in Table 1.   As a result of a substantially smaller cardiac mass in the 3-week old animals, a greater number of hearts (n=34) vs (n=10) was required for sampling in order to achieve comparable flow vector observation numbers.

TABLE 1. Percentages of concurrent flow according to a sequence of capillary rankings recorded for IN VIVO and IN VITRO (ADULT)and (3-WEEK) groups. Each group further subdivided according to MID and SUB-E regions.

CAPILLARY RANKING:	1	2	3	4	5
IN VIVO (n=9)					
% Concurrent (MID)	86%	84%	82%	79%	77%
% Concurrent (SUB-E)	72%	61%	64%	56%	52%
IN VITRO: ADULT (n=10)					
% Concurrent (MID)	87%	82%	81%	78%	75%
% Concurrent (SUB-E)	79%	74%	63%	65%	58%
IN VITRO: 3-WEEK (n=34)					
% Concurrent (MID)	83%	78%	73%	75%	70%
% Concurrent (SUB-E)	80%	74%	66%	69%	63%

To investigate possible differences between the in vivo and present adult isolated heart data, a four-way ANOVA for proportions was selected to examine the contributions and potential significance for the independant variables of capillary ranking, in vivo/in vitro, midmyocardium versus subendocardium (MID/SUB-E) and the individual hearts to the flow vector observations.   In both experimental models, results indicate a predominance in concurrent flow direction, which decreased (p< 0.001) with capillaries increasingly removed from an individual reference vessel (Table 1). A regional comparison between the two experimental groups is illustrated in Figure 2. Almost identical values were seen in midmyocardium. With respect to subendocardial regions, significant group differences were revealed (p < 0.05), with higher percentages of concurrent flow in the isolated heart. Both groups revealed significant differences (p < 0.01) in percentages of concurrent flow between mid- and subendocardium.

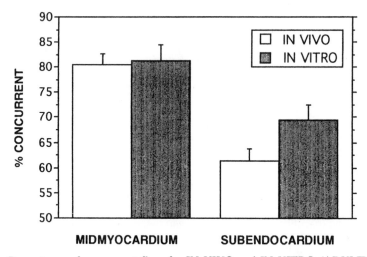

Figure 2. Percentages of concurrent flow for IN VIVO and IN VITRO (ADULT) groups in midyocardial and subendocardial regions. Both groups revealed higher percentages of concurrent flow in midmyocardium (p<0.01). The IN VITRO group depicted higher percentages of concurrent flow in subendocardium compared to the IN VIVO group (p<0.05).

The same statistical model was utilized to test for possible differences between the (ADULT) isolated heart group vs the (3-Week) group. The 3-week old group also demonstrated a preponderance in the percentage of concurrent flow, which declined significantly (P < 0.001) with capillaries further removed from a reference vessel (Figure 3A). Figure 3B illustrates a regional comparison between the isolated heart experiments in adult and 3-week old rats. Although regional differences within groups were found to be statitistically significant (P < 0.05), comparisons between groups were not significantly different in either midmyocardium or subendocardium.

DISCUSSION

The preeminent finding of this investigation was that coronary capillary flow direction can be characterized reliably in the isolated perfused heart model. This finding resulted from application of our previously described technique of sequential in vivo infusion of different colored microspheres into rat myocardium (see Reeves and Rakusan, 1988; Cicutti and Rakusan, 1992).

The isolated perfused heart according to Langendorff remains 95 years after its first description, one of the most popular and useful techniques available for studying the hemodynamics, metabolism, and histological structure of the heart. Nevertheless,

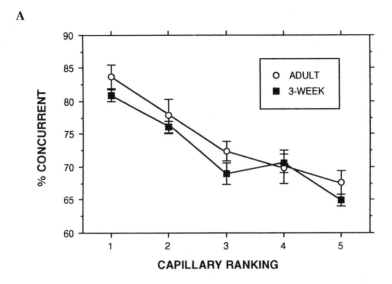

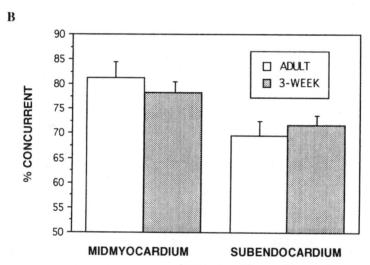

Figure 3. (A) Graphical representation of the effect of capillary ranking on the percentages of concurrent flow in isolated ADULT and 3-WEEK old hearts. In both groups the overall effect of capillary ranking is significant (p<0.01). (B) Regional differences within the ADULT and 3-WEEK old hearts were significanly different (p<0.05). However, regional comparisons between groups were not statistically significant.

preparations such as the Langendorff heart have been criticized periodically because they are lacking a normal neural and humoral background, and do not function mechanically as does the intact heart. Consequently, the results obtained from this model are often regarded as somewhat "non-physiological". Such potential shortcomings must be taken into account when proposing an investigation. On the other hand, the comparative ease of the technical set-up, surgical preparation, with the ability to precisely control various parameters should not be undervalued. Ultimately, the ability of the isolated heart to provide potentially useful information required an evaluation on the basis of results from previously worked out standards. For the present study, these standards for comparison were provided from our earlier in vivo study of capillary flow vectors in myocardium.

Overall, flow vector data obtained from the isolated heart model do not appear appreciably different from results obtained in previous in vivo experimentation. As with the in vivo model, results indicate a predominance in concurrent flow direction, with, however a progressive decrease in the percentage of concurrent flow with capillaries increasingly removed from an individual reference vessel. This has been postulated to be representative of a distinctive geometric arrangement of arteriolar units; individual arteriolar units being characterized by a predominantly concurrent internal flow pattern, which, however may be oriented in countercurrent fashion to adjacents arteriolar units. Therefore, as one expands the area of analysis away from a reference capillary, the greater the possibility of capturing capillaries originating from a separate arteriolar unit. In addition, the percentage of concurrent flow was significantly lower in subendocardium than in midmyocardium. Overall levels over the range of capillary rankings in subendocardium were higher in the isolated heart than in vivo. This apparent discrepancy may be related to basic differences in mechanical function between the two models. Although regional capillary flow direction in myocardium is largely dictated by an intrinsic microvascular architecture, temporal variability in flow pattern may be produced by changes in contractile state, driving pressure, vasomotion, etc. In the Langendorff preparation, although the heart contracts (isovolumetrically), its mechanical performance and metabolic requirements do not approach those of the intact heart in vivo. In the intact heart, the balance between oxygen supply and demand is more critical in the subendocardial layers than in subepi- or midmyocardium (Griggs et al.,1973; Eng et al., 1987). Such regional differences would be expected to be minimized in the Langendorff model, where a depressed myocardial contractile state is less likely to influence microvascular flow pattern.

A further objective of this study was to compare regional capillary flow direction in developing versus adult hearts. Our rationale behind this objective is based on findings that the capillary network in developing hearts depicts systematic differences in geometric organization relative to adult hearts. For example, a lateral expansion of the capillary set with myocardial growth is evidenced by an increase in the number of adjacent capillaries traversing the path from arteriole to venule (Batra and Rakusan, 1992). In terms of flow direction, this conceivably increased the possibility of encountering countercurrent flow observations in the developing heart if "individual" capillary sets were to display a uniform internal flow pattern. Despite slight qualitative differences, results were not significantly different from those obtained in adult myocardium. This would suggest that overall capillary flow pattern does not differ appreciably between the two age groups. Thus, the typical lateral expansion of the coronary capillary set with age is not reflected by adaptations or changes in flow direction.

In conclusion, this investigation indicates that the isolated heart model according to Langendorff is a suitable and useful tool for the determination of capillary flow vectors in rat myocardium. Despite slight differences noted in subendocardial regions between the two preparations, the overall uniformity of results obtained is encouraging. Indeed, the Langendorff heart forms the basis of current work in determining capillary flow direction during conditions of experimental anoxia using our colored microsphere technique. Preliminary results reveal a higher percentage of countercurrent flow observations among neighboring capillaries subsequent to the anoxic intervention than during an earlier period of normoxia.

[Supported by the Medical Research Council of Canada]

REFERENCES

Batra, S., and Rakusan, K., 1992, Capillary network geometry during postnatal growth in the rat heart, Am. J. Physiol. (in press)

Cicutti, N., and Rakusan, K., 1992, Microvascular flow vectors in normal and hypertrophic myocardium as determined by the method of colored microspheres, Microvasc. Res. 43: 267-275.

Diemer, K., 1965, Über die Sauerstoffdiffusion im Gehirn. I. Räumliche Vorstellung und Berechnung der Sauerstoffdiffusion, Pflügers Archiv. 285: 99-108.

Eng, C., Cho, S., Factor, S.M., and Kirk, E.S., 1987, A nonflow basis for the vulnerability of the subendocardium, Am. Coll. Cardiol. 9: 374-379.

Griggs, D.M., Chen, C.C., and Tchokoev, V.V., 1973, Subendocardial metabolism in experimental aortic stenosis, Am. J. Physiol. 224: 607-613

Lübbers, D.W., 1976, Quantitative measurement and description of oxygen supply to the tissue, in "Oxygen and Physiological Function " F.F. Jobsis, ed., Professional Information Library, Dallas.

Reeves, W.J., and Rakusan, K., 1988, Myocardial capillary flow pattern as determined by the method of colored microspheres, in "Oxygen Transport to Tissue- X", M. Machizuki, C. R. Honig, T. Koyama, T.K. Goldstick, D.F. Bruley, eds., Plenum Press, New York and London, pp. 13-19.

MYOCARDIAL OXYGENATION IN IMMATURE AND ADULT RATS

Zdenek Turek, Sanjay Batra,
and Karel Rakusan

Departments of Physiology, Faculty of Medicine
Catholic University, Nijmegen, The Netherlands
and Faculty of Medicine, University of Ottawa
Ottawa, Ontario, Canada

INTRODUCTION

Blood oxygen capacity is one of the most important determinants of myocardial oxygenation (Rakusan, 1971). Immature rats have a lower blood oxygen carrying capacity than the adult animals due to a lower hemoglobin (Hb) concentration (Dhindsa et al., 1981). They also have a lower myocardial myoglobin (Mb) concentration (Rakusan et al., 1965). We are not aware of any direct measurement of the other important myocardial oxygen pressure determinants, such as coronary blood flow and myocardial oxygen consumption in immature rats. Estimations of coronary blood flow (in ml/g of tissue) based on cardiac output and rubidium clearance measurements (Vizek and Albrecht, 1973; Rakusan and Marcinek, 1973) indicate no significant difference between immature and adult rats.

Similar levels of coronary blood flow, combined with a low Hb concentration, suggest a lower O_2 delivery to cardiac muscle in immature animals when compared to adults. This apparent handicap may be partly or entirely compensated for by the improved geometrical conditions for O_2 transport due to a specific arrangement of the capillary bed. Our recent measurements confirm more advantageous geometrical configuration of coronary capillaries in young rats. They have a higher capillary density and a more homogeneous capillary spacing than adult animals. This has been demonstrated for both the arteriolar and the venular segments of the capillary bed (Batra and Rakusan, 1992).

In the present communication we evaluated quantitatively the effect of these differences in determinants of myocardial oxygenation between immature and adult animals. In particular, we wanted to elucidate to what degree a more advantageous

Oxygen Transport to Tissue XV, P. Vaupel,
et al., Plenum Publishing, New York, 1994

geometrical configuration of the capillary bed in the hearts of young animals can compensate for the concomitantly occurring lower hemoglobin concentration.

METHODS

The myocardial P_{O_2} histograms were computed using the truncated cone model, presented at the last ISOTT Meeting. This model uses the morphometric data on arteriolar and venular segments of coronary capillaries. The principles and limitations of the model have been described previously (Turek et al., 1992). Basically, the model consists of sets of parallel Kroghian tissue cylinders. Radii of these cylinders within the arteriolar capillary section have a distribution that is different from that corresponding to the venular section. Morphometric data on capillarization in rats of various age were taken from Batra and Rakusan (1992). In general, both the average radius and its variability are smaller at the venular then at the arteriolar portion of the capillaries. These values are also lower in younger then in older animals (see Table 1). Data on hemoglobin concentration and P_{50} were taken from Dhindsa et al. (1981). For coronary blood flow, we used the same value as previously used for the adult animals (Turek et al., 1992) for reasons explained in the Introduction. Regrettably, we were not able to find any data on myocardial O_2 consumption in immature and adolescent rats and therefore here also the value identical to those in adult animals were used. Myoglobin concentration from Rakusan et al. (1965) was used for the calculation of myoglobin facilitation pressure, and the remaining input data are taken from Turek et al. (1992). In addition, a capillary barrier corresponding to a P_{O_2} drop of 10 mm Hg in average-sized tissue cylinder was used.

Table 1.

Morphometric input data.

Age:	3 w	4 w	8 w	Adult
Arteriolar section:				
R (μm)	9.8	10.7	12.6	13.0
logSD	0.063	0.057	0.066	0.073
percentage of total length	53	56	69	81
Venular section:				
R (μm)	9.1	10.1	12.1	12.0
logSD	0.066	0.069	0.067	0.071
percentage of total length	47	44	31	19

w = weeks; R = average radius of the Kroghian tissue cylinder;
logSD = logarithmic standard deviation, index of heterogeneity

RESULTS

Fig. 1 depicts the myocardial P_{O_2} histograms in adult rats, calculated using their normal capillary geometry and hemoglobin concentration (14.2 g/100 ml blood). Fig. 2 shows myocardial tissue P_{O_2} histograms computed using the entry data for adult hearts, except for hemoglobin

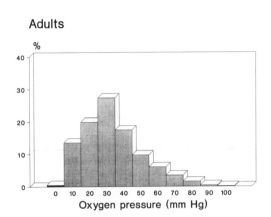

Adults

Fig. 1. Myocardial tissue P_{O_2} histograms in adult rats calculated using their normal Hb concentration and capillary geometry.

concentration: values corresponding to measurements in 3, 4, and 8 weeks old animals were entered in this case (9.7 g/100 ml; 10.3 g/100 ml; 14.2 g/100ml, respectively). Evidently, with decreasing Hb concentration the histograms shift increasingly towards the lower values. Thus, the percentage of anoxic tissue ($P_{O_2} < 0.005$ mm Hg) and that of tissue with P_{O_2} lower than 10 mm Hg gradually increases. This demonstrates the important role of hemoglobin concentration as one of the principal myocardial P_{O_2} determinants. On the other hand, the effect of Mb concentration was rather small and the P_{O_2} histograms with Mb concentration of adult animals were practically indistinguishable from those calculated with a Mb concentration corresponding to values found in young animals. Therefore, they were not shown separately.

Fig. 3 shows myocardial P_{O_2} histograms computed using the hemoglobin and myoglobin concentrations as observed in young rats but this time we used their real capillary geometry (see Table 1.). Clearly, the capillary geometry of young rats compensates almost completely for the lower hemoglobin concentration. Again, the effect of differing Mb concentrations was negligible and is not shown here.

DISCUSSION

To our knowledge, this is the first attempt to evaluate the potential differences in P_{O_2} histograms between immature and adult hearts. Unfortunately, only some of the important input data are based on direct measurements: Hb and Mb concentrations as

Hb concentr. of 3 weeks old

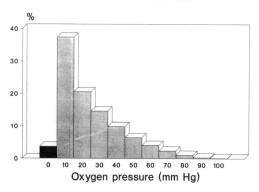

Hb concentr. of 4 weeks old

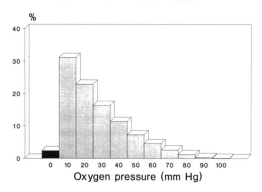

Hb concentr. of 8 weeks old

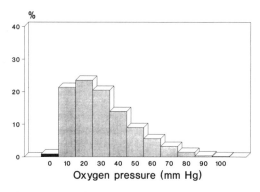

Fig. 2. Myocardial tissue P_{O_2} histograms computed using the entry data for adult hearts except for Hb and Mb concentrations. Values corresponding to the measurements in 3, 4 and 8 weeks old animals were entered in this case.

3 weeks old

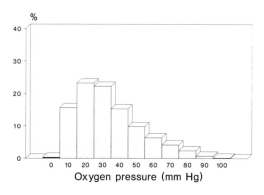

4 weeks old

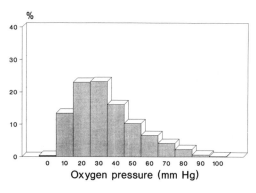

8 weeks old

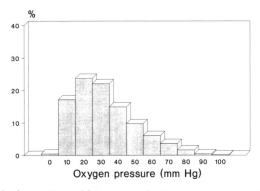

Fig. 3. Myocardial tissue P_{O_2} histograms in immature rats calculated using their normal Hb and Mb concentration and capillary geometry.

well as coronary capillary morphometric data. Our results on myocardial tissue oxygenation indicate that the capillary geometry of immature rat hearts can compensate to a large degree for the low Hb concentration occurring during postnatal development.

Our current computations also confirm the previous estimates of Rakusan (1971) on the importance of the blood O_2 carrying capacity for myocardial oxygenation. His deductions, which were based on a model of homogeneous capillary geometry, are also valid for the more realistic geometric arrangement. In this case, the heterogeneity in capillary spacing is also taken into account.

The obtained results should be interpreted with caution. The presented myocardial P_{O_2} histograms were calculated while using a model of myocardial tissue oxygenation that is based on several assumptions.[7] In addition, some input data had to be assumed. Another important point is that the hematological parameters and the morphometric data were not measured in the same animals. Therefore, while the trend of the differences is probably valid, the absolute values of P_{O_2} histograms are not necessarily accurate. Nevertheless, it is clear that the actual myocardial capillary geometry in immature animals helps to improve myocardial oxygenation and can, at least in part, compensate for the deleterious effect of low hemoglobin concentration naturally occurring in immature aninals.

REFERENCES

Batra, S., and Rakusan,K., 1991, Capillary network geometry during postnatal growth in rat hearts. *Am. J. Physiol.* 262: H635-H640.

Dhindsa, D.S., Metcalfe, J., Blackmore D.W., and Koler R.D., 1981, Postnatal changes in oxygen affinity of rat blood. *Comp. Biochem. Physiol.* 69A: 279-283.

Rakusan, K., 1971, "Oxygen in the Heart Muscle", C.C. Thomas, Springfield, Illinois.

Rakusan, K., and Marcinek, H., 1973, Postnatal development of the cardiac output distribution in rat. *Biol. Neonate* 22: 58-63.

Rakusan, K., Radl, J., and Poupa O., 1965, The distribution and content of myoglobin in the heart of the rat during postnatal development. *Physiol. Bohemoslov.* 14: 317-319.

Turek, Z., Rakusan, K., Olders, J., Hoofd, L., and Kreuzer, F. 1991, Computed myo cardial P_{O_2} histograms: effects of various geometrical and functional conditions. *J. Appl. Physiol.* 70: 1845-1853.

Turek, Z., Hoofd, L., Batra, S., and Rakusan, K., 1992, The effect of realistic geometry of capillary networks on tissue P_{O_2} in hypertrophied rat heart. *In*: Oxygen Transport to Tissue-XIV, in press.

Vizek, M., and Albrecht, I., 1973, Development of cardiac output in male rats. *Physiol. Bohemoslov.* 22: 573-580.

ISCHEMIC AREAS IN HYPERTROPHIC LANGENDORFF RAT HEARTS VISUALIZED BY NADH VIDEOFLUORIMETRY

J.F. Ashruf[1], C. Ince[1],
H.A. Bruining[1] and W.C. Hulsmann[2]

[1]Department of Surgery and [2]Thorax Center
Erasmus University Rotterdam
Dr. Molewaterplein 40
3015 GD Rotterdam
The Netherlands

INTRODUCTION

Reduced nicotinamide adenine dinucleotide (NADH) is a naturally occuring intracellular fluorophore which plays a key role in the transfer of reducing equivalents from the tricarboxylic acid cycle to the respiratory chain in mitochondria. Inhibition of the respiratory chain due to inadequate oxygen supply is reflected by increased NADH levels. Upon illumination of tissue with light around 360 nm, NADH (and not NAD^+) fluoresces around 460 nm. Ischemic myocardium is therefore characterized by a high intensity of NADH fluorescence, whereas adequately oxygenated myocardium is low fluorescent (Chance 1976; Chance et al. 1978).

Hypertrophia is caused by the addition of sarcomeres. Since during this process intercapillary distances increase (Roberts et al. 1941) and the number of transverse capillary profiles decreases (Anversa et al. 1980), problems in oxygen- and substrate supply to the myocytes may arise. Heterogeneity of blood supply in hypertrophic hearts has been recognized by others and interpreted as the difference in ratio of vascular supply to muscle mass in different areas. In this study we investigated whether it was possible to evoke ischemic areas (as witnessed by increased NADH fluorescence) in hypertrophic Langendorff hearts by perfusion with O_2-saturated tyrode. We hypothesized that in hypertrophic Langendorff hearts areas with decreased vascularization, in contrast to adequately vascularized areas, would become ischemic due to the poorer oxygen-carrying capacity of tyrode compared to blood.

MATERIALS AND METHODS

5 male Wistar rats weighing about 150 g were operated for subdiaphragmatic and

Oxygen Transport to Tissue XV, Edited by P. Vaupel
et al., Plenum Press, New York, 1994

suprarenal aortic narrowing to produce hypertrophic hearts 5-6 weeks later. Hypertrophic hearts had a total ventricle wet weight of 1.6 $\pm$ 0.1 g (n = 5) (non-hypertrophic hearts weighed 1.0 $\pm$ 0.1 g (n = 5). The hearts were removed, cooled in ice-cold tyrode, and rapidly arranged for retrograde perfusion with O_2-saturated tyrode via the aorta. Coronary flow was measured with a electromagnetic flow probe (Skalar Medical, Delft, The Netherlands).

The tyrode consisted of 128 mM NaCl, 4.7 mM KCl, 1 mM $MgCl_2$, 0.4 mM NaH_2PO_4, 20.2 mM $NaHCO_3$, 1.3 mM $CaCl_2$, 11 mM glucose and was equilibrated with 5% CO_2 in O_2. Once ischemic spots developed, the effect of adenosine (final concentration in tyrode: 10 μM) on these spots was observed.

The video fluorimeter (Ince et al. 1992) consisted of a fluorescence unit B2-RFCA of an Olympus BH2 microscope, a 100 W mercury arc lamp and an image-intensified CCD video camera (MXRi 5051 camera, HCS Vision Technology, Eindhoven, The Netherlands) fitted with a C-mount, to which a 105 mm Micro-Nikkor macrolens was attached. The B2-RFCA unit housed a dichroic mirror with an UG-1 barrier filter providing the 360 nm light needed for NADH excitation (Fig. 1). A band-pass filter allowed transmission of the NADH fluorescence centered around 460 $\pm$ 20 nm. Fluorescence images were recorded continuously on a VHS recorder (Panasonic Type AG 7330) and printed on a Mitsubishi Video Copy Processor. Images could be analyzed off-line for quantification of the fluorescence intensity.

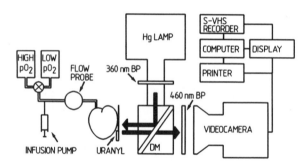

Figure 1. The experimental set-up consisted of a Langendorff set-up with two reservoirs for tyrode. In this study only the left reservoir was used ("HIGH pO_2"). An infusion pump allowed infusion of adenosine into the perfusate. A small piece of uranyl fluorescence calibration glass is placed next to the heart as a fluorescence reference.

RESULTS AND CONCLUSIONS

Within 5 min after the onset of perfusion, high fluorescent areas appeared on the epicardial surface of hypertrophic hearts, which were clearly demarcated from the surrounding low fluorescent myocardium (Fig. 2), whereas normal hearts remained low fluorescent for at least 3 hours (Fig. 3) (Ince et al. 1992). The NADH fluorescence intensity of the high fluorescent areas was at least 4 times that of the low fluorescent areas. Addition of adenosine to the tyrode resulted in a 2 to 3-fold increase of the coronary flow. The high fluorescent spots disappeared within 2 minutes after addition of adenosine, indicating improved transport of oxygen to these areas. These results suggest the exsistence of areas in hypertrophic rat myocardium which are relatively

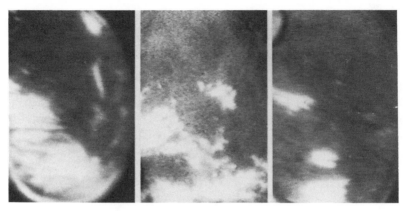

Figure 2. Images of three hypertrophic Langendorff rat hearts during oxygen saturated perfusion. Ischemic areas (high fluorescent, white areas) can be clearly seen. Images were taken 5 minutes after the onset of the Langendorff perfusion.

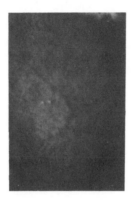

Figure 3. Image of a control, non-hypertrophic, Langendorff heart. This image was taken after 2 hours of Langendorff perfusion, and as can be seen, no ischemic high fluorescent areas are present.

hypoperfused (the high fluorescent areas in Fig. 2). Application of the above described optical method enables identification of hypoperfused areas in hypertrophic hearts and may prove to be a powerful tool in further investigation of oxygen transport and hypertrophia induced alterations therein.

REFERENCES

Anversa, P., Olivetti, G., Melissari, M. and V. Loud, A., 1980, Stereological measurement of cellular and subcellular hypertrophy and hyperplasia in the papillary muscle of adult rat, J. Mol. Cel. Card., 12: 781 - 795.

Chance, B., 1976, Pyridine nucleotide as an indicator of the oxygen requirements for energy-linked functions of mitochondria, Circ. Res., 38 (suppl I): 31 - 38.

Chance, B., Barlow, C., Nakase, Y., Takeda, H., Mayevsky, A., Fischetti, R., Graham, N. and Sorge, J., 1978, Heterogeneity of oxygen delivery in normoxic and anoxic states: a fluorimeter study, Am. J. Physiol., 235 (6): H809 - H820.

Ince, C., Coremans, J.M.C.C. and Bruining, H.A., 1992, In vivo NADH fluorescence, In: Advances in Experimental Medicine and Biology: Oxygen Transport to Tissue XIV: 267 - 275, Editors: W. Erdmann and D.F. Bruley, Publishers: Plenum Press.

Ince, C., Ashruf, J.F., Avontuur, J.A.M., Wieringa, P.A., Spaan, J.A.E. and Bruining, H.A., 1992, Heterogeneity of the hypoxic state in the rat heart is determined at capillary level, Am. J. Physiol., (in press).

Roberts, J.T. and Wearn, J.T., 1941, Quantitative changes in the capillary-muscle relationship in human hearts during normal growth and hypertrophy, Am. Heart. J., 21: 617 - 633.

POTENTIAL OF NITROIMIDAZOLES AS MARKERS OF HYPOXIA IN HEART

W.L. Rumsey, B. Patel, B. Kuczynski, R.K. Narra, Y-W. Chan, K.E. Linder,
J. Cyr, N. Raju, K. Ramalingam, and A.D. Nunn

Bristol-Myers Squibb Pharmaceutical Research Institute
New Brunswick, NJ 08903

INTRODUCTION

It is well known that cardiac muscle has a high and continuous requirement for oxygen. Oxygen is primarily needed, i.e., over 95%, to maintain flux through mitochondrial oxidative phosphorylation for synthesis of ATP. Oxygen is delivered to the working cardiac myocytes at levels consistent with the prevailing metabolic demands established by the various ATP-dependent reactions, principally cycling of the contractile myofilaments. When oxygen delivery is diminished, for example during ischemia, electron flux within the respiratory chain is impeded by the lack of appropriate electron acceptor at the cytochrome oxidase reaction. Consequently, the concentration of reducing equivalents (NADH and $FADH_2$) increases. This condition establishes the opportunity for these and other sources of biological reductants to interact with exogenously supplied molecules having high electron affinity.

Nitroheterocycles are electron affinic compounds that have been used for treatment of certain bacterial infections and as radiosensitizers in cancer therapy (for review, see Rauth, 1984). Cytotoxicity of these compounds is thought to result from reduction of the nitro group and subsequent binding to various intracellular constituents, such as lipids (Raleigh et al., 1981), nucleic acids and protein (Varghese and Whitmore, 1980). Misonidazole (1-[2-nitroimidazol-1-yl]-3-methoxy-2-propanol), originally developed as a radiosensitizer, undergoes reduction in hypoxic tissue (see for example, Stratford, 1982). It has been suggested that radiolabeled nitroheterocycles could be useful for demarcation and imaging of hypoxic tissue (Chapman et al., 1989). Fluorinated derivatives (^{18}F) of misonidazole may have potential for identifying regions of hypoxia in myocardium using positron emission tomography (Martin et al., 1989; Shelton et al., 1989). We have been engaged in the development of a ^{99m}Tc-labeled nitroimidazole suitable for imaging hypoxia in tissue using the gamma camera. In this report, we provide preliminary evidence that a PnAO derivative containing a 2-nitroimidazole and complexed with technetium, is retained preferentially in hypoxic cardiac myocytes and that retention requires the presence of the nitro group. Comparison with ^{3}H-fluoromisonidazole, [131]Iodo-vinyl-misonidazole and other ^{99m}Tc-PnAO-nitroimidazole derivatives indicates that uptake is dependent, in part, on the lipophilicity of the respective compounds.

Oxygen Transport to Tissue XV, Edited by P. Vaupel
et al., Plenum Press, New York, 1994

METHODS AND MATERIALS

In Vitro Experiments

Calcium-tolerant ventricular myocytes were isolated from hearts of adult Sprague Dawley rats (175-225 gm) according to the procedure of Wittenberg and Robinson (1981) as described previously (Rumsey et al., 1990). The rats were anesthetized with sodium pentobarbital (50 mg/kg IP, Nembutal, Abbott, Chicago, IL) and heparinized (500 IU, Invenex, Chagrin Falls, OH) via the caudal vena cava. Hearts were excised quickly and were perfused retrogradely at 72 cm H_2O and 37o C with a calcium-free Hepes-Ringer buffer supplemented with 14 mM glucose and insulin (10 mU/ml). The perfusate was gassed with 100% O_2. After 3 minutes, the hearts were perfused via recirculation with the same medium plus 0.1% collagenase (231 U/mg) at a constant flow of 6 ml/min/heart. The ventricles were minced and incubated for 10 min in similar medium containing 0.15% collagenase, 0.7% BSA and 0.3 mM $CaCl_2$ using a Dubnoff Metabolic Shaker water bath at 37o C. Four additional incubations were used to collect the remaining cell population. The cells were washed and resuspended in Hepes-Ringer buffer containing 0.7% BSA and 0.3 mM $CaCl_2$. Viability of the dissociated cells was analysed using a hemocytometer. Immediately following morphological analysis, the cells were used for experiments. The number of quiescent, rod shaped cells ranged from 65-85% within a total population of 5-9 X 10^6 cells. Cells were suspended at a concentration of 4-6 mg dry wt/ml of media.

Cells were incubated in 25 ml erlhenmeyer flasks (2 ml of cell suspension/flask) with each compound for a period of one hour under conditions of normoxia (exposed to room air) or hypoxia. Preliminary results (data not shown) indicated that maximal levels of retention were obtained with an incubation period of 60 min, therefore, all samples were quenched at this time by centrifugation through a layer of 100% dibutylphthalate. In order to produce hypoxia, the cells were subjected to an atmosphere of argon. To ensure that these cells were incubated in a low oxygen environment, glucose oxidase (final concentration = 65 U/ml) and catalase (final concentration = 1300 U/ml) were added to the suspending media. The cells suspensions were were maintained at 37o C. The amounts of radiopharmaceutical added to each reaction vessel were considered to be tracer quantities (3-5 μCi/ ml or about 0.1 nM for the technetium compounds and 0.5 mM for ^{3}H-Fluoromisonidazole). Triplicate aliquots (100 ul) were sampled and were centrifuged (12,000 rpm X 1 min; Beckman Microfuge 11, Irvine CA) using 400 μl polypropylene microfuge tubes containing 50 μl of 100% dibutylphthalate. Radioactivity arising from technetium or iodine labelled compounds within the separated fractions was counted in a LKB gamma counter (Pharmacia, Gaithersburg, MD). ^{3}H-Fluoromisonidazole was counted (Beckman LS 7500) after suspension of the pellet fraction in saturated NH_4Cl and subsequent addition of 3 ml of scintillant (Scintiverse II; Fisher Chemical, Fairlawn, NJ). The remaining fractions were similarly treated with scintillant for counting of radioactivity. Retention in cells was expressed as a percentage of the total radioactivity in the sampled aliquot.

In Vivo Experiments

Mongrel dogs (15-18 kg) were anaesthetized with sodium pentobarbital (50 mg/kg IP, Nembutal, Abbott, Chicago, IL) and instrumented for measurements of arterial and left intraventricular pressures. Both femoral veins were cannulated for administration of additional anesthesia (when needed), $^{99m}TcO(PnAO-1-2-nitro)$ and isoproterenol. A tracheal cannula was inserted and the animal was respirated at rates sufficient to produce normoxemia (arterial pO_2 = 85-95 Torr) and arterial pH values in the normal range (7.3-7.38, pCO_2 = 37-42 Torr). The heart was exposed via thoracotomy. The left anterior descending artery (LAD) was isolated near its origin and partially occluded with a hydraulic occluder. An electromagnetic flow probe (Carolina Medical Electronics, King, NC) was placed proximal to the occluder. The animal was sacrificed using a standard euthanasia solution (Euthanasia-5; Schein, Port Washington, NY) after sufficient residence time had elapsed (40 min) to clear the complex from the normoxic region. The latter was estimated from data on blood clearance rates (data not shown).

The heart was freed from the great vessels, removed from the thorax, and rinsed in ice-cold saline. The tissue was sliced into 2 cm thick slabs, frozen in liquid freon and sectioned (40 micron slices) using a cryostat thermostated at -15° C (Lipshaw Corp., Detroit, MI). The mounted sections were exposed for 24 hrs (XAR film; Kodak, Rochester, NY). Image analysis was performed using commercially available software (M1, Imaging Research, INC., Toronto, Canada).

Preparation of Radiopharmaceuticals

Table 1 provides a summary description of the compounds used in the present study. Synthesis of BMS 181321 (Oxo [[3,3,9,9-tetramethyl-1-(2-nitro-1H-imidazol-1-yl)-4,8-diazaundecane-2, 10-dione dioximato] (3-)-N, N', N'', N''']technetium) has been described previously (Linder et al., 1992). In brief, BMS 181321 was prepared by dissolving 2.0 mg of PnAO-1,2-nitroimidazole ligand in 1.5 ml of saline, 0.5 ml of 0.1N $NaHCO_3$ and 0.5 ml of generator eluant (up to 100 mCi $^{99m}TcO_4^-$). The reaction was initiated by addition of 50 μl of a deoxygenated saturated stannous tartrate solution. The reaction was completed within 10 min at room temperature. The complex was then separated from nonradioactive components and purified by adsorption onto PRP-1 reversed phase resin, following a modification of the procedure of Jurisson et al. (1991). The product was eluted with 100% ethanol, brought to dryness, and dissolved in saline. BMS 181409, BMS 180902, and BMS 181004 were prepared in similar fashion as described for BMS 181321. For the preparation of BMS 181031, PnAO-6-Me was dissolved in 0.1 mL of MeOH and then used to prepare the technetium complex as described above. The radiochemical purity of the Tc-complexes was >90% as determined by High Pressure Liquid Chromatography (HPLC) using a Hamilton PRP-1 column eluted with acetonitrile/0.1M NH_4OAc, pH 4.6.

Table 1. Summary of nitroimidazole compounds.

Compound			6-OH	6-amide-2-nitro	1,4-nitro	6-CH3	1,2-nitro
R group	-	-	6-OH	6-amide-2-nitro	1,4-nitro	6-CH3	1,2-nitro
Name/BMS Number	Fluoro-misonidazole	Iodovinyl-misonidazole	180 902	181 004	181 409	183 603	181 321
Label*	1	4	2	3+	5+	6+	7

*Label refers to the identification numbers (+ = ligand only) used throughout text and for symbols in Figure 1.

For synthesis of [131]Iodovinylmisonidazole, a 0.2 mg sample of Sn (n-butyl)$_3$ vinyl misonidazole (generously provided by J. Biskupiak, University of Washington) was labelled with [131]Iodine, following the procedure of Biskupiak et al. (1991) The reaction mixture was partially purified by adsorption onto PRP-1 reversed phase resin as described above. The product was eluted from the resin with 100% ethanol and evaporated to dryness. The complex was then redissolved in ethanol:saline (50:50) and purified by (HPLC) on a Whatman ODS-3 Partisil Column as described previously (Biskupiak et al., 1991). The radiochemical purity was greater than 90%.

The specific activity of ^{3}H-Fluoromisonidazole (generously provided by Dr. K. Krohn, University of Washington) was 63 μCi/mg. The compound was dissolved in 100% ethanol. On the day of the experiment, an aliquot was evaporated to dryness using an atmosphere of nitrogen and redissolved in saline.

The lipophilicity of the compounds was measured using HPLC (Feld and Nunn, 1989). This procedure provides a correlate to log P; where P = octanol/water partition coefficient, in the form of a log k' value; where k' = HPLC capacity factor.

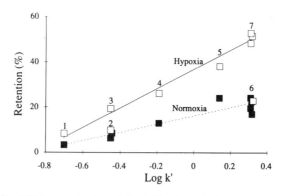

Figure 1. Effect of lipophilicity on retention of nitroimidazoles in isolated cardiac myocytes. The values (means; n = 3 except where noted below) refer to radioactivity in the pellet expressed as a percent of its total in the sampled aliquot. For each compound, open symbols represent hypoxic values and closed ones aligned directly below indicate the nomoxic counterpart. The lines represent the line of best fit of the data. Numbers directly above each hypoxic value identify the compound: 1 = 3H-Fluoromisonidazole, 2 = BMS 180902 (n = 1), 3 = BMS 181004 (n = 1), 4 = ^{131}Iodovinylmisonidazole, 5 = BMS 181409, 6 = BMS 181031 (n = 1), 7 = BMS 181321. The latter compound was compared to other radiopharmaceuticals using the same preparations of cells, thus, three means are provided for both normoxic and hypoxic cells.

RESULTS AND DISCUSSION

Figure 1 shows that quiescent cardiac myocytes incubated with nitroimidazole compounds retain greater levels of radioactivity when suspended in media at very low oxygen pressures (< 0.1 Torr) than do cells suspended in media exposed to room air.

In most cases, i.e., those compounds having the nitro group linked to the 2- position of the imidazole ring, the differences in retention between hypoxic and normoxic cells were about 2 to 1. The lone exception was compound 5 (BMS 181409) in which the nitro group was in the 4- position of the imidazole ring. When the nitro moiety is in the 4- position, the difficulty of reducing this compound increases relative to the 2-nitroimidazoles (Greenstock et al., 1976). For compound 5, the hypoxic to normoxic ratio was 1.7 ± 0.1 (n =3) as compared to a value of 2.3 ± 0.3 (n = 3) for compound 7 (BMS 181321) obtained with the same preparations of myocytes.

It can also be seen in Figure 1 that the retention of compound 7 was greater than that of the other nitroimidazoles in cells suspended in both normoxic and hypoxic media, about 22 and 50%, respectively. The log k' value of this compound, 0.31, was the highest measured for this group of compounds. On the other hand, compound 1 (3H-Fluoromisonidazole), which was the least lipophilic (log k' = -0.7), resulted in the lowest level of retention for both normoxic and hypoxic cells, about 3 and 8%, respectively.

The results indicate that the nitro group is a necessary substituent of the compounds to affect selective retention in hypoxic cells. For example, retention of compound 6 (BMS 181031), a PnAO derivative which lacks the nitroimidazole group was 17.4% in normoxic cells and 22.7% in hypoxic cells (Figure 1) , resulting in an hypoxic/normoxic ratio of 1.3. The latter results were confirmed with compound 2 (BMS 180902; hypoxic/normoxic ratio = 1.3) which similarly lacks the nitroimidazole moiety and is less lipophilic than the former compound. It was posssible that the low oxygen environment of the media in which these cells were suspended may have resulted in changes in plasma membrane stability, thereby permitting greater uptake of compound. The absence of a marked difference in retention between normoxic and hypoxic cells incubated with compounds 2 or 6 argues against the latter possibility.

The findings above indicate that misonidazole and like compounds linked to a gamma emitter (either ^{131}I or ^{99m}Tc) are retained more so in hypoxic cardiac myocytes than in normoxic ones. Moreover, the level of retention is dependent, at least in part, on the relative lipophilicity of the compound, being greater for the more lipophilic compounds. The latter finding suggests that radioactivity associated with the normoxic cells is due primarily to non-specific binding of the compounds to cellular constituents. This suggestion is supported by the finding that incubation of a broken cell preparation with BMS 181321 under normoxic and hypoxic conditions resulted in equivalent levels of radioactivity associated with the particulate fraction which were similar to those data obtained with an intact normoxic preparation. The greater lipophilicity of BMS 181321 would provide over time a higher level of signal intensity (over background values) when administered in vivo for imaging with a gamma camera. The amount of radioactivity within a hypoxic region would remain "trapped" within these cells whereas that within normoxic regions would clear eventually of non-specifically bound material.

Figure 2 shows an autoradiogram produced from a section obtained midway between the base and apex of the left ventricle (the right ventricle was removed) from a dog injected with BMS 181321. In this case, flow within the LAD was reduced from 21 to 4 ml/min, a change of about 75%. The animal then received isoproterenol to increase cardiac work and metabolic demand. Increases in dp/dt (from 3250 to 6250 mm Hg/sec), mean arterial pressure (from 117 to 142 mm Hg), and heart rate (from 168 to 240 bpm) indicated that cardiac work was markedly enhanced by administration of isoproterenol. Although myocardial oxygen consumption was not determined, it was likely that oxygen demand was increased under these conditions. It can be seen in Figure 2 that the optical density is markedly higher, indicating an enhanced level of radioactivity and thus retention of compound, in a large section of the outer wall of the left ventricle (right side of the image). When a region of interest was obtained from the latter area and compared to one from the septal wall of the heart (left side of image), the difference in optical density was about 4 to 1. The latter result indicates that BMS 181321 can localize in tissue in which oxygen delivery has been markedly limited.

This hypoxia/normoxia ratio is greater than that found for isolated cardiac myocytes (2:1) and likely reflects the clearance capacity of the intact heart.

For the most part, the enriched region of radioactivity within the ventricular wall is restricted to the endo- and mesocardium with little accumulation occurring in the epicardium. It is apparent that under such conditions, myocytes within the endocardial region were rendered hypoxic more so than those within the epicardial territory. These findings are consistent with what is commonly termed "coronary steal syndrome" in which coronary flow is shunted away from the endocardium and directed towards the epicardial tissue during periods of enhanced cardiac work.

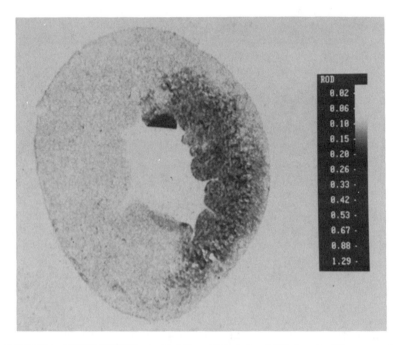

Figure 2. Retention of BMS 181321 in canine left ventricle during LAD stenosis. Flow was reduced in the LAD from 21 to 4 ml/min using a hydraulic occluder. The animal was stabilized for 35 min. Isoproterenol was then infused stepwise from 0.1 to 0.4 mg/kg/min permitting each increment in delivery of drug to result in appropriate changes in dp/dt, heart rate and arterial pressure. After the animal had reached a new steady state (25 min from start of isoproterenol infusion), BMS 181321 was administered as a bolus injection within the femoral vein. Residence time of the radiopharmaceutical was 40 min, after which the heart was removed quickly from the thorax. The right ventricle was removed for ease of processing.

In the intact dog heart, oxygen pressure in the cardiac myocytes is low, less than about 5 Torr, during normoxemia (Coburn et al., 1973). Although myoglobin may serve as a temporary resevoir of intracellular oxygen, cardiac myocytes are particularly vulnerable to even brief periods of oxygen deprivation due, in part, to the sensitivity of mitochondrial oxidative phosphorylation to oxygen in these cells (Rumsey et al., 1990). These characteristics indicate that cardiac myocytes are a likely target for trapping of the nitro complex, *in vivo*. It is evident that these cells contain the necessary intracellular components to complete the biochemical trapping process since these compounds were found to localize in isolated hypoxic cardiac myocytes. It is conceivable, however, that other cells types, for example, fibroblasts, smooth muscle cells or endothelial cells, may also "trap" nitroimidazoles during hypoxic conditions and contribute to the overall signal emitted from a hypoxic region *in vivo*.

The mechanism of 2-nitroimidazole retention in hypoxic tissue has not been completely elucidated (for review, see Rauth, 1984). Misonidazole is readily reduced to a radical anion in both normoxic and hypoxic environments, however, this species reacts with oxygen to produce the superoxide anion and to regenerate the initial form of the nitroimidazole. In hypoxic tissue, misonidazole is thought to be reduced further (a total 4 electron stoichiometry) to yield a hydroxylamine derivative (McClelland et al., 1984) and to covalently bind to intracellular macromolecules (Kedderis et al., 1989; Varghese et al., 1980; Varghese and Whitmore, 1981). Electron transfer may be catalyzed by any number of intracellular reductases. It is interesting to speculate that, in cardiac myocytes, the enzymes of oxidative phosphorylation may play a role in intracellular trapping of these compounds. Limitation of oxygen availability, even in small amounts, results in increased levels of reduction of the cytochromes of the respiratory chain and thus increases the level of reducing equivalents (for example, see Wilson et al., 1988; Rumsey et al., 1990). The interplay between the levels of oxygen pressure and reducing equivalents and nitroimidazole may serve to provide a sensitive measure of myocardial oxygenation.

The findings of the present report support the notion that radiolabeled nitroheterocycles, in particular, nitroimidazoles complexed with a technetium ligand, can be used as markers of hypoxic cells in the heart. These data confirm and extend those reported recently (DiRocco et al., 1992). In the latter study, it was reported that BMS 181321 was preferentially retained in a manner similar to that of ^{3}H-Fluoromisonidazole in a region bordering an ischemic zone in rabbit heart. In this animal model, the LAD was fully occluded. These studies indicate that technetium-labeled nitroimidazoles may have clinical utility. Further work with BMS 181321 may therefore fulfill the potential of 2-nitroimidazoles and thus, provide the clinician with a qualitative probe of tissue oxygenation status.

Acknowledgments   The authors are grateful for the skilled technical assistance of Ms Christine Hood.

REFERENCES

Biskupiak, J.E., Grierson, J.R., Rasey, J.S., Martin, G.V., and Krohn, K.A., 1991, Synthesis of an (Iodovinyl)misonidazole derivative for hypoxia imaging, *J. Med. Chem.* 34: 2165.

DiRocco, R.J., Bauer, A., Kuczynski, B.L., Pirro, J.P., Linder, K.E., Narra, R.K., and Nunn, A.D., 1991, Imaging regional hypoxia with a new technetium-labeled imaging agent in rabbit myocardium after occlusion of the left anterior descending coronary artery. *J. Nucl. Med.* 33 Suppl (5): 865 (abstr.).

Chapman, D., Lee, J., and Meeker, B.E., 1989, Cellular reduction of nitroimidazole drugs: Potential for selective chemotherapy and diagnosis of hypoxic cells, *Int. J. Radiation Oncology Biol. Phys.* 16: 911.

Coburn, R.E., Ploemaker, F., Gondric, P., and Abboul, R., 1973, Myocardial myoglobin oxygen tension, *Am. J. Physiol.*, 224: 870.

Greenstock, C.L., Ruddock, G.W., and Neta, P., 1976, Pulse radiolysis and ESR studies of the electron affinic properties of nitroheterocyclic radiosensitizers, 66: 472.

Feld, T., and Nunn, A.D. 1989, A chromatographic method for the measurement of lipophilicity of lipophilic technetium complexes, *J. Labeled Compd. Radiopharm.* 26: 274.

Jurisson. SS.; Hirth, W., Linder, K.E., Di Rocco R.J., Narra, R.K., Nowotnik, D.P., Nunn, A.D., 1991, Chloro-hydroxy substitution of technetium BATO [TcCl(dioxime)3BR] complexes, *Nucl. Med. Biol.* 18: 735.

Kedderis, G.L., Argenbright, L.S., and Miwa, G.T., 1989, Covalent interaction of 5-nitroimidazoles with DNA and protein in vitro: Mechanism of reductive activation, *Chem. Res. Toxicol.* 2: 146.

Linder, K.E., Cyr, J., Chan, Y.-W., Raju, N., Ramalingam, K., Nowotnik, D.P., and Nunn, A.D., 1992, Chemistry of a Tc-PnAO-nitroimidazole complex that localizes in hypoxic tissue, *J. Nucl. Med.* 33 Suppl (5): 919 (abstr.)

Martin, G.V., Caldwell, J.H., Rasey, J.S., Grunbaum, Z., Cerqueira, M., and Krohn, K.A. Enhanced binding of the hypoxic cell marker [^{3}H]fluoromisonidazole in ischemic myocardium. *J. Nucl. Med.* 30:194-201, 1989.

McClelland, R.A., Fuller, J.R., Seaman, N.E., Rauth, A.M., and Battistella, R. 1984, 2-Hydroxylaminoimidazoles-Unstable intermediates in the reduction of 2-nitroimidazoles, *Biochem. Pharmacol.* 33: 303.

Raleigh, J.A., Shum, F.Y., and Lu, S.F., 1981, Nitroreductase-induced binding of nireoaromatic radiosensitizers to unsaturated lipids. Nitroxyl adducts, *Biochem. Pharmacol.* 30 (21): 2921.

Rauth, A.M., 1984, Pharmacology and toxicology of sensitizers: Mechanism studies, *Int. J. Radiation Oncology* 10: 1293.

Rumsey, W.L., Schlosser, C., Nuutinen, E.M., Robiolio, M., and Wilson, D.F., 1988, Cellular Energetics and the oxygen dependence of respiration in cardiac myocytes isolated from adult rat. *J. Biol. Chem.* 265 (26): 15392.

Shelton, M.E., Dence, C.S., Hwang, D.-R., Welch, M.J., and Bergmann, S.R., , 1989, Myocardial kinetics of fluorine-18 misonidazole: A marker of hypoxic myocardium. *J. Nucl. Med.* 30: 351-358.

Stratford, I.J., 1982, Mechanisms of hypoxic cell radiosensitization and the development of new sensitizers, *Int.J. Radiation Oncology Biol. Phys.* 8: 391.

Varghese, A.J., Gulyus, S., Mohindra, J.K., 1976, Hypoxia-dependent reduction of 1-(2-nitro-1-imidazoyl)-3-methoxy-2-propanol by Chinese hamster ovary cells and KHT tumor cells in vitro and in vivo., *Cancer Res.* 36: 3761.

Varghese, A.J., and Whitmore, G.F., 1980, Binding to cellular macromolecules as a possible mechanism for the cytotoxicity of misonidazole, *Cancer Res.* 40: 2166.

Varghese, A.J., and Whitmore, G.F., 1981, Cellular and chemical reduction products of misonidazole, *Chem. Biol. Interactions*, 36: 141.

Wilson, D.F., Rumsey, W.L., Green, T.J., and Vanderkooi, J.M., 1988, The oxygen dependence of mitochondrial oxidative phosphorylation measured by a new optical method for measuring oxygen concentration, *J. Biol. Chem.* 263 (6): 2712.

Wittenberg, B.A., and Robinson, T.F., 1981, Oxygen requirements, morphology, cell coat and membrane permeability of calcium-tolerant myocytes from hearts of adult rats, *Cell. Tissue Res.* 216: 231.

METHOD FOR SIMULTANEOUS DETERMINATION OF THE DISTRIBUTION OF CAPILLARY PLASMA FLOW AND MYOCYTE REDOX STATE (NADH-FLUORESCENCE) IN THE HYPOPERFUSED MYOCARDIUM OF THE ANESTHETIZED RAT

Friedrich Vetterlein, Michael Prange, Phuong-Nga Tran, and
Gerhard Schmidt

Zentrum Pharmakologie und Toxikologie der Universität, Robert-Koch-Str. 40
D-3400 Göttingen

INTRODUCTION

Narrowing of a coronary artery does not induce ischemia to the same degree throughout the affected myocardium but leads to significant spatial differences in the depression of local supply conditions (e.g. Jennings et al, 1975). One indication for the development of such a regional heterogeneity in tissue supply on even a rather low scale comes from topographic analyses of the blue NADH-fluorescence on the surface of isolated hearts perfused under ischemic conditions (Steenbergen et al, 1977). While it can be safely assumed that this blue fluorescence indicates extreme degrees of oxygen deficiency in the myocytes due to accumulation of mitochondrial NADH, the question whether this signal is indicative for a loss of local blood flow as well, could only insufficiently be answered until now.

This knowledge, however, appears to be quite important. The chance of the cells to survive conditions of anoxic perfusion or ischemic conditions differs significantly because local metabolites accumulate to quite a different degree. This question may gain importance for the hypoperfused myocardium during incomplete coronary obstruction and also for the borderzone around complete myocardial infarcts.

Different attempts have been made in order to correlate perfusion and redox state. Steenbergen et al (1980) photographed the heart surface during uv-illumination and subsequently added thioflavine S to the perfusion medium; its distribution was again photographed. From these studies they concluded that NADH is increased in areas lacking capillary flow. Simon et al (1979) used fluorescein to mark the perfused vascular system and found hints for a non-perfused, but non-anoxic zone between normal and infarcted tissue.

The reason why these studies revealed only rough estimates of the distribution of perfused areas in relation to NADH-fluorescences comes from the fact that the dyes used diffuse out of the vascular system (Simon et al, 1979), making studies on time dependent changes in blood distribution impossible. In addition, surface fluorescence is blunted by fluorescence from underlying tissue, with the additional drawback that the latter influence changes with varying hemoglobin content of the deep tissue (Chance et al, 1962). For this reason mostly organs perfused with hemoglobin-free media have been studied.

The present contribution describes a method which circumvents most of these disadvantages. It describes a technique whereby flow distribution and NADH-fluorescence may be observed even in histological sections obtained from flow-restricted hearts of anesthetized rats.

Oxygen Transport to Tissue XV, Edited by P. Vaupel
et al., Plenum Press, New York, 1994

METHODS

The experiments were performed on male rats anesthetized with 50 mg/kg sodium-pentobarbital i.p., an N_2O/O_2 inhalation and maintenance doses of ketamine (1.25 mg/kg i.v.). Systemic pressure was measured in the left femoral artery. The animals were ventilated with a positive pressure respirator and the thoracic cavity opened by transsection of clavicula and ribs 1-6. The left and the right common carotid arteries were dissected free and, after heparinization, the left one was connected with an anastomosis which diverted the blood via the right carotid artery to the left coronary ostium. The anastomosis consisted of the following elements: a proximal glass tube of 10 mm length, a flow probe of 0.95 mm int.diam. (Carolina Med. Electr., Mod. EP 103), and a distal glass tube of 25 mm length with a tip which exactly fitted to the ostium of the left coronary artery. A side branch allowed to measure the coronary perfusion pressure. An occlusor was placed around the left carotid artery for control of the arterial inflow pressure. A double catheter was introduced into the left atrial appendage for registration of left atrial pressure and infusion of one of the indicator dyes (see below).

In separate experimental groups, the perfusion pressure was left unchanged, adjusted to 60, 50 or 40 mm Hg for 10 min. At the end of this period, FITC-albumin as an intravascular label (Vetterlein et al, 1982) was injected i.v., 40 s later the infusion of lissamine-rhodamin B200 (RB200)-albumin into the left atrium was begun. After additional 20 s a biopsy cylinder of 2.0 mm diameter was cut from the affected myocardium and rapidly transferred into precooled (-130°C) isopentane by application of vacuum. The tissue was then transferred into liquid nitrogen.

For demonstration of the intravascular dyes and the myocyte NADH-fluorescence, frozen sections were prepared. The 5 μm thick slices were freeze-substituted by placing them on frozen alcohol and waiting until the alcohol had penetrated the tissue. They were then floated in alcohol of room temperature and covered by a cover glass. The artificial medium Histokit[R] was placed around the cover glass in order to prevent evaporation of the alcohol.

The preparation was transferred to a cold stage which maintained a temperature of -150°C. This measure was necessary in order to avoid temperature-induced changes in NADH-fluorescence (Chance et al, 1979). The low temperature was attained with the aid of liquid nitrogen. As a maximal optical magnification a x40 dry objective could be used.

The intravascular dyes FITC and RB200 could be observed by application of the filter combinations 465/515/520 nm for FITC and 546/590/590 nm for RB200. In these sections NADH could also be observed by applying a third combination: 365/395/420 nm. A short-pass filter was additionally used which cut off light with wave lengths longer than 500 nm.

For quantification of the distribution of dye-labeled capillaries in areas of cross sectioned capillaries, the "concentric-circles method" was used (Kayar et al, 1982). For quantification of the NADH-fluorescence in the measuring points, a diaphragm of 10 μm diameter was placed into the center of the circle system (slightly shifted to the nearest myocyte if necessary). The illumination was switched to NADH-excitation and the intensity of the blue fluorescent light measured with the aid of a highly sensible television camera (CCD camera, Mod. STM, ICCD-03, SIM, Security and Electronic System).

Calibration of the NADH-fluorescence intensity was enabled by the fact that the outermost layers of myocytes laying just below the endocardium are oxygenated by the intraventricular blood and are thus normoxic even during cessation of coronary blood flow. The fluorescence intensity of these cells was taken as the reference value (factor 1).

RESULTS AND DISCUSSION

With the presented method we observed that the reduction in coronary perfusion pressure led to an incomplete vascular labeling after 20 s and 60 s. The distribution of areas to which no dye had gained access during these times increased with reduction in perfusion pressure. The distribution of areas showing an increased NADH-fluorescence was not congruent with the non-labeled zones, however. Especially in the 60 mm Hg and 50 mm Hg groups, regions were found with complete vascular labeling and spotlike distributed zones of NADH-fluorescence in the myocytes. In most regions without FITC or RB200, NADH was found increased, in some areas, however, a lacking rise in NADH could be observed despite a failing intravascular staining.

The method which enabled the performance of these experiments was developed in a great number of preliminary trials. They should overcome the above mentioned drawbacks of the established methods for NADH-detection. The main improvement in this respect was achieved when finding out that NADH may be preserved by the method of section freeze-substitution, in the same way as the intravascular marker proteins. This principle works because NADH is also insoluble in abs. alcohol. In this way the optical resolution could greatly be increased and errors due to hemoglobin-induced fluorescence quenching could be eliminated. Due to the small size of the applied diaphragm vascular elements and myocytes could be separated from each other.

A sufficiently rapid freezing of the tissue was another problem. Freezing of the whole heart proved to be too slow even when applying snap-freezing-tongs. With the biopsy cutting system we found no significant difference in the intensity of NADH-fluorescence in the marginal layer as compared to central zones in tissue obtained from non-occluded myocardium.

SUMMARY

A method is described which allows to observe the pattern of capillary plasma filling simultaneously with the redox state (NADH-fluorescence) of the myocytes in the hypoperfused myocardium. In anesthetized rats the coronary perfusion pressure was reduced to a defined level, the blood plasma labeled with dye-conjugated albumin and a myocardial biopsy sampled. Freeze-substitution of histological sections allowed to detect the intravascular plasma label as well as the myocyte NADH-fluorescence on a microscopic level. It was found that areas showing increased cellular NADH-fluorescence did not arise in a distribution congruent with zones of failing capillary plasma flow in the hypoperfused myocardium.

Acknowledgement

This study has been supported by the Deutsche Forschungsgemeinschaft, SFB 330 (Organprotektion)

REFERENCES

Chance, B., Cohen, P., Jöbsis, F.F., and Schoener, B., 1962, Intracellular oxidation-reduction states in vivo, Science 137: 499-508.

Chance, B., Schoener, B., Oshino, R., Hshak, F., Nakase, Y., 1979, Oxidation-reduced ratio studies of mitochondria in freeze-trapped samples. NADH and flavoprotein fluorescence signals, J.Biol.Chem. 254: 4764-4771.

Jennings, R.B., Ganote, C.E., and Reimer, K.A., 1975, Ichemic tissue injury, Am.J.Pathol. 81: 179-198.

Kayar, S., Archer, P.G., Lechner, A.J., and Banchero, N., 1982, Evaluation of the concentric-circles method for estimating capillary-tissue diffusion distances, Microvasc.Res., 24: 342-353

Simon, M.B., Harden, W., Barlow, C., and Harken, A.H., 1979, Visualization of the distances between perfusion and anoxia along an ischemic border, Circulation, 5: 1151-1155.

Steenbergen, C., Deleeuw, G., Barlow, C., Chance, B., and Williamson, J.R., 1977, Heterogeneity of the hypoxic state in perfused rat heart, Circ.Res. 41: 606-615.

Steenbergen, C., and Williamson, J.R., 1980, Heterogeneous coronary perfusion during myocardial hypoxia. Adv. in Myocardiology, Vol. 2, eds. M.v.Tajuddin, B. Bhatia, H.H. Siddiqui, G. Rona, University Park Press, Baltimore, pp 271-284.

Vetterlein, F., dal Ri, H., and Schmidt, G., 1982, Capillary density in rat myocardium during timed plasma staining, Am.J.Physiol. 242: H133-H141

THE INFLUENCE OF FLOW REDISTRIBUTIONS ON
THE CALCULATED pO$_2$ IN RAT HEART TISSUE

Louis Hoofd, and Zdenek Turek

Department of Physiology
University of Nijmegen
The Netherlands

INTRODUCTION

Calculations of muscle tissue pO$_2$ from models that take into account realistic geometrical capillary distributions have shown a resulting considerable range in pO$_2$ values (broad histograms), due to the heterogeneity in capillary spacing. In these models, however, only few selected blood flow types were considered, most often, equal flow through each capillary. The question is addressed here, what the influence is of different flow patterns on calculated tissue pO$_2$ and particularly whether the resulting pO$_2$ histograms can be made more uniform, i.e., less variation in pO$_2$ values.

METHODS

Mathematical treatment

The mathematical treatment was the same as in our previous publications (Multicapillary model; Hoofd et al., 1989; Hoofd et al., 1990; Hoofd and Turek, in press), in where a variety of different data can be substituted for each individual capillary, including flow. In each consecutive slab of the volume (a block, here), tissue oxygen pressure p is calculated from:

$$p + p_F s = C_p + \frac{M}{4 \wp} \left\{ \Phi(x,y) - \sum_{i=1}^{N} \frac{A_i}{\pi} \ln\left(\frac{(x-x_i)^2 + (y-y_i)^2}{r_{ci}^2} \right) \right\} \tag{1.a}$$

$$\Phi(x,y) = \sum_{n=1}^{4} \left[\Delta x_n \Delta y_n \ln(\Delta x_n^2 + \Delta y_n^2) + \Delta x_n^2 \arctan\left(\frac{\Delta y_n}{\Delta x_n} \right) + \Delta y_n^2 \arctan\left(\frac{\Delta x_n}{\Delta y_n} \right) \right] \tag{1.b}$$

Oxygen Transport to Tissue XV, Edited by P. Vaupel
et al., Plenum Press, New York, 1994

where p_F is facilitation pressure, s is myoglobin (Mb) oxygen saturation, M is tissue oxygen consumption, $\mathcal{P}$ is tissue oxygen permeability (product of diffusion coefficient D and solubility α), C_p is a constant, x and y are rectangular coordinates in the slab, x_i, y_i, A_i, r_{ci} are coordinates, supply area and radius of the ith capillary respectively, and Δx_n, Δy_n are the distances of the nth corner to the actual point (x,y). The "background function" $\Phi(x,y)$ is written slightly different from previous publications but mathematically equivalent. The constants C_p, A_i are determined by matching to capillary oxygen pressure p_i and total slab consumption. The link to the next slab is:

$$c_{i,z+\Delta z} = c_{i,z} - \frac{M}{F_i}\left(A_i - \pi r_{ci}^2\right)\Delta z \tag{2}$$

where $c_{i,z}$ is total oxygen concentration of the ith capillary in the slab at vertical coordinate z, F_i is its blood flow and Δz is the thickness of the slab - note, that F_i may be negative which implies countercurrent flow. $c_{i,z}$ and p_i are linked through the hemoglobin saturation curve. In matching tissue p to p_i, a flux-dependent extra pericapillary pO_2 drop was accounted for; the mean drop value is called *Extraction Pressure* (EP), often also referred to as *Capillary Barrier* (CB).

Model layout

The capillaries in the tissue block run in parallel and the slabs were perpendicular to them, leading to identical capillary locations in each slab. Two situations were considered. A rat heart block, 100 layers of 177×140 μm^2 250 μm deep, and a block of dog gracilis muscle, 110 layers of 80×80 μm^2 500 μm deep. The rat heart layers contained 71 capillaries, locations read from an actual photomicrograph, divided in six zones of 59×70 μm^2, alternately staggered by taking as initial capillary pO_2 the arterial pressure (13.3 kPa = 100 mm Hg) in three zones and "half-way" in the other zones, i.e., with a pO_2 distribution equal to that that the other capillaries reached at the end of the block (Hoofd and Turek, 1992). In the dog gracilis muscle block there were 4 capillaries laid out in a configuration as depicted by Groebe (1990), in his figure 2: two capillaries were supplied from an arteriole half-way, the other two drained into a venule at the end of the block. This was modelled here by reversing the flow after passing arteriole or venule.

Model data

Data used are shown in table 1. For some input values, only composite data have to be used; these were: consumption divided by permeability $M/\mathcal{P}$, overall blood flow

Table 1. Summary of input data; for symbols see text.

	EP	p_F	p_{50Mb}	$M/\mathcal{P}$	F/D	C_{Hm}/α_e	p_{50Hb}	n
	kPa	kPa	kPa	$kPa \cdot \mu m^{-2}$	μm	kPa	kPa	
Rat	1.40	1.87	0.707	0.0253	10.56	844	4.93	2.70
Dog	1.40	5.28	0.707	0.0121	28.65	1336	3.52	2.65

divided by tissue diffusion coefficient F/D, and heme concentration divided by erythro-cytic O_2 solubility C_{Hm}/α_e.

Data for EP were derived from a companion paper (Hoofd et al., this volume) slightly higher to account for O_2 transport within the erythrocyte. Other data were as in our former calculations (Hoofd et al., 1990) for the rat heart and from Groebe (1990) for the dog gracilis muscle. Hemoglobin saturation was calculated from the Hill equation $s = p^n/(p_{50Hb}{}^n + p^n)$ and myoglobin saturation as $s = p/(p_{50Mb} + p)$.

The histograms were constructed by calculating p in the same rectangular grid for each layer. For the rat heart, the grid spacing was 5 μm; for the dog gracilis, it was 4.5 μm in order to avoid grid points at the centres of the capillaries (all four placed at offsets of 20 μm in x- and y- direction from the centre). A tissue zone of 2 μm around each capillary was left out from the calculations in order to avoid occasional high pO_2's close to the capillary. Furthermore, for the rat heart a 10 μm zone was left out from top and sides of the block, avoiding high arteriolar pO_2's and zones possibly depending on capillaries that would have laid just outside the block. All this leaves between 27000 and 65000 points for the histograms, depending on the actual situation.

RESULTS

As a first step, pO_2 histograms were calculated for the data given above. Then, different situations were considered and compared against these "basic" histograms. Bar histograms are shown in the figures, frequency f on the left axis, as well as cumulative histograms by connected symbols, totalling 100% as scaled on the right axis. Histogram class width was chosen as 0.5 kPa [3.75 mm Hg] for all cases.

Rat heart muscle

The following cases were considered for the rat heart:

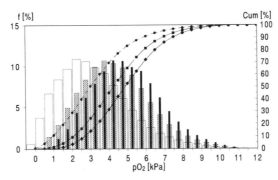

Figure 1. Rat heart, basic histogram (open bars, ●), flow increased by 50% (crossed bars, ■) and flow increased by 100% (filled bars, ◆).

Increasing overall flow, without changing flow pattern, so equal flow through each capillary still. Flow was increased by 50% and by 100% respectively. The resulting histograms are shown in figure 1. Increasing flow shift the histograms towards higher pO_2 values, mean values of 3.22 kPa [24.2 mm Hg], 4.38 kPa [32.9 mm Hg] and 4.98 kPa [37.4 mm Hg] respectively, but the width of the histogram hardly changed leaving high variation in pO_2 - the standard deviation in pO_2, SDp, decreased by less than 5%.

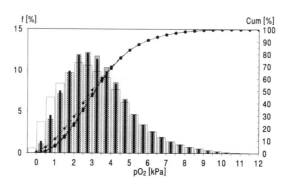

Figure 2. Rat heart, basic histogram (open bars, ●), matched capillary flow (crossed bars, ■) and overcompensated by 30% (filled bars, ♦).

Matching individual capillary flow. Now, capillaries with a large O_2 supply had correspondingly higher flow such that the end-capillary pO_2 was uniform. The resulting histogram was shifted slightly towards higher pO_2 but still very broad, as can be seen from figure 2 - SDp decreased only from 1.91 kPa [14.3 mm Hg] to 1.77 kPa [13.2 mm Hg]. So, the question arose, whether an overcompensation could lead to more uniform pO_2. However, any overcompensation tried out yielded broader histograms again; a case is shown for 30% more respectively less flow in each capillary than needed for the "matched" case, in figure 2. It is in between the other two cases.

Countercurrent flow. The central area of the tissue slabs (so, the 2 middle zones) was assigned countercurrent flow. The resulting histogram hardly was different from the basic case, as seen from figure 3. So, also a case was computed in where each second capillary in the data listing was given a countercurrent flow, in fact, resulting in random capillary flow direction. As seen from figure 3, now the high tissue pO_2 values had disappeared, and the histogram seems more random; but still very broad - SDp of 1.57 kPa [11.8 mm Hg]. The skewness of the histogram (defined as the cubic root of $(p_i\text{-}p_{mean})^3$ averaged) was considerably decreased, from 1.73 kPa [12.9 mm Hg] to 1.18 kPa [8.8 mm Hg].

Random flow. Finally, since all these flow patterns turned out to have so little influence, a case was constructed in where the capillary flows of the "matched flow" case were taken and now were randomly distributed. So, a flow distribution with a standard deviation of 28% was added to the existing heterogeneity in capillary spacing. The resulting histogram was very near the basic one; the largest deviation in f was 0,5%, and the cumulative histogram shifted to lower pO_2 by less than 0.1 kPa (0.7 mm Hg).

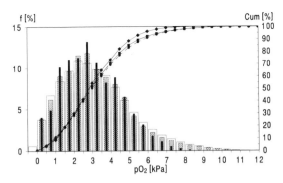

Figure 3. Rat heart, basic histogram (open bars, ●), 2-zone countercurrent flow (crossed bars, ■) and random countercurrent flow (filled bars, ◆).

Dog gracilis muscle

The basic histogram here was of the semi-staggered semi-countercurrent layout of Groebe (1990). Though pO_2's calculated here were much lower, class scaling is the same as in the former figures, for easier comparison.

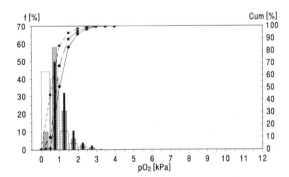

Figure 4. Dog gracilis muscle, basic histogram (open bars, ●), flow increased by 50% (crossed bars, ■) and flow increased 100% (filled bars, ◆).

Increasing overall flow, again each capillary 50% more and 100% more flow respectively. All histograms were sharply peaked - note the different scale for the left axis! The shift towards higher pO_2 is much less pronounced than in the rat heart case, mean values of pO_2 were 0.66 kPa [4.9 mm Hg], 0.93 kPa [7.0 mm Hg] and 1.12 kPa [8.4 mm Hg] respectively.

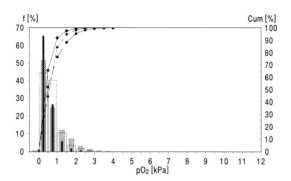

Figure 5. Dog gracilis muscle, basic histogram (open bars, ●), parallel flow (crossed bars, ■) and counter current, antiparallel flow (filled bars, ◆).

Non-staggered flow. Identical capillary flows all in the same direction, shown as "parallel flow" in figure 5, and 2 of them opposite flow direction, denoted "antiparallel flow" in figure 5. All histograms were sharply peaked again, with pO_2's not very different. The basic case largely is in between the other two. The parallel case has some more high and low values (SDp 50% higher), pO_2 now up to 4 kPa [30 mm Hg] instead of 3 kPa [23 mm Hg]. Additionally, a calculation was done for a Krogh cylinder with a radius of 22.6 μm - equivalent to the O_2 supply area of the capillaries here; the resulting histogram was nearly identical to the "parallel" case (differences of less than 1%).

DISCUSSION

Most remarkable in all the calculations shown above is the limited influence of flow patterns, i.e., changing individual capillary flow while keeping total flow the same. For the rat heart case, the explanation must be found in the influence of the heterogeneity in capillary spacing. It is this heterogeneity that renders the histogram so broad (Hoofd and Turek, 1992); a histogram calculated for the same 71 capillaries now regularly spaced in a rectangular grid had a mean pO_2 of 4.26 kPa [31.9 mm Hg] and an SDp of 1.54 kPa [11.5 mm Hg] which is 1 kPa higher and 0.4 kPa lower respectively than in the heterogeneous case here - so, vastly different. Obviously, this geometrical influence is so large, that additional flow heterogeneity or redistributions are of very limited importance.

It was found already earlier, that flow matching did very little to the histogram (Hoofd and Turek, 1992). Matching was such, that the end-capillary pO_2 was the same - note that the changing size of the supply area along the capillary does not allow the conclusion that capillary pO_2 is the same at every level! Then, the pO_2 drop into the tissue will be larger for large supply areas than for small ones and the question arises whether this could be counteracted by over-matching the flow, rendering more homogeneous tissue pressures. Obviously, that is not the case. The explanation must be found in that the high-flow capillaries now will have higher capillary pO_2 but consequently an even larger supply area leading to a larger drop in tissue pO_2. Already a small overmatching of 10% made the histogram a little bit broader. We were not able to imagine any other flow pattern that would render the histograms smaller. Also, going the other way, randomizing capillary flow was of very little importance. All this goes through the adaptation of supply area sizes of the individual capillaries. Altogether, this leads to the conclusion that in the multicylinder models of tissue oxygenation (tissue represented by a set of Krogh cylinders - e.g., Turek et al., 1991) specific flow is the better alternative.

It should be added here that, although the flow distribution had little effect on the histogram as a whole, local effects might be marked. For example, tissue portions with low pO_2 or with high pO_2 could be markedly reduced in size - examples found in the "matched" and "random countercurrent" cases. So, flow redistribution might be of local importance.

The situation is different for dog gracilis case - data taken from Groebe (1990). Here, the histograms were confined to low pO_2 values and there were no large differences, due to a combination of factors. First of all, arteriolar pO_2 is much lower, 8 kPa against 13.3 kPa for the rat heart. Then, the combination of low M and large R leads to shallow tissue gradients over larger areas. Last but not least, p_F is almost three times higher, leading to a much larger share of myoglobin facilitation in the O_2 transport. Without the latter, adequate O_2 supply would be impossible: the Krogh model predict a capillary-tissue pO_2 drop of 5.52 kPa [41.4 mm Hg]. With maximum facilitation (i.e., down to zero pO_2), this is reduced to 1.76 kPa [13.2 mm Hg]. Consequently, most tissue pO_2's will be not far from the p_{50} of Mb, leading to histograms mainly below 1 kPa [7.5 mm Hg], not much dependent on capillary supply. This is confirmed by figure 4, where increasing overall flow does very little (increase in mean pO_2 of only 0.46 kPa [3.4 mm Hg]).

The regular capillary pattern in the dog gracilis case also contributes to the smallness and steepness of the histogram. However, it is difficult to speculate what the influence of geometrical heterogeneity in this case would be, because the very different set of data used for this case. With only 4 capillaries, no realistic heterogeneous pattern could be investigated. In the multicylindrical model, where only a single value of heterogeneity of capillary spacing is needed, adding such heterogeneity resulted in some portion of anoxic tissue (Turek et al., 1988). It would be very interesting to have information about realistic capillary locations in this type of tissue so that calculations with the present model could be performed.

REFERENCES

Groebe, K., 1990, A versatile model of steady state O_2 supply to tissue; application to skeletal muscle, *Biophys. J.* 57: 485 - 498.

Hoofd, L., Bos, C.G., and Turek, Z., in press, Modelling erythrocytes as point-like O_2 sources in a Kroghian cylinder model, this volume.

Hoofd, L., Olders, J., and Turek, Z., 1990, Oxygen pressures calculated in a tissue volume with parallel capillaries, *in*: "Oxygen Transport to Tissue - XII", J. Piiper, T.K. Goldstick, and M. Meyer, eds., Plenum Press, New York & London, pp.21-29.

Hoofd, L., and Turek, Z., 1992, Oxygen pressure histograms calculated in a block of rat heart tissue, *in*: "Oxygen Transport to Tissue - XIV", W. Erdmann et al., eds., Plenum Press, New York & London, pp.561-566.

Hoofd, L., Turek, Z., and Olders, J., 1989, Calculation of oxygen pressures and fluxes in a flat plane perpendicular to any capillary distribution, *in*: "Oxygen Transport to Tissue - XI", K. Rakusan, G. Biro, T.K. Goldstick, and Z. Turek, eds., Plenum Press, New York & London, pp.187-196.

Turek, Z., Kreuzer, F., Hoofd, L., and Rakusan, K., 1988, Effects of Mb-facilitated diffusion and

pO_2 dependent oxygen consumption on the calculated pO_2 profiles and histograms in skeletal muscle. *FASEB J.* 2: A1523.

Turek, Z., Rakusan, K., Olders, J., Hoofd, L., and Kreuzer, F., 1991, Computed myocardial pO_2 histograms: effects of various geometrical and functional conditions. *J. Appl. Physiol.* 70: 1845-1853.

DOES COLD BLOOD CARDIOPLEGIA OFFER ADEQUATE OXYGEN DELIVERY TO THE MYOCARDIUM DURING CORONARY ARTERY BYPASS GRAFTING?

G. Nollert, H.O. Vetter, K. Martin, C. Weinhold, E. Kreuzer, W. Schmidt, and B. Reichart

Dept. of Cardiac Surgery, Ludwig-Maximilians-University, Munich, Germany

INTRODUCTION

Many investigations have shown the superiority of cold blood cardioplegia (BCP) to crystalloid cadioplegic solutions (CCP) in myocardial protection, especially in cardiac operations with a long ischemic time, in order to perform the distal coronary anastomoses on a quiescient, bloodless heart. In animal experiments, parameters of myocardial protection with BCP have been the left ventricular contractile function, the myocardial contents of high energy phosphates and the histological integrity of the myocardial cells[1,2,3,4]. Clinical investigations have shown the advantages of BCP with respect to operative mortality, perioperative infarction, incidence of heart rhythm disturbances and need for positive inotropic substances[5,6,7].

The reasons for the cardioprotective effects of BCP are uncertain. Three factors are thought to play a major role: pH buffering capacity, endogenous oxygen free radical scavenging capacity and oxygen content. With regard to the latter, the oxygen content of saturated BCP is much higher than that of oxygenated CCP, in which oxygen is only physically dissolved. Thus BCP is assumed to provide a superior oxygen delivery to the myocardium during ischemia. The myocardial oxygen pressure (pmO_2) is determined by the oxygen delivery and the oxygen consumption of the myocardium. The pmO_2 would therefore seem to be a reasonable parameter with which to evaluate the reduction of myocardial metabolism and the oxygen delivery by the cardioplegic solution. In the following study, the pmO_2 was measured in patients during coronary artery bypass grafting (CABG) in order to decide whether a better oxygen delivery is the reason for improved postoperative hemodynamic results of patients receiving BCP.

PATIENTS AND METHODS

Eighteen patients with coronary artery disease were prospectively randomized into two groups: eight patients received multi-dose blood cardioplegia according to Buckberg[8] and

Oxygen Transport to Tissue XV, Edited by P. Vaupel
et al., Plenum Press, New York, 1994

ten patients, 100 % oxygenated crystalloid cardioplegia according to Kirklin. Hemodynamic and myocardial oxygen pressure measurements were performed in these 18 patients. Another 42 patients underwent only hemodynamic measurements. The preoperative clinical data of all 60 patients are shown in Table 1.

Table 1. Preoperative clinical data

	BCP	CCP
Number of patients	28	32
Age (years)	63.1 ± 8.5	60.7 ± 11.0
Sex (male/female)	27/1	24/8
1-vessel disease	2	1
2-vessel disease	7	11
3-vessel disease	19	20
Ejection fraction (%)	61.3 ± 2.6	63.4 ± 2.6

Except for the male/female ratio there were no statistically significant differences between the blood cardioplegia group (BCP) and the crystalloid cardioplegia group (CCP).

General Anesthesia and Surgical Management

Anesthesia was induced with etomidate (0.2 mg/kg), fentanyl (5-10 g/kg) and pancuronium (8 mg). Repeated doses of fentanyl and the addition of nitrous oxide and isoflurane to the ventilation gas sustained anesthesia. A balloon-tipped Swan-Ganz-catheter (CritiCath, Spectramed, Germany) was introduced into the pulmonary artery.

After median sternotomy the right atrium and the aorta were cannulated and extracorporeal circulation (ECC) started. Systemic cooling to 27 ± 1 °C begun together with ECC. The aorta was then crossclamped and the cardioplegic solution infused into the aortic root. All peripheral anastomoses were done during one aortic crossclamp. Whenever possible an A. mammaria interna graft was used to bypass the LAD. After construction of the final peripheral saphenous vein anastomosis, the aorta was unclamped and the reperfusion continued until all proximal anastomoses were completed and the rectal temperature reached at least 35 °C.

In both groups cardioplegia was flow-controlled infused as long as the aortic root pressure of the cardioplegia was below 80 mmHg and the temperature of the perfusate monitored. The cardioplegic solutions are described in detail in Table 2. The BCP consists of the following two solution - one for induction and one for maintainance of cardiac arrest. The relation of 4:1 between blood and cardioplegic solution was achieved by a cardioplegic delivery system. The cardioplegic record is shown in Table 3.

Table 2. Characteristics of the cardioplegic solutions

Blood Cardioplegia according to Buckberg	Solution 1	Solution 2	Crystalloid Cardioplegia according to Kirklin	1000 ml
Glucose 5 %	250 ml	250 ml	Glucose	27.75 mmol/l
Citrate-phosphate-dextrose	50 ml	50 ml	Sodium-hydrogen-carbonate	26.80 mmol/l
TRIS-buffer	20 ml	20 ml	Mannitol	54.33 mmol/l
Glutamate / Aspartate	250 ml	250 ml	CaCl	0.50 mmol/l
KCl 1mol/ml	60 ml	40 ml	KCl	30.02 mmol/l
NaCl 0.9 %	180 ml	180 ml	NaCl	82.47 mmol/l

Table 3. Cardioplegia management according to Buckberg[8].

	Temperature [°C]	Max.pressure [mmHg]	Flow [ml/min]	Duration [min]
Initial Dose: Solution 1 after cardiac arrest:	8-10	80	300	
Solution 2	8-10	80	200	3
Multiple Reinfusions: Solution 2, every 20 min	8-10	80	200	2
Warm Reperfusion Solution 2	37	50	150	2

Measurement of Hemodynamic Parameters

Mean arterial pressure (MAP), mean pulmonary artery pressure (MPAP), heart rate (HR), pulmonary capillary wedge pressure (PCWP), and central venous pressure (CVP) were continuously monitored intraoperatively and throughout the following 24 hours after

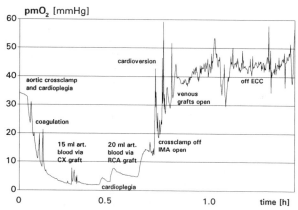

Figure 1. Original registration of continuously measured intramyocardial oxygen pressure. In this graph the pmO2 during CABG of a 60-year-old patient with a three-vessel disease is shown. The patient received two venous grafts and one A. mammaria interna graft. The pmO2 decreases continuously to minimum values of 2 mmHg during ischemia. Each infusion of blood into the grafts (via the Ramus circumflexus (CX) or the right coronary artery (RCA)) or of the oxygenated crystalloid cardioplegic solution into the aortic root results in a rising pmO2. After unclamping the IMA-bypass the pmO2 in the measurement area is raised and further increases after unclamping the aorta. During reperfusion there is a dependence between the pmO2 and the flow of the ECC. Measurements in patients receiving blood cardioplegia showed qualitatively same results as shown in this figure.

termination of the ECC. Cardiac output (CO) was measured with the thermodilution method twice before ECC and 0.5h, 1h, 2h, 3h, 4h, 8h, 12h, and 24h after ECC. Cardiac index (CI = CO/BSA [l/min/m2]; BSA: body surface area) and left ventricular stroke work index (LVSWI = CO MAP x 0.0136 / BSA x HR [g x m/m2]) were calculated.

Continuous Measurement of the Intramyocardial Oxygen Pressure

The myocardial oxygen pressure was continuously measured intraoperatively with a flexible electrode[9] (Clark-Type, 0.55 mm diameter, Shiley Inc.). The polarographic sensor was connected to a computer controlled device[10] (LICOX, GMS mbH, Kiel, Germany) which polarizes the cathode with -630 mV against the anode. The data were taken every two seconds and immediately shown on the monitor of the device.

Before every measurement the system was adjusted by a two-point-calibration using N_2 and air. Oxygen pressure measurement was started before onset of the ECC. The area chosen for the probe should not show any coronary vessels and any pathologically altered myocardium. The sensor was inserted in a silastic tube fastened to an atraumatic needle, which was pulled through the puncture channel of about 4 cm length. The tube was removed from the sensor, a clip placed at the sensor tip, and the measurement area of the sensor, 0.5 cm from the sensor tip, pulled back into the myocardium. The correct intramyocardial location of the sensor was verified by the measured values. If there was macroscopic bleeding or if the values indicated a misplacement of the sensor, the sensor was removed and reinserted at a different site. The temperature probe was inserted by means of the same technique at a distance of 1 cm. The whole procedure was finished in less than 3 minutes. All events suspected of influencing the pmO_2 were registrated. The computer stored temperature and pmO_2 values. Measurements were continued until chest closure.

Methods of Statistical Evaluation

All data are expressed as mean values and standard deviations. Univariate statistics for categorical data used the chi-square test and continuous variables were compared with use of Student's t-test. All analyses consisted of two-tailed tests, with an alpha level of 0.05 used to demonstrate statistical significance.

RESULTS

The two groups did not differ significantly with regard to age, coronary status, number of grafts per patient, ECC-time, aortic crossclamp time, spontaneous defibrillations, and electrical defibrillations. There was no difference in the demand of positive inotropic drugs between the two groups. Clinical and operative data are summarized in Tables 1 and 4.

Table 4. Operative data

	BCP; n=28	CCP; n=32
Number of venous grafts per patient	1.97 ± 1.25	1.79 ± 0.84
Number of IMA-grafts per patient	0.96	0.71
Extracorporeal circulation time (min)	83.9 ± 25.8	78.3 ± 20.0
aortic crossclamp time (min)	52.0 ± 16.4	45.3 ± 12.6
Spontaneous defibrillation after declamping	8 (29 %)	11 (34 %)
Electrical defibrillations after declamping	0.9 ± 0.7	1.3 ± 1.3
transitory pacing due to av-block °III	5	6
Duration of av-block °III: 0-1h	4	4
>1h	1	2
Mortality (%)	0	0

mean ± standard deviation. No statistically significant differences between the blood cardioplegia group (BCP) and the crystalloid cardioplegia group (CCP) were found.

Results of Hemodynamic Measurements

The preoperative hemodynamic values did not differ statistically between the two groups. Hemodynamic results are summarized in Table 5. There was a tendency for the cardiac index in the CCP group to rise slowly after ECC from 2.3 ± 0.4 l/min/m^2 to 2.8 ± 0.8 l/min/m^2. In the BCP group the CI increased from 2.3 ± 0.5 l/min/m^2 to 3.5 ± 0.9 l/min/m^2 ($p<0.05$); one hour after ECC a significantly higher level was reached in the BCP group ($p<0.01$). The LVSWI after ECC was significantly lower in the CCP group (0.5h: 32 ± 10 g*m/m^2 vs.41 ± 13 g*m/m^2 ($p < 0.05$) 1h: 33 ± 9 g*m/m^2 vs. 41 ± 9 g*m/m^2 ($p < 0.01$)).

Table 5. Hemodynamic results

Parameter		Control	0.5h	1h	2h	4h	8h	24h
CI	BCP	2.3 ± 0.5	3.5 ± 0.9**	3.5 ± 0.6**	2.9 ± 0.6	3.1 ± 0.8	3.2 ± 0.8	3.1 ± 0.8
(l/min/m^2)	CCP	2.3 ± 0.4	2.8 ± 0.8	2.6 ± 0.6	2.7 ± 0.8	2.8 ± 0.7	2.9 ± 0.7	2.9 ± 0.5
LVSWI	BCP	4 ± 10	41 ± 13*	41 ± 9**	37 ± 9	36 ± 10	36 ± 0	39 ± 8
(g*m/m^2)	CCP	44 ± 11	32 ± 10	33 ± 9	34 ± 11	34 ± 11	33 ± 9	36 ± 10

Mean ± standard deviation, * = p<0.05, ** p<0.01. Control values were taken before thoracotomy, the other values are measured 0.5 - 24 h after the end of extracorporeal circulation. BCP: blood cardioplegia group. CCP: crystalloid cardioplegia group.

Results of Myocardial Temperature and Myocardial Oxygen Pressure Measurements

The tissue temperature did not differ significantly between the groups at any time. Before onset of extracorporeal circulation the average temperature in the CCP group was 32.1 °C and 34.1 °C in the BCP group. Minimum temperature values were measured after five minutes of ischemia: 17.8 °C in the BCP and 18.6 °C in the CCP group. In the reperfusion period 5 minutes after opening the aortic crossclamp, the average temperature was 35.2 °C in the BCP group and 34.2 °C in the CCP group.

Before ECC the pmO$_2$ in the BCP group was 32.7 ± 4.1 mmHg; in the CCP group, 32.8 ± 6.7 mmHg. Five minutes after starting ischemia by crossclamping the aorta and induction of cardioplegia, the pmO$_2$ decreased to 9.5 ± 4.3 mmHg in both groups. The minimum values of 2.4 ± 1.5 mmHg in the CCP group and 2.6 ± 1.8 mmHg in the BCP group were at the same level. At the first postischemic measurement, five minutes after ECC, the BCP values were 23.0 ± 9.8 mmHg. The CCP values were 27.1 ± 10.0 mmHg, but this difference was not statistically significant. Five minutes after opening the constructed grafts the BCP values increased to 27.9 ± 11.9 mmHg and the CCP values to 29.1 ± 12.4 mmHg. The maximum values during ECC in the BCP group were 38.5 ± 14.6 mmHg, in the CCP group, 38.5 ± 13.3 mmHg.

DISCUSSION

The mean pmO$_2$ values of 32 ± 3.5 mmHg in the right ventricle before extracorporeal circulation were within the range of pmO$_2$ values (15 - 55 mmHg) reported by other authors. This was shown in animal experiments[11,12,13,14], measurements in man[15,16] and by calculation[17]. Most investigators used surface or microneedle probes. Our oxygen measurements were performed with a relatively large probe not measuring the local pmO$_2$ as microprobes do but integrating the pmO$_2$ values of a tissue cylinder. The size of the probe may lead to bleeding within the tissue. If there was macroscopic bleeding, the probes were repositioned. However micro-bleeding cannot be ruled out. In addition, the probe might compress capillaries or arterioles in the surrounding tissue resulting in a lowered perfusion and pmO$_2$.

A comparison of this probe with microneedle probes showed no differences in mean pmO₂ values in skeletal muscle[28]. Methodological differences in pmO₂ values might appear in the perfused beating heart; they are, however, not likely in the non-perfused resting myocardium.

The advantages of the probes used for the present study are flexibility and ease of fixation in the myocardium. Surgery was not delayed, and no problems arose.

The patients in the BCP group showed benefits in their hemodynamic outcome in the early postoperative period. LVSWI and CI were significantly higher than in the patients receiving CCP. These results were expected and are also described by several other authors[19,20,21,22].

There were, however, no differences in the average pmO₂ between the BCP and the CCP group, and in both groups the pmO₂ decreased in only 5 min after aortic crossclamping to ischemic values below 10 mmHg. These results show that neither oxygenated CCP nor saturated cold BCP provide an adequate oxygen offer to the myocardium. In the first

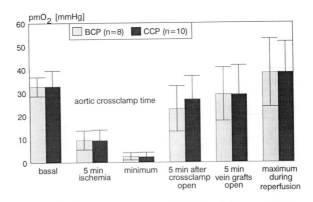

Figure 2. Myocardial oxygen pressure measurement. This figure shows the average values ± standard deviation of the pmO₂ at defined points of time during coronary artery bypass grafting. Basal values were obtained in the beating heart before aortic crossclamping. A statistically significant difference between the blood cardioplegia group (BCP) and the crystalloid cardioplegia group (CCP) could not be found at any point of time, but there was a trend to higher pmO₂ values in the CCP group during the early reperfusion period.

minutes of reperfusion the pmO₂ in the CCP group was slightly higher than in the BCP group. Since there is no hint for a higher oxygen offer in the CCP group, the lower pmO₂ levels in the BCP group may be interpreted as a higher myocardial oxygen utilisation during reperfusion.

The oxygenated CCP contains 3 ± 1 Vol % oxygen at 7° C, and BCP 10 ± 0.5 Vol % at 9° C with a hematocrit of 30 %[23,24]. The BCP is applied at a temperature of 8-10 °C. Compared with values at 37 °C, the oxygen binding curve of hemoglobin is shifted to the left, resulting in an increased oxygen affinity of hemoglobin[25]. At this temperature only very little oxygen can be released in the myocardium from the hemoglobin[26,27,28]. The plasma contains approximately the same amount of physically dissolved oxygen as CCP. This oxygen may diffuse to the tissue. The fact that there is no difference in pmO₂ between the BCP and the CCP group indicates that only the physically dissolved oxygen contributes to the oxygen supply of the myocardium in cold BCP.

Consequently, the temperature of BCP should be elevated to increase the oxygen offer. Since the myocardial metabolism rises with the temperature, the temperature for optimal balance between oxygen offer and oxygen uptake must therefore be found. In recent investigations encouraging results are reported using continuous applications of warm BCP[29].

Our results have, however, been confirmed by an animal study that used cold BCP at different hematocrit levels. The investigators did not see a correlation between oxygen content and efficacy of cold BCP[30]. By contrast, a more recent study[24] has shown a dependency between the protective effect of BCP and oxygen saturation using BCP with different saturation levels of hemoglobin. In the desaturated group the plasma was not oxygenated.

From all these findings one may may draw the following conclusions:

(1) Cold BCP does not offer more oxygen to the myocardium than oxygenated CCP.

(2) The physically dissolved oxygen has got a protective effect in cold BCP.

(3) The hemoglobin bounded oxygen does not correlate with the protective effect of cold BCP.

(4) The physically dissolved oxygen in combination with blood is more protective than the dissolved oxygen in a crystalloid cardioplegic solution.

This study was supported by grants of Walter Schulz Foundation, Munich, Germany.

REFERENCES

1. F.P. Catinella, E.A. Knopp, and J.N. Cunningham, Preservation of myocardial ATP during cardioplegia: comparison of techniques. J Cardiovasc Surg 25:296 (1984)
2. R.J. Novick, H.J. Stefaniszyn, R.P. Michel, F.D. Burdon, and T.A. Salerno, Protection of the hypertrophed pig myocardium. J Thorac Cardiovasc Surg 89:547 (1985)
3. D.M. Follette, D.G. Mulder, J.V. Malony, and G.D. Buckberg, Advantages of blood cardioplegia over continuous coronary perfusion or intermittent ischemia. J Thorac Cardiovasc Surg 76:604 (1978)
4. A.K. Singh, R. Farrugia, C. Teplitz, and K.E. Karlson, Electrolyte versus blood cardioplegia: randomized clinical and myocardial ultrastructural study. Ann Thorac Surg 33:218 (1982).
5. S.E. Fremes, G.T. Christakis, R.D. Weisel D.A.G. Mickle, M.M. Madonik, J. Ivanov, R. Harding, and S.J. Seawright, A clinical trial of blood and crystalloid cardioplegia. J Thorac Cardiovasc Surg 88:726 (1984)
6. S.R. Gundry, A. Sequeira, T.R. Coughlin, and J.S. McLaughlin, Postoperative conduction disturbances: a comparison of blood and crystalloid cardioplegia. Ann Thorac Surg 47:384 (1989)
7. W.M. Daggett, J.D. Randolph, M. Jacobs, D.D O'Keefe, G.A. Geffin, L.A. Swinski, B.R. Boggs, and W.G. Austen, The superiority of cold oxygenated blood cardioplegia. Ann Thorac Surg 43:397 (1987)
8. G.D. Buckberg, Recent progress in myocardial protection during cardiac operations. Cardiovasc Clin 17:291 (1987)
9. P. Eberhard, W. Fehlmann, and W. Mindt, An electrochemical sensor for continuous intravascular oxygen monitoring. Biotelem Patient Monit 6:16 (1979)
10. W. Fleckenstein, A.I.R. Maas, G. Nollert, and D.A. de Jong, Oxygen pressure in cerebrospinal fluid. In: Clinical Oxygen Measurement II., Ehrly, Hauss, editors, Blackwell Ueberreuter Verlag London, Berlin (1990)
11. C.S. Angell, E.G. Lakatta, M.L. Weisfeldt, and N.W. Shock, Relationship of intramyocardial oxygen tension and epicardial ST segment changes following acute coronary ligation: effects of coronary perfusion pressure. Cardiovasc Res 9:12 (1975)
12. P. Boeckstegers, J. Diebold, and C. Weiss, Selective ECG synchronised suction and retroinfusion of coronary veins: First results of studies in acute myocardial ischaemia in dogs. Cardiovasc Res 24:456 (1990)
13. J.W. Brantigan, V.L. Gott, and M.N. Martz, A teflon membrane for measurements of blood and intramyocardial gas tensions by mass spectroscopy. J Appl Physiol 32:276 (1972)
14. H. Forst, J. Racenberg, R. Schosser, and K. Messmer, Right ventricular Tissue O_2 in dogs. Effects of hemodilution and acute right coronary artery occlussion. Resp Exp Med 187:159 (1987)
15. L. Wiener, M. Feola, and J.Y. Templeton, Monitoring Tissue oxygenation of the heart after myocardial revascularization. Am J Cardiol 38:38 (1976)
16. N. Mendler, S. Schuchhardt, and F. Sebening, Measurements of intramyocardial oxygen tension during cardiac surgery in man. Res Exp Med 159:231 (1973)

17. G. Thews, Die Sauerstoffdrucke im Herzmuskelgewebe. Pflügers Arch. ges Physiol. 276:166 (1962)
18. P.Boeckstegers, pers. comm. (1992)
19. S.F. Khuri, K.G. Warner, M. Josa, M. Butler, A. Hayes, R. Hanson, S. Siouffi. and E.M. Barsamian, The superiority of continuous cold blood cadioplegia in the metabolic protection of the hypertrophied human heart. J Thorac Cardiovasc Surg 95:442 (1988)
20. F. Beyersdorf, E. Krause, K. Sarai, B. Sieber, N. Deutschländer, G. Zimmer, L. Mainka, S. Probst, M. Zegelmann, W. Schneider, and P. Satter, Clinical evaluation of hypothermic ventricullar fibrillation, multi-dose blood cardioplegia, and single-dose Bretschneider cardioplegia in coronary surgery. Thorac Cardiovasc Surg 38:20 (1990)
21. R.M. Engelmann, J.H. Rousou, W. Dobbs, M.A. Pels, and F. Longo, The superiority of blood cardioplegia in myocardial preservation. Circulation 62:162 (1980)
22. O.M. Feindel, G.A. Tait, G.J. Wilson, P. Kleman. and D.C. MacGregor, Multidose blood versus crystalloid cardioplegia. J Thorac Cardiovasc Surg 87:585 (1984)
23. K. Tabayashi, P.P. McKeown, M. Miyamoto, A.E. Luedtke, R. Thomas, D.G. Breazeale, G.A. Misbach, M. Allen, and T.D. Ivey, Myocardial preservation: a comparison of oxygenated crystalloid and blood cardioplegia. Tohoku J Exp Med 161:185 (1990)
24. J. Vinten-Johanson, J.S. Julian, H. Yokoyama, W.E. Johnston, T.D. Smith, D.S. McGee, and A.R. Cordell, Efficacy of myocardial protection with hypothermic blood cardioplegia depends on oxygen. Ann Thorac Surg 52:939 (1991)
25. J.W. Severinghaus, Oxyhemoglobin dissociation curve correction for temperature and pH variation in human blood. J Appl Physiology 12:485 (1957)
26. R.A. Guyton, L.M.A. Dorsey, J.M. Craver, D.K. Bone, E.L. Jones, D.A. Murphy, and C.R. Hathcer, Improved myocardial recovery after cardioplegic arrest with an oxygenated crystalloid solution. J Thorac Cardiovasc Surg 89:877 (1985)
27. J.D. Randolph, K.W. Toak, G.A. Geffin, L.M. DeBoer, D.D. O'Keefe, S.F. Khuri and W.M. Dagget, Improved myocardial preservation with oxygenated cardioplegic solutions as reflected by on-line monitoring of intramyocardial pH during arrest. J Vasc Surg 3:216 (1986)
28. J.A. Rousou, R.M. Engelman, R.H. Breyer, H. Otani, S. Lemeshow, and D. K. Das, The effect of temperature and hematocrit level of oxygenated cardioplegic solutions on myocardial preservations. J Thorac Cardiovasc Surg 95:625 (1988)
29. S.V. Lichtenstein, J.G. Abel, and T.A. Salerno, Warm heart surgery and results of operation for recent myocardial infarction. Ann Thorac Surg 52:455 (1991)
30. R.W. Illes, N.A. Silverman, I.B. Krukenkamp, R.D. Yusen, D.D Chausow, and S. Levitzky, The efficacy of blood cardioplegia is not due to oxygen delivery. J Thorac Cardiovasc Surg 98:1051 (1989)

FUNCTION OF ISOLATED RABBIT HEARTS PERFUSED WITH ERYTHROCYTE SUSPENSION IS NOT STABLE BUT IMPROVEMENT MAY BE FEASIBLE WITH HEMOGLOBIN SOLUTION

J.B. Hak[1], P.T.M. Biessels[2], J.H.G.M. van Beek[1], J.C. Bakker[2] and N. Westerhof[1]

[1] Laboratory for Physiology
Free University
1081 BT Amsterdam
[2] Central Laboratory of The Netherlands Red
Cross Blood Transfusion Service
1006 AK Amsterdam
The Netherlands

INTRODUCTION

In order to study cardiac function many investigators use isolated heart preparations perfused with saline solutions. In isolated rabbit heart perfused with a Tyrode solution at 37 °C it has been shown that oxygen supply is partially limiting oxygen consumption[1]. Experiments with isolated Tyrode perfused rabbit hearts at 28 °C proved that oxygen supply was not limiting. This finding has been explained by increased oxygen solubility and decreased metabolic demand at the lower temperature[2].

To study the isolated rabbit heart preparation at 37 °C oxygen supply has to be improved to prevent partial limitation of cardiac metabolism by oxygen supply. To achieve this many investigators added human erythrocytes[3,4] or sheep erythrocytes[5] to the perfusion medium or used heparinized rabbit blood[6], while others chose for blood from a support animal to perfuse the isolated heart[7]. However, it has also been reported that perfusion with erythrocyte suspensions in artificial perfusion systems are unsuccessful probably due to obstruction of capillaries[8]. Perfusion of the isolated rabbit heart with a low concentration of purified stroma-free hemoglobin (3 g/l) shows that cardiac function can be increased, probably due to the increased oxygen transporting capacity of the perfusate[9]. Due to thorough purification of the hemoglobin little vasoconstriction was found in these preparations.

In this study we investigated cardiac function of the isolated rabbit heart, perfused at

Oxygen Transport to Tissue XV, Edited by P. Vaupel
et al., Plenum Press, New York, 1994

37 °C according to Langendorff with a Tyrode solution containing human erythrocytes or with cell-free hemoglobin solutions. Since carefully purified and chemically modified cell-free hemoglobin solutions are still in very short supply, we had to restrict ourselves to a limited number of preliminary experiments with cell-free solutions.

MATERIALS AND METHODS

Preparation Procedures

Ten New Zealand white rabbits, weighing 3.1 ± 0.1 kg (mean ± S.E.M.), were anesthetized with 9.3 mg/kg fluanisone and 0.3 mg/kg fentanyl citrate (Hypnorm®, Janssen Pharmaceutica, Beerse, Belgium), injected intramuscularly. Supplementary anesthesia, 10 mg/kg pentobarbital, was given in the ear vein just before opening the thorax. Heparin (at least 2500 IU, Leo Pharmaceutical Products, Weesp, The Netherlands) was given in the ear vein. The aorta was then cannulated *in situ* and perfusion according to Langendorff was started whereafter excision of the heart followed. From the beginning of the artificial perfusion to the beginning of perfusion with erythrocyte suspension, hearts were perfused with a modified Tyrode solution (in mM: NaCl, 128.3; KCl, 4.7; $CaCl_2$, 1.36; $MgCl_2$, 1.05; $NaHCO_3$, 20.2; NaH_2PO_4, 0.42; and glucose, 11.1) containing 25 g/l bovine serum albumin (Sigma A-7030 or A-9647, St. Louis MO, USA). The perfusate was filtered before use with a 1.2 μm filter (Millipore, Bedford MA, USA). A water-filled latex balloon was placed in the left ventricle. Hearts were paced with electrodes placed on the right atrium. The preparation procedures have been described in detail before[2]. The temperature was kept constant during the entire experiment at 37 °C.

Experimental Setup

A schematic drawing of the experimental setup is given in Figure 1. The perfusate was pumped out of a blood bag, placed in a water bath kept at 37 °C, with a roller pump and recirculated through a membrane oxygenator (VPCML, Cobe Laboratories, Lakewood CO, USA). Just after the oxygenator a line branched off to a second pump which perfused the heart at constant flow. The perfusate first passed a bubble catcher and a heat exchanger before entering the heart. Only if the hearts were perfused with erythrocyte suspensions a blood filter (40 μm transfusion filter, Fenwal, Deerfield IL, USA) was placed in the perfusion line. All tubes used in the setup were of medical grade silicon. During erythrocyte and stroma-free hemoglobin perfusion the perfusate was recirculated.

Blood and Stroma-Free Hemoglobin Solution Preparation

Human erythrocytes were supplied by the Central Laboratory of The Netherlands Red Cross Blood Transfusion Service. Blood was filtered to remove all white blood cells whereafter the erythrocyte suspension was washed three times with saline (0.154 M NaCl) so that only erythrocytes remained. Then the erythrocytes were resuspended in the Tyrode solution to a hematocrit of 21.5 ± 0.5 %, which corresponded to a hemoglobin concentration of 7.6 ± 0.1 g/dl. Before the experiment we examined the erythrocytes under the microscope. If forms of erythrocytes other than normal, e.g. echinocytes, were detected, the erythrocytes were not used. For each experiment erythrocytes of a single human donor were used.

In four experiments stroma-free hemoglobin was used at a concentration of 4-7 g/dl in

Tyrode solution. Three types were used: carefully purified but unmodified stroma-free hemoglobin (SFHb), cross-linked HbNFPLP, i.e. a chemically modified Hb molecule which does not dissociate in dimers and whose oxygen affinity is considerably lowered to blood-like values[10], and polyHbNFPLP which is a polymer consisting of several HbNFPLP molecules linked together[11]. All hemoglobin solutions were prepared by the Central Laboratory of The Netherlands Red Cross Blood Transfusion Service.

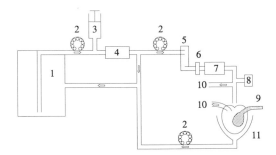

Figure 1. Experimental setup for perfusion of the isolated rabbit heart with erythrocyte suspension or hemoglobin solution. 1: blood bag was placed in a water bath at 37 °C; 2: roller pump; 3: windkessel; 4: membrane oxygenator; 5: bubble trap + Windkessel; 6: blood filter; 7: heat exchanger; 8: pressure transducer; 9: balloon connected to pressure transducer; 10: to arterial and venous oxygen electrodes; 11: cup.

Oxygen tension was measured with Clark-type oxygen electrodes which were calibrated before and after the experiment[1]. Oxygen saturation during erythrocyte perfusion was continuously measured with a fiber-optic densitometer (Schwarzer, Munich, FRG). The oxygen concentration (cO_2) was calculated according to equation (1)[12]:

$$cO_2(\mu M) = 60.7(\mu mol/g) \cdot cHb(g/l) \cdot sO_2(\%/100) + 1.34(\mu M/mmHg) \cdot PO_2(mmHg) \quad (1)$$

where cHb is the hemoglobin concentration, sO_2 the oxygen saturation of hemoglobin and PO_2 the partial oxygen pressure in the suspension. The saline perfusate was oxygenated with gas containing 95% O_2 / 5% CO_2, the erythrocyte suspension or hemoglobin solutions with 20% O_2 / 5% CO_2 / 75% N_2. Oxygen consumption was calculated from the product of coronary flow and the arterio-venous oxygen concentration difference.

Data are presented as mean ± S.E.M.. Trends in pressures and oxygen consumption during perfusion with erythrocyte suspension were statistically analyzed with linear regression analysis. The significance ($P < 0.05$) of the slope of the regression analysis was determined with an F-test.

RESULTS

Wet weight of the hearts, determined just after the experiment, was 13.3 ± 1.1 g. Dry weight, determined after 2 days of dehydration at 60 °C was 2.9 ± 0.2 g. The heart rate during six experiments with erythrocyte suspension was set at 158 ± 10 beats.min[-1] and flow was 1.8 ± 0.3 ml.min^{-1}.g^{-1}$_{\text{wet weight}}$. During the experiments with erythrocyte suspensions perfusion pressure increased significantly over the course of the experiment as shown in Figure 2A. Because flow was constant this implies that the vascular resistance increased. Also left ventricular diastolic pressure as shown in Figure 2B increased significantly during the experiment. Left ventricular systolic pressure increased significantly and reached a steady state after about 60 minutes (Fig 2B). Oxygen consumption decreased significantly with time (Fig. 2C). In all hearts, within half an hour, dark spots appeared on the surface. Development of these spots started on the right ventricle just under the pulmonary artery whereafter the spots spread over the remaining part of the right ventricle and the left ventricle. Histology showed large numbers of erythrocytes in the interstitial space outside the blood vessels after 2 hours of perfusion, suggesting that the macroscopically visible dark spots were the result of extravasation of erythrocytes.

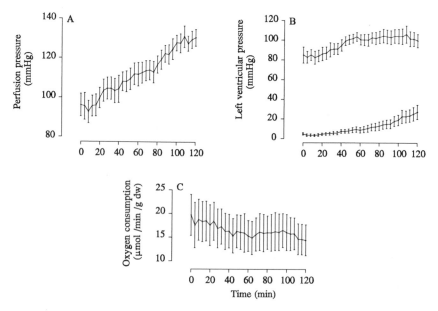

Figure 2. Perfusion pressure (*panel A*), systolic and diastolic left ventricular pressure (*panel B*) and oxygen consumption (*panel C*) during 2 hours of perfusion with erythrocyte suspension at constant flow. Bars indicate S.E.M. (n=6).

The hearts perfused with stroma-free hemoglobin solutions showed an increased left ventricular developed pressure directly after switching from Tyrode solution to hemoglobin solutions. Perfusion pressure, systolic and diastolic pressure of the two hearts perfused with SFHb at a constant flow, remained constant for 2 hours (Fig 3), whereafter perfusion pressure and diastolic left ventricular pressure increased markedly. The heart perfused with HbNFPLP performed reasonably for more than 2 hours and the heart perfused with polyHbNFPLP performed reasonably for more than 4 hours. In these hearts perfused with the two modified hemoglobin solutions, HbNFPLP and polyHbNFPLP, we found that left ventricular developed pressure increased when heart rate was increased. The increase in left ventricular developed pressure with heart rate is known as a positive staircase. This finding is in contrast with findings in hearts perfused with saline solution where left ventricular developed pressure usually decreases when heart rate is increased[1,2]. Perfusion pressure decreased with heart rate indicating intact regulatory vasodilation during perfusion with hemoglobin solution.

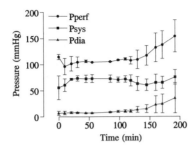

Figure 3. Preliminary experiments on hearts perfused with SFHb. Diastolic (Pdia) and systolic left ventricular pressure (Psys), and perfusion pressure (Pperf) during perfusion with SFHb (n = 2).

DISCUSSION

Because we found in pilot experiments that metal-erythrocyte suspension contact resulted in an increased amount of echinocytes, we omitted all metal parts from the experimental setup. Stirring the perfusate in a bottle gave aggregation of erythrocytes. Therefore the perfusate was kept in a blood bag (Fig. 1) placed in a water bath which was used for maintaining the temperature of the setup, and the suspension was stirred by the turbulent water. This arrangement reduces air-suspension contact which has negative effects on the condition of the erythrocytes. Only limited contact with air remained in the bubble-trap (5 in Fig. 1) and in the cup which collects the perfusate leaving the heart (11 in Fig. 1). All glassware was siliconized to improve smoothness of the surface. All these improvements in the setup reduced the formation of echinocytes.

However, despite these precautions we still found that perfusion of the isolated rabbit heart with the human erythrocyte suspension resulted in a progressive decrease in performance of these hearts. Because the blood was filtered and washed before the experiment only erythrocytes remain. Due to the absence of the coagulation system and of thrombocytes extravasation of the erythrocytes may no longer be prevented. The dark spots seen on the surface of the heart apparently were the result of extravasation of erythrocytes. This phenomenon resembles petechiae[13] or the disease purpura[14]: because of a decreased amount of blood platelets or a dysfunction of plasma factors involved in coagulation, small lesions in the capillary wall are not closed and erythrocytes can leave the blood vessels and form small bleedings known as petechiae. It has been hypothesized before that petechiae occurring in the isolated heart preparation are the result of the complete absence of thrombocytes[15]. In humans it is found that lesions of the vascular wall are the result of muscular activity or increased vascular pressure[14]. This suggests that in our preparation vascular lesions might be the result of cardiac contraction or that venous pressure is elevated. Because of the absence of the coagulation system and of thrombocytes in our case these lesions are not closed and extravasation of erythrocytes is the result. Coronary vessels might be compressed by the increased extravascular volume due to the extravasation of the erythrocytes. Consequently, the decrease in cardiac function may be the result of a decreased supply of substrates and oxygen to the myocardial cells.

In the literature many apparently successful studies of isolated hearts perfused with erythrocyte suspensions have been reported[3,4,5]. However, other investigators report that perfusion with erythrocyte suspensions is unsuccessful[8]. For the rabbit heart perfused with sheep erythrocyte suspension it has been reported that coronary flow decreases by 35 % during 6 hours of perfusion[16]. However, heart function was good during 6 hours in that study[16], although in another study[5] no data on heart function after 90 minutes of perfusion were reported. Perfusion of isolated hearts from a donor animal seems often successful although a large amount of experimental animals is required for this method[7]. From the present study we conclude that the isolated hearts perfused with an erythrocyte suspension form a difficult and sometimes unstable preparation and may not always be so trouble-free as implied in some of the literature. To rule out the possibility that our findings were based on the combination of human erythrocytes and rabbit heart we also perfused the isolated hearts with heparinized rabbit blood (unpublished data) since this was reported in the literature to be successful[6]. However, with this perfusion medium we also found an increase in perfusion pressure and development of dark spots with a similar time course as for human erythrocyte suspensions.

The function of hearts perfused with SFHb solutions was stable for a longer period than in hearts perfused with erythrocytes. However, after two hours cardiac function started to decline. During perfusion with SFHb solutions formation of small particles was found. Although their concentration was low it might be possible that they obstruct the capillaries. The formation of these small particles is probably due to dissociation of the hemoglobin tetramer (2 α and 2 β - units) in two α-β dimers which are not stable under these perfusion conditions. The decline of cardiac function of the SFHb perfused hearts might thus be explained by formation of particles. With the modified hemoglobin solutions the β chains are chemically cross-linked, thereby preventing the dissociation in α-β dimers[10]. The formation of particles was less when HbNFPLP or polyHbNFPLP was used which suggests that cardiac function may be maintained longer. In hearts perfused with stroma-free hemoglobin solutions, lesions of the vascular wall may also appear. Although hemoglobin might enter the extravascular space, it will presumably not compress the blood vessels. In the present experiments the hemoglobin solutions were available in small amounts only which limited the possibilities to study their effects. However, in the near future cell-free hemoglobin solutions will probably be available in larger amounts so that experiments can be done to study these perfusates for the isolated heart perfusion more carefully. Our preliminary conclusion is that hemoglobin solutions may prove suitable to provide adequate oxygen supply during artificial perfusion provided the hemoglobin is carefully purified[9]. This may be especially true for the chemically cross-linked hemoglobins.

SUMMARY

In the present study isolated rabbit hearts were perfused with erythrocyte suspensions (hematocrit 21.5 ± 0.5 %) or hemoglobin solutions according to Langendorff with a constant flow at 37 °C. In preliminary experiments three types of stroma-free hemoglobin were used: unmodified, but carefully purified, stroma-free hemoglobin (SFHb), HbNFPLP which is a chemically modified Hb molecule and polyHbNFPLP which is a polymer of HbNFPLP.

In hearts perfused with erythrocyte suspensions left ventricular developed pressure and oxygen consumption decreased and perfusion pressure increased steadily from the beginning of the perfusion. Dark spots appeared on the surfaces of these hearts, which were the result of extravasation of erythrocytes. As a consequence capillaries probably became obstructed, leading to reduced cardiac function. Hearts perfused with stroma-free hemoglobin solutions showed an initial increase in left ventricular developed pressure after switching from Tyrode perfusion to perfusion with hemoglobin solutions. Left ventricular developed pressure and perfusion pressure were stable for about 2 hours in hearts perfused with SFHb and were reasonable for 2 hours when the heart was perfused with HbNFPLP or more than 4 hours with polyHbNFPLP. More extensive experiments with stroma-free hemoglobin solutions when these become available in sufficient quantities have, according to the results from preliminary experiments, the potential of showing good oxygen supply resulting in reasonable cardiac function.

This study was supported, in part, by the Dutch Organization for Scientific Research (NWO) and, in part, by the Ministry of Defense of The Netherlands.

REFERENCES

1. J.H.G.M. van Beek, P. Bouma, and N. Westerhof. Oxygen uptake in saline-perfused rabbit heart is decreased to a similar extent during reductions in flow and in arterial oxygen concentration. *Pflügers Arch.* 414:82 (1989).

2. J.B. Hak, J.H.G.M. van Beek, M.H. van Wijhe, and N. Westerhof. Influence of temperature on the response time of mitochondrial oxygen consumption in isolated rabbit heart. *J. Physiol. (Lond)* 447:17 (1992).

3. C.S. Apstein, R.C. Dennis, L. Briggs, W.M. Vogel, J. Frazer and C.R. Valeri. Effect of erythrocyte storage and oxyhemoglobin affinity changes on cardiac function. *Am. J. Physiol.* 248:H508 (1985).

4. J.F. Baron, E. Vicaut, X. Hou and M. Duvelleroy. Independent role of arterial O_2 tension in local control of coronary blood flow. *Am. J. Physiol.* 258:H1388 (1990).

5. S.R. Bergmann, R.E. Clark and B.E. Sobel. An improved isolated heart preparation for external assessment of myocardial metabolism. *Am. J. Physiol.* 236:H644 (1979).

6. J.A. Leppo and D.J. Meerdink. Comparison of the myocardial uptake of a technetium-labelled isonitrile analogue and thallium. *Circ. Res.* 65:632 (1989).

7. Y. Goto, B.K. Slinker, and M.M. LeWinter. Similar normalized Emax and O_2 consumption-pressure-volume area relation in rabbit and dog. *Am. J. Physiol.* 255:H366 (1988).

8. K. Nishiki, M. Erecinska, and D.F. Wilson. Energy relationships between cytosolic metabolism and mitochondrial respiration in rat heart. *Am. J. Physiol.* 234:C73 (1978).

9. P.T.M. Biessels, J.B. Hak, W.K. Bleeker, J.H.G.M. van Beek, and J.C. Bakker. Effects of modified hemoglobin solutions on the isolated rabbit heart. *Biomaterials, Artificial Cells and Immobilization technology*, in press.

10. J. van der Plas, A. de Vries-van Rossen, J.J. Koorevaar, A. Buursma, W.G. Zijlstra and J.C. Bakker. Purification and physical characteristics of a hemoglobin solution modified by coupling to 2-nor-2-formylpyridoxal 5'-phosphate (NFPLP). *Transfusion* 28:525 (1988).

11. G.A.M. Berbers, W.K. Bleeker, P. Stekkinger, J. Agterberg, G. Rigter, and J.C. Bakker. Biophysical characteristics of hemoglobin intramolecularly cross-linked and polymerized. *J. Lab. Clin. Med.* 117:157 (1991).

12. R.W. Baer, G.J. Vlahakes, P.N. Uhlig, and J.I.E. Hoffman. Maximum myocardial oxygen transport during anemia and polycythemia in dogs. *Am. J. Physiol.* 252:H1086 (1987).

13. L.E.H. Whitby, and C.J.C. Britton. Disorders of the blood: Diagnosis, Pathology, Treatment, Technique. Ninth edition, Churchill, London (1963).

14. W.J. Williams, E. Beutler, A.J. Erslev and M.A. Lichtman. Hematology. Third Edition, McGraw-Hill, New York, USA (1983).

15. P.H. Huisman and J.J. Schipperheyn. The isolated heart-lung preparation. Martinus Nijhoff Medical Division. The Hague (1978).

16. L.D. Segel, J.L. Ensunsa and W.A. Boyle III. Prolonged support of working rabbit hearts using fluosol-43 or erythrocyte media. *Am. J. Physiol.* 252:H349 (1987).

CLASSICAL KROGH MODEL DOES NOT APPLY WELL TO CORONARY OXYGEN EXCHANGE

Catharina P.B. Van der Ploeg[1], Jenny Dankelman[1], Jos A.E. Spaan[1,2]

[1] Laboratory for Measurement and Control
University of Technology Delft, Mekelweg 2
2628 CD Delft, The Netherlands
[2] Department of Medical Physics and Informatics
University of Amsterdam, Meibergdreef 15
1105 AZ Amsterdam, The Netherlands

INTRODUCTION

Description of especially the dynamics of tissue oxygen control and coronary flow requires an oxygen exchange model (Dankelman et al, 1989). A manageable model, taking into account the complex capillary anatomy and all convective and diffusive processes, is not available. A classical model for oxygen exchange between blood and tissue is the Krogh cylinder model (Krogh, 1919). In this model oxygen leaves blood when flowing through a capillary, gradually decreasing oxygen saturation from arterial to venous values. A weak point of this model is that averaged capillary oxygen saturation is higher than venous saturation while experiments show that both saturations are about equal or that the former is even lower than the latter. A simple alternative model is based on the assumption of a well-mixed compartment in which average blood Po_2 is essentially equal to venous Po_2. The purpose of this study is to further assess the applicability of the two models in estimating intramyocardial blood volume involved in oxygen exchange. This information is contained within the transient in arteriovenous oxygen saturation difference induced by a sudden flow step (Van der Ploeg et al, 1992, 1993). Extraction of this information is model dependent. It will be assessed whether the volume is better determined by either the single mixed compartment or a series array of these compartments that has the characteristics of a Krogh model.

METHOD

Description of the Models

Both models are based on the O_2 mass balance. For the model with a single mixed compartment (figure 1A) the time response of the venous O_2 content to a flow step can be calculated from the following differential equation:

$$V^* \cdot d/dt([O_2]_v(t)) = Q_a \cdot [O_2]_a(t) - Q_a \cdot [O_2]_v(t) - MVO_2(t)$$

where: V^* = volume mixed compartment
$[O_2]_v$ = O_2 content in mixed compartment
$[O_2]_a$ = arterial O_2 content
Q_a = arterial flow
MVO_2 = O_2 consumption

The distributed model consisted of n mixed compartments in series (figure 1B). The volumes of the compartments were equal. Oxygen consumption is homogeneously distributed over the compartments. Of each compartment j, the O_2 content time course can be calculated by:

$$(V/n) \cdot d/dt([O_2]_{v,j}(t)) = Q_a \cdot [O_2]_{v,j-1}(t) - Q_a \cdot [O_2]_j(t) - (MVO_2(t)/n)$$

The response of the last compartment is the output of the model. With n=30 this response resembled the response of a continuously distributed model (n=∞). Note that the single mixed compartment model is a special case of the distributed model: for n=1 both models are equal.

The main distinction between the models is the distribution of oxygen. While in a single mixed compartment Po_2 is distributed homogeneously, in an array of mixed compartments with oxygen consumption the Po_2 declines in the direction of the flow. In this respect the latter model resembles the classical Krogh model.

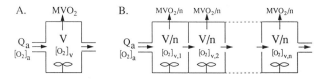

Figure 1. Models: A. Single mixed compartment and B. Series array of mixed compartments

Simulated Intervention

In the calculations flow was changed stepwise and MVO_2 and $[O_2]_a$ were assumed to be constant. Since $[O_2]_a$ is constant, the responses of the arteriovenous oxygen content difference and $[O_2]_v$ have the same shape (AVox = $[O_2]_a$ -$[O_2]_v$), only the direction of the change and offset are different. Responses of the distributed model were calculated for the sum of the mixed compartment volumes V being equal to 10 ml/100 g.

Comparison of the Model Simulations

The effect of model choice on the volume estimations from experimental data was determined indirectly: the two models were compared by fitting the response to a flow step of the model with a single mixed compartment to the response of the distributed model. The response of a single mixed compartment after a step in flow is exponential when oxygen consumption is constant. When the flow after the flow step ($Q_{a,after}$) is fixed, the time constant of the exponential response is determined by the volume of the mixed compartment ($\tau = V^*/Q_{a,after}$).

In both models the venous O_2 content starts to change at the same moment as the change in flow. However, when measured responses of the arteriovenous oxygen content difference (AVox) are examined, a time delay is apparent (figure 2). This time delay can be interpreted as being the result of transport vessels, which can be included in the model as an unmixed compartment distal of the oxygen exchange part of the model. The volume of this compartment, probably representing the larger veins, can be estimated from time delay and flow after the flow step: Vunm = time delay * $Q_{a,after}$. Since for the estimation of this volume the model response was fitted by shifting it on a time scale, we also used a variable time delay when the exponential response from the single mixed compartment was fitted to the distributed model response. In this way we could determine whether there would be a <u>difference</u> in estimated time delay, and thus unmixed volume, when the different models are used for data analysis.

Thus, the exponential curve was fitted to the distributed model response by varying time constant and time delay. The moments at which the response of the distributed model had changed relatively 10 and 90 % determined the time period for which the sum of squared differences between distributed model response and exponential curve was minimized. With this method the estimated volume V^* could be calculated and compared to the volume of the distributed model V. Furthermore, from the apparent time shift the difference in estimated unmixed volume (ΔVunm) between the two models could be calculated.

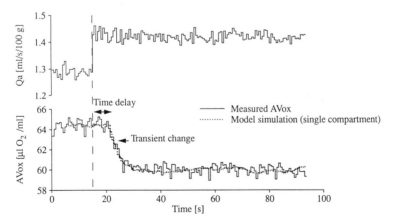

Figure 2. Measured coronary arterial flow (Q_a) and arteriovenous O_2 content difference (AVox), averaged per heart beat. Interpretation of the AVox response with a model for the coronary circulation results in an estimation of coronary blood volume distribution.

The same fitting procedure as described here was also used for the estimation of the coronary volume distribution from the measured response of the arteriovenous oxygen content difference after a flow step. The model consisting of a single mixed compartment in series with an unmixed compartment was used in this data analysis (figure 2).

RESULTS

The model responses of the venous oxygen content to a step change in flow are shown in figure 3. Because O_2 consumption was constant, the response of the single mixed compartment model (n=1) to a flow step was exponential with $\tau = V^*/Q_{a,after}$. Increase of the number of compartments in series (n) in the distributed model results in a deviation of the exponential curve: with many mixed compartments in series the response of the distributed model is an almost straight rise to another value. The slope of this rise depends on the volume assumed in the model.

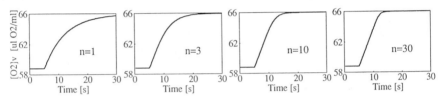

Figure 3. Model responses of the venous oxygen content $[O_2]_v$ to a flow step. The response of the single mixed compartment model (n=1) is exponential. Increment of the number of compartments (n) results in a more straight response.

For n=30 the response of the distributed model resembled the response of a continuously distributed model (n=∞). This response and the exponential curve fitted to it are shown in figure 4. Fitting of the single mixed compartment response to the distributed model response resulted in an underestimation of the oxygen exchange volume. The magnitude of this underestimation depended on the number of mixed compartments in series n (figure 5A). The estimated mixed volume is about 50 % of the total volume in the

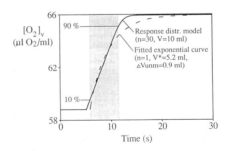

Figure 4. The response of a model with a single mixed compartment and an unmixed compartment is fitted to the response of the distributed model (n=30).

distributed model. Though no time delay existed in the distributed model, fitting of its response with an exponential curve resulted in an apparent time delay. From this time delay the apparent difference in unmixed volume between the two models could be calculated. The unmixed volume was overestimated by 1 ml/100 g when the single compartment model response was fitted to the distributed model response (figure 5B).

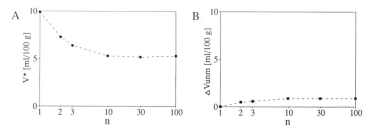

Figure 5. Volumes found by fitting an exponential curve to the response of a series array of n mixed compartments with V = 10 ml/100 g and Vunm = 0 ml/100 g.
A. Oxygen exchange volume V^*. Oxygen exchange volume appeared to be underestimated.
B. Difference in unmixed volume between the two models. Unmixed volume is overestimated.

DISCUSSION

In this study two models for coronary oxygen exchange were compared: A. a single well-mixed compartment and B. a distributed cylinder having Krogh characteristics. In the former model partial oxygen pressure is distributed homogeneously. Therefore, the Po_2 of blood leaving the compartment (venous Po_2) is equal to the Po_2 in the compartment (average capillary Po_2). In the latter model Po_2 declines gradually in the direction of the flow, which results in a venous Po_2 being less than the average capillary Po_2. However, measurements of capillary and tissue Po_2 revealed low values: e.g. Whalen (1971) measured an average Po_2 of 6-9 mmHg in a beating cat heart. Furthermore, model analysis of O_2 exchange in capillary networks revealed that tissue and capillary Po_2 might be less than venous Po_2 (Wieringa, 1985). These findings indicate that a single Krogh-like cylinder is a less realistic model for coronary O_2 exchange than a single mixed compartment.

The effect of model choice on the volume estimations was investigated. From the results it is clear that when measured data are fitted with a single mixed compartment the estimates of oxygen exchange and total volume will be less than when a continuously distributed model is applied. In previous examinations, measured AVox responses to a flow step were fitted with a single mixed compartment in series with an unmixed compartment (Van der Ploeg et al, 1993). The estimated volumes (mixed volume of 9.9 ml/100 g, unmixed volume of 3.8 ml/100 g) were within the range of coronary volumes which have been previously published, although they were rather high. When the described series array of mixed compartments would have been applied to these data, the resulting mixed volume estimations would even have been about twice as large. Since this is not likely, these results also indicate that the small oxygen exchanging coronary vessels can be represented better by a single mixed compartment than by a distributed cylinder.

We realize that both models that were compared are only global approximations of the coronary circulation. E.g. microvascular heterogeneity in partial oxygen pressure (Weiss and Sinha, 1978) and flow (Bassingthwaighte et al, 1989) have been demonstrated and were not taken into account. However, experimental and theoretical studies of tissue Po_2 and coronary volume indicate that, as a global approximation, the coronary O_2 exchange vessels of the beating heart can be represented better by a single mixed compartment than by a series array of mixed compartments having Krogh characteristics.

SUMMARY

By fitting of simulations with an oxygen exchange model to measured responses of the arteriovenous oxygen content difference after a flow step, coronary volumes can be estimated. In this study the dependence of the volume estimates on the choice of the oxygen exchange model for the coronary circulation was investigated. A model consisting of a single well-mixed compartment results in smaller volume estimates than a series array of mixed compartments in which Po_2 declines gradually (Krogh-like model). Use of the former model for data analysis resulted in realistic volume estimates. Thus, these results indicate that the oxygen exchange vessels are better represented by a single mixed compartment than by a cylinder having Krogh characteristics. This conclusion agrees with capillary Po_2 being equal to or smaller than venous Po_2 which cannot be explained by a Krogh model.

From these arguments we conclude that though both models are rough representations of the coronary circulation, the coronary O_2 exchange vessels of the beating heart can be represented better by a single mixed compartment than by a series array of mixed compartments which has Krogh characteristics.

REFERENCES

Bassingthwaighte, J.B., King, R.B. and Roger, S.A., 1989, Fractal nature of regional myocardial blood flow heterogeneity, *Circ.Res.* 65:578-590.

Dankelman, J., Spaan, J.A.E., Stassen, H.G. and Vergroesen, I., 1989, Dynamics of coronary adjustment to a change in heart rate in the anaesthetized goat, *J.Physiol.* 408:295-312.

Krogh, A., 1919, The number and distribution of capillaries in muscles with calculations of the oxygen pressure head necessary for supplying the tissue, *J.Physiol.* 52:409-415.

Van der Ploeg, C.P.B., Dankelman, J. and Spaan, J.A.E., 1992, Effect of heart rate on the functional distribution of the coronary vascular volume in the goat, *FASEB J.* 6:A1505.

Van der Ploeg, C.P.B., Dankelman, J. and Spaan, J.A.E., 1993, Functional distribution of coronary vascular volume in beating goat hearts, *Am.J.Physiol.* 264 (*Heart Circ.Physiol.* 33): in press.

Weiss, H.R. and Sinha, A.K., 1978, Regional oxygen saturation of small arteries and veins in the canine myocardium, *Circ.Res.* 42:119-126.

Wieringa, P.A., 1985, "The Influence of the Coronary Capillary Network on the Distribution and Control of Local Blood Flow", PhD thesis, Delft University of Technology, The Netherlands.

Whalen, W.J., 1971, Intracellular Po_2 in heart skeletal muscle. *Physiologist* 14, 69-82.

OXYGEN CONSUMPTION, OXYGEN TRANSPORT, AND LEFT VENTRICULAR FUNCTION IN SEVERE SEPSIS IN MAN

Luigi S. Brandi [1], Daniela Laudano [2], Armando M.R. Cuttano [2], Patrizia Baldi [2], and Francesco Giunta [3]

[1] Researcher in Anesthesiology and Intensive Care
[2] Staff Anesthesiologist
[3] Associate Professor in Anesthesiology and Intensive Care
Department of Anesthesiology and Intensive Care, University of Pisa, Italy

INTRODUCTION

Sepsis and septic shock remain a major cause of mortality among critically ill patients [1]. Even with effective therapeutic regimens (antibiotics, surgical drainage, hemodynamic support) and advanced hemodynamic monitoring, sepsis and septic shock remain the most prevalent clinical problem in Intensive Care Units and a common cause of death [1]. Death is frequently caused by a refractory hypotension with a low systemic vascular resistance, due to a derangement in regulation of peripheral vasomotor tone.

Recently, investigators have stressed the presence of global myocardial dysfunction in experimental, as well as in human sepsis [2,3,4]. In one of these studies, that examined the effect of a volume challenge in patients with septic shock, the observed increases in left ventricular stroke work index were smaller in non survivors than in survivor [2]. Besides, patients with sepsis and septic shock have an impaired ability to utilize oxygen by peripheral tissues [5,6], even when cardiac output is elevated, causing a condition of oxygen supply dependency. Pathologic oxygen supply dependency is an abnormal situation in which oxygen consumption varies directly with oxygen delivery. Its presence in patients with sepsis has been associated with particularly high mortality rates [7] that may be the results of tissue hypoxia that cause multiple organ failure. This pathologic dependency between oxygen

Oxygen Transport to Tissue XV, Edited by P. Vaupel
et al., Plenum Press, New York, 1994

consumption and oxygen delivery also has been showed in patients with sepsis and septic shock who have high lactate levels, whereas those with normal lactate levels show no variations in oxygen consumption when oxygen delivery is raised with fluid loading [8,9]. But, the clinical significance of this condition of pathologic supply dependency in sepsis is still debated, and its presence has been recently challenged [10,11].

The purpose of this study was to describe the timed-honored traditional oxygen derived variables together with the acid-base status of 41 patients with severe sepsis admitted to a postsurgical intensive care unit. We focused the attention on the differences related to the inICU outcome of these patients.

PATIENTS AND METHODS

We analyzed the hemodynamic data and blood gases of 41 patients (26 male, 15 female; age from 18 to 87 years, mean body weight 69.8 ± 14, mean body surface area 1.77 ± 0.2) admitted to ICU with diagnosis of severe sepsis. Severe sepsis was defined by the presence of positive blood culture or a documented site of infection (positive bacterial cultures or surgical laparatomy identification), and three of the following criteria: hyperthermia (> 38 °C) or hypothermia (< 36 °C), heart rate (> 100 beats/min), tachypnea (> 20 breath/min), leukocytosis (> 14,000/mm^3) or leukopenia (< 3,500/mm^3), thrombocytopenia (< 150,000/mm^3). In each patient the severity of the sepsis was assessed by a Simplified Acute Physiologic Score (SAPS).

Each patient was monitored using a 7 Fr, flow-directed thermistor-tip catheter, and an indwelling radial or femoral artery catheter. Systemic arterial, pulmonary arterial, and central venous pressures, along with heart rate (HR) were monitored continuously by a monitoring system (RM 300, Honeywell, Best, Holland). All pressure values were recorded using a strain-gauge transducer (Novotrans TM, Medex Inc, Hilliar, Ohio, USA) leveled to the mid-chest position, zeroed to atmosphere and calibrated to a known mercury standard. Cardiac output was determined by standard thermodilution technique and cardiac computer at least every six hours. Injections of 10 mL of a room-temperature (21 to 24 °C) solution of 5% dextrose in water were used. Injection times were always < 4 sec, thus eliminating possible effects of varying injection rates on calculations. The reported cardiac output was the average of three serial measurements obtained within 2 to 3 mins, providing that the intermeasurement variance was < 10%. If variance was >10%, two additional measurements were made, and high and low values rejected. Every effort was made to spread the indicator injection equally over the respiratory cycle. Immediately after cardiac output measurement, arterial and mixed venous blood samples were obtained simultaneously from the catheter in the radial or femoral artery and from the distal port of the pulmonary artery catheter. Air bubbles in the samples were carefully avoided, and an appropriate amount of heparin in the samples was used. Blood gases were measured immediately by an automated blood gas laboratory (IL System 1312 Instrumentation Laboratory, Lexington, Ma, USA). Hemoglobin concentration and oxyhemoglobin saturation were measured directly using a cooximeter (IL 282 Instrumentation Laboratory). From these values we derived values for arterial and mixed venous oxygen content (CaO_2 and CvO_2) and total arterial mixed-venous oxygen content [$C(a-v)O_2$] as follows:

$$CaO_2 = (1.39 * Hgb * SaO_2) + 0.0031 * PaO_2$$

$$CvO_2 = (1.39 * Hgb * SvO_2) + 0.0031 * PvO_2$$

$$C(a-v)O_2 = CaO_2 - CvO_2$$

in which Hgb (g/dL) is the hemoglobin concentration, SaO_2 and SvO_2 (%) the arterial and mixed venous oxygen saturation, and PaO_2, and PvO_2 (torr) the arterial and mixed venous oxygen tension, 1.39 is the amount of oxygen/g Hgb, and $(0.0031) * (PO_2)$ is the amount of oxygen dissolved in plasma. Oxygen delivery (DO_2)was calculated as:

$$DO_2 = CO * CaO_2$$

and oxygen consumption (VO_2) was measured as:

$$VO_2 = CO * C(a-v)O_2$$

All patients received appropriate antibiotics depending on the presumed site of infection and suspected bacteriology. Once an organism was identified, the antinfective therapy was given according to the bacteriological results. Every effort was made to identify and drain infected sites (CAT, echography). Initial treatment included fluid administration (colloid or plasma) to achieve a pulmonary artery occlusion pressure between 12 and 15 mmHg. Persisting hypotension was treated with dopamine up to 15 μg/kg/min. When pulmonary artery occlusion pressure was in the range between 12 and 15 mmHg, and when low flow persisted (oliguria, cardiac index < 3 L/min, systolic blood pressure < 90 mmHg, dobutamine was added up to 20 μg/kg/min). Supplemental oxygen by nasal prong or mechanical ventilation (19 patients [46 %]) were used to maintain arterial saturation > 90%. A total of 694 measurements (survivors 261, nonsurvivors 433) was obtained during the time-course of sepsis. Initial measurements were obtained immediately after the admission in ICU and before the use of vasoactive drugs. Final measurements were obtained after recovery of sepsis (clinical judgment and no infusion of vasoactive drugs), or two or four hours before the death. All data were presented as mean ± SD. Statistical analysis was performed using the two-tail Student t test for unpaired data to compare all the measurements between survivors and non survivors. The two-way analysis of variance (ANOVA) for repeated measurements was used to compare the initial and final measurements between

Table I. Hemodynamics and acid-base status in 41 patients during severe sepsis. The values reported are the means of all measurements obtained for survivors (n = 261) and for nonsurvivors (n = 433) during their course of sepsis[1].

	SURVIVORS	NONSURVIVORS
SAPS	12.9 ± 3	15.6 ± 2.8 *
LVSWI (g.m/m^2)	53.7 ± 17	42.2 ± 15 *
SVR (dynes/sec/cm^{-5})	952 ± 305	711 ± 263 *
CI (L/min/m^2)	4.1 ± 1.1	4.2 ± 1.2
CaO$_2$ (mg/dL)	14.1 ± 1.8	14.1 ± 2.0
VO$_2$ (mL/min/m^2)	138 ± 47	129 ± 31 *
DO$_2$ (mL/min/m^2)	575 ± 184	586 ± 168
O$_2$ER (%)	24. 8 ± 7.2	23.3 ± 7.3 *
pHa (Units)	7.45 ± 0.06	7.39 ± 0.11 *
HCO$_3$a (mmol/L)	27.8 ± 3.6	25.5 ± 5.3 *
[H$^+$] (nmol/L)	36. 2 ± 5	42.0 ± 13 *

[1] * $p < 0.05$ or less

survivors and nonsurvivors. For all the data collected, linear regression was used to find the correlation coefficient between oxygen delivery and oxygen consumption. Statistical significance is reported at a $p < 0.05$.

RESULTS

Of the 41 patients 18 survived (43%) and twenty-three patients (57%) died. Table I summarized the all hemodynamic and acid-base status data of those who died and survived.

For all the data collect, the survivors had a significantly higher left ventricular stroke work index (LVSWI) (p < 0.001), systemic vascular resistance (SVR) (p < 0.001), oxygen consumption (VO_2) $(p < 0.01)$, oxygen extraction index (O_2ER) $(p < 0.05)$, arterial bicarbonate (HCO_3a) $(p < 0.001)$, pH $(p < 0.001)$, and significantly lower arterial hydrogenions concentration $([H^+])$ $(p < 0.001)$. There was no significant difference in cardiac index (CI), oxygen delivery (DO_2), and total arterial oxygen content (CaO_2) between survivors and nonsurvivors.

Table II summarizes the hemodynamic and acid-base status data of those who died and survived, according to the initial and final values.

Table II. Hemodynamics and acid-base status in the 41 patients (18 survivors and 23 nonsurvivors) according to the initial and final phase of sepsis [1].

	SURVIVORS		NONSURVIVORS	
	Initial	Final	Initial	Final
LVSWI $(gm.m^2)$	54.6 ± 23	55.8 ± 20	38.2 ± 16 [*]	32.9 ± 14 [*]
SVR $(dynes/sec/cm^{-5})$	896 ± 281	1050 ± 251 [†]	692 ± 301 [*]	569 ± 288 [*]
CI $(L/min/m^2)$	4.12 ± 1.4	3.69 ± 0.8	4.15 ± 1.6	3.99 ± 1.6
CaO_2 (mL/dL)	13.9 ± 2.7	14.2 ± 1.5	13.7 ± 2.3	13.5 ± 2.6
VO_2 $(mL/min/m^2)$	139 ± 40	134 ± 31	117 ± 34 [*]	122 ± 31 [*]
DO_2 $(mL/min/m^2)$	575 ± 218	519 ± 85	554 ± 203	543 ± 250
O_2ER (%)	26.7 ± 11	26.1 ± 6	22.4 ± 7	26.5 ± 12
pHa (Unit)	7.41 ± 0.1	7.46 ± 0.01 [†]	7.35 ± 0.1 [*]	7.30 ± 0.2 [*]
HCO_3a (mmol/L)	25.4 ± 5.1	28.7 ± 3.1 [†]	22.5 ± 5.5 [*]	22.1 ± 6.3 [*]
$[H^+]$ (nmol/L)	38.9 ± 6.1	34.3 ± 3.1 [†]	46.2 ± 17 [*]	51.9 ± 26 [*]

[1] * p-value between survivors and nonsurvivors; † p-value between initial and final phase of sepsis; $p < 0.05$ or less.

The survivors had a significantly higher LVSWI $(p < 0.001)$ (Fig. 1), and VO_2 $(p < 0.05)$, either initially or in the final phase of sepsis. There were no significant differences in CI, CaO_2, DO_2, and ERO_2 neither initially nor in the final phase of the sepsis between survivors and non survivors. Survivors had significantly higher SVR $(p < 0.001)$, both in the initial phase and in the final phase. Only the survivors had a significant increase $(p < 0.05)$ in SVR during the evolution of sepsis (Fig.2). Other differences were observed in HCO_3a, pH, and $[H^+]$. Nonsurvivors had a significantly lower pH and HCO_3a (both $p < 0.005$), and higher $[H^+]$ $(p < 0.01)$ than survivors both initially and in the final phase of their illness. Only survivors have a significant increase in arterial pH and HCO_3a (both < 0.005) (Fig. 3 and Fig. 4), and a significant decrease in arterial $[H^+]$ $(p < 0.005)$.

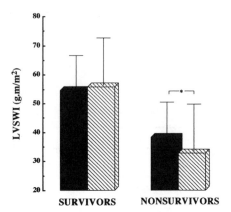

Figure 1. Mean left ventricular stroke work index (LVSWI) in the 18 patients survived and the 23 patients nonsurvived during the initial and the final phase of sepsis. The black bars refer to the initial values, the dotted bars refer to the final values. * Significant *vs* survivors' values.

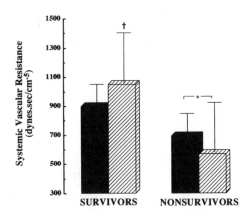

Figure 2. Mean SVR in the 18 patients survived and the 23 patients nonsurvived during the initial and final phase of sepsis. The black bar refers to the initial values, the dotted bar refers to the final values. * Significant *vs* survivors; † significant *vs* initial.

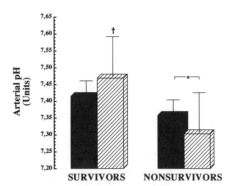

Figure 3. Mean arterial pH in the 18 patients survived and the 23 patients nonsurvived during the initial and final phase of sepsis. The black bar refers to the initial values, the dotted bar refers to the final values. * Significant *vs* survivors; † significant *vs* initial.

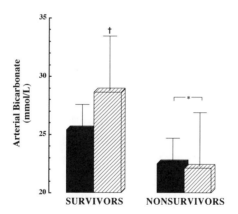

Figure 4. Mean arterial bicarbonate in the 18 patients survived and the 23 patients nonsurvived during the initial and final phase of sepsis. The black bar refers to the initial values, the dotted bars refer to the final values. * Significant *vs* survivors; † Significant *vs* initial.

For all the data collect in the survivors there was a significant linear relationship between oxygen delivery and oxygen consumption (r = 0.76, p < 0.001), while in the nonsurvivors the linear relationship had a significantly lower slope (r = 0.35, p < 0.01) (Fig. 5).

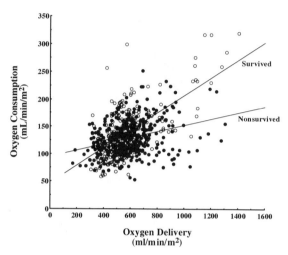

Figure 5. Relation between oxygen delivery and oxygen consumption for all the observations in the nonsurvivors (n = 433) and survivors (n = 261).

DISCUSSION

The first finding of our study is that survivors had either initially or in the final phase of sepsis a higher left ventricular stoke work index than nonsurvivors. Myocardial depression and dysfunction in sepsis is well established and is a generally accepted finding demonstrated by early [12] and recent works [13]. Besides, the role of myocardial dysfunction in sepsis has been considered above all in septic shock than in initial stage of sepsis. The importance of myocardial dysfunction to mortality in sepsis is still controversial. Some investigators have observed no differences in indices of cardiac performance between survivors and non survivors [13]. Several studies have reported depressed myocardial performance in nonsurvivors compared with survivors. Artucio and coworkers [4], by using noninvasive method (systolic time intervals and preejection period/left ventricular ejection time ratio) to assess left ventricular function during early phase of sepsis, noted that patients who died had significantly greater ventricular dysfunction than patients who survived (75% *vs* 35%). Ognibene and coworkers [14] in a study that examined the effect of a volume challenge in patients with and without sepsis, the observed increase in left ventricular stroke work index was smaller in the septic group, although the pulmonary artery wedge pressure was similar in both group at the end of the fluid challenge. In our group of patients, we observed that nonsurvivors had left ventricular stroke work index either initially or in the final phase of their illness significantly lower than survivors, despite no significant difference in cardiac index. This parameter has some limitations in evaluation of myocardial contractlity, as a volume measurement of preload should be used instead of a pressure measurement (wedge pressure). Therefore, the differences in left ventricular stroke work index between survivors and non survivors may be due to differences in ventricular contractility but could be also due to differences in ventricular compliance. Even though with these limitations, our data are in agreement with Artucio's data [4], who used a non invasive method to assess left ventricular performance, which bears a strong correlation with the internal indices of ventricular function as well as with the ejection fraction as determined by contrast venticulography.

The second finding is that nonsurvivors had lower systemic vascular resistance either initially or in the final phase, and that only survivors had an evolution toward normal at the end of sepsis. In the survivors this probably means a tendency toward the normalization of the peripheral vascular abnormalities and suggests that the patients are clinically improving. These results are in agreement with those reported by previous studies [14, 16]. These Authors documented that the derangement in peripheral vascular resistance was the major determinant of mortality, since peripheral vascular resistance was lower in nonsurvivors as compared to survivors, without difference in cardiac index in both groups. This suggests that either abnormalities of regional or organ blood flow, or alteration in vascular control, are more likely causes of inadequate tissue utilization of oxygen than could be an inadequate cardiac index.

The third finding is the time evolution of acid base status (pH, hydrogenions concentration, and bicarbonate) in these patients. We did not measure blood lactate levels that recently has been considered superior to hemodynamic variables in predicting outcome in human septic shock [17]. But, these Authors reported a significant correlation between bicarbonate and blood lactate levels [17]. On this basis, it could be supposed that in both nonsurvivors and survivors bicarbonate levels were an indirect expression of blood lactate levels. In contrast to cardiac index and oxygen delivery, initial pH and bicarbonate clearly separated the survivors from the nonsurvivors. The nonsurvivors had significantly lower arterial pH, and bicarbonate than the survivors both in the initial and in the final phase of sepsis. Only the survivors had a significant increase in pH and in bicarbonate during sepsis. This suggests that the extent of organ and tissue ischemia producing anaerobic metabolism is greater at the onset of sepsis in non survivors, in whom the hemodynamic abnormalities (low oxygen consumption, low systemic vascular resistance, and low left ventricular stroke work index) persist until the patients died.

The fourth finding is the relationship observed for all the data collect in the 41 patients, between oxygen consumption and oxygen delivery. Some explanation for this relationship could result from the manner by which oxygen consumption was obtained (*i.e.*, calculated by Fick method than measured by indirect calorimetry) [10, 11]. First, by using the Fick method, random errors in values for shared measurements may cause an apparently dependent relationship between oxygen delivery and oxygen consumption in a static situation [10,11]. Second, misinterpretation of the data may result from a failure to consider the effect of treatments on oxygen consumption (e.i., sedation, vasoactive drugs), and to control for the effect of between-subject variability in metabolic rate [18]. Third, pooling of data collected in different period, can lead to a false relationship between oxygen delivery and oxygen consumption [18]. While previous study [16,17] have found no significant differences in cardiac index, oxygen delivery, and in oxygen consumption between survivors and non survivors during septic shock, a recent study [19] have shown that elevation of cardiac output and oxygen delivery improves outcome in septic shock. Our data do not match with these results, as we observed in nonsurvivors a lower oxygen consumption, despite similar values in cardiac index and oxygen delivery both in the initial and in the final phase. This finding means that the capability to increase oxygen extraction is great different between nonsurvivors and survivors both initially and in the final phase of sepsis.

In summary, this study shows that patients with severe sepsis had a significant hyperdynamic cardiovascular state togheter with a myocardial dysfunction that is more pronounced in non survivors. Outcome is principally related to the time course of pH and bicarbonate levels, rather than to the traditional oxygen transport variables.

REFERENCES

1. J.E. Parrillo, Septic shock in humans: Clinical evaluation, pathophysiology, and therapeutic approach, *in*:: "Textbook of critical care", *ed*. W.C.Shomaker, W.L. Thompson, P.R. Holbrook, Saunders, Philadelphia, pp 1006 (1989).

2. R.D. Weisel, L. Vito, R.C. Dennis, C.R. Valeri, H.B. Hechtman, Myocardial depression during sepsis, Arch Surg. 133:512 (1977).

3. C. Natason, M.P. Fink, H.K. Ballantine, T.J. MacVittie, J.J. Conklin, J.E. Parrillo, Gram negative bacteriemia produces both severe systolic and diastolic cardiac dysfunction in a canine model that simulates human septic shock, J Clin Invest. 78:259 (1986).

4. H. Artucio, A. Digenio, M; Pereira, Left ventricular function during sepsis, Crit Care Med. 17:323 (1989).

5. D.P. Nelson, C. Beyer, R.W. Samsel, L.D.H. Wood, P.T. Shumaker, Pathologic supply dependence of O2 uptake during bacteriemia in dogs, J Appl Physiol. 63:1487 (1988).

6. Y.G. Wolf, S. Cotev, A. Perel, J. Manny, Dependence of oxygen consumption on cardiac output in sepsis, Crit Care Med. 15:198 (1987).

7. D.J. Bihari, M. Smithies, A. Gimson, J. Tinker, The effect of vasodialtation with prostacyclin on oxygen delivery and uptake in critically ill patients, New Engl Med. 317:397 (1987).

8. M.T. Haupt, E.M. Gilbert, R.W. Carlson, Fluid loading increases oxygen consumption in septic shock with lactate acidosis, Am Rev Resp Dis. 131:912 (1985).

9. B.S. Kaufman, R.C. Rackow, J.L. Falk, The relationship between oxygen delivery and consumption during fluid resuscitation of hypovolemic and septic shock, Chest. 85:336 (1984).

10. C.G. Vermeij, Feenestra BWA, H.A. Bruinung, Oxygen delivery and oxygen uptake in postoperative and septic patients, Chest. 98:415 (1990).

11. M. Wysocki, M. Besbes, E. Roupie, C. Brun-Buisson, Modification of oxygen extraction ratio by change in oxygen transport in septic shock, Chest. 102:221 (1992).

12. JH Siegel, M. Greenspan, L.R.M. Del Guercio, Abnormal vascular tone, defective oxygen transport and myocardial failure in human septic shock, Ann Surg. 165:504 (1967).

13. M.M. Parker, J.H. Shelhamer, S.L. Bacharach, Profound but reversible myocardial depression in patients with septic shock, Ann Int Med. 100:483 (1984).

14. F.P. Ognibene, M.M. ParkerC. Natason, Depressed left ventricular performance response to volume infusion in patients with sepsis and septic shock, Chest. 93:903 (1988).

15. A.B.J. Groenelved, W. Bronsveld, L.G. Thiijs, Hemodynamic determinants of mortality in human septic shock. , Surgery. 99:140 (1986).

16. M.M. Parker, J.M. Shelhamer, C. Natanson, D.W. Alling, J.E. Parrillo, Serial cardiovascular variables in survivors and nonsurvivors of human septic shock: heart rate as an early predictor of prognosis, Crit Care Med. 15:923 (1987).

17. J. Bakker, M. Coffernils, M. Leon, P. Gris, J.L. Vincent, Blood lactate levels are superior to oxygen-derived variables in predicting outcome in human septic shock, Chest. 99:956 (1991).

18. O. Boyd, E.B. Bennett, Is oxygen consumption an important clinical target ? in, "Year book of intensive care and emergency medicine" ed, J.L. Vincent, Springer-Verlag, Berlin, pp 310 (1992).

19. J. Tuchschmidt, J. Fried, M. Astiz, E. Rackow, Elevation of cardiac output and oxygen delivery improves outcome in septic shock, Chest. 102:216 (1992).

EFFECTS OF HIGH ARTERIAL OXYGEN TENSION ON CORONARY BLOOD FLOW REGULATION AND MYOCARDIAL OXYGEN DELIVERY

Brian A. Cason[1], Helen J. Gordon[2], Carla B. Shnier[1],
Anne F. Horton[1], Reed P. Hickey[1], Robert F. Hickey[1]

[1]University of California, San Francisco, CA 94143 at the
Veterans Affairs Medical Center, San Francisco, CA 94121 and
[2]Veterans Affairs Medical Centers of Palo Alto, CA 94305

INTRODUCTION

The effects of high oxygen tension, or hyperoxia, on the control of myocardial blood flow are both complex and controversial. Substantial evidence suggests that high arterial oxygen tension has a direct vasoconstrictor effect (Baron et al., 1990; Bourdeau-Martini et al., 1974; Ishikawa et al., 1984; Lammerant et al., 1969; Sobol et al., 1962), similar to the vasoconstrictor effects oxgyen demonstrates in other tissues (Daugherty et al., 1967; Duling and Pittman, 1975; Sullivan and Johnson, 1981). It is often difficult, however, to distinguish direct vasoconstrictor effects from other, indirect effects of oxygen which also cause coronary vasoconstriction. For example, increasing arterial oxygen tension causes multiple direct and reflex hemodynamic effects, including reduced heart rate Ganz et al., 1972; Kenmure et al., 1971; Whalen et al., 1965) and decreased ventricular wall tension (Ishikawa et al., 1984; Ishikawa et al., 1982), both of which may reduce myocardial oxygen demand and which may therefore lead to coronary vasoconstriction by metabolic regulation mechanism. Additionally, higher oxygen tension is generally associated with higher oxygen content, so it might expected that when arterial oxygen tension is raised beyond the normal range (raising oxygen content slightly), that the metabolic regulation mechanisms of the heart would induce vasoconstriction, reducing blood flow slightly, but maintaining constant oxygen delivery.

Although the role of arterial oxygen tension in control of regional myocardial blood flow remains controversial, no studies to date have determined the effect of high arterial PO_2 on the normal coronary pressure-flow relationship. Coronary autoregulation normally adjusts vascular tone to keep myocardial blood flow relatively constant over a wide range of perfusion pressures. We hypothesized that if the direct vasoconstrictor effects of oxygen predominate, then coronary arterial hyperoxia should reduce regional myocardial blood flow at all levels of coronary pressure. As an alternative to this hypothesis, arterial hyperoxia may exert its effects indirectly: increasing oxygen content of blood may allow O_2 needs to be met with less blood flow, inducing a metabolically-mediated vasoconstriction. If so, then the effects of hyperoxia on coronary blood flow should be accounted for by the changes in delivered oxygen, and myocardial oxygen delivery should remain constant. In order to further clarify the direct vasoconstrictor effects versus the metabolically-mediated vasoconstrictor effects of arterial oxygen on coronary blood flow, we used a swine model of isolated coronary perfusion in which regional coronary arterial PO_2 could be independently controlled. In 15 swine, we measured the effects coronary hyperoxia on the regional myocardial blood flow–coronary pressure relationships and on regional myocardial oxygen delivery.

METHODS

General Methods

Anesthesia. This experimental protocol was approved by our Animal Welfare Committee, and follows the guidelines for animal use provided by the American Physiological Society. Studies were performed under general anesthesia, in 15 open-chest domestic swine weighing 40–50 kg. Swine were premedicated with ketamine (10 mg/kg s.c.), then anesthesia was induced by mask using oxygen and isoflurane (1–4%). A tracheostomy was performed under deep general anesthesia, ventilation was controlled, and anesthesia was maintained with isoflurane 0.8–1.5%. Ventilation was controlled to keep P_aCO_2 at 35–40 mmHg. After completion of the surgical preparation, isoflurane was discontinued and anesthesia was converted to a high-dose narcotic technique to avoid the potentially confounding coronary vasodilator effects of isoflurane anesthesia (Cason et al., 1987). Each animal received 25 mg/kg pentobarbital over a 30-minute period, and a loading dose of fentanyl (50 mg·kg^{-1}) followed by a continuous fentanyl infusion (0.5 mg·kg^{-1}·min^{-1}). Temperature was maintained at 36.5–37°C by use of a heating blanket and by warming humidified inhaled gases. Inspired gas concentration was measured by mass spectrometry. Arterial blood gases were measured using a Radiometer ABL-II blood gas laboratory. Hemoglobin and oxyhemoglobin saturation are measured using a Radiometer OSM-2 hemoximeter with electronic correction made for swine hemoglobin absorption characteristics..

Surgery and Hemodynamic Instrumentation. Through a neck dissection, 16-gauge catheters were inserted into the internal jugular vein and carotid artery. A median sternotomy was performed and a pressure transducer-tip (Millar) catheter was inserted through the left atrium into the left ventricle for measurement of left ventricular pressure and its first derivative with respect to time (dP/dt).

Epicardial pacing electrodes were attached to the right atrium, and pacing was instituted at a rate 20% higher than the intrinsic heart rate in order to maintain constant heart rate throughout the experiment.

After all surgery and instrumentation was completed, the animal was heparinized systemically (10,000 u heparin i.v. bolus, and 5,000 u/hour continuous infusion).

Sonomicrometry. In all experiments, myocardial contractile function was quantified by using subendocardial segment shortening measurements. A small epicardial incision was made and (2 mm) lensed piezoelectric crystals were inserted, using a Teflon guide tube, to a position within 3 mm of the subendocardium. These crystals were inserted 10–15 mm apart, facing each other, and oriented parallel to the minor axis of the heart. Crystal position was confirmed by direct inspection at dissection of the heart, and function data was used only if crystals are confirmed to be within 3 mm of the endocardium, and properly oriented facing each other.

Systolic segment shortening was calculated as segment shortening during systole, averaged over at least 5 heartbeats:

$$\text{Systolic Shortening (\%)} = \frac{(\text{end-diastolic length} - \text{end-systolic length})}{\text{end-diastolic length}} \times 100$$

End-diastole was defined as the onset of positive left ventricular dP/dt; end-systole was defined as the time of peak negative dP/dt (Abel, 1981).

LAD coronary cannulation and perfusion. Initial measurements of segmental function and coronary pressure were made, then the LAD coronary artery was cannulated proximally using a plastic cannula manufactured in our laboratory (3mm o.d.). Coronary pressure was measured just distal to the tip of this cannula by a 25-gauge catheter which passed through the cannula. Oxygenated blood was withdrawn from a carotid artery and pumped through a membrane oxygenator (Sci-Med) into the LAD coronary artery, using a Masterflex digital roller pump (Cole-Parmer). Flow was measured both by an in-line ultrasonic flowmeter (Transonic). Coronary flow was initially set to provide a mean intracoronary pressure equal to mean aortic pressure. Adequacy of perfusion was assessed by the quick return of segmental function to pre-cannulation values. If function did not return to pre-cannulation levels within 3 minutes the animal was excluded from study.

Determination of normal or "control" coronary flow. After return of segmental function to pre-cannulation values and a 20-minute stabilization period, "control flow" was defined as that coronary flow at which mean coronary pressure equals mean aortic pressure.

Cardiac dissection. At the end of each experiment, the area of myocardium perfused by the cannulated LAD artery was defined by a dye infusion technique: blood stained with Evans blue dye is infused into the root of the aorta at normal aortic pressures, while the LAD artery is perfused at the same pressure with undyed blood from a reservoir. The unstained myocardial area is sharply demarcated in swine, and represents the area of LAD perfusion.

Coronary pressure-flow plots and autoregulation measurements. To determine the baseline coronary pressure-flow relationship, 4–6 paired values of CBF and pressure were obtained over the pressure range of 90–120 mm Hg. To determine each point, CBF was altered slightly (2–4 ml/min), then held constant until coronary pressure stabilized and remained stable for 45 seconds. The average time required to obtain each pressure-flow point was approximately 2 minutes. Then, coronary flow was altered again, and a new pressure-flow point was obtained. After all the initial paired values of coronary pressure and flow were obtained at one level of arterial oxygen tension, the coronary arterial oxygen tension was changed by manipulating the oxygenator gas flows. Coronary flow was servo-controlled to keep coronary pressure equal to MAP. After several minutes of coronary pressure-flow stability at the new level of oxygen tension, a new set of paired measurements of coronary pressure and flow was obtained.

Regional myocardial oxygen consumption. MVO_2 was calculated for the LAD-perfused zone, using the Fick Principle, as the product of LAD blood flow and the (coronary arterial–coronary venous) oxygen content difference.

Protocols

The LAD coronary artery was initially perfused, via the membrane oxygenator, with arterial blood having normal $PaCO_2$ and PaO_2. Coronary pressure-flow relationships were measured during two randomized experimental periods: a) coronary normoxia (paO_2 = 90–100), and b) coronary hyperoxia (paO_2 >400 mmHg). At each level of oxygen tension, we measured hemodynamic indices of myocardial oxygen demand (arterial pressure, heart rate, filling pressures), regional myocardial function (sonomicrometry), regional coronary pressure–flow plots, and regional MVO_2.

Data Analysis

Data are expressed as mean ± standard deviation. Comparisons were made between normoxia and hyperoxia measurement periods, where appropriate, using paired t-tests.

In each experiment, and under each experimental condition, plots of the measured values of coronary pressure and flow were constructed over the pressure range of 90–120 mm Hg and the best-fit relationship between pressure and flow was determined by least-squares linear regression. To obtain, for purposes of comparison, the flow and oxygen delivery values at 90, 100, 110 and 120 mm Hg, each pressure-flow regression equation was solved for the flow values at these pressures. Since each individual regression plot was very well described by a straight line (r^2>.95 in all cases), this method was considered appropriate.

The degree of coronary autoregulation was then quantitated by two methods. The slope of the pressure-flow relationship provided one measure of coronary autoregulation. A second measure of autoregulation was obtained by use of an autoregulation index (ARI) (Norris et al., 1979) which compares the measured change in coronary vascular conductance (delta F/delta P) to the ideal change in coronary vascular conductance which would be expected if autoregulation had been perfect and CBF had remained constant. Mathematically, the index is calculated as:

$$\text{Autoregulatory gain} = \left[\frac{F_i}{P_i} - \frac{F}{P}\right] \times \left[\frac{F_i}{P_i} - \frac{F_i}{P}\right]^{-1}$$

where F_i = CBF at starting pressure P_i, and F = CBF at a new steady-state reduced pressure, P. Autoregulatory gain was calculated for each autoregulation plot over the range of 80 to 120 mm Hg.

RESULTS

Hemodynamics: Heart rate was held constant by atrial pacing. Mean arterial pressure, left ventricular end-diastolic pressure (LVEDP), and left anterior descending zone systolic shortening were unaffected by regional hyperoxia.

Table 1. Hemodynamics and regional contractile function.

CONDITION:	NORMOXIA	HYPEROXIA
Heart Rate (beats/min)	119 ± 14.7	118 ± 13.2
Mean Arterial Pressure (mm Hg)	85.3 ± 15.5	82.8 ± 15.6
LAD Systolic Shortening (%)	22.7 ± 4.8	21.7 ± 4.9
LVEDP (mm Hg)	4.7 ± 2.3	5.0 ± 2.5

(No significant differences at the P<.05 level, by paired t-test.)

Coronary Pressure-flow Relationships and Oxygen Delivery: The effects of hyperoxia on the coronary pressure-flow relationship are described in **Table 2**, and are illustrated **Figure 1**.

Table 2. Effects of hyperoxia on coronary pressure-flow relationships and regional oxygen delivery.

	At Coronary Pressure:	90 mmHg	100 mmHg	110 mmHg	120 mmHg
Normoxia:	Coronary Blood Flow (ml/100g/min)	62.8 ± 27.5	65.8 ± 28.7	68.9 ± 29.8	71.9 ± 31.0
	Oxygen Delivery (ml /100g/m)	10.5 ± 2.3	11.0 ± 2.4	11.5 ± 2.5	12.0 ± 2.6
Hyperoxia:	Coronary Blood Flow (ml/100g/min)	56.0 ± 24.3*	58.9 ± 25.4*	61.7 ± 26.6*	64.6 ± 27.9*
	Oxygen Delivery (ml /100g/m)	9.3 ± 1.8*	9.8 ± 1.9*	10.3 ± 2.0*	10.7 ± 2.1*

(*=P<.05 vs. corresponding normal O_2 period, by paired t-test.)

High PaO2 decreased coronary flow (**Fig. 1**) and myocardial oxygen delivery (**Fig. 2**) at all levels of coronary pressure.

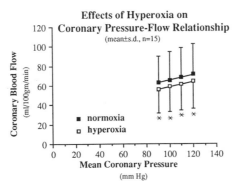

Figure 1. Regional hyperoxia decreased coronary blood flow across a wide range of coronary pressures, despite no change in systemic hemodynamics. (*=P<.05 vs. corresponding normal O2 period, by paired t-test).

Derived indices of coronary pressure-flow regulation: The slope of the coronary pressure-flow relationship, within the pressure range of 80-120 mm Hg, was not affected by regional coronary hyperoxia. In addition, the autoregulation index was unaffected by coronary hyperoxia. (**Table 3**)

Table 3. Indices of coronary autoregulation.

CONDITION:	NORMOXIA	HYPEROXIA
Coronary Pressure-Flow Slope (ml . min-1 . mm Hg -1)	.36 ± .143	.31 ± .128
Autoregulation Index	.488 ± .159	.472 ± .207

(No significant differences at the P<.05 level, by paired t-test.)

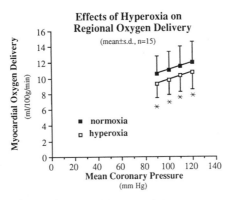

Figure 2. Regional coronary hyperoxia decreased myocardial oxytgen delivery across a wide range of pressures, despite no significant change in systemic hemodynamics. (*=P<.05 vs. corresponding normal O2 period, by paired t-test.)

Myocardial Oxygen Balance: Despite the fact that regional coronary hyperoxia increased coronary arterial oxygen content 9.7%, regional hyperoxia also increased the coronary A-V O_2 content difference, and decreased myocardial oxygen delivery. (**Table 4**) Regional coronary hyperoxia decreased oxygen delivery over a wide range of pressures (**Fig. 2**). Regional myocardial oxygen consumption, calculated by the Fick method, decreased 9.5% during regional coronary hyperoxia (**Table 4**), although there were no significant changes in systemic hemodynamics.

Table 4. Myocardial oxygen balance.

CONDITION:	NORMOXIA	HYPEROXIA
P_aO_2 (mm Hg)	88.3 ± 17.7	415.5 ± 59.8[*]
Content$_a$ O_2 (ml O_2/dl)	13.56 ± 0.81	14.88 ± 1.04[*]
$P_{cv}O_2$ (mm Hg)	30.7 ± 4.5	34.3 ± 4.5[*]
Content$_{cv}$ O_2 (ml O_2/dl)	3.79 ± 1.09	4.25 ± 1.07[*]
MVO_2 (ml O_2/100 gm/min)	7.35 ± 1.69	6.57 ± 1.48[*]
O_2 delivery (ml O_2/100 gm/min)	10.28 ± 2.57	9.20 ± 1.96[*]
A-V O_2 content (ml O_2/dl)	9.77 ± 1.27	10.62 ± 1.15[*]

([*]=P<.05 vs. corresponding normal O_2 period, by paired t-test.)

DISCUSSION

In this swine model, moderate regional hyperoxia (PaO_2 = 415.5 ± 59.8) decreased coronary flow over a wide range of coronary pressures, and in this respect acted as a coronary vasoconstrictor. In addition, coronary hyperoxia actually decreased myocardial oxygen delivery at all levels of coronary pressure. Although coronary hyperoxia decreased regional oxygen delivery, no detrimental effects on contractile function were observed. Interpretation of these results is complicated, however, with respect to the direct vs. indirect vasoconstrictor effects of hyperoxia. Because we found that regional coronary hyperoxia decreased regional myocardial oxygen consumption, (despite no evidence for diminished regional work), an indirect, metabolically-mediated vasoconstrictor effect of hyperoxia is not excluded by these experiments.

The observation that high oxygen tension can diminish myocardial MVO_2, in absence of significant changes in myocardial work, has been previously noted in experiments utilizing the isolated, blood perfused rabbit heart (Baron et al., 1990). Although we did not measure regional myocardial work in the current study, we controlled one major determinant of work (heart rate), and measured another (MAP), finding it to be constant. Our confirmation of the finding that hyperoxia decreases MVO_2 is somewhat surprising, in that myocardial MVO_2 is not generally considered to be determined by arterial tension except under conditions of oxygen deficiency. Several potential explanations for this finding exist, all of which require further investigation.

First, there is the possibility of altered substrate usage. Hyperoxia may induce a shift in the substrates used for myocardial metabolism. A shift from primary use of free fatty acids to use of more heavily oxidized substrate such as carbohydrates could theoretically yield a small increase in the efficiency of aerobic metabolism.

Alternatively, we speculate that coronary hyperoxia could change MVO_2 by its direct vasoconstrictor effects, causing shutdown of arteriolar blood supply to some contractile units which are not necessary for normal mechanical function but which would, in absence of hyperoxia, contribute to basal metabolic oxygen consumption. There is known to be some normal temporal heterogeneity of myocardial blood flow (Marcus et al., 1977), attributed to microvascular vasomotion, as it does in other tissues (Bertuglia et al., 1991; Sullivan and Johnson, 1981). This hypothesis is also suggested by whole-organ inert gas washout studies which show that hyperoxia increases myocardial blood flow heterogeneity (Wolpers et al., 1990).

Finally, it is possible that some aspect of the biochemical machinery of contraction is PO_2-dependent, so that hyperoxia increases the biochemical efficiency of contraction. We are unaware of any such PO_2-dependence of the described biochemistry of myocardial contraction, so this possibility remains speculative.

REFERENCES

Abel, F, 1981, Maximal negative dP/dt as an indicator of end of systole. *Am J Physiol* 240: H676-H679.

Baron, J. F., Vicaut, E., Hou, X. and M. Duvelleroy, 1990, Independent role of arterial O_2 tension in local control of coronary blood flow. *Am J Physiol* 258: H1388-H1394.

Bertuglia, S., Colantuoni, A., Coppini, G. and M. Intaglietta, 1991, Hypoxia- or hyperoxia-induced changes in arteriolar vasomotion in skeletal muscle microcirculation. *Am J Physiol* 260:H362-H372.

Bourdeau-Martini, J., Odoroff, C.L. and Honig, C.R., 1974, Dual effect of oxygen on magnitude and uniformity of coronary intercapillary distance. *Am J Physiol* 226: 800-810.

Cason, B. A., Verrier, E.D., London, M.J., Mangano, D.T. and Hickey, R.F, 1987, Effects of isoflurane and halothane on coronary vascular resistance and collateral myocardial blood flow: Their capacity to induce coronary steal. *Anesthesiology* 67(5): 665-675.

Daugherty, J., Scott, J.B., Dabney, J.M. and Haddy, F.J., 1967, Local effects of O_2 and CO_2 on limb, renal, and coronary vascular resistances. *Am J Physiol* 213: 1102-1110.

Duling, B. and Pittman, R., 1975, Oxygen tension: dependent or independent variable in local control of blood flow? *Fed Proc* 34: 2012-2019.

Ganz, W., Donoso, R., Marcus, H. and Swan, H.J.C, 1972, Coronary hemodynamics and myocardial oxygen metabolism during oxygen breathing in patients with and without coronary disease. *Circulation* 45: 763-768.

Ishikawa, K., Hayashi, T., Kohashi, Y., Otani, S., Kanamasa, K., Yamakado, T., Yashi, M., Osato, S. and Katori, R., 1984, Reduction of left ventricular size following oxygen inhalation in patients with coronary artery disease as measured by biplane coronary cineangiograms. *Jpn Circ J* 48: 225-232.

Ishikawa, K., Kanamasa, K., Yamakado, K. and Katori, R., 1982, Reduction of left ventricular epicardial segment length by 100% oxygen breathing in open-chest dogs. *Tohoku J Exp Med* 136: 313-318.

Kenmure, A. C. F., Beatson, J.M., Cameron, A.J.V. and Horton, P.W., 1971,Effects of oxygen on myocardial blood flow and metabolism. *Cardiovasc Res* 5: 483-489.

Lammerant, J., Schryver, C.D., Becsei, I., Camphyn, M, and Mertens-Strijthagen, J., 1969, Coronary circulation response to hyperoxia after vagotomy and combined alpha and beta adrenergic receptors blockade in the anesthetized intact dog. *Pflugers Arch* 308: 185-186.

Marcus, M. L., Kerber, R.E., Erhardt, J.C., Falsetti, H.L., Davis, D.E. and Abbound, F.M., 1977, Spatial and temporal heterogeneity of left ventricular perfusion in awake dogs. *Am Heart J* 94(6): 748-754.

Norris, C. P., Barnes, G.E., Smith, E.E. and Granger, H.J., 1979, Autoregulation of superior mesenteric flow fasted and fed dogs. Am J Physiol 237: H174-H177.

Sobol, B. J., Wanlass, S.A., Joseph, E.B. and Azarshahy, I., 1962, Alteration of coronary blood flow in the dog by inhalation of 100 percent oxygen. *Circ Res* 11: 797-802.

Sullivan, S. M. and Johnson, P.C., 1981, Effect of oxygen on blood flow autoregulation in cat sartorius muscle. *Am J Physiol* 241: H807-H815.

Whalen, R. E., Saltzman, H.A., Holloway, D.H. Jr., McIntosh, H.D., Sieker, H.O. and Brown, I.W., Jr., 1965, Cardiovascular and blood gas responses to hyperbaric oxygenation. *Am J Cardiol* 15: 638-646.

Wolpers, H. G., Hoeft, A., Korb, H., Lichtlen, P.R. and Hellige, G., 1990, Heterogeneity of myocardial blood flow under normal conditions and its dependence on arterial PO2. *Am J Physiol* 258: H549-H555.

OXYGEN SUPPLY TO TUMORS

GLUCOSE-, ENERGY-METABOLISM AND CELL PROLIFERATION IN TUMORS

Christian Streffer

Institut für Med. Strahlenbiologie
Universitätsklinikum Essen
Hufelandstr. 55
D-4300 Essen 1, Germany

INTRODUCTION

The malignancy of a tumor is determined by its unlimited invasive growth and metasizing potential through cell proliferation. Therefore the main goals of metabolism in tumors are the production of energy and of precursors for the synthesis of macromolecules which are needed for cell proliferation. Since the studies of Warburg (1925) it has often been stated that glycolysis with the production of lactate is most important for energy production in tumors and it has been neglected that oxidative metabolism can take place in tumors to an appreciable extent. Although it has been found in most tumors that the glycolytic rates are high, it also has been demonstrated that the enzymes of the citrate cycle are present in tumor cells and oxygen supply regulates the number of proliferating cells and therefore oxidative metabolism is apparently necessary for cell proliferation in tumors (Newsholme and Board 1991; Monschke et al. 1991; Tannock et al. 1968). The regulation of metabolic fluxes is essential in this connection. It is the aim of this paper to discuss these phenomena in more details.

FLUX-REGULATING REACTIONS

Several possibilities for flux-regulations exist in metabolic pathways, between them are non-equilibrium reactions and branched pathways (Newsholme and Board 1991). In the case of non-equilibrium reactions the activity of the enzyme that catalyzes the specific reaction is low in comparison to the other enzyme activities of that metabolic pathway in direction of the end product P (cf E_2 in Fig. 1). On the other hand the forward reaction (v_f) is much faster than the reverse reaction (v_r) (Fig. 1) and this leads consequently to a drive of the overall reaction towards the product P but to a smaller concentration of the product B than that of the substrate A. In the case of glycolysis in tumors the glucose uptake measured as the uptake of 2-deoxyglucose (2-DG) is much faster than in other tissues cf. brain (Table 1), phosphorylation of glucose to glucose-6-phosphate (again as

$$E_1 \qquad E_2\ (v_f) \qquad E_3\ E_4\ E_5$$
$$S \longrightarrow A \underset{(v_r)}{\overset{}{\rightleftharpoons}} B \longrightarrow \longrightarrow \longrightarrow P$$

Non-equilibr.: 1) E_1 (v), $> E_2$ (v), $< E_3$ (v), E_4 (v), E_5 (v)

2) $v_f > v_r$

3) $[A] > [B]$

Figure 1.   Principles of Non-equilibrium Reaction

Table 1. Uptake of Tritiated Deoxyglucose (^{3}H-DG) after Intraperitoneal Injection of ^{3}H-DG into Mouse Brain and Adenocarcinoma: Total Radioactivity (dpm g^{-1} Tissue) and Unphosphorylated ^{3}H-DG in these Tissues (Percent). Control: Uptake in Untreated Animals; Sensitizer: Uptake 2 Hours after Intraperitoneal Injection of MISO (1 g kg^{-1} Body Weight)

	Control	Sensitizer
Tumor		
Total Activ. (dpm x g^{-1})	88×10^3	34×10^3
Unphosphor. DG (percent)	10	38
Brain		
Total Activ. (dpm x g^{-1})	49×10^3	27×10^3
Unphosphor. DG (percent)	9	26

2-DG) occurs faster than dephosphorylation. Therefore the 2-DG which has been taken up into the tumor cell has been driven very quickly to phosphorylated 2-DG; the flux is very fast in the direction of glucose phosphorylation on the other hand the concentration of glucose is higher than that of glucose-6-phosphate (Table 2) as further glucose is taken up very fast from the high glucose levels in blood (Streffer and Tamulevicius 1991). The enzymatic measurements have shown that the hexokinase/glucokinase activity is much higher than the activity of glucose-6-phosphatase in tumors. These studies were performed with human tumors which grew as xenografts on nude mice (Table 3). In

Table 2. Metabolites in Xenograft of Human Tumors on Nude Mice and in Mouse Liver(μMoles/g μMoles/g Tissue)

	Gluc.	G-6-P	Lact.	Pyr.	L/P
MeWo	1.20	0.19	6.4	0.23	28
Adeno	1.60	0.55	4.0	0.14	28
Mo	0.80	0.18	3.2	0.10	32
4197	0.76	-	5.9	-	-
Liver	10.9	0.38	2.2	0.16	13.7

Table 3. Maximal Enzyme Activities in Human Tumor Xenografts and Normal Tissues of Mice (μMoles/min/g Tissue)

Tumor/Tissue	Hexokin.	Glucokin.	G-6-Pase
Adeno	1.06	1.92	0.24
Mo	0.38	0.58	0.04
SW-480	0.52	1.11	0.03
4197	0.26	0.38	0.15
Liver	0.72	0.80	1.22
Brain	0.31	0.58	0.03

contrast to the data in tumors the glucose-6-phosphatase activity is quite high in liver. This enzyme is needed for hepatic gluconegenesis.

Besides non-equilibrium reactions branched pathways are a further possibility for metabolic flux-regulation. Glucose-6-phosphate (G-6-P) can be used for the further glycolytic pathway. Besides energy production through glycolysis and further degradation through the citrate cycle triosephosphates are needed for biosynthesis of phospholipids for membrane formation necessary for cell proliferation, these metabolites are formed in the pathway of the G-6-P shunt. Furthermore G-6-P can be metabolized to ribose-phosphate and deoxyribose-phosphate which are needed for the biosynthesis of nucleic acids. These data show that G-6-P plays a key role for energy metabolism as well as for the provision of precursors for the synthesis of macromolecules and this is widely used in tumors.

Under these circumstances G-6-P and the hexokinase/glucokinase reaction are very important regulatory steps for metabolic fluxes in proliferating tumor cells. Enzymatic studies in some tumorigenic and non-tumorigenic cell lines show that hexokinase is in the same range in the cell lines, however phosphofructokinase and lactate dehydrogenase activities (two further enzymes of anaerobic glycolysis) tend to be higher in tumorous than in normal cells (Table 4).

Studies of glycolytic metabolites in human xenografts on nude mice show that the glucose level is about 3 to 10 times higher than the G-6-P level in tumors but in liver this factor is about 25 (Table 2). On the other hand the lactate levels as well as the

Table 4. Maximum Activities of Some Glycolytic Enzymes in Various Cell Lines Enzyme activities (nmol/min per mg of protein) (Newsholme and Board 1991)

Cells	Hexokinase	Phospho-fructokinase	Pyruvate-kinase	Lactate dehydrogenase	Citrate synthase	Isocitrate dehydro-genase
MRC5	11.0	44.9	547	221	86.4	43.2
ESH P6	20.0	6.71	28.4	416	39.7	1.6
2B1	14.7	10.9	314	1078	38.6	12.1
rcc-1	62.5	0.96	174	28.5	-	-
H.Ep.2+	12.8	42.6	1627	3775	179.0	24.3
ESH TR1.2*	11.5	21.6	899	2590	71.2	8.2
rcc-1t*	84.7	40.4	1280	7978	74.1	50.5

lactate/pyruvate ratios are higher in all xenografts of human tumors than in the murine liver tissue. This finding is apparently caused by hypoxic regions in the tumors which will be discussed later. Such a situation is apparently not due to a metabolic condition which is characteristic for tumor cells, as it has not been found in melanoma cells in vitro. Under these conditions the lactate/pyruvate ratio is about the same as it has been observed in liver tissue (Tables 2 and 5). Preliminary studies with biopsies from human brain tumors have resulted in very similar values for the levels of glucose, G-6-P and lactate as they have been found in the human tumor xenografts (unpublished data).

Table 5. Lactate and Pyruvate Levels in Human Melanoma Cells (MeWo) in vitro and their Xenografts on Nude Mice after Hyperthermia

	MeWo Cells in vitro μmoles/10^9 cells		MeWo-Tumor μmoles/g tissue	
	Control	1 h after 44^0 C, 1 h	Control	2 h after 43^0 C, 1 h
Lactate	19.5	12.5	6.6	7.8
Pyruvate	1.6	1.8	0.25	0.20
Lact./Pyr.	12.1	6.9	26.4	39.0

It has been observed that all enzymes of the citrate cycle and oxidative energy production are present in tumor cells (Board et al. 1990) (Table 4). These enzyme activities are not lower in tumor cells than in normal cells. These data clearly demonstrate that tumor cells possess all the necessary enzymatic machinery in order to perform oxidative energy metabolism.

GLUCOSE METABOLISM AND BLOOD FLOW

Although all enzymatic activities are present for oxidative energy metabolism in tumor cells the question arises to which extent does such a metabolism occur in tumors in situ. A necessary presupposition for this metabolism is the presence of oxygen. Therefore blood supply and oxygen transport are most important. Recent studies have demonstrated that tumor tissues differ considerably from normal tissues with respect to vascularization. While normal tissues have a very regular distribution and architecture of blood vessels. This is quite different in tumors where vascularization is very irregular with a heterogeneous distribution of blood vessels (Konerding et al. 1989 and 1989b). Studies by means of corrosion cast techniques and electron microscopy showed in xenotransplants from human melanomas and sarcomas that the vascular system lacks a vascular hierarchy with respect to vessel distribution and development. Structurally complete arteries or veins cannot be seen. Frequently different cell types and even tumor cells are part of the vessel walls. Endothelial cells vary very much with respect to their structure and have immature cell contacts. The distribution of vessels is very irregular and leads to regions with a very low density or absence of blood vessels. The heterogeneity is seen within the same tumor (intraindivual) and between tumors (interindividual). Investigations on the density of blood vessels have demonstrated that such heterogeneities are also observed in human breast cancers (Monschke et al. 1991). It has been shown that the blood vessels in tumors can be more vulnerable to exogenous factors, cf. heat, than vessels in normal tissues (Vaupel and Kallinowski 1987).

Such phenomena also influence glucose metabolism. If lactate levels are measured in MeWo cells after a heat treatment in vitro, a decrease of the lactate level and especially of the lactate/pyruvate ratio is observed. This can be explained by an increased metabolic turnover during the heat treatment. However, the opposite occurs if xenografts of the same human melanoma cells are heated on nude mice (Table 5). Under these conditions a considerable increase of the lactate/pyruvate ratio is observed. The effect is apparently due to an increased heat-induced hypoxia in the tumor tissue which may be due to a reduced blood flow in the xenograft and/or to an increased oxygen consumption after the heat treatment. However this is not a general phenomenon. A treatment of xenografts even from the same tumor entity (melanomas) can lead to very different reactions. This interindividual heterogeneity has also therapeutic consequences. The comparison of two human melanoma xenografts shows a doubling of the lactate level and of the lactate/pyruvate ratio in one xenograft, while these effects are much smaller in the second tumor. In this connection it is interesting that the radiosensitizing effect of heat is much higher in the first tumor than in the second tumor (Table 6). The increased

Table 6. Metabolites (μmoles/g tissue) and Cell Survival in Xenografts of Melanoma after Hyperthermia (Ht) at 43°C for 1 hour.

	Bo		MeWo	
	Contr.	Ht	Contr.	Ht
Glucose	1.8	1.1	1.9	1.9
Lactate	5.8	12.1	6.6	7.8
Pyruvate	0.19	0,17	0.25	0.20
Lact./Pyruvate	30.5	71.2	26.4	39.0
Cell Survival after 4 Gy X-Rays	0.32	0.005	0.21	0.009
TER	3.16		2.27	

lactate/pyruvate ratio is a good indicator for the heat-induced hypoxia in the tumor, as a consequence the pH decreases and these changes of the micromilieu increase heat sensitivity which has a great significance for tumor regression after therapeutic treatments.

These metabolic effects can be further enhanced by a combined treatment of heat plus hypoxic cell sensitizers. Under these conditions the glucose level is also increased in the tumor, as total metabolism is disturbed under these conditions. A reduced blood flow leads to an increased lactate/pyruvate-ratio but apparently also the glycolytic rate is reduced by inhibition of glucose phosphorsylation through the sensitizer (Table 1) which causes the higher glucose level. Further studies have shown that such a treatment enhances the damaging effect on tumors. Cytogenetic damage and tumor regression increased (George et al. 1989). A tremendous extent of necrosis was observed in the tumors after such treatments. Cell proliferation studies showed a formation of cells with an doubled DNA content which did not go into mitosis but started again DNA synthesis and underwent mitosis after a second cell cycle. After these processes apparently expression of cytogenetic damage and necrosis occurred (George et al. 1989). Some of these cells arrested in S-phase which contributed to cell killing. These studies were performed after incorporation of 5'-bromodeoxyuridin (BUdR) into the DNA and labelling of these cells with an antibody against BUdR which is labelled with a fluorescent dye. In the same cells the DNA is stained with a second fluorescent dye. Thus it is possible to determine by flow cytometry not only the distribution of the cells in the various cell cycle phases but also the number of DNA synthesizing cells (Wilson et al. 1988).

CELL PROLIFERATION AND METABOLISM

The above described data show that cell proliferation is closely connected to energy metabolism. With a decreasing pH, which is frequently observed in tumors and which can be provoked by increased glucose metabolism or reduced oxygen supply, energy metabolism is reduced and cell proliferation goes down. Under these conditions DNA synthesis is stopped even in those cells which are in S-phase. These quiescent S-phase cells can start proliferation again when the pH returns to normal values.

In human xenografts on nude mice it was oberved that the volume doubling time of the tumor was dependent on the oxygen concentration, the glucose concentration and the number of S-phase cells (Table 7). Such a correlation was not only found in transplantable xenografts but also in human primary breast carcinomas. In biopsies from such tumors a clear correlation existed between the proportion of proliferating cells and

Table 7. Volume doubling time (VDT, days), number of S-phase cells (%), partial oxygen pressure (mm Hg) and glucose levels (μmoles/g tissue) in two tumor xenografts on nude mice.

	VDT	S-phase	pO_2	Gluc.
Morz.	2.1	10	6.8	0.27
Adeno Ca	1.1	37	11.0	1.55

the vascular density. No proliferating cells were found in distances larger than 130 µm from a blood vessel. Similar correlations have been observed in human rectum and ovary cancers. Thus a close correlation apparently exists between cell proliferation and blood flow as well as oxygen supply. This means oxidative metabolism is necessary for tumor growth.

CONCLUSIONS

1) In tumor cells and tumors in situ high glycolytic rates are possible. However high inter- as well as intraindividual heterogeneities exist.
2) Hexokinase activity and glucose-6-phosphate are regulating factors in these processes.
3) Tumors have the whole enzymatic machinery for the citrate cycle and oxidative energy production. Therefore these processes are used in tumors for energy production.
4) The flux in these metabolic pathways is coupled to blood flow and oxygen supply.
5) Blood supply is essential for cell proliferation and tumor growth.
6) In hypoxic regions and conditions the lactate formation and level is increased. The lactate/pyruvate-ratio is a good indicator for this situation.
7) These metabolic conditions alter the micromilieu of tumors and have a strong impact on tumor therapy.
8) First studies with primary human tumors in brain, breast, ovary and rectum confirm the data with human tumor xenografts and cells in vitro.

REFERENCES

Board, M., Humm, S., and Newsholme, E.A., 1990, Maximum activities of key enzymes of glycolysis, glutaminolysis, pentose phosphate pathway and tricarboxylic acid pathway in normal neoplastic and suppressed cells, Biochem. J. 265: 503.

George, K.C., Streffer, C., and Pelzer, T., 1989, Combined effects of X-rays, Ro 03-8799, and hyperthermia on growth, necrosis, and cell proliferation in a mouse tumor, Int. J. Radiat. Oncol. Biol. Phys. 16: 1119.

Konerding, M.A., Steinberg, F., and Streffer, C., 1989, The vasculature of xenotransplanted human melanomas and sarcomas on nude mice. I. Vascular corrosion casting studies, Acta Anat. 136: 21.

Konerding, M.A., Steinberg, F., and Streffer, C., 1989, The vasculature of xenotransplanted human melanomas and sarcomas on nude mice. II. Scanning and transmission electron microscopic studies, Acta Anat. 136: 27.

Monschke, F., Müller, W.-U., Winkler, U., and Streffer, C., 1991, Cell proliferation and vascularization in human breast carcinomas, Int. J. Cancer 49: 812.

Newsholme, E.A., and Board, M., 1991, Application of metabolic-control logic to fuel utilization and its significance in tumor cells, Adv. Enzyme Reg. 31: 225.

Streffer, C., and Tamulevicius, P., 1990, Metabolic effects of hypoxic cell sensitizers, in: "Selective Activation of Drugs by Redox Processes", G.E. Adams, A. Breccia, E.M. Fielden, and P. Wardman, eds., Plenum Press, 159.

Tannock, J.F., 1968, The relation between cell proliferation and the vascular system in a transplanted mouse mammary tumour, Brit. J. Cancer 22: 258.

Vaupel, P., and Kallinowski, F., 1987, Physiological effects of hyperthermia, in: "Hyperthermia and the Therapy of Malignant Tumors", C. Streffer, ed., Springer-Verlag, Berlin, Heidelberg, New York, London, Paris, Tokyo, Vol. 104, pp. 71.

Warburg, O., Wind, F., and Negelein, E., 1926, Über den Stoffwechsel von Tumoren im Körper. Klin. Wochenschr. 5: 829.

Wilson, G.D., McNally, N.J., Dische, S., Saunders, M.I., Des Rochers, C., Lewis, A.A., and Bennett, M.H., 1988, Measurement of cell kinetics in human tumours in vivo using bromodeoxyuridine incorporation and flow cytometry. Br. J. Cancer 58: 423.

RATES OF OXYGEN CONSUMPTION FOR PROLIFERATING AND QUIESCENT CELLS ISOLATED FROM MULTICELLULAR TUMOR SPHEROIDS

James P. Freyer

Life Sciences Division
Los Alamos National Laboratory
Los Alamos, NM 87545

INTRODUCTION

Multicellular tumor spheroids have proven to be valuable models of the interactions between the extracellular microenvironment and the metabolism, proliferation and viability of tumor cells (1,2). Studies on a variety of cell systems have shown that the supply of oxygen and glucose is critical to the maintenance of cellular viability (2-5). The role of oxygen and other energy-related nutrients in the development of proliferation arrest is considerably less well established. While it is generally believed that hypoxia is related to cellular quiescence, there is evidence that proliferation arrest in spheroids occurs at relatively high oxygen concentrations (4,6,7). Recent work also indicates that restricted cellular energy metabolism is not the mechanism behind quiescence in spheroids, either at small diameters or during the saturation phase of growth (8,9).

Whatever the mechanism of growth arrest in spheroids, entry into a quiescent state correlates with alterations in many physiological and morphological parameters (2,6,10-12). The rates of both oxygen and glucose consumption decrease with increasing spheroid size (13-15) and upon reaching the plateau phase of the growth of monolayers (12,16). This reduction has been correlated with the development of quiescence and the committant decrease in mean cell volume. Although the induction of quiescence in spheroids is probably not causally related to limitations on energy metabolism, the concurrent reduction in nutrient consumption will have a large effect on the spheroid microenvironment. In addition, the cellular physiology and energy metabolism of quiescent cells must affect the kinetics of re-entry into the cell cycle once growth inhibiting signals have been interrupted.

Previous studies have only measured the mean rates of nutrient consumption for the total spheroid cell population. The uniform volume rate of consumption throughout the viable cell region (17,18) could indicate that all cells decrease their consumption uniformly with spheroid growth. However, we have shown a decrease in glucose consumption for inner versus outer region cells in spheroids (11). Recent morphometric work has demonstrated a reduction in the number of mitochondria per cell with increasing depth in the cell rim for EMT6/Ro spheroids, but a concurrent increase in the cell packing, resulting in a uniform rate of consumption per volume in the viable zone (19). The objective of this study was to directly measure the oxygen consumption rates of proliferating and quiescent cells isolated from different regions in spheroids of two different tumor cell types.

Oxygen Transport to Tissue XV, Edited by P. Vaupel
et al., Plenum Press, New York, 1994

METHODS

Cell and Spheroid Culture

EMT6/Ro mouse mammary carcinoma and 9L rat glioma cells and spheroids were cultured in α-MEM (Grand Island Biologicals) supplemented with 10% bovine calf serum (Hyclone Laboratories) and antibiotics (referred to hereafter as complete medium). Details of monolayer and spheroid culture have been provided previously (3,8,9). Spinner cultures were maintained such that the oxygen and glucose concentrations and the pH were within 5% of initial values (20.9% oxygen, 5.5 mM glucose, pH 7.4) throughout the culture period.

Spheroid Selective Dissociation

Selective dissociation of spheroids was carried out essentially as described previously (11). Briefly, 150 spheroids were exposed to 0.25% trypsin in HEPES-buffered balanced salt solution containing 25 mM EDTA at pH 7.4 and 37°. Dissociation was performed in a flow-through chamber in which cells separated from the spheroids were continuously removed from the chamber into tubes containing complete medium on ice. For both EMT6/Ro and 9L spheroids, careful control of the mixing speed and chamber temperature results in the dissociation of cells only from the exposed spheroid surface in a uniform manner (11). Four fractions of released cells were collected in 25-30 minutes with the time of collection controlled such that each fraction represented approximately 25% of the total spheroid cell population. The original location of each fraction in the viable rim was estimated by geometrical calculations considering the cell number in each fraction, the thickness of the viable cell rim, and the assumption of a uniform packing of cells throughout the cell rim (11). A fraction representing the entire spheroid cell population was created by combining equal amounts of each of the dissociated fractions.

Rates of Oxygen Consumption

The method for measuring oxygen consumption rates has been described in detail previously (13,14). Cell suspensions isolated from monolayers or spheroids were centrifuged and resuspended in complete medium at 4°. The oxygen tension in a sealed glass chamber containing 8 mls of air-equilibrated complete medium with no gas overlayer was monitored with a Clarke-type polarographic electrode (Yellow Springs Instruments) until a steady current ($\pm 0.5\%$ of the signal) was observed for 5-10 minutes. Then 2-3 x 10^6 cells in 200 μl of medium were injected into the chamber, and the rate of oxygen disappearance was continuously recorded with a strip chart for 10-15 minutes (final oxygen tension was 80-90% of saturation). The suspension was stirred throughout equilibration and measurement (200 rpm) and maintained at 37 $\pm$ 0.2°. Rates of oxygen consumption were determined from the slopes of linear equations best fit to 10 concentration values extracted from the chart recording ($r^2 > 0.97$ in all cases). These slopes were converted to rates of cellular consumption by consideration of the oxygen concentration in complete medium at 37° (0.16 mM) and the total number of cells in the chamber. The oxygen concentration of medium was determined in the same apparatus using the method of Robinson and Cooper (20). Total cell number in the chamber was determined from cell counts of a sample taken after completion of the measurement. There was no significant effect of the measurement on mean cell volume, growth fraction, or clonogenic efficiency.

Multiple cell samples obtained from the selective dissociation of spheroids were held at 4° until measurement; the total elapsed time between resuspending the samples and completing consumption rate measurements was <2 hours. A separate experiment with cells from exponential monolayer cultures of both cell lines demonstrated that the oxygen consumption rate was essentially constant (± 2-3%) for cells held for up to 2 hours at 4°. Maintaining cells in complete medium at 4° also had no significant effect on the mean cell volume, growth fraction or clonogenic efficiency.

Consumption rates of intact spheroids were determined similarly, except that the equilibrated chamber was unsealed for the addition of 50 spheroids and then resealed with no gas overlayer. This resulted in a 1-2 minute disruption in the temperature and electrode current, but linear oxygen disappearance rates were obtained and fit after this period.

Cell Counting and Volume

Cells were counted with an electronic particle counter (Coulter Electronics) equipped with a pulse height analyzer (3,13). All counts were based on a region selected from the particle volume distribution to exclude acellular debris. Mean volumes of cell populations were determined by analysis of distributions of >10,000 cells, as calibrated with polystyrene microspheres. Coefficients of variation within the cell volume distributions were 25-40%.

DNA Content and Growth Fraction

DNA contents of individual cells were measured by flow cytometric analysis of fixed and stained cells (6,14). DNA content histograms of >20,000 cells were analyzed to yield estimates of the percentages of cells in the G_1-, S- and G_2-phases of the cell cycle using commercial software (Multicycle). Growth fractions were estimated from ratios of the S-phase fraction in a given sample to the S-phase fraction of an exponentially-growing monolayer culture ($55 \pm 2.3\%$ and $43 \pm 3.6\%$ for EMT6/Ro and 9L cells, respectively).

Clonogenic Efficiency and Viability

Clonogenic efficiency was measured using a standard monolayer colony formation assay (6) employing 10 dishes per experimental measurement. The thickness of the viable cell rim in spheroids was determined by measurements on eosin and hematoxalin stained histological sections cut through the centers of 20-25 spheroids as described in detail elsewhere (6,14).

RESULTS

Spheroids were hand-selected for these experiments at a diameter of approximately 1200 µm. The mean sizes of the populations used for the three experiments were 1218 ± 32 and 1224 ± 54 µm for the EMT6/Ro and 9L spheroids, respectively. The spheroid diameter size distributions within an experiment had coefficients of variation <5%. EMT6/Ro and 9L spheroids contained $2.54 \pm 0.15 \times 10^5$ and $2.31 \pm 0.22 \times 10^5$ total cells per spheroid, respectively. Measurement of histological sections prepared on spheroids after oxygen consumption determination gave viable rims of 223 ± 13 and 182 ± 28 µm. The selective dissociations of cells from EMT6/Ro spheroids resulted in populations containing 24 ± 1.2, 23 ± 0.9, 27 ± 1.3 and 26 ± 1.8 percent of the total cell population (from the outer to inner fraction). The corresponding values for 9L spheroids were 21 ± 2.2, 24 ± 0.4, 24 ± 1.6 and 31 ± 1.4 percent. For EMT6/Ro spheroids, the distances from the spheroid surface for these cell fractions were 0-41, 42-88, 89-117 and 118-223 µm. For 9L spheroids, these values were 0-35, 36-75, 76-122 and 123-182 µm, respectively. Figure 1 illustrates the locations of the various fractions within a spheroid for each of the cell lines. Taking account of variations within and between experiments, these estimates are accurate to within 10 µm for each individual spheroid. Consumption rate measurements were also performed on monolayer cultures which were prepared at 2 (exponentially-growing) and 5 (plateau-phase) days after inoculating 1×10^5 cells into 100 mm culture dishes. Plateau-phase cultures were not replenished with medium prior to use.

The results of oxygen consumption measurements are shown in Tables 1 and 2, along with mean cell volumes, growth fractions and clonogenic efficiencies. For each of the cell lines, there were reductions in cell volume, growth fraction, clonogenic capacity, and rate of oxygen consumption per cell with increasing distance into the spheroid. Total spheroid cell populations had intermediate values of each of these parameters, whether measured on cells

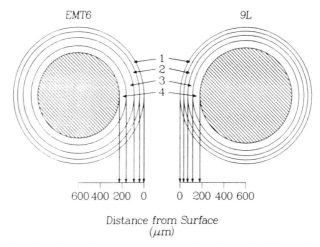

Figure 1. Illustration of locations of the cell fractions dissociated from EMT6/Ro (left) and 9L (right) spheroids 1200 μm in diameter. The shaded circle in each case represents the extent of the necrotic center.

obtained from recombination of cell fractions from different spheroid locations or by complete dissociation of a separate group of spheroids. There were no significant differences in the rates of oxygen consumption for the total spheroid cell populations measured on dissociated or intact spheroids. Monolayer cells also showed reductions in all of these parameters when comparing plateau-phase cells to exponentially-growing cultures.

Table 1. Cell volume, growth fraction and oxygen consumption of cells from EMT6/Ro spheroids and monolayers. Values are means ± standard deviations for 3-5 experiments.

Sample	Cell Volume (μm³)	Growth Fraction (percent)	Clonogenic Efficiency (percent)	Oxygen Consumption[1] (x 10^17 M/c-s)
Spheroids				
Fraction 1	1750 ± 63	87 ± 3.9	75 ± 3.4	6.78 ± 0.22
Fraction 2	1540 ± 55	53 ± 2.7	72 ± 4.5	4.47 ± 0.12
Fraction 3	1480 ± 76	21 ± 2.3	64 ± 3.7	2.92 ± 0.10
Fraction 4	1380 ± 36	8.2 ± 1.4	59 ± 3.3	2.41 ± 0.16
Total	1520 ± 56	45 ± 3.3	69 ± 5.5	3.53 ± 0.16
Intact	1540 ± 72	48 ± 2.6	63 ± 4.9	3.55 ± 0.28
Monolayers				
Exponential	2200 ± 81	100 ± 2.2	82 ± 3.1	8.98 ± 0.45
Plateau	1490 ± 43	7.8 ± 1.1	77 ± 4.3	5.95 ± 0.28

[1]Consumption rates are given in units of moles consumed per cell per second.

Table 2. Cell volume, growth fraction and oxygen consumption of cells from 9L spheroids and monolayers. Values are as described in Table 1.

Sample	Cell Volume (μm^3)	Growth Fraction (percent)	Clonogenic Efficiency (percent)	Oxygen Consumption[1] ($\times 10^{17}$ M/c-s)
Spheroids				
Fraction 1	1300 ± 46	77 ± 3.7	65 ± 4.4	5.17 ± 0.13
Fraction 2	1150 ± 37	46 ± 2.5	57 ± 3.6	3.45 ± 0.09
Fraction 3	1020 ± 40	18 ± 1.0	49 ± 2.5	1.91 ± 0.07
Fraction 4	1010 ± 51	6.7 ± 1.4	51 ± 5.3	1.71 ± 0.11
Total	1180 ± 39	35 ± 2.1	55 ± 4.2	3.05 ± 0.18
Intact	1160 ± 43	31 ± 0.9	59 ± 5.9	3.15 ± 0.09
Monolayers				
Exponential	1470 ± 82	100 ± 3.4	68 ± 3.2	6.65 ± 0.19
Plateau	1190 ± 53	2.8 ± 0.7	57 ± 5.1	3.95 ± 0.10

The rates of oxygen consumption per cell for cells isolated from spheroids were correlated with the mean cell volume and the growth fraction for both EMT6/Ro and 9L cells (r^2=0.97-0.91). The correlations were not as good between the consumption rate and the clonogenic capacity for either cell line (r^2=0.91-0.78). When the values for the exponentially-growing monolayer cells were added to the correlation analysis, the correlation

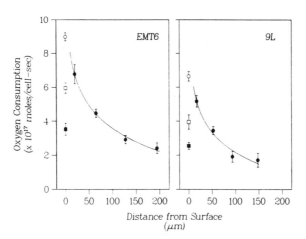

Figure 2. Rates of oxygen consumption per cell as a function of distance from the spheroid surface for cells isolated from EMT6/Ro (left) and 9L (right) spheroids. Solid circles indicate cells from different locations in spheroids, solid squares show the total spheroid cell population, open circles represent exponential monolayers, and open squares indicate plateau monolayers. Each value represents the mean ± standard deviation; lines are best fits of the data from different locations in spheroids to a logarithmic equation.

339

was improved in all but two cases. However, addition of the data for plateau-phase monolayer cells resulted in a worse correlation (e.g.., from r^2 values of 0.97 to 0.28).

The rates of oxygen consumption per cell are illustrated in Figure 2 as a function of location within the spheroid cell rim. For ease of comparison, the rates of consumption for the total spheroid cell population (determined on intact spheroids) as well as the monolayer consumption rates are plotted at a distance of zero micrometers from the spheroid surface. The data for the total spheroid populations reconstructed from the different cell fractions were not different from those for the intact spheroids, and are thus omitted from Figure 2 for clarity. For each cell line, there was a continuous decline in consumption rate with increasing depth of location within the cell rim. These data were well described by a logarithmic equation ($r^2 > 0.95$) which, when extrapolated back to the spheroid surface, gave values very close to those measured for exponentially-growing monolayer cultures.

To determine the influence on cellular oxygen consumption of the change in cell size, the rates of consumption per cell were divided by the mean cell volume for each sample. If the changes in consumption observed were merely due to a smaller cell size, the rate of

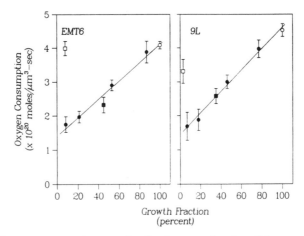

Figure 3. Rates of oxygen consumption per unit cell volume as a function of the growth fraction for EMT6/Ro (left) and 9L (right) cells. Symbols are as described in Figure 2; lines represent best fits of all data (except for plateau monolayers, open squares) to a linear equation

consumption per unit cell volume should have been relatively constant for all samples. However, the rate of oxygen consumption per unit cell volume showed a significant decline across the spheroid rim, being 2.2 (EMT6/Ro) to 2.3 (9L) times lower for the inner fraction compared to the outer fraction. This was not true when comparing the different monolayer cultures: the rates of oxygen consumption per unit cell volume were not significantly different ($p > 0.05$) when comparing exponentially-growing to plateau-phase monolayer cultures. Note that while the rates of oxygen consumption per cell differ by 20-40% for these cell types (Figure 2), the rates of consumption per unit cell volume differ by only 10% at most (Figure 3). The rates of consumption per unit volume for cells from spheroids were strongly correlated ($r^2 > 0.95$) with the growth fraction for both cell lines, as illustrated in Figure 3. Addition of the data for exponentially-growing monolayer cultures improved the correlation coefficients in each case ($r^2 > 0.97$). It is also interesting that the slopes of the lines for the two cell types differ by only 20%. As can be clearly seen from Figure 3, the data for plateau-phase monolayer cultures did not fit the same relationship for either cell line. Rates of oxygen consumption per unit cell volume were also correlated with clonogenic capacity, but the correlations were worse ($r^2 = 0.91$ for EMT6/Ro and 0.78 for 9L).

DISCUSSION

The rates of oxygen consumption for cells from different spheroid regions are consistent with previous reports (13,14,16,19). There was also a close similarity for two very different tumor cell types, implying that the mechanisms of microenvironmental regulation of cellular respiration in tumor cells are general and fundamental. This may not be true for differentiating cell systems, in which unusual patterns of oxygenation and proliferation have been reported (21,22). The rate of oxygen consumption is clearly not constant across the cell rim, so that the decreasing consumption rate as a function of spheroid growth (13-16,19) is due to an increasing fraction of cells with low consumption in a mixed population. One can only reconcile these results with the uniform volume rate of consumption across the cell rim (15,17,18) by postulating that the cell packing varies with position in the spheroid (19).

The present results are also internally consistent. Mean rates of consumption calculated by proportional addition of the rates for the four different cell fractions are essentially identical to the measured rates for the whole spheroid cell population. Also, there was no difference in the mean rates of consumption when comparing measurements made on intact spheroids to for single cells from dissociated spheroids (13,14). This implies that the effect of the spheroid microenvironment on cellular respiration is indirect (i.e. through induction of quiescence). A final internal consistency is that when the change in consumption rate as a function of depth in the spheroid was extrapolated back to the spheroid surface, a value similar to that for proliferating cells was obtained. Assuming that the consumption rate for inner fraction cells represents that of a purely quiescent population, one can predict the data shown in Figure 2 by mathematically constructing mixed cell populations using the measured growth fractions and consumption rates for proliferating and quiescent cells. Thus, there is no intrinsic difference in cellular respiration between spheroid and monolayer cells.

Perhaps the most interesting finding is the apparent difference in cellular respiration between quiescent monolayer cells and inner-region spheroid cells. Even when comparing the rates of consumption per unit of cell volume, plateau-phase cells perform at twice the rate of inner-region spheroid cells. The difference may be the length of time a cell spends in the quiescent state. We have shown a similar result when comparing short- and long-term plateau-phase monolayer cells (14). A reduced rate of consumption within the cell must be due to a lower number of mitochondria, a reduced mitochondrial function, or both. Recent morphometric analysis of spheroids showed a constant number of mitochondria across the viable rim of EMT6/Ro spheroids, but an increase in cell packing with depth (19). This implies an lower number of mitochondria per cell in the inner spheroid region, consistent with the present results. Little is known about the regulation of mitochondrial number in mammalian cells, and the spheroid model may be valuable in investigating this basic aspect of cellular physiology in tumor cells.

Finally, these results have some implications concerning the recovery of cells from the quiescent state. Quiescent cells from both EMT6/Ro and 9L spheroids show a 20-30 hour lag period between separation from the spheroid and resumption of cell division (23). This delay is 2.5-times as long as the time required to transit the cell cycle once proliferation begins, with most of this period spent in the G_1-phase (23). The data presented here suggest that at least part of the delay in resumption of proliferation may be due to the restricted energy metabolism of the quiescent cells. The decreased rate of oxygen consumption implies a reduction in ATP production, which could seriously hamper the macromolecular synthesis necessary for traversal of the cell cycle. If the lower rate of respiration is due to a reduced number of mitochondria, then the long growth lag observed when quiescent cells are separated from the spheroid may be partly due to the time needed to replicate mitochondria. A preliminary experiment with EMT6/Ro cells has shown that the rate of oxygen consumption of inner region spheroid cells begins to increase within 4 hours after separation from the spheroid, and reaches rates comparable to proliferating cells at 8-12 hours after separation. This would support the concept that cells need to re-establish their ATP generating capacity prior to recovery from quiescence. Potentially, inhibition of mitochondrial replication could have therapeutic application through preventing the entry of quiescent cells into the proliferating population.

The assistance of Drs. Stephan Wallenta and Wolfgang Mueller-Klieser of the Institute of Physiology and Pathophysiology, University of Mainz, is gratefully acknowledged. This work was supported by National Cancer Institute grant CA-51150.

REFERENCES

1. Mueller-Klieser, W., Multicellular spheroids: a review on cellular aggregates in cancer research, J. Cancer Res. Clin. Oncol. 113: 101 (1987).
2. Sutherland, R.M., Cell and environment interactions in tumor microregions: the multicell spheroid model, Science 240: 177 (1988).
3. Freyer, J.P. and R.M. Sutherland, Regulation of growth saturation and development of necrosis in EMT6/Ro multicellular spheroids by the glucose and oxygen supply, Cancer Res. 46: 3504 (1986).
4. Tannock, I.F. and I. Kopelyan, Variation of PO_2 in the growth medium of spheroids: Interaction with glucose to influence spheroid growth and necrosis, Br. J. Cancer 53: 823 (1986).
5. Hlatky, L., R.K. Sachs and E.L. Alpen, Joint oxygen-glucose deprivation as the cause of necrosis in a tumor analog, J. Cell. Physiol. 134, 167 (1988).
6. Freyer, J.P. and R.M. Sutherland, Proliferative and clonogenic heterogeneity of cells from EMT6/Ro multicellular spheroids induced by the glucose and oxygen supply, Cancer Res. 46: 3513 (1986).
7. Mueller-Klieser, W., J.P. Freyer and R.M. Sutherland, Influence of glucose and oxygen supply conditions on the oxygenation of multicellular tumor spheroids, Br. J. Cancer. 53: 345 (1985).
8. Freyer, J.P., P.L. Schor, K.A. Jarrett, M. Neeman and L.O. Sillerud, Cellular energetics measured by phosphorous nuclear magnetic resonance spectroscopy are not correlated with chronic nutrient deficiency in multicellular tumor spheroids, Cancer Res. 51: 3831 (1991).
9. Freyer, J.P., Role of necrosis in regulating the growth saturation of multicellular spheroids, Cancer Res. 48: 2432 (1988).
10. Freyer, J.P. and R.M. Sutherland, Selective dissociation and characterization of cells from different regions of multicell tumor spheroids, Cancer Res. 42: 72 (1980).
11. Freyer, J.P. and P.L. Schor, Automated selective dissociation of cells from different regions of multicellular spheroids, In Vitro Cell. Develop. Biol. 25: 9 (1989).
12. Walenta, S., A. Bredel, U. Karbach, L. Kunz, L. Vollrath and W. Mueller-Klieser, Interrelationship amoung morphology, metabolism and proliferation of tumor cells in monolayer and spheroid culture, Adv. Exp. Med. Biol. 248: 847 (1989).
13. Freyer, J.P., E. Tustanoff, A.J. Franko and R.M. Sutherland, In situ oxygen consumption rates of cells in V-79 multicellular spheroids during growth, J. Cell. Physiol. 118: 53 (1984).
14. Freyer, J.P. and R.M. Sutherland, A reduction in the in situ rates of oxygen and glucose consumption of cells in EMT6/Ro spheroids during growth, J. Cell. Physiol. 124: 516 (1985).
15. Mueller-Klieser, W., B. Bourrat, H. Gabbart and R.M. Sutherland, Changes in O_2 consumption of multicellular spheroids during development of necrosis, Adv. Exp. Med. Biol. 191: 775 (1985).
16. Walenta, S. and W. Mueller-Klieser, Oxygen consumption rate of tumor cells as a function of their proliferative status, Adv. Exp. Med. Biol. 215: 389 (1987).
17. Mueller-Klieser, W., Method for the determination of oxygen consumption rates and diffusion coefficients in multicellular spheroids, Biophys. J. 46: 343 (1984).
18. Goldstruck, T.K., W. Mueller-Klieser, B. Borrat and L.A. Jurman, Oxygen consuming regions in EMT6/Ro multicellular tumor spheroids determined by nonlinear regression analysis of experimental PO_2 profiles, Adv. Exp. Med. Biol. 215: 381 (1987).
19. Bredel-Giessler, A., U. Karbach, S. Walenta, L. Vollrath and W. Mueller-Klieser, Proliferation-associated oxygen consumption and morphology of tumor cells in monolayer and spheroid culture, J. Cell. Physiol., in press (1992).
20. Robinson, J. and J.M. Cooper, Method of determining oxygen concentrations in biological media suitable for calibration of oxygen electrodes, Anal. Biochem. 33: 390 (1970).
21. Sutherland, R.M., B. Sordat, J. Bamat, H. Gabbart, B. Bouratt and W. Mueller-Klieser, Oxygenation and differentiation in multicellular spheroids of human colon carcinoma, Cancer Res. 46: 5320 (1986).
22. Karbach, U., C.-D. Gerhartz, K. Groebe, H.E. Gabbert and W. Mueller-Klieser, Rhabdomyosarcoma spheroids with central proliferation and differentiation, Cancer Res. 52: 474 (1992).
23. Freyer, J.P. and P.L. Schor, Regrowth kinetics of cells from different regions of multicellular spheroids of four cell lines, J. Cell. Physiol. 138: 384, (1989).

THE RELATIONSHIP OF RADIATION SENSITIVITY AND MICROENVIRONMENT OF HUMAN TUMOR CELLS IN MULTICELLULAR SPHEROID TISSUE CULTURE

A. Görlach and H. Acker

Max-Planck-Institut für Systemphysiologie
Rheinlanddamm 201, 4600 Dortmund 1, FRG

INTRODUCTION

Despite many publications describing a correlation between radioresistance and radiobiological hypoxia (Adams, 1990; Hill and Pallavicini, 1984; Rockwell and Moulder, 1990) the importance of this phenomenon is still under discussion as well as the mechanisms relevant for the outcome to radiotherapy (Deacon et al., 1984; Steel and Peacock, 1989).

Radiobiological hypoxia is described to occur at pO_2 values below 10 mm Hg. Radiosensitivity becomes half maximal at 3-4 mm Hg (Hill and Pallavicini, 1984). The evidence for radiobiological hypoxia leading to radioprotection, however, is mainly derived from survival curves of tumor systems in vitro. Hypoxia in vivo develops in areas where the supply of oxygen, nutrients and other substances like growth factors becomes insufficient. Multicellular spheroids as avascular tumor cell aggregates have been shown as valuable model system in radiobiology (Sutherland, 1988). Due to their threedimensional structure they exhibit diffusion gradients for oxygen, nutrients, H^+ ions and other substances. Such gradients are able to modify the proliferative status, viability, clonogenicity, cell cycle distribution, differentiation, antigen expression etc. of malignant cells (Freitas and Baronzio, 1989). The resulting heterogeneity in tumor metabolism and tumor microenvironment might be an important factor responsible for differences in therapeutic sensitivity of tumors. For evaluating these interactions spheroids of two human tumor cell lines HT29, a colonic adenocarcinoma, and U118MG, a malignant glioma, have been investigated regarding their microenvironment and metabolism, their growth behavior and their response to fractionated irradiation therapy.

MATERIALS AND METHODS

Cell culture

Cells of two human tumor cell lines U118MG, a malignant glioma, and HT29, a colonic adenocarcinoma, grown as multicellular spheroids were used in this study. These cell lines have been described previously (Carlsson and Acker, 1988). Both cell lines were cultivated in Ham's F10 medium (ICN Flow, Meckenheim, FRG)

Oxygen Transport to Tissue XV, Edited by P. Vaupel
et al., Plenum Press, New York, 1994

supplemented with 10% fetal calf serum (Boehringer, Mannheim, FRG), 2 mM L-glutamine, 100 IU/ml penicillin and 100 μg/ml streptomycin (ICN Flow). Spheroids were grown using the spinner flask technique. Agarose coated petri dishes were seeded with $1*10^5$ (HT29) or $5*10^5$ (U118MG) cells. After initial aggregation the small cell clusters were inoculated in 250 ml containing spinner flasks (Tecnomara, Fernwald, FRG) together with 150 ml complete medium and agitated with 40 rpm using a Techne stirrer system (MCS-104S, Techne Ltd., Cambridge, UK). Medium was changed three times a week. The cultures were free of mycoplasms as was controlled by a DAPI fluorescence assay (kindly performed by H. Loehrke, DKFZ Heidelberg, FRG).

Growth curves

Spheroids were individually cultivated in agarose coated 24 multiwell plates (Costar, Fernwald, FRG) containing 2 ml complete medium. Maximal and minimal radii were determined using an inverted microscope supplied with a microscale (Olympus, Hamburg, FRG) and volumes were calculated according to the equation
$$V = 4/3*\pi*(a*b)^{3/2}$$
where a and b were the maximal and minimal radii measured at right angles.

Irradiation

Spheroids were individually irradiated in an IC 900 irradiation apparatus (Scanditronix-AB, Uppsala, Sweden) with two $1.7*10^{13}$ Bq (450 Ci) ^{137}Cs sources above and below the sample with a dose rate of 0.63 Gy/minute. The spheroids were kept in a small glass incubator installed in the irradiation chamber during the irradiation for maintaining the same conditions as in the incubator (37°C, 5% CO_2, 95% air). Single spheroids were irradiated in precoated culture dishes using a fractionated scheme with 5 Gy on 8 consecutive days starting on day 0. Control spheroids were transferred to the irradiation chamber for shamirradiation.

LDH activity

LDH activity in spheroids was determined spectrophotometrically according to the method of Bergmeier and Bernt (1974). Spheroids were homogenized with 100 μl 50 mM phosphate buffer (pH 7.5). In the presence of 11.3 mM ß-NADH and of Na-pyruvate in a concentration range between 0.05 and 0.63 mM LDH activity was determined at 25°C in 10 μl spheroid homogenates by following the reaction spectrophotometrically (DU62, Beckman, Munich, FRG) for 3 minutes. The K_m and the maximal turnover rates V_{max} were estimated by analysis in the Lineweaver-Burk plot.

Microelectrode measurements

Double barrelled pO_2 or pH sensitive microelectrodes with tip diameters of about 3 μm were used for pO_2 and pH measurements inside the spheroids. Details of the manufacturing procedure of these microsensors have been described previously (Holtermann and Acker, 1992). Microelectrode measurements were carried out in spheroids with a diameter range between 500 and 900 μm. In this size range no dependence between volume and central pH or pO_2 values could be observed (results not shown here). A little bench with holes in the size of the spheroids was mounted inside the superfusion chamber and spheroids were placed in an appropriately sized hole as can be seen schematically in figure 1. For superfusing a physiological solution was used containing 128 mM NaCl, 5.6 mM KCl, 2.1 mM $CaCl_2$, 5.5 mM D-glucose, 10 mM $NaHCO_3$ and 7 mM Hepes (all reagents from

Sigma, Munich, FRG). The microelectrode was positioned with a 15° deviation from the vertical axis and was penetrated stepwise (50 μm) through the spheroids by a micromanipulator until it reached the lower surface of the spheroids. An example of a penetration procedure is given in figure 1. Using this setup almost symmetric pO_2 and pH profiles could be obtained with lowest values near the center. During the measurements stable conditions were maintained in the superfusion chamber with a pO_2 of about 145 mm Hg, pH of about 7.34 and a temperature of 37°C. Microelectrodes were calibrated before and after the experiments and only measurements from stable electrodes were considered.

Oxygen consumption

According to the method of Grossmann (1984) the oxygen consumption of the spheroids has been estimated from the measured pO_2 gradients. Under the assumptions of oxygen transport into the spheroid by diffusion and simultaneous oxygen consumption the measured pO_2 values in the spheroids could be fitted to the adapted Henry-Dalton law:

$$P(r) = P_0 - (V_{O2} * (R^2 - r^2)/6 * D * \alpha)$$

$P(r)$	:	oxygen partial pressure at r
P_0	:	oxygen partial pressure at the surface
V_{O2}	:	oxygen consumption [ml O_2/(100g*min)]
R	:	radius of the spheroid
r	:	distance from the center
D	:	oxygen diffusion coefficient
α	:	oxygen solubility coefficient

Values for D and α were assumed as described by Grote et al. (1979). As a measure for the reliability of the fit the pO_2 gradients predicted by the calculation were compared to the measured pO_2 gradients. Variation coefficients were 2.5 ± 1% for the estimations.

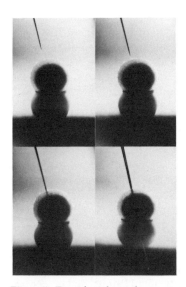
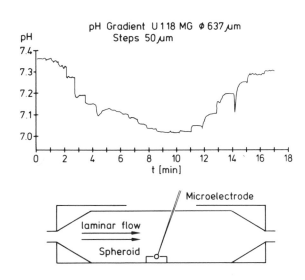

Figure 1. For microelectrode measurements spheroids were placed on an appropriately sized hole of a little bench in the superfusion chamber. With this set up almost symmetric pO_2 and pH gradients were obtained as is demonstrated by the original pH recording. The photographs at the left side show an example of a pO_2 gradient measurement in an HT29 spheroid.

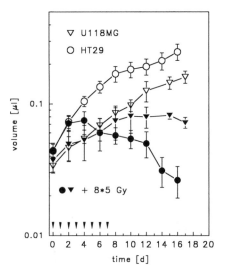

Figure 2. Growth curves of spheroids of the two cell lines were derived from volume measurements. Each point represents mean value ± standard deviation of 10 spheroids investigated in one experiment. Three experiments were performed on each cell line with comparable results. Fractionated irradiation with 8 daily fractions à 5 Gy started on day 0.

RESULTS

Grown as multicellular spheroids the tumor cell lines investigated exhibited a Gompertzian growth behavior with initial doubling times of 74.1 ± 6.2 h (HT29; $n = 27$) and 133.8 ± 2.3 h (U118MG; $n = 15$) (figure 2).

For irradiation experiments a fractionated treatment schedule with a daily fraction of 5 Gy for 8 consecutive days was used starting on day 0. After initial volume increases HT29 spheroids showed growth inhibition and severe volume reductions by the 4th day. U118MG spheroids were not affected in their growth during the radiation treatment. After the fractionated radiation therapy, however, growth retardation without degenerative changes took place (figure 2).

To elucidate reasons for the different radiosensitivity of these spheroid types pO_2 and pH measurements were carried out inside the spheroids to investigate the microenvironmental conditions.

In HT29 spheroids steep pO_2 gradients could be obtained with pO_2 values in the center of about 5 mm Hg leading to a hypoxic fraction with pO_2 values below 10 mm Hg of almost 20% and a median pO_2 of 23 mm Hg. No pO_2 values below 10 mm Hg could be registered in U118MG spheroids with a median pO_2 of 60 mm Hg, however, and pO_2 gradients showed high central pO_2 values of about 40 mm Hg (figure 3 c, d).

pH measurements revealed steeper pH gradients in U118MG spheroids with central values of about 6.93 and more than 25% of the recordings being below pH 7 whereas pH profiles of HT29 spheroids showed about 0.15 pH units higher central values. Only 5% of the pH measurements were below pH 7 in this spheroid type (figure 3 a,b).

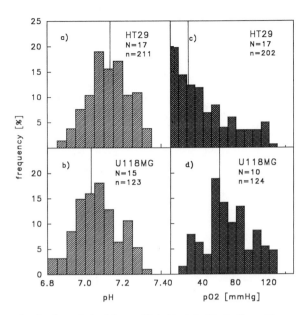

Figure 3. Frequency distributions derived from pH (a,b) and pO_2 (c,d) profile measurements of HT29 and U118MG spheroids. Median values of pO_2 determinations were 23 mm Hg (HT29) and 60 mm Hg (U118MG). Median pH values were pH 7.13 (HT29) and pH 7.04 (U118MG).

For describing the microenvironmental state in spheroids pO_2 and pH gradients were normalized i.e. the measured pO_2 and pH gradients were related to the relative distance from the surface. Now pO_2 and pH values at relative distances inside the spheroids, for example halfway between surface and center (50%), could be determined. Relating pO_2 and pH values at the same relative distances from the surface of the spheroids led to characteristic pO_2 - pH curves (figure 4). Whereas U118MG spheroids exhibited an almost linear decrease of pO_2 - pH couples towards the center HT29 spheroids showed relative higher pO_2 decreases in the outer cell layers whereas towards the center the pO_2 decreases diminished.

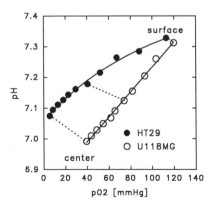

Figure 4. The curves represent pO_2-pH couples at the same relative distance from the spheroid surfaces showing an almost linear relationship between pO_2 and pH decreases in U118MG spheroids and a hyperbolic pO_2-pH curve in HT29 spheroids.

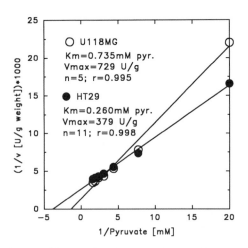

Figure 5. Lineweaver-Burk plot of lactate dehydrogenase kinetics in U118MG and HT29 spheroid homogenates. K_m is the Michaelis-Menten constant, V_{max} the maximal turnover rate, r the correlation coefficient of the linear regression performed.

As pH gradients are determined by lactate production to a high extent (Carlsson and Acker, 1988) lactate dehydrogenase (LDH) activity was measured in homogenates of both spheroid types. U118MG spheroids showed a low affinity but high capacity LDH with a K_m value of about 0.735 mM pyruvate and a maximal turnover rate (V_{max}) of 729 U/g wet weight whereas HT29 spheroids exhibited a high affinity but low capacity LDH with a K_m value of 0.260 mM pyruvate and a V_{max} value of 379 U/g wet weight (figure 5). These different enzyme characteristics might be one reason for variations in the pH profiles in the both spheroid types.

Using the method of Grossmann (1984) for calculation of oxygen consumption values from the measured pO_2 profiles in the spheroids a significant difference in the amount of oxygen consumed in the two spheroid types could be observed (figure 6). HT29 spheroids exhibited significantly higher oxygen consumption values of 1.78 ± 0.33 ml O_2/(100g*min) compared to 1.35 ± 0.21 ml O_2/(100g*min) calculated in U118MG spheroids.

DISCUSSION

Irradiation experiments performed on a fractionated schedule with 8 daily doses à 5 Gy in multicellular spheroids derived from two human tumor cell lines showed differences in the radioresponse of these spheroid types. Whereas HT29 spheroids exhibited a high radiosensitivity with strong degenerations starting during radiation treatment U118MG spheroids did not show decreased growth rates during the radiation schedule. However, after the treatment volume increases were retardated but no degenerative changes could be observed. Thus U118MG revealed a markedly lower radiosensitivity. These results are in good agreement with a previous publication by Nylen et al. (1989).

Hypoxia has been claimed an important reason for the lack of radioresponse of tumors (Adams, 1990; Hill and Pallavicini, 1984; Rockwell and Moulder, 1990). pO_2 measurements inside the two different spheroid types, however, did not show a correlation between the oxygenation state of the spheroids and their radiosensitivity.

HT29 spheroids exhibited markedly lower pO_2 values than U118MG spheroids but showed a higher radiosensitivity. These results are in agreement with observations by Nylen et al. (1989) as well as by Schwachöfer et al. (1991) who reported a higher radiosensitivity of spheroids from a neuroblastoma cell line with steeper pO_2 gradients compared to spheroids from a squamous cell carcinoma cell line with a better oxygenation state.

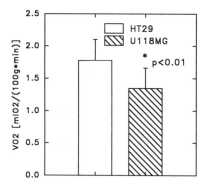

Figure 6. Oxygen consumption values were calculated from pO_2 profiles measured in spheroids according to the method of Grossmann (1984). U118MG spheroids (n=11) exhibited significant (p<0.01) lower oxygen consumption values than HT29 spheroids (n=15). p was determined by t-test.

Murine mammary carcinoma cells exhibited decreased radiation sensitivity when irradiated under low pH conditions (Haveman, 1980). These results have been confirmed in human glial cells for fractionated radiotherapy in an acidotic environment (Röttinger and Mendonca, 1982). The radioprotective effect seemed to be especially important during fractionated radiotherapy. Low pH values have been shown to inhibit cell proliferation, DNA synthesis and glycolysis and affect the cell cycle distribution leading to a shift to G1 (for review see Wike-Hooley et al., 1984). In U118MG spheroids with low radiosensitivity more than 25% of the pH measurements were below pH 7 compared to only 5% in HT29 spheroids. pH gradients are mainly the result of glycolysis with concomitant lactate production. High glycolysis often occurs under anaerobic conditions. In tumor cells as well as in some other cell types, however, high aerobic glycolysis is described (Murray, 1987). pO_2 - pH relationships inside the spheroids revealed characteristic patterns for the different spheroid types resulting in steep pH gradients despite good oxygenation in U118MG spheroids as well as in steep pO_2 gradients with concomitantly flat pH gradients in HT29 spheroids. These different patterns might be the result of different metabolic characteristics as LDH activity measurements and the variations in oxygen consumption suggest a more glycolytic metabolism in U118MG spheroids compared to HT29 spheroids. Carlsson and Acker (1988) also demonstrated a higher lactate production in U118MG spheroids and a higher oxygen consumption of HT29 spheroids measured by a haemoglobin dilution method. Thus the lower growth rate found in U118MG spheroids might be in part due to a higher acidotic fraction. A linkage between high growth rates due to high metabolic activity and higher radiosensitivity was suggested by Schwachöfer et al. (1990) based on observations on several tumor cell lines. This might also explain in part the higher radiation response of HT29 spheroids with a faster growth rate and higher oxygen consumption values.

Summarizing these findings the role of tissue oxygenation alone as a predictive parameter for outcome to radiotherapy remains questionable at least in the spheroid model. As the microenvironment is determined by metabolic factors beside diffusion conditions investigations about the interaction between metabolic characteristics and radiotherapy might be necessary to further understand heterogenous growth behaviour and therapeutic response in tumors.

REFERENCES

Adams, G.E., 1990, The clinical relevance of tumour hypoxia, *Eur. J. Cancer*, 26:420-421.

Bergmeyer, H.U., and Bernt, E., 1974, Lactate dehydrogenase, *in*: "Methods of Enzymatic Analysis," H.U. Bergmeyer, ed., Academic Press, New York-London.

Carlsson, J., and Acker, H., 1988, Relations between pH, oxygen partial pressure and growth in cultured cell spheroids, *Int. J. Canc.* 42:715-720.

Deacon, J., Peckham, M.J., and Steel, G.G., 1984, The radioresponsiveness of human tumours and the initial slope of the cell survival curve, *Radioth. Oncol.* 2:317-323.

Freitas, I., and Baronzio, G.F., 1991, Tumor hypoxia, reoxygenation and oxygenation strategies: possible role in photodynamic therapy, *J. Photochem. Photobiol. B: Biol.* 11:3-30.

Grossmann, U., 1984, Profiles of oxygen partial pressure and oxygen consumption inside multicellular spheroids, *Rec. Res. Cancer Res.* 95:150-161.

Grote, J., Süsskind, R., and Vaupel, P., 1977, Oxygen diffusivity in tumor tissue (DS-Carcinosarcoma) under temperature conditions within the range of 20-40°C, *Pflügers Arch.* 372:37-42.

Haveman, J., 1980, The influence of pH on the survival after X-irradiation of cultured malignant cells. Effects of carbonylcyanide-3-chlorophenylhydrazone, *Int. J. Rad. Biol.* 37:201-205.

Hill, R.P., and Pallavicini, M.G., 1983, Hypoxia and the radiation response of tumors, *Adv. Exp. Med. Biol.* 159:17-35.

Holtermann, G., and Acker, H., 1992, Easy producible amperometric and voltametric glass microsensors with tip-diameters between 0.3 and 3 μm, *in*: "Biosensors: Fundamentals, Technologies and Applications," F. Scheller, R.D. Schmid, eds., VCH, Weinheim, FRG.

Murray, R.K., 1987, Biochemical properties of cancer cells, *in*: "The Basic Science of Oncology," I.F. Tannock, R.P. Hill, eds., Pergamon Press, New York.

Nylen, T., Acker, H., Bölling, B., Holtermann, G., and Carlsson J., 1989, Influence of ionizing radiation on oxygen profiles in different types of multicellular spheroids, *Rad. Res.* 120:213-226.

Rockwell, S., and Moulder, J.E., 1990, Hypoxic fractions of human tumors xenografted into mice, *Int. J. Rad. Onc.* 19:197-202.

Röttinger E.M., and Mendonca, M., 1982, Radioresistance secondary to low pH in human glial cells and Chinese hamster ovary cells, *Int. J. Rad. Onc.* 8:1309-1314.

Schwachöfer, J.H.M., Crooijmans, R.P.M.A., Hoogenhout, J., Jerusalem, C.R., Kal, H.B., and Theeuwes, A.G.M., 1990, Radiosensitivity of human melanoma spheroids influenced by growth rate, *Int. J. Rad. Onc.* 19:1191-1197.

Schwachöfer, J.H.M., Acker, H., Crooijmans, R.P.M.A., van Gasteren, R.P.M.A., Holtermann, G., Hoogenhout, J., Jerusalem, C.R., and Kal, H.B., 1991, Oxygen tension in two human tumor cell lines grown and irradiated as multicellular spheroids, *Anticancer Res.* 11:1365-1368.

Steel, G.G., and Peacock, J.H., 1989, Why are some tumors more radiosensitive than others? *Radioth. Oncol.* 15:63-72.

Sutherland, R.M., 1988, Cell and environment interactions in tumor microregions: The multicell spheroid model, *Science* 240:177-184.

Wike-Hooley, J.L., Haveman, J., and Reinhold, H.S., 1984, The relevance of tumor pH to the treatment of malignant disease, *Radiother. Oncol.* 2:343-366

OXYGENATION STATUS OF RHABDOMYOSARCOMA SPHEROIDS WITH DIFFERENT STAGES OF DIFFERENTIATION

H. Stier, U. Karbach, C.-D. Gerharz, H. Gabbert, and W. Mueller-Klieser

Institute of Physiology and Pathophysiology, University of Mainz
D-6500 Mainz, Germany

INTRODUCTION

Multicellular tumor spheroids with regional heterogeneities of proliferation and substrate concentrations have been investigated recently to study the biological properties of small tumor nodules prior to onset of vascularization (for reviews see: Mueller-Klieser, 1987; Sutherland, 1988).

A novel spheroid system with three phenotypically different cell clones (A, B, and C) of the rat rhabdomyosarcoma cell line BA-HAN-1 has been established to evaluate the influence of genetic and epigenetic factors in the regulation of proliferation and differentiation in tumor cell aggregates (Karbach et al., 1992). These cell clones abortively recapitulate stages of normal embryonic rhabdomyogenesis, but differ in their clone specific differentiation capacity. In this report, spheroids of these three clones were analyzed with regard to their oxygen tension (pO_2) distribution, volume growth kinetics, and histology.

MATERIALS AND METHODS

Cell Line

The three cell clones (A, B, and C) with different differentiation patterns were derived from the dimethylbenzanthracene-induced rat rhabdomyosarcoma cell line BA-HAN-1 as previously described by Gerharz et al., 1988 and Gabbert et al., 1988.

Culture Conditions

Culturing of all three cell clones was performed in Dulbecco's modified Eagle's medium (DMEM) supplemented with 10% (v/v) heat-inactivated fetal calf serum (FCS), antibiotics

(100 IU/ml penicillin and 100 μg/ml streptomycin), and 4,5 g/l glucose. The cell cultures were incubated in a humidified atmosphere of 5% (v/v) CO_2 and air in 37° C.

Spheroid Culture

After initiation of spheroid growth in microbiological Petri dishes, spheroids were transfered into spinner flasks and cultivated in stirred media as described previously (Mueller-Klieser, 1987). The spheroid volume growth as a function of time in suspension culture was quantified by standardized procedures (Freyer and Sutherland, 1980) and was analyzed by fitting the Gompertz function to the measured volume data (Winsor, 1932; Laird, 1964).

Spheroid Histology

Spheroids of different sizes were fixed in 2.5 % (v/v) glutaraldehyde, wax embedded and serially sectioned into 5μm thick slices. The sections were stained with hematoxylin and eosin. Spheroid diameter and the thickness of the viable cell layer were determined in central sections of individual spheroids, taking into account an average shrinkage of 20 % as a result of the histological processing.

Oxygen Microelectrode Measurements

pO_2 values within the spheroids were determined under conditions matching those to which spheroids were exposed during growth. A Whalen-type pO_2-sensitive microelectrode (Whalen et al.,1967) was inserted by micromanipulation into a spheroid within stirred medium (= Lock's solution; Acker et al., 1983) and values were recorded on a radial track through the spheroid center as described previously (Mueller-Klieser and Sutherland, 1982).

RESULTS AND DISCUSSION

Spheroids of the different cell clones investigated showed differences in volume growth with Gompertz kinetics that were similar to those described for solid tumors. As illustrated in Fig. 1, volume growth stagnated at day 22, 26 and 20 at final volumes (mean ± SD) of $(1.53 \pm 0.5) \cdot 10^{-3}$ cm^3, $(1.19 \pm 0.27) \cdot 10^{-3}$ cm^3 and $(8.13 \pm 2.11) \cdot 10^{-4}$ cm^3 for spheroids of clones A, B, and C, respectively. A reduction in oxygen supply from 20 % (v/v) to 5 % (v/v) leads to a considerable retardation in volume growth of clone C spheroids with a final volume of $(3.00 \pm 1.26) \cdot 10^{-4}$ cm^3 at day 24.

At diameters of 700 - 900 μm, spheroids of clone A and B consisted of a viable cell rim (mean ± SD) of 184 ± 31 μm and 301 ± 27 μm thickness, respectively, containing mononuclear morphologically undifferentiated sarcoma cells surrounding a central necrotic area. In contrast, spheroids of clone C of the same size exhibited mononuclear cells and postmitotic differentiated myotube-like giant cells with multiple nuclei. These giant cells were found predominantly in central spheroid regions where no necrosis could be detected.

The central pO_2 in clone A, B, and C spheroids as a function of spheroid size is shown in Fig.2 a,b and Fig.3 a,b. At similar sizes, different spheroids of clone A and B exhibited relatively uniform central pO_2 values that decreased with increasing spheroid diameter. pO_2 values < 5 mm Hg were found in spheroids of clone A with diameters larger than 750 µm

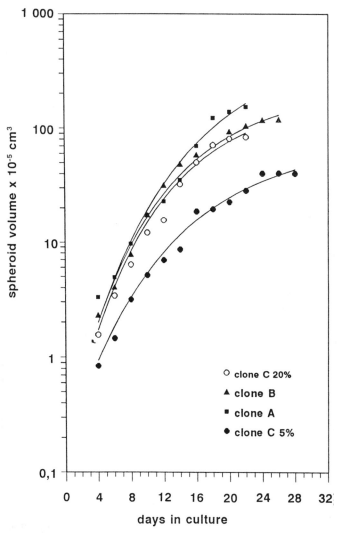

Fig. 1 Spheroid volume of clone A, B, and C as a function of time in spinner culture. The lines represent the results of fitting the Gompertz equation to the measured data. Clone C spheroids were cultured in 20% or 5% oxygen.

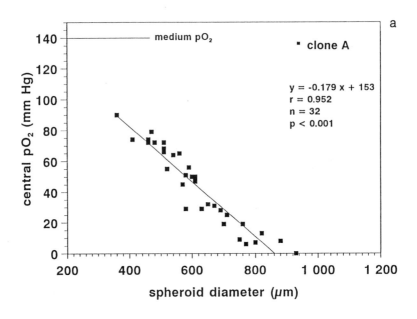

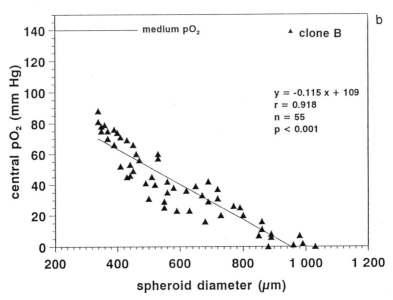

Fig. 2 a, b   Central oxygen tension (pO_2) in spheroids of clone A (a) and B (b) as a function of spheroid size with 20 % (v/v) oxygen in the external gas phase.

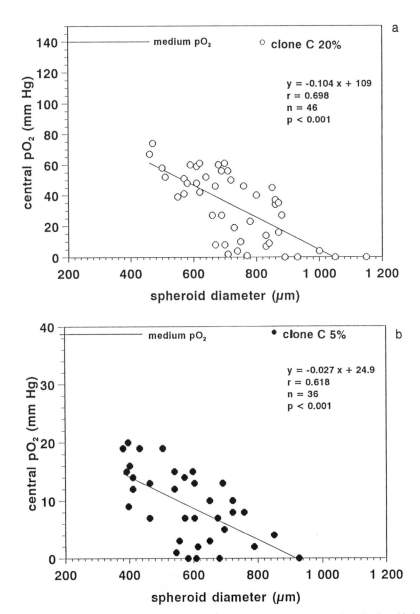

Fig. 3 a, b Central oxygen tension (pO₂) in spheroids of clone C as a function of spheroid size with 20 % (v/v) (a) and 5 % (v/v) (b) of oxygen in the external gas phase.

(Fig. 2 a). Therefore, increased resistence to ionizing radiation and oxygen-depend antitumor agents may be expected in these aggregates. Such low central pO_2 values were present in clone B spheroids only at sizes larger than 850 µm (Fig.2 b). In contrast, spheroids of clone C exhibited a pronounced variability in their central pO_2 values particularly in the size range of 600-900 µm (Fig.3 a). This is correlated with the variable volume proportion of myotube-like giant cells in these spheroids: Low central pO_2 values are associated with a high proportion of differentiated and vice versa.

As expected, a reduction of oxygen in the external gas phase from 20 % (v/v) to 5 % (v/v) leads to an increased proportion of low oxygen tensions in clone C spheroids with a substantial number of pO_2-recordings less than 1 mm Hg at relatively small spheroid sizes (Fig.3 b).

The results of the pO_2 measurements indicate that the oxygen consumption of cells of the differentiated clone C is reduced compared to cells of clone A and B. Low central pO_2-values are associated with myotube-like cells preferentially located in the spheroid center.

pO_2 measurements of clone C spheroids demonstrate that mononuclear sarcoma cells of these rhabdomyosarcoma clone can maintain viability and even proliferation at pO_2 values of < 25 mm Hg. Thus, we assume that the central necrosis in spheroids of clone A and B (occurring at pO_2 values of 40 - 80 mm Hg) may not be caused by lack of oxygen, which has been demonstrated in several other tumor cell spheroids (Bourrat-Floeck et al., 1991).

Upon further characterization of the microenvironment in spheroids of these cell clones, the role of genetic and epigenetic factors in cell differentiation may be studied systematically in future investigations.

ACKNOWLEDGEMENT

This work was supported by the Deutsche Forschungsgemeinschaft (Mu 576/4-1).

REFERENCES

Acker H., Holtermann G., Carlsson J., and Nederman T., 1983, Methodological aspects of microelectrode measurements in cellular spheroids. *Adv. Exp. Med. Biol. 159: 445-462.*

Bourrat-Floeck, B., Groebe, K., and Mueller-Klieser, W., 1991, Biological response of multicellular EMT6 spheroids to exogenous lactate. *Int. J. Cancer* 47: 792-799.

Freyer , J.P., and Sutherland, R.M., 1980, Selective dissociation and characterization of cells from different regions of multicell tumor spheroids. *Cancer Res.* 40: 3956-3965.

Gabbert, H.E., Gerharz, C.D., Engers, R., Mueller-Klieser, W., and Moll, R., 1988, Terminally differentiated postmitotic tumor cells in a rat rhabdomyosarcoma cell line. *Virchows Arch. B Cell Pathol.* 55: 255-261.

356

Gerharz, C.D., Gabbert, H.E., Moll, R., Mellin, W., Engers, R., and Gabbiani, G., 1988, The intraclonal and interclonal phenotypic heterogeneity in a rhabdomyosarcoma cell line with abortive imitation of embryonic myogenesis. *Virchows Arch. B Cell Pathol. 55: 193-206.*

Karbach, U.,Gerharz, C.D., Groebe, K., Gabbert, H.E., and Mueller-Klieser, W., 1992, Rhabdomyosarcoma spheroids with central proliferation and differentiation. *Cancer Res.* 52: 474-477.

Laird A.K., 1964, Dynamics of tumor growth. *Br. J. Cancer* 18: 490-501.

Mueller-Klieser, W., 1987, Multicellular spheroids. A review on cellular aggregates in cancer research. *J. Cancer Res. Clin. Oncol. 113: 101-122.*

Mueller-Klieser, W., and Sutherland R.M., 1982, Influence of convection in the growth medium on oxygen tension in multicellular tumor spheroids.*Cancer Res.* 42: 237-242.

Sutherland, R.M., 1988, Cell and environment interactions in tumor microregions: The multicell spheroid model. *Science* 240: 177-184.

Whalen W.J., Riley J., and Nair P., 1967, A microelectrode for measuring intracellular PO_2. *J Appl. Physiol.* 23: 798-801.

Winsor, C.P., 1932, The Gompertz curve as a growth curve. *Proc. Natl. Acad. Sci. USA,* 18: 1-7.

ONCOGENE-ASSOCIATED GROWTH BEHAVIOR AND OXYGENATION OF MULTICELLULAR SPHEROIDS FROM RAT EMBRYO FIBROBLASTS

Leoni A. Kunz, Karlfried Groebe, and Wolfgang Mueller-Klieser

Institute of Physiology and Pathophysiology, Univ. of Mainz, D-6500 Mainz, Germany

INTRODUCTION

It is now well documented that naturally occurring and experimentally induced tumors develop by a multistep process involving different stages such as unlimited growth, metastasis, and invasiveness. There is much evidence that malignant transformation involves activation of oncogenes and/or loss of suppressor genes (= anti-oncogenes). The former fundamental class of genes, including the ras and myc families, are associated with cell proliferation and differentiation and may mediate tumor initiation, promotion and progression (for reviews see: Spandidos, 1985; Spandidos and Anderson, 1987, Weinberg, 1989).

For the last few years an in vitro model of rat embryo fibroblasts with different extents of transformation has gained practical importance to investigate the oncogene-dependent carcinogenesis. Since tumorigenic conversion of Fisher 344 rat embryo fibroblasts requires two cooperating oncogenes, one can study separately the stage of immortality by single oncogene transfection and further alterations leading to a tumorigenic cell phenotype by cotransfection (Land et al., 1983). To evaluate the emergence of cellular heterogeneity during tumor formation in a well-defined microenvironment, we have established a two-stage carcinogenesis in vitro model as multicellular spheroids. In order to gain further insight into the influence of genetic alterations on relevant parameters, we have studied growth behavior, morphology and oxygenation state of the differently transformed fibroblasts in threedimensional culture.

MATERIALS AND METHODS

Cell Lines

A total of four Fisher 344 rat embryo fibroblast cell lines were included in this study. Spontaneously immortalized, poorly tumorigenic **Rat1** and c-myc-transfected, non-tumorigenic **M1** cells represent the first step towards malignant conversion. Ras-transfection of these two parental cell clones resulted in the creation of the the two other types, **Rat1-T1** and **MR1**, which are highly tumorigenic in vivo (Simm et al, 1987; Simm and Adam, 1988).

Plasmids used for oncogene-transfection via calcium phosphate precipitation were pSV2neo (antibiotics resistance gene) and pSVc-myc1 (Shen-Ong et al, 1982, Land et al., 1983) inducing the step of immortalization, and a point mutated ras-gene plasmid pHO6T1 (= T24Ha-ras; Spandidos and Wilkie, 1984), cooperating with the myc gene in the transformation of early passage rat embryo cells.

Culture Conditions

All cell lines were routinely cultured in Dulbecco's modified Eagle's medium (DMEM) supplemented with 5 % (v/v) fetal calf serum (FCS), antibiotics (10,000 IU/ml penicillin and 10 mg/l streptomycin), and 4.5 g/l glucose. The cell cultures were incubated in a humidified atmosphere of 5 % (v/v) CO_2 in air at 37° C.

Spheroid Growth

Spheroid formation was initiated by inoculating $1 - 2 \cdot 10^5$ T24Ha-ras-transfected Rat1-T1 or MR1 cells and $1 - 2 \cdot 10^6$ Rat1 or M1 cells per non-adhesive petridish. After an initiation phase of 4 days, aggregates were transferred into spinner flasks and cultivated in stirred medium, that was replenished daily (Freyer and Sutherland, 1980, Mueller-Klieser, 1987). Spheroid volume growth was quantified by standardized procedures (Freyer and Sutherland, 1980) and was analyzed by fitting the Gompertz function to the experimental data (Winsor, 1932; Laird, 1964).

Spheroid Histology

Spheroids of various sizes were fixed in 2.5 % (v/v) glutaraldehyde, wax embedded, and prepared for serial paraffin slicing (thickness of the sections: 5 μm). Paraffin thin sections were stained with hematoxylin and eosin for histologic observation. Central sections were used to assess the distribution of viable and necrotic areas, taking into account an average shrinkage of 19 % resulting from histological processing. The thickness of the viable cell layer within individual spheroids was obtained from the geometric mean of 4 orthogonal measurements of the radial distance between the spheroid surface and the edge of necrosis. The average thickness of the viable rim within one spheroid type was determined by calculating the arithmetic mean of $\geq$ 50 individual values.

Oxygen Tension Distributions

Oxygen tension measurements were carried out using O_2-sensitive microelectrodes according to Whalen et al. (1967). Lock's solution was used as a measuring medium (Acker et al., 1983). The special technique of determining the pO_2 in spheroids on radial tracks through the spheroid center has been described previously (Mueller-Klieser and Sutherland, 1982). The measured pO_2 profiles were evaluated by fitting model functions to the experimental data via non-linear regression analysis based upon a Quasi-Newton algorithm (Gill and Murray, 1972) to obtain cell line specific Krogh's diffusion coefficients, volume-related oxygen consumption rates Q_VO_2 within the viable parts of the spheroids, and cellular oxygen uptake rates Q_CO_2.

RESULTS AND DISCUSSION

Tab. 1 displays the Gompertz parameter values of the four spheroid types describing the spheroid volume as a function of the cultivation time in spinner flasks. Myc/ras-cotransfected MR1 fibroblasts and spontaneously immortalized, ras-transfected Rat1-T1 cells seem to be characterized by a different aggregation and proliferation behavior during the initiation phase resulting in a varying initial volume. For this reason, MR1 spheroids already reach maximum spheroid diameters of 1421 $\pm$ 208 μm at day 12 - 14, whereas Rat1-T1 spheroids grow somewhat slower reaching maximum diameters of about 1237 $\pm$ 92 μm at day 20. In contrast, non- or poorly tumorigenic Rat1 and M1 cells form spheroids that can be initiated exclusively by inoculating a 10-fold higher cell concentration. Both ras-free spheroid types remain small in size with average maximum diameters of 150 - 200 μm.

Tab. 1   Parameter values of spheroid growth by fitting the Gompertz function to measured spheroid volumes as a function of culturing time (correlation r > 0.992).

CELL LINE	A (day^{-1})	B (day^{-1})	V_0 (cm^3)	dt$_S$ (h)	V_{pot} (cm^3)	N
Rat1	0.462	0.339	$2.2 \cdot 10^{-7}$	50.3	$8.5 \cdot 10^{-7}$	10
Rat1-T1	0.827	0.094	$5.9 \cdot 10^{-7}$	21.0	$3.9 \cdot 10^{-3}$	21
M1	0.458	0.264	$2.3 \cdot 10^{-7}$	46.4	$1.3 \cdot 10^{-6}$	10
MR1	0.908	0.155	$8.9 \cdot 10^{-6}$	19.5	$3.2 \cdot 10^{-3}$	14

$$V_t = V_0 \cdot e^{A/B \, (1 - e^{-Bt})}$$

V_t	: spheroid volume at t	(cm^3)
V_0	: initial spheroid volume at $t_0 = 0$	(cm^3)
t	: time	(day)
A, B	: Gompertz parameter	(day^{-1})
dt$_S$	: initial spheroid volume doubling time	(h)
V_{pot}	: calculated spheroid volume at t = ∞	(cm^3)

Although the non-ras-transfected Rat1 and M1 aggregates show very similar growth kinetic, they differ drastically in their histological structure and cellular viability. Rat1 spheroids consist of viable cells only, whereas multiple myc-transfected M1 aggregates of the same size contain a few outer layers of viable cells and an inner region with cellular debris under the same culture conditions. Therefore, M1 spheroids show a 7 - 10-fold lower cell content than the other three spheroid types at equal sizes.

T24Ha-ras-transfected Rat1-T1 spheroids exhibit central necrosis with dense pycnotic nuclei at diameters of 500 - 600 μm. The viable cell rim is characterized by two layers of morphologically different fibroblast cells and measures 210 ± 34 μm. In contrast to this spontaneously immortalized, tumorigenic cell type, there is a striking change in three-dimensional MR1 cell morphology. Epithelium like cells form spheroids with a viable cell rim of 304 ± 28 μm and a centrally located necrosis developing at diameters above 800 μm. In addition, cell density in the viable part is significantly less in MR1 as compared to Rat1-T1 spheroids ($p < 0.001$). The data obtained show that the ability of forming multicellular spheroids with tumor-like growth is correlated with tumorigenicity, at least in this oncogene-transformed fibroblast system.

Representative pO_2 profiles of the four spheroid types are shown in Fig. 1 a-d. All profiles are characterized by a decrease of O_2 in the medium directly surrounding the spheroid, thus lowering the pO_2 at the surface of the spheroid below the level in the bulk medium. Within small spheroids (Fig. 1 a), oxygen tension profiles are parabolic in shape indicating that there is a small oxygen consumption even within the necrotic, i.e., structurally degenerated area of the non-tumorigenic M1 spheroids. Gradients of oxygen tensions are very shallow in these M1 aggregates with central pO_2 values of 115 ± 9 mmHg ($n = 10$), contrasted by steep pO_2 profiles with an average central pO_2 value of 85 ± 15 mmHg ($n = 13$) in Rat1 aggregates (pO_2 in the medium: 140 mmHg). This result is partly due to the different cell counts per spheroid. We conclude that the emergence of necrosis within M1 spheroids is not elicited by a lack of oxygen.

A central pO_2 plateau can be observed within larger spheroids of the highly tumorigenic cell clones Rat1-T1 and MR1 (Fig. 1 c/d). In all cases, the oxygen tension decreases faster within Rat1-T1 as compared to MR1 spheroids and central pO_2-values are consistently less in Rat1-T1 spheroids up to diameters of 600 - 700 μm. This is demonstrated in Fig. 2 a/b showing the central pO_2 as a function of the spheroid diameter. This observation might at least partially be explained by the lower cell density of the myc-transfected spheroids. The viable cell rim of MR1 spheroids as determined by histological investigation has a width of about 300 μm, whereas the layer of oxygen consuming cells identified by the presence of pO_2 gradients has a thickness of only 225 ± 45 μm. In the course of spheroid growth, central pO_2 values drop to 0 mmHg prior to the emergence of necrosis in MR1 spheroids, whereas the development of necrosis coincides with the depletion of oxygen in Rat1-T1 spheroids. These results indicate that in the malignant fibroblast spheroid types oxygen might play a different role in the mechanisms underlying the development of necrosis.

pO_2 distributions were evaluated with the aim of obtaining cell line specific O_2 diffusion coefficients and rates of oxygen consumption within the viable parts of the spheroid types investigated. The results ($\pm$ SD) are listed in Tab. 2. All values lie within the range known from previous studies on other spheroid types (e.g. Freyer et al., 1984; Freyer and Sutherland, 1985; Mueller-Klieser 1984, Mueller-Klieser et al., 1986; Bourrat-Floeck et al., 1991).

The data shown in Tab. 2 illustrate that ras-transfection and tumorigenicity in vivo are associated with a higher oxygen diffusivity (significant for MR1 spheroids: $p < 0.02$) and a significantly lower cellular respiration rate ($p < 0.001$) in the spheroid system of oncogene-related fibroblasts. Furthermore, the results show that the volume-related oxygen uptake rate rather than the cellular respiration rate is relevant for the different oxygenation states of the four spheroid types. Thus, M1 aggregates are characterized by an extremely low

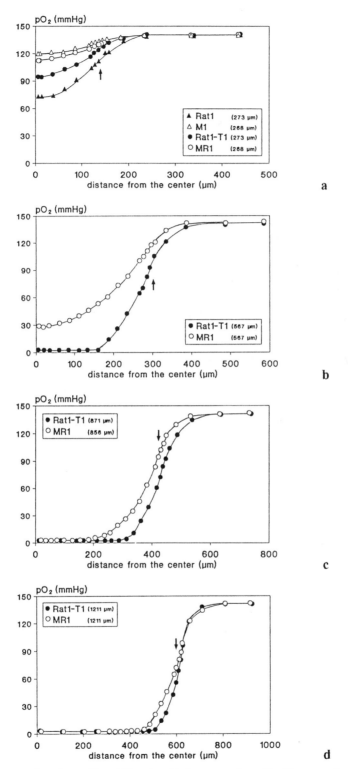

Fig. 1 Representative pO_2 profiles within spheroids from rat embryo fibroblasts transformed to different extents in 4 different ranges of spheroid size   (arrow: spheroid surface)

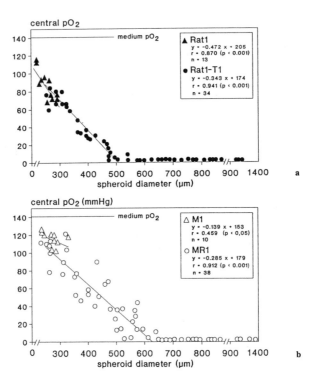

Fig. 2 Central pO$_2$ in spheroids from rat embryo fibroblasts transformed to different extents as a function of the spheroid size

cell lines: **(a)** Rat1 and Rat1-T1   **(b)** M1 and MR1

volume-related O_2 consumption, although single M1 cells possess cellular respiration rates that are significantly higher than that of the other cells investigated. Conversely, ras-transfected Rat1-T1 and MR1 spheroids do not differ in their oxygenation status, yet show a significantly different cellular O_2 uptake rate. This illustrates the histological significance of cellular packing density for tissue oxygenation.

Tab.2 Krogh's diffusion constant K_S, volume-related oxygen consumption rate $Q_V O_2$, and cellular O_2 uptake rate $Q_C O_2$ in the viable part of spheroids from rat emryo fibroblasts transformed to different extents

CELL LINE	K_S ml O_2 (s · cm · mmHg)$^{-1}$	$Q_V O_2$ ml O_2 · (s · cm^3)$^{-1}$	$Q_C O_2$ mol O_2 · (s · cell)$^{-1}$
Rat1	$(5.11 \pm 1.56) \cdot 10^{-10}$	$(7.70 \pm 1.78) \cdot 10^{-4}$	$(6.6 \pm 1.6) \cdot 10^{-17}$
Rat1-T1	$(5.72 \pm 1.45) \cdot 10^{-10}$	$(5.95 \pm 1.58) \cdot 10^{-4}$	$(3.5 \pm 1.5) \cdot 10^{-17}$
M1	$(4.40 \pm 1.75) \cdot 10^{-10}$	$(2.19 \pm 0.64) \cdot 10^{-4}$	$(15.2 \pm 4.7) \cdot 10^{-17}$
MR1	$(6.32 \pm 1.31) \cdot 10^{-10}$	$(5.00 \pm 1.33) \cdot 10^{-4}$	$(6.3 \pm 1.5) \cdot 10^{-17}$

SUMMARY

The basis of the present investigation was the establishment of an oncogene-dependent, genetically determined two-stage carcinogenesis in vitro model as multicellular spheroids. Spheroid formation was achieved with four rat embryo fibroblast cell lines, two of which represent the first step of malignant transformation, known as stage of immortalization. The ras-transfected counterparts of these two parental cell clones represent fully transformed phenotypes. The data obtained show that spheroid volume growth and cellular viability reflect the degree of tumorigenicity in vivo of the different fibroblast types investigated. In addition, ras-transfection alters not only the growth kinetics but also the cellular oxygen metabolism. Furthermore, the results demonstrate very clearly that different fibroblast clones at the same stage of malignant transformation may be characterized by an entirely different growth behavior, morphology and metabolic activity in spheroid culture. This is true, although these cells originate from the same primary cells, differ only in the step of immortalization, and were cultured as spheroids under identical environmental conditions.

ACKNOWLEDGEMENTS

All cell lines were kindly provided by Dr. G. Adam and Dr. G. Simm, Faculty of Biology, University of Konstanz, D-7750 Konstanz, Germany.

This work was supported by the DFG (Mu 576/2-4; Mu 576/4-1)

REFERENCES

Acker H. Holtermann G., Carlsson J., and Nederman T., *1983*, Methodological aspects of microelectrode measurements in cellular spheroids, *Adv. Exp. Med. Biol. 159: 445 - 462*

Bourrat-Floeck B., Groebe K., and Mueller-Klieser W., *1991*, Biological response of multicellular EMT6 spheroids to exogenous lactate, *Int. J. Cancer 47: 792 - 799*

Freyer J.P. and Sutherland R.M., *1980*, Selective dissociation and characterization of cells from different regions of multicell tumor spheroids, *Cancer Res. 40: 3956 - 3965*

Freyer J.P. and Sutherland R.M., *1985*, A reduction in the in situ rates of oxygen and glucose consumption of cells in EMT6/Ro spheroids during growth, *J. Cell. Physiol. 124: 516 - 524*

Freyer J.P., Tustanoff E., Franco A.J., and Sutherland R.M., *1984*, In situ oxygen consumption rates of cells in V-79 multicellular spheroids during growth, *J. Cell. Physiol. 118: 53 - 61*

Gill P.E. and Murray W., *1972*, Quasi-Newton methods for unconstrained optimization, *J. Inst. Maths. Applics. 9: 91 - 108*

Laird A.K., *1964*, Dynamics of tumor growth, *Br. J. Cancer 18: 490 - 501*

Land H., Parada L.F., and Weinberg R.A., *1983*, Tumorigenic conversion of primary embryo fibroblasts requires at least two cooperating oncogenes, *Nature 304: 596 - 602*

Mueller-Klieser W., *1984*, Methods for the determination of oxygen consumption rates and diffusion coefficients in multicellular spheroids, *Biophys. J. 46: 343 - 348*

Mueller-Klieser W., *1987*, Multicellular spheroids. A review on cellular aggregates in cancer research, *J. Cancer Clin. Oncol. 113: 101 - 122*

Mueller Klieser W. and Sutherland R.M., *1982*, Influence of convection in the growth medium on oxygen tension in multicellular tumor spheroids, *Cancer Res. 42: 237 - 242*

Mueller-Klieser W., Freyer J.P., and Sutherland R.M., *1986*, Influence of glucose and oxygen supply conditions on the oxygenation of multicellular spheroids, *Br. J. Cancer 53: 345 - 353*)

Shen-Ong G.L.C., Keath E.J., Piccoli S.P., and Cole M.D., *1982*, Novel myc oncogene RNA from abortive immunoglobulin-gene recombination in mouse plasmacytomas, *Cell 31: 161 - 169*

Simm A. and Adam G., *1988*, Cell-biological characterization of the action of c-myc and T24Ha-ras oncogenes in transfected secondary rat embryo fibroblasts, *Biol. Chem. Hoppe-Seyler 369: 918*

Simm A., Gruber F., and Adam G., *1987*, Cell-biological characterization of different clones of Rat1 cells transfected by plasmids carrying c-ras and T24-ras oncogene, *Europ. J. Cell. Biol. 43: 56; S Suppl. 17*

Spandidos D.A., *1985*, Mechanisms of carcinogenesis: The role of oncogenes, transcriptional enhancers and growth factors, *Anticancer Res. 5: 485 - 498*

Spandidos D.A. and Anderson M.L.M., *1987*, A study of mechanisms of carcinogenesis by gene transfer of oncogenes into mammalian cells, *Mutation Res. 185: 271 - 291*

Spandidos D.A. and Wilkie N.M., *1984*, Malignant transformation of early passage rodent cells by a single mutated human oncogene, *Nature 310: 469 - 475*

Weinberg R.A., *1989*, Oncogenes, antioncogenes, and the molecular bases of multistep carcinogenesis, *Cancer Res. 49: 3713 - 3721*

Whalen W.J., Riley J., and Nair P., *1967*, A microelectrode for measuring intracellular pO$_2$, *J. Appl. Physiol. 23: 798 - 801*

Winsor C.P., *1932*, The Gompertz curve as a growth curve, *Proc. Natl. Acad. Sci. USA 18: 1-7*

CHARACTERISATION OF THE MICROCIRCULATION OF TUMOURS WHERE THE BLOOD SUPPLY ORIGINATES FROM A SINGLE ARTERY AND VEIN

Gillian M. Tozer[1], Paul L. Sensky[1], Katija M. Shaffi[1], Vivien E. Prise[1] and Vincent J. Cunningham[2]

[1]CRC Gray Laboratory
P.O. Box 100
Mount Vernon Hospital
Northwood
Middlesex, HA6 2JR

[2]MRC Cyclotron Unit
Hammersmith Hospital
Ducane Road
London, W12 OHS

INTRODUCTION

Gullino and his colleagues were the first to develop methods for growing transplanted and primary rat tumours so that they were supplied by a single artery and drained by a single vein (Gullino & Grantham, 1961, Grantham et al., 1973). Subsequently, this type of preparation has been used for a variety of studies of in vivo tumour pathophysiology and biochemistry, including the study of oxygen utilisation (Gullino et al., 1967, Gullino, 1976, Vaupel et al., 1985). Further developments on the original method have been the use of human tumours growing in nude rats (Steinau et al., 1981, Vaupel et al., 1985) and tumour perfusion ex vivo, using physiological buffers or donor blood (Sevick and Jain, 1989a, 1989b, Sensky et al., 1992).

Tumour preparation involves surrounding the growing tumour in a material which prevents ingrowth of new vessels other than those arising from a specific artery and vein. We are particularly interested in using these "isolated" tumours for investigating the effects of blood flow modifiers on the tumour microcirculation. Access to the tumour artery allows administration of vasoactive agents directly to the tumour without their entry into the systemic circulation and access to the tumour vein allows for a direct determination of tumour blood flow as well as venous sampling of metabolites. It is well known that the heterogeneous delivery of oxygen as well as chemotherapeutic drugs is a major problem in cancer therapy. Modification of tumour blood flow is a possible means of alleviating this problem.

This paper describes experiments to characterise blood flow and vascular resistance in isolated, transplanted tumours growing in the inguinal fat pad of rats in order to determine the suitability of this system for further studies with blood flow modifiers.

Oxygen Transport to Tissue XV, Edited by P. Vaupel
et al., Plenum Press, New York, 1994

METHODS

Tumour

A transplanted rat carcinosarcoma, designated P22, was used for these experiments. Details of maintenance of this tumour are described elsewhere (Tozer & Shaffi, 1992). Experiments were performed on 5th to 10th passage tumours growing subcutaneously in the left flank of 10 to 12 week old male BD9 rats or growing as isolated preparations in the right inguinal fat pad of 12 to 13 week old male BD9 rats (see below).

Preparation of Isolated Tumours

Rats were anaesthetised with Hypnorm (Crown Chemical Co. Ltd.) and midazolam (Roche) and a small incision was made in the skin over the right hind leg. The inguinal fat pad receives the majority of its blood supply from the epigastric artery and vein which branch from the femoral artery and vein. A small section (≈ 0.2 g) of the fat pad was surgically isolated together with the proximal portion of the epigastric artery and vein. Branches of the artery and vein distal to the isolated fat were ligated or cauterised to prevent bleeding during this procedure.

Donor tumour was implanted into the isolated fat either as small pieces (1-2 mm diameter) or as a slurry prepared by mincing the donor tumour with scissors followed by aspiration through hypodermic needles of decreasing sizes. Moulded silicon chambers made from Silastic MDX4-4210 medical grade elastomer (Dow Corning) were used to enclose the fat and growing tumour and prevent ingrowth of new blood vessels from surrounding fat, skin or muscle. The chambers were constructed so as not to constrict the vascular pedicle supplying the tumour and to allow drainage of fluids. Wounds were stitched and teeth were clipped to prevent the animals from interfering with their stitches. Lost fluid was replaced by s.c. injection of several millilitres of dextrose/saline solution and rats were placed on a heated blanket until partial recovery from the effects of anaesthesia. They were subsequently housed in separate cages with free access to both soft and regular diet and water.

Surgical Preparation for *in vivo* Experiments

Two to three weeks following surgery, animals were re-anaesthetised with Hypnorm and midazolam and the skin overlying the tumour re-opened. The saphenous artery was catheterised such that the catheter tip passed along the femoral artery until it was just distal to the tumour (epigastric) artery. The femoral vein was catheterised such that the catheter tip was just distal to the tumour (epigastric) vein. A piece of suture thread was placed under the femoral vein proximal to the catheterisation site. All other vessels near the catheterisation site, including the saphenous vein and muscular artery and vein were ligated or cauterised. This catheterisation procedure means that systemic circulation through the tumour is maintained and also permits both the administration of agents to the tumour via the arterial catheter and the selective collection of venous outflow from the tumour. The tumour was kept warm and moist throughout the surgical procedure. The tail artery and vein were also catheterised and the wounds strapped. The preparation was left undisturbed for approximately half an hour before blood flow measurements. Top-up doses of anaesthetic were administered intraperitoneally at 45 minute intervals and mean arterial blood pressure (MABP) was monitored continuously via a pressure transducer (Gould) connected to the tail artery catheter. Rats were kept warm using a thermostatically-controlled heating blanket.

Surgical Preparation for *ex vivo* Experiments

Ex vivo tumour perfusion was also performed after 2 - 3 weeks of tumour growth. The saphenous artery was catheterised as for the *in vivo* experiments, acting as the route of perfusate administration. Unlike the *in vivo* surgery, the femoral vein was catheterised on the proximal side of the tumour vein and ligated on the distal side. This less complicated catheterisation is possible since maintaining the systemic circulation through the tumour is not required for *ex vivo* perfusion. Perfusion of a modified, well-oxygenated Krebs-Henseleit (KH) buffer was initiated via the arterial catheter, at ≈ 0.20 ml min^{-1} immediately prior to ligating the femoral artery proximal to the tumour artery, so that the perfusate flowed through the tumour and out through the venous catheter (Sensky *et al.*, 1992). Flow to the tumour was never interrupted during the procedure. The tumours were then excised with the arterial and venous catheters intact and placed in a humidified perfusion chamber maintained at 37°C. Tumour perfusion pressure was recorded at different perfusion rates between 0.05 ml min^{-1} and 0.5 ml min^{-1}.

Blood Flow Measurements in Subcutaneous Tumours

Blood flow to subcutaneous tumours was measured using the uptake, over a short infusion time, of the inert, readily diffusible compound, iodo-antipyrine labelled with ^{14}C or ^{125}I (^{14}C-IAP (Amersham) or ^{125}I-IAP (Institute of Cancer Research, U.K.)). IAP was administered i.v. via a catheterised tail vein. Arterial samples were collected, over the infusion time, from free-flowing blood from a catheterised tail artery in order to obtain an arterial input function. Tumours were excised at the end of infusion for measurement of radioactivity. Details of this technique have been published elsewhere (Tozer *et al.*, 1990, Tozer & Shaffi, 1992).

Blood Flow Measurements in the *in vivo* Preparation

Rats were heparinised by i.v. injection of 0.2 ml 1000 units ml^{-1} heparin. The suture around the femoral vein was tied off such that blood entered the tumour from the femoral artery, left the tumour via the tumour vein and flowed down the femoral vein catheter where it was collected at intervals using a fraction collector. Donor blood, obtained by cardiac puncture of syngeneic rats, was replaced at the same rate as the loss from the venous catheter, by infusion via the tail vein catheter. The flow rate of blood from the tumour vein was monitored and designated "total flow".

Tumour blood flow was also measured using the uptake of ^{125}I-IAP. IAP was infused directly into the tumour circulation via the arterial catheter at 5% of the rate of the total flow. Tumour levels of IAP were measured continuously using external gamma counting and suitable shielding of the tumour. Venous levels of IAP were measured from timed venous samples counted in a well-counter. At the end of the experiment (1 to 2 hours after the start of infusion of IAP) rats were killed using bolus i.v. injection of Euthatal (May & Baker) and the tumour rapidly excised and counted in the well-counter. These counts were used to determine a factor for expressing the relationship between counts in the well-counter and counts measured by the external counter.

Blood flow (designated "fitted flow") was calculated from radioactivity in the arterial blood and tumour during the first 300 seconds of IAP infusion, using a modification of the relationships described by Kety (1960). The model includes a correction for dispersion of blood along the plastic catheter such that the final model equation is

$$C_{tiss} = (k_1 k_d) / (k_d - k_2) C_i * \{e^{-k_2 t} - e^{-k_d t}\} \qquad 1)$$

where * denotes convolution

$C_{tiss}(t)$ is concentration of label in the tumour as a function of time in cpm ml^{-1};

k_1 is fitted blood flow per g of whole tumour in ml g^{-1} min^{-1};

$k_2 = k_1 / \alpha.\lambda$ where α is the fraction of tumour effectively perfused and λ is the equilibrium partition coefficient of the tracer between tissue and blood ($\alpha.\lambda$ is equivalent to V_d, the *apparent* volume of distribution of the label in the tissue relative to the blood);

$C_i(t)$ is the concentration of label in the arterial blood calculated from the infusion rate of IAP into the artery and the total flow rate from the tumour;

k_d is a dispersion constant.

λ was measured, where possible, from the ratio of label in tumour and venous blood after allowing sufficient time for equilibration. Calculated values for fitted blood flow (k_1) and effectively perfused fraction (α) were compared with total flow for different tumours.

RESULTS

Figure 1 illustrates the relationship between tumour size and flow rate for the P22 tumour growing subcutaneously (a) and as isolated *in vivo* and *ex vivo* preparations in the inguinal fat pad (b). Flow is measured by uptake of systemically administered IAP for the subcutaneous tumours, by venous outflow (total flow) for the *in vivo*, inguinal tumours and by infusion rate of KH-buffer required to sustain a perfusion pressure of 85 mmHg for the *ex vivo*, inguinal tumours. This pressure is equivalent to the mean MABP for all the animals used in the *in vivo* experiments (85 ± 2.9 mmHg). Mean MABP for all the animals with subcutaneous tumours was similar (92 ± 1.6 mmHg).

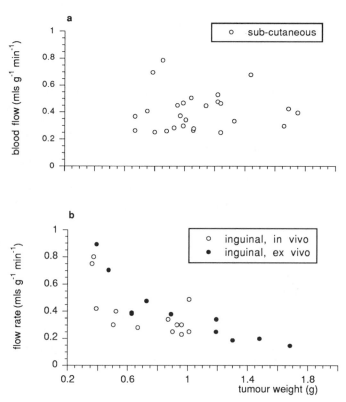

Figure 1. Relationship between flow rate and tumour size for subcutaneous (a) and inguinal (b) P22 tumours. Each point represents an individual tumour.

These results show that there is no relationship between blood flow and tumour size for the subcutaneous tumours within the weight range studied (Figure 1a). This lack of correlation is probably associated with a very low necrotic fraction, reported for the P22 tumour growing in this site (Tozer & Shaffi, 1992). On the other hand, flow rate in the isolated tumours decreases significantly with increase in tumour size (Figure 1b). Figure 2 shows that tumour vascular flow resistance is also independent of size for the subcutaneous tumours but tends to increase with size for the isolated tumours. This increase is significant for the *ex vivo* tumours ($r^2 = 0.875$) but is not significant for the *in vivo* tumours which cover a smaller weight range. Blood flow tends to be lower and flow resistance higher in the *in vivo* isolated tumours relative to the *ex vivo* tumours. Although this would be expected considering the different viscosities of blood and KH-buffer, the difference is rather small and not significant for the number of animals used (p = 0.303 that the difference has occurred by chance, using the student's t-test for unpaired data and excluding the three largest *ex vivo* tumours).

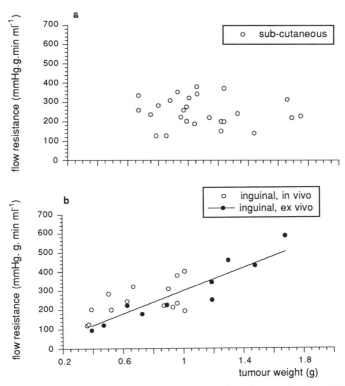

Figure 2. Relationship between flow resistance and tumour size for subcutaneous (a) and inguinal (b) P22 tumours. Each point represents an individual tumour.

There are several possible explanations for the differences between the flow characteristics of tumours growing in the subcutaneous and inguinal sites. One possibility is that there are physical pressures restraining the growth of tumours in the inguinal fat pad resulting in vascular collapse and possibly the development of necrosis which would lead to an increase in vascular resistance as the tumour grows. Alternatively, blood flow as measured by tracer uptake may not be equivalent to blood flow as measured by total flow methods.

In order to investigate these possibilities further, blood flow was measured using the uptake of IAP (fitted flow) and using the collected venous outflow (total flow) in the same tumours perfused *in vivo*. Two small tumours (< 0.4 g) and two larger tumours (> 0.6 g) were used in this study. Figure 3 shows two examples, from individual rats, of the arterial input and the tumour uptake of 125I-IAP, which were used for calculations of fitted flow. The total flow throughout the time course of each experiment is also shown. There are obvious differences between the two tumours. IAP in the small tumour rapidly equilibrated with the blood giving a value of 0.92 for λ. In the larger tumour, equilibration was much slower and was not complete by the end of the experiment so that no accurate estimation of λ could be made. Total flow was much higher in the small tumour than in the large tumour.

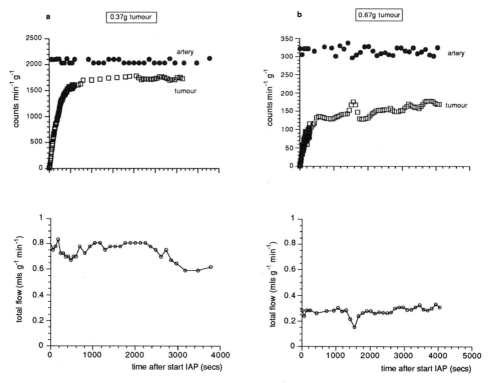

Figure 3. Upper panel: Arterial input and tumour uptake of ^{125}I-IAP following intra-arterial infusion of ^{125}I-IAP for a small tumour (a) and a larger tumour (b). Lower panel: total flow measured from the venous outflow for the same tumours.

Figure 4 shows the relationship between fitted flow, total flow, effectively perfused fraction (α) and tumour size, assuming a value of 1.0 for λ in the larger two tumours. Fitted flow was lower than the total flow for all tumours and decreased less, if at all, with increase in tumour size. Thus total flow was approximately 3 times higher than fitted flow in the small tumours and twice as high in the larger tumours. Figure 4b shows that the effectively perfused tumour fraction also decreased with tumour size such that only a third of the tumour volume in the large tumours was effectively perfused in the first 300 seconds of the experiment.

DISCUSSION

Apparent differences in blood flow and flow resistance in the P22 tumour growing in the subcutaneous and inguinal sites were at least partially due to the different methods of measuring blood flow in each case. Total blood flow as measured by the venous outflow method was consistently higher than the fitted flow as measured by tracer uptake. This suggests that there was a large blood fraction which passed through the tumour without significant exchange with the tumour interstitium. This "shunting" of blood was particularly large for the small tumours and could account for the very steep increase in total flow rate at low tumour weights observed for both *in vivo* and *ex vivo* tumours in Figure 1. It may be that arteriovenous anastomoses between the epigastric artery and vein develop early after tumour transplantation and that tumour growth progressively displaces them. The results suggest examination of tumours weighing about 1 g to determine whether shunting is negligible by this stage of tumour growth.

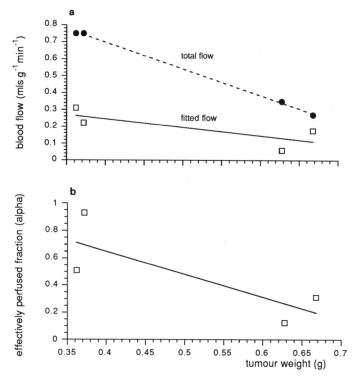

Figure 4. The relationship between total flow, fitted flow and tumour size (a) and effectively perfused fraction and tumour size (b) for the same four inguinal tumours perfused *in vivo*.

Measurements of fitted flow in the *in vivo* tumours tended to be lower than fitted flow for the subcutaneous tumours (comparing Figure 4a and Figure 1a). This suggests that the necrotic fraction may be higher for tumours in the inguinal site. We were not able to measure necrotic fractions in tumours infused with IAP. However, a qualitative assessment of other inguinal tumours, which have not undergone the catheterisation procedure, suggests that the necrotic fraction is higher than for subcutaneous tumours but not high enough to account for α values of around 20% in 0.6 to 0.8 g tumours. Similarly, measurements of the spatial distribution of blood flow in these tumours using the uptake of ^{14}C-IAP have revealed no large non-perfused regions (results not shown). It is possible that the catheterisation procedure required for isolating the tumour circulation for the *in vivo* and *ex vivo* preparations caused blood vessels to collapse. We are currently seeking ways to improve the surgery so that there is minimal disturbance of the tumour vasculature.

We have found a significant degree of shunting and a significant proportion of poorly perfused tissue in the isolated tumour model. Shunting is more apparent in the smaller tumours than in the larger tumours but the reverse is true for the poorly perfused fraction. It was not possible to accurately quantitate shunting using IAP but it may be no more than is present in other tumours where assessment is much more difficult. Radioactively-labelled microspheres would provide a means of quantitation in the isolated tumours where there is ready access to the tumour vein. The poorly perfused fraction, on the other hand, was much greater than expected in the larger tumours and may be due to the experimental procedure. Further experiments should clarify this point.

Acknowledgement

We would like to thank Mr P. Russell and his staff for care of the animals and Dr B. Vojnovic and his staff for development of some of the electronic instrumentation. This work is supported by the Cancer Research Campaign.

REFERENCES

Grantham, F.H., Hill, D.M. and Gullino, P.M., 1973, Primary mammary tumors connected to the host by a single artery and vein, *J. Natl. Cancer Inst.* 50:1381.

Gullino, P.M., 1976, *In vivo* utilization of oxygen and glucose by neoplastic tissue, *in*: "Oxygen Transport to Tissue II," J. Grote, D. Reneau and G. Thews, eds., Plenum Publishing Corporation, New York.

Gullino, P.M. and Grantham, F.H., 1961, Studies on the exchange of fluids between host and tumor. I. A method for growing "tissue-isolated" tumors in laboratory animals, *J. Natl. Cancer Inst.* 27:679.

Gullino, P.M., F.H., G. and Courtney, A.H., 1967, Utilization of oxygen by transplanted tumors *in vivo*, *Cancer Res.* 27:1020.

Kety, S.S., 1960, Theory of blood tissue exchange and its application to measurements of blood flow, *Methods Med. Res.* 8:223.

Sensky, P.L., Prise, V.E., Tozer, G.M., Shaffi, K.M. and Hirst, D.G., 1992, Resistance to flow through tissue-isolated tumours located in two different sites, *Br. J. Cancer* (submitted).

Sevick, E.M. and Jain, R.K., 1989, Geometric resistance to blood flow in solid tumors perfused *ex vivo*: effects of tumor size and perfusion pressure, *Cancer Res.* 49:3506.

Sevick, E.M. and Jain, R.K., 1989, Viscous resistance to blood flow in solid tumors: effect of hematocrit on intratumor blood viscosity, *Cancer Res.* 49:3513.

Steinau, H.U., Bastert, G., Eichholz, H., Fortmeyer, H.P. and Schmidt-Matthiesen, H., 1981, Epigastric pouching technique: human xenografts in rnu/rnu rats, *in*: "Thymusaplastic Nude Mice and Rats in Clinical Oncology," G.B.A. Bastert, *et al.*, eds., Gustav Fischer Verlag, Stuttgart, New York.

Tozer, G. M., Lewis, S., Michalowski, A. and Aber, V., 1990, The relationship between regional variations in blood flow and histology in a transplanted rat fibrosarcoma, *Br. J. Cancer* 61:250.

Tozer, G.M. and Shaffi, K.M., 1992, Modification of tumour blood flow using the hypertensive agent, angiotensin II, *Br. J. Cancer* (submitted).

Vaupel, P., Kallinowski, F., Dave, S., Gabbert, H. and Bastert, G., 1985, Human mammary carcinomas in nude rats - a new approach for investigating oxygen transport and substrate utilization in tumor tissues, *Adv. Exp. Med. Biol.* 191:737.

RELATIVE PERFUSION OF TUMOURS IN TWO SITES FOR UP TO 6 HOURS AFTER THE INDUCTION OF ANAEMIA

Paul L. Sensky, Vivien E. Prise, and David G. Hirst

CRC Gray Laboratory
P.O. Box 100
Mount Vernon Hospital
Northwood
Middlesex, HA6 2JR

INTRODUCTION

Anaemia in the cancer patient is widely recognised as an important factor in determining the outcome of various forms of treatment. Animal studies have shown in several tumour lines that acute reductions in haematocrit produce a significant increase in the hypoxic fraction of tumour cells, thus rendering the tumour cells more resistant to radiotherapy (Hirst *et al.*, 1984; Siemann *et al.*, 1975). Where inspired air of low oxygen content has been used to induce anaemia, the reduced radiosensitivity has been attributed to a reduction in O_2 availability resulting from the low pO_2 in the arterial blood, whilst induction by phlebotomy, with subsequent plasma replacement, directly reduces the Hb concentration of the blood, thus reducing the O_2 carrying capacity. It may be expected that compensatory mechanisms act to increase the cardiac output to maintain the supply of oxygen to tissues. The way in which any such increase affects the relative distribution of blood between tumours and normal tissues has not been closely investigated as yet. This study examines how the cardiac output is distributed between 5 minutes and 6 hours after the onset of anaemia.

METHODS

Animals and Tumours

The NT carcinoma, a transplantable mammary adenocarcinoma, was used in syngeneic CBA male 8 week old mice in all experiments. A single suspension of tumour cells was prepared in physiological saline. $1 - 2 \times 10^5$ cells were inoculated intradermally (i.d.) on the back in a volume of 50 µl under metofane anaesthesia. 6 - 8 days post-transplant a similar quantity of cells were implanted in the abdominal fat pad after exposing the tissue with a 10 mm incision in the body wall. The muscle was sutured with silk and the skin closed with

Oxygen Transport to Tissue XV, Edited by P. Vaupel
et al., Plenum Press, New York, 1994

autoclips. Relative perfusion measurements were undertaken 12 - 18 days later, once the i.d. tumours had grown to 300 - 600 mg.

Induction of Anaemia

Anaemia was induced under metofane anaesthesia by the withdrawal of ≈ 0.7 ml blood from the suborbital sinus into heparinised pasteur pipettes, followed by transfusion of 0.7 - 1 ml freshly prepared plasma from syngeneic donors via the tail vein in order to maintain the blood volume. Packed cell measurements were made on blood samples from the tail or suborbital sinus before and after the exchange transfusion procedure to assess the degree of anaemia induced. Haematocrit readings were also taken immediately prior to the measurement of relative blood flow (Microhaematocrit centrifuge, Patterson Scientific).

Measurement of Relative Blood Flow

The relative blood flow (RBF) to both tumours and several normal tissues (gastocnemius muscle, liver, kidney, spleen, gut and tail) was measured at various timepoints between 5 minutes and 6 hours after the induction of anaemia, using the ^{86}Rb extraction technique (Sapirstein, 1958). 185 kBq [86]RbCl (Amersham International, UK) was injected in a volume of 100 µl into the tail vein. After 1 minute the mouse was killed and the tail, tumours and selected tissues were excised and weighed in individual tubes. The radioactivity of each tissue was counted in a gamma-counter (1282 CompuGamma Gamma Counter, LKB Wallac) over a 15 minute period, or until 1000 counts were measured, and the % injected activity in 1 gram of tissue was calculated by comparing with the activity of 100 µl aliquots of the isotope. Where more than 20% of the injected activity remained in the tail, the results were discarded and not included in any analysis.

RESULTS

Throughout the period of anaemia, haematocrit values remained below 30% with no significant variations (Figure 1). The distribution of the cardiac output to the tumours and other tissues of untreated animals (haematocrit = 42.62 ± 0.50 (SEM), $n = 61$) is shown in table 1. Relative perfusion of the i.d. and abdominal tumours was found to be very similar and significantly lower than the perfusion of the non-neoplastic tissues selected. Preliminary experiments in which blood was withdrawn from the suborbital sinus and retransfused into the tail vein indicated that the exchange transfusion procedure had no significant effect on relative tissue perfusion.

Table 1. Relative perfusion of intradermal and abdominal tumours and several normal tissues in untreated male CBA mice.

Tissue	n	% injected activity/g tissue (mean ± SEM)
id Tumour	61	0.751 ± 0.049
abd Tumour	42	0.727 ± 0.052
Muscle	61	1.864 ± 0.074
Liver	61	2.196 ± 0.108
Kidney	61	22.064 ± 1.025
Spleen	61	1.716 ± 0.088
Gut	54	8.733 ± 0.365

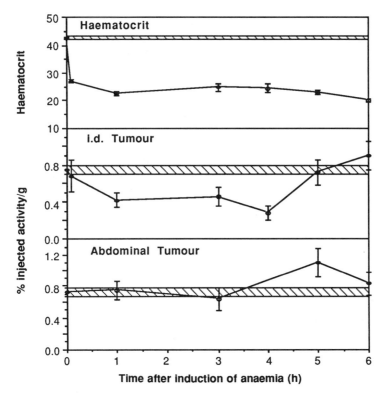

Figure 1. The effect of inducing anaemia on the haematocrit of CBA male mice and the changes in the relative perfusion of intradermal (i.d.) (464 ± 14 mg) and abdominal tumours (648 ± 57 mg) over a period of 6 hours. Shaded areas represent the SEM of control values.

Table 2. Relative perfusion of intradermal tumours, abdominal tumours and several normal tissues 5 minutes, 1, 3, 4, 5 and 6 hours after the induction of anaemia.

Duration of Anaemia	n	Relative Blood Flow (% Control values)						
		Tumours		Normal Tissues				
		Intradermal	Abdominal	Muscle	Liver	Kidney	Spleen	Gut
5 min	11	90.3±22.9	-	44.5±4.9‡	168.4±27.1†	149.1±25.3*	221.1±28.8‡	121.9±13.8
1 h	19	55.8±10.3†	102.6±15.9[1]	70.3±7.0†	121.2±14.1	126.4±11.5*	172.5±21.1‡	91.0±9.2
3 h	9	61.0±13.5*	87.0±20.5	64.6±10.9*	145.8±13.4†	153.5±21.7†	159.6±20.8†	117.8±13.6
4 h	6	37.4±10.1†	-	83.9±7.5	144.3±17.9*	128.0±15.4	190.2±35.6†	-
5 h	17	96.3±18.3	150.9±25.6†[2]	80.9±8.3	144.0±20.3‡	148.1±15.7‡	197.3±26.5‡	118.2±14.2
6 h	15	119.4±20.2	114.8±20.3[3]	86.9±11.6	159.7±22.4†	133.7±24.5	178.2±23.9‡	132.2±19.7

* p < 0.05; † p < 0.01; ‡ p < 0.001
[1] n = 16
[2] n = 11
[3] n = 14

Immediately following the induction of anaemia, there was a sharp decrease in RBF to the gastrocnemius muscle (p < 0.001) and a large increase in the relative perfusion of the liver (p < 0.01), kidney (p < 0.05) and spleen (p < 0.001). Relative perfusion of the i.d. tumour did not change significantly (Table 2). However, 1 hour after the onset of anaemia, the cardiac output distribution to the i.d. tumour was significantly reduced to 55.8 ± 10.34% control values (p < 0.01). The RBF of the muscle was still below normal, but to a lesser extent than immediately following the reduction in the haematocrit. Similarly, the increased perfusion of the liver, kidney and spleen was less marked. The RBF of the abdominal tumour remained at normal levels. The relative perfusion of the i.d. tumours remained low in anaemic mice for up to 5 hours (Figure 1). The distribution of the cardiac output to the abdominal tumours did not vary significantly from control levels except when the mice had been anaemic for 5 hours, by which time the RBF of the i.d. tumours had returned to normal, increasing to 150.85 ± 25.59% control values (p < 0.01). The RBF of the gastrocnemius muscle returned to control levels within 4 hours following the induction of anaemia, whilst the relative perfusion of the liver, kidney and spleen remained elevated throughout the 6 hours of induced anaemia (Figure 2). No significant changes in gut perfusion were noted in anaemic conditions (Table 2).

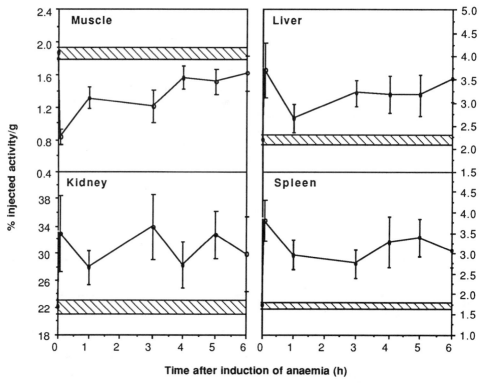

Figure 2. Changes in the relative perfusion of several non-cancerous tissues during a 6 hour period of induced anaemia.

DISCUSSION

Induction of acute anaemia in tumour-bearing mice produces several changes in the distribution of the cardiac output over a 6 hour period. Initially, there is a homeostatic response resulting in an increase in the relative blood flow to the liver, kidney and spleen at the expense of muscle perfusion. This is followed by a period where the relative perfusion of the muscle is re-established to pre-anaemic levels at a cost to the percentage of the cardiac output being directed to the i.d. tumour. Within 6 hours, the relative perfusion of all tissues and both tumours returns to control values indicating a short-term effect, despite the haematocrit remaining below 30%. This indicates that there are several adaptive responses affecting the systemic and tumour circulation during the first 6 hours of acute anaemia.

Anaemia results in a reduction in the O_2 carrying capacity of the blood. Thus, in order to maintain the supply of O_2 to tissues, tissue perfusion must increase, and, in the case of those vital organs in which RBF was measured, this was found to occur immediately after anaemia had been induced. Since the relative perfusion of some tissues increases, the percentage of the cardiac output reaching less vital tissues is likely to be reduced, as was seen in the gastrocnemius muscle. This effect appears to be fully compensated for within 6 hours, so that relative perfusion returns to pre-anaemic values. The fact that the haematocrit is still low suggests that either the cardiac output is significantly raised, so that absolute blood flow is greater than normal, or that the concentration of 2,3-diphosphoglycerate (2,3-DPG) in the red cells has been increased sufficiently to improve tissue O_2 extraction. However, increases in 2,3-DPG don't occur until 24 - 48 hours after the exposure of mice to low O_2 tensions (Siemann *et al.*, 1979).

The reduced perfusion of the i.d. tumour during the first few hours of anaemia suggests that the hypoxic fraction of the tumour should be increased under anaemic conditions. A decrease in O_2 delivery to the tumour means that fewer cells around the tumour vessels can be supported, resulting in an increase in the resistance of the tumour to radiotherapy. Such an effect has been demonstrated in several other murine tumours (Hirst *et al.*, 1984; Siemann *et al.*, 1975).

It has been suggested that the return to tumour control sensitivity whilst the haematocrit remains low may reflect the rate of death of the hypoxic cells furthest from the tumour vessels (Hirst *et al.*, 1984). However, recent work has demonstrated that the tumour cord radius, i.e. the thickness of the viable tumour cells surrounding the blood vessels, does not vary significantly over a 48 hour period following the induction of anaemia (Hirst *et al.*, 1991*a*). Consequently another mechanism must be operating and this appears to be a blood flow effect, since the return of tumour perfusion to pre-anaemic levels would re-establish tumour oxygenation, thereby reducing the hypoxic fraction.

The lack of response of the relative perfusion of the abdominal tumours to anaemia indicates that tumour response is site dependent. The response of NT tumours implanted in i.d., intra-abdominal and intramuscular sites to various vasoactive drugs has also been shown to affect the relative perfusion of each tumour in different ways (Hirst *et al.*, 1991*b*). Consequently, the response of tumours to reductions in haematocrit cannot always be predicted. Thus tumour site is an important factor when considering how anaemia might affect the outcome of radiotherapy.

Acknowledgement

This work is supported entirely by the Cancer Research Campaign.

REFERENCES

Hirst, D.G., Hazelhurst, J.L. and Brown, J.M., 1984, The effect of alterations in haematocrit on tumour sensitivity to X-rays, *Int. J. Radiat. Biol.* 46:345.

Hirst, D.G., Hirst, V.K., Joiner, B., Prise, V.E. and Shaffi, K.M., 1991, Changes in tumour morphology with alterations in oxygen availability: further evidence for oxygen as a limiting substrate, *Br. J. Cancer* 64:54.

Hirst, D.G., Hirst, V.K., Shaffi, K.M., Prise, V.E. and Joiner, B., 1991, The influence of vasoactive agents on the perfusion of tumours growing in three sites in the mouse, *Int. J. Radiat. Biol.* 60:211.

Sapirstein, L.A., 1958, Regional blood flow by functional distribution of indicators, *Am. J. Physiol.* 193:161.

Siemann, D.W., Bronskill, M.J., Hill, R.P. and Bush, R.S., 1975, The effect of chronic reductions in the arterial partial pressure of oxygen on the radiation response of an experimental tumour, *Br. J. Radiol.* 48:662.

Siemann, D.W., Hill, R.P., Bush, R.S. and Chabra, P., 1979, The in vivo radiation response of an experimental tumor: the effect of exposing tumor-bearing mice to a reduced oxygen environment prior to but not during irradiation, *Int. J. Radiat. Oncol. Biol. Phys.* 5:61.

INTERMITTENT BLOOD FLOW IN THE CANT AND CARH TUMOURS IN TWO DIFFERENT SITES

Carrie E. Peters

CRC Gray Laboratory
PO Box 100
Mount Vernon Hospital
Northwood, Middx.   HA6 2JR

INTRODUCTION

Based on both his own studies of tumour cell radioresistance and those of others, Brown (1979) suggested that solid tumours contained a population of transiently, acutely hypoxic cells.   This was in addition to the tumour cells that are chronically hypoxic because they are beyond the diffusion distance of oxygen from blood vessels. Previously, Reinhold et al. (1977) and Intaglietta et al. (1977) observed in sandwich tumours that blood flow slowed down or stopped temporarily, which Brown proposed as the mechanism behind both transient acute hypoxia and reoxygenation in tumours. Hypoxia resulting from transient nonperfusion of blood vessels in solid tumours was first demonstrated by Chaplin et al. (1986, 1987).   Temporal heterogeneity in tumour blood flow may have important implications for both radiotherapy and chemotherapy (Coleman, 1988).   If a proportion of the tumour cells is hypoxic at the time of irradiation, the efficacy of radiotherapy will be reduced.   Alternatively, the delivery of blood-borne chemotherapeutic agents will be compromised if there are some nonperfused vessels within the tumour.   Due to its potential importance to therapy, a detailed examination of the incidence of intermittent blood flow in solid tumours is needed.

It is possible that the level of vessel nonperfusion varies with tumour type. Nonperfusion may also be influenced by the transplantation site of the experimental tumour. Past histological studies have looked at intermittent perfusion in subcutaneous and intramuscular tumours only (Chaplin and Trotter, 1991; Horsman et al., 1990; Trotter et al., 1989; Zwi et al., 1989). Using a histological double-staining technique developed by Trotter et al. (1989), I have compared the level of vessel nonperfusion in two adenocarcinomas with different growth characteristics. I have also compared vessel nonperfusion in tumours grown in two different sites; intradermally and non-superficially on the caecum.

Oxygen Transport to Tissue XV, Edited by P. Vaupel
et al., Plenum Press, New York, 1994

METHODS

Mice and Tumour

The CaNT adenocarcinoma was grown intradermally over the sacral region of the back and internally on the caecum in female CBA mice. The CaRH adenocarcinoma was grown in the same two sites in female Wht mice. The two tumours were chosen for contrast; the CaNT tumour is rapidly-growing and poorly differentiated, while the CaRH tumour is slowly-growing and moderately differentiated.

For growing intradermal tumours, a donor tumour was mechanically digested and a cell suspension prepared with saline. Recipient mice were anaesthetized with metofane and 0.05 ml of suspension was injected over the sacral region using a 27 gauge needle.

The technique for growing tumours on the caecum of the gut has been developed recently in our laboratory and is fully described elsewhere (Hirst et al, in press). Briefly, a donor tumour was cut into 1 mm^3 pieces. The recipient mouse was anaesthetized with metofane, an incision was made on the left abdominal wall, and the caecum was withdrawn from the body cavity. A circle of 0.22 μm millipore filter paper carrying a piece of tumour was placed tumour side down onto the exposed caecum, and secured with several drops of histoacryl tissue adhesive (Davis and Geck). After allowing the adhesive to dry for one minute, the caecum was replaced in the body cavity. The abdominal wall was sutured and the skin opening was closed with autoclips.

Tumours were used when they were between 300 and 800 mg in size. For the CaNT tumour this was approximately 3 weeks after transplantation. The CaRH tumour took 8 to 14 weeks to reach the appropriate size.

Double-Staining

A double-staining technique as developed by Trotter et. al. (1989) was used to visualize intermittent blood flow within the tumours. Hoechst 33342 (Sigma) was dissolved at 9 mg/ml in sterile saline, and sonicated to ensure complete dissolution. DiOC$_7$(3) was dissolved at 0.6 mg/ml in 75% DMSO 25% saline. For experiments in which the stains were given simultaneously, they were made up together in the DMSO/saline solution at the above concentrations.

Hoechst 33342 was injected intravenously at a dose of 15 mg/kg. After twenty or sixty minutes, DiOC$_7$(3) was injected intravenously at a dose of 1 mg/kg. Alternatively, the stains were given simultaneously at the above doses in a single intravenous injection. Five minutes after injection of DiOC$_7$(3) the mouse was sacrificed, and the tumour excised, weighed, and frozen in OCT embedding compound. 10μm thick tumour sections were examined using a fluorescence microscope; Hoechst was visualized using a 400 nm filter and DiOC$_7$(3) with a 510 nm filter. 400 to 1000 vessels were counted in a random cross section of each tumour. Perfusion mismatch, that is the percentage of vessels in a tumour section stained with only one of the two dyes, was determined.

Statistics

The student's unpaired t-test was used to compare groups of data.

RESULTS

The percentage perfusion mismatch versus size was examined for each combination of the tumour, site, and time between stains and the R^2 value describing the fit of the data to a straight line was calculated (data not shown). For the CaNT tumour, $R^2 \leq 0.14$ for both sites and all time combinations. For the CaRH tumour $R^2 \leq 0.16$ for all time combinations in sacral tumours. However, for CaRH tumours grown on the caecum, R^2 was between 0.5 and 0.6. This was likely due to the low number of animals used (4-6). The slopes of all the curves were ≤ 0.02 in absolute value, indicating no relationship between the level of perfusion mismatch and tumour size for 300 to 800 mg tumours.

Perfusion mismatch in the CaNT tumour is shown in Figure 1. Levels of perfusion mismatch are significantly higher when the stains are given 20 or 60 minutes apart than when they are given simultaneously, regardless of site ($p<.05$ for all cases). The level of perfusion mismatch does not vary significantly if the stains are given 20 or 60 minutes apart. Perfusion mismatch tends to be higher for tumours grown on the caecum than for intradermal tumours, but there is no significant difference for any individual time point between tumours grown in the two different sites.

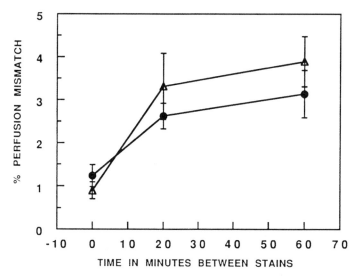

Figure 1. Perfusion mismatch (±s.e.m.) in the CaNT tumour. ● sacral tumours Δ caecum tumours

Perfusion mismatch in the CaRH tumour is shown in Figure 2. Levels of perfusion mismatch are not significantly different between any time points in either sacral tumours or those grown on the caecum. As for the CaNT tumours, perfusion mismatch tends to be higher in caecum than in intradermal tumours, but none of the individual points show a significant difference.

For any given tumour site and time between stains, there was no significant difference between CaNT and CaRH tumours.

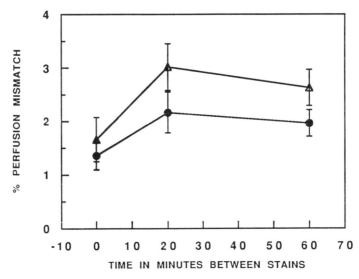

Figure 2. Perfusion mismatch (±s.e.m.) in the CaRH tumour. ● sacral tumours △ caecum tumours

DISCUSSION

Transient nonperfusion occurs in the CaNT tumour. Using the double-staining technique, similar levels of tumour vessel nonperfusion were detected whether the two stains were given 20 or 60 minutes apart, and were significantly higher than when the stains were administered simultaneously. (The perfusion mismatch seen when stains are administered simultaneously indicates the level of error inherent in the method.) In the CaRH tumour, levels of nonperfusion appeared higher when the stains were given separately than when they were given simultaneously, but the differences were not found to be statistically significant. This may reflect that fact that fewer experiments were performed with the CaRH tumour, particularly with caecum tumours, or that transient nonperfusion does not occur universally.

Transient nonperfusion has not, in fact, been found in all tumour types examined (Table 1). Using the histological double-staining technique or a modification, six other tumours have been examined. The level of perfusion mismatch found varies between 9% in the SCCVII tumour to no detectable levels in the Colon 38 and EMT-6/Ak tumours. The CaNT and CaRH tumours fall within the range of perfusion mismatch found in other tumours.

There was no significant difference between the level of perfusion mismatch in the two different tumours for any combination of transplantation site and time between stains. This is despite the fact that the CaNT tumour grows much more rapidly than the CaRH tumour (3 weeks versus 8-14 weeks to reach experimental size), and the CaNT tumour is very poorly differentiated, while the CaRH tumour is moderately differentiated.

No correlation was found between the level of perfusion mismatch and tumour size in either tumour or site. Thus, tumours between 300 and 800 mg are all suitable for examining intermittent perfusion and its modification using this method. Previous work by Trotter (1990) using the SCCVII tumour transplanted subcutaneously did show a relationship between tumour size and the level of perfusion mismatch over a larger size range (Table 1). Transient nonperfusion was very low in tumours smaller than 200 mg and increased with increasing tumour size up to 500 mg. However, it is doubtful that there were significant differences between tumours in the 300 to 800 mg size range.

Table 1. Perfusion Mismatch in Different Tumours

TUMOUR	SITE	SIZE (mg)	NUMBER	TIME	% MISMATCH
SCCVII	sc	100-200	n/a	20 min	4.2±1.7(SD)*
	sc	200-400	n/a	20 min	5.1±3.1(SD)*
	sc	400-600	n/a	20 min	8.6±2.9(SD)*
	sc	600-800	n/a	20 min	8.4±2.8(SD)*
	sc	500-1000	25	20 min	8.9±2.4(SD)**
	im	500-1000	14	20 min	6.6±6.0(SD)*
FaDu	sc	n/a	6	20 min	3.68±2.67(SD)†
Na11	sc	n/a	8	20 min	6.80±4.41(SD)†
C3H/Tif	foot	200 mm3	7	20 min	7.73††
Colon 38	sc	200-900	3	60 min	0†††
EMT-6/Ak	im	200-900	3	60 min	0†††
CaNT	id	300-800	14	20 min	2.6±0.3(sem)
	caecum	300-800	8	20 min	3.3±0.8(sem)
CaRH	id	300-800	11	20 min	2.2±0.4(sem)
	caecum	300-800	6	20 min	3.0±0.4(sem)

FaDu = head and neck squamous cell carcinoma; Na11 = malignant melanoma; Both are human tumour xenografts grown in athymic nude mice. sc=subcutaneous grown over sacral region of back; im=intramuscular; id=intradermal; caecum=on caecum portion of gut.
*Trotter, 1990; **Trotter et al, 1989; †Chaplin and Trotter, 1991; ††Horsman et al, 1990; †††Zwi et al, 1989.

The level of perfusion mismatch did not vary significantly with transplantation site, although it tended to be higher in the caecum tumours for both CaNT and CaRH tumours. Thus tumours in either transplantation site may be appropriate for studying the heterogeneity of vessel perfusion.

Both the CaNT and the CaRH adenocarcinomas exhibit low levels of perfusion mismatch. The level of perfusion mismatch did not vary with size for tumours between 300 and 800 mg, nor did it vary with transplantation site. Despite variable growth characteristics, the level of perfusion mismatch also did not vary between the two tumours. Thus either tumour, in either site, would be a suitable model for further investigation of heterogeneous vessel perfusion.

Although transient nonperfusion has been demonstrated in a variety of murine tumours and in two human tumour xenografts, whether or not it occurs in human tumours *in situ* is unknown. If tumour blood vessel perfusion is heterogeneous in humans, both radiotherapy and chemotherapy may be compromised. In the first case, acutely hypoxic cells resulting from the temporary nonperfusion of nearby blood vessels will be radioresistant. In the latter case, chemotherapeutic drugs may not reach all tumour cells if sections of the vasculature are not perfused. However, the importance of transient nonperfusion and the resultant acute hypoxia, even in murine tumours, remains unclear. More work is required to determine the magnitude of its importance, relative to other factors such as chronic hypoxia, to therapy.

ACKNOWLEDGMENTS

I wish to thank Dr. David Chaplin, Dr. Gillian Tozer, and Dr. David Hirst for helpful discussions and comments. This work is supported entirely by the Cancer Research Campaign.

REFERENCES

Brown, J.M., 1979, Evidence for acutely hypoxic cells in mouse tumours, and a possible mechanism of reoxygenation. *Br. J. Radiol.* 52:650.

Chaplin, D.J., Durand, R.E., and Olive, P.L., 1986, Acute hypoxia in tumours: implications for modifiers of radiation effects. *Int. J. Radiat Oncol. Biol. Phys.* 12:1279.

Chaplin, D.J., Olive, P.L., and Durand, R.E., 1987, Intermittent blood flow in a murine tumour: radiobiological effects. *Cancer Res.* 47:597.

Chaplin, D.J. and Trotter, M.J., 1991, Chemical modifiers of tumour blood flow, *in* "Tumor Blood Supply and Metabolic Microenvironment. Characterization and Implications for Therapy," P. Vaupel and R.K. Jain, eds., Gustav Fischer Verlag: Stuttgart.

Coleman, C.N., 1988, Hypoxia in tumours: a paradigm for the approach to biochemical and physiologic heterogeneity. *J. Natl.Cancer Inst.* 80:310.

Hirst, D.G., Joiner, B., and Hirst, V.K., in press, Blood flow modification by nicotinamide and metoclopramide in mouse tumours growing in different sites. *Br. J. Cancer*

Horsman, M.R., Chaplin, D.J., and Overgaard, J., 1990, Combination of nicotinamide and hyperthermia to eliminate radioresistant chronically and acutely hypoxic tumour cells. *Cancer Res.* 50:7430.

Intaglietta, M., Myers, R.R., Gross, J.F., and Reinhold, H.S., 1977, Dynamics of microvascular flow in implanted mouse mammary tumours. *Bibl. Anat.* 15:273.

Reinhold, H.S., Blachiwiecz, B., and Blok,A., 1977, Oxygenation and reoxygenation in"sandwich" tumours. *Bibl. Anat.* 15:270.

Trotter, M.J., Chaplin, D.J., Durand, R.E., and Olive, P.L., 1989, The use of fluorescent probes to identify regions of transient perfusion in murine tumours. *Int. J. Radiat. Oncol. Biol. Phys.* 16:31.

Trotter, M.J., 1990, Intermittent Tumour Blood Flow, PhD. Thesis, University of British Columbia, Canada.

Zwi, L. J., Baguley, B.C., Gavin, J.B., and Wilson, W.R., 1989, Blood flow failure as a major determinant in the antitumour action of flavone acetic acid. *J. Natl Cancer Inst.* 81:1005.

CORRELATION BETWEEN REGIONAL ATP AND BLOOD FLOW IN TUMORS AND SURROUNDING NORMAL TISSUE

S. Walenta[1], M. Dellian[2], A.E. Goetz[3], and W. Mueller-Klieser[1]

[1] Institute of Physiology and Pathophysiology
University of Mainz, D-6500 Mainz, Germany

[2] Institute of Surgical Research and [3]Institute of Anesthesiology
Ludwig-Maximilians-University, D-8000 Munich, Germany

INTRODUCTION

Various experimental and human tumors are characterized by a marked heterogeneity in the pathophysiologic micromilieu (1, 2). An inadequate and heterogeneous nutritional blood supply has been suggested to explain the non-uniform distribution of oxygen, pH, and high energy phosphates as it has been observed by many investigators (3, 4). Although there is a distinct understanding of the general interrelationships between these parameters (5), little is known about their actual regional correlation, which cannot be assessed by global measurements. With the autoradiographic method for measurement of blood flow (6, 7) and the metabolic imaging with ATP-induced bioluminescence (8, 9) it has become possible to evaluate the distribution of these physiological parameters in cryosections at an almost cellular level. In the present study both methods were combined to correlate regional blood flow with ATP values in the amelanotic hamster melanoma A-Mel-3. Locoregional measurements were obtained in mostly viable and mostly necrotic tumor areas, and in adjacent normal tissue as classified by histological investigation.

MATERIALS AND METHODS

Initiation of Tumor Growth and Preparation of the Animals

Experiments were carried out on 71 tumors of the amelanotic hamster melanoma A-Mel-3 (10). Tumor growth was initiated by implanting 5×10^6 cells subcutaneously into the dorsum of male Syrian golden hamsters. At a median tumor volume of around 150 mm^3 animals were anesthetized (Na-pentobarbital, i.p., 60 mg/kg), and the common carotid artery and jugular vein were cannulated. An additional catheter in the femoral artery served for continuous monitoring of arterial blood pressure.

Blood Flow Measurements

Blood flow was measured with an autoradiographic method (6, 7) using the tissue uptake of the inert and readily diffusible radioactive tracer 4-N-methyl-^{14}C-iodoantipyrine (IAP, NEC 712; Du Pont NEN, Dreieich, Germany). 40 µCi IAP in 500 µl saline was injected into the jugular vein, and blood samples of 15-25 µl were withdrawn from the carotid artery every 5 s for a period of 30 s. Then tumors were surgically removed from the animals and immediately frozen in liquid nitrogen. IAP concentrations in the blood samples were determined by a liquid scintillation counter (Rack Beta 1219; LKB Wallace, Turku, Finland). For autoradiographic measurements of regional blood flow, 20 µm thick cryosections were made that were picked up on a glass cover slip and put on an autoradiographic film (NMC, Kodak, Rochester, N.Y.) together with ^{14}C-methylmethacrylate standards (Amersham Buchler GmbH, Braunschweig, Germany). After an exposure of 14 days and conventional processing, autoradiographs were registered with a CCD-camera (XC-77; Sony, Cologne, Germany) and calibrated with a specially designed image analysis system (IBAS 2.0; Kontron, Eching, Germany). By taking into account the blood concentration and the blood/tissue partition coefficient of IAP, the volume-related blood flow [ml/(100g min)] could be derived from the calibrated autoradiographs.

ATP Determination

Images of the ATP distribution in the melanomas were assessed by quantitative bioluminescence and imaging photon counting as described previously (8, 9). Briefly, 5 µm thick cryosections adjacent to those used for autoradiography were picked up on a cover glass and were put upside down on a casting mold that was filled with a frozen solution containing firefly luciferase and luciferin to use the tissue ATP for the luminescence. The light reaction started by raising the temperature above the melting point of the enzyme solution. The emitted photons were registered through a microscope (Axiophot, Zeiss, Oberkochen, Germany) and by a special video system with image analysis (Argus 100, Hamamatsu, Herrsching, Germany). The distribution of light intensity was calibrated in absolute terms (µmole/g wet weight) using appropriate standards.

Histological Investigations

Cryosections adjacent to those used for autoradiography and bioluminescence were stained with hematoxylin and eosin, allowing for the differentiation of viable and necrotic tumor areas. In general, the tumor area was surrounded by normal tissue, consisting of skin, muscle, fatty tissue, and connective tissue. Using a scanning pattern of $30 \times 30 \ \mu m^2$ squares, the mostly viable tumor area of the sections was expressed as a relative part of the total tumor area. By overlaying the histological section with the images obtained, the median ATP and blood flow values in mostly viable or mostly necrotic areas of the tumor and in surrounding normal tissue were evaluated.

RESULTS

The data presented in this paper are based on 71 animals. The mean volume of the tumors entering the study was $147 \pm 7 \ mm^3$, possessing a mean viable tumor fraction of $72 \pm 3 \ \%$. Fig. 1 summarizes median $\pm$ standard error of the median of blood flow (a) and ATP (b) data obtained in the tumors investigated. There was no significant difference between the blood flow values obtained in the total tumor area and the surrounding normal tissue (35.0 ± 2.9 and 35.0 ± 3.0 ml/(100g min), respectively), whereas the mostly viable tumor parts showed significantly higher blood perfusion rates than the former data (42.1 ± 3.4 ml/(100g min). In contrast, very low blood flow values were measured in the mostly necrotic parts of the tumors. Registered ATP concentrations were significantly higher in normal tissue, compared to tumor data. Mostly viable tumor areas consisted of higher, mostly necrotic tumor areas of lower ATP values, compared to the values obtained for the total tumor.

The correlation of ATP and blood flow values in designated tissue areas is depicted in Fig.2. Each dot represents data averaged over one individual tumor. A significant correlation, as expressed by the SPEARMAN rank correlation coefficient, could be found in the total tumor (a), the surrounding normal tissue (b), and the mostly viable tumor (c). There was no significant correlation between these parameters in mostly necrotic tumor areas (d).

DISCUSSION AND SUMMARY

Nutritional blood flow and high-energy phosphate content have been proposed to be of significant importance in tumor response to treatment (1, 11, 12). The interrelation of both parameters has been studied in differently sized tumors, in tumors of identical volume after treatment and within experimental brain tumors (13, 14, 15). These global

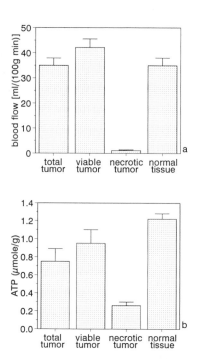

Fig.1. Median (a) blood flow [ml/(100g min)] and (b) ATP (µmole/g) values ± standard error of the median in designated tissue areas of A-Mel-3 tumors.

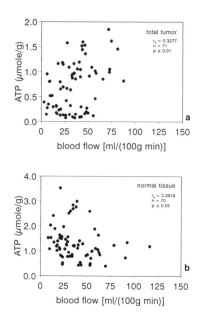

Fig.2a+b. Correlation of the local ATP concentration as a function of the local blood flow in designated tissue areas of A-Mel-3 tumors: (a) total tumor, (b) normal tissue, (Each dot represents the values of an individual tumor; r_S: SPEARMAN rank correlation coefficient)

measurements, however, do not reveal any information about the intra-tumor variability of the parameters in relation to the histology.

In the present study the autoradiographic visualization of blood flow and ATP imaging bioluminescence of consecutive tumor sections was combined with histological investigations and subsequent digital image processing and analysis. Tumor sections

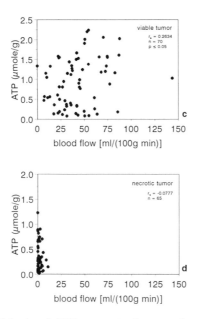

Fig.2c+d. Correlation of the local ATP concentration as a function of the local blood flow in designated tissue areas of A-Mel-3 tumors: (c) mostly viable tumor proportion , (d) mostly necrotic tumor proportion.

adjacent to those used for the imaging techniques were stained with hematoxylin and eosin, and subsequently classified into normal tissue, mostly viable and mostly necrotic tumor tissue, respectively. The histological pattern obtained was overlaid on the ATP and blood flow images, allowing for the regional evaluation of the local ATP concentration and the local blood flow in designated tissue areas.

A significant correlation was found between overall ATP and blood flow values regarding total tumor areas, as expressed by SPEARMAN′s rank correlation coefficient r_s. A weaker correlation was registered in viable tumor areas and in surrounding normal tissue, whereas these parameters were uncorrelated in mostly necrotic parts of the tumors (Fig.2). Mostly necrotic tumor regions had both lower flow and ATP values than mostly viable tissue areas. In contrast, the statistically significant correlation between ATP and perfusion in the normal tissue was somewhat weaker. This may be due to the variable composition of different tissue types in the respective normal tissue area. Nevertheless, the pronounced variation of the data does not allow a prediction for one individual tumor.

The data provide evidence for the viability and the energetic state of cancer cells being strongly influenced by the efficiency of the tumor microcirculation in several but not in all malignancies investigated. The experimental procedure established in the present study may therefore be used to evaluate the amenability of tumor microcirculation and energetic state to manipulation for the improvement of cancer therapy.

ACKNOWLEDGEMENTS. Supported by the Bundesministerium fuer Forschung und Technologie (01 ZO 8801 and 0706903A5) and by the Kurt-Koerber-Stiftung

REFERENCES

1. Vaupel, P., Kallinowski, F., and Okunieff, P., Blood flow, oxygen, and nutrient supply, and metabolic microenvironment of human tumors: a review. *Cancer Res.*, 49: 6449 (1989).
2. Jain, R. K., Determinants of tumor blood flow: a review. *Cancer Res.*, 48: 2641 (1988).
3. Mueller-Klieser, W., Schaefer, C., Walenta, S., Rofstad, E. K., Fenton, B. M., and Sutherland, R. M., Assessment of tumor energy and oxygenation status by bioluminescence, nuclear magnetic resonance spectroscopy, and cryospectrophotometry. *Cancer Res.*, 50: 1681 (1990).
4. Tozer, G. M., Lewis, S., Michalowski, A., and Aber, V., The relationship between regional variations in blood flow and histology in a transplanted rat fibrosarcoma. *Br. J. Cancer*, 61: 250 (1990).
5. Atkinson, D. E., Cellular Energy Metabolism and its Regulation. Academic Press, New York (1977).
6. Kety, S., Measurement of local blood flow by the exchange of an inert, diffusible substance. *Methods Med. Res.* 8: 228 (1960).
7. Sakurada, O., Kennedy, C., Jehle, J., Brown, J. D., Carbin, G. L., and Sokoloff, L., Measurement of local cerebral blood flow with iodo(^{14}C)antipyrine. *Am. J. Physiol.*, 234: H59 (1978).
8. Mueller-Klieser, W., Walenta S., Paschen, W., Kallinowski, F., and Vaupel, P., Metabolic imaging in microregions of tumors and normal tissues with bioluminescence and photon counting. *J. Natl. Cancer Inst.*, 80:842 (1988).
9. Walenta, S., Doetsch, J., and Mueller-Klieser, W., ATP concentrations in multicellular tumor spheroids

assessed by single photon imaging and quantitative bioluminescence. *Eur. J. Cell Biol.*, 52: 389 (1990).

10. Fortner, J. G., Mahy, A. G., and Schrodt, G. R., Transplantable tumors of the Syrian (Golden) hamster. Part I: Tumors of the alimentary tract, endocrine glands, and melanomas. *Cancer Res.*, 21: 161 (1961).

11. Denekamp, J., Hill, S., and Hobsen, B., Vascular occlusion and tumor cell death. *Eur. J. Cancer Clin. Oncol.* 19:271 (1983).

12. Horsman, M. R., Chaplin, D. J., and Overgaard, J., The use of blood flow modifiers to improve the treatment response of solid tumors. *Radiother. Oncol.* 20 (Suppl.1):47 (1991).

13. Vaupel, P., Okunieff, P., and Neuringer, L. J., Blood flow, tissue oxygenation, pH distribution, and energy metabolism of murine mammary adenocarcinomas during growth. *Adv. Exp. Med. Biol.* 248:835 (1989).

14. Lilly, M. B., Katholi, C. R., and Ng, T. C., Direct relationship between high-energy phosphate content and blood flow in thermally treated murine tumors. *J. Natl. Cancer Inst.* 75:885 (1985).

15. Mies, G., Paschen, W., Ebhardt, G., and Hossmann, K.-A., Relationship between blood flow, glucose metabolism, protein synthesis, glucose and ATP content in experimentally induced glioma (RG1 2.2) of rat brain. *J. Neuro-Oncol.*, 9: 17 (1990).

THE EFFECT OF NICOTINAMIDE ON MICROCIRCULATORY FUNCTION, TISSUE OXYGENATION AND BIOENERGETIC STATUS IN RAT TUMORS

Debra K. Kelleher and Peter Vaupel

Institute of Physiology and Pathophysiology
University of Mainz, D-6500 Mainz, Germany

INTRODUCTION

The failure of many attempts to improve tumor oxygenation - and thus the outcome of standard radiotherapy - may be due to the fact that the occurrence of hypoxia in tumors is not solely a result of diffusion-limited "chronic" hypoxia but is also due to temporary flow cessations in microregional tumor perfusion which have been shown to occur in tumor tissue[1]. As a result, attempts have more recently been made to reduce hypoxia in tumors through the reduction of tumor perfusion fluctuations. The benzamide analog nicotinamide is an agent which has recently received attention in this respect. It has been reported to be an effective, tumor-specific radiosensitizer in several tumor models, an effect thought to be mediated through an increase in tumor blood perfusion[2]. To date, little is known about the mechanism by which nicotinamide brings about its radiosensitizing effect. The aim of this study therefore was to investigate nicotinamide-induced changes in tumor and muscle microcirculatory function, tumor oxygenation, and tumor and muscle metabolism in an attempt to try and elucidate possible mechanisms for nicotinamide's actions.

MATERIALS AND METHODS

Animals and Tumors

Sprague Dawley rats (200 - 350 g) were used in this study. They received a standard diet and water *ad libitum*. Tumors were grown subcutaneously after injection of DS-sarcoma ascites cells into the dorsum of the hind foot. Tumors were used in experiments when they reached a volume of approximately 1 ml.

Drugs

Nicotinamide (Sigma Chemical Co., St. Louis, MO.) was dissolved in 0.9 % NaCl to give a 5 % solution (freshly prepared before each experiment) and administered intraperitoneally (i.p.) at a dose of 500 mg/kg over a 10 min infusion period. Control animals received an equivalent volume of 0.9 % NaCl (10 ml/kg).

Surgical Procedures

When the tumors had reached the desired size, rats were anaesthetized with sodium pentobarbital (40 mg/kg i.p., Nembutal, Ceva, Paris, France). Polyethylene catheters were surgically placed into the thoracic aorta via the left common carotid artery (for measurement of the mean arterial blood pressure, MABP, using a Statham pressure transducer), and i.p. (for administration of test substances). Blood coagulation was prevented by i.v. injection of heparin (350 USP-units/kg). Rectal temperature was maintained at 37.5°C. Arterial blood gas and pH status was monitored using a pH/Blood Gas Analyzer (type 178, Ciba Corning).

Laser Doppler Flowmetry

A Periflux model PF 2B laser Doppler flowmeter (Perimed, Stockholm, Sweden) was used to measure red blood cell flux (RBC flux) in central locations within the tumors or in the hind leg adductor muscle. Data were expressed as relative RBC flux (rel. RBC flux), which represent percentage values related to the RBC flux read-out at the start of the experiments. The additional measurement of total backscattered light served to optimize probe positioning, avoid tissue compression, and ensure a constant probe location.

After the surgical procedure, animals were allowed to stabilize and measurements commenced once constant baseline readings for MABP and RBC flux were obtained for at least 20 min. MABP and RBC flux were then continuously recorded for 10 min before i.p. administration of NaCl or nicotinamide and 120 min thereafter. Subsequently, an arterial blood pressure/laser Doppler flux ratio (MABP/LDF ratio) was estimated. This ratio provides a measure of resistance to flow.

Tumor Oxygen Tension

Tumor O_2 tension values were determined using polarographic needle electrodes (recessed gold in glass electrode; shaft diameter 250 µm; diameter of the cathode 12 µm) and pO_2 histography (model KIMOC-6650, Eppendorf, Hamburg, Germany) as described by Vaupel et al[3]. Measurements were made 60 min following the commencement of nicotinamide or NaCl infusion.

Metabolic and Bioenergetic Status

One hour following the commencement of nicotinamide or NaCl administration, tumors and resting skeletal muscle were rapidly frozen in liquid nitrogen, ground to a fine powder and freeze-dried. After extraction with 0.66 M perchloric acid and neutralisation with 2 M potassium hydroxide, ATP, ADP and AMP concentrations were determined using reverse phase HPLC techniques. Tissue glucose and lactate levels were measured using standard enzymatic assays for tissue extracts (Gluco quant glucose; Lactate, Boehringer-Mannheim, Mannheim, Germany).

Statistical Analysis

Results are expressed as means ± SEM with the numbers of experiments indicated in brackets. Significance was assessed using the paired or unpaired Student's t-test, as appropriate, or in the case of pO_2 histogram comparisons, with the White test.

RESULTS

Intraperitoneal infusion of nicotinamide (500 mg/kg) caused a significant decrease in MABP from a pretreatment value of 125 ± 3 mmHg (8) to a minimum pressure of 94 ± 5 mmHg, 20 min after the start of infusion (p < 0.001), with partial recovery thereafter to 100 ± 3 mmHg at the end of the measurement period. The MABP in control animals receiving a saline infusion did not significantly change (Fig. 1, upper panel).

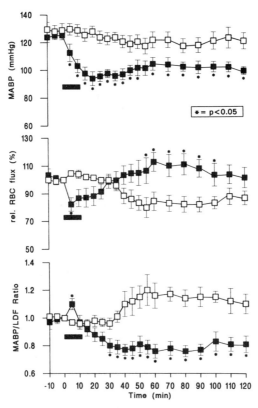

Figure 1. Mean arterial blood pressure (MABP, upper panel), tumor relative red blood cell flux (rel. RBC flux, center panel) and MABP/LDF ratio (lower panel) in DS-sarcoma-bearing rats as a function of time following i.p. administration of nicotinamide (500 mg/kg, n = 8) (■) or 0.9 % NaCl (10 ml/kg, n = 9) (□). The time of i.p. nicotinamide or NaCl infusion is indicated by the black rectangle.

Nicotinamide infusion resulted in an initial rapid decrease in tumor RBC flux which reached a minimum of 82 ± 5 % (8) of the pretreatment value during the first 5 min following the start of infusion. Thereafter, tumor RBC flux steadily rose until it reached a maximum level 113 ± 7 % (8) of the pretreatment value 60 min after the commencement of nicotinamide infusion. Following this peak, tumor RBC flux gradually decreased to pre-infusion levels by the end of the 120 min measurement period (101 ± 7 % (8); Fig. 1, center panel). Since, under control conditions, the tumor RBC flux at t = 60 min was reduced to 84 ± 7 % (7) of the pretreatment value, the effective maximum rise in tumor RBC flux following nicotinamide infusion was approximately 34% (p < 0.05).

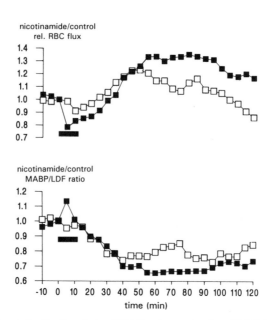

Figure 2. Treatment/control ratios for relative RBC flux (upper panel) and MABP /LDF ratio (lower panel) in adductor muscle (□) and tumor tissue (■) as a function of time. The time of i.p. nicotinamide (500 mg/kg) or 0.9 % NaCl (10 ml/kg) infusion is indicated by the black rectangle. Each point represents ratios obtained from measurements in at least 15 animals.

When these changes in MABP and RBC flux were converted into a pressure-to-flux ratio (MABP/LDF ratio), changes induced by nicotinamide application could again be seen. Following nicotinamide infusion, a short-lived initial rise in the MABP/LDF ratio was observed, followed by a more prolonged fall to values approximately 24% below initial values by 60 min following the start of nicotinamide infusion. This significant reduction in the MABP/LDF ratio was maintained for the remainder of the measuring period. When changes in control animals were taken into account, the effective decrease in MABP/LDF ratios at t = 60 min following nicotinamide infusion was 34% (p < 0.01) (Fig. 1, lower panel). These changes indicate therefore that nicotinamide effectuates a decrease in the resistance to flow within tumor tissue while at the same time increasing tumor blood circulation.

In order to ascertain whether these effects of nicotinamide were preferential or even specific to the tumor circulation, RBC flux was also measured in the adductor muscle of the rat. Similar trends to those seen in tumor tissue were also seen in muscle tissue following i.p. administration of nicotinamide, although the extent of these changes (when considered together with changes seen in the muscle tissue of control animals) was not as pronounced as those seen in tumor tissue. None of the changes in muscle RBC flux were significantly different to control measurements. These results therefore suggest a preferential, but not specific, effect of nicotinamide on tumor circulatory function which reaches its maximum approximately 60 min following nicotinamide application. This preferential effect can be seen in Fig. 2 where treatment/control (nicotinamide treatment/NaCl treatment) ratios are shown for RBC flux and the MABP/LDF ratio in muscle and tumor tissue simultaneously.

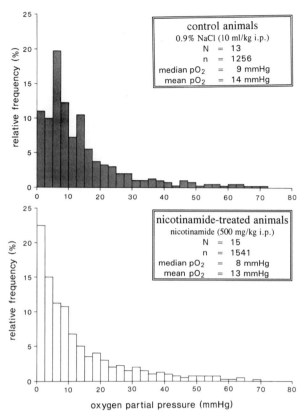

Figure 3. Frequency distributions of oxygen partial pressures (pO_2 histograms) measured in tumors 60 min following 0.9 % NaCl (10 ml/kg i.p., upper panel) or nicotinamide application (500 mg/kg i.p., lower panel). N = number of tumors, n = number of pO_2 measurements.

Table 1. Arterial blood O_2 (pO_2) and CO_2 (pCO_2) tensions and pH values in control (saline-treated) and nicotinamide-treated animals, immediately before drug application (t = 0) and 60 min thereafter (t = 60).

	No. of animals	pO_2 (mmHg)		pCO_2 (mmHg)		pH	
		t=0	t=60	t=0	t=60	t=0	t=60
Control (0.9% NaCl, 10 ml/kg i.p.)	15	79 ± 1	77 ± 1	43 ± 1	38 ± 1	7.44 ± 0.01	7.45 ± 0.01
Nicotinamide (500 mg/kg i.p.)	17	79 ± 1	86 ± 2 p < 0.001	41 ± 1	40 ± 1	7.44 ± 0.01	7.46 ± 0.01

Using computerized pO_2 histography, pO_2 values were recorded in tumor tissue 60 min following i.p. nicotinamide or NaCl application (to coincide with the time of maximum increase in RBC flux seen following nicotinamide administration).

pO_2 frequency distributions from pooled measurements plotted with class widths of 2.5 mmHg are shown in Fig. 3. No significant differences were seen on comparison of pO_2 histograms or mean or median pO_2 values from tumors in nicotinamide- and NaCl-treated animals. Thus although nicotinamide application results in an increased RBC flux through tumor tissue, an associated improvement in tissue oxygenation could not be detected.

Arterial blood gas and pH status from animals in this study, measured immediately before drug application and 60 min thereafter are shown in Table 1. One hour after nicotinamide application, a significant improvement in arterial blood pO_2 ($p < 0.001$) was observed, while no changes were seen in arterial blood pCO_2 and pH.

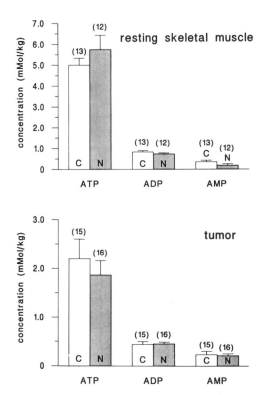

Figure 4. ATP, ADP and AMP concentrations, as measured by HPLC in resting skeletal muscle (upper panel) and tumor tissue (lower panel), 60 min following 0.9 % NaCl (10 ml/kg i.p.; C) or nicotinamide (500 mg/kg i.p.; N) application.

Biochemical analyses were performed in tumors and resting skeletal muscle frozen in liquid nitrogen 60 min following nicotinamide or NaCl treatment. ATP, ADP and AMP concentrations are shown in Fig. 3, glucose and lactate concentrations in Fig. 4. No significant changes were seen in the concentrations of ATP, ADP, AMP or glucose in either tumor or muscle tissue following nicotinamide application. However, lactate concentrations in tumors from animals treated with nicotinamide were found to be significantly higher than those found in tumors from control animals.

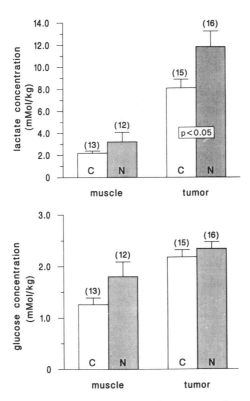

Figure 5. Lactate (upper panel) and glucose (lower panel) concentrations, as measured by standard enzymatic assays in resting skeletal muscle and tumor tissue, 60 min following 0.9 % NaCl (10 ml/kg i.p.; C) or nicotinamide (500 mg/kg i.p.; N) application.

DISCUSSION

This study has shown that nicotinamide induces changes in MABP and microcirculatory function (measured as RBC flux) and increases lactate concentration in tumor tissue. The described changes in RBC flux support findings previously reported by Horsman et al. who observed increases in [86]RbCl uptake and increases in Hoechst 33342 fluorescent labelling in SCCVII/ST carcinomas in mice[4]. The time span over which radiosensitization has been reported to occur correlates temporally with the increase in RBC flux observed[5] This increase in RBC flux through tumor tissue could bring about an increase in O_2 delivery which might explain the radiosensitization brought about by this agent. In the present study however, no improvement in tumor oxygenation could be detected following nicotinamide administration. Since no deterioration (but rather an improvement) in arterial blood pO_2 was seen following nicotinamide application, and since the RBC flux through tumor tissue was significantly increased the amount of oxygen being delivered to the tumor (which is dependent on these two parameters) must also accordingly be increased. It therefore seems possible that the lack of measurable oxygenation improvement in the tumor tissue following nicotinamide application may be the result of an increase in oxygen consumtion within the tumor tissue, which is known to be - up to a "saturation level" - dependent on oxygen availability[6].

A present "working hypothesis" aimed at explaining the alterations in lactate concentrations, seen following nicotinamide application is shown in Fig. 5.

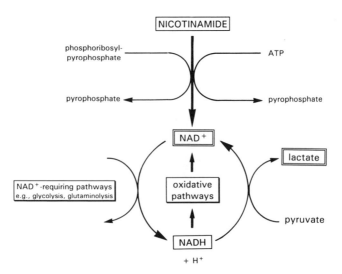

Figure 6. Metabolic pathway explaining the increase in tissue lactate concentration following nicotinamide application.

The first step in this hypothesis, the conversion of nicotinamide to NAD⁺, is supported by the work of Calcutt et al[7]. who showed that nicotinamide injected i.p. into mice, led to an increase in the concentration of NAD⁺ in lymphomas. This increase in NAD⁺ was accompanied by an increased radiosensitization in this tumor line. Were NAD⁺ levels to increase in tissues following nicotinamide application, then NAD⁺-requiring reactions such as glycolysis or glutaminolysis would be stimulated. The NADH thus formed would be reconverted to NAD⁺ in most cells by oxidative pathways or, as characteristically occurs in tumor cells, additionally by the conversion of pyruvate to lactate, thus explaining the higher lactate levels found in tumor but not in skeletal muscle following nicotinamide administration. The reconversion of NADH to NAD⁺, occurring via the oxidative pathways would additionally cause a higher oxygen consumption rate, and therefore, an improvement in tumor oxygenation at a time when RBC flux is increased may not be observed. The mechanism triggering an increase in RBC flux through tumors may be the build up of lactic acid levels within the tumor which would result in a local lactacidosis, and subsequently a local vasodilation, which might be observed as an increase in RBC flux concomitant with a decrease in the MABP/LDF ratio. Further investigations are currently being planned to measure NAD⁺ levels in this tumor model in an attempt to further test this hypothesis.

REFERENCES

1. D.J. Chaplin, P.L. Olive and R.E. Durand. Intermittent blood flow in a murine tumor: Radiobiological effects, *Cancer Res.* 47:597 (1987).
2. M.R. Horsman, D.J. Chaplin and J.M. Brown. Tumor radiosensitization by nicotinamide: a result of improved perfusion and oxygenation, *Radiat. Res.* 118:139 (1989).
3. P. Vaupel, K. Schlenger, C. Knoop and M. Höckel. Oxygenation of human tumors: evaluation of tissue oxygen distribution in breast cancers by computerized O₂ tension measurements. Cancer Res. 51:3316 (1991).
4. M.R. Horsman, D.J. Chaplin, V.K. Hirst, M.J. Lemmon, P.J. Wood, E.P. Dunphy and J. Overgaard. Mechanism of action of the selective tumor radiosensitizer nicotinamide. *Int. J. Radiat. Oncol. Biol. Phys.* 15:685 (1988).
5. M.R. Horsman, P.J. Wood, D.J. Chaplin, J.M. Brown and J. Overgaard. The potentiation of radiation damage by nicotinamide in the SCCVII tumor in vivo. *Radiother. Oncol.* 18:49 (1990).
6. P. Vaupel, H.P. Fortmeyer, S. Runkel and F. Kallinowski. Blood flow, oxygen consumption, and tissue oxygenation of human breast cancer xenografts in nude rats, *Cancer Res.* 47:3496 (1987).
7. G. Calcutt, S.M. Ting and A.W. Preece. Tissue NAD levels and the response to irradiation or cytotoxic drugs, *Br. J. Cancer* 24:380 (1970).

TUMOUR RADIOSENSITIZATION BY NICOTINAMIDE: IS IT THE RESULT OF AN IMPROVEMENT IN TUMOUR OXYGENATION?

Michael R. Horsman, Marianne Nordsmark, Azza Khalil, David J. Chaplin, and Jens Overgaard

Danish Cancer Society
Department of Experimental Clinical Oncology
Nörrebrogade 44
DK - 8000 Aarhus C, Denmark

INTRODUCTION

Nicotinamide is an agent that has been shown to be capable of enhancing radiation damage in a variety of murine tumours with both single and fractionated radiation treatments (Horsman et al., 1989b; Kjellen et al., 1991). The mechanism of action of this drug is not entirely understood, but it has been demonstrated that nicotinamide can increase tumour perfusion (Horsman et al., 1988; 1989a), decrease ^{14}C-misonidazole binding in tumours (Horsman et al., 1988; 1989a), and increase tumour metabolic activity as measured by both biochemical analysis (Horsman et al., 1992), and ^{31}P-NMR (Wood et al., 1991), all of which strongly suggest that nicotinamide works by improving tumour oxygenation at the time of irradiation.

Probably the most clinically applicable method for directly estimating tumour oxygenation is to determine oxygen partial pressure (pO_2) distributions using microelectrodes (Vaupel et al., 1989). In the current study we have used an Eppendorf microelectrode to measure pO_2 levels in a C3H/Tif mouse mammary carcinoma after treatment with nicotinamide, in an attempt to confirm whether or not nicotinamide does improve tumour oxygenation.

MATERIALS AND METHODS

Animal and Tumour Model. All experiments were performed on 10-14 week-old female CDF1 mice. The tumour model used was the C3H/Tif mouse mammary carcinoma. Its derivation and maintenance have been described previously [Overgaard 1980]. Experimental tumours were produced following sterile dissection of large flank tumours. Macroscopically viable tumour tissue was minced with a pair of scissors, and 5-10 μl of this material were injected into the foot of the right hind limb of the experimental animals. This location ensured easy access to the tumour for treatment without involvement of critical normal tissue in the treatment fields. In addition, anaesthetization of the animals during treatment could be avoided. Treatments were carried out when tumours had reached a tumour volume of 200 mm^3, which generally occurred within 2-3 weeks after challenge. Tumour size was determined by the formula: D_1 x D_2 x D_3 x $\pi/6$, (where the D values represent three orthogonal diameters).

Drug Preparation. Nicotinamide (Sigma Chemical Co., St. Louis, MO) was dissolved at a concentration of 50 mg/ml in a sterile saline (0.9% NaCl) solution immediately before each experiment. It was injected intraperitoneally (i.p.) into mice at a constant injection volume of 0.02 ml/g body weight.

Radiation Treatment. Irradiations were given with a conventional therapeutic X-ray machine (250 kV; 15 mA; 2 mm Al filter; 1.1 mm Cu half-value layer; dose rate, 2.3 Gy per min). Dosimetry was accomplished by use of an integrating chamber. All treatments to tumour-bearing feet were administered to non-anaesthetized mice placed in a Lucite jig. Their tumour-bearing legs were exposed and loosely attached to the jig with tape, without impairing the blood supply to the foot. Tumours only were irradiated, the remainder of the animal being shielded by 1 cm of lead. To secure homogeneity of the radiation dose, tumours were immersed in a water bath with about 5 cm of water between the X-ray source and the tumour. Tumour response to treatment involved measuring tumour volume 5 times each week following irradiation and calculating the tumour growth time, which was the time taken for tumours to reach 3 times the treatment volume.

Measurements with the pO$_2$ Histograph. Unanesthetized mice were restrained in Lucite jigs with the tumour-bearing leg exposed and taped to the jig as described earlier. A fine needle autosensitive microelectrode probe (Eppendorf, Hamburg, Germany) was inserted about 1 mm into the tumour and then moved through the tumour in 0.7 mm increments, followed each time by a 0.3 mm backward step prior to measurement. The response time was 1.3 seconds. Parallel repeated insertions were performed in each tumour until a total of 35 to 100 measurements were made. The relative frequency of the pO$_2$ measurements was automatically calculated and displayed as a histogram.

RESULTS

The effect of nicotinamide on the response of a C3H/Tif mouse mammary carcinoma to radiation is illustrated in Figure 1. Nicotinamide clearly enhances the radiation effect with the maximal sensitization occurring between 30-120 minutes following drug injection.

Figure 2 illustrates typical pO$_2$ histograms obtained in this tumour model in control animals or 90 minutes after nicotinamide injection. The various pO$_2$ parameters obtained from this data are summarized in Figure 3, along with the results for other time intervals up to 150 minutes after administration of the drug. It is clear that this large single dose of nicotinamide has no apparent influence on the pO$_2$ values less than or equal to 5 mmHg, nor on the median and mean pO$_2$ results.

Table 1 summarizes all the available data relevant to the mechanism of the nicotinamide affect in this C3H/Tif mouse mammary carcinoma. The enhancement of radiation damage by nicotinamide 30 to 120 minutes after drug injection is significant. Nicotinamide, however, has no significant influence on tumour pO$_2$ measurements, nor on tumour perfusion estimated using the RbCl uptake procedure. On the other hand, there is an increase in tumour metabolic activity shown by the ratio of ATP to inorganic phosphate (Pi), as well as a significant decrease in fluorescent staining mismatch. This latter assay involved a histological fluorescent staining technique to visualise tumour vasculature at 2

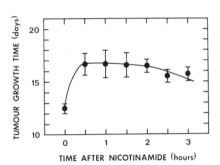

Figure 1. Modification of the radiation response of a C3H/Tif mouse mammary carcinoma by nicotinamide. Mice were injected with nicotinamide (1000 mg/kg; i.p.) at various times before local tumour irradiation with 15 Gy X-rays. Results show means (± 1 S.E.) of the time taken for tumours to regrow to 3 times the treatment volume.

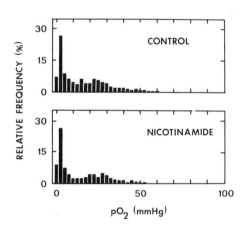

Figure 2. Representative pO_2 histograms showing the oxygen profiles from C3H/Tif mouse mammary carcinomas in either control mice or 90 minutes after injection with nicotinamide (1000 mg/kg; i.p.).

intervals in time. Histological tumour sections were prepared from mice which had been injected with 2 fluorescent stains separated by an interval of 20 minutes. Vessels shown to be stained with one stain but not both were recorded as mismatched. The results demonstrated that almost 8% of vessels in this tumour were functional at one time but not the other, but after nicotinamide treatment only about 3% of vessels showed these transient stoppages in blood flow.

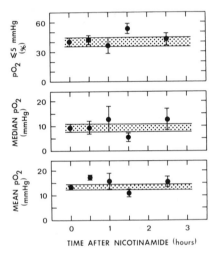

Figure 3. Effect of nicotinamide on tumour oxygenation. Measurements of pO_2 were made in C3H/Tif mouse mammary carcinomas at different times after nicotinamide (1000 mg/kg; i.p.) injection and from data similar to that of Figure 2 the pO_2 values less than or equal to 5 mmHg, median pO_2 and mean pO_2 were determined. Results show mean values ($\pm$ 1 S.E.). The shaded region represents control mice.

DISCUSSION

A single i.p. injection of nicotinamide at a dose of 1000 mg/kg significantly enhanced radiation damage in this C3H/Tif mouse mammary carcinoma when the irradiation was given within 2 hours after drug administration. However, using a pO_2 microelectrode we were unable to directly demonstrate any improvement in tumour oxygenation at any time up to 150 minutes after injection of this same drug dose.

Previous studies in other tumours had found that large single doses of nicotinamide could increase blood perfusion (Horsman et al., 1988; 1989a) and metabolism (Wood et al., 1991), as well as decrease the binding of ^{14}C-misonidazole (Horsman et al., 1988;

1989a). All of these results are consistent with nicotinamide improving tumour oxygenation. In this C3H/Tif tumour we did not see any significant change in tumour perfusion, but did find an increase in tumour metabolism, which although indicative of an improved oxygen status, could be explained by some other mechanism. These results coupled with the pO_2 measurements suggest that the enhancement of radiation damage by nicotinamide in this tumour may therefore not actually involve an increase in oxygenation.

Table 1. Summary of the effects of nicotinamide (1000 mg/kg; i.p.) in a C3H/Tif mouse mammary carcinoma[1].

Assay	Control	Nicotinamide	Level of significance[5]
Tumour Growth Time after 15 Gy X-rays (days)[2]	12.50 (12.07-12.93)	16.60 (16.10-17.11)	p<0.001
pO_2 values ≤5 mmHg (%)[2]	40.02 (35.42-44.61)	44.51 (40.87-48.15)	NS
Median pO_2 (mmHg)[2]	9.28 (7.90-10.67)	8.96 (7.01-10.92)	NS
Mean pO_2 (mmHg)[2]	13.35 (12.33-14.37)	14.43 (13.16-15.70)	NS
ATP: Pi ratio[3]	0.11 (0.10-0.12)	0.21 (0.20-0.23)	p<0.001
RbCl uptake (% injected/g of tumour)[3]	4.48 (4.10-4.85)	3.75 (3.51-3.99)	NS
Fluorescent staining mismatch (%)[4]	7.73 (6.65-8.82)	2.80 (2.42-3.18)	p<0.001

[1]Values show means (± 1 S.E.) for all results obtained between 30-120 minutes after nicotinamide injection.
[2]Results obtained from this study.
[3]Results taken from Horsman et al., 1992.
[4]Results taken from Horsman et al., 1990a.
[5]Level of significance estimated from a Students t-test. NS indicates no significant effect (p>0.05).

However, we also found that almost 8% of blood vessels in this C3H/Tif tumour were temporarily closed at any one time. Such transient fluctuations in blood flow are known to result in the development of perfusion limited acute hypoxia (Chaplin et al., 1986; 1987). More importantly, nicotinamide decreased the number of vessels closing, an effect which has been reported for nicotinamide and its structurally related analogue pyrazinamide in the SCCVII tumour (Chaplin et al., 1990a; 1990b). Nicotinamide must therefore be reducing the level of acute hypoxia and as such would be expected to increase tumour oxygenation. Even though some vessels are opening up there does not necessarily have to be any change in overall perfusion through the tumour and this may explain why we found no increase in RbCl uptake. It is also likely that the transient fluctuations in flow are occurring in only small areas. Hence the effect of nicotinamide is more likely to be detected by any technique which looks at the tumour as a whole, such as occurs with the measurement of metabolic activity, but could be missed by the pO_2 microelectrode as it passes through the tumour.

A similar failure to change tumour pO_2 was observed in a rat DS-sarcoma after treatment with 500 mg/kg nicotinamide (D.K. Kelleher, personal communication), although Lee and Song (1992) also using 500 mg/kg in various mice tumours did see a nicotinamide induced change in pO_2. It is possible that in those mouse tumours the nicotinamide effects are being detected because they are more prevalent and not restricted to acute hypoxia alone. In fact, our own studies have shown that although nicotinamide primarily influences acute hypoxia in the C3H/Tif and can result in an enhancement ratio (ER) of between 1.2 to 1.4 (Horsman et al., 1990a), in the SCCVII tumour it seems to affect both acute and chronic hypoxia, giving rise to ERs as large as 1.7 (Horsman et al., 1990b).

In conclusion, our results with pO_2 measurements are not inconsistent with nicotinamide improving tumour oxygenation. It is possible that the pO_2 microelectrode is simply unable to detect such small changes which occur at the microregional level, yet such changes could have a profound influence on radiation response.

ACKNOWLEDGEMENTS

The authors would like to thank Ms. I.M. Johansen for expert technical help, and Ms. D. Rasmussen for the manuscript preparation. This work was supported by a grant from the Danish Cancer Society.

REFERENCES

Chaplin, D.J., Durand, R.E., and Olive, P.L., 1986, Acute hypoxia in tumors: implication for modifiers of radiation effects, *Int.J.Radiat.Oncol.Biol.Phys.* 12:1279.

Chaplin, D.J., Horsman, M.R., and Trotter, M.J., 1990a, Effect of nicotinamide on the microregional heterogeneity of oxygen delivery within a murine tumour, *J.Natl. Cancer Inst.* 82:672.

Chaplin, D.J., Olive, P.L., and Durand, R.E., 1987, Intermittent blood flow in a murine tumor: radiobiological effects, *Cancer Res.* 47:597.

Chaplin, D.J., Trotter, M.J., Skov, K.A., and Horsman, M.R., 1990b, Modification of tumour radiation response in vivo by the benzamide analog pyrazinamide, *Br.J. Cancer* 62:561.

Horsman, M.R., Brown, J.M., Hirst, V.K., Lemmon, M.J., Wood, P.J., Dunphy, E.P., and Overgaard, J., 1988, Mechanism of action of the selective tumor radiosensitizer nicotinamide, *Int.J.Radiat.Oncol.Biol.Phys.* 15:685.

Horsman, M.R., Chaplin, D.J., and Brown, J.M., 1989a, Tumor radiosensitization by nicotinamide: a result of improved blood perfusion and oxygenation, *Radiat.Res.* 118:139.

Horsman, M.R., Chaplin, D.J., and Overgaard, J., 1990a, Combination of nicotinamide and hyperthermia to eliminate radioresistant chronically and acutely hypoxic tumor cells, *Cancer Res.* 50:7430.

Horsman, M.R., Hansen, P.V., and Overgaard, J., 1989b, Radiosensitization by nicotinamide in tumors and normal tissues: the importance of tissue oxygenation status, *Int.J. Radiat.Oncol.Biol.Phys.* 16:1273.

Horsman, M.R., Kristjansen, P.E.G., Mizuno, M., Christensen, K., Chaplin, D.J., Quistorff, B., and Overgaard, J., 1992, Biochemical and physiological changes induced by nicotinamide in a C3H mouse mammary carcinoma and CDF1 mice, *Int.J.Radiat.Oncol. Biol.Phys.* 22:451.

Horsman, M.R., Wood, P.J., Chaplin, D.J., Brown, J.M., and Overgaard, J., 1990b, The potentiation of radiation damage by nicotinamide in the SCCVII tumour in vivo, *Radiother.Oncol.* 18:49.

Kjellen, E., Joiner, M.C., Collier, J.M., Johns, H., and Rojas, A., 1991, A therapeutic benefit from combining normobaric carbogen or oxygen with nicotinamide in fractionated X-ray treatments, *Radiother.Oncol.* 22:81.

Lee, I., and Song, C.W., 1992, The oxygenation of murine tumor isografts and human tumor xenografts by nicotinamide, *Radiat.Res.* 130:65.

Overgaard, J., 1980, Simultaneous and sequential hyperthermia and radiation treatment of an experimental tumor and its surrounding normal tissue in vivo, *Int.J.Radiat.Oncol. Biol.Phys.* 6:1507.

Vaupel, P., Kallinowski, F., and Okunieff, P., 1989, Blocd flow, oxygen and nutrient supply, and metabolic micro-environment of human tumors: a review, *Cancer Res.* 49:6449.

Wood, P.J., Counsell, C.J.R., Bremner, J.C.M., Horsman, M.R., and Adams, G.E., 1991, The measurement of radiosensitizer-induced changes in mouse tumour metabolism by 31-P magnetic resonance spectroscopy, *Int.J.Radiat.Oncol.Biol.Phys.* 20:291.

" UPSTREAM" MODIFICATION OF VASOCONSTRICTOR RESPONSES IN RAT EPIGASTRIC ARTERY SUPPLYING AN IMPLANTED TUMOUR

G.D.Kennovin,[1] F.W.Flitney,[1] and D.G.Hirst[2]

[1]Cancer Biology Research Group
Cell Biology & Neuroscience Research Division
University of St. Andrews
St. Andrews, Fife, KY16 9TS
[2]CRC Gray Laboratory
P.O. Box 100
Mount Vernon Hospital
Northwood, Middlesex, HA6 2JR

INTRODUCTION

Malignant tumours are known to exert a powerful influence on neighbouring blood vessels (Coman & Sheldon, 1946), as well as releasing factors which stimulate the proliferation of neovasculature (Folkman & Cotran, 1976). Haemodynamic studies suggest that the vasculature within solid tumours is much less responsive to vasodilators than that in normal tissues (see Hirst & Wood, 1989, for review). The reduction in tumour blood flow seen after systemic administration of these agents is thought to be mainly passive as a result of local changes in perfusion pressure (Brown, 1987; Chaplin, 1987). The suggestion has been made that this mechanism might be exploited to create a more hypoxic enviroment within tumours and so enhance the potency of bioreductive cytotoxins (Brown, 1987; Chaplin, 1987; Stratford et al, 1987). The major arteries that supply tumours are recruited vessels, which unlike vessels within the tumour, possess well defined intimal, medial and adventitial structure, and are responsive to vasoactive agents (Hirst et al, 1991; Hirst & Tozer, in press). It is not known whether tumour growth affects the properties of these vessels. Here we report on a study of the vasoconstrictor responses of isolated rat epigastric arteries which had supplied implanted tumours, compared to contralateral (control) arteries which supplied normal tissue.

METHODS

Small pieces (2-3mm) of P22 carcinosarcoma from a donor animal were implanted into

Oxygen Transport to Tissue XV, Edited by P. Vaupel
et al., Plenum Press, New York, 1994

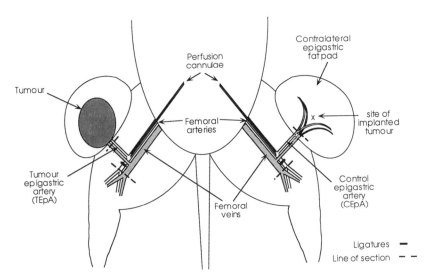

Figure 1. Diagram of the vascular supply to the implanted tumour in the rat hindlimb (see text for details).

the inguinal fat pads of isogeneic BD9 rats under general anaesthesia (90mg.kg^{-1} Ketamine: 10mg.kg^{-1} Xylazine), close to the first bifurcation of the epigastric artery (see figure 1). The location of the implant ensured that the developing tumour was supplied primarily through the epigastric artery. Three or four weeks later, when the tumours were of sufficient size, the femoral and epigastric arteries on both legs were cleared under anaesthesia. After the side branches of the femoral arteries were ligated, the animal was heparinised (1unit.g^{-1}, i.p.) and a perfusion cannula inserted into each femoral artery until its tip was adjacent to the junction with the epigastric artery (see fig.1). The femoral arteries were then ligated

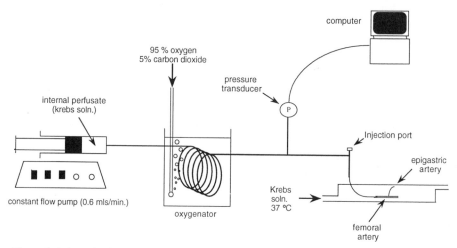

Figure 2. Schematic diagram of the perfusion apparatus. There were two such set-ups run in parallel.

distal to the cannula tip, and each epigastric artery was isolated, removed and mounted in a perfusion apparatus, schematically described in figure 2. The animal was then killed by anaesthetic overdose. Both arteries were simultaneously perfused internally with Krebs solution at a constant flow rate of 0.6 mls.min.$^{-1}$, while the temperature was maintained at

37°C by an external Krebs perfusate. The vasoconstrictor tone of each artery was monitored by recording the pressure of the internal perfusate. Any vasoconstriction in the artery resulted in an increase in perfusion pressure whereas a vasodilation caused the pressure to fall. After the preparations had been left for 1 hour to stabilise, bolus injections (10µl) of phenylephrine (PE) were introduced into the internal perfusate, and the responses of tumour and control epigastric arteries were compared.

RESULTS

Spontaneous pressure oscillations in tumour epigastric arteries. The epigastric artery that had supplied the tumour (TEpA) differed from the contralateral control artery (CEpA) in that it was prone to spontaneous activity. Over 60% of TEpAs (24/38)

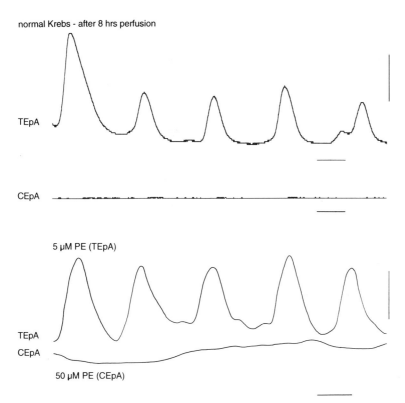

Figure 3. Spontaneous rythmic oscillations in vasoconstrictor tone in tumour arteries (TEpA) after constant perfusion of Krebs' solution or Krebs' containing 5µM phenylephrine (PE). Note that the control artery (CEpA) does not exhibit any spontaneous activity despite being perfused with a 10 fold higher PE concentration (50µM). (vertical scale bars: 50mmHg , time scale bars: 5 minutes (drawn at 0mmHg))

exhibited fluctuations in vasoconstrictor tone, but this was never observed in any CEpA preparation. These fluctuations were initially small (5-15 mmHg) and fairly infrequent (i.e. every 30 min.) but longer term (>200mins) infusions of Krebs' solutions or constant infusions of phenylephrine (PE) increased both their size (e.g. to 40-85 mmHg) and frequency (e.g. every 10 min.) (see fig.3). These procedures could also induce previously quiescent TEpA preparations to become spontaneously active.

Sensitivity of arteries to phenylephrine. Figure 4 shows log dose response curves to PE for TEpAs and CEpAs that were measured early in the experiment (fig. 4a) and after longer perfusion durations (fig. 4b). The size of the vasoconstrictor responses of TEpAs and CEpAs were not significantly different at PE doses below 1-2mM. Larger PE concentrations failed to increase the TEpA response (max. pressure: 170 ± 19 mmHg, (n=28)) but continued to increase the initial CEpA response (max. pressure: 250 ± 16 mmHg, (n=22)) (see fig. 4a). The difference between the two types of artery gradually disappeared as the perfusion time increased, such that after 400 min there were no significant differences throughout the [PE] range (see fig.4b). This was due to a time dependent decrease in the size of the CEpA response (max. pressure: 175 ± 19mmHg) to higher [PE] (>2mM).

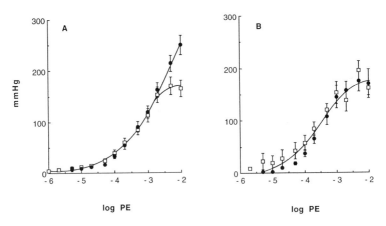

Figure 4. These graphs show the mean rise in perfusion pressure in response to injecting increasing concentrations of phenylephrine (PE) into the internal perfusate of tumour (TEpA: ☐) and control (CEpA: ●) epigastric arteries, at 126-246 ($\pm$16)mins (fig. 4a) and 400-508 ($\pm$43) mins (fig. 4b) after the onset of perfusion.

Effect of a nitric oxide synthase inhibitor on the sensitivity of arteries to PE. The time dependent reduction in sensitivity of CEpAs to PE could be due to expression of the inducible form of nitric oxide synthase (NOS), as described by Rees et al (1990a) in similar pharmacological preparations. This hypothesis was tested by adding a competitive inhibitor of NOS, N^G-monomethyl-L-arginine (L-NMMA), to the internal perfusate. L-NMMA ($40\mu M$) increased the sensitivity of both TEpAs and CEpAs to PE (see fig.5a,b). The effect was greater for TEpAs than CEpAs, so that there were no longer any significant differences between the two. The action of L-NMMA was fully reversed by perfusing vessels with Krebs' solution containing L-arginine (1mM), the endogenous substrate for NOS (Palmer et al, 1987) (fig. 5a,b). This re-established the difference in sensitivity to higher PE. A further dose response curve in normal Krebs' at later times (526-583 min) again demonstrates the time dependent decrease in CEpA sensitivity to PE. The PE sensitivity of TEpA preparations in normal Krebs did not change significantly throughout the duration of the experiment (up to 583 min).

DISCUSSION

Our experiments reveal clear differences between TEpAs and CEpAs which imply that tumour growth can influence the properties of the main supply vessel. The underlying mechanism is not yet understood, though it seems possible that tumour arteries may differ from normal arteries in the extent to which the constitutive and inducible isoforms of nitric

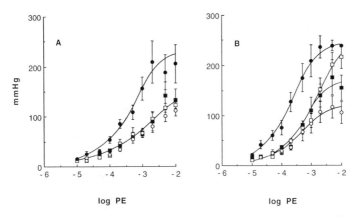

Figure 5. This figure shows the effect of constantly perfusing 40μM L-NMMA (●) and 1mM l-arginine (■) on the PE dose response curves of TEpAs (fig.5a) and CEpAs (fig.5b). Key : (❑)-Normal Krebs' (136-228 min. after onset of perfusion); (●)- 40μM L-NMMA (248-332 min.); (■)- 1mM L-arginine (363-438 min.); (O)- Krebs' (526-583 min.)

oxide synthase (NOS) are expressed. The time dependent decrease of sensitivity to PE in control arteries is consistent with the expression of inducible NOS (Rees et al, 1990a). This is known to occur in vitro, over several hours, in response to bacterial endotoxins and cytokines (Rees et al, 1990a; Fleming et al 1991). If this is happening in our experiments, then it raises the question: why is the PE sensitivity of tumour arteries independent of perfusion time ? One possible explanation currently being investigated, is that both isoforms of NOS are already elevated in tumour preparations. Indirect evidence for this comes also from their tendency to spontaneously constrict. It has been demonstrated that endogenous nitric oxide induces spontaneous rhythmic vasoconstrictions in hamster aorta during continuous exposure to PE (Jackson et al, 1991). If a similar mechanism occurs in our preparations, then it could expain the marked tendency for tumour arteries to spontaneously constrict, especially after long perfusion durations and constant exposure to PE. The occurence of spontaneous rhythmic activity in vivo, might be a contributory factor in the temporal heterogeneity of microregional blood flow in tumours demonstrated by Trotter et al (1989). Further elucidation of the mechanisms underlying these observations could prove to be important in developing new strategies for controlling tumour bloood flow.

This work is supported by a grant from the Cancer Research Campaign.

REFERENCES

Brown, J.M., (1987), Hypoxia-targeted chemotherapy: a role for vasoactive drugs, *Proceedings of the 8th International Congress of Radiation Research, Edinburgh, U.K.*, E.M.Fielden et al , ed., Taylor &Francis,London,vol. 2, 719-724

Chaplin, D.J., (1987), Hypoxia-targeted chemotherapy: a role for vasoactive drugs, *Proceedings of the 8th International Congress of Radiation Research, Edinburgh, U.K.*, E.M.Fielden et al , ed., Taylor & Francis, London,vol. 2,731-736

Coman D.R. & Sheldon, W.F., (1946) The significance of hyperemia around tumour implants, *Am. J. Pathol.*, **22**: 821-826

Folkman, J. & Cotran, R., (1976) Relation of vascular proliferation to tumour growth, *Int. Rev. Exp. Pathol.*, **16** : 207-248

Fleming, I., Gray, G.A., Schott, C. & Stoclet, J.C. (1991), Inducible but not constitutive production of nitric oxide by vascular smooth muscle cells, *Eur. J. Pharmacol.*, **200**:375-6.

Hirst, D.G., & Tozer, G.M., Pharmacological manipulation of blood flow, *Br. J. Radiol.* (in press)

Hirst, D.G. & Wood, P.J., (1989) The control of tumour blood flow for therapeutic benefit, *Scientific basis of modern therapy (BIR london)*, **19**:76-80

Hirst, D.G., Hirst, V.K., Shaffi, K.M., Prise, V.E. & Joiner, B., (1991) The influence of vasoactive agents on the perfusion of tumours growing in three sites in the mouse, *Int. J. Radiat. Biol.* **60**: 211-218

Jackson, W.F., Mulsch, A. & Busse, R. (1991), Rhythmic smooth muscle activity in hamster aortas is mediated by continuous release of NO from the endothelium, *Am. J. Physiol.*, **260**: H248-253

Palmer, R.J., Ashton, D. & Moncada, S. (1987), Vascular endothelial cells synthesise nitric oxide from L-arginine. *Nature*, **333**; 664-666

Rees, D.D., Cellek, S., Palmer, R. J. & Moncada, S. (1990a), Dexamethasone prevents the induction by endotoxin of a nitric oxide synthase and the associated effects on vascular tone. *Biochem. Biophys.Res.Commun.* **173**: 541-547

Rees, D.D., Palmer, R.J., Schultz, R., Hodson, H.F. & Moncada, S. (1990b), Characterisation of three inhibitors of nitric oxide synthase in vitro and in vivo. *Br. J. Pharmacol.*, **101**: 746-752

Trotter, M.J., Chaplin, D.J., durand, R.E., & Olive, P.L. (1989) The use of flourescent probes to identify regions of transient perfusion in murine tumours. *Int. J. Radiat. Oncol. Biol. Phys.* **16**:3 1

THE EFFECT OF VINCA ALKALOIDS
ON TUMOUR BLOOD FLOW

S.A. Hill, S.J. Lonergan, J. Denekamp and D.J. Chaplin

Vascular Targeting Group
CRC Gray Laboratory
Northwood
Middlesex, U.K.

INTRODUCTION

Vascular insufficiency, induced by damage to the tumour vasculature, or closure of individual blood vessels, can lead to a dramatic increase in tumour hypoxia. This may be exploited therapeutically by combination therapy with bioreductive agents. Alternatively, if vascular function remains chronically impaired, the lack of oxygen becomes critical, resulting in ischaemic cell death. Since all of the cells supplied by an individual vessel will be affected by its closure, the potential for extensive tumour destruction exists.

Increasingly, it is emerging that therapies already in use mediate their action, to some extent via the induction of ischaemia. As well as hyperthermia and photodynamic therapy, the cytokines TNFα and Interleukin 1 have been shown to cause profound reductions in tumour blood flow (Song, 1984; Star et al., 1986; Watanabe et al., 1988; Constantinidis et al., 1989). Flavone acetic acid (FAA) created great interest when it too was found to produce similar effects (Evelhoch et al., 1988; Bibby et al., 1989; Hill et al., 1989; Zwi et al., 1989).

Although both FAA and TNF have produced rapid blood flow reductions and necrosis in a wide range of murine solid tumours, the therapeutic dose window is narrow and limited by toxicity (Asher et al., 1987; Hill et al., 1991). Toxic side effects have also limited the dose of drug that can be given clinically and this may, to some extent, account for the lack of antitumour effectiveness so far observed with these tumour necrotizing agents. The potential benefits associated with such drugs make it important to identify other agents which may either work via a different mechanism or show significantly less toxicity.

The search for agents which have anti-vascular effects in tumours is hampered by the absence of an appropriate *in vitro* evaluation process. In the absence of a large scale *in vivo* screening programme, other approaches for identifying suitable candidate agents have to be sought. One approach is to identify from the literature those agents which produce changes within tumours characteristic of vascular damage and/or ischemia. One of the hallmarks of ischaemic cell death is a reduction in cell survival or the yield of live cells from a treated tumour when excision is delayed (Denekamp, 1989). Some years ago, Stephens and Peacock (1978) measured the cell yield from B16 melanomas excised 20-24hr after treatment with a comprehensive range of cytotoxic agents. We have plotted their data in Fig.1. It was on the basis of these data that we identified the vinca alkaloids as warranting further investigation.

Oxygen Transport to Tissue XV, Edited by P. Vaupel
et al., Plenum Press, New York, 1994

MATERIALS AND METHODS
Tumour model

The CaNT is a poorly differentiated mammary carcinoma which has been maintained for many generations in the murine strain of origin. Tumours were grown subcutaneously on the backs of 12 to 16 week old female CBA/Gy f TO mice from an inoculum of 0.05ml of a crude tumour cell suspension. For assessment of tumour growth and response to treatment, animals were selected when their tumours reached a geometric mean diameter (GMD) of 5.5 to 6.5mm (150-300mg).

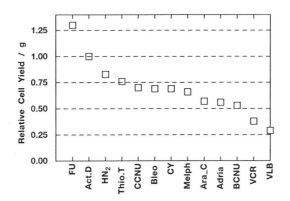

Fig.1: The relative cell yield from B16 melanomas excised 20-24hr after treatment with a range of chemotherapeutic agents. Data redrawn from Stephens and Peacock (1978).

Drug treatment

Vincristine and vinblastine were dissolved in the bacteriocide diluent supplied by the manufacturers (Eli Lilly and Co.). Further dilutions were made using sterile water or 0.9% saline respectively. The two drugs were compared at both equimolar and equitoxic doses. Thus groups of at least 5 mice were injected with 3mg/kg vincristine (the maximum tolerated dose) or 3 or 10mg/kg vinblastine. All drug doses were injected i.p. in 0.1ml per 10g body weight.

Tumour Response

Tumours were measured regularly after treatment and mean growth curves were produced for each group of animals. Alternatively, tumour perfusion was measured at successive times after treatment, using ^{86}RbCl extraction (Sapirstein, 1958). Tissue radioactivity measured 1min. after an i.v. injection can be used to calculate relative blood flow as a proportion of cardiac output (Hill and Denekamp, 1982).

RESULTS

We have determined the maximum tolerated dose (MTD) of drug in our mice to be 3mg/kg vincristine and 10mg/kg vinblastine. Compared on this basis, vinblastine is more effective at inhibiting the growth of the CaNT than is vincristine, as illustrated in Fig.2. To allow comparison at equimolar drug doses also, the tumour growth response to 3mg/kg vinblastine was measured. On this basis, vincristine is the more effective drug.

The relative changes in tumour blood flow induced by single i.p. injections of vincristine and vinblastine are shown in Fig.3, as measured by [86]RbCl extraction. At equitoxic doses, both drugs produced a 60% reduction in tumour perfusion within 30min. of injection. After vinblastine, blood flow continued to fall to at least 6hr after injection,

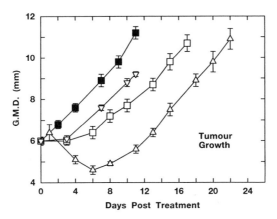

Fig.2: The effect of vincristine and vinblastine on the growth of the CaNT. Untreated tumours ■; 3mg/kg vincristine □; 3 and 10mg/kg vinblastine ▽, △. Errors are ± 1 sem.

reaching a level of less than 10% of that measured in control tumours. Even at 24hr, no significant recovery was seen. A less pronounced effect was measured after vincristine; blood flow was reduced by approximately 70% at 6hr and although remaining depressed at 24hr, some recovery was apparent. Also plotted is the response to 3mg/kg vinblastine. A rapid decrease in perfusion was again measured, a 70% reduction at 1hr. Although this was followed by some recovery, tumour perfusion remained significantly below control levels at 24hr.

The effects of drug treatment on normal tissue perfusion were also measured. The greatest changes were seen after 10 mg/kg vinblastine and data for kidney and skin are plotted in Fig.4. Maximum blood flow changes of approximately 40% were seen in both tissues, perfusion increasing in the kidney but decreasing in skin at 2hr after treatment. Blood flow had returned to control levels by 6hr. Vincristine had less effect on the vascular function of the normal tissues tested (liver, kidney, skin, muscle) and caused a transient decrease, rather than an increase in kidney perfusion.

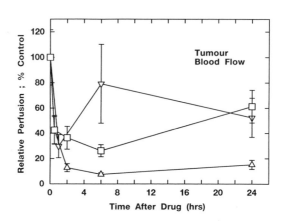

Fig.3: The time course of changes in relative blood flow in CaNT tumours treated with 3mg/kg vincristine □; 3mg/kg vinblastine ▽ or 10mg/kg vinblastine △. Errors are ± 1 sem.

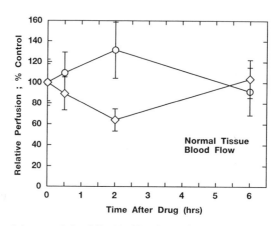

Fig.4: Changes in normal tissue perfusion following 10mg/kg vinblastine. Kidney ○; skin ◇. Errors are ± sem.

DISCUSSION

The vinca alkaloids, widely used in cancer chemotherapy, are potent inhibitors of cell proliferation. By binding to tubulin and interfering with the formation of the mitotic spindle, cell division is prevented. The data presented in this study suggest that, at the doses used, additional tumour cell killing may occur *in vivo* as the result of an indirect mechanism.

The dramatic reductions in tumour blood flow measured after both vincristine and vinblastine are accompanied by the histological appearance of haemorrhagic necrosis, similar to that seen following treatment with TNFα and FAA (Old, 1985; Smith *et al.*, 1987). By 24hr, large areas of treated tumours appear totally necrotic, particularly after vinblastine (data not shown). Vinblastine is also the more effective drug at both decreasing tumour blood flow and inhibiting tumour growth. These data together suggest that the antitumour activity measured is mediated at least in part via prolonged impairment of tumour blood flow and thus oxygen delivery.

Unlike normal tissues, tumours have an inadequate vascular supply, showing structural and functional heterogeneity. As a consequence, many tumour cells already exist at the limits of diffusion for nutrients and oxygen and are thus particularly susceptible to any further deterioration in perfusion. That a prolonged reduction in blood flow can cause significant tumour cell death has been demonstrated by artificially occluding the vascular supply with a metal clamp (Denekamp *et al.*, 1983). However, tumour eradication could only be achieved when complete occlusion was maintained for more than 15hr. Thus, unless a treatment can induce permanent cessation of flow in all tumour vessels, individual drugs with antivascular properties will not be useful as sole agents. Indeed, in this study, the massive and prolonged decrease in blood flow induced by vinblastine resulted in only a relatively modest delay in tumour growth. However, by combining antivascular therapies with other agents which exploit the microenvironmental changes (e.g. reduced oxygenation and increased acidity) resulting from a reduction in blood flow, more profound antitumour effects may be achieved. Another approach would be to combine anti-vascular agents which mediate their action via different mechanisms or have different normal tissue toxicity to facilitate a more complete vascular shutdown in the tumour.

The mechanism by which the vinca alkaloids reduce tumour blood flow is unknown. However, previous studies have indicated that agents which interfere with microtubule formation can alter vascular function within tumours. As early as 1954, it was reported that the microtubule inhibitor podophyllotoxin caused vascular stasis and haemorrhage, leading to ischaemia and ultimately necrosis (Algire *et al.*, 1954). More recently, Baguley *et al.* (1991) reported the ability of a number of tubulin-binding agents, including vincristine and vinblastine, to induce haemorrhagic necrosis and suggested that, in common with FAA, cytokine induction may be involved. The current study has added to these data by demonstrating that tumour responsiveness to vincristine and vinblastine at the doses studied appears to be correlated with the extent and duration of the induced changes in tumour blood flow. In their study with podophyllotoxin, Algire and colleagues attributed the blood flow changes to the induction of hypotension by the agent. However, hypotension is not reported to be dose-limiting for the vinca alkaloids and the normal tissue data presented do not suggest the widespread peripheral vasodilation which might indicate such an effect in the treated animals; however, direct measurements have not been made.

Whether the mechanism of action of the vinca alkaloids is similar to that of FAA or not, it is important that another group of agents has been identified as having long term effects on tumour blood flow. Clinically, as with FAA and TNF, antivascular effects of vincristine and vinblastine are unlikely to be seen since the doses used are outside the clinical range and close to the toxic limit in mice. We therefore intend to investigate other tubulin-binding agents and different analogues of the vinca alkaloids which may show less toxicity and a wider therapeutic window of dose.

REFERENCES

ALGIRE, G.H., LEGALLAIS, F.Y. & ANDERSON, B.F. (1954). Vascular reactions of normal and malignant tissues *in vivo*. VI. The role of hypotension in the action of components of Podophyllin on transplanted sarcomas. *J.N.C.I.*, **14**, 879-893.

ASHER, A., MULÉ, J.J., REICHERT, C.M., SHILONI, E. & ROSENBERG, S.A. (1987). Studies on the anti-tumour efficacy of systemically administered recombinant tumour necrosis factor against several murine tumours *in vivo*. *J. Immunol.*, **138**, 963-974.

BAGULEY, B.C., HOLDAWAY, K.M., THOMSEN, L.L., ZHUANG, L. & ZWI, L.J. (1991). Inhibition of growth of colon 38 adenocarcinoma by vinblastine and colchicine: Evidence for a vascular mechanism. *Eur. J. Cancer*, **27**, 482-487.

BIBBY, M.C., DOUBLE, J.A., LOADMAN, P.M. & DUKE, C.V. (1989). Reduction of tumor blood flow by flavone acetic acid: a possible component of therapy. *JNCI*, **81**, 216-220.

CONSTANTINIDIS, I., BRAUNSCHWEIGER, P.G., WEHRLE, J.P., KUMAR, N., JOHNSON, C.S., FURMANSKI, P. & GLICKSON, J.D. (1989). ^{31}P-NMR studies of the effect of recombinant human interleukin-1α on the bioenergetics of RIF-1 tumors. *Cancer Res.*, **49**, 6379-6382.

DENEKAMP, J. (1989). Induced vascular collapse in tumours: a way of increasing the therapeutic gain in cancer therapy. In: 'The Scientific Basis of Modern Radiotherapy'. Ed. N.J. McNally, *BIR Report*, **19**, 63-70.

DENEKAMP, J., HILL, S.A. & HOBSON, B. (1983). Vascular occlusion and tumour-cell death. *Eur. J. Cancer & Clin. Oncol.*, **19**, 271-275.

EVELHOCH, J.L., BISSERY, M-C, CHABOT, G.C., SIMPSON, N.E., MCCOY, C.L., HEILBRUN, L.K. & CORBETT, T.H. (1988). Flavone acetic acid (NSC 347512)-induced modulation of murine tumor physiology monitored by *in vivo* nuclear magnetic resonance spectroscopy. *Cancer Res.*, **48**, 4749-4755.

HILL, S.A. AND DENEKAMP, J. (1982). Site dependent response of tumours to combined heat and radiation. *Br. J. Radiol.*, **55**, 905-912.

HILL, S.A., WILLIAMS, K.B. & DENEKAMP, J. (1989). Vascular collapse after flavone acetic acid: a possible mechanism of its antitumour action. *Eur. J. Cancer, Clin. Oncol.*, **25**, 1419-1424.

HILL, S.A., WILLIAMS, K.B. & DENEKAMP, J. (1991). Studies with a panel of tumours having a variable sensitivity to FAA, to investigate the mechanism of action. *Int. J. Radiat. Biol.*, **60**, 379-384.

OLD, L.J. (1985). Tumour necrosis factor (TNF). *Science*, **230**, 630-633.

SAPIRSTEIN, L.A. (1958). Regional blood flow by fractional distribution of indicators. *Am. J. Physiol.*, **193**, 161-168.

SMITH, G.P., CALVELEY, S.B., SMITH, M.J. & BAGULEY, B.C. (1987). Flavone acetic acid (NSC 347512) induces haemorrhagic necrosis of mouse colon 26 and 38 tumours. *Eur. J. Cancer, Clin. Oncol.*, **23**, 1209-1211.

SONG, C.W. (1984). Effect of local hyperthermia on blood flow and microenvironment. *Cancer Res. (Suppl.)*, **44**, 4721S-4730S.

STAR, W.M., MARIJNISSEN, H.P.A., VANDEN BERG-BLOK, A.E., VERSTEEG, J.A.C., FRANKEN, K.A.P. & REINHOLD, H.S. (1986). Destruction of rat mammary tumour and normal tissue microcirculation by hematoporphyrin derivative photoradiation observed *in vivo* in sandwich observation chambers. *Cancer Res.*, **46**, 2532-2540.

STEPHENS, T.C. & PEACOCK, J.H. (1978). Cell yield and cell survival following chemotherapy of the B16 melanoma. *Br. J. Cancer*, **38**, 591-598.

WATANABE, N., NIITSU, Y., UMENO, H., KURIYANA, H., NEDA, H., YAMAUCHI, Y., MAEDA, M. & URUSHIZAKI, I. (1988). Toxic effect of tumour necrosis factor on tumour vasculature in mice. *Cancer Res.*, **48**, 2179-2183.

ZWI, L.J., BAGULEY, B.C., GAVIN, J.B. & WILSON, W.R. (1989). Blood flow failure as a major determinant in the antitumor action of flavone acetic acid (NSC 347512). *JNCI*, **81**, 1005-1013.

USE OF THE HYPERTENSIVE AGENT ANGIOTENSIN II FOR MODIFYING OXYGEN DELIVERY TO TUMOURS

Gillian M. Tozer, Katija M. Shaffi and David G. Hirst

CRC Gray Laboratory
P.O. Box 100
Mount Vernon Hospital
Northwood
Middlesex, HA6 2JR

INTRODUCTION

Ischaemia-induced tumour hypoxia can limit the effectiveness of radiotherapy. Regions of deficient blood flow within tumours also limit the access of blood-borne anti-cancer agents. Vasoconstrictor drugs, such as angiotensin II, have potential for improving the oxygen status of tumours via an increase in their blood flow. This would occur if the tumour perfusion pressure could be increased without increasing tumour vascular resistance. An increase in absolute tumour blood flow following i.v. infusion of angiotensin II has been reported in the literature (Hori et al., 1991, Tanda et al., 1991, Tokuda et al., 1990). The aims of this study were 1) to determine the relationship between blood flow response to angiotensin II and perfusion pressure and 2) to investigate whether angiotensin II induces any improvement in blood flow to very poorly perfused tumour regions which are critical for the outcome of both radiotherapy and chemotherapy.

METHODS

Tumour

A transplanted rat carcinosarcoma, designated P22, was used for these experiments. Details of maintenance of this tumour are described elsewhere (Tozer & Shaffi, 1992). Experiments were performed on 1st to 10th passage tumours growing subcutaneously in the left flank of 10 to 12 week old male BD9 rats. Tumours were used for experiments when they reached 1-2g (all 3 orthogonal diameters 10-15mm including skin thickness).

Blood Flow

All blood flow measurements were made at 20 minutes after the start of i.v. infusion of different doses of angiotensin II (Sigma) or 0.9% saline. Blood flow was measured using the uptake, over a short infusion time, of the inert, readily diffusible compound, iodo-antipyrine (IAP). Sampling of arterial blood over the infusion time, measurement of tissue levels of IAP

Oxygen Transport to Tissue XV, Edited by P. Vaupel
et al., Plenum Press, New York, 1994

at the end of the infusion time and a knowledge of the relative solubility of IAP in tissue and blood allows calculation of the specific blood flow to a tissue (Kety, 1960).

Details of this technique are described elsewhere (Tozer & Shaffi, 1992). Briefly, all procedures were carried out under Hypnorm (Crown Chemical Co. Ltd.) and midazolam (Roche) anaesthesia. Two tail veins and one tail artery were catheterised using polyethylene catheters (external diameter 0.96mm: internal diameter 0.58mm). Catheterised tail veins were used for i.v. infusion of angiotensin II or saline, i.v. infusion of IAP and rapid killing of the rats at the end of IAP infusion using i.v. injection of 0.2ml Euthatal (May & Baker). The catheterised tail artery was used for monitoring mean arterial blood pressure (MABP) via a physiological pressure transducer (Gould) and sampling arterial blood during IAP infusion.

IAP was labelled with [125]I (Institute of Cancer Research, England) or [14]C (Amersham). Radioactivity in timed arterial blood samples, collected over the IAP infusion time, was measured using scintillation counting. Radioactivity in tissue samples, excised after killing the animals at the end of IAP infusion, was measured using scintillation counting or autoradiography (^{14}C only). Scintillation counting provided a single value for blood flow to each tissue whereas autoradiography provided a means of investigating spatial heterogeneity of blood flow.

Tumours for autoradiography were excised at the end of experimentation and immediately frozen in isopentane cooled to -30 C to -40 C. Autoradiograms were produced from 20μm thick cryostat sections together with plastic standards of known ^{14}C activity using autoradiographic film (Hyperfim-βmax, Amersham) and an exposure time of several weeks. Adjacent frozen sections were fixed and stained with haematoxylin and eosin for histological analysis.

Mathematical Analysis and Autoradiography

Arterial input curves (concentration of IAP in arterial blood versus time after start of infusion of IAP) were deconvolved to account for delay and dispersion of blood along the plastic catheters. Tissue curves (concentration of IAP in tissue versus time after start of infusion of IAP) were obtained by convolution of the arterial input using the relationships derived by Kety (1960). For each blood flow determination, convolutions were repeated for 200 possible blood flow values in order to produce a look-up table for tissue concentration of IAP versus blood flow.

Autoradiograms from sections cut from the centre of tumours were analysed using an Applied Imaging image analysis system and "WBA" software. Autoradiographic images were captured by camera as optical density images and transformed, pixel by pixel, into blood flow images, using the mathematical procedure described above. Thus, transformed images consisted of approximately 10,000 separate blood flow measurements. Results were expressed as mean blood flow ± standard deviation for all the pixel measurements in whole sections or in "peripheral" or "central" regions of each section. "Peripheral" regions were defined as a rim of tissue around the edge of a tumour section whose width equalled one tenth of the largest diameter of the section. A rim of this size around the whole tumour would be roughly equivalent to half of the tumour volume. "Central" tumour regions were defined as the area within the rim.

RESULTS

A dose response for the hypertensive effect of angiotensin II, in BD9 rats, has been found for doses between 0 and 0.2 μg kg[-1] min[-1] (Tozer & Shaffi, 1992). Doses above 0.2 μg kg[-1] min[-1] caused no further increase in MABP. MABP was 91 ± 2 mmHg in control rats and 155 ± 2 mmHg in the most hypertensive group.

Figure 1 shows the effect of different doses of angiotensin II on the overall blood flow to the P22 tumour and to normal skin from the contralateral flank, plotted against perfusion pressure which is assumed to be equivalent to MABP. Blood flow is plotted relative to blood flow in untreated (saline-infused) rats, such that a relative value of 1.0 represents no effect of angiotensin on tissue blood flow. Blood flow to both skin and the P22 tumour is significantly reduced by angiotensin II infusion. A previous study has shown that the tumour response is of the same order as that of normal skeletal muscle, kidney and ileum and represents a significant rise in tumour vascular resistance (Tozer & Shaffi, 1992). This suggests that the P22 tumour is responding directly to the vasoconstrictive effects of angiotensin II.

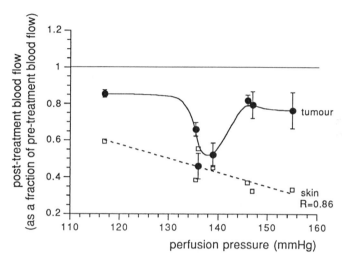

Figure 1. Effect of 20 minutes i.v. infusion of angiotensin II on blood flow to whole tumours and skin from the contralateral flank measured by scintillation counting. Angiotensin doses between .02 µg kg[-1] min[-1] and .5 µg kg[-1] min[-1] were used to induce varying degrees of hypertension. Each point represents mean ± 1 S.E.M. for at least 6 test animals and 6 controls animals. All points for skin and 3 out of 7 points for tumour represent a significant reduction in blood flow (P<.05 for student's t-test for unpaired data).

Response of normal skin blood flow to angiotensin II can be represented by a straight line through the data in Figure 1 (R=0.86). A similar dose response has been found for normal muscle, kidney, ileum and skin overlying the tumour (Tozer &Shaffi, 1992). However, the response of the tumour, in Figure 1, follows no well-defined pattern.

A significant inter-transplant variation in blood flow has been found for the P22 tumour (Tozer & Shaffi, 1992). In order to minimise the effects of this variation, angiotensin effects were always assessed relative to control tumours from the same transplant group. Despite this precaution, tumour blood flow response to angiotensin II was found to be dependent upon pre-treatment blood flow. If tumour blood flow in the control, saline-treated rats was below around 0.5 mls g[-1] min[-1] for a particular transplant group, angiotensin caused a moderate decrease in flow (to around 0.8 of controls). However, if pre-treatment blood flow was higher than 0.6 mls g[-1] min[-1], the response to angiotensin was larger (Figure 2). This dependence of angiotensin effect on pre-treatment blood flow is the most likely explanation for the variation in tumour response shown in Figure 1, where the 3 points showing the biggest drop in blood flow originated from transplant groups where control flow was the highest (Figure 2). Tumours from the first passage away from the primary tumour (open symbols in Figure 2), represent the largest angiotensin-induced decrease in flow.

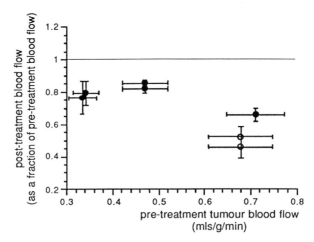

Figure 2. Dependence of tumour blood flow response to angiotensin II on pre-treatment blood flow. Each point represents mean ± 1 S.E.M. for at least 6 test animals and 6 controls. Open symbols: 1st passage away from primary tumour.

Blood flow to peripheral tumour regions was found to be 1.34 ± 0.15 times as high as blood flow to central regions in untreated tumours (Figure 3). This was true for both high and low flow tumours and is similar to that found for the LBDS$_1$ tumour in a previous study (Tozer et al., 1990). This differential between flow to the periphery and centre was partially due to the development of central coagulative necrosis. However, the necrotic fraction we observed in these tumours was low (never more than 12% of the sectional surface area) and central flow tended to be lower than peripheral flow even when there was no significant necrosis in the section. Angiotensin II tended to normalise tumour blood flow such that flow to the periphery was approximately equal to that to the centre (Figure 3).

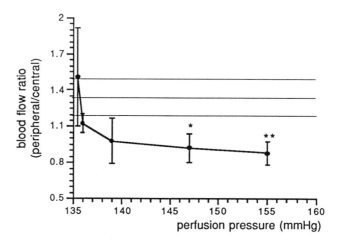

Figure 3. Relationship between regional tumour blood flow and perfusion pressure. Results obtained by autoradiography. Each point represents mean ± 1 S.E.M for at least 3 test animals and 3 controls. * represents P=.06 and ** represents P=.03 for the probability that these points are not significantly different from controls (student's t-test for unpaired data). Horizontal lines represent mean ± 1 S.E.M. for control tumours.

Figure 4 is an attempt to determine whether the angiotensin-induced equalisation of blood flow between the periphery and the centre is due to a decrease in blood flow to the periphery or an increase to the centre. Results in Figure 4 are pooled data for two angiotensin doses where blood flow equalisation is significant or near-significant (the two highest perfusion pressures in Figure 3). The first column in Figure 4 shows that angiotensin, at these doses, was able to significantly reduce tumour blood flow to whole tumours (measured by scintillation counting) to around 0.8 of the control flow (as also shown in Figure 1). However, the second column shows that this reduction was not apparent if only sections cut from the centre of the tumours were analysed (measured by autoradiography). This suggests that angiotensin is preferentially vasoconstricting in the tumour periphery. The last two columns in Figure 4 suggest further, that angiotensin may be having opposite effects in the tumour periphery and the tumour centre. That is, angiotensin tends to decrease flow to the periphery whilst simultaneously tending to increase flow to the centre. Although neither of these results are significant, for the number of animals used so far (P = 0.28 and P = 0.29 for the effect of angiotensin on peripheral and central blood flow respectively), the trends are worthy of further study.

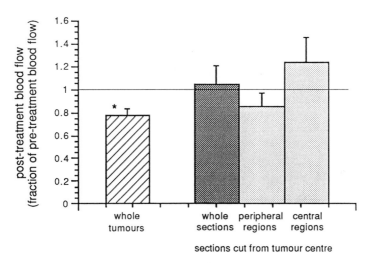

Figure 4. Comparison of tumour blood flow response to angiotensin II for whole tumours (measured by scintillation counting and for sections cut from the centre of tumours (measured by autoradiography). Columns represent means and bars represent 1 S.E.M. Data is pooled for tumours from the 2 highest perfusion pressure groups shown in Figure 3. * represents a significant difference (P = .004) between blood flow in angiotensin-treated animals and control animals, using student's t-test for unpaired data.

DISCUSSION

The angiotensin-induced reduction in overall blood flow to the P22 tumour, found in this study and in a previous study (Tozer & Shaffi, 1992), suggests that these tumours can respond directly to the vasoconstrictive effect of angiotensin II and that, for the tumours as a whole, this vasoconstriction overcomes any tendency for blood flow to increase as a result of an increase in perfusion pressure. This follows from the relationship,

tissue vascular resistance = perfusion pressure ÷ tissue blood flow.

This result is in agreement with the findings of Jirtle et al. (1978). However, other studies have found that angiotensin II induced an increase in absolute tumour blood flow in their systems (Hori et al., 1991, Tanda et al., 1991, Tokuda et al., 1990). We found that the response of tumours was dependent on the pre-treatment level of blood flow, with reduction in flow tending to be highest for tumours with the highest pre-treatment blood flow. Blood flow to tumours in the Jirtle study was even higher than for the P22 tumour (1.3 mls g-1 min-1). Conversely, the subcutaneous tumours used in the studies which showed a consistent improvement in blood flow following angiotensin II administration (Hori et al., 1991, Tanda et al., 1991, Tokuda et al., 1991), had rather low pre-treatment blood flow (around 0.2 mls g-1 min-1 for the AH109A tumour and the LY80 tumour). Therefore, the discrepancy between results in the different studies could be explained by differences in pre-treatment blood flow.

It is not clear why angiotensin II should be particularly efficient at reducing blood flow in tumours with high initial flow. It is possible that low flow tumours have a higher fraction of collapsed vessels (perhaps induced by high interstitial fluid pressure) than high flow tumours. The high perfusion pressures induced by angiotensin II would tend to re-open these vessels, thus off-setting any direct vasoconstrictive effects of angiotensin II (from the relationship shown above). Alternatively, high flow tumours may possess more vascular smooth muscle receptors for angiotensin II. We are currently investigating these possibilities.

We also noted that tumours from a first generation transplant away from the primary P22 tumour were particularly sensitive to angiotensin-induced vasoconstriction. Angiotensin increased tissue vascular resistance by a factor of more than three in these tumours, which is similar to that induced in the most sensitive normal tissues studied in a previous report (Tozer & Shaffi, 1992). Again, the reasons for this finding are unclear but it certainly does not support the proposal that tumours have very little capacity for responding directly to vasoactive agents.

Autoradiography showed that the angiotensin-induced decrease in overall tumour blood flow concealed a differential response between the tumour periphery and centre. Most of the overall reduction in flow was due to vasoconstriction in the higher flow tumour periphery. There was even a suggestion, although it was not statistically significant, that, at high enough perfusion pressures, blood flow may be increased in the tumour centre. If this finding can be confirmed by further experiments, it is consistent with either 1) opening up of collapsed vessels in the tumour centre where interstitial fluid pressure is probably high (Wiig et al., 1982, Boucher et al., 1990, Less et al., 1991) or 2) a heterogeneous distribution of angiotensin II receptors between the tumour periphery and centre.

These results have implications for cancer radiotherapy and chemotherapy. Our recent findings (Tozer & Shaffi, 1992) and those of others, have shown that angiotensin II increases tumour blood flow *relative* to several normal tissues. Thus, angiotensin II has potential as an adjuvant to chemotherapy (Sasaki et al., 1985, Takematsu et al., 1985, Noguchi et al., 1988, Anderson et al., 1991, Kobayashi et al., 1990 & 1991). On the other hand, the decrease in *absolute* tumour blood flow would decrease oxygen delivery to tumours. This would decrease the efficacy of radiotherapy but may improve the efficacy of bioreductive drugs (Brown, 1987) if oxygen levels fall far enough. The tendency for angiotensin to equalise the blood flow between the tumour periphery and centre is beneficial for all forms of therapy.

Generally, the application of blood flow modifiers in the clinic is limited by the unpredictability of the tumour response. Hirst et al. (1991 & 1992) have shown that even the same tumour growing in different sites in the mouse can respond very differently to angiotensin II, for instance. The present study has shown that pre-treatment blood flow may be one predictive factor for the response of tumours to vasoactive agents. Such factors are urgently required for a rational approach to modifying tumour blood flow and oxygen delivery in the clinic.

Acknowledgement

We would like to thank Mr P Russell and his staff for care of the animals. We would also like to thank Dr P Carnochan for some free samples of 125I-IAP, Dr V Cunningham for his blood flow program and Dr B Vojnovic and his staff for providing some of the electronic equipment. This work was funded by the Cancer Research Campaign.

REFERENCES

Anderson, J.H., Willmott, N., Bessent, R., Angerson, W.J., Kerr, D.J. & McArdle, C.S., 1991, Regional chemotherapy for inoperable renal carcinoma: a method of targeting therapeutic microspheres to tumour, *Br. J. Cancer* 64:365.

Brown, J. M. Exploitation of bioreductive agents with vasoactive drugs, *in*: "Proc. 8th International Congress of Radiation Research, Edinburgh, U.K., 1987" Taylor & Francis, London. Vol. 2, p 719.

Boucher, Y., Baxter, L.T. & Jain, R.K., 1990, Interstitial pressure gradients in tissue-isolated and subcutaneous tumors: implications for therapy, *Cancer Research* 50:4478.

Hirst D. G, Hirst, V.K., Shaffi, K.M., Prise, V.E. & Joiner, B., 1991, The influence of vasoactive agents on the perfusion of tumours growing in three sites in the mouse, *Int. J. Radiat. Biol.* 60:211.

Hirst, D.G. & Tozer, G.M., 1992, Pharmacological manipulation of blood flow, *Br. J. Radiol., in press.*

Hori, K., Suzuki, M., Tanda, S., Saito, S., Shinozaki, M. & Zhang, Q.H., 1991, Fluctuations in tumor blood flow under normotension and the effect of angiotensin II-induced hypertension, *Jpn. J. Cancer Res.* 82:1309.

Jirtle, R., Clifton, K.H. & Rankin, J.H.G., 1978, Effects of several vasoactive drugs on the vascular resistance of MT-W9B tumors in W/Fu rats, *Cancer Res.* 38:2385.

Kety, S.S., 1960, Theory of blood tissue exchange and its application to measurements of blood flow, *Methods Med. Res.* 8:223.

Kobayashi, H., Hasuda, K., Aoki, K., Taniguchi, S. & Baba, T., 1990, Systemic chemotherapy in tumour-bearing rats using high-dose cis-diamminedichloroplatinum (ii) with low nephrotoxicity in combination with angiotensin II and sodium thiosulfate, *Int. J. Cancer* 45:940.

Kobayashi, H., Hasuda, K., Taniguchi, S. & Baba, T., 1991, Therapeutic efficacy of two-route chemotherapy using cis-diamminedichloroplatinum (II) and its antidote, sodium thiosulfate, combined with the angiotensin-II-induced hypertension method in a rat uterine tumor, *Int. J. Cancer* 47:893.

Less, J.R., Possner, M.C., Boucher, Y., Wolmark, N. & Jain, R.K., 1991, Elevated interstitial fluid pressure in human tumors, *Pro. Am. Assoc. Cancer Res.* 32:59.

Noguchi, S., Miyachi,K., Nishizawa, Y., Sasaki, Y., Imaoka, S., Iwanaga, T., Koyama, H. and Terasawa, T., 1988, Augmentation of anti-cancer effect with angiotensin II in intra-arterial infusion chemotherapy for breast carcinoma, *Cancer* 62:467.

Sasaki, Y., Imaoka, S., Hasegawa, Y., Nakano, S., Ishikawa, O., Ohigashi, H., Taniguchi, K., Koyama, H., Iwanaga, T. and Terasawa, T., 1985, Changes in distribution of hepatic blood flow induced by intra-arterial infusion of angiotensin II in human hepatic cancer, *Cancer* 55:311.

Takematsu, H., Tomita, Y. & Kato, T., 1985, Angiotensin-induced hypertension and chemotherapy for multiple lesions of malignant melanoma, *Brit. J. Dermatol.* 113:463.

Tanda, S., Hori, K., Saito, S., Shinozaki, M., Zhang, Q.H. & Suzuki, M., 1991, Comparison of the effects of intravenously bolus-administered endothelin-1 and infused angiotensin II on the subcutaneous tumor blood flow in anaethetized rats, *Jpn. J. Cancer Res.* 82:958.

Tokuda, K., Abe, H., Aida, T., Sugimoto, S. & Kaneko, S., 1990, Modification of tumor blood flow and enhancement of therapeutic effect of ACNU on experimental rat gliomas with angiotensin II, *J. Neurooncol.* 8:205.

Tozer, G.M., Lewis, S., Michalowski, A. & Aber, V., 1990, The relationship between regional variations in blood flow and histology in a transplanted rat fibrosarcoma, *Br. J. Cancer* 61:250.

Tozer, G.M. & Shaffi, K. M., 1992, Modification of tumour blood flow using the hypertensive agent, angiotensin II, *Submitted to Br. J. Cancer.*

Wiig, H., Tveit, E., Hultborn, R., Reed, R.K. and Weiss, L., 1982, Interstitial fluid pressure in DMBA-induced rat mammary tumours, *Scand. J. Clin. Lab. Invest.* 42:159.

IS OXYGEN THE LIMITING SUBSTRATE FOR THE EXPANSION OF CORDS AROUND BLOOD VESSELS IN TUMOURS?

David G. Hirst, Barbara Joiner and V. Kate Hirst

CRC Gray Laboratory
P.O. Box 100, Mount Vernon Hospital
Northwood
Middx. HA6 2JR
England

INTRODUCTION

The supply of metabolic substrates to the cells of most tissues is achieved entirely by perfusion with blood via the vascular system. In most normal tissues the spatial relationship between supplying vessels and the dependent parenchymal cells is precisely regulated so that no cell is further from the vessel than the oxygen diffusion distance for that tissue. The distance between supplying vessels may vary depending on the metabolic requirements of particular cells. Thus, in normal healthy tissues necrosis due to nutrient deprivation is rarely seen. In tumours, however, parenchymal proliferation is often so rapid that proliferation and geometric organization of vascular elements is inadequate (Hirst, 1980; Tannock,1970), even under the influence of tumour angiogenesis factors, and regions of necrosis develop as the tumour grows.

In many rodent and some human tumours (Thomlinson & Gray, 1955) necrosis arises in a clearly identifiable pattern, with cords of viable tumour cells surrounding individual blood vessels. Thomlinson and Gray (1955) suggested that the width of these cords represents the maximum diffusion distance of the limiting substrate which their calculations lead them to believe is oxygen. More direct evidence for the importance of oxygen as the limiting factor in the expansion of cords away from blood vessels was obtained by Tannock, 1970. He demonstrated that the thickness of cords was reduced in the tumours of mice that had been exposed to an oxygen-poor (10%) atmosphere for 48hr. The ability of cells to survive at a distance from blood vessels depends not only on the nutrient supply but also on the metabolic consumption of substrates. We will show in this paper the importance of both nutrient supply and demand on tumour cord radius.

Oxygen Transport to Tissue XV, Edited by P. Vaupel
et al., Plenum Press, New York, 1994

MATERIALS AND METHODS

Tumour System

The techniques for passaging the RH carcinoma and implanting it in its syngeneic host, the WHT/GyfBSVS mouse have been described previously (Hirst et al, 1991). Briefly, 2×10^5 tumour cells were implanted intradermally on the dorsum and allowed to grow to the experimental size of 500-800mg which took about 3 months in this slow growing carcinoma.

Environmental Alterations

In some experiments mice were exposed to an atmosphere with either higher (100%) or lower (10%) oxygen levels as previously described (Hirst, et al 1991). In others, the mice were placed in a cold room (4°C), four animals to a cage for varoius periods up to 48hr.

Measurement of Cord Radius

After exposure to the altered environments the mice were killed by neck fracture and the tumours excised and prepared for histology. 4μm paraffin sections were cut and stained with haematoxylin and eosin. Sections were scanned at a magnification of 400x and the distance between blood vessels and necrosis measured according to a strict protocol as previously described (Hirst et al., 1991). No selection of fields or individual vessels was made.

RESULTS

The mean radius of tumour cords in animals exposed to either increased or decreased levels of inspired O_2 is shown in Fig.1. The mean radius in animals breathing 10% O_2 did not change significantly from the control value of 105±2μm (m±1s.e.; n=23) for the first 15hr of exposure, but fell rapidly over the following 9hr to reach a significantly lower value of 93±2μm (p<0.005; n=10) after 15hr of exposure. This reduction in radius remained very consistent over the following 53hr, a new steady state having been established.

Cord radius in the animals breathing 100% oxygen changed more abruptly than in oxygen deprived animals. It was increased significantly (p<0.05) after only 3hr of exposure and reached a maximum value of 117±3μm. Further exposure to 100% O_2 did not lead to wider cords, rather, there was slight reduction possibly reflecting the toxicity of high pO_2 in the lungs.

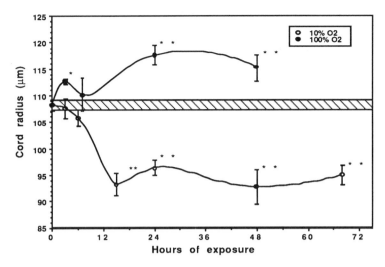

Figure 1. The effect of breathing 100% O2 (●) or 10% O2 (O) on the width of tumour cords around blood vessels in the RH carcinoma growing in mice. The mean width (±1 s.e.) of cords in the tumours of air-breathing animals is shown by the hatched bar. All error bars show ± 1 s.e. Values statistically different from control are indicated (* , p<0.05; **, p<0.005). Reproduced from Hirst et al. (1991) with permission.

Oxygen delivery to tissue can also be increased by promoting its release from haemoglobin. The antihyperlipidaemia drug clofibrate has been shown to reduce the binding affinity of haemoglobin for oxygen and to reduce the radiobiologically hypoxic fraction in tumours (Hirst et al, 1987; Hirst & Wood, 1989). As shown in Fig. 2, a single clofibrate dose of 2mmole/kg did not produce a significant change in cord radius, however, 4hr after a second dose cord radius was significantly increased (p=0.02) from 106.6±1.2 to 110.4±1.3.

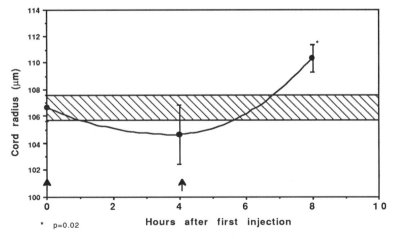

Figure2. The influence of one or two oral oral doses of clofibrate (1mmole/kg), a haemoglobin/O_2 bindingaffinity modifier, on the radius of tumour cords in the RH carcinoma. The arrows mark the timing of drug administration.

When animals were placed in a cold room at 4°C they could tolerate prolonged exposure (up to 24hr) provided four animals were placed in a cage together. Significant changes in cord radius were observed (Fig. 3). Under those circumstances, tumour core temperature fell by an average of 3.5°C to 33.1±0.36 (±1s.e.)°C. Cord radius rose significantly (p<0.01) from 101.3±2.2μm to 108.5±0.6μm within 4hr and reached a maximum of 109.2±1.2 after 8hr. At later times up to 24hr radii remained elevated though at no individual time was this significant.

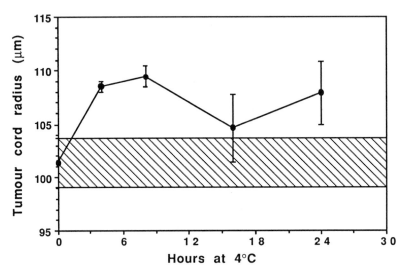

Figure 3. Cord radius in the RH tumour as a function of time at low temperature. Data points are means ±1s.e., hatched bar shows control range in this experiment (±1 s.e.).

DISCUSSION

In both of the experiments where cord radius increased either in response to additional O_2 availability or reduced O_2 consumption, the effect occurred in less then 4hr. At first sight, this might seem to be a remarkably rapid response. We wished to know whether this change was a result of an increase in the size of individual tumour cells or a consequence of accelerated cell division leading to more cells per cord. We counted the number of tumour cell nuclei per cord radius for the control and 4 hr groups shown in Fig.3. Between 0 and 4hr the number of cells/cord increased by 6.5% while the cord radius increased by 7.1% so that there was no significant increase in mean cell diameter. We might assume that this reflects more rapid proliferation under conditions of improved oxygenation. However, it does seem highly unlikely that an increased rate of entry into mitosis could yield a significant increase in cord radius in as short a time as 4hr, because most cells that are out of cycle must first undergo DNA synthesis in preparation for cell division.

A careful consideration of the cell kinetics of this tumour suggests a more plausible explanation. The pressure of cell proliferation in tumour cords leads to a constant outward migration of cells towards the necrotic zone, which in the RH carcinoma proceeds at the rate of about 2μm/hr (Hirst, et al. 1982). This migration does not normally lead to cord expansion because the cells die at some point after they pass the limit for oxygen diffusion. Thus the cord is not a static structure but rather comprises cells that are in constant radial motion. When the O_2 diffusion distance is altered either by increasing inspired pO_2 or by lowering the rate of tumour cell metabolism, cell migration can continue immediately to the new diffusion limit. At a rate of 2μm/hr we can calculate that the migrating cells would cover a distance of 8μm in 4hr, almost exactly the amount of cord expansion seen in this study (Fig. 3). Thus, cord expansion can be a very rapid process when conditions are favourable and we should be aware that any intervention that improves tumour oxygenation may very rapidly increase the diffusion distance required for chemotherapy drugs and even O_2 itself to reach the most distant cells.

We have shown clearly (Fig.1) that the process of cord shrinkage under O_2 deprivation is much slower than cord expansion. This phenomenon has been discussed in detail previously (Hirst, et al. 1991). Briefly, cord shrinkage following exposure to low O_2 must be a consequence of the death of the outermost tumour cell layers, no longer able to survive at very low pO_2. Typically tumour cells take at least 8hr to die when they are deprived of O_2 (Denekamp et al., 1983) so that the onset of cord shrinkage will be delayed to an extent that is dependent on the hypoxia tolerance of the particular cell line.

ACKNOWLEDGMENTS

This work is supported by the Cancer Research Campaign.

REFERENCES

Denekamp, J., Hill, S.A. and Hobson, B., 1983, Vascular occlusion and tumour cell death. *Eur. J. Cancer Clin. Oncol.*, 19: 271.

Hirst, D.G. and Denekamp, J., 1979, Tumor cell proliferation in relation to the vasculature. *Cell Tissue Kinet.* 12: 31.

Hirst, D.G., Denekamp, J. and Hobson, B., 1982, Proliferation kinetics of endothelial cells in three mammary carcinomas. *Cell Tissue Kinet..*, 15: 251.

Hirst, D.G., Hirst, V.K., Joiner, B., Prise, V. and Shaffi. K.M., 1991, Changes in tumour morphology with alterations in oxygen availability: further evidence for oxygen as a limiting substrate. *Br. J. Cancer,* 64: 54.

Hirst, D.G. and Wood, P.J., 1989, Chlorophenoxyacetic acid derivatives as hemoglobin modifiers and tumor radiosensitizers. *Int. J. Radiat. Oncol. Biol. Phys.*, 16: 1183.

Hirst, D.G., Wood, P.J. and Schwartz, H.C., 1987, The modification of hemoglobin affinity for oxygen and tumor radiosensitivity by antilipidemic drugs. *Radiat. Res.* 112: 164.

Tannock, I.F., 1970, Effects of pO$_2$ on cell proliferation kinetics. In *Time and DoseRelationships in Radiation Biology as Applied to Therapy*, Bond, V.P., Suit, H.D. & Marcial, V. (eds), p.215, Brookhaven National Laboratory, Upton.

THE EFFECT OF ARTIFICIALLY INDUCED ISCHEMIA ON TUMOUR CELL SURVIVAL

D.J. Chaplin[1,2] and M.R. Horsman[3]

[1]Vascular Targeting Group, CRC Gray Laboratory, Northwood, Middx, U.K.
[2]Medical Biophysics Unit, B.C. Cancer Research Centre, 601 West 10th Avenue, Vancouver, Canada
[3]Danish Cancer Society, Department of Experimental Clinical Oncology Norrebrogade 44, DK-8000, Aarhus, Denmark

INTRODUCTION

There has been much recent interest in the therapeutic potential of reducing blood flow and thus oxygenation selectively within tumours[1,2]. Transient reductions in tumour blood flow induced by agents such as hydralazine and serotonin have been exploited to enhance the anti-tumour efficacy of drugs known to be more toxic in a hypoxic environment[3-5]. Long term or permanent reductions in tumour blood flow can be induced by a number of cytokines (e.g. TNF), drugs (e.g. FAA and vinca alkaloids), and modalities such as hyperthermia and photodynamic therapy. These agents have anti-tumour efficacy in experimental tumours when used alone. Indeed for such treatment modalities, the major part of their anti-tumour effects are attributed to ischemia induced cytotoxicity as a result of the chronic blood flow reductions they induce[6,7].

For both transient reductions of blood flow to enhance cytotoxic drugs and chronic reductions to induce ischemic cell death, one physiological parameter which will be of major importance in determining therapeutic outcome will be tumour temperature. Reductions in temperature can reduce drug toxicity and protect against ischaemic cell death. This is particularly relevant since most of the studies with blood flow modifiers have been performed in superficially located rodent tumours. In such tumours reductions in blood flow would be expected to decrease tumour temperature.

In order to address the importance of tumour temperature on therapeutic potential of blood flow, we have evaluated the effects of temperature on ischemia induced cell death in two tumour systems.

MATERIALS AND METHODS

Mice and Tumours

SCCVII tumour cells obtained by enzymic disaggregation were implanted subcutaneously over the sacral region of the back in 6-12 week old C$_3$H/He mice (Charles River Inc. Quebec, Canada). Tumours were used in the size range 350-500mg. Derivation and Maintenance or this line has been described previously[8]. The C$_3$H/Tif mammary carcinoma was implanted into the foot of the right hind limb of 10-14 week old female

Oxygen Transport to Tissue XV, Edited by P. Vaupel
et al., Plenum Press, New York, 1994

$C_3D_2F_1$/Bom mice. The derivation, maintenance and implantation of this tumour has been described previously[9]. Treatments were carried out when the tumours had reached a tumour size of 200mm^3.

Ischemia

Ischemia was induced in SCCVII tumours either by application of D-shaped metal clamps as described previously[10] or by nitrogen asphyxiation of the host animal. Vascular occlusion in the C_3H/Tif mammary carcinoma was achieved by using a rubber tube tightened around the leg[11].

Tumour Temperature

Measurement. Tumour temperatures were measured by inserting a microprobe thermocouple into the tumour. The technique has been described in detail previously[11].

Temperature Maintenance

Tumour temperatures between 27°C and 37°C were attained for SCCVII tumours by placing the tumour-bearing animal in a water-jacketed incubator. To attain a temperature of 4°C a cold room was used. For the C_3H/Tif tumour, all tumour temperatures were reached and maintained by placing the tumour-bearing foot in a circulating water bath. For this procedure tumour-bearing legs were exposed and loosely attached to the jig with tape prior to insertion of the leg into the water bath. The water bach was covered with a lucite plate with holes allowing immersion of the foot approximately 1cm below the water surface. Previous measurements of intratumoural temperature have shown stabilization within a few minutes to 0.2°C below the water bath temperature.

Tumour Response

The response of the SCCVII tumour was assessed immediately following the termination of vascular occlusion by clonogenic assay as described previously[12].

For the C_3H/Tif mammary carcinoma treatment response was assessed using a regrowth delay assay. This procedure has been described previously[13]. Basically tumour volume was measured on a daily basis following treatment. The time taken to reach 5 times the treatment volume was determined and from this value the mean (±1 S.E.) calculated for all the mice in each treatment group.

RESULTS

The effect of vascular occlusion on tumour temperature is shown in Table 1. It can be seen that 60 minutes following the induction of ischemia, the temperature in subcutaneous SCCVII tumours falls to a value of only 2°C above ambient temperature from a pretreatment temperature of 35.2°C. Similar results are obtained with the C_3H/Tif tumour although in this tumour the resting temperature is only 26.6°C, it is reduced to 21.9°C after 60 minutes of ischemia. The effect of temperature on the survival of cells within SCCVII tumours subject to a 3-hour period of ischemia is shown in Figure 1. It can be seen that cell survival is dependent on the temperature maintained during the ischemia insult. No cell kill is observed if the environmental temperature is maintained at 4°C during the ischemia yet if tumours are maintained at a temperature of 37°C over 3 decades of cell kill are evident. It can also be seen that methods of induction of ischemia, i.e. either by clamping or asphysiation of the host animal, does not affect the level of cell survival. The time course

Table 1

The effect of ischemia induced by vascular occlusion on the tumour temperature in SCCVII and C_3H/Tif tumours. Values are the mean [±1.S.E.] from 4 to 5 animals. Room temperatures are also indicated.

Tumour	Tumour	temperature	Room temperature
	Pre	60' Post	
SCCVII	35.2[±0.2]	24.0[±0.5]	22.3[±0.2]
C_3H/Tif	26.6[±0.2]	21.9[±0.4]	21.9[±0.1]

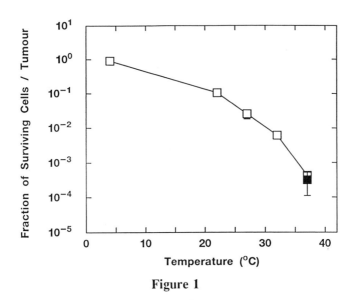

Figure 1

The effect of a 3-hour period of ischemia under different external temperatures on the survival of SCCVII tumour cells. Open symbols: ischemia induced by death of the host animal. Closed symbol: ischemia induced by clamping. Results are the mean [±1.S.E.] of 4 to 5 experiments.

of tumour cell death as a result of ischemia at temperatures of 4°C, 22°C and 37°C is shown in Figure 2. It can be seen that amount of cell death increases with increasing duration of ischemia for all temperatures examined. The results confirm the temperature dependence of cell survival indicated from Figure 1.

The effect of temperature on ischemia-induced growth delay induced in C₃H/Tif tumours is shown in Figure 3. If the tumours are allowed to cool to room temperature (21.9°C) following vascular occlusion, no significant effects on growth delay can be

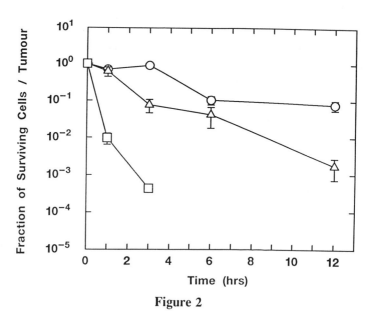

Figure 2

The effect of duration of ischemia on tumour cell survival. Ischemic insult carried out at temperatures of 37°C(□), 22°C (Δ) and 4°C (O).

observed for periods of ischemia up to 6 hours. However if tumours are maintained at a temperature of 37°C during the ischaemic insult, significant growth delay is observed for all occlusion times exceeding one hour. In the lower panel in Figure 3, the effect of varying tumour temperature during a fixed ischaemic insult of 4 hours is shown. Significant growth delays are observed for temperatures of 31°C or higher.

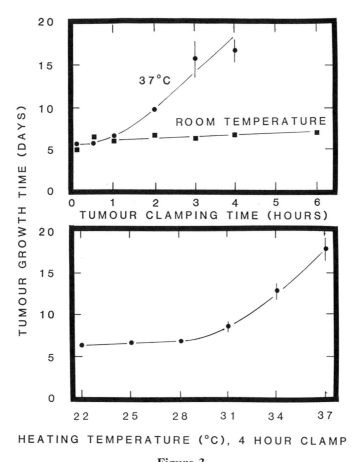

Figure 3

(Upper panel) Growth delay induced in C_3H/Tif mammary carcinoma by varying periods of ischemic insult at room temperature and at 37°C.

(Lower panel) Growth delay induced by different temperatures maintained during a 4-hour ischemic insult. Each point represents the mean (±S.E.) from at least 5 individual tumours.

DISCUSSION

The results show that induction of ischemia in tumours implanted subcutaneously in the back or foot produces a rapid fall in tumour temperature. For both SCCVII and C₃H/Tif tumours, temperature alters a value close to ambient following 60 minutes of ischemia. Moreover the study demonstrates that this cooling of the tumour tissue can reduce the rate of tumour cell death resulting from the ischemic insult.

The effect of external temperature on the survival of SCCVII tumour to a three-hour period of ischemia indicates that cell survival increases with decreasing environmental temperature. Of particular importance is the reduction in cell kill observed over the temperature range 22°C to 37°C. For example if an experimental therapeutic intervention produced a complete cessation in blood flow with subcutaneous SCCVII tumour for 3 hours, it would, based on results from Figure 1, produce 1 decade of cell kill. However if a similar blood flow reduction was produced but the tumour maintained at 37°C which would be close to the temperature of a tumour located within the body, 3 decades of cell kill would be produced. By analogy a less dramatic or shorter blood flow reduction may produce the same cell killing in centrally located tumour masses than that in superficially located tumours. This may be particularly relevant since some chemical agents are known to produce smaller blood flow reductions in centrally located tumours when compared to subcutaneously located ones[14].

Qualitatively similar temperature dependence of ischemic cell death is seen in C₃H/Tif tumours. Results shown in Figure 3 illustrate that if tumours are allowed to cool following vascular occlusion, no significant growth delay is seen even after 6 hours of ischemia. In contrast significant growth delay is observed for all periods of vascular occlusion greater than one hour if the tumours are maintained at 37°C.

The mechanism of ischemia-induced cell death in the tumours studied has not been directly investigated. However it is known that cell survival is greatly reduced *in vitro* under combination of anoxia and acidic pH[15]. Since anaerobic glycolysis is a temperature dependent process, it is possible that the protection from ischemic cell death afforded by reduced temperature is due at least in part to a less dramatic build up of acidic catabolites.

Whatever the mechanism of ischemia-induced tumour cell death, the protective effect of reduced temperatures is obvious. This finding is not novel since the preservation of the integrity of normal tissues for transplant purposes is known to be enhanced by hypothermia[16, 17]. However as far as we are aware, little or no work has been previously reported on the influence of temperature on ischemic cell death in malignant tissue. Based on the studies reported here, tumour temperature is an important factor to be considered when therapeutic strategies which induce blood flow reduction are used in mice bearing superficially located tumour masses.

ACKNOWLEDGEMENTS

This work was funded in part by grants from the Medical Research Council of Canada and the Danish Cancer Society. We would like to thank Ms Sandy Lynde and Ms Inger-Marie Johanson for their excellent technical support.

REFERENCES

1. Denekamp, J. The current status of targeting tumour vasculature as a means of cancer therapy: an overview. *Int. J. Radiat. Biol.* 60: 401 (1991).
2. Chaplin, D.J. and Trotter, M.J. Chemical Modifiers of Tumour Blood Flow. *In:* "Tumour Blood Supply and Metabolic Microenvironment". Vaupel, P. and Jain, R.K., eds., Gustav Fischer Verlag, Stuttgart (1991).

3. Chaplin, D.J. Potentiation of RSU-1069 tumour cytotoxicity by 5-hydroxytryptamine (5-HT). *Br. J. Cancer* 54: 727 (1986).
4. Chaplin, D.J. Hydralazine induced tumour hypoxia: a potential target for cancer chemotherapy. *J. Natl. Cancer Inst.* 81: 618 (1989).
5. Stratford, I.J., Godden, J., Howells, N., Embling, P. and Adams, G.E. Manipulation of tumour oxygenation by hydralazine increases the potency of bioreductive radiosensitisers and enhances the effect of melphalan in experimental tumours. *In:* "Proceedings of the 8th International Congress of Radiation Research". Eds. Fielden, E.M., Fowler, J.F., Hendry, J.H. and Scott, D. Taylor and Frances, London (1987).
6. Chaplin, D.J. The effect of therapy on tumour vascular function. *Int. J. Radiat. Biol.* 60: 311 (1991).
7. Vaupel, P., Mueller-Klieser, W., Otte, J., Manz, R., Kallinowski, F. Blood flow, tissue oxygenation and pH distribution in malignant tumours upon localised hyperthermia. *Strahlentherapie* 159: 73 (1983).
8. Olive, P.L., Chaplin, D.J. and Durand, R.E. Pharmacokinetics binding and distribution of Hoechst 33342 in spheroids and murine tumours. *Br. J. Cancer* 51: 569 (1985).
9. Overgaard, J. Simultaneous and sequential hyperthermia and radiation treatment of an experimental tumour and its surrounding normal tissue in vivo. *Int. J. Radiat. Oncol. Biol. Phys.* 6: 1507.
10. Denekamp, J., Hill, S.A. and Hobson, B. Vascular occlusion and tumour cell death. *Eur. J. Cancer. Clin. Oncol.* 19: 271 (1983).
11. Horsman, M.R., Christenson, K.L. and Overgaard, J. Hydralazine induced enhancement of hyperthermic damage in a C_3H mammary carcinoma in vivo. *Int. J. Hyperthermia* 5: 123 (1989).
12. Chaplin, D.J., Olive, P.L., Durand, R.E. Intermittent blood flow in a murine tumour: radiobiological effects. *Cancer Res.* 47: 597 (1987).
13. Kamura, T., Nielsen, O.S., Overgaard, J. and Anderson, A.H. Development of thermotolerance during fractionated hyperthermia in a solid tumour in vivo. *Cancer Res.* 42: 1744 (1982).
14. Hirst, D.G., Hirst, V.K., Shaffi, K.M., Prise, V.E. and Joiner, B. The influence of vasoactive agents on the perfusion of tumours growing in three sites in the mouse. *Int. J. Radiat. Biol.* 60: 211 (1991).
15. Rotin, D., Robinson, B., and Tannock, I.F. Influence of hypoxia and an acidic microenvironment on the metabolism and viability of cultured cells: potential implications for cell death in tumours. *Cancer Res.* 46: 2821 (1986).
16. Fuller, B.J. Storage of cells and tissues at hypothermia for clinical use. *Symp. Soc. Exp. Biol.* 41: 341 (1987).
17. Collste, H. Preservation of kidneys for transplantation: experimental studies. *Acta. Chir. Scand.* Suppl.425: 1 (1972).

INTRATUMORAL pO_2 HISTOGRAPHY AS PREDICTIVE ASSAY IN ADVANCED CANCER OF THE UTERINE CERVIX[*]

Michael Höckel[1], Claudia Knoop[1], Karlheinz Schlenger[1], Birgit Vorndran[1], Paul Georg Knapstein[1], and Peter Vaupel[2]

[1] Department of Obstetrics and Gynecology, and
[2] Institute of Physiology and Pathophysiology
University of Mainz
D-6500 Mainz, Germany

INTRODUCTION

Experimental evidence suggests that the hypoxic fraction in a solid tumor may increase its malignant potential and reduce its sensitivity towards non-surgical treatment modalities such as standard irradiation and certain anticancer agents[1-5]. However, the clinical importance of tumor hypoxia remains uncertain since valid methods for the routine measurement of intratumoral O_2-tensions in patients have so far been lacking.

METHODS AND PATIENTS

A **prospective clinical trial** for the evaluation of intratumoral pO_2 distribution in advanced cervical carcinomas has been initiated at the Department of Obstetrics and Gynecology, University of Mainz, in June 1989.

[*]Supported by Deutsche Krebshilfe, Grant M 40/91/Va 1

Up until September 1991, thirtyone patients with advanced cervical cancers have entered the study. The median age of the patients was 57 years with a range of 27 - 80 years. The macroscopic and microscopic tumor features as well as the treatment modalities are listed in Table 1.

Table 1. Patient and tumor characteristics, treatment modality, and tumor oxygenation

	Number of patients (N = 31)	Median $pO_2 \leq 10$ mmHg (n = 15)	Median $pO_2 > 10$ mmHg (n = 16)
Tumor stage			
FIGO Ib (bulky)	1	-	1
FIGO IIa,b	17	8	9
FIGO IIIb	12	6	6
FIGO IV a	1	1	-
Clinical tumor size (maximum diameter)			
< 40 mm	6	3	3
40 - 60 mm	13	5	8
> 60 mm	12	7	5
Histological type			
Squamous cell carcinoma	28	14	14
Adenocarcinoma	3	1	2
Histological grading			
I	3	1	2
II	23	11	12
III	5	3	2
Treatment			
RT	15	6	9
RT + CT	7	5	2
RT + surg	1	1	-
RT + CT + surg	3	1	2
Surg	1	1	-
Surg + CT	4	1	3

RT = radiotherapy, CT = chemotherapy, surg = surgery

Intratumoral pO_2 measurements using the Eppendorf computerized histography system (Eppendorf-Netheler-Hinz, Hamburg, Germany) have been carried out in untreated conscious patients as described earlier[6]. Since position may influence pO_2 readings, all patients were placed in a defined lithotomy position during the measurements (thigh flexion 45°, abduction 90°, lower leg horizontal).

25 - 30 pO_2 measurements along each of two linear tracks at the 12 o'clock and 6 o'clock positions (50 - 60 measurements in total) were obtained from each patient. The tracks were directed parallel to the cervical canal or - in case of distortion by the tumor - parallel to the vaginal axis. The measurements were performed 1 to 5 days before initiation of the oncologic therapy. Using an on-line computing system the pO_2 data were expressed as relative frequencies within a pO_2 histogram between 0 and 100 mmHg with a class width of 2.5 mm Hg. The **median pO_2**, the two lowest pO_2 classes (i.e. 0 - 5 mmHg) which are designated as the **"hypoxic fraction"** and the **range between the 10th**

and 90th percentiles of the pooled histograms of each tumor were used for **statistical analysis.** The Mann-Whitney-Wilcoxon test ("U-test") was applied to detect possible differences between groups. Survival and recurrence-free survival was calculated with the Kaplan-Meier life table method. Variables influencing survival were evaluated by use of the Cox proportional hazards model.

RESULTS

The pO_2 histograms characterizing each tumor showed marked intra- and intertumoral heterogeneity. **Median pO_2** ranged from 2 to 34 mmHg. Fifteen patients had tumors with median pO_2 lower or equal to 10 mmHg. In 21 patients "hypoxic fractions" were detected. The relative amount of the "**hypoxic fraction**" varied from 2 to 96%. The intratumoral **range of the pO_2 distribution** between the 10th and 90th percentiles was 5 mmHg to 72 mmHg with a mean of 37 mmHg. Both "hypoxic fraction" and 10% - 90% pO_2 range significantly correlate with the median pO_2. **Tumor oxygenation** as expressed by median pO_2, "hypoxic fraction" and 10% - 90% pO_2 range was **independent** of patient age, menopausal status, use of oral contraceptives, smoking habits and arterial hemoglobin concentration. Moreover, tumor stage, clinical tumor size, growth pattern, tumor tissue consistency, histologic type and grading had no influence on tumor oxygenation as calculated by the Mann-Whitney-Wilcoxon test from the data of this study.

At a median follow up of 19 months (range 5 to 31 months) 10 patients relapsed and 9 patients died. Recurrent or progressing tumors have been confirmed in the pelvis in all these cases, in one patient distant metastases have been detected also.

Kaplan-Meier survival analysis stratified for median intratumoral pO_2 showed that patients with median **intratumoral $pO_2 \leq$ 10 mmHg** had a significantly **lower survival** and **recurrence-free survival** compared to patients with tumors of >10 mmHg median pO_2 (Fig. 1). Nine of the 10 patients with tumor progression or relapses had median intratumoral $pO_2 \leq$ 10 mmHg. Tumor stage, size, histologic grading and treatment modality were not significantly different in both groups stratified for median pO_2 (Table 1).

Similar results were obtained when the survival analyses were conferred to the subgroups of patients whose treatment included radiation (n = 26, p = 0.005) or those receiving radiotherapy exclusively (n = 15, p = 0.03).

Stratification of the Kaplan-Meier survival analysis of the whole patient cohort for the two other characteristics of the pO_2 histogram, i.e. "hypoxic fraction" and 10% - 90% pO_2 range also showed statistically significant differences with somewhat higher p-values compared to median pO_2. Of the

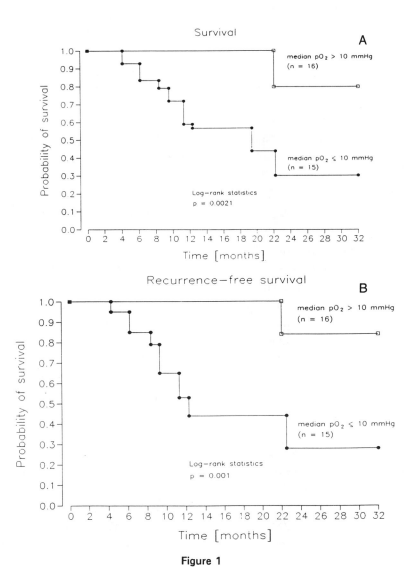

Figure 1

Survival probability (A) and recurrence-free survival probability (B) for patients with advanced cancer of the uterine cervix influenced by tumor oxygenation.

other analyzed oncologic parameters only tumor stage had a significant influence on survival and recurrence-free survival. The Cox proportional hazards model revealed median pO_2 and the correlated "hypoxic fraction" as highly predictive factors for recurrence-free survival and survival respectively, independent of tumor stage, size, histopathologic grading and treatment modality (Table 2).

Table 2. Cox regression analysis

	Influence on survival	Influence on recurrence-free survival
Univariate procedure	"Hypoxic fraction" p = 0.0017 Tumor stage p = 0.0038 Median pO_2 p = 0.0093	Tumor stage p = 0.014 Median pO_2 p = 0.023
Multivariate procedure	"Hypoxic fraction" p = 0.0017 Tumor stage p = 0.0056	Tumor stage p = 0.014 Median pO_2 p = 0.014

Variables tested: Tumor stage, tumor size, histologic grading, median pO_2, "hypoxic fraction", 10 % - 90 % pO_2-range, treatment modality

DISCUSSION AND CONCLUSIONS

The preliminary analysis of the ongoing clinical trial revealed that intratumoral pO_2 as determined with the standard procedure strongly predicts survival and recurrence-free survival in advanced cervical cancer.

The data of this study do not definitively answer the question as to whether the poor prognosis of "hypoxic" cervical cancers is related to the therapeutic approach or represents the malignant potential of the tumor itself in terms of locoregional and distant spread. However, since the majority of the patients have been treated with some form of pelvic radiation and all patients had tumor recurrences in the pelvis, the results of this study may support the assumption that hypoxic tumors are less radiocurable than well oxygenated neoplasms.

The determination of tumor oxygenation with computerized pO_2 histography might become an important **new oncologic parameter** for **advanced cervical cancers** and probably other solid tumors as well[7,8]. The possibility of identifying "hypoxic tumors" could be used to select patients for new clinical trials with the goal to achieve **radiosensitization**[9,10].

Alternatively, radiation might be substituted by **ultraradical surgery** and **pelvic reconstruction** in these patients. Moreover, further knowledge concerning tumor oxygenation may additionally influence cytotoxic drug selection and/or decisions relating to adjunctive oncological treatment at all.

REFERENCES

1. J.M. Brown, Tumor hypoxia, drug resistance, and metastases, *J. Natl. Cancer Inst.* 82:338 (1990).

2. L.H. Gray, A.D. Conger, M. Ebert, S. Hornsey, and O.C.A. Scott, The concentration of oxygen dissolved in tissues at the time of irradiation as a factor in radiotherapy, *Brit. J. Radiol.* 26:638 (1953).

3. G.C. Rice, C.A. Hoy, and R.T. Schimke, Transient hypoxia enhances the frequency of dihydrofolate reductase gene amplification in Chinese hamster ovary cells, *Proc. Natl. Acad. Sci. USA* 83:5978 (1986).

4. B.A. Teicher, S.A. Holden, A. Al-Achi, and T.S. Herman, Classification of antineoplastic treatments by their differential toxicity toward putative oxygenated and hypoxic tumor subpopulations in vivo in the FSaIIC murine fibrosarcoma, *Cancer Res.* 50:3339 (1990).

5. R.H. Thomlinson, L.H. Gray, The histologic structure of some human lung cancers and the possible implications for radiotherapy, *Br. J. Cancer* 9:537 (1955).

6. M. Höckel, K. Schlenger, C. Knoop, and P. Vaupel, Oxygenation of carcinomas of the uterine cervix: evaluation by computerized O_2 tension measurements, *Cancer Res.* 51:6098 (1991).

7. M. Höckel, C. Knoop, K. Schlenger, B. Vorndran, E. Baußmann, M. Mitze, P.G. Knapstein, and P. Vaupel, Intratumoral pO_2 predicts survival in advanced cancer of the uterine cervix, *Radiother. Oncol.* in press (1992).

8. R.A. Gatenby, H.B. Kessler, J.S. Rosemblum, L.R. Coia, P.J. Moldofsky, W.H. Hartz, and G.J. Broder, Oxygen distribution in squamous cell carcinoma metastases and its relationship to outcome of radiation therapy, *Int. J. Radiat. Oncol. Biol. Phys.* 14:831 (1988).

9. H. Bartelink, and J. Overgaard, Tumour hypoxia, *Radiother. Oncol. Suppl.* 20:1 (1991).

10. M. Höckel, P.G. Knapstein, J. Kutzner, A novel combined operative and radiotherapeutic treatment approach for recurrent gynecologic malignant lesions infiltrating the pelvic wall, *Surg. Gyn. Obstet.* 173:297 (1991).

OXYGENATION OF MAMMARY TUMORS AS EVALUATED BY ULTRASOUND-GUIDED COMPUTERIZED-pO₂-HISTOGRAPHY

S. Runkel[1], A. Wischnik[1], J. Teubner[2], E. Kaven[1], J. Gaa[2] and F. Melchert[1]

Departments of [1] Obstetrics and Gynecology and [2] Radiology
Clinical Faculty Mannheim, University of Heidelberg
Mannheim, Germany

INTRODUCTION

Many solid tumors are known to possess inadequate and heterogeneous vascular networks (1,2) which by influencing the nutrient supply to the tissue determine the tumor micromilieu such as the pH and the O_2 partial pressure in the tissue. The resulting tissue hypoxia further modifies the response of non-surgical modalities such as radiation (3) and cytotoxic therapy (4) of these tumors.

As hypoxic cells make up a significant fraction of the total cell population in solid tumors (5-7), determination of the degree of hypoxia by measuring the distribution of pO_2 could help in predicting the tumor response to these various therapies. Many reports are available on measurement of oxygenation in different tumor systems using various methods (8). However until recently oxygenation in human tumors could only be obtained using biopsy material (9,10) or using indirect methods such as positron emission tomography (11). Technological advances in recent years now allow measurement of pO_2 directly in human tissues in situ. The method known as computerized pO_2 histography was first described by Weiss and Fleckenstein (12) and has already been used in normal tissues as well as in various human tumors (13-16). In the present study we evaluated the pO_2 in human breast tumors in situ using an ultrasonographically guided fine needle for the puncture of the tumors. Mammary tumors were selected because radiation and chemotherapy are important therapy options.

The aim of this study was to correlate the pO_2 pattern in mammary tumors of various clinical stages and gradings and in normal breast tissue. The ultrasound location technique enabled the evaluation of the pO_2 gradient from the periphery to the center of the tumor and also allowed measurements in small, non-palpable tumors.

MATERIALS AND METHODS

Patients: As a part of an ongoing study, pO_2 measurements were carried out in a total of 26 patients (aged 32- 81 years, 7 pre- and 19 postmenopausal) admitted with a lump in the breast to the Department of Gynecology at the University Hospital Mannheim, Germany. PO_2 was measured in 18 mammary carcinomas and in 9 benign mammary tumors (one patient with bilateral fibroadenomas). All measurements were performed under sterile conditions immediately prior to surgery in unmedicated, awake patients. Location of tumors followed clinical examination, mammography, and sonography whereby insertion of the pO_2 needle electrode was performed under direct ultrasound guidance. Patient consent prior to measurement and total excision of the examined tissue were mandatory. Relevant systemic parameters such as mean arterial blood pressure, hemoglobin concentration, hematocrit and systemic oxygen saturation were monitored in all patients.

Evaluation of pO_2: Using the pO_2 histograph (KIMOC 6650, Eppendorf, Germany) measurements were performed with sterile polarographic needle electrodes of 300 μm outer diameter and containing a recessed membrane covered electrode of 12 μm in diameter. For the detailed description of the technical data and calibration cycle of the electrode see reference 12. In unanesthetized patients the tumor was located using ultrasonography (5 MHz LS3000 or 7.5 MHz CS9200, Picker International, Germany). Under direct visual control a plastic trocar (0.8 mm outer diameter) containing a hypodermic needle was inserted in to the skin and advanced up to the periphery of the tumor. After removing the needle the pO_2 electrode was inserted slightly beyond the tip of the trocar. The total measurement path was adjusted according to tumor size, so that measurements were only performed in the tumor tissue. The electrode automatically penetrated the tissue in forward steps of 1.0 mm and a subsequent backward step of 0.3 mm, such that measurements were taken effectively at every 0.7 mm. At the end of the measurement the pO_2 electrode was automatically withdrawn from the tissue. The contralateral normal breast tissue in each patient served as control values whereby measurements were performed in same location in the normal breast as the site of tumor in diseased breast.

Statistical analyses: The values are given as mean $\pm$ S.E.M. Statistical significance was obtained using either the student T-test or the Mann-Whitney-U Test.

RESULTS

Using the KIMOC pO_2- histography a total of 26 patients were investigated, of whom 7 were pre- and 19 in the postmenopausal age. Of the 18 mammary carcinomas evaluated 6 were classified as T_1, 5 tumors as T_2 and 7 as T_4 carcinomas. Histologically the majority of carcinomas (n=10) were invasive ductal, 5 were invasive lobular and 3 were ductolobular. 17 of the 18 breast cancers arose in postmenopausal patients. The diameters of the smallest and the largest tumors investigated were 0.6 cm and 9.0 cm respectively.

The average pO_2 in breast carcinomas in situ evaluated in this study was 31.5 ± 4.8 mmHg and is significantly lower than the average pO_2 in the normal breast tissue, namely 58.0 ± 4.3 mmHg ($p<0.001$). The mean pO_2 values in the various clinical stages did not differ significantly from each other and was noted to be 32.8 ± 10.0 mmHg for T_1 tumors, 31.6 ± 8.5 mmHg for T_2 and 30.4 ± 7.6 mmHg for T_4 tumors respectively. Considering the histological classification the average pO_2 value for the invasive lobular carcinomas was 21.7 ± 6.6 mmHg and was found to be lower than the value for ductolobular carcinomas (44.8 ± 18.6 mmHg) but was similar to the average pO_2 of invasive ductal carcinomas (32.5 ± 5.7 mmHg). These differences were however not significant.

Of the 9 benign breast tumors measured, 7 were histologically classified as fibroadenomas, one was a ductal papilloma and one hamartoma. For statistical analyses these were pooled together. The mean pO_2 in these benign tumors was 43.8 ± 6.4 mmHg and thus lies not only significantly higher than the mean value for breast cancers (31.5 ± 4.8 mmHg, $p<0.05$) but is also significantly lower than the mean value for the normal breast tissue (58.0 ± 4.3 mmHg, $p<0.05$).

The patterns of pO_2 distribution observed in mammary carcinomas were distinctly more heterogeneous in comparison to those in the normal breast tissue and in benign tumors. In breast cancers at least 26% of pO_2 values were in the hypoxic region of below 10 mmHg; whereby 15.5 % were below 5 and 7.5 % below 2.5 mmHg. In the normal breast tissue only 4% of the total pO_2 values were found to lie below 10 mmHg, 1.5% below 5 and none below 2.5 mmHg. Thus pooling all the measured values for each group, the pO_2 distribution curve for breast cancers is shifted towards the hypoxic region as compared to benign tumors and to normal breast tissue (fig. 1)

There was a widespread tumor to tumor variability such that individual tumors of the same clinical stage showed a contrasting pattern of pO_2 distribution (fig.2). On the other hand very similar histograms were obtained for some tumors of different stages and different histology. We also studied the change in pO_2 values from the periphery to the center of the tumor tissue. Taking all breast cancers it was observed that the average pO_2 value at the tumor periphery lies in the normoxic range and decreases considerably towards the center of the cancer tissue (fig.3). This pattern of decrease remains the same for the T_1, T_2 and T_4 breast cancers.

Comparing the average pO_2 values of the normal breast tissue for the pre- and postmenopausal patients, a significantly higher mean value was observed for the pre- than for the postmenopausal women (75.9 ± 6.2 vs 53.8 ± 5.1 mmHg, $p<0.05$).

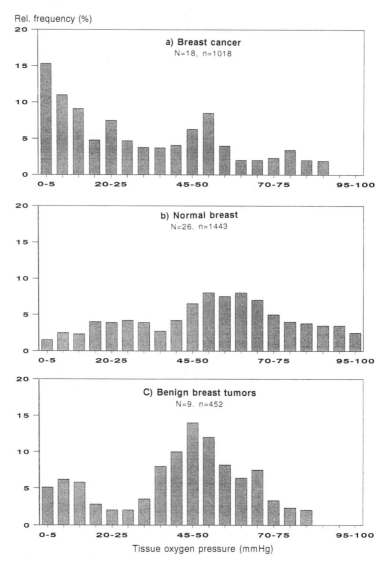

Fig. 1. pO_2 distribution in a) breast cancer, in b) normal breast tissue and in c) benign breast tumors. N represents the number of cases and n the total number of pO_2 measurements.

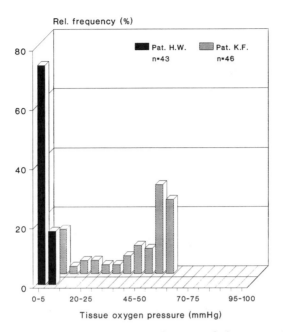

Fig. 2. pO$_2$ frequency distribution in two carcinomas of the same clinical stage and histological classification; T$_2$ carcinoma of the invasive ductal type, a) and b).

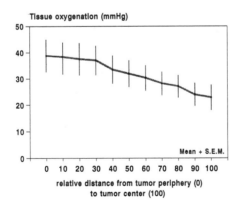

Fig. 3. The average pO$_2$ values (± S.E.M.) in all breast cancers as a function of distance in to the tumor tissue. The unit 0 represents the tumor periphery and the distance of 100 units the center of the tumor.

DISCUSSION

Using the pO_2- histography, measurements of pO_2 were performed in 18 breast cancers of different clinical staging and histology and in 9 benign breast tumors in situ. We report the first series of measurements in breast tumors without the use of local anesthesia prior to measurement and ultrasonographically guided punction of the tumors. The results reported here show that the average pO_2 in normal breast tissue is comparable to the values obtained in other "normoxic" tissues such as the subcutis and oral and gastric mucosa (5,7,21). Due to deficiency in tumor vascularization which is frequent in malignant neoplasms, hypoxic compartments are created within the tumors (5,18), such that the pO_2 distribution shifts to the hypoxic region thus giving rise to significantly lower pO_2 values in breast cancers as compared to normal tissue, as reported here. Our results are similar to those obtained by Vaupel et al. (15) using the same method. We differ however, in the evaluation of the average pO_2 value of benign breast tumors; the previous study quotes a value for fibroadenomas which is similar to that of the normal breast tissue whereas in our report the normal breast pO_2 value was significantly higher than the mean value for the benign breast tumors. Considering that benign tumors are mostly composed of fibrous tissue and or cystic components, one would expect that these tumors are not as well vascularized as the functioning normal breast tissue and thus would reflect oxygen partial pressures lower than that of the normal tissue as reported in our study.

The known heterogeneity within tumors (15,19) make it a difficult task to predict the pO_2 values for the tumors of the same clinical stage and the same histology (figs.2). In human carcinomas the correlation of hypoxia to the clinical staging, grading and histology is disputed. Earlier studies in other human cancers such as the cervical cancer report a decrease in the mean oxygen partial pressure with advancing tumor stage (20) but previous studies using the pO_2-histography show no correlation between these two parameters (15,16). In agreement with the latter authors we too did not observe any differences for the 3 stages investigated. Although we did find the average pO_2 values to differ considerably with the 3 histological types, statistical significance is not observed at present, probably due to the small numbers involved in two of the groups. Thus the reported extensive heterogeneity within a tumor and from tumor to tumor make it necessary that each tumor be evaluated individually so that specific treatment protocols can be designed for each patient in order to improve the tumor response to therapy and to aim for a longer disease free interval.

When comparing the mean pO_2 values of malignant tumors from the periphery to the center of the tumor, a decrease in pO_2 is observed with increasing distance from the periphery (fig.3); the value nearing the center of the tumor being almost half of that at the periphery. This pattern of decrease is also observed in other human tumors (14) and correlates well with the fact that centers of solid tumors are deprived of adequate blood supply and thus in turn oxygenation, giving rise to the well known "necrotic centers" of solid malignancies.

The differences in average pO_2 values observed in pre- and postmenopausal patients reported in this study reflect the non functional, atrophic status of the normal breast tissue found in postmenopausal women due to lack of hormonal stimulation. Using the pO_2 - histography method, important pathophysiological parameters can be evaluated in human tumors in situ. The similar results obtained in breast carcinomas (15 and this study) show the reasonable accuracy and reproducibility of this method. Although the method is invasive, it is clinically applicable with the minimum of discomfort to the patient and allows direct assessment of tissue pO_2. The unique movement of the electrode avoids tissue compression and bleeding at the site. The use of ultrasonography further ensures accurate measurement and allows evaluation of tissue pO_2 in small non palpable tumors.

SUMMARY

The average pO_2 in breast carcinomas in situ is significantly lower than that in the normal breast tissue.

The mean pO_2 value for benign breast tumors is significantly higher than that of the breast cancers but lies significantly lower than the corresponding normal breast.

No significant differences are found in the mean pO_2 values when comparing cancers of different stages and histology.

A decrease in the mean pO_2 value is measured from the periphery to the center of the breast tumors investigated.

The average pO_2 values for pre- and postmenopausal patients differ significantly.

The described method provides a reliable assessment of tissue pO_2 in situ with a minimum of discomfort.

Due to extensive inter tumor heterogeneity, prediction of pO_2 values for tumors of same stage and same histology is not possible, so that measurement of individual tumor is mandatory for determining therapy response.

REFERENCES

1. P. Vaupel, H.P. Fortmeyer, S. Runkel and F. Kallinowski, Blood flow, oxygen consumption and tissue oxygenation of human breast cancer xenografts in nude rats, Cancer Res. 47: 3496 (1987).
2. P. Vaupel and F. Kallinowski, Microcirculation and metabolic micromilieu in malignant tumors, Funktionsanal. Biol. Syst. 18: 265 (1988).
3. R.S. Bush, R.D.T. Jenkin, W.E.C. Allt, F.A. Beale, H. Bean, A.J.Dembo and J.F.Pringel, Definitive evidence for hypoxic cells influencing cure in cancer therapy, Br. J. Cancer. 37(3): 302 (1978).
4. B.A. Teicher, S.A. Holden, A. Al-Achi and T.S. Herman, Classification of antineoplastic treatments by their differential toxicity toward putative oxygenated and hypoxic tumor subpopulations in vivo in the FSaIIc murine fibrosarcomas, Cancer Res. 50: 3339 (1990).

5. P. Vaupel, F. Kallinowski and P. Okunieff, Blood flow, oxygen and nutrient supply and metabolic microenvironment of human tumors: a review, <u>Cancer Res.</u> 49: 6449 (1989).

6. J.E. Moulder and S. Rockwell, Tumor hypoxia: its impact on cancer therapy, <u>Cancer Metastasis Rev.</u> 5: 313 (1987).

7. P. Vaupel, P. Okunieff, F. Kallinowski and L.J. Nuringer, Correlation between ^{31}P-NMR spectroscopy and tissue O_2-tension measurements in a murine fibrosarcoma, <u>Radiat. Res.</u> 120: 477 (1989).

8. W. Müller-Klieser, K-H. Schlenger, S. Walenta, M. Gross, U. Karbach, M. Höckel and P. Vaupel, Pathophysiological approaches to identifying tumor hypoxia in patients, <u>Radiotherapy and oncology,Suppl.</u> 20: 21 (1991).

9. W. Müller-Klieser, P. Vaupel, R. Manz and R. Schmidseder, Intracapillary oxyhemoglobin saturation of malignant tumors in humans, <u>Int. J. Radiat. Oncol. Biol. Phys.</u> 7: 1397 (1981).

10. P. Wendling, R. Manz, G. Thews and P. Vaupel, Inhomogeneous oxygenation of rectal carcinomas in humans. A critical parameter for preoperative irradiation? <u>Adv. Exp. Med. Biol.</u> 180: 293 (1984).

11. R.P. Beaney, A.A. Lammertsma, T. Jones, C. McKenzie and K.E. Halnan, Positron emission tomography for in vivo measurement of regional blood flow, oxygen utilisation and blood volume in patients with breast carcinoma, <u>Lancet.</u> 1: 131 (1984).

12. C. Weiss and W. Fleckenstein, Local tissue pO_2 measured with "thick" needle probes, <u>Funktionsanal. Biol. Syst.</u> 15: 155 (1986).

13. P. Boeckstegers, R. Riessen and W. Seyde, Oxygen partial pressure fields within the skeletal muscle : indicator of the systemic oxygen delivery in patients? <u>Adv. Exp. Med.Biol.</u> in press (1990).

14. W. Fleckenstein, J.R. Jungblut, M. Suckfüll, W. Hoppe and C. Weiss, Sauerstoffdruckverteilungen in Zentrum und Peripherie maligner Kopf-Hals Tumoren, <u>Dtsch. Z. Mund-Kiefer-Gesichts-Chir.</u> 12: 205 (1988).

15. P. Vaupel, K. Schlenger, C. Knoop and M. Höckel, Oxygenation of human tumors: evaluation of tissue oxygen distribution in breast cancers by computerised O_2 tension measurements, <u>Cancer Res.</u> 51: 3316 (1991).

16. M. Höckel, K.Schlenger, C. Knoop and P. Vaupel, Oxygenation of carcinomas of the uterine cervix: evaluation by computerised O_2 tension measurements, <u>Cancer Res.</u> 51: 3316 (1991).

17. G.H. Fletcher. "Textbook of Radiotherapy", Lea and Febiger, Philadelphia (1980).

18. R.K. Jain, Determinants of tumor blood flow: a review, <u>Cancer Res.</u> 48: 2641 1988).

19. P.J. Bergsjö and C. Evans, Oxygenation of cervical carcinoma during the early phase of external irradiation, <u>Scand. J. Clin. Lab. Invest.</u> 27: 71 (1971).

OXYGENATION OF LOCALLY ADVANCED RECURRENT RECTAL CANCER, SOFT TISSUE SARCOMA AND BREAST CANCER

M. Molls[1], H.J. Feldmann[2], J. Füller[2]

[1]Department of Radiooncology, Technische Universität München, 8000 München 80
FRG
[2]Department of Radiooncology, West German Tumor Centre, University Hospital, 4300
Essen 1, FRG

INTRODUCTION

Hypoxia is regarded to be an important factor for radioresistance. In general, approximately 2 to 3 times higher radiation doses are needed to kill hypoxic cells when compared with well oxygenated cells (Gray et al. 1953, Evans and Naylor 1963). However, the clinical importance of tumor hypoxia remains uncertain due to methodological problems for routine measurements of intratumoral O_2 tensions in patients. Considerable advances have been made in the investigation of tissue oxygenation in patients using a novel technique developed by Fleckenstein (1986). This technique has been shown to be valid in measuring the O_2 tension distribution in normal tissues (Weiss and Fleckenstein 1986, Kallinowski et al. 1990) and tumors (Höckel et al. 1991, Vaupel et al.1991).

The objective of this study was to investigate the oxygenation pattern in locally advanced recurrent tumors of different histologies, in which radiotherapy plays a major role as treatment modality.

MATERIALS AND METHODS

A total of 20 patients with recurrences of soft tissue sarcomas (n=8), recurrences of breast cancer (n=9) and recurrences of rectal cancer (n=3) were pretherapeutically investigated. Patients suffered from locally advanced tumors with a mean tumor volume of 230 cc. (range 4-540 cc.). The age ranged from 48 to 82 years with a mean of 68.1 years. All patients were referred to the Department of Radiooncology for irradiation alone or in combination with hyperthermia. In most of the patients two independent measurements could be performed pretherapeutically.

Measurements of tissue oxygenation:
Tissue oxygen tension was measured using sterile polarographic needle electrodes (pO_2 histograph, Eppendorf, Hamburg, FRG). The outer tip of the probes has a diameter of 200-300 um. Technical data of the needle electrodes, the calibration procedure and the data display have been recently described (Höckel et al. 1991, Vaupel et al. 1991).

3 radial electrode tracks were evaluated in each tumor. After local anesthesia (Scandicain 1%, Astra chemicals) a plastic trocar (0.8 mm outer diameter, Fa.Abbott, Ireland) with a hypodermic needle was inserted into the tumor periphery. The hypodermic needle was then removed and the O_2 sensor (needle electrode) was placed into the tumor tissue via the plastic trocar. Measurements were performed from the

Tab. 1a Characteristic of patients with recurrent tumors and oxygen tension in the tumors

Patient	G. J.	S. W.	L. M.	K. V.	M. L.	R. K.	B. H.	W. L.	F. H.	M. U.
Age	66	70	62	82	71	77	65	71	55	66
Sex	male	male	female	female	female	male	female	female	male	female
Tumor	Rectal cancer	Rectal cancer	Rectal cancer	Chondrosarcoma	Soft t. sarcoma	Soft t. sarcoma	Soft t. sarcoma	Soft t. sarcoma	Soft t. sarcoma	Soft t. sarcoma
Site	Presacral	Presacral	Presacral	Presacral	Upper leg	Scapula	Chestwall	Chestwall	Upper leg	Chestwall
Volume (cc)	400	383	374	374	325	125	179	172	213	63
Arterial blood pressure (mmHg)	140/85	150/80	130/80	180/90	150/75	140/70	140/80	110/70	100/60	100/60
Heart rate (1-min)	96	98	60	72	100	62	72	76	80	60
Hemoglobin (g%)	13.5	12.2	12.9	11.9	10.5	13.6	12.5	10.2	10.3	12.5
Arterial HbO2 saturation (%)	98	97	--------	99	99	--------	-------	-------	99	95
Mean pO2 (mmHg)	36.7	26.6	23.1	23.7	44	27.5	50.4	2.5	23.2	32.8
10% percentile (mmHg)	1.9	7.1	3.6	4.5	5.7	2.8	27.6	0.9	5.0	10.8
90% percentile (mmHg)	73.6	73.5	63.3	51.9	105.9	59.7	69.1	5.4	66.1	53.3
pO2 readings ≤ 2.5 mmHg (%)	14	0	0	1	0	2.5	0	35	2	17
No. of measured tumor sites	116	117	71	140	129	200	129	116	115	200

460

Tab. 1b Characteristic of patients with recurrent tumors and oxygen tension in the tumors

Patient	B. M.	S.-H. D.	J. B.	S. M.	H. M.	W. I.	W. K.	S. W.	K. M.	O. E.
Age	48	64	79	55	61	63	74	77	76	79
Sex	female	female	female	female	female	female	female	female	female	female
Tumor	Soft t. sarcoma	Breast cancer	Breast cancer	Breast cancer	Breast cancer	Breast cancer	Breast cancer	Breast cancer	Breast cancer	Breast cancer
Site	Chestwall	Chestwall	Chestwall	Arm	Chestwall	Chestwall	Chestwall	Chestwall	Chestwall	Chestwall
Volume (cc)	540	32	14	256	365	108	498	69	117	4
Arterial blood pressure (mmHg)	130/95	120/80	160/95	130/85	135/75	170/110	160/90	110/70	140/65	140/80
Heart rate (1-min)	78	104	66	104	120	60	96	64	76	95
Hemoglobin (g%)	11.9	13.7	17.2	11.5	11.2	12.2	12.7	13.5	10.4	11.9
Arterial HbO2 saturation (%)	-------	-------	-------	-------	99	-------	-------	-------	-------	96
Mean pO2 (mmHg)	20.3	19.7	62.9	12.1	9.0	24.9	50.4	4.4	69.4	49.6
10% percentile (mmHg)	16.8	1.3	53.2	7.9	0.5	6.5	8.8	3.8	61.8	15.8
90% percentile (mmHg)	22.6	45.5	79.9	20.9	42.1	46.4	71.7	5.1	76.1	76
pO2 readings ≤ 2.5 mmHg (%)	0	32	0	0	32	0	6	0	0	9
No. of measured tumor sites	155	86	64	100	71	88	188	129	69	105

periphery to the central part of the tumor. The electrode was automatically moved through the tissue. Each rapid forward movement was followed by a backward step of 0.3 mm in order to minimize the compression effects. The resulting overall forward step length was 0.7 mm. The local pO_2 was measured 1.4 sec after the backward motion.

Monitoring of systemic parameters:
   Systemic parameters (e.g. heart rate, blood pressure) and factors related to the arterial O_2 concentration (e.g. hemoglobin concentration, arterial oxyhemoglobin saturation) were monitored during measurements.

RESULTS

   A total of 35 measurements could be performed in 20 patients. In 4 measurements relatively high pO_2 values were obtained due to clinical relevant bleeding. In addition, in 4 measurements there were some uncertainties with the localization of the normal tissue / tumor boundary.
   Patient characteristics, systemic parameters and the results of the pO_2 measurements are given in Table 1a/b. There is a marked tumor-to-tumor variability even for tumors of the same histology. The occurence of radiobiological hypoxia does not correlate with tumor volume or histology. 5 of 8 soft tissue sarcomas, 1 of 3 recurrent rectal cancers, 4 of 9 recurrent breast cancers exhibited pO_2 values between zero and 2.5 mmHg, i.e. tissue areas with less than half-maximum radiosensitivity. 35% of the values measured in rectal cancer, 25 of the values measured in breast cancer and 17% of the values measured in soft tissue sarcomas were lower than 5 mmHg (Table 2).

Table 2. Hypoxia in recurrent tumors

Tumor	No. of tumors	No. of measurements ≤ 5 mmHg (%)
Breast cancer	9	25
Soft tissue sarcoma	8	17
Rectal cancer	3	35

DISCUSSION

   The existence of tumor areas with pO_2 values between 0 and 5 mmHg in approximately 17 to 35% of pO_2 readings is a finding which has not been addressed previously in recurrent malignant tumors of different histologies. It is remarkable that the oxygenation status of individual tumors cannot be predicted by tumor volume and histology. This is in agreement with the clinical studies of other investigators (Höckel et al. 1991, Vaupel et al. 1991).
   However, coming from clincal experience we would like to point out that besides hypoxia also other biological properties such as cell kinetics and inherent radiosensitivity significantly influence the response to radiotherapy. In future, it will be useful to prove if the determination of the oxygenation status of individuel tumors can predict treatment outcome.

SUMMARY

   Oxygen tension distributions (pO_2) were measured in 20 patients with recurrent soft tissue sarcoma (n=8), recurrent breast cancer (n=9) and recurrent rectal cancer (n=3) using computerized pO_2 histography. A total of 35 measurements could be performed pretherapeutically. In 8 measurements there exist some problems with
regard to clinical relevant bleeding or uncertainties of the tumor / normal tissue boundary. In general, there is a marked tumor-to-tumor variability even for tumors of the same histology. 5 of 8 soft tissue sarcomas,

1 of 3 recurrent rectal cancers, 4 of 9 breast cancersexhibited pO_2 values between zero and 2.5 mmHg, i.e. tissue areas with less than half-maximum radiosensitivity.

REFERENCES

1. Tumor hypoxia: Proceedings of a Consensus Meeting . Radiotherapy and Oncology Suppl. 20 (1991)

2. N.T.S. Evans and P.F.D. Naylor, The effect of oxygen breathing and radiotherapy upon tissue oxygen tension of some human tumors. Br.J.Radiol. 36: 418-425 (1963)

3. W. Fleckenstein, C. Weiss, R. Heinrich, H. Schomerus, T. Kersting, A new method for the bed-side recording of tissue pO_2 histograms. Verh. Dtsch. Ges. Inn. Med. 90: 439-443 (1984)

4. L.H. Gray, A.D. Conger, M. Ebert, S. Hornsey, O.C.A. Scott, The concentration of oxygen dissolved in tissue at the time of irradiation as a factor in radiotherapy. Br. J. Radiol. 26: 638-642 (1953)

5. M. Höckel, K. Schlenger, C. Knoop, P. Vaupel, Oxygenation of carcinomas of the uterine cervix: Evaluation by computerized O_2 tension measurements. Cancer Res. 51: 6098-6102 (1991)

6. F. Kallinowski, R. Zander, M. Höckel, P. Vaupel, Tumor tissue oxygenation as evaluated by computerized pO_2 histography. Int. J. Radiat. Ocol. Biol. Phys. 19: 953-962 (1990)

7. P. Vaupel, F. Kallinowski, P. Okunieff, Blood flow, oxygen and nutrient supply, and metabolic microenvironment of human tumors: a review. Cancer Res. 49:6449-6465 (1989)

8. P. Vaupel, K. Schlenger, C. Knoop, M. Höckel, Oxygenation of human tumors: Evaluation of tissue oxygen distribution in breast cancers by computerized O_2 tension measurements. Cancer Res. 51:3316-3322 (1991)

9. C. Weiss, W. Fleckenstein, Local tissue pO_2 measured with "thick" needle probes. Funktionsanalyse biologischer Systeme 15: 155-166 (1986)

DIRECT MEASUREMENT OF THE PO2 DISTRIBUTION
IN HUMAN MALIGNANT BRAIN TUMOURS

G.S. Cruickshank[1], R.P. Rampling[2], W. Cowans[3]

1. Institute of Neurological Sciences, Glasgow
2. Beatson Oncology Centre, Western Infirmary, Glasgow
3. Sterling Health, Philadelphia

INTRODUCTION

Malignant brain tumours are known to have a faster rate of recurrence and increased resistance to radiotherapy and chemotherapy than other solid tumours.[1] One of the related causes is thought to be focal hypoxia,[2] however the presence of hypoxic areas in malignant brain tumours has been disputed by PET studies and by the marginal effect of the hypoxic cell sensitisers such as Misonidazole.[3] Low pO_2 areas ($<2.5mmHg$) provide a source of radiobiological resistance,[4] whereas pO_2 levels less than 10-15 mmHg may provide conditions for the activation of new classes of bioreductive agents.[5] These agents require metabolic reduction under conditions of low oxygen tension to generate a cytotoxic species. In this study the oxygen status of peritumoural brain and tumour tissue has been measured to determine the presence of hypoxic regions and conditions for drug activation.

METHOD

The Eppendorf-pO_2-Histograph was utilised peroperatively to investigate the tissue Oxygen Tension in and around malignant brain tumours in 18 patients.
In open craniotomy a 300 micrometre needle probe was inserted under direct vision and tracked using peroperative ultrasound at 6MHz. Probe calibration was performed before and after readings. At least six tracks of 32 readings were made in each tissue. Anaesthesia was under a standardised procedure with either Isoflurane and Nitrous Oxide or Intravenous Propofol, with an inspired oxygen of 40% to produce adequate blood oxygenation. This gave arterial saturations of better than 98.3% in all cases. The arterial pCO_2 was maintained between 3.5 and 4.5 KPa. Peroperative tissue samples were sent for pathological assessment.

RESULTS AND DISCUSSION

1. Peritumoural Brain

Multiple track measurements were made in peritumoural brain areas in 8 patients. The pooled results, regardless of degree of oedema or histological grade, are shown in Fig.1. The pO_2 values were lower than expected by comparison with multiwire surface methods.[6] This reflects the technical improvements possible with this type of fine-needle polarography.[8] It also reflects the lower oxygen supply of white matter (around tumour) compared with that of grey matter,[7] as well as the effect of peritumoural conditions on O_2 diffusion path, blood supply and local pO_2 consumption.

The graph shows the effect of tumour decompression on peroperative peritumoural pO_2. The shift of the histogram to the right suggests improved tissue oxygenation, implying improved blood supply within this time span. Recovery of peritumoural brain tissue would agree with the observed improvement in function of patients undergoing surgical decompression.

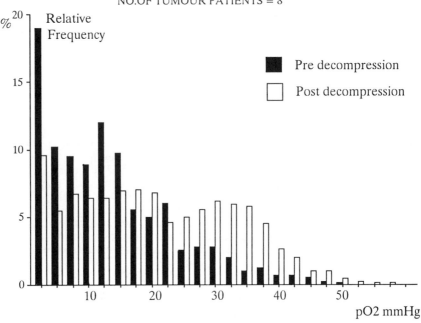

Figure 1.Pooled histograms from eight patients. Pre-decompression (median pO_2=10.5mmHg. n=1536) and post-decompression (median pO_2=17.8mmHg. n=1536) frequency histograms recorded during open craniotomy, recorded before and after tumour removal, in the peritumoural penumbra at 2cm from the tumour edge. The difference in values achieved p<.024 by the Wilcoxon signed ranks test.

Bioreductive agents activated at low pO_2 levels may be more likely to be neurotoxic in the peritumoural area if given too soon in relation to operation, before peritumoural oxygenation has recovered. Conversely, residual tumour cell-kill may be enhanced in the peritumoural area during this time.

Table 1. Summary table of pO_2 histography recordings from intracranial tumours.

No	Age	Sex	Location	Size mm	Oedema	Pathology	Necrosis	Mean pO_2	Median pO_2	%pO_2 <2.5mmHg	%pO_2 <15mmHg
1	52	F	L.Frontal	46	+++	Glioblastoma	Yes	11.1	3.2	43.7	68.0
2	62	M	R.Frontal	32	++	Glioblastoma	Yes	20.8	19.3	22.5	43.0
3	58	M	R.Occipital	34	+++	Glioblastoma	Yes	7.7	5.4	35.5	35.5
4	53	M	R.Parietal	36	++	Glioblastoma	Yes	25.2	24.3	9.5	33.0
5	68	F	L.Parietal	39	++	Glioblastoma	Yes	12.8	15.8	84.5	92.3
6	49	F	L.Temporal	64	++++	Glioblastoma	Yes	8.8	2.2	20.0	38.5
7	53	M	L.Parietal	30	++	Anaplastic	No	12.3	10.0	19.5	63.3
8	70	M	R.Temporal	45	++++	Anaplastic	No	33.1	42.3	9.0	21.0
9	50	F	L.Temporal	39	++++	Intermediate	No	23.0	13.7	22.5	48.0
10	32	F	R.Frontal	41	+	Low Grade	No	7.3	6.4	0.0	73.5
11	54	M	L.Occipital	58	+++	Oligocytoma	No	22.6	13.8	18.5	53.0
12	53	M	R.Parietal	43	+	Bronchus	Yes	15.0	14.1	1.5	65.5
13	72	F	R.Frontal	46	++	Bronchus	Yes	2.9	3.0	29.5	81.0
14	63	M	L.Parietal	37	+++	Bronchus	Yes	2.9	0.3	87.3	94.0
15	36	F	R.Occipital	36	++	Breast	Yes	6.9	4.3	46.5	58.0
16	62	F	L.Frontal	26	+++	Melanoma	Yes	14.8	9.7	71.0	81.3
17	30	M	L.Temporal	30	++	Melanoma	Yes	22.5	23.7	20.0	38.5
18	17	F	R.Parietal	73	+++	Sarcoma	No	8.6	3.8	34.0	73.0

2. Malignant Brain Tumours

a. **Astrocytomas** (Fig. 2)   The presence of low pO_2 (less than 2.5mmHg) was demonstrated in nine out of ten patients with astrocytomas and in one patient with a recurrent oligodendrocytoma. (Table 1.) The sample frequency of these low pO_2 values varied widely from 9 to 84%. The frequency did not obviously relate to histological grade. Low pO_2 values were seen in patients with glioblastoma, a highly malignant, necrotic tumour but were also seen with anaplastic astrocytomas without necrosis. (Fig.2b) In glioblastomas and anaplastic astrocytomas the number of values below 15mmHg occurred more frequently in the metastases. The incidence of low pO_2 values in these intracranial tumours was much higher than that recorded by others using a similar technique, in extracranial tumours (breast, cervix).[9]

b. **Metastatic Tumours** (Fig. 3)   Three bronchial metastases had between 29.5 and 87.3% pO_2 values below 2.5mmHg. Two melanomas had a pooled mean of 16.9mmHg with a median of 10.1mmHg reflecting a high proportion (40%) of low pO_2 values. Results are also shown for a breast metastasis and a highly malignant, fast growing non-necrotic sarcoma in a young patient.

c. **Tumour heterogeneity versus spatial resolution (Fig. 4)**   Although the pattern of O2 measurements along any particular track suggests gradients of tissue pO_2 within the tumour parenchyma the gradients appear to vary unpredictably in similar tumours using the same orientation eg. surface to core. A high degree of spatial information can be obtained when measurements are combined with ultrasound. This allows correlation of tissue pO_2 with, for example, the boundary areas of cystic tumours. (Fig. 4)

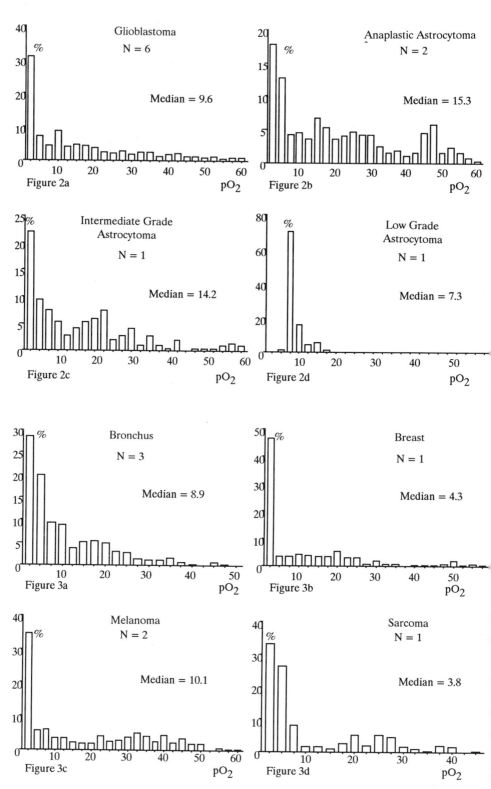

Figures 2 and 3. % refers to the percentage of values recorded within each level of pO$_2$ (mmHg). See text for explanation of figures.

From these results High Grade astrocytomas have a 22-30% sample volume "hypoxic", and potentially resistant to radiation therapy. By comparison the appropriate Bioreductive Agent should, if the required activating enzyme is present, capable and accessible, have an effect on a greater tumour volume, with nearly 50% of the tumour with a pO_2 of less than 10mmHg. This would include the radiobiologically resistant "hypoxic cell fraction" and thus enhance the effect of current therapy.

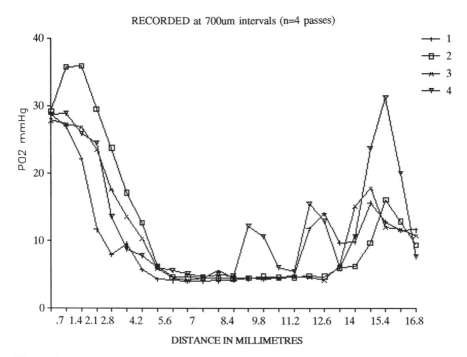

RECORDED at 700um intervals (n=4 passes)

Figure 4. Ultrasound directed recordings of pO_2 along four probe tracks across the wall of a deep-lying cystic astrocytoma. Probe passage was from the cystic cavity, through the wall and shows a reproducible pattern of values. Note the elevation in levels of pO_2 at the outer edge before falling to peritumoural levels.

CONCLUSIONS

These results suggest that a high proportion of malignant brain tumours contain areas of low oxygenation. In addition, these areas are present in greater proportions than have been recorded in other solid tumours. These features may be related to the relative treatment resistant nature of these tumours, but may also offer an environment for cytotoxic activation.[5]

REFERENCES

1. Bloom H.J.G. Intracranial tumours: Response and resistance to therapeutic endeavours 1970-1980. Int.J. Radiation Oncol. Biol. Phys. 8:1083-1113, 1982
2. Gray L.H, Conger A.D, Ebert M, Hornsey S, Scott O.C.A. Concentration of oxygen dissolved in tissues at time of irradiation as a factor in Radiotherapy. Br.J.Radiol 26:638-648,1953
3. Brooks D.J, Beaney R.P, Thomas D.G. The role of Positron Emission Tomography in the study of Cerebral Tumours. Seminars in Oncology, 13:83-93, 1986
4. Bush R.S, Jenkin R.D.T, Allt W.E.C, Beale F.A, Bean H, Dembo A.J, Pringle J.F. Definitive evidence for hypoxic cells influencing cure in cancer therapy. Br.J.Cancer, 37(Suppl.3):302-306, 1978
5. Workman P, Walton M.I. Enzyme-directed bioreductive drug development. In:Adams E, Breccia A, Fielden E, Wardman P. eds: Selective activation of drugs by Redox processes. New York, NY:Plenum;1991:173-191
6. Schultheiss R, Leuwer R, Leniger-Follert E, Wassmann H, Wullenweber R. Tissue pO_2 of Human Brain Cortex-Method, Basic Results and Effects of Pentoxifylline Angiology 38 : 3 221-225.
7. Grote J. In: Schmidt R.F, Thews G. eds. Physiologie des Menschen. Springer,Berlin 23 ed: p635
8. Fleckenstein W, Schaffler A, Heinrich R, Petersen M, Gunderoth-Palmowski M Nollert G. On the Differences between Muscle pO_2 measurements obtained with Hypodermic Needle Probes and with Multiwire Surface Probes. Parts 1 & 2, In: Clinical Oxygen Pressure Measurement II eds: Ehrly A.M, Fleckenstein W, Hauss J, H Huch R. Blackwell Ueberreuter Wissenschaft. Berlin, 1990
9. Vaupel P, Schlenger K, Knoop C, Hockel M. Oxygenation of Human Tumours: Evaluation of Tissue Oxygen Distribution in Breast Cancers by Computerised O_2Tension Measurements. Cancer Research 51:3316-3322, 1991

MEASUREMENT OF OXYGEN PARTIAL PRESSURE IN BRAIN TUMORS UNDER STEREOTACTIC CONDITIONS

Jean R. Moringlane

Department of Neurosurgery
Saarland University
Homburg/Saar, Germany

Introduction

Oxygenation is assigned an important influence in the response of malignancies to radiation therapy [1]. Oxygen distribution and regional blood flow in malignant experimental tumors show considerable variations [2]. Another field of interest is the role which hypoxic areas in a tumor could play in the cascade of events that lead to the proliferation and migration of endothelial cells and to the sprouting of new capillaries. Extensive neovascularization can be observed in malignant brain gliomas [3]. Not enough data exists about oxygen distribution in brain tumors. The polarographic method [4] seems to offer a new possiblity of pO_2 measurement in brain tumors. The present study was undertaken in order to evaluate whether measurement of pO_2 distribution in brain tunours is feasible under surgical conditions using the stereotactic methodology.

Material and Methods

Measurement of pO_2 values was performed in brain tumors of twelve patients undergoing stereotactic biopsy. CT - guided stereotactic sereial biopsy is routinely used to establish the histologic diagnosis of cerebral lesions. Initially superficially located tumors (frontal and occipital) were considered suitable, and in the following measurement was undertaken in lesions located in the basal ganglia, the suprasellar region and in the level of the skull base.

All stereotaxic biopsy procedures were carried out under local anesthesia and mild sedation (Midazolam). The stereotaxy head ring was firmly fixed to the head of the patients with the aid of four pins which were positioned at previously anesthetized points (Scandicain 0.5 %) of the frontal and occipital region (figure1). An intravenous infusion of contrast medium (Omnipaque) at the rate of 1ml / kg. body weight was applied. A CT scan was performed with the stereotaxy headring (Riechert/ Mundinger) fixed to the table by means of a special adapter. The axis of the stereotaxy headring are made to coincide with those of the CT scan unit, so that stereotactic coordinates of any point of the CT images can be automatically obtained. The coordinates of the " target point " and those of the entry point in the skull bone are entered into a PC which calculates the angles of insertion   and the

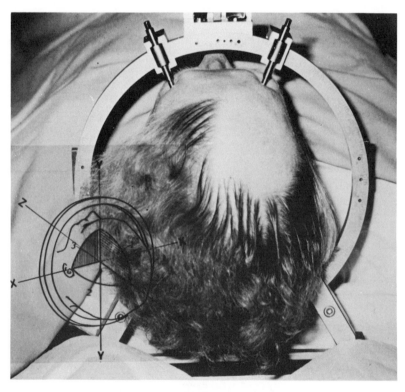

Figure 1. The stereotaxy head ring is firmly attached to the skull of the patient. The localization of any intracranial structure can be described as coordinates in the three planes.

required distance. A small area (5 x 5 cm) of the scalp was shaved. Following surgical desinfection and draping a small incision was made and a burr hole with a diameter of 6 mm was drilled. A small incision in the dura allowed to coagulate the entry point on the brain cortex. Measurement of pO_2-values was intended to be carried out along the same trajectory as planned for biopsy.

The polarographic principle of pO_2-measurement in tumor tissue is the electrochemical reduction of oxygen molecules. A negative voltage being applied to a platine or gold electrode O_2 molecules are reduced to H_2O. The extent of oxygen diffusion in the tissue depends on the difference in partial pressure between the electrode and the tissue. The increase in current is proportional to the oxygen partial pressure in the tissue.

The Sigma pO_2-Histograph (Netheler Hinz/ Eppendorf, Hamburg, Germany) was used for the study with a specially designed electrode* (diameter 0. 35 mm, length 30 cm) made to fit the stereotaxy system. Inside the teflon covered oblique cut end of the electrode (shaped similar to a hypodermic needle) was a glas isolated gold-microcathode with a diameter of 12 um). Following calibration the sterilized probe was positioned to pass through the guiding channel of the stereotactic set and inserted through the burr hole and advanced manually through the coagulated point of the cortex towards the tumor. A plain stereotactic teleradiographic X-Ray film was made in order to verify the position of the electrode and facilitate later correlation with CT scan and histologic findings (figure 2). Then the distance to traverse was determined according to the volume of the tumor. Stepwise with the aid of a motor drive pO_2 measurements were carried out at 1 mm intervals. Following the last measurement the probe automatically slid back into starting position. A listing of single pO_2 values was obtained immediately. Histograms were delivered as soon as the procedure was finished.

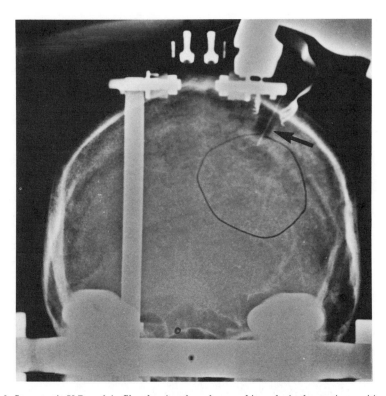

Figure 2. Stereotactic X-Ray plain film showing the polarographic probe in the starting position (arrow).

Before and during the pO_2 measurement capillary oxygenation was monitored continuously with a infrared oxygen sensor and an Oxy-Shuttle (Critikon) connected to a finger of the patient.

Through the same path tissue samples were taken at intervalls of 3 - 4 mm beginning at the periphery of the tumor, through the tumor, to the opposite side. Generally six to nine tissue samples were taken. Lightmicroscopic examination of a few samples was performed intraoperatively in order to be sure that the tissue samples were of tumoral origin [5].

Results

All procedures were carried out without any complications; in particular there was no bleeding or infection due to the use of the polarographic electrode.

Histologic diagnosis, localization and number of pO_2- values measured in each tumor are listed on table 1.

Table 1: Measurement of Oxygen Partial Pressure in Brain Tumors under Stereotactic Conditions.

Pat.	sex	Age	Histology	Localization	pO_2-values
Si	F	64	Glioblastoma	right frontal	200
Ke	F	41	Anaplastic Astrocytoma	left occipital	61
Sh	M	68	Anaplastic Astrocytoma	left occipital	41
Gu	F	66	Glioblastoma	basal ganglia	68
Ha	M	46	Oligo-astro-cytoma	left frontal	52
Gr	M	57	Cranio-pharingioma	suprasellar	36
Ha	F	63	Chordoma	clivus	43
Ga	F	60	Melanoma	left frontal	51
He	M	58	Anaplastic Astrocytoma	left occipital	40
Kr	M	31	Glioblastoma	left frontal	47
Ah	M	24	Astrocytoma	left frontal	39
Hd	M	65	Glioblastoma	left occipital	49

Histograms of 3 different glioblastomas with areas of necrosis showed very low pO_2 values close to zero. In two low grade astrocytomas and in a vascularized melanoma metastasis pO_2 values were higher (figure 3).

With the position of the polarographic probe visualized on the X-ray film under stereotactic conditions and thanks to the possibility to transpose the outlines and the position

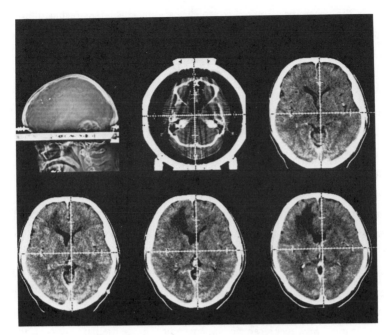

Figure 3 a. CT scans of an intracerebral low grade astrocytoma.

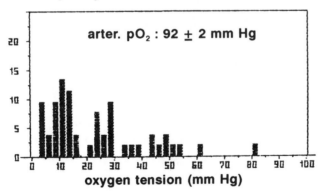

Figure 3 b. p-O$_2$ histogram of the astrocytoma (see fig. 2)

of the slices of the tumor from the CT-images it was possible to correlate the pO_2-values with the corresponding regions of the tumor. Areas with very low levels of pO_2 corresponded to hypodense zones of edema or of tissue necrosis.

Apart from the necessity of being extremely careful while transferring the probe from the calibration chamber to the tumor, in order to keep the electrode sterile, no further difficulty was encountered with the probe under stereotactic conditions.

Conclusion

This study shows that pO_2- measurement in individual brain tumors is technically feasible under surgical conditions. The present data collected from a small group of patients suggests that a wide range of variation is to be expected, corresponding to morphological findings and imaging data. It can be assumed that every brain tumor has its own individual pO_2 distribution pattern which may be determined by the histologic nature, the volume, the degree of malignancy, the blood supply, and the topographic localization.

The stereotactic technique offers several advantages: minimal invasiveness, integration and point to point correlation of data from different sources like CT, MRI, angiography, PET scan, pO_2 and pH values.

Many questions, however, remain unanswered, in particular how is the oxygen distribution in brain tumors regulated? How can it be successfully modified and in which cases it may be useful?

Further investigation is necessary in order to understand which role hypoxic areas of a tumor play in the release of mitogenic growth factors for endothelial cells, like for example the vascular endothelial cell growth factor (VECGF), fibroblast growth factor (FGF) and which role they play in the phenomenon of endothelial cell and capillary proliferation which are characteristics of malignant brain tumors [6].

Acknowledgements

The author thanks Dr. M. Günderoth-Scheuregger for technical assistance and Dr. G. Vince and Dr. S. Felber for editorial assistance.

References

1. L.H. Gray, A.D. Langer, M. Ebert, S. Hornsey, O.C.A. Scott. The concentration of oxygen dissolved in tissues at the time of irradiation as a factor of radiotherapy. Br. J Radiol 26:638 - 648 (1953).

2. P. Vaupel, S. Frinak, H.I. Bicher. Heterogenous oxygen partial pressure and pH distribution in C3H mouse mammary adenocarcinoma. Cancer Res 41 : 2008 - 2013 (1981).

3. D.S. Russel, L.J. Rubinstein. Pathology of tumors of the nervous system. Baltimore, Williams and Wilkins 4th ed. (1977).

4. W. Fleckenstein, J.R. Jungblut, M. Suckfill. Distribution of oxygen pressure in the periphery and centre of malignant head and neck tumors. In : Clinical Oxygen Pressure Measurment II. A.M. Ehrly, W. Fleckenstein, J. Hauss, R. Huch (Eds.) Blackwell Ueberreuter Wissenschaft Berlin S. 81 -90 (1990).

5. J.R. Moringlane, C.B. Ostertag. La definition spatiale des tumeurs cerebrales. Revue d`EEG Neurophysiol clin 17 :45 - 53 (1987).

6. J.R. Moringlane, R. Spinas, P. Bhlen. Acidic fibroblast growth factor is present in the fluid of brain tumor pseudocysts. Acta Neurochir. 107 : 88 - 92 (1990).

CHANGES IN OXYGENATION PATTERNS OF LOCALLY ADVANCED RECURRENT TUMORS UNDER THERMORADIOTHERAPY

Horst Jürgen Feldmann[1], Michael Molls[2], Jürgen Füller[1], Georg Stüben[1], Horst Sack[1]

[1]Department of Radiooncology, West German Tumor Centre, University Hospital
4300 Essen 1, FRG
[2]Department of Radiooncology, Technische Universität München, 8000 München 80, FRG

INTRODUCTION

The metabolic micromilieu (including blood flow and oxygenation) is an important research topic in clinical oncology (Vaupel et al. 1989, Molls and Feldmann 1991, Feldmann et al. 1992). The sensitivity to radiation is positively correlated with the concentration of free oxygen (Gray et al. 1953, Evans and Naylor 1963). Well oxygenated tumor cells are more sensitive to radiation than anoxic tumor cells. Considerable advances have been made in the investigation of tissue oxygenation using a novel technique (Fleckenstein), which allows for the systematic evaluation of the tissue oxygen status. The aim of this study was to evaluate changes in oxygenation patterns of recurrent tumors under extreme treatment conditions, in particular under hyperthermic conditions.

MATERIALS AND METHODS

A total of 10 patients with recurrent soft tissue sarcomas (n=4), recurrent breast cancer (n=3), recurrent rectal cancer (n=2) and recurrent neck nodes (n=1) were investigated pretherapeutically and 24 hours after the 1 st. hyperthermic treatment. All patients were treated with conventional fractionated radiotherapy and hyperthermia.

Measurements of tissue oxygenation

Tissue oxygen tension was measured using sterile polarographic needle electrodes (pO_2 histograph, Eppendorf, Hamburg, FRG). The outer tip of the probes has a diameter of 200-300 um. Technical data of the needle electrodes, the calibration procedure and the data display have been recently described (Höckel et al. 1991, Vaupel et al. 1991).

3 radial electrode tracks were evaluated in each tumor. After local anesthesia (Scandicain 1%, Astra chemicals) a plastic trocar (0.8 mm outer diameter, Fa. Abbott, Ireland) with a hypodermic needle was inserted into the tumor periphery. The hypodermic needle was then removed and the O_2 sensor was placed into the tumor tissue via the plastic trocar. Measurements were performed from the periphery to the central part of the tumor. The electrode was automatically moved through the tissue. Each rapid forward movement was followed by a backward step of 0.3 mm in order to minimize the compression effects. The resulting overall forward step length was 0.7 mm. The local pO_2 was measured 1.4 sec after the backward motion.

Oxygen Transport to Tissue XV, Edited by P. Vaupel
et al., Plenum Press, New York, 1994

Monitoring of systemic parameters

Systemic parameters (e.g. heart rate, blood pressure) and factors related to the arterial O_2 concentration (e.g. hemoglobin concentration, arterial oxyhemoglobin saturation) were monitored during measurements.

Hyperthermia, thermometry and thermal parameters

Patients with superficial tumors were treated using the Mono-Horn or Dual-Horn applicator of the BSD 1000 system, patients with deep seated tumors were treated using the annular phased array (APA) or Sigma-60 applicator of the BSD 1000 / 2000 system (Fa. BSD Medical Corporation, Salt Lake City, Utah, USA). Temperatures were monitored by high resistance lead thermistor probes (Gibbs). The temperature distribution in the tumor was recorded along the length of the inserted catheters by thermal mapping (Gibbs). The minimum, maximum and mean tumor temperature and the time-averaged temperatures reported in terms of T20, T50 and T90, which are temperatures above 20%, 50% and 90% of the monitored points resided, were determined for the hyperthermic treatment (Oleson).

Statistical analysis

Differences in pO_2 distributions before and after hyperthermia were checked using the Spearman rank non-parametric test.

Table 1. Thermal parameters in 10 tumors

Parameter	Mean ± S.D. (°C)	Range (°C)
T max.	45.1 ± 1.0	41.0 - 50.0
T mean	41.9 ± 0.7	39.5 - 46.3
T min.	39.0 ± 0.4	37.7 - 41.0
T 20	43.3 ± 0.8	40.3 - 47.7
T 50	41.6 ± 0.8	38.9 - 46.9
T 90	40.2 ± 0.5	38.0 - 43.3

RESULTS

In 9 from 10 patients cytotoxic temperatures (≥ 42.5 °C) could be reached in nearly 50% of the treatment volume. The mean thermal parameters for all 10 tumors are given in Table 1. Patient characteristics, systemic parameters and the results of the pO_2 measurements are given in Table 2. 5 of 10 patients developed a clinical relevant edema within the treatment volume 24 hours after hyperthermia. In 9 patients a decrease in the mean pO_2 was observed 24 hours after the first cytotoxic hyperthermic treatment. In addition, a decrease in the 50% percentiles was evident in 9 patients (Table 2). Only in patient O.E. (Table 2) an increase in the mean pO_2 and the 10, 50 and 90% percentiles were evident. This patient developed a decrease of the tumor volume after the first hyperthermic treatment. Significant differences (p=0,01) in pooled pO_2 distributions are evident between measurements before and measurements 24 hours after a cytotoxic hyperthermic treatment (Fig. 1). The median pO_2 from 1248 measurements before

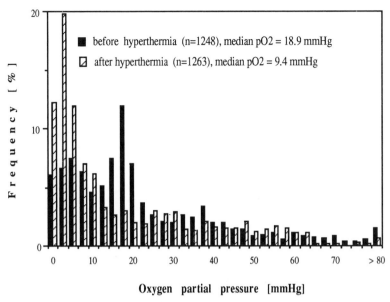

Oxygen partial pressure [mmHg]

Fig. 1   Pooled data before and after hyperthermia in 10 tumors

hyperthermia is 18.9 mmHg, whereas the median pO_2 from 1263 measurements after hyperthermia is 9.4 mmHg.

DISCUSSION

In the literature there exist some data that tumor oxygenation could be improved during radiation therapy. This will be predominantly the effect of partial tumor regression with relieved pressure on the capillaries and restored normal blood flow and oxygen diffusion to the hypoxic parts of the tumor (Badib and Webster, Cater and Silver, Evans and Naylor). In one patient with an early tumor response an increase in the mean pO_2 could be observed in our series. The significant decrease of the mean pO_2 values after hyperthermia in the other patients, who showed no change in tumor volume, might be the result of a higher interstitial pressure after hyperthermia due to edema.

In summary, we are able to demonstrate that initial changes of oxygen tension distributions under extreme treatment conditions may occur. In future, it will be necessary to evaluate changes under fractionated thermoradiotherapy or radiotherapy in more detail using this novel technique.

SUMMARY

Oxygen tension distributions (pO_2) were measured in 10 patients with recurrent soft tissue sarcoma (n=4), recurrent rectal cancer (n=2), recurrent breast cancer (n=3) and recurrent neck nodes (n=1) using computerized pO_2 histography. Measurements were performed pretherapeutically and 24 hours after the first cytotoxic hyperthermic treatment. In one patient an increase of the mean pO_2 value was evident after hyperthermia. The other 9 patients showed a significant decrease in the mean pO_2 values after hyperthermia. Pooled pO_2 distributions of measurements before and after hyperthermia differ statistically significant (p<0,01). The median pO_2 from 1248 measurements before hyperthermia is 18.9 mmHg, whereas the median pO_2 from 1263 measurements after hyperthermia is 9.4 mmHg.

Table 2. Characteristic of patients undergoing oxygen tension measurements before and after hyperthermia

Patient	O. E.		H. M.		W. I.		S. W.		G. J.		K. V.		B. M.		M. U.		F. H.		B. A.	
Age	79		61		63		70		66		82		48		66		55		55	
Sex	female		female		female		male		male		female		female		female		male		male	
Tumor	Rec. breast cancer		Rec. breast ca.		Rec. breast ca.		Rec. rectal cancer		Rec. rectal ca.		Chondrosarcoma		Rec. soft t. sarc.		Rec. soft t. sarc.		Rec. soft t. sarc.		Rec. lymphnode	
Site	Chestwall		Chestwall		Chestwall		Presacral		Presacral		Presacral		Chestwall		Chestwall		upper leg		Neck	
Volume (cc)	4		384		112		383		400		374		144		108		212		118	
Investigation	I	II	I	II	I	II	I	II	I	II	I	II	I	II	I	II	I	II	I	II
Arterial blood pressure (mmHg)	140/80	140/80	135/75	125/80	170/110	130/80	150/80	140/85	140/85	150/75	180/90	140/80	130/95	120/80	100/60	110/65	120/70	110/65	115/80	140/75
Heart rate (1-min)	101	98	120	107	60	64	98	72	96	90	72	72	78	68	60	56	64	60	88	88
Hemoglobin (g%)	11.9	11.7	11.2	11.5	12.2	11.8	12.2	11.9	13.5	13.2	11.9	11.9	11.9	12.2	12.5	12.5	10.3	10.5	14.0	14.2
Arterial HbO2 saturation (%)	96	97	99	100	------		97	97	98	97	99	95	------		------		99	98	------	
Mean pO2 (mmHg)	49.6	80.3	9.0	6.4	24.9	17.0	26.6	17.2	36.7	18.2	23.7	15.7	20.3	7	32.8	23.8	23.2	6.8	23.5	17.0
10% percentile (mmHg)	15.8	22.2	0.5	1.0	6.5	10.5	7.1	6.1	1.9	2.5	4.5	4.9	16.8	2.4	10.8	3.4	5.0	3.4	9.2	1.0
50% percentile (mmHg)	54.2	90.9	2.4	1.7	22.3	13.1	11.8	9.0	36.0	4.7	17.1	12.8	19.5	4.0	28.0	26.7	9.4	4.1	19.4	14.4
90% percentile	76	99	42.1	17.9	46.4	25.5	73.5	43.9	73.6	58.2	51.9	30.6	22.6	11.7	53.3	45.6	66.1	16.4	40.9	40.1
No. of measured tumor sites	105	98	71	71	88	133	117	129	116	108	140	108	155	132	200	200	115	113	141	171

REFERENCES

1. A.O. Badib and J.H. Webster, Changes in tumor oxygen tension during radiation therapy. Acta Radiologica Therapy Physics Biology 8: 247-257 (1969)

2. R.R. Bowman, A probe for measuring temperatures in radiofrequency heated material. IEEE Trans. Microw. Theo. Tech. 24: 43-45 (1976)

3. D. Cater and I. Silver, Quantitative measurements of oxygen tension in normal tissues and in the tumors of patients before and after radiotherapy. Acta radiol. 53: 233-256 (1959)

4. N.T.S. Evans and P.F.D.Naylor, The effect of oxygen breathing and radiotherapy upon tissue oxygen tension of some human tumors. Br.J.Radiol. 36: 418-425 (1963)

5. H.J. Feldmann, M. Molls, A. Hoederath, S. Krümpelmann and H. Sack, Blood flow and steady state temperatures in deep seated tumors and normal tissues. Int. J. Radiat. Oncol. Biol. Phys. 23: 1003-1008 (1992)

6. W. Fleckenstein, C. Weiss, R. Heinrich, H. Schomerus, T. Kersting, A new method for the bed-side recording of tissue pO_2 histograms. Verh. Dtsch. Ges. Inn. Med. 90: 439-443 (1984)

7. F.A. Gibbs Jr., "Thermal mapping" in experimental cancer treatment with hyperthermia: Description and use of a semiautomatic system. Int. J. Radiat. Oncol. Biol. Phys. 9: 1057-1063 (1983)

8. L.H. Gray, A.D. Conger, M. Ebert, S. Hornsey, O.C.A. Scott, The concentration of oxygen dissolved in tissue at the time of irradiation as a factor in radiotherapy. Br. J. Radiol. 26: 638-642 (1953)

9. M. Höckel, K. Schlenger, C. Knoop, P. Vaupel, Oxygenation of carcinomas of the uterine cervix: Evaluation by computerized O_2 tension measurements. Cancer Res. 51: 6098-6102 (1991)

10. M. Molls and H.J. Feldmann, Clinical investigations on blood flow in malignant tumors of the pelvis and the abdomen. In: Tumor blood supply and metabolic microenvironment: characterization and implications for therapy, eds. P. Vaupel, R.K. Jain, 1st edition, Fischer Verlag, Stuttgart, Funktionsanalyse biologischer Systeme 20: 143-153 (1991)

11. J.R. Oleson, M.W. Dewhirst, J.M. Harrelson, K.A. Leopold, T.V. Samulski, C.Y. Tso, Tumor temperature distributions predict hyperthermia effect. Int. J. Radiat. Oncol. Biol. Phys. 16: 559-570 (1989)

12. P. Vaupel, F. Kallinowski, P. Okunieff, Blood flow, oxygen and nutrient supply, and metabolic microenvironment of human tumors: a review. Cancer Res. 49:6449-6465 (1989)

13. P. Vaupel, K. Schlenger, C. Knoop, M. Höckel, Oxygenation of human tumors : Evaluation of tissue oxygen distribution in breast cancers by computerized O_2 tension measurements. Cancer Res. 51:3316-3322 (1991)

14. C. Weiss, W. Fleckenstein, Local tissue pO_2 measured with "thick" needle probes. Funktionsanalyse biologischer Systeme 15: 155-166 (1986)

THE ROLE OF OXYGEN TENSION DISTRIBUTION ON THE RADIATION RESPONSE OF HUMAN BREAST CARCINOMA

Paul Okunieff[1]* , Eamonn P. Dunphy[2], Michael Hoeckel[5], David J. Terris[3], and Peter Vaupel[4]

[1]Radiation Oncology Branch, Natl. Cancer Inst., Bethesda, MD, USA

[2]Dept. Radiation Oncology and [3]Div. Head and Neck Surgery Stanford Univ., Stanford, CA, USA

[4]Inst. Physiology and Pathophysiology, and [5]Dept. Obstetrics and Gynecology, Univ. of Mainz, Mainz, Germany

INTRODUCTION

The response of tumors to radiation is heterogeneous even in animal tumor systems where tumors all originate from the same cell culture, are implanted in genetically similar age-matched animals in a constant anatomic location[1]. Hence great heterogeneity of response exists even in situations where intrinsic genetic or epigenetic factors are minimally variable. Several metabolic factors are known to influence the probability of tumor control after radiation. These metabolic factors are also known to vary widely between tumors in humans[2,3] and even in animal tumor models. Heterogeneous variables include tumor oxygen tension distribution, glutathione content, glucose delivery and utilization rate, pH, and blood flow. In addition, radiation response can be modified by intrinsic radiation sensitivity, rate of repopulation, and tumor size. The relative importance of oxygen in this list of modifiers of treatment response is unclear, but has been of major concern since the 1950's[4,5]. In animal tumors treated with a few radiation fractions, oxygen tension distribution is probably the most powerful predictor of radiation response[6]. The impact of oxygen on human tumor response, however, is controversial particularly in the treatment of human disease wherein treatment is delivered in many fractions. Recently it has been pos-

*This work supported in part by NIH grants CA48096 and CA13311, and by the American Cancer Society Career Development Award.

sible to measure the oxygen tension distributions of human breast carcinoma[3,7]. Using well established modeling techniques and classical radiation biology it is therefore possible to predict the heterogeneity of radiation treatment response expected secondary to the oxygen tension distribution. The purpose of this analysis is to determine to what extent the known shape of the radiation response curve for human breast cancers treated in situ can be predicted by the tumor oxygenation status.

MATERIALS AND METHODS

Human Breast Carcinoma Dose Response Data

The dose response curve was calculated based on pooled data published by Hellman[8]. Tumor control probability (TCP) as a function of radiation dose was estimated by fitting the data to a probit curve. The slope of the tumor control curve measured in % increase in TCP for a % increase in dose at a given TCP is called the γ_x (where x is the TCP at which the slope is calculated). For most calculations, the slope at TCP=50% was used (γ_{50}).

Model of Oxygen Response

pO_2 values under 5 mmHg are well tolerated by tumor cells. Oxygen tensions at this level, however, confers substantial radiation protection that can be predicted using the relation:

$$OER = (K + m*pO_2)/(K + pO_2).$$

OER is the oxygen enhancement ratio, m is the maximum OER (assumed a conservative 2.5), K has units of mmHg and defines the pO_2 at half maximum OER (6.81 mmHg). Assuming patients are treated with daily radiation doses of 2 Gy, that the breast cancer α/β ratio of normoxic tumor cells is 10 Gy, and tumors have M stem cells, the linear-quadratic formula predicts a survival fraction of:

$$S/So = \exp([-2\alpha*[OER/m]-4\beta*[OER/m]^2])$$

where β under fully oxygenated conditions is $(1/TCD_{50}) * (\ln(M/2) / ([\alpha/\beta] + 2))$, α is therefore 10β [9,10]. For the purpose of this study we assume there is no difference of the intrinsic radiation resistance between tumors. Hence all cells from any dose response curve have the same OER curve, and same α and β. Since oxygenation can modify the effective α and β, the above equation is only an estimate of β and the value used was determined by iteration driven by the oxygen tension distributions of all patients and the known clinical TCD_{50} (62.9 Gy). γ_{50} is independent of α/β and of α and β. The TCD_{50} is the dose of radiation that cures 50% of patients. Based on the work of Hellman[8] this dose can be calculated to be 62.9 Gy (Figure 1). The mean M is always assumed to be 10^8 stem cells for all calculations. The mean tumor volume of the 22 patients with pO_2 histograms was 84 mL hence the density of clonogenic cells in tumor is assumed to be approximately 10^6 cell/mL.

Model of TCP

Based on the Poisson approximation of binomial statistics, the tumor control probability for a tumor with a homogeneous oxygen tension distribution is simply[11]:

$$TCP(2\ Gy) = \exp(-M*[S/So]).$$

The TCP for a single tumor with a pO_2 histogram made up of I (i=1..I) categories and with a density function F(i) would be:

$$TCP(2\ Gy) = \exp(-M*\Sigma_i F(i)*[S/So])$$

Finally the TCP for a group of N (n=1..N) tumors, each with its own pO_2 histogram, $F_n(i)$, has a TCP after one 2 Gy fraction of:

$$TCP(2\ Gy) = (1/N)\Sigma_n \exp(-M*\Sigma_i F_n(i)*[S/So]).$$

For a fractionated course of treatment, with j fractions (total dose of 2j Gy) in which no redistribution of oxygenation occurs between fractions, the TCP is:

$$TCP(2j\ Gy) = (1/N)\Sigma_n \exp(-M*\Sigma_i F_n(i)*[S/So]^j).$$

If full reoxygenation occurs the TCP of a fractionated course of treatment becomes:

$$TCP(2j\ Gy) = (1/N)\Sigma_n \exp(-M*[\Sigma_i F_n(i)*[S/So]]^j).$$

Since [S/So] is a function of radiation dose (D=2j Gy) the TCP can be plotted as a function of dose and compared to the clinical data.

Human Breast Carcinoma pO_2 Histography

Twenty two women with breast cancer at either the University of Mainz (19 patients) or at Stanford University (3 patients) had pO_2 measurements made of their breast cancers using the Eppendorf pO_2 histograph. An average of 87 ± 58 (range 21 to 300) measurements were made from each patient and histograms were individually entered into the computer data base. The details of the methods can be found elsewhere[3,7]. Tumor dimensions were recorded and volumes were calculated based on an ellipsoid approximation and ranged 1.4 to 747 mL (mean ± SD = 84 ± 173 mL.)

RESULTS

The data of Hellman[8] along with the probit fit of that data are shown in Figure 1. The slope, measured in percent control per percent increase in dose at TCP = 50%, is the γ_{50}, and was 1.46.

Assuming typical adenocarcinomas of the breast are 0.1 to 1000 mL, M would be approxmimately 10^6 to 10^{10} stem cells and the maximum theoretical γ_{50}s are therefore 4.9 to 8.1[1]. For our calculations we used a mean M of 10^8, thus the maximum possible γ_{50} is 6.5. Some reoxygenation is expected between radiation fractions. The effect of reoxygenation to the baseline state between each fraction (full reoxygenation) would reduce the importance of hypoxia and thus steepen the dose response toward the maximum.

The predicted TCP for the 22 tumors studied is analyzed in Fig. 2. For these calculations tumors are all assumed to be of the same size (10^8 stem cells), α was 0.36 and 0.44 Gy^{-1}, and β was 0.036 and 0.044 Gy^{-2} for full reoxygenation and non-reoxygenation conditions respectively. As expected reoxygenation steepens the slope of the dose response curve, but it still deviates considerably from the theoretical maximum. The γ_{50} of the two curves are 2.37 and 1.43, both of which are close to the clinically observed value of 1.46.

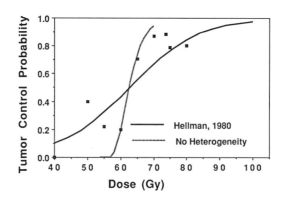

FIGURE 1. Probit fit of the clinical dose response data[8]. The theoretical steep TCP-curve would occur if there was no inter- or intra- tumor heterogeneity of radiation sensitivity.

Figure 3 shows the effect of tumor size on the dose response curve. Tumor size, though important clinically does not add significantly to the shape of the dose response curve despite the very large range of sizes of clinical breast cancers treated here and in the data reported by Hellman[8]. The values of α and β were 0.35 Gy^{-1} and 0.035 Gy^{-2} for reoxgenating conditions and 0.42 Gy^{-1} and 0.042 Gy^{-2} for conditions where there is no reoxygenation. The tumor size distribution caused the γ_{50} values to change from 2.37 to 2.00 in the fully reoxygenated tumors. Under conditions of no reoxygenation the γ_{50} went from 1.43 to 1.23. The theoretical effect of tumor size distribution alone is shown in Figure 4. Here it is assumed that all tumor cells in all patients have identical radiation sensitivities and are well oxygenated. The tumor sizes of the 22 patients was used

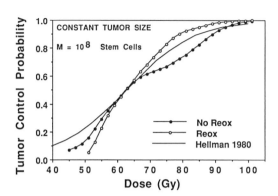

FIGURE 2. Calculated dose response curves for the 22 patients with pO_2 histograms. Full inter-fraction reoxygenation (Reox), or no reoxygenation between fractions (No Reox) are shown. The clinical data from Figure 1 are plotted for comparison.

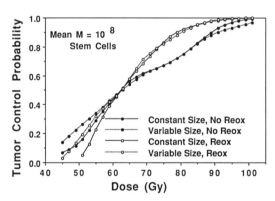

FIGURE 3. Calculated dose response curves with full inter-fraction reoxygenation (Reox), or no reoxygenation between fractions (No Reox), assuming either all tumors have 10^8 stem cells (Constant Size) or that the tumors have their measured volumes with an average of 10^8 cells.

as the size distribution. The effect of tumor size is significantly less than that of the pO_2 distribution. The γ_{50} due to a 500-fold variation in tumor size is 3.34, and is still far steeper than the clinical data shown in Figure 1. Tumor size does however impact on the shape of the dose response curve and the γ_{50} is significantly less than the maximum value of 6.5. Tumor size distributions, unlike the oxygen tension distribution is not sufficient to explain the clinical variability seen in Figure 1.

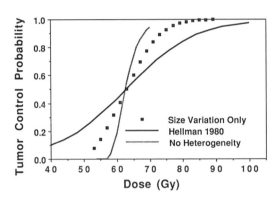

FIGURE 4. The dose response curve that would occur if all aspects of radiation response were constant except the measured size distribution among the 22 patients studied. The clinical dose response data and theoretical steep TCP-curves from Figure 1 are shown for comparison.

DISCUSSION

Tumor oxygenation is an extremely important modifier of treatment response of animal tumor models. It is arguably the most important determinant of response among tumors of the same type treated with a single fraction of radiation[12]. The importance of hypoxia is decreased during a course of fractionated radiation due to processes including reoxygenation, natural redistribution of the cell cycle, repopulation (tumor growth during a fractionated course of treatment) and repair of radiation damage between fractions[6]. Hence the impact of hypoxia on the fractionated treatment of human tumors has been controversial.

Proponents of pO_2 as a major determinant of radiation treatment response argue that reoxygenation between fractions is rarely complete and that hypoxic cells being greatly protected from radiation effects will be responsible for many or most treatment failures. Indeed the hypoxia present in human tumors[2,3,13,14] is similar to that observed in animal tumor models[12,15,16], particularly when considering only those animal tumors that are of clinically relevant sizes.

The alternate argument suggests that intrinsic heterogeneity of response within clones in a given tumor and certainly between different patients will dominate as a cause for failure and that the impact of hypoxia might be negligible[10].

The dominant cause of local failure of fractionated radiation is unknown. The purpose of this investigation was to determine to what extent observed clinical heterogeneity of radiation treatment response can be explained by the distribution of oxygenation measured in patients with breast cancer.

The slope of the dose response curve is a measure of the clinical heterogeneity of response. Great heterogeneity of radiation sensitivity causes a shallow slope (eg. a low γ_{50}), if all the cells in all the tumors have identical sensitivities the slope is maximally steep. The maximal steepness is dependent on the log of the number of stem cells and is independent of intrinsic sensitivity (eg. $[\alpha/\beta]$). Poisson statistics and reasonable tumor sizes suggest that γ_{50} is unlikely to be greater than approximately 6.5[1]. We found the oxygen tension distribution was an important modifier of the slope of the dose response curve and alone was sufficient to account for the shape of the known dose response curve for human breast carcinoma. Tumor size distribution had only a minimal effect of the shape of the curve suggesting it is significantly less important than oxygen for predicting treatment outcome. Two models of radiation induced reoxygenation were tested, one that allowed full reoxygenation to the baseline state between the daily radiation fractions and another with no reoxygenation between fractions. The clinical data fell between these two models in accordance with the expected incomplete reoxygenation between treatments. The results support the conclusion that in human breast carcinoma, as in animal tumor models, tumor oxygen tension distribution is a critical modifier of radiation treatment response. The role of tumor oxygen tension distribution in the radiation treatment of other cancer sites deserves further evaluation.

REFERENCES

1. H.D. Suit, S. Skates, A. Taghian, P. Okunieff, et al, Clinical implications of heterogeneity of tumor response to radiation therapy, *Radiother. Oncol.* 25:251-260 (1992).
2. P. Vaupel, F. Kallinowski and P. Okunieff, Blood flow, oxygen and nutrient supply, and metabolic microenvironment of human tumors: a review, *Cancer Res.* 49:6449 (1989).
3. P. Vaupel, K. Schlenger and M. Hoeckel, Blood flow and tissue oxygenation of human tumors: an update, *Adv. Exp. Med. Biol.* 277:895-906 (1990).
4. R.H. Thomlinson, Changes of oxygenation in tumors in relation to irradiation, *Front. Radiat. Ther. Oncol.* 3:109 (1968).

5. H.D. Suit, Hyperbaric oxygen in radiotherapy of four mouse tumors, *Proc. Intern. Conf. Radiation Biology & Cancer* 1:39 (1966).

6. H.D. Suit, R. Sedlacek, G. Silver, C-C. Hsieh, et al, Therapeutic gain factors to fractionated radiation treatment of spontaneous murine tumors using fast neutrons, photons plus O_2 at 1 or 3 ATA, or photons plus misonidazole, *Radiat. Res.* 116:482 (1988).

7. P. Vaupel, K. Schlenger, C. Knoop and M. Hoeckel, Oxygenation of human tumors: evaluation of tissue oxygen distribution in breast cancers by computerized O_2 tension measurements, *Cancer Res.* 51:3316 (1991).

8. S. Hellman, Improving the therapeutic index in breast cancer treatment: The Richard and Hinda Rosenthal Foundation Award lecture, *Cancer Res.* 40:4335 (1980).

9. H.D. Thames and H.D. Suit, Tumor radioresponsiveness versus fractionation sensitivity, *Int. J. Radiat. Oncol. Biol. Phys.* 12:687 (1986).

10. J.H. Hendry and H.D. Thames, Fractionation sensitivity and the oxygen effect, *Br. J. Radiol.* 63:79 (1992).

11. S.S. Tucker, H.D. Thames and J.M. Taylor, How well is the probability of tumor cure after fractionated irradiation described by Poisson statistics, *Radiat. Res.* 124:273 (1990).

12. J.E. Moulder and S. Rockwell, Hypoxic fractions of solid tumors: experimental techniques, methods of analysis and a survey of exist-ing data, *Int. J. Radiat. Oncol. Biol. Phys.* 10:695 (1984).

13. J. Denekamp, J.F. Fowler and S. Dische, The proportion of hypox-ic cells in a human tumor, *Int. J. Radiat. Oncol. Biol. Phys.* 2:1227 (1977).

14. R.A. Gatenby, H.B. Kessler, J.S. Rosenblum, L.R. Coia, et al, Oxygen distribution in squamous cell carcinoma metastases and its relationship to outcome of radiation therapy, *Int. J. Radiat. Oncol. Biol. Phys.* 14:831 (1988).

15. P. Okunieff, M. Urano, F. Kallinowski, P. Vaupel, et al, Tumors growing in irradiated tissue: Oxygenation, metabolic state, and pH, *Int. J. Radiat. Oncol. Biol. Phys.* 21:667 (1991).

16. P. Vaupel, P. Okunieff, F. Kallinowski and L.J. Neuringer, Correlations between ^{31}P-NMR spectroscopy and tissue O_2 tension measurements in a murine fibrosarcoma, *Radiat. Res.* 120:477 (1989).

MEASUREMENT OF pO$_2$ IN A MURINE TUMOUR AND ITS CORRELATION WITH HYPOXIC FRACTION

Michael R. Horsman, Azza A. Khalil, Marianne Nordsmark, Cai Grau, and Jens Overgaard

Danish Cancer Society
Department of Experimental Clinical Oncology
Nörrebrogade 44
DK - 8000 Aarhus C, Denmark

INTRODUCTION

Radiation resistant hypoxic cells, found to exist in most animal and human solid tumours (Moulder and Rockwell, 1984; Vaupel et al., 1989), are now believed to compromise the success of clinical radiotherapy (Dische, 1989; Overgaard, 1989). Numerous attempts have been made to try and identify those human tumours which contain hypoxic regions and therefore are most likely to benefit from therapies which can overcome hypoxia (for review see Horsman, 1993). These techniques have included measurements of tumour vascularization, cryospectrophotometric estimates of intercapillary haemoglobin oxygen saturations, tumour metabolic activity, the binding of radioactive or fluorescently labelled nitroimidazole compounds and the determination of oxygen partial pressure (pO$_2$) distributions using microelectrodes.

Measurements of tumour oxygenation using microelectrodes is probably the most direct method currently available for estimating hypoxia in tumours and one that has clinical applicability (for review see Vaupel et al., 1989). In fact, three small clinical studies using microelectrodes to measure pO$_2$ in cervical cancers (Kolstad, 1968; Höckel et al., 1993) as well as head and neck tumours (Gatenby et al., 1988) have found that the less well oxygenated tumours showed the poorest response to radiation therapy. However, as yet there have been no direct correlations between the microelectrode measurements of tumour oxygenation and the actual level of hypoxia in tumours.

The aim of our current study was to use a variety of treatments to both increase and decrease the normal hypoxic fraction in a C3H mouse mammary carcinoma, to estimate the hypoxic fraction from the radiation response under these different treatment conditions, and then attempt to correlate these results with tumour oxygenation measurements obtained using a pO$_2$ microelectrode.

Oxygen Transport to Tissue XV, Edited by P. Vaupel
et al., Plenum Press, New York, 1994

MATERIALS AND METHODS

Animal and tumour model. All experiments were performed on 10-14 week-old male or female CDF1 mice. The tumour model used was the C3H mouse mammary carcinoma. Its derivation and maintenance have been described previously (Overgaard, 1980). Experimental tumours were produced following sterile dissection of large flank tumours. Macroscopically viable tumour tissue was minced with a pair of scissors, and 5-10 μl of this material were injected into the foot of the right hind limb of the experimental animals. This location ensured easy access to the tumour for treatment without involvement of critical normal tissue in the treatment fields. In addition, anaesthetization of the animals during treatment could be avoided. Treatments were carried out when tumours had reached a tumour volume of about 200 mm^3, which generally occurred within 2-3 weeks after challenge. Tumour size was determined by the formula: D_1 x D_2 x D_3 x $\pi/6$, (where the D values represent three orthogonal diameters).

Drug Preparation. Hydralazine (HDZ) was obtained from Ciba-Geigy Co., Copenhagen, Denmark, and dissolved in a sterile saline (0.9% NaCl) solution immediately before each experiment. It was injected intravenously (i.v.) into mice at a constant injection volume of 0.02 ml/g body weight.

Gassing Procedures. Mice were restrained in Lucite jigs and flushed with either carbogen (95% O_2 + 5% CO_2) or carbon monoxide (CO; 220 ppm) at a flow rate of 2.5 l/min. The period of exposure to the gas prior to any subsequent treatment was at least 5 minutes for carbogen and 35 minutes for carbon monoxide. Flow was also maintained during the subsequent treatment.

Radiation Treatment. Irradiations were given with a conventional therapeutic X-ray machine (250 kV; 15 mA; 2 mm Al filter; 1.1 mm Cu half-value layer; dose rate 2.3 Gy/min). Dosimetry was accomplished by use of an integrating chamber. All treatments to tumour-bearing feet were administered to non anaesthetized mice placed in a Lucite jig. Their tumour-bearing legs were exposed and loosely attached to the jig with tape, without impairing the blood supply to the foot. Tumours only were irradiated, the remainder of the animal being shielded by 1 cm of lead. To secure homogeneity of the radiation dose, tumours were immersed in a water bath with about 5 cm of water between the X-ray source and the tumour. Irradiation of hypoxic tumours involved clamping the tumour-bearing leg 5 min before and during the period of irradiation. Clamping was achieved by constriction of the blood flow using a rubber tube tightened around the leg. Following radiation treatment tumour-bearing mice were observed at weekly intervals up to 90 days post treatment. Tumour response was calculated as the percentage of animals in each treatment group showing local tumour control at 90 days. From logit analysis of the data the TCD-50 doses (radiation doses required to control 50% of treated tumours) were calculated and from these values the hypoxic fractions were determined by direct analysis (Bentzen and Grau, 1991).

Measurements with the pO$_2$ Histograph. Unanesthetized mice were restrained in Lucite jigs with the tumour-bearing leg exposed and taped to the jig as described earlier. A fine needle autosensitive microelectrode probe (Eppendorf, Hamburg, Germany) was inserted about 1 mm into the tumour and moved through the tissue in 0.7 mm increments, followed each time by a 0.3 mm backward step prior to measurement. The response time was 1.4 seconds. Parallel repeated insertions were performed in each tumour until a total of 35 to 100 measurements were obtained. The relative frequency of the pO$_2$ measurements was automatically calculated and displayed as a histogram.

RESULTS

Figures 1 and 2 show typical examples of both the radiation dose response curves and pO$_2$ histograms obtained in this study. Clamping tumours substantially modifies the radiation response such that the normal TCD-50 dose of around 54 Gy is increased to 66 Gy. Measurements of tumour oxygenation demonstrates that clamping results in a much larger percentage of lower pO$_2$ values.

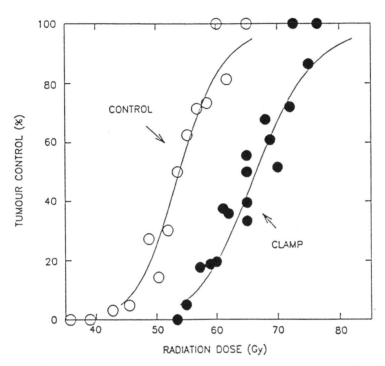

Figure 1. Representative examples of the radiation dose response curves as measured in a C3H mouse mammary carcinoma under either normal air breathing control conditions or in clamped tumours.

The various pO$_2$ parameters obtained from the histograms, along with the TCD-50 values and calculated hypoxic fractions from the radiation dose response curves, are summarized in Table 1. Also shown in this table are the results obtained under all other treatment conditions used in this study.

The TCD-50 radiation doses after HDZ or CO treatment were found to increase, as did the hypoxic fraction. In those mice breathing carbogen there was a decrease in both TCD-50 and hypoxia. Similar changes for the different treatments were observed with the pO$_2$ values obtained, although these are more clearly seen when plotted against the respective hypoxic fraction as shown in Figure 3.

Linear relationships were seen between hypoxic fraction and the pO$_2$ measurements when the latter was expressed as either the percentage of values ≤5 mmHg, the median or mean pO$_2$. The respective correlation coefficients were calculated to be 0.97, - 0.99, and -0.97. When the oxygenation results were represented by the pO$_2$ value below which 10% of the measurements were recorded no clear correlation with hypoxic fraction was observed.

Table 1. Summary of the radiation response and pO_2 values measured in a C3H mouse mammary carcinoma under a variety of treatment conditions.

Treatment[1]	TCD50[2] (Gy)	Hypoxic[2] Fraction	% ≤5 mmHg	pO_2 values (mmHg)[2] Median	Mean	10 percentile
Control	53.8±0.7	16.1±2.5	47.8±5.4	8.4±2.4	13.0±2.1	0.1±0.4
Clamped	65.9±0.9	100	96.8±2.0	0.9±0.2	1.4±0.1	0.0±0.1
HDZ (1 h)	61.8±2.7	55.4±21.7	85.4±2.0	1.3±0.1	2.6±0.4	-0.2±0.2
HDZ (6 h)	57.4±2.3	29.4±11.0	63.4±4.5	3.3±0.8	7.7±0.8	0.5±0.1
CO (220 ppm)	61.2±3.9	51.5±29.0	71.7±5.8	2.3±0.5	5.9±1.5	0.2±0.2
Carbogen	43.9±3.5	4.3±1.7	24.1±2.9	45.1±8.7	78.4±10.6	1.2±0.2

[1]Results were measured in mice under normal air breathing control conditions; in clamped tumours; 1 or 6 hours after injecting mice with HDZ (5 mg/kg; i.v.); after breathing CO (220 ppm)for at least 35 minutes; or following carbogen breathing for at least 5 minutes.

[2]Errors for the TCD-50 and hypoxic fraction results are 95% confidence intervals, while for the pO_2 values they represent ±1 S.E.

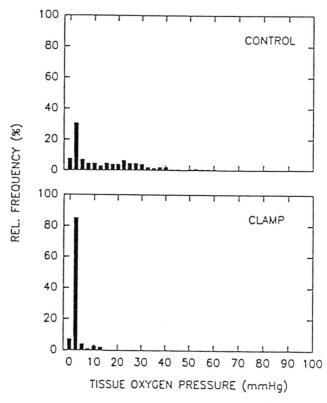

Figure 2. Representative examples of the pO_2 histogram as measured in a C3H mouse mammary carcinoma under either normal air breathing control conditions or in clamped tumours. Results show the relative frequency of each pO_2 value obtained.

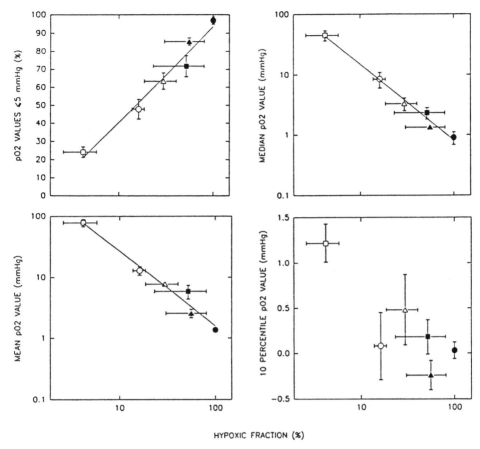

HYPOXIC FRACTION (%)

Figure 3. Relationship between pO$_2$ measurements and the radiobiological hypoxic fraction in a C3H tumour. Results were obtained from normal air breathing mice (○); in clamped tumours (●); in mice 1 hour (▲) or 6 hours (△) after injecting HDZ (5 mg/kg; i.v.); or in mice allowed to breathe CO (220 ppm) for at least 35 minutes (■); or carbogen for at least 5 minutes (□). Lines were fitted by regression analysis.

DISCUSSION

This study has shown that radiobiological hypoxia measured under a variety of treatment conditions in this C3H mouse mammary carcinoma can be clearly correlated with microelectrode oxygen measurements provided that the appropriate end point is selected. Vaupel and colleagues had previously demonstrated that median pO$_2$ values in animal tumours decreased with increasing tumour size (Vaupel 1979; Vaupel et al., 1987; Kallinowski et al., 1990), which strongly suggested a correlation between pO$_2$ measurements and tumour hypoxia since the level of radiobiological hypoxia is known to increase with tumour volume (Rofstad et al., 1989). But, as far as we know our study is the first to show a direct relationship between pO$_2$ and hypoxia.

The treatments used to change hypoxia in this tumour model were very different. Hydralazine is an antihypertensive drug which can substantially reduce tumour blood flow (Horsman et al., 1989b) to a level sufficient to enhance the cytotoxic action of agents which are specifically cytotoxic to hypoxic cells such as hyperthermia (Horsman et al., 1989b) and bioreductive drugs (Chaplin and Acker, 1987). Carbon monoxide breathing can also decrease tumour blood flow, but its ability to increase tumour hypoxia is primarily the result of an increase in carboxyhaemoglobin, which ultimatively reduces the amount of oxygen that can be transported to the tumour (Grau et al., 1992b). With carbogen the reverse is true, in that breathing this gas increases the amount of physically dissolved oxygen in the blood and thereby improves tumour oxygen delivery (Grau et al., 1992a). This would suggest that the effect of any agent that can change tumour hypoxia should be detected by measurements of pO_2.

However, this may not be true in all situations. Nicotinamide is an agent that can enhance radiation damage in murine tumours, and indirect evidence strongly suggests that this enhancement is primarily the result of an improvement in tumour oxygenation (Horsman et al., 1988; 1989a; 1992). Yet we have been unable to demonstrate this effect directly using the pO_2 histograph (unpublished observations). Since more recent data suggests that this effect may only be occurring at the microregional level in tumours (Chaplin et al., 1990; Horsman et al., 1990) it is possible that it is not being detected by a procedure like the pO_2 microelectrode which only measures oxygenation along specific tracts through the tumour, but is detected by techniques in which analysis is based on the whole tumour (Horsman et al., 1988; 1989a; 1992).

Nevertheless, it would appear that in most situations microelectrode pO_2 measurements could be used as a reliable prognostic indicator of tumour hypoxia. Measurements of tumour oxygenation in those human tumours in which hypoxia is believed to influence the response to radiation, similar to previous studies in cervical cancers and tumours of the head and neck region (Kolstad, 1968; Gatenby et al., 1988; Höckel et al., 1993), are now strongly recommended prior to the start of radiotherapy.

ACKNOWLEDGEMENTS

The authors thank Ms. A.Baden, Ms. I.M. Johansen, and Ms. M.H. Simonsen for excellent technical assistance, and Ms. D. Rasmussen for the manuscript preparation. This study was supported by a grant from the Danish Cancer Society.

REFERENCES

Bentzen, S.M., and Grau, C., 1991, Direct estimation of the fraction of hypoxic cells from tumour-control data obtained under aerobic and clamped conditions, *Int.J.Radiat. Biol.* 59:1435.

Chaplin, D.J., and Acker, B., 1987, The effect of hydralazine on the tumor cytotoxicity of the hypoxic cell cytotoxin RSU-1069: evidence of therapeutic gain, *Int.J.Radiat. Oncol.Biol.Phys.* 13:579.

Chaplin, D.J., Horsman, M.R., and Trotter, M.J., 1990, Effect of nicotinamide on the microregional heterogeneity of oxygen delivery within a murine tumour, *J.Natl. Cancer Inst.* 82:672.

Dische, S,. 1989, The clinical consequences of the oxygen effect, *in:* "The Biological Basis of Radiotherapy," G.G. Steel, G.E. Adams, and A. Horwich, eds., Elsevier Science Publishers, Amsterdam, The Netherlands.

Gatenby, R.A., Kessler, H.B., Rosenblaum, J.S., Coia, L.R., Moldofsky, P.J., Hartz, W.H., and Broder, G.J., 1988, Oxygen distribution in squamous cell carcinoma metastases and its relationship to outcome of radiation therapy, *Int.J.Radiat. Oncol.Biol.Phys.* 14:831.

Grau, C., Horsman, M.R., and Overgaard, J., 1992a, Improving the radiation response in a C3H mouse mammary carcinoma by normobaric oxygen or carbogen breathing, *Int.J. Radiat.Oncol.Biol.Phys.* 22:415.

Grau, C., Horsman, M.R., and Overgaard, J., 1992b, Influence of carboxyhemoglobin level on tumor growth, blood flow and radiation response in an experimental model, *Int.J. Radiat.Oncol.Biol.Phys.* 22:421.

Horsman, M.R., 1993, Hypoxia in tumours: its relevance, identification and modification, *in:* Current Topics in Clinical Radiobiology of Tumours, H.P. Beck-Bornholt, ed., Springer Verlag, Heidelberg (in press).

Horsman, M.R., Brown, J.M., Hirst, V.K., Lemmon, M.J., Wood, P.J., Dunphy, E.P., and Overgaard, J., 1988, Mechanism of action of the selective tumor radiosensitizer nicotinamide, *Int.J.Radiat.Oncol.Biol.Phys.* 15:685.

Horsman, M.R., Chaplin, D.J., and Brown, J.M., 1989a, Tumor radiosensitization by nicotinamide: a result of improved blood perfusion and oxygenation, *Radiat.Res.* 118:139.

Horsman, M.R., Chaplin, D.J., and Overgaard, J., 1990, Combination of nicotinamide and hyperthermia to eliminate radioresistant chronically and acutely hypoxic tumor cells, *Cancer Res.* 50:7430.

Horsman, M.R., Christensen, K.L., and Overgaard, J., 1989b, Hydralazine-induced enhancement of hyperthermic damage in a C3H mammary carcinoma in vivo, *Int.J. Hyperthermia* 5:123.

Horsman, M.R., Kristjansen, P.E.G., Mizuno, M., Christensen, K., Chaplin, D.J., Quistorff, B., and Overgaard, J., 1992, Biochemical and physiological changes induced by nicotinamide in a C3H mouse mammary carcinoma and CDF1 mice, *Int. J.Radiat.Oncol.Biol.Phys.* 22:451.

Höckel, M., Knoop, C., Schlenger, K., Vorndran, B., Mitz, M., Knapstein, P.G., and Vaupel, P., 1993, Intratumoral pO2 predicts survival in advanced cancer of the uterine cervix, *Radiother.Oncol.* (In Press)

Kallinowski, F., Zander, R., Höckel, M., and Vaupel, P., 1990, Tumor tissue oxygenation as evaluated by computerised - pO2 - histography, *Int.J.Radiat.Oncol. Biol. Phys.* 19:953.

Kolstad, P., 1968, Intercapillary distance, oxygen tension and local recurrence in cervix cancer, *Scand.J.Clin.Lab. Invest.* 106:145.

Moulder, J.E., and Rockwell, S., 1984, Hypoxic fractions of solid tumors, *Int.J.Radiat. Oncol.Biol.Phys.* 10:695.

Overgaard, J., 1980, Simultaneous and sequential hyperthermia and radiation treatment of an experimental tumor and its surrounding normal tissue in vivo, *Int.J.Radiat. Oncol. Biol.Phys.* 6:1507.

Overgaard, J., 1989, Sensitization of hypoxic tumour cells - clinical experience, *Int.J. Radiat.Biol.* 56:801.

Rofstad, E.K., DeMuth, P., Fenton, B.M., Ceckler, T.L., and Sutherland, R.M., 1989, 31-P NMR spectroscopy and HbO2 cryospectrophotometry in prediction of tumor radioresistance caused by hypoxia, *Int.J.Radiat.Oncol. Biol.Phys.* 16:919.

Vaupel, P., 1979, Oxygen supply to malignant tumors, *in:* "Tumor Blood Circulation: Angiogenesis, Vascular Morphology and Blood Flow of Experimental and Human Tumors," H.I. Peterson, ed., CRC Press Inc., Boca Raton, Florida.

Vaupel, P., Fortmeyer, H.P., Runkel, S., and Kallinowski, F., 1987, Blood flow, oxygen consumption and tissue oxygenation of human breast cancer xenografts in nude mice, *Cancer Res.* 47:3496.

Vaupel, P., Kallinowski, F., and Okunieff, P., 1989, Blood flow, oxygen and nutrient supply, and metabolic micro-environment of human tumors: a review, *Cancer Res.* 49:6449.

ACUTE EFFECTS OF TUMOR NECROSIS FACTOR-α OR LYMPHOTOXIN ON OXYGENATION AND BIOENERGETIC STATUS IN EXPERIMENTAL TUMORS

Tina Engel and Peter Vaupel

Institute of Physiology and Pathophysiology
University of Mainz
D-6500 Mainz, Germany

INTRODUCTION

Recombinant human tumor necrosis factor-α (rhTNF-α) exerts direct cytolytic and cytostatic effects on tumor cells in vitro (Fiers, 1991). In vivo, indirect actions on the tumor microvasculature have been described, such as the formation of fibrin thrombi (Nawroth et al., 1988), which cause stasis and damage of tumor microvessels with subsequent hemorrhagic necrosis.

Recombinant human lymphotoxin (rhLT or TNF-ß) shows a large structural homology with TNF-α and shares many of its biologic activities (Nedwin et al., 1985; for a recent review see Balkwill, 1989).

Previous studies on rat tumors have shown that i.v. administration of both cytokines at a dose of 1 mg/kg leads to a significant increase in tumor vascular resistance (TVR) and, as a result of this, to a significant decrease in tumor blood flow (TBF) without any changes of these parameters in normal tissues (Kluge et al., 1992).

The key question of the present study was to clarify whether these changes in tumor perfusion upon i.v. administration of the cytokines have an impact on therapeutically relevant parameters such as tissue oxygenation, bioenergetic and metabolic status of tumors and normal tissues. Subcutaneously implanted DS-sarcomas, resting thigh muscle and the subcutis of the hind foot dorsum of SD-rats were investigated over an observation period of 2 h.

MATERIALS AND METHODS

Animals and Tumors

DS-sarcoma ascites cells were serially passaged in the peritoneal cavity of Sprague-Dawley rats (200-400 g). Approximately $4 \cdot 10^6$ tumor cells were implanted subcutaneously into the hind foot dorsum of the rats. Tumors were used in experiments when they reached volumes of 0.7 to 1.0 ml.

Oxygen Transport to Tissue XV, Edited by P. Vaupel
et al., Plenum Press, New York, 1994

Cytokines

rhTNF-α (Knoll, Ludwigshafen, Germany) used in experiments had a specific activity of $6.6 \cdot 10^6$ U/mg protein (determined by a L 929 bioassay without actinomycin D). The purity of rhTNF-α was > 99% and the mean endotoxin level was < 2.7 pg/mg protein (determined by Limulus amebocyte lysate assay). rh lymphotoxin (Knoll, Ludwigshafen, Germany) had a specific activity of $4.27 \cdot 10^7$ U/mg protein. The purity was > 99% and the mean endotoxin level was < 0.5 ng/mg protein. Cytokines were applied i.v. at a dose of 1 mg/kg. Control animals received an equivalent volume of phosphate buffered saline (PBS, 1 ml/kg).

Surgical Procedures

After anaesthesia with sodium pentobarbital (40 mg/kg i.p.; Nembutal, Ceva, Paris, France), polyethylene catheters (inside diameters 0.5 mm, outside diameters 1.0 mm) were surgically placed into the thoracic aorta via the left common carotic artery and into the left external jugular vein. The animals were placed on a heated operation pad and the rectal temperature was maintained at 37.5 °C.

Mean arterial blood pressure was monitored continuously. The arterial catheter was connected to a Statham pressure transducer (type P 23 ID; Gould, Oxnard, CA). Arterial blood gas and acid base status were monitored by a pH/Blood Gas Analyzer (type 178, Ciba Corning, Fernwald, Germany).

Tissue Oxygenation

Tissue oxygenation was investigated polarographically in tumors and in the subcutis of the hind foot dorsum using pO_2 needle electrodes (recessed gold in glass electrode; shaft diameter 250 μm; diameter of the cathode 12 μm; Sigma pO_2 Histography, Eppendorf, Hamburg, Germany, for details see Vaupel et al., 1989). pO_2 values were obtained immediately before and (in the contralateral tumor or subcutis) 2 h after i.v. application of cytokines or PBS.

Metabolic and Bioenergetic Status

Two hours after i.v. administration of TNF-α, LT or PBS, tumors and resting skeletal muscle were rapidly frozen in liquid nitrogen, ground to a fine powder and freeze-dried. Tissue glucose and lactate levels were measured using standard enzymatic assays for tissue extracts (Boehringer-Mannheim, Mannheim, Germany).

After extraction with 0.66 M perchloric acid and neutralisation with 2 M KOH, ATP, ADP and AMP concentrations were determined by reverse phase HPLC techniques (Krueger et al., 1991). The energy charge (ECh) was calculated using the absolute concentrations of the adenylate phosphates:

$$ECh = \frac{[ATP] + 0.5\,[ADP]}{[ATP] + [ADP] + [AMP]}$$

Statistical Analysis

The results are expressed as means ± SEM, the numbers of experiments are indicated in brackets. Significant differences between histograms were assessed using a modified White test (Raatz, 1966), the unpaired Student's t-test was used to test for differences between means.

RESULTS

Mean arterial blood pressure, arterial blood gas and acid base status remained almost constant over the 2 h observation period following i.v. PBS or cytokine application.

Effects of Cytokines on Normal Tissues

Tissue Oxygenation. In the subcutis of the hind foot dorsum **pO$_2$ values** remained unchanged during the 2 h observation period after i.v. application of PBS, TNF-α or lymphotoxin (LT) as compared to pretreatment values (Fig. 1).

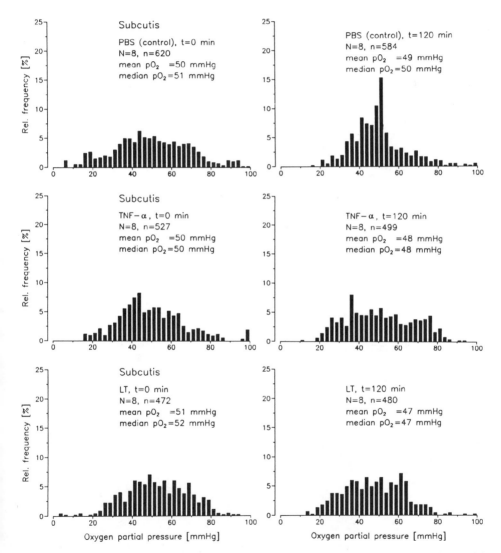

Fig. 1. Frequency distributions of measured oxygen partial pressures (pO$_2$ histograms) of the subcutis of the hind foot dorsum before (left panels) and 2 h after i.v. application of 1 ml/kg PBS (controls, upper right panel), TNF-α (1 mg/kg, center right panel) or LT (1mg/kg, lower right panel). N = number of experiments, n = number of pO$_2$ measurements.

Metabolic and Bioenergetic Status. After i.v. application of TNF-α **glucose concentrations** in skeletal muscle significantly increased (2.57 ± 0.21 mMol/kg) when compared to control values (PBS, 1.94 ± 0.09 mMol/kg) whereas LT treatment only led to a slight increase (2.14 ± 0.17 mMol/kg). **Lactate concentrations** in resting skeletal muscle increased following i.v. application of TNF-α (5.89 ± 0.56 mMol/kg) but remained unchanged upon LT treatment (4.86 ± 0.45 mMol/kg) when compared to PBS treated animals (4.82 ± 0.51 mMol/kg; Fig. 2). **ATP concentrations** in resting skeletal muscle did not differ significantly from control values (PBS, 4.82 ± 0.23 mMol/kg) following i.v. application of TNF-α (5.20 ± 0.27 mMol/kg) or LT (5.05 ± 0.23 mMol/kg). As a result of marginal decreases in ADP and AMP concentrations the **energy charge** increased following administration of the cytokines (Fig. 3).

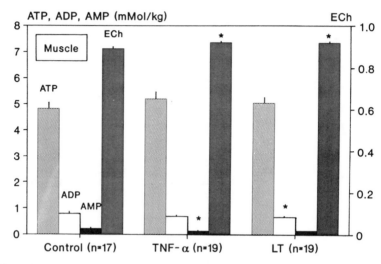

Fig. 2. Mean glucose and lactate concentrations (mMol/kg) in resting skeletal muscle 2 h after i.v. application of PBS (controls, 1 ml/kg), TNF-α or lymphotoxin (LT, 1 mg/kg). Number of experiments is indicated in brackets ($*$ p < 0.05).

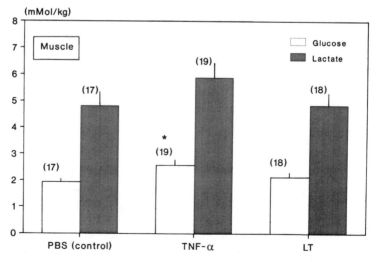

Fig. 3. Mean ATP, ADP and AMP concentrations (mMol/kg) and energy charge (ECh) in resting skeletal muscle 2 h after i.v. administration of PBS (controls, 1 ml/kg), TNF-α or lymphotoxin (LT, 1 mg/kg). Number of observations is indicated in brackets ($*$ p < 0.05).

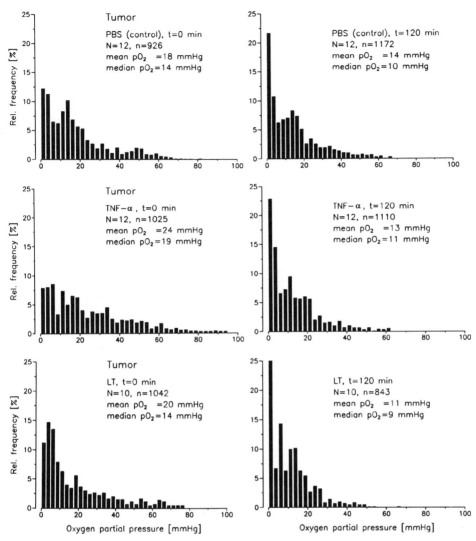

Fig. 4. pO$_2$ histograms obtained from tumors before (left panels) and 2 h after i.v. administration of 1 ml/kg PBS (controls, upper right panel), TNF-α (1 mg/kg, center right panel) or LT (1mg/kg, lower right panel).

Effects of Cytokines on Tumor Tissues

Tumor Oxygenation. In control tumors **pO$_2$ values** declined only marginally whereas cytokines led to a significant deterioration of the tumor oxygenation within 2 h after i.v. administration, as compared to pretreatment values (Fig. 4).

Metabolic and Bioenergetic Status. Mean tumor **glucose concentrations** significantly declined following i.v. administration of TNF-α (1.41 ± 0.16 mMol/kg) or were slightly reduced 2 h after application of LT (1.74 ± 0.11 mMol/kg) when compared to controls (PBS, 2.08 ± 0.33 mMol/kg). Mean tumor **lactate levels** increased following cytokine treatment (7.98 ± 1.36 mMol/kg 2 h after application of TNF-α, 8.06 ± 0.50 mMol/kg after administration of lymphotoxin) when compared to control values (PBS, 5.76 ± 0.38 mMol/kg; Fig. 5).

Despite the distinct drop in tumor oxygenation, no significant alterations were observed in mean tumor **ATP concentrations** following i.v. administration of TNF-α (0.77 ± 0.06 mMol/kg) or LT (0.99 ± 0.11 mMol/kg) when compared to control values (PBS, 0.68 ± 0.10 mMol/kg; Fig. 6). Likewise no changes in the energy charge were seen upon cytokine treatment.

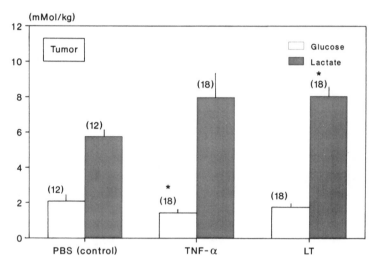

Fig. 5. Glucose and lactate concentrations (mMol/kg) in tumors 2 h after i.v. application of PBS (controls, 1 ml/kg), TNF-α or lymphotoxin (LT, 1 mg/kg). Number of experiments is indicated in brackets (∗ p < 0.05).

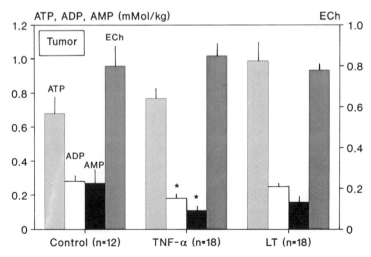

Fig. 6. ATP, ADP and AMP concentrations (mMol/kg) and energy charge (ECh) in tumors 2 h after i.v. administration of PBS (controls, 1 ml/kg), TNF-α or lymphotoxin (LT, 1 mg/kg). Number of experiments is indicated in brackets (∗ p < 0.05).

Table 1. Differential effects of TNF-α or lymphotoxin on tumor (DS-sarcoma) and normal tissues (resting skeletal muscle, subcutis of the hind foot dorsum).

		BLOOD FLOW	pO$_2$	[GLUCOSE]	[LACTATE]	[ATP]
TNF-α	skeletal muscle			↑ (glycogenolysis↑)	↑ (glycogenolysis ↑)	Ø
	subcutis	Ø	Ø			
	DS-sarcoma	↓	↓	↓ (glycolysis ↑)	↑ (glycolysis ↑)	Ø
LT (TNF-ß)	skeletal muscle			(↑)	Ø	Ø
	subcutis	Ø	Ø			
	DS-sarcoma	↓	↓	(↓) (glycolysis ↑)	↑ (glycolysis ↑)	Ø

DISCUSSION AND CONCLUSIONS

The effects of TNF-α and LT on DS-sarcomas and normal tissues in the rat are summarized in Table 1.

In acute experiments, the two cytokines show differential effects on tumor and normal tissues. In tumors, blood flow (Kluge et al., 1992) and tissue oxygenation declined significantly whereas no changes of these parameters occurred in normal tissues. According to earlier studies (Kallinowski et al., 1989), a 60% drop in the cellular respiration rate of DS-sarcoma cells ex vivo upon repeated application of TNF-α (every 12 h over 6 days) is evident. This reduction in the respiration rate seems to play a minor role in solid tumors in situ in acute experiments, otherwise tumor tissue oxygenation would have remained unchanged.

Cytokine treatment had a differential impact also on energy metabolism: tumor ATP concentrations remained unchanged following i.v. application of TNF-α or lymphotoxin with no changes in the energy charge, most probably due to a stimulation of glycolysis in tumors upon cytokine treatment (Jäättelä, 1991). Decreased tumor glucose concentrations and increased lactate levels support this notion. In resting skeletal muscle glucose concentrations increased following TNF-α treatment, probably due to a stimulation of glycogenolysis in muscle cells as previously reported for in vitro conditions (Lee et al., 1987). Similar to these results obtained in vitro, muscle lactate concentrations also increased following i.v. administration of TNF-α (for a recent review see Jäättelä, 1991). After LT application these latter effects were less pronounced, i.e., stimulation of glycogenolysis in muscle cells upon LT treatment may only occur to a minor extent, if at all. ATP concentrations in skeletal muscle remained stable following cytokine application but, as a result of slight decreases in ADP and AMP concentrations, energy charge increased.

REFERENCES

Balkwill, F.R., 1989, Tumor necrosis factor, Br. Med. Bull. **45**: 389.

Fiers, W., 1991, Tumor necrosis factor- characterization at the molecular, cellular and in vivo level, FEBS letters **285**: 199.

Jäättelä, M., 1991, Biology of disease-biologic activities and mechanisms of action of tumor necrosis factor-α/cachectin, Lab. Invest. **64**: 724.

Kallinowski, F., Schaefer, C., Tyler, G., and Vaupel, P., 1989, In vivo targets of recombinant human tumour necrosis factor-α: blood flow, oxygen consumption and growth of isotransplanted rat tumours, Br. J. Cancer **60**: 555.

Kluge, M., Elger, B., Engel, T., Schaefer, C., Seega, J., and Vaupel, P., 1992, Acute effects of tumor necrosis factor-α or lymphotoxin on global blood flow, laser Doppler flux, and bioenergetic status of subcutaneous rodent tumors, Cancer Res. **52**: 2167.

Krueger, W., Mayer, W.K., Schaefer, C., Stohrer, M., and Vaupel, P., 1991, Acute changes of systemic parameters in tumor-bearing rats, and of tumor glucose, lactate, and ATP levels upon local hyperthermia and/or hyperglycemia, J. Cancer Res. Clin. Oncol. **117**: 409.

Lee, M.D., Zentella, A., Pekala, P.H., and Cerami, C., 1987, Effect of endotoxin-induced monokines on glucose metabolism in the muscle cell line L6, Proc. Natl. Acad. Sci. USA **84**: 2590.

Nawroth, P., Handley, D., Matsueda, G., De Waal, R., Gerlach, H., Blohm, D., and Stern, D., 1988, Tumor necrosis factor/cachectin induced intravascular fibrin formation in Meth A fibrosarcomas, J. Exp. Med. **168**: 637.

Nedwin, G.E., Naylor, S.L., and Sakaguchi, A.Y., 1985, Human lymphotoxin and tumor necrosis factor genes: structure, homology and chromosomal location, Nucleic Acids Res. **13**: 6361.

Raatz, U., 1966, Eine Modifikation des White-Tests bei großen Stichproben, Biometr. Zeitschrift **8**: 42.

Vaupel, P., Okunieff, P., Kallinowski, F., and Neuringer, L., 1989, Correlation between ^{31}P-NMR spectroscopy and tissue O_2 tension measurements in a murine fibrosarcoma, Radiat. Res. **120**: 477.

THE EFFECT OF IFOSFAMIDE ON TUMOR OXYGENATION
AT DIFFERENT TEMPERATURES

M. Mentzel [*], G. Wiedemann [+], A.S. Mendoza [°]

Dept. of Physiology[*], Dept. of Internal Medicine[+]
and Dept. of Anatomy[°]
Medical University of Lübeck, Germany

INTRODUCTION

A broad range of human tumors respond to the oxaza-
phosphorine compound ifosfamide (IFO), an analogue of the
well-established alcylating agent cyclophosphamid (CP) [for
review: 1]. IFO, like CP, may be regarded as a prodrug which
undergoes a complex metabolism in vivo [2-4]. The initial
metabolism of IFO consists of two different pathways: An
enzymatic hydroxylation at carbon-4 forms 4-OH-IFO which is
probably the major biologically active compound, and a side
chain oxydation leading to the liberation of chloroacetaldehyde, a compound with possible neurotoxic properties.
Tumor temperature may vary greatly depending on the topo-
graphical situation (from core to skin). This fact is important because the effectiveness of IFO is steeply temperature
dependent increasing with raising tumor temperatures from
26°C to 41°C [5]. Since different tumor temperatures change
tumor blood supply, tumor oxygenation and tumor blood flow
[6-9], it is of special interest to measure tumor oxygenation, tumor pH, laser Doppler flow and lactic acid concentration in tumor tissue during treatment with IFO under different tumor temperatures. For histological studies tumors were
shockfrozen or fixed with formalin or glutaraldehyde.

MATERIALS AND METHODS

Tumor tissue of MX1, a human breast cancer cell line, was
transplanted to the right hind paw of female athymic, 6-8
weeks old nude mice. When the tumors had grown within 3-4
weeks to a volume of 180 mm^3, the mice were treated with IFO
or saline [5]. IFO at a concentration of 25 mg/ml was injected i.v. in a dosage of 250 mg/kg b.w.. The control group was
treated with the same volume of physiological saline. The
anaesthesized animals, fixed with tape on special carriers,
were immersed immediately after IFO or saline injection in a
thermostatically controlled waterbath for one hour [10].
Temperatures were measured with a microthermo-couple with 0.3

mm tip diameter inserted into the tumor center. Tumor-pH and pO_2 were measured with semimicro needle probes with 0.3 mm (pO_2) or 0.5 mm (pH) tip diameters before and 15', 30', 60' and 120' after beginning of treatment [11, 12]. Laser doppler flow was measured continuously. The laser probe was fixed with an excentric fitting ring on the tumor surface. For determination of lactic acid concentration the tumor was dissected and immediately shockfrozen in liquid nitrogen. The frozen tumor was then pulverized and stored in liquid nitrogen until lactic acid concentration was determined enzymatically. Routine procedures were used for histological studies.

RESULTS

pH and pO_2

Controls. At room temperature, prior to the water bath, tumor temperatures lay between 26°C and 28°C, mean intratumoral pO_2 was then 5 mm Hg (fig.1), the intratumoral pH 6.7 (fig.5). After 15 min. in the water bath at a tumor temperature of 37°C mean pO_2 was 9 mm Hg, the pH still 6.7. After 15 min in the water bath at a temperature of 41°C mean pO_2 was 9 mm Hg (fig.2), pH was 6.6.(n.s.) There was no significant change of intratumoral concentration of lactic acid.

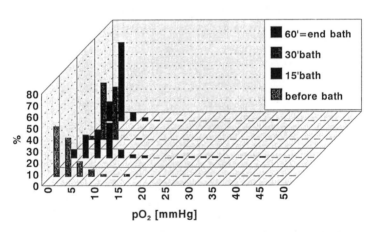

Intratumoral pO_2
Bath 1h 37°C, Mx1

Fig. 1. Frequency distribition of local pO_2 values in MX1 tumors in the control group before and during water bath application for 1 h at 37°C.

Ifosfamide. After the application of 250 mg/kg b.w. IFO mean intratumoral pO_2 at 26°C to 28°C was 4 mm Hg (fig.3), intratumoral pH 6.7. After 15 min. in the water bath at a tumor temperature of 37°C, mean pO_2 was 2 mm Hg and pH 6.4. After 15 min. at 41°C mean pO_2 was 2 mmHg (fig.4), pH 6.3 (fig.5). There was a significant increase of intratumoral lactic acid concentration at 32°C, 37°C and 41°C tumor tempe-

rature that showed a close correlation to the decrease of pH
(fig.6).

Laser Doppler Flow

The variability range of laser doppler flow values in MX1

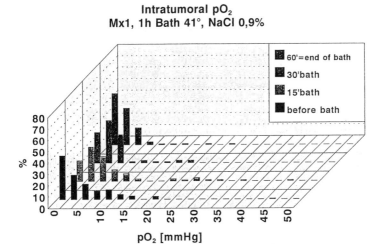

Intratumoral pO₂
Mx1, 1h Bath 41°, NaCl 0,9%

Fig. 2. Frequency distribution of local pO₂ values in MX1 tumors in the control group before and during water bath application for 1 h at 41°C.

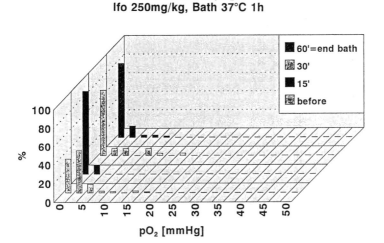

Intratumoral pO₂
Ifo 250mg/kg, Bath 37°C 1h

Fig. 3. Frequency distribution of local pO₂ values in MX1 tumors in the IFO group before and during water bath application for 1 h at 37°C.

tumors were similar to the variability range of other
investigators laser doppler flow values [6]. At 37°C there
was no significant difference in laser doppler flow between
controls and Ifo groups. In the controlgroups at 41°C the
laser doppler flow increased by 40 % with a maximum after 20

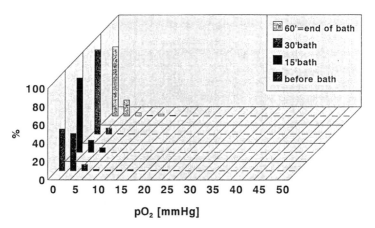

Fig. 4. Frequency distribution of local pO$_2$ values in MX1 tumors in the IFO group before and during water bath application for 1 h at 41°C.

- 30' and then slowly decreased to starting values. In the IFO group the laser doppler flow slowly decreased irreversibly by 70 % (p<0.05) (fig.7).

Histology

The ongoing light microscopical investigation does not show significant differences between IFO and control groups.

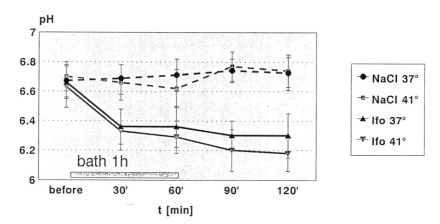

Fig. 5. Intratumoral pH in MX1 tumors before and during treatment with IFO or NaCl combined with water bath application for 1 h at 37°C or 41°C.

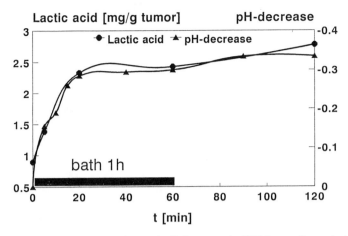

Fig. 6. Lactic acid concentration and pH decrease in MX1 tumor tissue before and during treatment with IFO combined with water bath application at 37°C.

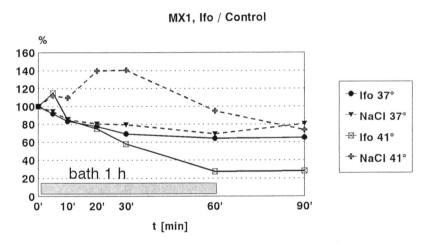

Fig. 7. Laser Doppler flow in MX1 tumor tissue before and during treatment with IFO or NaCl combined with water bath application for 1 h at 37°C or 41°C.

DISCUSSION

The cytostatically inactive drug ifosfamide is hydroxylized mostly in the liver to the active cytostatic agent 4-OH-ifosfamide. On the other hand a small fraction of IFO is oxidized to chloroacetaldehyde, a neurotoxic agent which causes spasm of the skeletal muscle. This suggests that IFO metabolites may have a similar effect on the blood vessels smooth muscle cells and may thus explain, at least in part, the observed decrease of tumor laser doppler flow and tissue

pO_2. The rapid changes of laser doppler flow and tissue pO_2 caused by IFO treatment could not be correlated so far with early changes in the tumor morphology at the light microscopical level. However it is still unproven whether IFO or one of the metabolites cause the decrease of laser doppler flow in tumor.

SUMMARY

In MX1 human breast cancer xenografts grown on the hind paw of thymusaplastic nude mice the effect of ifosfamide on tumor oxygenation, tumor pH and the concentration of lactic acid have been determined at mean tumor temperatures of 32°C, 37°C and 41°C. For histological studies tumors were shock-frozen or fixed with formalin or glutaraldehyde. Treatment with Ifosfamide (250 mg/kg b.w.) reduced intratumoral laser Doppler flow, oxygenation and pH. This suggests that ifosfamide or its metabolites may have an effect on tumor vasculature.

ACKNOWLEDGEMENTS

This study was supported by grants from the Deutsche Forschungsgemeinschaft (DFG, grant Wi 1152/1-1).

REFERENCES

1. Berger, D.P., Fiebig, H.H., Winterhalter, B.R., Wallbrecher, E., Henss, H., Preclinical phase II study of ifosfamide in human tumor xenografts in vivo. Cancer Chemother. Pharmacol. 26 (suppl):7-11 (1990).

2. Kurowski, V., Cerny, T., Küpfer, A., Wagner, T., Metabolism and pharmacokinetics of oral and intravenous ifosfamide. J.Cancer Res.Clin.Oncol. 117:148-153 (1991).

3. Wagner, T., Peter, G., Voelcker, G., Hohorst, H.J. Characterization and quantitative estimation of activated cyclophosphamide in blood and urine. Cancer Res. 37:2592-2596 (1977).

4. Wagner, T., Mittendorff, F., Walter, E., Intracavitary chemotherapy with activated cyclophosphamides and simultaneous systemic detoxification with protector thiols in sarcoma 180 ascites tumor. Cancer Res. 46:2214-2219 (1986).

5. Wiedemann, G., Knox, D., Mentzel, M., Weiss, C., Wagner, T., Effects of temperature on metabolism and action of cyclophosphamide and ifosfamide, J. Cancer Res. Clin. Oncol., 118:149 (1992).

6. Vaupel, P., Kallinowski, F., Okunieff, P., Blood flow, oxygen and nutrient supply, and metabolic microenvironment of human tumors: a review. Cancer Res. 49:6449-6465 (1989).

7. Kallinowski, F., Schlenger, K.H., Kloes, M., Stohrer, M., Vaupel, P., Tumor blood flow: The principal modulator of oxidative and glycolytic metabolism, and of the metabolic micromilieu of human tumor xenografts in vivo. Int. J. Cancer 44;266-272 (1989).

8. Kallinowski, F., Schlenger, K.H., Runkel, S., Kloes, M., Stohrer, M., Okunieff, P., Vaupel, P., Blood flow, metabolism, cellular micro-environment, and growth rate of human tumor xenografts. Cancer Res. 49:3759-3764 (1989).

9. Vaupel, P., Fortmeyer, H.P., Runkel, S., Kallinowski, F., Blood flow, oxygen consumption, and tissue oxygenation of human breast cancer xenografts in nude rats. Cancer Res. 7:3496-3503 (1987).

10. Wiedemann, G., Roszinski, S., Biersack, A., Mentzel, M., Weiss, C., Wagner, T., Treatment efficacy, intratumoral pO_2 and pH during thermochemotherapy in xenotransplanted human tumors growing in nude mice. Contr. Oncol. 42:556-565 (1992).

11. Roszinski, S., Wiedemann, G., Jiang, S.Z., Baretton, G., Wagner, T., Weiss, C., Effects of hyperthermia and /or hyperglycemia on Ph and pO_2 in well oxygenated xenotransplanted human sarcoma. Int. J. Radiation Oncology Biol. Phys. 20:1273-1280 (1991).

12. Wiedemann, G., Roszinski, S., Biersack, A., Weiss, C., Wagner, T., Local hyperthermia enhances cyclophosphamide, ifosfamide and cis-diamminedichloroplatinum. J. Cancer Res. Clin Oncol. 118:129-135 (1992).

THE EFFECT OF ERYTHROPOIETIN ON TUMOR OXYGENATION
IN NORMAL AND ANEMIC RATS

D. K. Kelleher, E. Baussmann, E. Friedrich[*] and P. Vaupel

Institute of Physiology and Pathophysiology, Univ. of Mainz
D-6500 Mainz and [*]Inst. of Radiology and Pathophysiology
German Cancer Research Center, D-6900 Heidelberg, Germany

INTRODUCTION

Anemia associated with malignancy is a common clinical problem. Its etiology is varied and includes nutritional causes, hemorrhage, hemolysis, bone marrow metastasis and hypoplasia, paraneoplastic syndromes, and chemotherapy[1], with many patients presenting with anemia even before they receive cytotoxic therapy and even if their bone marrow is not invaded by tumor cells[2]. The response of tumors to standard radiotherapy and oxygen-dependent chemotherapy in these patients is often less satisfactory than in subjects with normal hemoglobin levels[3]. This is presumed to be due to the worsening of tumor oxygenation as a result of the decreased oxygen-carrying capacity of the blood in these anemic tumor patients. Blood transfusions for anemic patients undergoing radiotherapy have not been universally accepted on the ground of infection risks and non-specific immunosuppression, although beneficial effects of transfusions on radiotherapy in anemic patients have been reported[4]. As a result, interest has recently focused on the possible use of erythropoietin - a glycoprotein hormone regulating the differentiation and maturation of red blood cells - in the correction of malignancy-associated anemia. The aim of this study was to investigate the effects of recombinant human erythropoietin (rhEPO) on red blood cell-related parameters, tumor blood flow and tumor oxygenation, in anemic and non-anemic rats, in order to ascertain whether this more "physiological" approach could have implications for improving tumor oxygenation and subsequently radiotherapy outcome in anemic tumor patients.

MATERIALS AND METHODS

Animals

Sprague Dawley rats (160 - 210 g) were used in this study. They received a standard diet and water *ad libitum.*

Drugs

rhEPO (Recormon®, Boehringer-Mannheim, purity > 98%) was dissolved in buffered saline and administered (1000 IU/kg) three times per week, over 14 days, to animals by subcutaneous injection. Control animals received an equivalent volume of phosphate-buffered saline (PBS). Studies in rats have shown that there is no significant production of antibodies against rhEPO over this treatment period[5].

Tumors

Non-Anemic Animals: Solid tumors were induced on day 7 following commencement of rhEPO or PBS treatment by injection of DS-sarcoma ascites cells onto the hind foot dorsum.

Anemic Animals: Approximately 10^8 DS-sarcoma cells were injected i.p. on day 3 following commencement of rhEPO or PBS treatment to induce anemia which results primarily from the development of a hemorrhagic ascites. On day 7, solid tumors were induced on the hind foot dorsum as described above.

Measurements

Final investigations took place in all animals on day 14 following commencement of rhEPO or PBS treatment. Rats were anesthetized with sodium pentobarbital (40 mg/kg i.p., Nembutal, Ceva, Paris, France). Polyethylene catheters were surgically placed into the thoracic aorta via the left common carotid artery and connected to a Statham pressure transducer for mean arterial blood pressure measurement. Rectal temperature was maintained at 37.5°C. At the end of a 30 minute stabilization period, blood samples were taken and the arterial blood gas status, hematocrit, hemoglobin concentration and red blood cell-related parameters investigated. Tumors then underwent one of the following measurements:

a) Tumor oxygen tension: determined using polarographic needle electrodes (recessed gold in glass electrode; shaft diameter 250 µm; diameter of the cathode 12 µm) and pO_2 histography (model KIMOC-6650, Eppendorf, Hamburg, Germany). For more details see Vaupel et al[6].

b) Tumor blood flow: determined using the ^{85}Kr-clearance technique[7]. For calculation of tumor blood flow, the hematocrit-dependency of the blood/tissue partition coefficient was taken into account[8].

c) Metabolic and bioenergetic status: tumors and resting skeletal muscle were rapidly frozen in liquid nitrogen, ground to a fine powder and freeze-dried. After extraction with 0.66 M perchloric acid and neutralisation with 2 M potassium hydroxide, ATP, ADP and AMP concentrations were determined using reverse phase HPLC techniques. Tissue glucose and lactate levels were measured using standard enzymatic assays for tissue extracts (Gluco quant glucose; Lactate, Boehringer-Mannheim, Mannheim, Germany).

Statistical Analysis

Results are expressed as means ± SEM with the numbers of experiments indicated in brackets. Significance was assessed using the unpaired Student's t-test, or in the case of pO_2 histogram comparisons, with the White test. Significance levels for all tables and figures are: ★★★ $p < 0.001$; ★★ $p < 0.01$; ★ $p < 0.05$.

Key to Figures and Tables

RESULTS

At the end of the 14-day treatment period, rhEPO was found to induce significantly increased hematocrit values in non-anemic and anemic animals. The hematocrit in anemic animals receiving rhEPO (A + EPO) was found to be "corrected" in such a way that it was no longer significantly different from that found in non-anemic (N) rats (Figure 1). Red blood cell count and hemoglobin concentration were likewise significantly increased (Table 1).

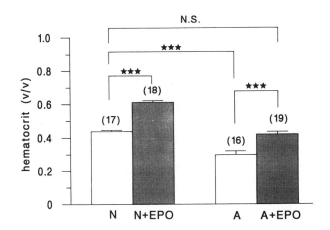

Figure 1. Hematocrit values in rhEPO- and PBS-treated non-anemic and anemic animals bearing s.c. DS-sarcomas.

The arterial blood gas and pH status, together with the oxygen saturation, oxygen content and tumor oxygen availability of animals in the four experimental groups are shown in Table 2. The oxygen content of the arterial blood was seen to be significantly increased following rhEPO treatment in both normal (N + EPO) and anemic (A + EPO) animals. The pO_2, and oxygen saturation were significantly lower in non-anemic animals receiving rhEPO. This effect was not evident in anemic animals receiving rhEPO.

Anemia was found to have a significant effect on tumor growth, with tumors in anemic animals (A) being smaller than those in non-anemic animals (N), 7 days after tumor implantation (p < 0.001). Tumors in untreated, non-anemic animals (N) were found to be significantly larger than those in rhEPO-treated, non-anemic animals (N + EPO) on day 7 following tumor implantation. rhEPO treatment did not significantly affect tumor growth in anemic animals, with tumor sizes on day 7 being comparable for both control (A) and rhEPO-treated (A + EPO) anemic animals. Growth curves for tumors in all four treatment groups are shown in Figure 2. The volume doubling times for the groups N, N+ EPO, A, and A + EPO are 1.8, 4.4, 6.2 and 4.7 days, respectively.

When tumors of the same size within the non-anemic and anemic groups were compared, rhEPO treatment did not affect tumor blood flow either in non-anemic or anemic animals. Likewise, no differences were found in mean arterial blood pressure or resistance to flow following rhEPO treatment in these animals (Table 3).

Table 1. Red blood cell-related parameters in rhEPO- and PBS-treated non-anemic and anemic animals bearing s.c. DS-sarcomas.

	N	N+EPO	A	A+EPO
number of observations	17	18	16	19
hematocrit (v/v)	0.44 ± 0.01	0.61 ± 0.01 ★★★	0.29 ± 0.02	0.42 ± 0.02 ★★★
red blood cell count ($10^6/\mu l$)	7.8 ± 0.2	10.3 ± 0.9 ★	3.9 ± 0.4	6.2 ± 0.3 ★★★
hemoglobin content (g/dl)	14.5 ± 0.3	19.2 ± 0.4 ★★★	8.5 ± 0.8	12.7 ± 0.7 ★★★
MCV (fl)	57.4 ± 1.7	63.3 ± 2.8	77.8 ± 3.2	67.9 ± 2.0 ★
MCH (pg)	19.0 ± 0.5	19.9 ± 0.9	21.9 ± 0.5	20.5 ± 0.5
MCHC (g/l)	331.0 ± 3.2	314.6 ± 3.9 ★★	286.0 ± 9.5	303.5 ± 5.0

The relationship between tumor size and mean tumor pO_2 in the four treatment groups can be seen in Figure 3. In non-anemic animals, a size-dependent reduction in tumor oxygenation was evident, irrespective of rhEPO treatment. This relationship was not found for tumors in anemic animals. The mean tumor pO_2 in rhEPO-treated animals was consistently higher than that measured in control animals, irrespective of anemia.

Table 2. Arterial blood gas, pH, oxygen saturation and oxygen content, and tumor oxygen availability (= art. $[O_2]$ • tumor blood flow) in rhEPO- and PBS-treated non-anemic and anemic animals.

	N	N+EPO	A	A+EPO
number of observations	17	17	16	19
pO_2 (mmHg)	76 ± 2	68 ± 3 ★★	74 ± 3	76 ± 2
pCO_2 (mmHg)	43 ± 2	45 ± 2	43 ± 3	42 ± 1
pH	7.43 ± 0.01	7.39 ± 0.01 ★	7.31 ± 0.03	7.34 ± 0.01
S_{O_2} (%)	93 ± 1	88 ± 2 ★	91 ± 2	94 ± 1
$[O_2]$ (ml/dl)	18.4 ± 0.4	23.1 ± 0.8 ★★★	10.5 ± 1.0	16.2 ± 0.8 ★★★
tumor O_2 availability ($ml.g^{-1}.min^{-1}$)	15.6 ± 0.8	16.3 ± 2.0	12.5 ± 2.5	16.3 ± 1.6

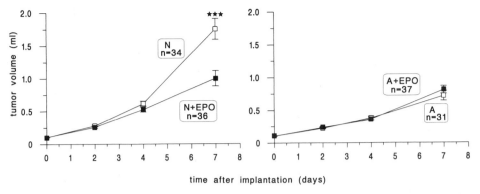

Figure 2. Growth curves for tumors in rhEPO- and PBS-treated non-anemic (left panel) and anemic (right panel) animals.

pO$_2$ histograms from tumors of comparable sizes within the non-anemic and anemic groups are shown in Figure 4. Parameters relevant to these histograms are presented in Table 4. Using the White test, the histogram from tumors in control anemic animals (A) was found to be significantly shifted to the left when compared to the histogram obtained from non-anemic control tumors (N; $p < 0.05$), indicating that the anemia in these animals led to a worsening of tumor oxygenation. The histogram from tumors in anemic animals treated with rhEPO (A + EPO) was found to be significantly shifted to the right when compared to the histogram obtained from control tumors (A; $p < 0.05$), indicating an improvement of tumor oxygenation following rhEPO treatment. Likewise, the mean tumor pO$_2$ in these animals was significantly higher (14 ± 2 mmHg; A + EPO) than in control anemic animals (9 ± 2 mmHg; A; $p < 0.05$). In anemic animals, rhEPO treatment was also found to reduce the number of measurements with pO$_2$ values less than 2.5 mmHg (i.e., at less than half maximum radiosensitivity), and to increase the number of measurements with pO$_2$ values greater than 30 mmHg (i.e., at full radiosensitivity).

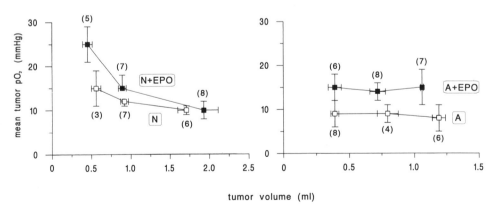

Figure 3. Mean tumor pO$_2$ as a function of tumor volume in rhEPO- and PBS-treated non-anemic (left panel) and anemic (right panel) animals.

Table 3. Tumor volume, mean arterial blood pressure, tumor blood flow and resistance to flow in rhEPO- and PBS-treated non-anemic and anemic animals.

	N	N+EPO	A	A+EPO
number of observations	10	11	8	11
tumor volume (ml)	1.33 ± 0.22	1.28 ± 0.18	0.75 ± 0.13	0.80 ± 0.12
mean arterial blood pressure (mmHg)	132 ± 4	130 ± 5	126 ± 8	130 ± 2
tumor blood flow (ml.g^{-1}.min^{-1})	0.90 ± 0.05	0.82 ± 0.11	0.92 ± 0.15	0.97 ± 0.09
resistance to flow (mmHg.g.min.ml^{-1})	147 ± 11	159 ± 28	137 ± 37	134 ± 21

Tumor and skeletal muscle concentrations of glucose, ATP, ADP and AMP were not significantly affected by either anemia or rhEPO treatment. Differences in lactate concentrations were only seen in the skeletal muscle from anemic animals where values were significantly higher (5.7 ± 1.4 mmol/kg) than in non-anemic animals (1.6 ± 0.2 mmol/kg; p < 0.01). The higher lactate levels were also evident in skeletal muscle tissue of anemic animals treated with rhEPO (A + EPO).

Table 4. Tumor volume and tumor oxygenation parameters in rhEPO- and PBS-treated non-anemic and anemic animals.

	N	N+EPO	A	A+EPO
number of observations	16	20	18	21
tumor volume (ml)	1.15 ± 0.13	1.20 ± 0.16	0.75 ± 0.09	0.74 ± 0.06
mean tumor pO$_2$ (mmHg)	12 ± 1	15 ± 2	9 ± 2 ★	14 ± 2
median tumor pO$_2$ (mmHg)	7 ± 1	11 ± 2	5 ± 1	9 ± 2
< half maximum radiosensitivity (% at 0 - 2.5 mmHg)	22	22	41	29
full radiosensitivity (% at ≥ 30 mmHg)	11	18	7	13

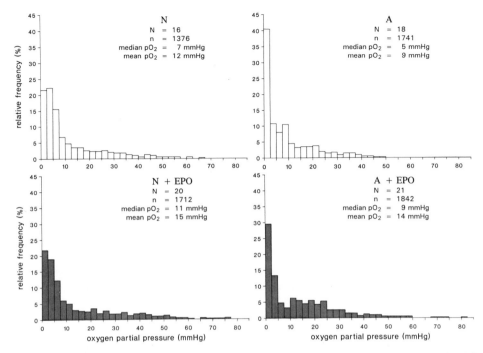

Figure 4. Frequency distributions of oxygen partial pressures (pO$_2$ histograms) measured in tumors in PBS-(upper panels) and rhEPO-treated (lower panels) in non-anemic (left side) and anemic (right side) animals. N = number of tumors, n = number of pO$_2$ measurements.

DISCUSSION

This study has shown the ability of rhEPO, at a dose of 1000 IU/kg, to cause significant increases in the hematocrit value in both non-anemic and anemic animals bearing s.c. DS-sarcomas, with a correction of the hematocrit value to pre-anemia levels in the latter group.

rhEPO treatment was found to cause no enhancement of tumor growth in any of the treatment groups (on the contrary, an inhibition of tumor growth was seen in non-anemic animals), a finding which is important with respect to the use of erythropoietin in the clinical setting. This finding is in agreement with a study by Mundt et al.[9] in which rhEPO was found to have no proliferative effects on the growth of human tumor cell lines *in vitro*.

Despite an improved release of oxygen to the tissue from erythrocytes in anemic animals (resulting from a right shift of the oxygen dissociation curve due to both anemia and arterial acidosis), the tumor oxygenation in these animals was significantly lower than in non-anemic animals, as indicated by a significant shifting to the left of the tumor pO$_2$ histogram. This confirms the work of McCormack et al.[10], who suggested that tumors grown in anemic mice have a higher hypoxic fraction than those grown in control mice. The improvement in tumor oxygenation seen in anemic animals following rhEPO treatment would suggest that rhEPO administration may sensitize tumors to standard radiotherapy and oxygen-dependent chemotherapy in anemic animals, although confirmation of such a sensitizing effect requires direct assessment of the effects of rhEPO on radiotherapy and oxygen-dependent chemotherapy outcome.

Although the main goal of this study was to evaluate tumor oxygenation following rhEPO administration in anemic and non-anemic animals, several other interesting observations concerning tumor oxygenation and blood flow were made. Firstly, the tumor volume following 7 days of tumor growth was significantly smaller than that in non-anemic animals. This increase in volume doubling time for tumors in anemic animals has also been reported in mice[8]. However, as a result of this smaller tumor volume, higher values for tumor blood flow and tumor oxygenation would be expected. Instead, tumor blood flow was similar to that found in non-anemic animals bearing larger tumors. In addition, although changes in whole blood viscosity would be expected following changes in hematocrit, no clear-cut alterations in tumor blood flow were detected following rhEPO treatment. While the poor oxygenation of tumors in anemic animals can be explained by the lower tumor oxygen availability in these animals, the disappearance of the size-dependency of tumor oxygenation is an unexpected finding. These "anomalies" in tumor blood flow and tumor oxygenation between non-anemic and anemic animals require further investigation.

ACKNOWLEDGEMENTS

The recombinant human erythropoietin used in this study was kindly donated by Boehringer-Mannheim. The authors wish to thank Monika Busse, Gabriele Berg and Anisa Kosan for their technical assistance in carrying out this study.

REFERENCES

1. J.L. Spivak. Application of recombinant human erythropoietin in oncology, *Cancer Invest.* 8:301 (1990).
2. C.B. Miller, R.J. Jones, S. Piantadosi, M.D. Abeloff and J.L. Spivak. Decreased erythropoietin response in patients with the anemia of cancer, *N.Engl.J.Med.* 322:1689 (1990).
3. D.G. Hirst. Anaemia: a problem or an opportunity in radiotherapy. *Int. J. Radiat. Oncol. Biol. Phys.* 12:2047 (1986).
4. S. Dische. Radiotherapy and anaemia - the clinical experience, *Radiother. Oncol.* Suppl 20:35 (1991).
5. G. Bode. Personal communication.
6. P. Vaupel, K. Schlenger, C. Knoop and M. Höckel. Oxygenation of human tumors: evaluation of tissue oxygen distribution in breast cancers by computerized O_2 tension measurements. *Cancer Res.* 51:3316 (1991).
7. F.E. Gump and R.L. White. Determination of regional tumor blood flow by krypton-85, *Cancer* 21:871 (1968).
8. K. Kitani. Solubility coefficients of ^{85}Kr and ^{133} xenon in water, saline, lipids, and blood, *Scand. J. Clin. Lab. Invest.* 29:167 (1972).
9. D. Mundt, M.R. Berger and G. Bode. Effect of recombinant human erythropoietin on the growth of human tumor cell lines in vitro, *Arzneim.-Forsch./Drug Res.* 42:92 (1992).
10. M. McCormack, A.H.W. Nias and E. Smith. Chronic anaemia, hyperbaric oxygen and tumour radiosensitivity, *Brit. J. Radiol.* 63:752 (1990).

INHIBITION OF ERYTHROPOIETIN PRODUCTION BY CYTOKINES AND CHEMOTHERAPY MAY CONTRIBUTE TO THE ANEMIA IN MALIGNANT DISEASES

W. Jelkmann, M. Wolff, and J. Fandrey

Institute of Physiology, University of Bonn
Nussallee 11, D- 5300 Bonn 1, Germany

INTRODUCTION

The kidneys and the liver are the main sites of synthesis of the hormone erythropoietin. Tissue hypoxia is the primary stimulus of its production. In general, plasma levels of erythropoietin increase exponentially with lowered O_2 carrying capacity of the blood. This response is missing in uremic patients. In addition, patients with malignant and inflammatory diseases often exhibit inappropriately low plasma erythropoietin levels[1].

The etiology of the anemia in tumor patients is multifactorial, as it can involve chronic bleeding, increased hemolysis and inhibition of the proliferation of erythrocytic progenitors by inflammatory cytokines and cytotoxic drugs. Because ineffective erythropoietin production is thought to contribute to the anemia in malignant diseases, clinical trials have been started to investigate the benefits of the prescription of recombinant human erythropoietin in tumor anemia[2-5].

The pathogenesis of the impaired production of erythropoietin in malignancy is only incompletely understood. Our working hypothesis is that inflammatory cytokines, primarily interleukin 1 (Il-1) and tumor necrosis factor α (TNF-α), inhibit the renal and the hepatic synthesis of the hormone [6,7]. Furthermore, the possibility needs to be considered that this inhibition is aggravated by certain cytotoxic drugs. Herein, we report studies of the effects of Il-1, TNF-α, and representatives of some of the major classes of anti-cancer drugs on the production of erythropoietin in human hepatoma cell cultures.

METHODS

Cell Cultures

Erythropoietin-producing human hepatoma cells of the line HepG2 were obtained from the American Type Culture Collection (ATCC No. HB 8065). They were grown in medium RPMI 1640 (Flow Laboratories) supplemented with 10% fetal bovine serum

Oxygen Transport to Tissue XV, Edited by P. Vaupel
et al., Plenum Press, New York, 1994

(Gibco). The cultures were kept in a humidified atmosphere (5% CO_2 in air, unless otherwise specified) at 37°C (Heraeus incubators). The experiments were carried out with confluent monolayers (about 0.5 x 10^6 cells/cm^2) in 24 -well polystyrene dishes (Falcon, Becton Dickinson). In some experiments, the pericellular pO_2 was continuously determined by polarographic O_2-sensitive solid state probes (Neocath; Biomedical Sensors, Shiley positioned in the monolayer. The data were processed on a microcomputer (Licox; GMS, Kiel). Erythropoietin was assayed in samples usually taken after 24 hours of incubation with the respective cytokine or drug added to the culture medium (1 ml/well).

Analytical Methods

Erythropoietin was measured in duplicate by radioimmunoassay[6]. Briefly, the assay system included ^{125}I-labeled recombinant human erythropoietin (rhu-Epo; 11-33 TBq/mmol; Amersham Buchler), rabbit antiserum against rhu-Epo, and human urinary erythropoietin standard calibrated by bioassay against International Reference Preparation B. The main parameters of performance were as follows: lower detection limit 5 U/l, intraassay variance <6% and interassay variance <12% in the range 20 to 100 U/l.

Cellular protein was measured in lysates prepared of washed cultures by the addition of SDS-NaOH (5g/l sodium dodecyl sulfate in 0.1 mol/l NaOH). A micro determination kit based on the phenol reagent method was used (Sigma).

Cytotoxicity was assessed by the colorimetric tetrazolium salt/formazan method[8]. The assay is based on the reduction of (3-(4,5-dimethylthiazol-2-yl)-2,5- diphenyl tetrazolium bromide (MTT; Sigma) to purple formazan by mitochondrial dehydrogenases in living cells. Confluent HepG2 cultures in 96-well dishes were used for these studies.

Cytokines and Anti-Cancer Drugs

The following human recombinant cytokines were used: Il-1 α, Il-1ß, Il-6, $\int$-interferon ($\int$-IFN), and TNF-α (Boehringer Mannheim). Anti-cancer drugs tested for their acute effect on hepatic erythropoietin production included: methotrexate (Medac), cytosine arabinoside (Mack), cyclophosphamide and ifosfamide (ASTA Pharma), daunorubicin and cis-diamminedichloroplatinum (Cis-DDP; Rhône-Poulenc Pharma) and vincristine (Lilly).

Statistics

Results are expressed as the mean $\pm$ S.D. Dunnett's test was applied to determine the significance of difference (P < 0.05) between the mean of a control group and several treatment means.

RESULTS

Steady-state production of erythropoietin

Confluent HepG2 cultures produced steadily 10-15 U immunoreactive erythropoietin per g cellular protein and hour when maintained in an atmosphere of 5% CO_2 in air. This high basal production rate is due to the cellular hypoxia (measured pericellular pO_2 < 1 mm Hg) typical for metabolically active cultures in the common gas-impermeable dishes made of polystyrene. Indeed, erythropoietin production decreased to 3.8 ± 0.6 U per hour and g protein (6 expt., pericellular pO_2 23 ± 21 mm Hg) and 1.1 ± 0.6 U per hour and g protein (5 expt., pericellular pO_2 205 ± 43 mm Hg), when 70 or 100% O_2 were used for incubation instead of air.

Effects of cytokines

Fig. 1 shows that Il-1α and Il-1ß produced a dose-dependent inhibition of the 24-hour rates of the production of erythropoietin (tested range 1 to 100 U/ml; half-maximal inhibition, I_{50}, at 5 U/ml and 2 U/ml, respectively). TNF-α also inhibited (tested range 1 to 1000 U/ml; I_{50} 20 U/ml). Cytotoxic effects were not induced by these compounds as judged from measurements of cellular protein, LDH release or tetrazolium salt/ formazan conversion. Il-6 and γ-IFN did not suppress the production of erythropoietin.

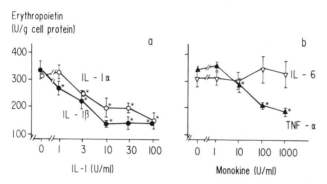

Fig. 1. Effects of (a) interleukin 1 (Il-1α, Il-1ß) and (b) Il-6 and tumor necrosis factor α (TNF-α) on the 24 h rate of the production of erythropoietin in HepG2 cultures. * indicates significant difference from respective control; P<0.05 (Dunnett's test). Reproduced from [7].

Washout experiments showed that the inhibition of the production of erythropoietin exerted by Il-1 and TNF-α was long-lasting and not reversed for at least 24 h following the removal of these cytokines. Since their action was neither lowered by the addition of glucocorticoids, phospholipase A_2-dependent mechanisms do not appear to play a major role in monokine-induced suppression of the in vitro production of erythropoietin (Fig. 2).

Effects of anti-cancer drugs

Major differences in the potency to lower the production of erythropoietin became apparent when representatives of some of the major classes of anti-cancer drugs were added to confluent HepG2 cultures in a dose range spanning the concentrations measured in plasma of cancer patients during treatment. As summarized in Table 1, compounds acting primarily on DNA-synthesis were ineffective, such as methotrexate or cytosine arabinoside. On the other hand, erythropoietin production was inhibited by compounds that act primarily on RNA-synthesis, translation or protein secretion. Lowered erythropoietin production was correlated partially with drug-induced cytotoxicity.

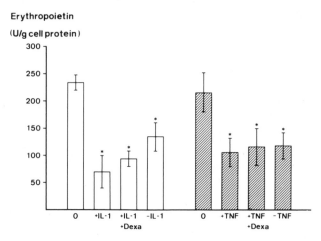

Fig. 2. Effects of interleukin 1ß (Il-1; 15 U/ml) and tumor necrosis factor α (TNF; 10 ng/ml) on the 24 h rate of the production of erythropoietin in HepG2 cultures. Studies were carried out with the respective monokine alone (+Il-1, +TNF), in combination with dexamethasone (+Dexa; 1 μg/ml), and washout experiments after 24 h preincubation with the monokines followed by their removal (-Il-1, -TNF). Values are the mean ± SD of 4 parallel cultures. * indicates significant difference from respective control; P <0.05 (Dunnett's test).

Table 1. Effects of anti-cancer drugs on the 24-hour rates of the production of erythropoietin in relation to cytotoxicity in HepG2 cultures.

Drug	Erythropoietin production I_{50}	Cytotoxicity I_{50}
Methotrexate	n.d. (>100 μg/ml)	n.d. (>100 μg/ml)
Cytosine arabinoside	n.d. (> 1 mg/ml)	n.d. (>1 mg/ml)
Daunorubicin	400 ng/ml	>10 μg/ml
Cyclophosphamide	400 μg/ml	>1 mg/ml
Ifosfamide	1 mg/ml	>1 mg/ml
Cis-DDP	5 μg/ml	>100 μg/ml
Vincristine	200 ng/ml	>100 μg/ml

I_{50}: Drug concentration resulting in half-maximal inhibition of the production of erythropoietin and tetrazolium salt/formazan formation, respectively. n.d.: no detectable inhibition even at the highest drug concentration

DISCUSSION

In this study various inflammatory cytokines and anti-cancer drugs were examined for their acute effects on the production of erythropoietin in confluent human hepatoma cultures of the line HepG2. The liver is considered the most important extra-renal site of the in vivo synthesis of the hormone. The cells elaborating erythropoietin in the kidney have not been clearly identified as yet[1]. Neither is an appropriate renal cell culture model available for study of erythropoietin synthesis. In contrast, HepG2 cells have the capacity to produce erythropoietin in large amounts and in dependence of the O_2 supply.

We have previously demonstrated Il-1 and TNF-α to inhibit the production of erythropoietin in hypoxic human hepatoma cell cultures[6,7]. In addition, the inhibition exerted by Il-1ß was confirmed in studies using isolated perfused rat kidneys[7]. The present experiments showed that the suppression of erythropoietin production is long-lasting and not lowered in the presence of glucocorticoids. In viability studies Il-1 and TNF-α exerted no cytotoxic effects on HepG2 cultures.

In all likelihood, Il-1, TNF-α, and related inflammatory cytokines play a role in the pathogenesis of erythropoietin deficiency in various diseases, including cancer. Indeed, Il-1 and TNF-α have been regarded as mediators of the anemia of chronic disorders[9,10]. The application of Il-1[11] and TNF-α [10,12] results in lowered red cell production in humans[13] and experimental animals[10-12].

In tumor patients the suppression of erythropoietin synthesis may be aggravated by certain anti-cancer drugs. The present studies show that the in vitro production of erythropoietin in confluent hepatoma cultures is lowered by compounds primarily blocking RNA synthesis (daunorubicin, cyclophosphamide, ifosfamide, cis-DDP) or protein secretion (vincristine), however not by compounds primarily acting in the DNA synthetic phase of the cell cycle (methotrexate, cytosine arabinoside). Viability studies also revealed major differences in the potency of these drugs to induce unspecific cellular damage, which was correlated only in part with the effect on erythropoietin formation.

Our findings appear of interest with respect to the use of recombinant human erythropoietin (rhu-Epo) in the treatment of tumor- and chemotherapy-associated anemia. In a rat model, high doses of rhu-Epo were required to correct 5-fluorouracil-induced anemia, while low doses sufficed to correct cis-DDP-induced anemia[14] being characterized by defect endogenous erythropoietin production. Patients with cis-DDP-induced anemia may also respond well to low-dose rhu-Epo treatment[15]. Usually rhu-Epo has been given in high doses in clinical trials aimed at correcting the anemia associated with hematologic malignancies[3-5]. Based on the present in vitro findings, more extensive clinical studies appear warrantable in regard to the effects of individual anti-cancer drugs on renal and extra-renal erythropoietin production.

REFERENCES

1. W. Jelkmann, Erythropoietin: structure, control of production, and function, Physiol. Rev. 72:449-489 (1992).
2. C.B. Miller, R.J. Jones, S. Piantadosi, M.D. Abeloff, and J.L. Spivak, Decreased erythropoietin response in patients with the anemia of cancer. New Engl. J. Med. 322:1689-1692 (1990).
3. C.B. Miller, L.C. Platanias, S.R. Mills, M.L. Zahurak, M.J. Ratain, D.S. Ettinger, and R.J. Jones, Phase I-II trial of erythropoietin in the treatment of cisplatin-associated anemia. J. Natl. Cancer Inst. 84:98-103 (1992).

4. H. Ludwig, E. Fritz, H. Kotzmann, P. Höcker, H. Gisslinger, and U. Barnas, Erythropoietin treatment of anemia associated with multiple myeloma. New Engl. J. Med. 322:1693-1699 (1990).

5. W. Oster, F. Hermann, H. Gramm, G. Zeile, A. Lindemann, G. Müller, T. Brune, H.-P. Kraemer, and R. Mertelsmann, Erythropoietin for the treatment of anemia of malignancy associated with bone marrow infiltration. J. Clin. Oncol. 8:956-962 (1990).

6. W. Jelkmann, M. Wolff, and J. Fandrey, Modulation of the production of erythropoietin by cytokines: In vitro studies and their clinical implications. Contrib. Nephrol. 87:68-77 (1990).

7. W. Jelkmann, H. Pagel, M. Wolff, and J. Fandrey, Monokines inhibiting erythropoietin production in human hepatoma cultures and in isolated perfused rat kidneys. Life Sci. 50:301-308 (1992).

8. M.B. Hansen, S.E. Nielsen, and K. Berg, Re-examination and further development of a precise and rapid dye method for measuring cell growth/cell kill. J. Immunol. Meth. 119:203-210 (1989).

9. J.C. Schooley, B. Kullgren, and A.C. Allison, Inhibition by interleukin-1 of the action of crythropoietin on erythroid precursors and its possible role in the pathogenesis of hypoplastic anaemias. Br. J. Haematol. 67:11-17 (1987).

10. K.J. Tracey, H. Wei, K.R. Manogue, Y. Fong, D.G. Hesse, H.T. Nguyen, G.C. Kuo, B. Beutler, R.S. Cotran, A. Cerami, and S.F. Lowry, Cachectin/tumor necrosis factor induces cachexia, anemia, and inflammation. J. Exp. Med. 167:1211-1227 (1988).

11. C.S. Johnson, D.J. Keckler, M.I. Topper, P.G. Braunschweiger, and P. Furmanski, In vivo hematopoietic effects of recombinant interleukin-1 α in mice: Stimulation of granulocytic, monocytic, megakaryocytic, and early erythroid progenitors, suppression of late-stage erythropoiesis, and reversal of erythroid suppression with erythropoietin. Blood 73:678-683 (1989).

12. C.S. Johnson, M.-J. Chang, and P. Furmanski, In vivo hematopoietic effects of tumor necrosis factor- in normal and erythroleukemic mice: Characterization and therapeutic applications. Bloood 72:1875-1883 (1988).

13. M. Blick, S.A. Sherwin, M. Rosenblum, and J. Gutterman, Phase I study of recombinant tumor necrosis factor in cancer patients. Cancer Res. 47:2986-2989 (1987).

14. T. Matsumoto, K. Endoh, K. Kamisango, K.-I. Akamatsu, K. Koizumi, M. Higuchi, N. Imai, H. Mitsui, and T. Kawaguchi, Effect of recombinant human erythropoietin on anticancer drug-induced anaemia. Br. J. Haematol. 75:463-468 (1990).

15. V. Gebbia, A. Russo, N. Gebbia, R. Valenza, L. Rausa, and S. Palmeri, Recombinant human erythropoietin accelerates recovery from cisplatin induced anemia in cancer patients: preliminary results. Cancer J. 4:343-347 (1991).

NON-INVASIVE ASSESSMENT OF TUMOR OXYGENATION STATUS BY INTEGRATED ^{31}P NMR SPECTROSCOPY AND ^{1}H NMR IMAGING

Einar K. Rofstad, Heidi Lyng, Dag R. Olsen, and Elin Steinsland

Department of Biophysics, Institute for Cancer Research
The Norwegian Radium Hospital, Oslo, Norway

INTRODUCTION

Tumors develop an abnormal vascular architecture during growth, resulting in poor perfusion and the occurrence of vessels with intermittent circulation, stasis, and thrombosis[1,2]. Local areas with hypoxic and anoxic cells, acid pH, and necrotic tissue arise gradually as a consequence of the insufficient blood supply[3,4]. These abnormal physiological conditions may cause resistance to radio- and chemotherapy, induce gene amplification, and lead to enhanced metastatic potential[5,6].

A method for assessment of tumor oxygenation status would be useful for providing prognostic information and for monitoring of tumor treatment response. Several methods are currently under development, including methods for measurement of tissue pO_2, intracapillary HbO_2 saturation, interstitial fluid pressure, and concentrations of ATP, glucose, and lactate[7,8]. These methods require biopsies or the insertion of needle probes. A non-invasive method would be preferable to invasive methods, particularly for routine clinical use. Moreover, the method should produce high spatial resolution since most tumors show physiological heterogeneity. ^{31}P NMR spectroscopy and ^{1}H NMR imaging are both potentially useful methods for non-invasive assessment of tumor oxygenation status and detection of tumor hypoxia[9-14].

Tumor hypoxia *per se* can not be detected by ^{31}P NMR spectroscopy or ^{1}H NMR imaging. However, physiological conditions which may be associated with tumor hypoxia can be detected. The purpose of the work reported here was to search for possible correlations between NMR parameters and physiological parameters related to tumor hypoxia. The NMR parameters that were measured included ^{31}P resonance ratios, ^{31}P spin-lattice relaxation times (phosphorus T_1s), ^{1}H spin-lattice relaxation times (proton T_1s), and ^{1}H spin-spin relaxation times (proton T_2s). The physiological parameters that were measured included tumor perfusion, blood supply per viable tumor cell, fraction of necrotic tumor tissue, and fractional tumor water content. Tumors from six human melanoma xenograft lines differing significantly in these physiological parameters were included in the study.

Oxygen Transport to Tissue XV, Edited by P. Vaupel
et al., Plenum Press, New York, 1994

MATERIALS AND METHODS

Male BALB/c-*nu/nu* mice, 8 - 10 weeks old, were used. They were bred at the animal department of our institute and kept under specific-pathogen-free conditions at constant temperature (24 - 26°C) and humidity (30 - 50%). The human melanoma xenograft lines (BEX-t, COX-t, HUX-t, ROX-t, SAX-t, WIX-t) were established in athymic mice from metastases of patients admitted to The Norwegian Radium Hospital[15]. The ROX-t and WIX-t tumors contained melanin whereas the tumors of the other four lines were amelanotic. Subcutaneous flank tumors in passages 15 - 25 were used in the work reported here. Tumor perfusion was determined by measuring the uptake of ^{86}Rb (% of ^{86}Rb injected/g of tumor tissue)[16]. Blood supply per viable tumor cell was calculated from the tumor perfusion and the tumor cell density. Tumor cell density and fraction of necrotic tumor tissue were determined by stereological analysis of histological sections[15,16]. Fractional tumor water content was measured by drying the tumor tissue at 50°C until a constant weight was reached.

Tumor ^{31}P NMR spectroscopy was performed in non-anaesthetized mice using solenoidal coils and a Bruker 4.7 T spectrometer operating at 81.025 MHz for phosphorus. The homogeneity of the magnetic field was optimized for each individual tumor by shimming on the water proton resonance. The acquisition parameters were: 90° pulse angle; 4 kHz sweep width; 1K data points per free induction decay (FID); 2,000 ms repetition time; 900 scans per spectrum. Phosphorus T_1s were measured using the one-shot superfast inversion recovery (SUFIR) technique described by Canet *et al*[17]. Spectral processing included 15 - 30 Hz matched exponential multiplication and convolution difference of 600 Hz. Peak heights were calculated from the best fits of Lorentzian line shapes to phased, resolution-enhanced, baseline-corrected spectra.

Tumor ^{1}H NMR imaging was performed to determine proton T_1 and T_2 distributions. The mice were anaesthetized with 0.01 ml/g body weight of a mixture containing 80% Sombrevin (Gedeon Richter, Hungary), 12% Hypnorm Vet (LEO, Sweeden), and 8% Stetsolid, 5 mg/ml (Dumex, Denmark). A General Electric 1.5 T whole-body NMR tomograph operating at 63.89 MHz for protons and a home-built parallel resonance mouse probe with a Q-factor of approximately 250 were employed for the imaging. Two different spin-echo pulse sequences were used, one with a repetition time (TR) of 600 ms and echo times (TE) of 20, 40, 60, and 80 ms and the other with a TR of 2,000 ms and TEs of 20, 40, 60, and 80 ms. T_1s and T_2s were calculated individually for each volume element corresponding to a pixel. A system of two equations summing up intensities (I) over four variables (the four TEs) formed the basis of the calculations:

$$\Sigma I_1^{i} = N_0(1 - \exp(-TR_1/T_1))\exp(-TE^i/T_2)$$

$$\Sigma I_2^{i} = N_0(1 - \exp(-TR_2/T_1))\exp(-TE^i/T_2)$$

where N_0 is spin density and $i \in [1,4]$. Histograms for T_1 and T_2 were generated from two imaged sections (3 mm thick and 2 mm apart) in each tumor.

A two-tailed *t*-test of correlation coefficients (r) determined by linear regression analysis was used to search for significant correlations between NMR parameters and physiological parameters of tumors. A significance level of $P = 0.05$ was used throughout.

RESULTS

^{31}P resonance ratios indicative of tumor bioenergetic status, *i.e.*, PCr/P_i, NTPβ/P_i, and (PCr + NTPβ)/P_i, as well as tumor perfusion and blood supply per viable tumor cell decreased with increasing tumor volume (Fig. 1). Significant correlations were found between the parameters for bioenergetic status and the blood flow parameters for individual tumors of the same melanoma line. However, there were no correlations between the NMR and the blood flow parameters across the six melanoma lines. This is illustrated in Fig. 2 which shows histograms for the (PCr + NTPβ)/P_i resonance ratio and the blood supply per viable tumor cell for tumors with volumes of 200 mm^3.

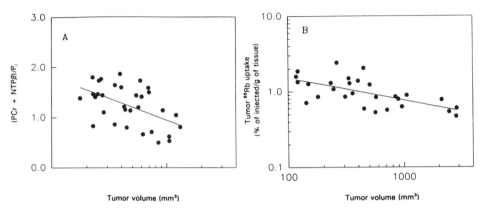

Figure 1. Tumor bioenergetic status (A) and tumor perfusion (B) *versus* tumor volume for SAX-t human melanoma xenografts. The resonance ratio (PCr + NTPβ)/P_i was used as parameter for tumor bioenergetic status. The uptake of ^{86}Rb (% of ^{86}Rb injected/g of tumor tissue) was used as parameter for tumor perfusion. *Points*, data from individual tumors. *Curves*, regression lines. The correlations are statistically significant: $r = 0.52$, $P < 0.01$ (A); $r = 0.64$, $P < 0.001$ (B). Data similar to those shown in (A) were obtained for the PCr/P_i, NTPβ/P_i, and (PCr + NTPβ)/P_i resonance ratios of the BEX-t, COX-t, HUX-t, ROX-t, SAX-t, and WIX-t lines. Data similar to those shown in (B) were also obtained for the BEX-t, COX-t, HUX-t, ROX-t, and WIX-t lines.

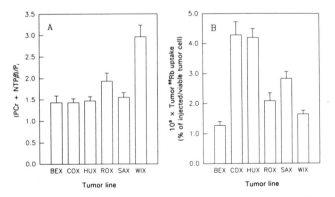

Figure 2. Histograms for tumor bioenergetic status (A) and blood supply per viable tumor cell (B) for human melanoma xenografts. The resonance ratio (PCr + NTPβ)/P_i was used as parameter for tumor bioenergetic status. The uptake og ^{86}Rb (% of ^{86}Rb injected/viable tumor cell) was used as parameter for blood supply per viable tumor cell. *Columns*, tumor bioenergetic status and blood supply per viable tumor cell at tumor volumes of 200 mm^3. *Bars*, standard errors. The data were derived from curves similar to those shown in Figs. 1A and B.

533

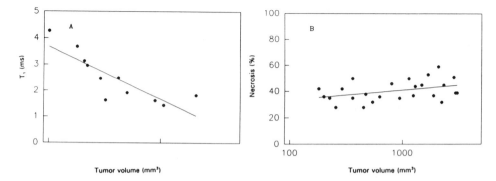

Figure 3. The T_1 of the P_i resonance (A) and fraction of necrotic tumor tissue (B) *versus* tumor volume for HUX-t human melanoma xenografts. *Points*, data from individual tumors. *Curves*, regression lines. The correlations are statistically significant: $r = 0.39$, $P < 0.0005$ (A); $r = 0.84$, $P < 0.05$ (B). Data similar to those shown in (A) were obtained for the T_1s of the PME, P_i, PDE, PCr, NTPγ, NTPα, and NTPβ resonances of the BEX-t, COX-t, HUX-t, and SAX-t lines. Data similar to those shown in (B) were also obtained for the BEX-t, COX-t, and SAX-t lines.

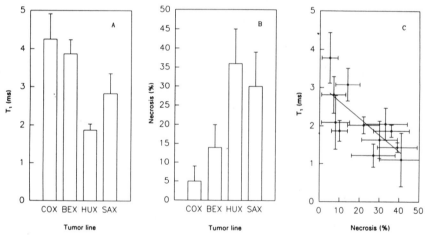

Figure 4. Histograms for the T_1 of the PCr resonance (A), histograms for fraction of necrotic tumor tissue (B), and the T_1 of the P_i resonance *versus* the fraction of necrotic tumor tissue (C) for amelanotic human melanoma xenografts. (A) *Columns*, T_1s at tumor volumes of 200 mm³. *Bars*, standard errors. The data were derived from curves similar to that shown in Fig. 3A. Similar histograms were also obtained for the PME, P_i, PDE, NTPγ, NTPα, and NTPβ resonances. (B) *Columns*, fractions of necrotic tumor tissue at tumor volumes of 200 mm³. *Bars*, standard errors. The data were derived from curves similar to that shown in Fig. 3B. (C) *Points*, mean values. The twelve data points refer to tumors with volumes of 200, 500, and 1,000 mm³ of the BEX-t, COX-t, HUX-t, and SAX-t lines. *Bars*, standard errors. *Curve*, regression line. The correlation is statistically significant: $r = 0.74$, $P < 0.005$. The data were derived from curves similar to those shown in Figs. 3A and B. Similar correlations were also obtained for the PME, PDE, PCr, NTPγ, NTPα, and NTPβ resonances.

534

The phosphorus T_1s for the BEX-t, COX-t, HUX-t, and SAX-t lines (amelanotic tumors) decreased with increasing tumor volume (Fig. 3A). The magnitude of the decrease differed significantly among the lines but not among the seven major resonances (PME, P_i, PDE, PCr, NTPγ, NTPα, NTPβ). Fraction of necrotic tumor tissue increased with increasing tumor volume (Fig. 3B). Significant correlations were found between the phosphorus T_1s and the fraction of necrotic tumor tissue across the four melanoma lines, irrespective of the phosphorus resonance considered. Thus, tumor lines showing long phosphorus T_1s showed low fractions of necrotic tumor tissue and *vice versa*. This is illustrated in Fig. 4 which shows histograms for the T_1 of the PCr resonance (Fig. 4A) and the fraction of necrotic tumor tissue (Fig. 4B) for tumors with volumes of 200 mm³. Moreover, Fig. 4C shows the correlation between the T_1 of the P_i resonance and the fraction of necrotic tumor tissue; tumors of the BEX-t, COX-t, HUX-t, and SAX-t lines with volumes of 200, 500, and 1,000 mm³ formed the basis of the analysis.

Tumors with volumes of approximately 1,000 mm³ of the BEX-t, COX-t, HUX-t, and SAX-t lines (amelanotic tumors) were subjected to ¹H NMR imaging for determination of proton T_1 and T_2 distributions. Significant correlations across the four melanoma lines were found for median T_1 and T_2 *versus* fractional tumor water content (Fig. 5) as well as for median T_1 and T_2 *versus* fraction of necrotic tumor tissue (Fig. 6). Both T_1 and T_2 increased with increasing fractional tumor water content and decreased with increasing fraction of necrotic tumor tissue; the correlations in Fig. 5 were stronger than the correlations in Fig. 6.

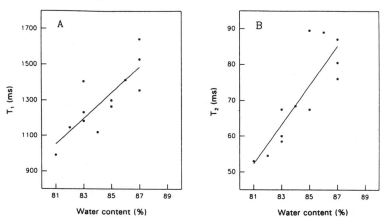

Figure 5. Median proton T_1 (A) and median proton T_2 (B) *versus* fractional tumor water content for amelanotic human melanoma xenografts. *Points*, data from individual tumors. *Curves*, regression lines. The regression analyses were based on three tumors from each of the BEX-t, COX-t, HUX-t, and SAX-t lines. The correlations are statistically significant: $r = 0.82$, $P < 0.005$ (A); $r = 0.85$, $P < 0.001$ (B).

DISCUSSION

A non-invasive method for assessment of tumor oxygenation status and detection of tumor hypoxia is needed in clinical oncology for prediction and monitoring of tumor treatment response. The potential usefulness of ³¹P NMR spectroscopy and ¹H NMR imaging was investigated in the present work. ³¹P NMR resonance ratios, phosphorus T_1s, and proton T_1s and T_2s are influenced simultaneously by a variety of biological and pathophysiological tumor parameters including those studied here; tumor perfusion, blood supply per viable tumor cell, fraction of necrotic tumor tissue, and fractional tumor water content. These four parameters are all related to tumor oxygenation status and may reflect the presence of hypoxic and/or anoxic tumor cells.

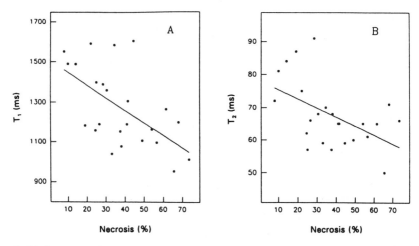

Figure 6. Median proton T_1 (A) and median proton T_2 (B) *versus* fraction of necrotic tumor tissue for amelanotic human melanoma xenografts. *Points*, data from individual tumor sections. *Curves*, regression lines. The regression analyses were based on three tumors from each of the BEX-t, COX-t, HUX-t, and SAX-t lines. Each tumor was imaged and examined histologically in two different sections. The correlations are statistically significant: $r = 0.58$, $P < 0.005$ (A); $r = 0.51$, $P < 0.05$ (B).

Tumor oxygenation is generally the resultant of the oxygen availability (nutritive tumor blood flow × arterial O_2 concentration) and the rate of oxygen consumption of the tumor cells[2]. Poor perfusion in tumors and hence low blood supply per viable tumor cell may thus be indicative of the presence of hypoxic regions. High fractions of necrotic tissue in tumors may be indicative of extensive chronic hypoxia since chronically hypoxic cells arise as a consequence of limited oxygen diffusion and are often found adjacent to necrosis[18-20]. Fractional tumor water content is correlated to tumor interstitial fluid pressure[21]. The interstitial fluid pressure is usually elevated in tumors, leading to reduced capillary blood flow and/or transient vascular occlusions[22,23]. High fractional water contents of tumors may thus be indicative of low oxygenation status and the presence of acutely hypoxic cells.

The resonance ratios PCr/P_i, NTPβ/P_i, and (PCr + NTPβ)/P_i were found to show significant correlations to tumor perfusion and blood supply per viable tumor cell within the melanoma lines. However, the correlations were different for the different lines, *i.e.*, there were no correlations across the melanoma lines. This observation is in agreement with data reported previously; tumor bioenergetic status measured by ^{31}P NMR spectroscopy was found to be correlated to intracapillary HbO$_2$ saturation within but not across tumor lines[24]. More importantly, significant correlations across the melanoma lines were found for phosphorus T_1s *versus* fraction of necrotic tumor tissue and for proton T_1s and T_2s *versus* fractional tumor water content and fraction of necrotic tumor tissue. These observations suggest that integrated ^{31}P NMR spectroscopy and ^{1}H NMR imaging may be a potentially useful non-invasive method for assessment of tumor oxygenation status and detection of tumor hypoxia.

However, further developments are required before integrated ^{31}P and ^{1}H NMR investigations can be utilized for clinical purposes. Deeper insight into the biological significance of ^{31}P and ^{1}H NMR signals is needed to facilitate the establishment of reliable criteria for identification of hypoxic regions in tumors. Technological developments are probably also needed; such developments may involve high-resolution chemical shift ^{31}P imaging[25] and diffusion-weighted ^{1}H imaging[26].

ACKNOWLEDGEMENTS

The technical assistance of Heidi Kongshaug, Berit Mathiesen, Hanne Stageboe Petersen, and Anne Wahl is gratefully acknowledged. Financial support was received from The Norwegian Cancer Society.

REFERENCES

1. R.K. Jain, Determinants of tumor blood flow: A review, *Cancer Res.* 48:2641 (1988).
2. P. Vaupel, F. Kallinowski, and P. Okunieff, Blood flow, oxygen and nutrient supply, and metabolic microenvironment of human tumors: A review, *Cancer Res.* 49:6449 (1989).
3. C.N. Coleman, Hypoxia in tumors: A paradigm for the approach to biochemical and physiologic heterogeneity, *J. Natl. Cancer Inst.* 80:310 (1988).
4. I.F. Tannock and D. Rotin, Acid pH in tumors and its potential for therapeutic exploitation, *Cancer Res.* 49:4373 (1989).
5. R.M. Sutherland, J.S. Rasey, and R.P. Hill, Tumor biology, *Am. J. Clin. Oncol.* 11:253 (1988).
6. R.P. Hill, Tumor progression: Potential role of unstable genomic changes, *Cancer Met. Reviews* 9:137 (1990).
7. J.D. Chapman, Measurement of tumor hypoxia by invasive and non-invasive procedures: A review of recent clinical studies, *Radiother. Oncol.* Suppl. 20:13 (1991).
8. W. Mueller-Klieser, K.-H. Schlenger, S. Walenta, M. Gross, U. Karbach, M. Hoeckel, and P. Vaupel, Pathophysiological approaches to identifying tumor hypoxia in patients, *Radiother. Oncol.* Suppl. 20:21 (1991).
9. P.F. Daly and J.S. Cohen, Magnetic resonance spectroscopy of tumors and potential *in vivo* clinical applications: A review, *Cancer Res.* 49:770 (1989).
10. E.K. Rofstad, NMR spectroscopy in prediction and monitoring of radiation response of tumours *in vivo*, *Int. J. Radiat. Biol.* 57:1 (1990).
11. C.T.W. Moonen, P.C.M. van Zijl, J.A. Frank, D. Le Bihan, and E.D. Becker, Functional magnetic resonance imaging in medicine and physiology, *Science* 250:53 (1990).
12. D.G. Gadian, Magnetic resonance spectroscopy as a probe of tumour metabolism, *Eur. J. Cancer* 27:526 (1991).
13. R.G. Steen, Characterization of tumor hypoxia by ^{31}P MR spectroscopy, *Am. J. Roentgenol.* 157:243 (1991).
14. R.G. Steen, Edema and tumor perfusion: Characterization by quantitative ^{1}H MR imaging, *Am. J. Roentgenol.* 158:259 (1992).
15. E.K. Rofstad, A. Wahl, T. Stokke, and J.M. Nesland, Establishment and characterization of six human melanoma xenograft lines, *Acta Pathol. Microbiol. Immunol. Scand.* 98:945 (1990).
16. H. Lyng, A. Skretting, and E.K. Rofstad, Blood flow in six human melanoma xenograft lines with different growth characteristics, *Cancer Res.* 52:584 (1992).
17. D. Canet, J. Brondeu, and K. Elbayed, Superfast T_1 determination by inversion-recovery, *J. Magn. Reson.* 77:483 (1988).
18. R.H. Thomlinson and L.H. Gray, The histological structure of some human lung cancers and the possible implications for radiotherapy, *Br. J. Cancer* 9:539, (1955).
19. R.C. Urtasun, J.D. Chapman, J.A Raleigh, A.J. Franko, and C.J. Koch, Binding of ^{3}H-misonidazole to solid human tumors as a measure of tumor hypoxia, *Int. J. Radiat. Oncol. Biol. Phys.* 12:1263 (1986).
20. D.G. Hirst, V.K. Hirst, B. Joiner, V. Prise, and K.M. Shaffi, Changes in tumour morphology with alterations in oxygen availability: Further evidence for oxygen as a limiting substrate, *Br. J. Cancer* 64:54 (1991).
21. I. Lee, Y. Boucher, and R.K. Jain, Nicotinamide can lower tumor interstitial fluid pressure: Mechanistic and therapeutic implications, *Cancer Res.* 52:3237 (1992).
22. R.K. Jain, Physiological barriers to delivery of monoclonal antibodies and other macromolecules in tumors, *Cancer Res.* 50:814s (1990).
23. H.D. Roh, Y. Boucher, S. Kalnicki, R. Buchsbaum, W.D. Bloomer, and R.K. Jain, Interstitial hypertension in carcinoma of uterine cervix in patients: Possible correlation with tumor oxygenation and radiation response, *Cancer Res.* 51:6695 (1991).

24. E.K. Rofstad, P. DeMuth, B.M. Fenton, and R.M. Sutherland, ^{31}P nuclear magnetic resonance spectroscopy studies of tumor energy metabolism and its relationship to intracapillary oxyhemoglobin saturation status and tumor hypoxia, *Cancer Res.* 48:5440 (1988).

25. T.R. Brown, S.D. Buchthal, J. Murphy-Boesch, S.J. Nelson, and J.S. Taylor, A multislice sequence for ^{31}P *in vivo* spectroscopy. 1D chemical-shift imaging with an adiabatic half-passage pulse, *J. Magn. Reson.* 82:629 (1989).

26. R.M. Henkelmann, Diffusion-weighted MR imaging: A useful adjunct to clinical diagnosis or a scientific curiousity?, *Am. J. Roentgenol.* 155:1066 (1990).

OXYGENATION OF TUMORS AS EVALUATED BY
PHOSPHORESCENCE IMAGING

David F. Wilson[1] and George J. Cerniglia[2]

Departments of Biochemistry and Biophysics[1] and of Radiation
Oncology[2], Medical School, University of Pennsylvania
Philadelphia, PA 19104

INTRODUCTION

Necrotic areas in tumors are generally considered to result from insuffi-
ciencies in nutrient delivery due to abnormal and/or poorly developed vasculature. This suggests that the levels of oxygen in tumors may be significantly
below those of normal tissue, at least in some local areas. It is also well recognized that the tissue oxygen concentration is of great importance in therapeutic
treatment of tumors by radiation and by some chemical antitumor agents. The
oxygen pressures in tumors has been difficult to quantitatate both because the
currently available technology is not well suited to measurements in tissue (for
review see Vaupel et al, 1989) and because of the heterogeneity in tumor development. Oxygen electrodes provide the most frequently used method for
measuring oxygen in tumors but they disrupt the tissue during insertion, are
difficult to appropriately calibrate, and both the oxygen sensitivity and zero
current drift with time in the tissue. Efforts to minimize measurement errors
have included the use of different routines for insertion of the electrode
(continuous insertion vs 1 mm advance followed by 0.5 mm withdrawl etc.).
Even with optimal performance, however, the electrodes make local measurements along the insertion track and only a tiny fraction of the tumor volume
can be sampled.

A new, non-destructive, optical method for measuring oxygen pressure,
oxygen dependent quenching of phosphorescence (see Wilson et al, 1987; 1988;
1989; 1990; Vanderkooi et al, 1987; Rumsey et al, 1989; 1990; Robiolio et al,
1989; Wilson and Cerniglia, 1992), has become available. In the present paper,
we will describe its application to study of tumors grown in rats. With this
method, it has been possible to obtain quantitative, two dimensional, maps of
the oxygen pressure in the blood contained in the surface 1 mm of tumor tissue
(Wilson and Cerniglia, 1992). These maps readily show heterogeneity in
oxygen distribution within the tumor and surrounding tissue. This permits not

Oxygen Transport to Tissue XV, Edited by P. Vaupel
et al., Plenum Press, New York, 1994

only accurate measurements of the oxygen levels in individual tumors, but also quantitation of the oxygen pressure in response to manipulations of the oxygen pressure in the inspired gas etc. by the investigator.

MATERIALS AND METHODS

Tumor Growth in Rats

Tumors were grown subcutaneously by either injecting approximately 10^6 cells from a culture of 9L glioma cells or using a trochar to inject a small piece of solid tumor grown from 9L cells onto the surface of muscle of the hind-quarter. The tumors were allowed to grow for 5 to 10 days. Measurements were made when the tumors had grown to from 0.2 to 1.5 cm diameter. On the day of the experiment, the rats were anesthetized using Ketamine (80 mg/kg), Xylazine (5 mg/kg) and Atropine (0.01 mg/kg) by intraperitoneal injection. The animals were placed on a heated pad and their temperature maintained at 38-39° C. Approximately 4 mg of Pd-meso-tetra-(4-carboxyphenyl) porphine (Porphyrin Products, Logan, Utah) was injected into the tail vein as a solution of 8.5 mg/ml in saline with 60 mg/ml bovine serum albumin (fraction V, ICN ImmunoBiologicals, Costa Mesa, CA), pH 7.4. The skin was folded back to expose the region of the tumor and a surrounding area of approximately 2.5 cm diameter. A small amount of saline was placed on the surface of the tissue and the tissue covered with a piece of clear plastic film. Measurements of the oxygen pressure in regions of tissue more than 1 cm from the tumors were used as the values for normal tissue.

Oxygen Dependent Quenching of Phosphorescence

Background: Oxygen dependent quenching of phosphorescence has been used to measure the oxygen dependence of respiration by suspensions of mitochondria and cells (see for example Wilson et al, 1987; 1988; Robiolio et al, 1989; Rumsey et al, 1990). Imaging of phosphorescence has been shown to be a valid method for obtaining two dimensional maps of oxygen pressure in tissues (see Rumsey et al, 1989; Wilson et al, 1989; 1991; Wilson and Cerniglia, 1992).

The oxygen dependence of the phosphorescence of the probes can be quantitatively described by the Stern-Volmer relationship:

$$I^o/I = T^o/T = 1 + k_Q T^o PO_2 \tag{1}$$

where, for the Pd complex of tetra-(4-carboxyphenyl) porphine bound to bovine serum albumin and at 38° C, k_Q has a value of 325 Torr^{-1} sec^{-1} and T^o is 600 μ sec (see 9). I^o and I are the phosphorescence intensities and T^o and T are the phosphorescence lifetimes at zero oxygen pressure and at an oxygen pressure of PO_2 respectively. Phosphorescence lifetime is a more reliable measure of oxygen pressure than is phosphorescence intensity. When the Pd-porphyrin is bound to albumin, it is in a defined environment and the lifetime measurements are independent of the concentration of probe and of the intensity of excitation light. Oxygen is the only compound in normal blood which quenches phosphorescence, and the result is a method which gives unambiguous measurements of oxygen pressure. Calibration of the probes is "absolute" in the sense that for any probe bound to albumin and at a given pH and temperature, the values of k_Q and T^o are characteristic of that probe. Thus, values of k_Q and T^o determined *in vitro* hold for measurements *in vivo* and are valid where ever and for as long as that particular probe is used. Lifetime measurements also have the advantage that they are essentially unaffected by changes in the absorbance of other chromophores in the tissue. Thus, for example, the measurements are independent of the degree of oxygenation of hemoglobin and myoglobin as well as of the state of reduction of cytochromes. There has been no detected toxicity of the Pd-porphyrins used and injection of the probes does not cause alterations in the blood pressure, PaO_2, $PaCO_2$, blood glucose or EEG in adult cats or newborn piglets.

Method. Observations were made using a Wild Macrozoom microscope with an epifluorescence attachment. The images were taken using a Xybion intensified CCD camera (Xybion Electronics Systems Corp., San Diego, CA). The optical filters for measuring phosphorescence (excitation through an interference filter with a center wavelength of 537 nm and a bandwidth at half height of 45 nm; emission through a 630 nm cutoff filter) were put in place and the room darkened. Under these conditions there was no detectable phosphorescence before the Pd-porphyrin was injected.

The illuminating light for the epifluorescence attachment was a EG&G 45 watt xenon flashlamp (EG&G, Salem, MA), with a flash duration of less than 5 µsec, mounted in a Leitz lamp housing. The flash lamp was controlled by a 80386 microcomputer which determined the timing of the flashes and the gating of the video camera intensifier using a 5 channel counter timer board. The frame grabber and image processing software were a customized version of the Image 1/AT system (Universal Imaging, Malvern, PA). A typical image collection protocol was as follows: Number of frames averaged for each delay time, 8; Delay times after the flash, 20 usec, 40 µsec, 80 µsec, 160 µsec, 300 µsec, 600 µsec, and 2,500 µsec; gate width in all cases, 2,500 µsec. The image processor averaged the frames for each delay time and this image was displayed and recorded. Between 1 and 1.5 seconds was required for the image for each delay time and about 40 seconds was required for a complete set of 7 images, including saving the images to the hard disk. A data analysis software system (Pawlowski and Wilson, licensed to Medical Systems Corp., Greenvale, N.Y.) was used to calculate the phosphorescence lifetime for each pixel location of the image sequence by best fit to a single exponential. This program also calculates the correlation coefficient of the fit and the oxygen pressure for each pixel.

RESULTS

Maps of the Distribution of Oxygen Pressures in Tumors

The phosphorescence lifetimes were calculated from sets of phosphorescence images taken with different delay times after the flash and then converted into oxygen pressure maps using equation 1. Oxygen pressure maps for four different tumor regions are shown in Figure 1A,B. The area of tissue was selected to include tumor and immediately surrounding tissue. The 9L tumors are in general quite hypoxic with much of the tumor area having oxygen pressures in the range of 1-4 Torr. The tumors were surrounded by tissue which is not part of the tumor *per se*, but in which the oxygen pressures were significantly altered from normal. This surrounding region was variable in size and oxygen pressure, but the latter were generally well below the 25 to 40 Torr

values of normal tissue (tissue more than 1 cm from the tumor). The oxygen
pressure map for R24OCS is for one side of a tumor approximately 1 cm in
diameter. There is an area hypoxic tissue extending from the side of the tumor.
R29OCS is of an area with a small tumor, less than 1 mm in diameter (central
right side of the map). In this case an area of relatively hypoxic tissue much
larger than the tumor extends to the central and upper region of the map.
Sequences of oxygen maps taken over a period of a few minutes often show
quite marked fluxuations in oxygen pressure in the otherwise normal tissue
near tumors. These oxygen pressure maps are representative of the tumor
regions observed in a total of about 15 animals and 20 different tumors.

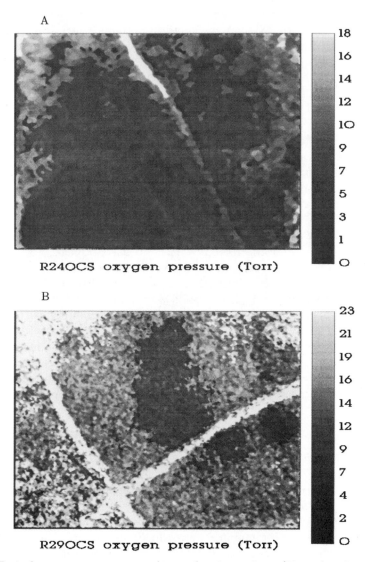

Figure 1. Typical oxygen pressure maps of tumor bearing regions of tissue in rats.
    The oxygen distribution maps are are representative of those obtained using at least 15
different rats and 20 different tumor bearing regions. The white lines are threads laid across
the tumor to aid imaging of the tumor area. The maps are for A: a tissue area 1.2 cm x 0.8 cm,
R24OCS, B: a tissue area 6.6 mm x 5.0 mm, R29OCS. In each case the oxygen pressure scale
in Torr is presented on the right side of the map.

Effect of Breathing Pure Oxygen on the Oxygen Pressure Maps of 9L Tumors

The effect of changing the inspired gas from air to 100% oxygen on the oxygen pressure in the tumors was determined by imaging the phosphorescence under control conditions (breathing air), changing to 100% oxygen and imaging the phosphorescence at various times during a 5-10 minute period of breathing oxygen, and then changing back to breathing air. In order to quantitate the changes in tumor oxygenation, histograms of the oxygen pressure distribution in the tumor area were prepared and integrated to give, for each oxygen pressure, the percent of the total tumor area with that oxygen pressure or less. The data for two tumors are graphed in Figure 2A,B. When breathing air, the oxygen pressures in the tumors were low, more than 50% of the values falling

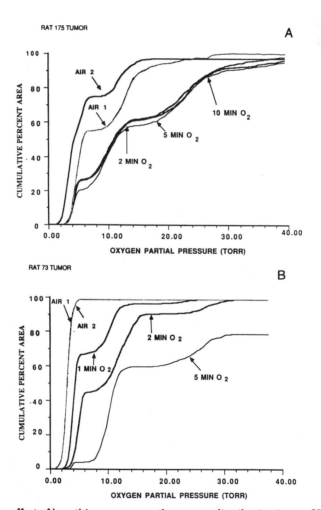

Figure 2A,B. The effect of breathing oxygen on the oxygen distribution in two 9L tumors.
The tumor region was observed during the control (Air 1) at the indicated times after giving the rat 100% O_2 to breath and 10 minutes after returning to breathing air (Air 2). Histograms of the tumor region of maps were integrated and the cumulative percent area plotted against oxygen pressure.

below about 4 Torr. When the inspired gas was changed to 100% oxygen, the oxygen pressures rapidly increased. When the oxygen pressure was returned to air, the oxygen pressures returned to the control values, although in some cases they may temporarily reached values below the control level. There is typically a large heterogeneity in the tumor with several distinctly different regions of oxygen pressure. The oxygen pressures in the tumor as well as the extent of increase when breathing oxygen are quite variable from tumor to tumor. Similarly, the time course of the changes in oxygen pressure, although the increase always occurs in less than 5 minutes, was significantly different from tumor to tumor.

DISCUSSION

Cells require a supply of oxygen at pressures sufficient to allow mitochondrial oxidative phosphorylation to synthesize ATP at the free energy level ([ATP]/[ADP][Pi] or energy state) necessary for growth and maintenance of the cell. For most cells, when the intracellular oxygen pressure falls below about 15 Torr there are metabolic changes, one of which is a decrease in the cellular energy state (Wilson et al, 1979; Wilson and Erecinska, 1982; Erecinska and Wilson, 1982). These alterations in cellular metabolism often include an increase in production of lactate from glucose, with glycolysis (sometimes given the misnomer "anaerobic glycolysis") partially compensating for the decreased capacity for oxidative phosphorylation. As long as the oxygen pressure does not fall too low, cellular metabolism is able to compensate sufficient for the cells to remain viable. The measured oxygen pressures in the vascular system of 9L tumors grown in rats (1-8 Torr) were substantially below those of normal tissue (25-40 Torr). Thus the tumor tissue was being supplied with oxygen, but the oxygen pressure in the internal vessels was lower than for normal tissue.

The measurements in this study were of the oxygen pressure in the vessels, although additional studies will be needed to rigorously exclude the possibility of some leakage of the albumin bound probe into the interstitial space. Tumor vasculature is known to be "leaky" compared to normal vessels and with longer times the Pd-porphyrins may enter the interstitial space. In the present work, however, significant leakage was unlikely because measurements began within a few minutes of probe injection and were completed within 1 hour. There was no evidence of progressive increase in phosphorescence and decrease in phosphorescence lifetime as would have occurred had probe been accumulating in the interstitial space.

The intracellular oxygen pressures must be lower than the values for the capillary bed. At vascular oxygen pressures of less than 10 Torr, at least some of the cells in the adjacent tissue will be very hypoxic compared to normal cells. In normal brain tissue, for example, decreasing the oxygen pressure even slightly below about 35 Torr results in increased neurotransmitter release (Pastuszko et al, this procedings). The observed oxygen pressures are for the surface 0.5 to 1 mm of tissue due to current limitations in the available oxygen probes. The currently available probes have absorption spectra which are confined to wavelengths less than about 580 nm and therefore must be excited with light of wavelengths shorter than about 580 nm. Pigments in the tissue, primarily hemoglobin, myoglobin and cytochromes, absorb strongly in this part of the spectrum and this limits penetration of the excitation light to about

1 mm. As oxygen probes are identified which have absorption at greater than about 630 nm, the lower tissue absorption at these longer wavelengths will make possible measurements to depths of several cm in tissue and greatly increase the efficiency of excitation of the probes.

The maps of phosphorescence lifetimes and of oxygen pressure indicate that even tumors less than 100 μm in diameter have low internal oxygen pressures relative to the surrounding tissue. The low oxygen pressures in tumors are consistent with the observation that ^{3}H-misonidazole binding was enhanced in tumors grown from 9L cells (Franko et al, 1992), measurements in other tumors using oxygen electrodes (see Vaupel et al, 1989) and general reports of hypoxic cells in tumors (for review see Vaupel et al, 1989; Franko et al, 1987; 1992; Chapman et al, 1983). Oxygen consumption by cells in solid tumors is dependent on the type of cell from which it is grown and the physical environment within the tumor structure. Measurements of the total oxygen consumption of solid tumors are consistent with the oxygen consumption being dependent on the rate of delivery (Gullino et al, 1967; Vaupel et al, 1987; Ito et al, 1982; Kairento et al, 1985). The increased respiratory rate of solid tumors as the oxygen pressure is increased would then be attributed to supply of oxygen to oxygen starved, but viable, cells. Kallinowski and coworkers (1989), however, pointed out that solid tumors contain a significant fraction of polymorphonuclear granulocytes, lymphocytes and monocytes. If these cells were activated (granulocytes and monocytes are reported to increase respiratory rate by up to 70 fold when activated) exposure to elevated oxygen pressures would be expected to greatly increase their oxygen consumption (predominantly through production of oxygen radicals). The authors concluded that increased oxygen consumption by nonmalignant cells in solid tumors could help to conceal possible beneficial effects of improved tumor oxygen supply by consuming the oxygen and keeping the oxygen pressure within the tumor low. It appears that poor tissue oxygenation can, in some cases, be a factor in failure of radiation therapy (Gray et al, 1953; Gatenby et al, 1988; Hall, 1988). Hyperbaric oxygen has been reported to improve radiotherapy in at least some clinical trials (van den Brenk, 1968; Henk and Smith, 1977). Anemia has been reported to play a significant negative role in the cure rate for carcinoma of the cervix (Bush et al, 1978) and on radiosensitivity of mouse tumors (Hirst et al, 1984).

It has been suggested that radiosensitizers such as misonidazole can serve as qualitative indicators of tissue hypoxia and evidence has been provided (see for examples Chapman et al, 1983; Franko et al, 1987; Koch et al, 1992) that this compound is incorporated into cells in an oxygen dependent reaction. The presence of regions of hypoxia in solid tumors and their possible role in determining the radiation sensitivity of the tumors can only be verified by quantitative measurements of oxygen pressure *in situ* since the effect of increased oxygen pressure in tumor is independent of the oxygen consumption rate *per se*.

Oxygen dependent quenching of phosphorescence provides an effective method for quantitatively measuring oxygen within tumors. Our data show that, at least for tumors grown from 9L cells, the oxygen pressure in even very small tumors is significantly below that of the surrounding tissue. The signal to noise of the measurements is excellent, allowing precise delineation of the limits of the hypoxic regions. The presence of hypoxic regions of similar appearance arising from causes other than tumors has not been, in the limited experiments carried out to date, observed. Extensive studies of different types of tumors will be required to determine the extent to which the hypoxia associated with the 9L tumors also holds for tumors of other cellular origin. Similarly, it will be important to make much more extensive measurements of normal tissue to determine the extent to which local regions of hypoxia may be present which would mimic the presence of tumors.

The oxygen dependent quenching of phosphorescence apppears to be an effective tool for examining the oxygen pressure in tumors and possible for identifying small tumors. The potential value of a high resolution and easily used method for quantitatively maping the oxygen pressure in tumors and other tissue to medical diagnosis and treatment is easily recognized. It remains to be seen the extent to which this potential can be realized.

Acknowledgements

This work was supported by grants NS-10939 (to D.F.W.) and CA-44982 (to Dr. John Biaglow). The authors are indebted to Drs. John Biaglow and Cameron Koch for their encouragement and support.

REFERENCES

Bush, R.S., Jenkin, R.D.T., Allt, W.E.C., Beale, F.A., Bean, H., Denko, A.J., and Pringle, J.F. , 1978, Definitive evidence for hypoxic cells influencing cure in cancer therapy. *Br. J. Cancer* 37: Suppl. III: 302-306.

Chapman, J.D., Baer, K., and Lee, J. , 1983, Characteristics of metabolism-induced binding of misonidazole to hypoxic mammalian cells. *Cancer Research* 43: 1523-1528.

Erecinska, M. and Wilson, D.F., 1982, Regulation of cellular energy metabolism. *J. Memb. Biol.* 70: 1-14.

Franko, A.J., Koch, C.J., and Boisvert, D.P.J., 1992, Distribution of Misonidazole adducts in 9L gliosarcoma tumors and spheroids: Implications for oxygen distribution. *Cancer Research,* 52: 3831-3837.

Franko, A.J., Koch, C.J., Garrecht, B.M., Sharplin, J., and Hughes, D., 1987, Oxygen concentration dependence of binding of misonidazole to rodent and human tumors *in vitro. Cancer Research* 47: 5367-5376.

Gatenby, R.A., Kessler, H.B., Rosenblum, J.S., Coia, L.R., Moldofsky, P.J., Hartz, W.H., and Broder, G.J., 1988, Oxygen distribution in squamous cell carcinoma metastases and its relationship to outcome of radiation therapy *Int. J. Radiat. Oncol. Biol. Phys.* 14: 831-838.

Gray, L.H., Conger, A.D., Ebert, M., Hornsey, S., and Scott, O.C.A., 1953, Concentration of oxygen dissolved in tissues at time of irradiation as a factor in radiotherapy. *Br. J. Radiol.* 26: 638-648.

Gullino, P.M., Grantham, F.H., and Courtney, A.H., 1967, Utilization of oxygen by transplanted tumors *in vivo. Cancer Res.* 27: 1020-1030.

Hall, E.J., 1988, Radiobiology for the Radiologist, 3rd Ed., Lippincott, Philadelphia (1988).

Henk, J.M. and Smith, C.W., 1977, Radiotherapy and hyperbaric oxygen in head and neck cancer: Interim report of the second clinical trial. *Lancet* 2: 104-105.

Hirst, D.G., Hazelhurst, J.L., and Brown, J.M., 1984, The effect of alterations in hematocrit on tumor sensitivity to x-rays. *Int. J. Radiat. Biol.* 46: 345-354.

Ito, M., Lammertsma, A.A., Wise, R.J.S., Bernardi, S., Frackowiak, R.S.J., Heather, J.D., McKenzie, C.G., Thomas, D.G.T., and Jones, T., 1982, Measurement of regional cerebral blood flow and oxygen utilization in patients with cerebral tumors using ^{15}O and positron emission tomography. *Neuroradiology* 23: 63-74.

Kairento, A.L., Brownell, G.L., Elmaleh, D.R., and Swartz, M.R., 1985, Comparative measurements of regional blood flow, oxygen and glucose utilization in soft tissue tumors of rabbit with positron imaging. *Br. J. Radiol.* 58: 637-643.

Kallinowski, F., Tyler, G., Mueller-Klieser, W., and Vaupel, P., 1989, Growth-related changes of oxygen consumption rates of tumor cells grown *in vitro* and *in vivo*. *J. Cellular Physiol.* 138: 183-191.

Koch, C.J., Stobbe, C.C., and Baer, K.A., 1992, Metabolism induced binding of ^{14}C-misonidazole to hypoxic cells: kinetic dependence on oxygen concentration and misonidazole concentration. *Int. J. Radiation Oncology Biol. Phys.* 10, 1327-1331.

Robiolio, M., Rumsey, W.L., and Wilson, D.F., 1989, Oxygen diffusion and mitochondrial respiration in neuroblastoma cells. *Amer. J. Physiol.* 256: C1207-C1213.

Rumsey, W.L., Schlosser, C., Nuutinen, E.M., Robiolio, M., and Wilson, D.F., 1990, Cellular energetics and the oxygen dependence of respiration in cardiac myocytes isolated from adult rats. *J. Biol. Chem.* 265: 15392-15399.

Rumsey, W.L., Vanderkooi, J.M., and Wilson, D.F., 1989, Imaging of phosphorescence: a novel method for measuring oxygen distribution in perfused tissue. *Science, Wash. DC* 241: 1649-1651.

van den Brenk, H.A., 1968, Hyperbaric oxygen in radiation therapy. An investigation of dose-effect relationships. *Am. J. Roentgenol.* 102: 8-26.

Vanderkooi, J.M., Maniara, G, Green, T.J., and Wilson, D.F., 1987, An optical method for measurement of dioxygen concentration based on quenching of phosphorescence. *J. Biol. Chem.* 262: 5476-5482.

Vaupel, P., Kallinowski, F., and Okunieff, P., 1989, Blood flow, oxygen and nutrient supply, and metabolic microenvironment of human tumors: a review. *Cancer Research* 49: 6449-6466.

Vaupel, P., Fortmeyer, H.P., Runkel, S., and Kallinowski, F., 1987, Blood flow, oxygen consumption, and tissue oxygenation of human breast cancer xenografts in nude rats. *Cancer Res.* 47: 3496-3503.

Vaupel, P., Manz, R., Muller-Kieser, W., and Grunewald, W.A., 1979, Intracapillary HbO_2 saturation in malignant tumors during normoxia and hyperoxia. *Microvas. Res.* 17: 181-191.

Wilson, D.F. and Cerniglia, G., 1992, Location of tumors and evaluation of their state of oxygenation by phosphorescence imaging. *Cancer Research* 52: 3988-3993.

Wilson, D.F. and Erecinska, M., 1982, Effect of oxygen concentration on cellular metabolism. *Chest* 88S: 229S-232S.

Wilson, D.F., Erecinska, M., Drown, C., and Silver, I.A., 1979, The oxygen dependence of cellular energy metabolism. *Arch. Biochem. Biophys.* 195: 485-493.

Wilson, D.F., Pastuszko, A., DiGiacomo, J.E., Pawlowski, M., Schneiderman, R., Delivoria-Papadopoulos, M., 1991, Effect of hyperventilation on oxygenation of the brain cortex of newborn piglets. *J. Appl. Physiol.* 70(6): 2691-2696.

Wilson, D.F., Rumsey, W.L., Green, T.J., and Vanderkooi, J.M., 1988, The oxygen dependence of mitochondrial oxidative phosphorylation measured by a new optical method for measuring oxygen concentration. *J. Biol. Chem.* 263: 2712-2718.

Wilson, D.F., Rumsey, W.L. and Vanderkooi, J.M., 1989, Oxygen distribution in isolated perfused liver observed by phosphorescence imaging. *Adv. Exptl. Med. Biol.* 248: 109-115.

Wilson, D.F., Vanderkooi, J.M., Green, T.J., Maniara, G., DeFeo, S.P., and Bloomgarden, D.C., 1987, A versatile and sensitive method for measuring oxygen. *Adv. Exptl. Med. Biol.* 215: 71-77.

NON-INVASIVE INFRARED-SPECTROSCOPIC MEASUREMENTS OF INTRAVASAL OXYGEN CONTENT IN XENOTRANSPLANTED TUMOURS ON NUDE MICE - CORRELATION TO GROWTH RATE

Fritz Steinberg, Monika Leßmann, and Christian Streffer

Institute of Medical Radiation Biology
University Clinics Essen
Essen, Germany

INTRODUCTION

Tumour cell proliferation is dependent on energy metabolism (Streffer et al., 1987), and in particular, on the oxygen supply available through the vascular system (Withers, 1987; Hall, 1988). Against others, the oxygen status is dependent on the tumour vascularity. Investigations up to now have shown intra- and interindividual heterogeneity in the vascularisation of experimental tumour models (Vaupel et al., 1987; Steinberg et al., 1990; Konerding et al., 1989) as well as in primary rectum carcinomas of the same grading und staging (Steinberg et al., 1991). Therefore, evaluation of the oxygenation status [oxygenated haemoglobin (HbO_2), deoxygenated haemoglobin (Hb), intratumoural total hemoglobin (TH)], cell proliferation (S-phase cells) and tumour growth rate in individual tumours might be most beneficial for specifically designing suitable individual treatment protocols for improving tumour treatment response.

Measurement of blood and tissue oxygenation by spectral analysis of transmitted or reflected light is a well established method (Chance, 1954; Mook, 1968; Wray et al.,

1988). Jöbsis et al. (1977) showed that near infrared light (NIR) at a wavelength of 700-1000 nm showed absorption characteristics low enough for spectral measurements to be carried out in tissues several cm in diameter. In this range absorption due to both oxyhaemoglobin (HbO_2) and deoxyhaemoglobin (Hb) can be observed. By means of near infrared spectroscopy it is possible to measure the oxygen status non-invasively in vivo. These data were correlated with tumour cell proliferation (% of S-phase-cells) and growth rate. In this study a slow growing leiomyosarcoma (MOR.) and a fast growing adenocarcinoma (E0771) transplanted on nude mice were compared.

MATERIAL AND METHODS

Animals and tumours

A slow growing human soft tissue sarcoma (leiomyosarcoma = MOR., n = 8) and a fast growing undifferentiated murine adenocarcinoma (E0771, n = 16) were transplanted on nude mice as previously described (Steinberg et al., 1990). The oxygenation status of the sarcoma was measured daily from day 14 to 28 after transplantation, and that of the adenocarcinoma from day 7 to 13. The measurements were carried out in vivo non-invasively within 20 sec using unanaesthetized and unrestrained animals. On the final measurement day the tumours were prepared and cell proliferation determined flow cytometrically as previously described (Steinberg et al., 1990). Tumour volume was measured three times a week.

Instrumentation

This prototype in vivo spectroscope (NIRO 500, Hamamatsu Photonics, Japan) has four semiconductor laser diodes (779, 828, 843, 913 nm) as light sources each pulsed sequentially at 4 KHz with a pulse length of 100 nsec and a peak diode power output of approximately 10 watt. Light from the diodes is transmitted to the tumour via a flexible fibre optic cable of 5 mm diameter attached to the skin. Light emerging laterally is collected by a similar cable and conveyed to a photomultiplier detector operating in a photon counting mode in excess of 100 MHz to ensure maximum sensitivity. This permits attenuated light from tumours to be detected within a few seconds by means of transillumination measurements. The photon counts detected are stored in a multichannel counter (one channel per laser diode). Stray light and the background can be substracted from the values measured by the photomultiplier on the opposite side. After the measurements the data are collected by a microprocessor from a defined time period and the change in transmitted intensity at each wavelength was calculated on a logarithmic scale in terms of optical density. For details see Edwards et al., 1988; Cope et al., 1988; Steinberg et al., 1992. Using correcting factors (Wyatt et al., 1990), concentration changes are expressed in μmol/l of path length. Assuming a tumour specific gravity of 1.05, the data can be converted to μmol x 100 g^{-1} of tissue. For this, a path length factor of 4.39 (Van der Zee et al., 1992) determined from measurements on adult brain were used since no real flight time measurements on tumours have been carried out up to now. Basal values for NIR measurements were established under standardized conditions. These are used to determine relative changes, but up to now cannot be quantified into absolute units. To compare the data measured, it is necessary to have the same defined level before each measurement. For this, a specially constructed grey filter (Balzers AG, Lichtenstein) was used. This filter possesses a uniform transmission at the wavelength used with < 5 % deviation. Then a first calibration measurement with this filter between the optodes was performed, used as baseline and followed by measurements with the animals. Based on this method they are now comparable in the case of serial measurements from one day to the other. The geometrical pathlength factor was between 10 and 14 mm. These differences in real flight time behaviour of photons were taken as equal. Oxygenated haemoglobin (HbO_2) and deoxygenated haemoglobin (Hb) are measured non-invasively in vivo. The total amount of hemoglobin in the blood (TH), i.e. the sum of Hb and HbO_2 is used as parameter for blood volume and expressed as relative units.

The overall sampling time is 5 sec involving a mean value of 5 x 10^6 measurements and three such periods were measured. All animals were measured at various times after transplantation and again a mean value was calculated. The optical pathlength per individual tumour (= diameter of the tumour) is measured with a vernier. The subcutaneousely localised tumour in the unanaesthetised and unrestrained animal was held between the two laser diodes, previously adjusted to the diameter of the tumour.

RESULTS

Fig 1 and 2 show the markedly different growth behaviour of the two tumour cell lines (left axis; note the different scaling on the x-axis). The proliferation rates measured on the final day are plotted (right axis = S-phase cells in %). Here, too, a significant difference is seen. Fig 3 and 4 show the development of the haemoglobin values with respect to tumour growth period. The means for the three parameters at the time of the first measurement are on the same level; the tumours have the same dimension on diameter at thus time. The HbO$_2$ value in both tumour lines increases by about 400 μmol/100 g. In the case of MOR., the HbO$_2$ distincly decreases at the end. The Hb value in both tumours is clearly enhanced, beeing significantly higher in the case of E0771. As a result there is an increase in TH, which is equally more marked in the E0771 than the MOR. At day 28 p.t., a decrease in all three parameters

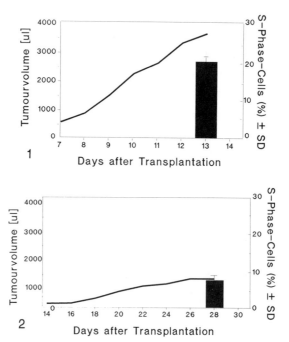

Figure 1 + 2. Growth curve of a xenotransplanted tumour on nude mice with % of S-phase cells (right axis). Fig 1 = adenocarcinoma (E0771, n = 16), fig 2 = leiomyosarcoma (MOR., n = 8).

is seen. An attempt was made to correlate the proliferation (S-phase cells) with the oxygen parameters (data not schown), but none were found. This was different when comparing the tumour growth rate and HbO$_2$. Here a statistical correlation between these two parameters was seen, and which was highly significant in the case of E0771 ($y = 1/(a+bx^2)$, r = 0.95). These correlations were also carried out for other days after transplantation and showed similar results.

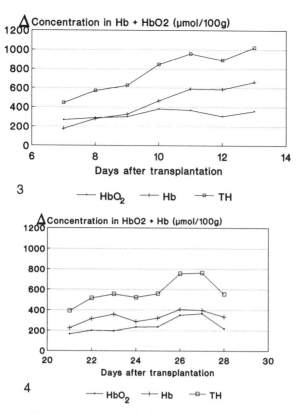

Figure 3 + 4. Changes (days after transplantation) in oxidised (HbO2), deoxidised (Hb) and total hemoglobin (TH) in xenotransplanted tumours. Fig 3 = adenocarcinoma (E0771, n = 16, N = 336), fig 4 = leiomyosarcoma (MOR., n = 8, N = 192).

DISCUSSION

A large body of literature exists concerning the role of oxygen as a parameter for tumour cell growth (Hall, 1988; Withers, 1987). Direct correlations between these two factors have been definitely shown from in vitro studies (Kallinowski et al., 1989), while experimental animal studies are more scarce (Kallinowski et al., 1990). Clinical studies, where oxygen was measured, have not attempted to correlate this data with tumour growth up to now (Gatenby et al., 1988; Vaupel et al., 1990). In the present study, the direct correlation between proliferating cells and oxygen tension could not be substantiated. By contrast, however, it could be shown that there was a direct relationship between tumour growth and oxygen supply, more explicitly the nutritive oxygen supply i. e. HbO_2. This relation occurred not only at the time of preparation but instead could also be seen in the individual animal serially over the entire growth period. A tumour showing a slow growth rate was also poorly supplied with oxygen ($=$ HbO_2) over this period. This relation could be demonstrated in both tumour lines. The growth rate was mainly determined by the level of HbO_2 but not by that of Hb or TH.

The difference in growth of xenotransplanted tumours on nude mice has been known for a long time, and also applies to cloned tumour cell lines. This effect may be based on the host animals which are also characterised by their own individually body status, immunology (Steinberg et al., 1992) which influence also the tumour microenvironment. This, in turn, may influence tumour behaviour as seen in this study. Cell and tissue growth is also regulated by very complex mechanisms and which, to a large extent, have up to now severly hindered all attempts to find an oncological factor in vivo determining tumour growth rate. In consideration of the central importance attached to oxygen and cellular performance, it is thus apparent from the tumour biological point of view that the relation between oxygen and tumor growth described in this study may be a general phenomenon. These statements need to be confirmed by further experimental models, in particular also with respect to the clinical situation.

REFERENCES

Chance, B. Spectrophotometry of intracellular respiratory pigments. *Science*, 120: 767-775, 1954.

Cope, M., Delpy, D.T. System for long-term measurement of cerebral blood and tissue oxygenation on newborn infants by near infra-red transillumination. *Med. & Biol. Eng. & Comp.*, 26: 289-294, 1988.

Edwards, AD., Wyatt, JS., Richardson, C., Delpy, DT., Cope, M., Reynolds, EOR., Cotside measurements of cerebral blood flow in ill preterm infants by near infrared spectroscopy. *Lancet*, 770-771, 1988.

Gatenby, R.A., Kessler, H.B., Rosenblum, J.S., Coia, L.R., Moldofsky, P.J., Hartz, W.H., Broder, G.J., Oxygen distribution in squamous cell carcinoma metastases and its relationship to outcome of radiation therapy. *Int. J. Rad. Oncol. Biol. Phys.*, 14: 831-838, 1988.

Hall, E.J., Radiobiology for the radiologist. 3rd ed. Philadelphia, Lippincott Co., 1988.

Jöbsis, F.F., Keizer, J.H., LaManna, J.C., Rosenthal, M., Reflectance spectrophotometry of cytochrome aa3 in vivo. *J. Appl. Physiol.: Respirat. Environ. Exercise Physiol.*, 43: 858- 872, 1977.

Kallinowski, F., Tyler, G., Mueller-Klieser, W., Vaupel, P., Growth-related changes of oxygen consumption rates of tumor cells grown in vitro and in vivo. *J. Cell Physiol.*, 138, 183-191, 1989.

Kallinowski, F., Zander, R., Hoeckel, M., Vaupel, P. Tumor tissue oxygenation as evaluated by computerized-pO_2-histography. *Int. J. Rad. Onc. Biol. Phys.*, 19: 953-961, 1990.

Konerding, M.A., Steinberg, F., Budach, V., The vascular system of xenotransplanted tumors - scanning electron and light microscopic studies. *Scanning Microsc.*, 3: 327-336, 1989.

Mook, G.A., Osypka, P., Sturm, R.E., Wood, E.H., Fibre optic reflection photometry on blood. *Cardiovasc. Res.* 2, 199-209, 1968.

Steinberg, F., Konerding, M.A., Streffer, C. The vascular architecture of tumors: Histological, morphometrical and ultrastructural studies. *J. Canc. Res. Clin. Oncol.*, 116: 517-524, 1990.

Steinberg, F., Konerding, M.A., Sander, A., Streffer, C., Vascularization, proliferation and necrosis in untreated human primary tumours and untreated human xenografts. *Int. J. Radiat. Biol.*, 60: 161-168, 1991.

Steinberg, F., Streffer, C., Non-invasive infrared spectroscopical method for the quantification of blood and cell oxygenation in tumours. (submitted) 1992.

Steinberg, F., Happel, M., Büttner, D., Konerding, MA., Grosse-Wilde, H., Streffer, C., Normal variations in B-, T-, NK cells and interleukin 2 receptors in the immune deficient mouse (NMRI nu/nu) and alterations after tumour transplantation. *In*: Fiebig and Berger (eds.): Immunodeficient Mice in Oncology, Contributions to Oncology, 42, 41-47, 1992.

Streffer, C., van Beuningen, D., The biological basis for tumour therapy by hyperthermia and radiation. *In*: Hyperthermia and the therapy of malignant tumours. C. Streffer (ed.). Springer, Berlin-Heidelberg-New York-London-Paris-Tokyo, pp 24-70, 1987.

Van der Zee, P., Cope, M., Arridge, S.R., Essenpreis, M., Potter, L.A., Edwards, A.D., Wyatt, J.S., McCormick, D.C., Roth, S.C., Reynolds, E.O.R., Delpy, D.T., Experimentally measured optical pathlengths for the adult head, calf and forearm and the head of the newborn infant as a function of inter optode spacing. *Adv.Exp.Med.Biol.* (in press), 1992.

Vaupel, P., Fortmeyer, HP., Runkel, S., Kallinowski, F., Blood flow, oxygen consumption and tissue oxygenation of human breast cancer xenografts in nude rats. *Cancer Res.* 47, 3496-3503, 1987.

Vaupel, P. Oxygenation of human tumors. *Strahlenther. Onkol.*, 166: 377-386, 1990.

Withers, H.R., Biologic basis of radiation therapy. *In*: Perez, C.A., Brady, L.W. (eds), Principles and practice of radiation oncology. Philadelphia, Lippincott, pp. 67-98, 1987.

Wray, S., Cope, M., Delpy, D.T., Wyatt, J.S., Reynolds, E.O.R. Characterization of the near infrared absorption spectra of cytochrome aa3 and haemoglobin for the non-invasive monitoring of cerebral oxygenation. *Biochem. Biophys. Act.*, 933: 184-192, 1988.

Wyatt, JS., Cope, M., Delpy, DT., van-der-Zee, P., Arridge, S., Edwards, AD., Reynolds, EOR., Measurement of optical path length for cerebral near-infrared spectroscopy in newborn infants. *Dev.Neurosci.*, 12, 140-144, 1990.

BRAIN

NONINVASIVE ASSESSMENT OF CEREBRAL HEMODYNAMICS AND TISSUE OXYGENATION DURING ACTIVATION OF BRAIN CELL FUNCTION IN HUMAN ADULTS USING NEAR INFRARED SPECTROSCOPY

A. Villringer[*][1], J. Planck[1], S. Stodieck[1],
K. Bötzel[1], L. Schleinkofer[2], U. Dirnagl[1]

[1]Department of Neurology, University of Munich
Klinikum Großhadern, 8000 Munich 70, and
[2]Hamamatsu Photonics, Germany

INTRODUCTION

Near Infrared Spectroscopy (NIRS) is an optical technique that measures tissue absorbance of light at several wavelengths in the 700-1000 nm spectral region. From the obtained values, changes in the concentration of oxygenated hemoglobin (HbO_2), deoxygenated hemoglobin (HbR), corpuscular blood volume (HbO_2 + HbR) and cytochrome C-oxidase oxygenation are determined. Since near infrared light penetrates biological tissue (and even bone) well, the method can be performed noninvasively through the intact skull as first proposed by Jöbsis in 1977 (Jöbsis 1977). Since this first report, most applications have focussed on neonates, in whom transmission studies through the entire head are possible (Brazy et al. 1985, Cope and Delpy 1988, Ferrari et al. 1986, Reynolds et al. 1988). The larger diameter of the adult head prevented such studies in adults with sufficient signal to noise ratio. However, using the signal reflected from the brain (instead of transilluminated through the brain) is another way to obtain measurements of light absorbance that follow the Lambert-Beer Law (Faris et al. 1991). This approach permits the examination of regions of the adult human brain (McCormick et al. 1991a, Elwell et al. 1992). Using this method, so far mainly severe global alterations in the general oxygenation state of the brain such as hypoxia have been assessed (McCormick et al. 1991b).

A.V. and U.D. are supported by the Deutsche Forschungsgemeinschaft, Gerhard-Hess-Programm

The aims of the present feasibility study were:
- to test whether NIRS-measurements are sensitive enough to follow changes in brain hemodynamics and oxygenation due to **physiological** changes in brain function
- to test whether the NIRS-method permits the assessment of changes due to transient **pathological changes in local brain function** such as during spontaneously occuring focal epileptic seizures

METHODS

The principles of transcranial near infrared spectroscopy (NIRS), have been described in detail elsewhere (Jobsis 1977, Cope and Delpy 1988). We used a Hamamatsu NIR0 500 NIRS system which uses wavelength at 775 nm, 825 nm, 850 nm, and 904 nm.

17 human subjects (age 23 - 75) were examined. The optodes were placed at a distance of 3.5 to 7 cm at various positions of the head.

Cognitive Stimulation (n = 12) was achieved by having the subject perform calculations. The optodes were placed over the left forehead avoiding the temporal muscle region at an interoptode spacing between 3.5 and 7 cm. The protocol included a period of rest with eyes closed (for baseline evaluation), a period of rest with eyes open (1 min), a period of calculation (1 min), followed by another period of rest with eyes closed.

For **visual stimulation** (n = 3), the optodes were placed over the occipital cortex at an interoptode distance between 3.5 and 5 cm. After a period of 10 min with eyes closed the subjects were exposed to a 1 min period of 10 Hz flash light (eyes open) followed by a period with eyes closed (5 min). Then, the subjects were asked to observe a picture and count the number of persons visible on the picture (duration 1 min). Again a period of rest with eyes closed followed.

Spontaneously occuring **epileptic seizures** were monitored in three patients. The optodes were placed at the right forehead in a patient with an epileptic focus in the right precentral region and in a patient with frontal seizures, and occipitally (and later frontally) in a patient with an epileptic focus presumably in the left parieto-occipital region.

RESULTS

The time course of the NIRS-parameters during cognitive stimulation (calculating) is given in **Figure 1**. In 10 of 12 subjects, an increase in the concentration of oxygenated hemoglobin [HbO$_2$] and in cerebral blood volume (= [HbO$_2$ + HbR]) was noted (in 2 a decrease was noted). Deoxygenated hemoglobin [HbR] either decreased (Figure 1 a), remained constant or increased slightly (Figure 1 b), however the increase was never comparable in size to the increase in [HbO$_2$].

Figure 2 gives an example of the effect of visual stimulation. During observation of a picture, the hemodynamic effects were similar to the results obtained frontally during calculation. In all three subjects examined [HbO$_2$] and blood volume increased and [HbR] decreased.

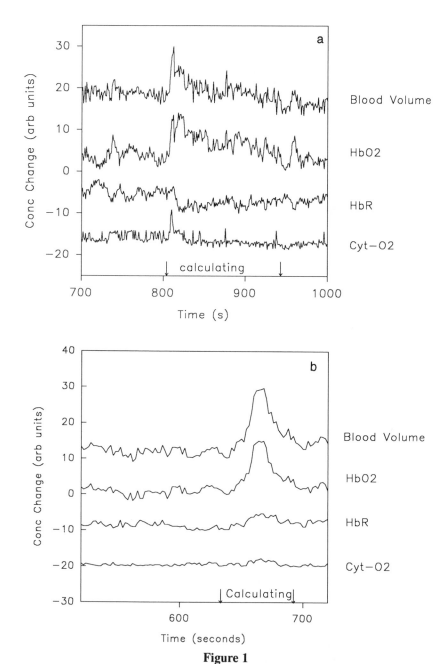

Figure 1

Influence of cognitive stimulation (calculating) on NIR-parameters. The optodes were placed over the left forehead at an interoptode distance of 7 cm (1a) and 4 cm (1b), respectively. The subject started calculating at the time point indicated by the first arrow mark, and stopped calculating and closed his eyes at the time point indicated by the second arrow. Please note the different behaviour of the [HbR] (concentration of deoxygenated hemoglobin) in the two experiments, and the different time course of the increase in [HbO$_2$] (concentration of oxygenated hemoglobin) and in blood volume ([HbR] + [HbO$_2$]). The time scale (X-axis) refers to the beginning of the experiment (at the beginning of the experiment x = 0 s).

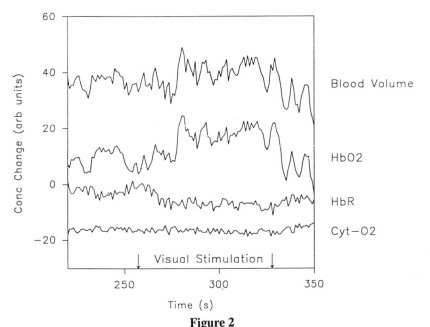

Figure 2

Influence of visual stimulation on NIR-parameters. The optodes were placed over the right occipital region with an interoptode spacing of 4 cm. At the time point indicated by the first arrow, the subject watched a picture and was asked to count the (large) number of people on the picture. The subject was asked to close his eyes at the time point indicated by the second arrow. The time scale (X-axis) refers to the beginning of the experiment (at the beginning of the experiment x = 0 s).

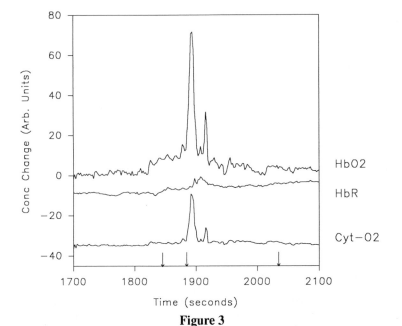

Figure 3

Time course of NIR-parameter during occurence of a complex-partial epileptic seizure. Optodes were positioned at the right forehead at an interoptode distance of 4.5 cm. The patient was sleeping. At the time point indicated by the first arrow, the patient stopped snoring, but did not wake up. At the time point indicated by the second arrow, the complex partial seizure began. At the time point indicated by the third arrow, the patient was alert again. The time scale (X-axis) refers to the beginning of the observation period (at the beginning of the observation period x = 0 s).

The effect of flash-light illumination was only visible when several subsequent 1-min stimulation periods were averaged (data not shown).

The measurements in **Figure 3** were performed during a frontal complex partial epileptic seizure. The optodes were positioned over the right forehead. A dramatic increase in [HbO$_2$] and blood volume occurred. A similar reaction during complex partial seizures was noted in another patient with a presumable epileptic focus in the left parieto-occipital region. In this patient, an increase in blood volume was seen in the parieto-occipital region as well as in the contralateral frontal region, however, the increase in the parieto-occipital region occurred earlier with respect to the seizure onset. In a third patient with a precentral epileptogenic focus on the right side (NIRS-measurement right forehead) a large drop in Cyt-O$_2$ occurred without a large change in [HbO$_2$] and [HbR].

DISCUSSION

In this feasibility study using a commercially available NIRS-system in a clinical setting we showed that NIRS permits the noninvasive assessment of changes in hemodynamics and tissue oxygenation during physiological and pathological stimulation of brain function in human adults.

The most frequent findings during physiological functional activation of brain tissue were an increase in local [HbO$_2$] and blood volume and an decrease in deoxgenated hemoglobin.
However, there were excemption from this In addition, the fact that [HbR] decreasd in most instances (in some instances it remained constant or increased only slightly, however, in any event its concentration relative to [HbO$_2$] decreased), indicates that during cognitive activation the increase in cerebral blood flow is larger than the increase in cerebral oxygen consumption.

During cognitive stimulation, usually only minor changes in [Cyt-O$_2$] (oxygenated cytochrome-oxidase) occurred which often paralleled the difference between oxygenated and deoxygeneate hemoglobin ([HbO$_2$]-[HbR]), but based on our data, at present we have no clear picture of its significance. However, the perspective of measuring not only intravascular ([HbO2] [HbR]) but also intracellular oxygenation status justifies further investigations.

During epileptic seizures a pronounced, spike-like increase in HbO$_2$ and blood volume occured. The temporal relationship of this increase to the onset of the epileptic seizure, the extent of the alteration, and the change in Cyt-O$_2$ (only seen in one patient) might be of localizing value with respect to the epileptic focus. Further studies are needed to evaluate this issue.

In conclusion, the results of our study indicate that NIRS has the potential of becoming a useful and simple technique to assess the functional state of the brain. However, a number of problems have to be addressed and overcome in the future:
- Exact quantitation depends on the knowledge of the optical pathlengths in each experiment. Thus, only when this is realized exact seems to be feasible.
- The contribution of extracranial tissue to the NIRS signal has to be defined more clearly and ideally eliminated. In preliminary studies, we have demonstrated that the

NIRS alterations after cognitive stimulation cannot be explained by changes in skin blood flow (as measured simultaneously by Laser Doppler flowmetry). When changes in skin blood flow were eliminated by maximizing skin blood flow with a local vasodilating agent, the NIRS-changes during cognitive stimulation still occured the same way (data not shown).
- Relatively simple to implement might be the use of several optode pairs simultaneously in order to improve spatial resolution of the method.

ABSTRACT

Near Infrared Spectroscopy (NIRS) was employed to noninvasively and continuously (temporal resolution 0.5 s) assess changes in cerebral hemodynamics and oxygenation during various functional states of the adult human brain. During cognitive stimulation (performing calculations) a frontal increase in local cerebral blood volume and oxygenated hemoglobin concentration was observed in most (10 of 12) subjects. During visual stimulation (observing a picture) this was demonstrated in the occipital region in all three subjects. Deoxygenated hemoglobin either decreased, remained unchanged or slightly increased during these procedures. Epileptic patients were examined during spontaneously occuring complex-partial seizures. During these seizures extremely large increases in blood volume and oxygenated hemoglobin concentration were measured. In conclusion, this feasibility study indicates that NIRS might become a useful and simple bedside tool to assess brain function.

REFERENCES

Brazy, J.E., Lewis, D.V., Mitnick, M.H., and Jöbsis, F.F., 1985, Noninvasive monitoring of cerebral oxygenation in preterm infants: preliminary observations, *Pediatrics*, 75:217

Copy, M. and Delpy, D.T. 1988. A system for long term measurement of cerebral blood and tissue oxygenation in newborn infants by near infrared trans-illumination, *Med. Biol. Eng. & Comp.*, 26,3:289

Elwell, C.E., Cope, M., Edwards, A.D., Wyatt, J.S., Reynolds, E.O.R., and Delpy D.T., 1992, Measurement of cerebral blood flow in adult humans using near infrared spectroscopy - methodology and possible errors, *Adv. Exp. Med. Biol.*, in press

Faris, F., Wickramasinghe, Y., Thorniley, M., Houston, R., and Rolfe, P., 1991, Influence of scattering on physiological measurement using laser light in vivo, *Biochem. Soc. Trans.*, 19:514

Ferrari, M., De Marchis, G., Nicola, A., Agostino, R., Nodari, S., and Bucci, G., 1986, Cerebral blood volume and haemoglobin oxygen saturation monitoring in neonatal brain by near infared spectroscopy, *Adv. Exp. Med. Biol.*, 200:203

Jöbsis, F.F., 1977, Noninvasive, infrared monitoring of cerebral and myocardial oxygen sufficiency and circulatory parameters, *Science*, 198:1264

McCormick, P.W., Stewart, M., Goetting, M.G., Dujovny, M., Lewis, G., and Ausman, J.I., 1991a, Noninvasive cerebral optical spectroscopy for monitoring cerebral oxygen delivery and hemodynmics, *Critical Care Medicine*, 19:89

McCormick, P.W., Stewart, M., Goetting, and Balakrishnan, G., 1991b, Regional Cerebrovascular oxygen saturation measured by optical spectroscopy in humans, *Stroke* 22:596

Reynolds, E.O.R., Wyatt, J.S., Azzopardi D., Delpy, D.T., Cady, E.B., Cope, M., and Wray, S., 1988, New nonivasive methods for assessing brain oxygenation and haemodynamics, Brit. Med. Bull. 44,4,1052

HETEROGENEITY AND STABILITY OF LOCAL PO$_2$ DISTRIBUTION WITHIN THE BRAIN TISSUE

D.W. Lübbers, H. Baumgärtl, W. Zimelka

Max-Planck-Institut für Systemphysiologie
Rheinlanddamm 201
4600 Dortmund 1, Germany

INTRODUCTION

Heterogeneity of tissue pO$_2$ is a necessary consequence of the fact that in order to supply living tissue with O$_2$, molecular oxygen has to be transported from the arterial blood to the intracellularly situated mitochondria. The O$_2$ delivery of the blood towards the tissue and the diffusional O$_2$ transport within the tissue produce an oxygen pressure field the heterogeneity of which characterizes quantitatively the tissue O$_2$ supply. On the basis of theoretical analyses it could be predicted[1,2] that for monitoring this heterogeneity small pO$_2$ sensors having diameters of only a few microns would be necessary. In 1948 using small needle-shaped pO$_2$ electrodes as developed by Davies and Brink[3] Rémond could measure directly such pO$_2$ profiles between two adjacent small vessels on the brain surface[4,5]. In a footnote[6] it was reported that G. Millikan suggested to use this electrode for intracerebral measurements. Distributions of parameters can be quantitatively presented by a frequency histogram. To our knowlegde Jamieson and van den Brenk[7] were the first who used in 1963 pO$_2$ frequency histograms of different organs (included brain tissue) to characterize tissue O$_2$ supply. pO$_2$ histograms are now widely used to describe the O$_2$ supply of the brain under normal and pathological conditions[8], but it is still difficult to decide by which means a histogram is measurable which can be considered as representative for the tissue O$_2$ supply. To answer this question a set of pO$_2$ profiles were measured under steady state conditions puncturing the brain cortex with small needle electrodes. It was found that there is a strong local heterogeneity which can be quite different in different punctures, but that by increasing the number of punctures it is possible to obtain a pO$_2$ histogram by which the O$_2$ supply of the brain tissue is characterized.

METHODS

Guinea pigs, weighing 200-400 g were pretreated with 0.5 ml heparin sodium (5000 I.E.) 30 min before starting the experiment. Pentobarbital (60 mg/kg) was used

Oxygen Transport to Tissue XV, Edited by P. Vaupel
et al., Plenum Press, New York, 1994

for anaesthesia. The animals were tracheotomized and ventilated with air. The skull was trephinated close to the middle line by drilling a hole of 5 mm into the skull. pO_2 measurements within the brain were performed using microcoaxial needle electrodes. The electrodes were made from 0.2 mm thick Pt-wires which were conically etched to a tip diameter of ca. 1 μm over a length of 15 to 25 mm using alternating current of controlled voltage. The wire is covered with glass. To improve mechanical stability the glass is treated by an ion exchange and/or by sputtering thin oxide layers on the glass surface. The Ag/AgCl reference electrode is directly sputtered on the shaft close to the tip[9]. Electrodes of similar size were successfully used to measure intracerebral pO_2[10]. The electrodes were calibrated before and after each experiment. To optimize calibration ethyleneglycol-borax-biphosphate-buffer solutions were used which simulate the oxygen conductivity of brain tissue. Before puncturing the dura was taken off. The surface of the cortex is covered by saline (37°C) in contact with air. The puncture was carried out by a nanostepper (type AM2M/HSG, Fa. Bachofer, Reutlingen, Germany). To minimize the pressure effect caused by puncturing, the electrode was perpendicularly pushed in by 2 steps of 50 μm and then immediately withdrawn by 1 step of 50 μm. One step was performed in 10 ms. The penetration depth amounted to ca. 3 mm, whereby the electrode tip passed the gray matter (ca. 2 mm thick). The pO_2 measuring signals were recorded continuously. Since tissue pO_2 stabilized within 10 s, pO_2 readings were taken every 10 s. In some punctures local pO_2 values oscillate, but by averaging a stable mean local pO_2 value is obtained. The experiments were carried out using 5 animals (#5, #7, #8, #9, #11). For the evaluation 452 single pO_2 values were obtained from 9 punctures penetrating the brain from the surface.

RESULTS

Fig. 1A shows as an example the sequence of local pO_2 values measured by perpendicularly penetrating the brain surface. In this pO_2 profile local pO_2 decreases in the uppermost layer rather steeply to values close to zero; then it varies between increases and decreases without a distinct dependance on the depth of the puncture.

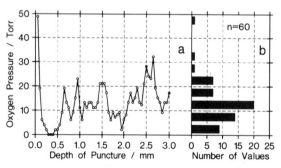 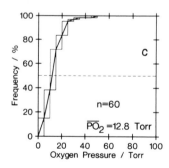

Fig. 1. Heterogeneity of local pO_2 within the brain tissue (guinea pig). The local pO_2 is measured by the polarographic microcoaxial needle electrode. (a) pO_2 profile measured by perpendicularly puncturing the brain surface. Local pO_2 varies between 49 Torr and 0 Torr. (b) pO_2 frequency histogram (class size 5 Torr). (c) Cumulative pO_2 histogram of the puncture (Puncture #11in).

There are 9 pO$_2$ peaks; the distance between the peaks varies between 150 and 300 μm (mean 238.9 $\pm$ 60.1 μm). The peaks characterize points at which the electrode tip is situated close to an oxygen source, i.e. a blood vessel. Similar pO$_2$ profiles were registered in 5 out of 9 punctures, the other 2 profiles showed besides the peaks large flat ranges and in 2 profiles were no distinct peaks at all.

The distribution of the local pO$_2$ values can be summarized and more quantitatively demonstrated by a pO$_2$ histogram in which the number of pO$_2$ values comprised in different classes is drawn. Fig. 1B shows the pO$_2$ histogram of this puncture using a class size of 5 Torr. About 70% of all values are smaller than 15 Torr, but only 5% close to zero (see Fig. 1A). In order to compare different pO$_2$ histograms the cumulative histogram is well suited (Fig. 1C). Here, the percentage values of the classes are consecutively drawn so that the diagonal forms a continuous line. It allows to present directly median and percentiles of the pO$_2$ distribution.

Fig. 2 and Table 1 show all the 9 punctures (#5a-#11in). They demonstrate that in the same brain region different punctures give quite different pO$_2$ histograms. The largest differences in mean pO$_2$ exist between histogram #5a and histogram #9a. The mean pO$_2$ amounts to 11.4 Torr in #5a and to 44.8 Torr in #9a.

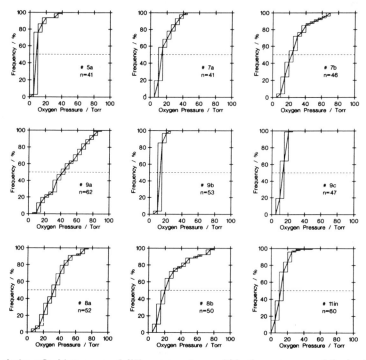

Fig. 2. Cumulative pO$_2$ histograms of different punctures within the same area of the brain cortex of the guinea pig. Although the same brain area is monitored the pO$_2$ histograms are quite different, e.g. #9a consists out of 17 classes of a similar size, whereas #9b has practically one large class.

Some histograms show distinct maxima of the frequency - in #5a 75% of all values are in the class of 10 Torr and in #9b 81% of the values-, whereas in other histograms a more even pO$_2$ distribution is seen - in #9a the pO$_2$ values are distributed with an almost similar frequency in 17 different pO$_2$ classes -. The histogram #9c consists practically only out of 3 pO$_2$ classes. These differences demonstrate that more than a single puncture is necessary to characterize the O$_2$ supply of the brain tissue. Fig. 3 shows in which way with increasing number of punctures (i.e. number of measured

Table 1. Data of the cumulative histograms of Fig. 2

Exp. Nr.	#5a	#7a	#7b	#8a	#8b	#9a	#9b	#9c	#11a	Mean*
Mean PO_2 [Torr]	11.4	18.1	27.4	34.7	27.1	44.8	13.7	13.9	12.8	23.3
Median [Torr]	9	14	22	32	20	42	13.5	14.5	13	16.0
Modal [Torr]	5-10	5-10	10-15	15-25 30-40	10-15	30-35	10-15	10-15	10-15	10-15
PO_2 min PO_2 max [Torr]	4 38	6 44	9 70	8 80	7 77	10 90	10 19	8 22	0 49	0 90
n	41	41	46	52	50	62	53	47	60	452

* Mean of the combined data of all punctures

pO_2 values) the mean value of the median approaches a final value if in each case the smallest or the largest values are selected and the corresponding mean values are calculated. With about 50 measuring values ($n_{min}=41$, $n_{max}=62$) the pO_2 difference amounts to 33 Torr, at about 200 values ($n_{min}=195$, $n_{max}=210$) to 17 Torr and at 300 values ($n_{min}=292$, $n_{max}=298$) to 7 Torr. This demonstrates clearly that a sufficient large number of measurig values are necessary to obtain a representative set of data.

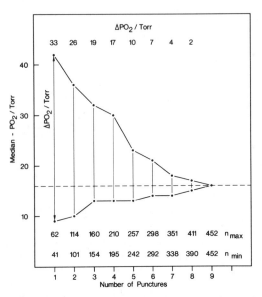

Fig. 3. Changes of the pO_2 median caused by increasing the number of punctures. The extreme values of the pO_2 median of the 9 punctures are 9 Torr for the minimum and 42 Torr for the maximum resulting in a pO_2 difference of 33 Torr. To obtain the largest possible differences the minimum or maximum values were selected and the corresponding mean median for 2 to 9 punctures calculated. To obtain a representative median at least 250 to 300 local pO_2 measurements are necessary. (n = number of the included pO_2 measurements selecting the largest (max) or the smallest values (min) of the median).

The data of all punctures are collected in Fig. 4. On the left side the local pO_2 values (n=452) measured at different depths are shown. Their distribution clearly demonstrates the strong local heterogeneity of tissue pO_2, but this heterogeneity coexists with a rather constant mean tissue pO_2: the mean profile (solid line) shows no systematic or large variations and also the mean pO_2 values within tissue layers of 500 μm thickness vary only between 19.7 and 27.1 Torr. The right side of Fig. 4 shows the frequency histogram of these pO_2 values and Fig. 5 their cumulative histogram. Only the small number of 2% of the values are less than 5 Torr (lowest class) and 2% larger than 65 Torr. About 80% of the values are smaller than 30-35 Torr which corresponds about to the pO_2 in the larger veins.

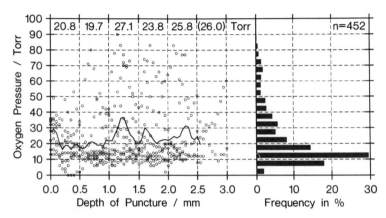

Fig 4. Combination of all measured local pO_2 values of the brain cortex of the guinea pig in dependance on the depth of the puncture. On the left side the solid line denotes the mean pO_2 profile obtained from all the data of Fig. 2. A single pO_2 value is marked by a circle. The distribution demonstrates the strong heterogeneity of tissue pO_2 whereas the mean pO_2 is constant and does not change in dependance of the depth of the puncture. Since in the frequency histogram (right side) only 2% of the values are in the lowest pO_2 class this histogram describes the pO_2 distribution of a well oxygenated tissue.

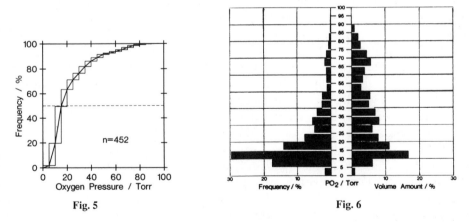

Fig. 5   Fig. 6

Fig. 5. Cumulative pO_2 histogram of all the 9 punctures of the brain cortex of the guinea pig.

Fig. 6. Relative amount of oxygen available in different pO_2 classes. The histogram (right side) demonstrates that in higher classes the amount of available oxygen is larger than the relative frequency of measured pO_2 values (left side) whereas in low pO_2 classes the opposite holds.

Assuming that the frequency of pO_2 values is representative of the tissue volume involved, the contours of the bars denote the relative tissue volume in which the pO_2 values of the corresponding class are found. The relative amount of oxygen available in the different pO_2 classes is obtained by multiplying the relative volume by the mean pO_2 of the class and the solubility coefficient of the tissue. Fig. 6 compares the relative frequency in the different pO_2 classes with the amount of oxygen available in this class. It demonstrates that the pO_2 frequency is not a sufficient measure to describe the amount of available oxygen: in higher pO_2 classes the amount of available oxygen is larger than the relative frequency of measured pO_2 values whereas in low pO_2 classes the opposite holds.

DISCUSSION AND CONCLUSION

The heterogeneity of local tissue pO_2 mirrors the heterogeneities of the vascular system, of the microcirculation and of the neuronal activity. Since the distance between 2 measuring points amounts to 50 μm and the mean capillary distance to ca. 60 μm the most of the measuring points are supplied by different vessels. To obtain information about pO_2 gradients within the tissue smaller measuring distances are necessary, e.g. 10 μm. Tissue pO_2 fluctuated corresponding to the oscillations of the microcirculation[11], but the calculated local mean pO_2 values proved to be so stable that they can be used to compare the pO_2 profiles of different tracks as well as to produce the corresponding histograms. It is known from other experiments, that because of effective regulatory processes tissue pO_2 remains rather stable, even if not too large changes of blood pressure or of neuronal activity occur[8].

Because of the large heterogeneity a sufficient number of single local pO_2 values are necessary to obtain a meaningful histogram. This is demonstrated in Fig. 3 using the pO_2 median as an example. By increasing the number of measurements the pO_2 difference between maximum and minimum decreases first rather steeply, than it approaches more gradually the final value of 16 Torr. These data show that at least 250 to 300 local pO_2 values are necessary to characterize the O_2 supply of the brain tissue and to obtain a sufficiently reliable representation of the data. Although in a single puncture (Fig. 2, #11in) the frequency of pO_2 values in the lowest class can amount up to 15%, in the mean of all punctures the frequency in this class is only 2% (Fig. 5). Since the critical pO_2 at which the function of the mitochondria is impaired is in the range of 1 to 2 Torr the measured data characterize an overall well oxygenated brain tissue. Obviously a setpoint for the O_2 supply is establisched in which blood flow is well adapted to metabolic needs.

For some analyses the relative amount of oxygen available within the tissue has to be known. Its frequency distribution as shown in Fig. 6 differs from the pO_2 distribution.

In Fig. 7 pO_2 histograms published in literature (A) are compared with the present data (B). For comparison experiments are selected in which the following methods are used: (1) pO_2 needle electrodes with a tip smaller than ca.3 μm (exception: in f a tip size of 150 μm and in i one of 10 μm is used), (2) pO_2 measurements by stepwise puncturing the surface of the brain, (3) spontaneous or artificial respiration of gas mixtures with an O_2 content of ca. 20% to 30% (exception: in f - probably - pure O_2 is used) and (4) presentation of the data by histograms with a class size of 5 Torr.

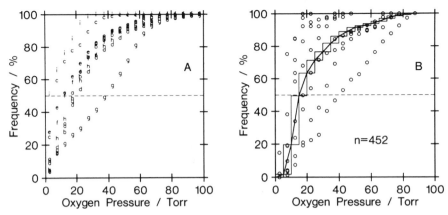

Fig. 7. Heterogeneity of local pO_2 values within the brain measured by pO_2 needle electrodes. Comparison of the present data and the data published in literature. The circles are drawn at the mean pO_2 of the different classes and at the corresponding frequency. (A) Compilation of published data about brain tissue pO_2 measured by polarographic microelectrodes. a: Baumgärtl et al. 1965, b: Baumgärtl et al. 1966, c: Sick et al. 1982, d: Seyde and Longnecker 1986, e: Aleksandrova et al. 1987, f: Crockard et al. 1975, g: Nair et al. 1975, h: Smith et al. 1977, i: Fennema et al. 1988. (B) The data are taken from Fig. 2 (cumulative histograms of the single punctures #5a to #11in) and Fig. 5 (cumulative histogram of all the punctures).- The heterogeneity in A and B is very similar, distinct differences exist in the lower classes.

Fig. 7A shows the selected histograms indicated by the letters a-i. The position of the letters marks the pO_2 class (2.5 Torr corresponds to class 5 Torr) and its percentage. The different experiments are denoted by different letters. It can be seen that the overall heterogeneity in Fig. 7A is similar to the heterogeneity in Fig. 7B. The cumulative histograms of the experiments a (guinea pig, n = 2010, pO_2 = 23.3 Torr[12]), b (rat, n = 854, pO_2 = 24.4 Torr[13]), d (rat, n (estimated) = 600-800, pO_2 = 29.5 Torr[15]), f (baboon, n = 48, pO_2 = 23,8 Torr[17]) and h (rabbit, n = 6363, pO_2 = 24.5 Torr[19]) are practically equal to the sum histogram in Fig. 7B, although they were measured in different animals. Three of the histograms, histogram c (rat, n = 136, pO_2 = 12.9 Torr[14]), e (rat, n (estimated) = 2000, pO_2 = 20.6 Torr[16]) and i (rabbit, n = ?, pO_2 = 9 Torr[20]), are left-shifted, i.e. they have a relative large amount of low pO_2 values. Because of the small number of pO_2 measurements histogram c may still be in the normal range, but this does not explain the other two results. It can not be decided wether the O_2 supply was different in these animals or some measuring problems occurred. The pO_2 histogram g[18] is similar to histogram #9a in Fig. 2, but it represents a large number of measurements (n = 627). Such a broad histogram with 2 peaks can be a sign of a special microcirculatory regulation (e.g. in hyperoxia) or of microcirculatory disturbances. In these experiments tissue pO_2 decreased from relative high values at the surface to lower values in a depth of 700 μm. A similar behavior is reported by Feng et al.[21], but this contradicts the other findings (a, b, c, h, i) and our own results. In conclusion, our experiments show that the oxygen of the supplying blood is well distributed and used within the tissue. We like to assume that the pO_2 histograms in Fig. 4 and 5 represent the O_2 supply of a normal well oxygenated tissue.

REFERENCES

1. A. Krogh, The rate of diffusion of gases through animal tissues with some remarks on the coefficient of invasion, *J. Physiol.* 52:391 (1919).
2. E. Opitz and M. Schneider, Über die Sauerstoffversorgung des Gehirns und den Mechanismus von Mangelwirkungen, *Ergeb. Physiol.* 46:126 (1950).
3. P.W. Davies and F. Brink, Microelectrodes for measuring local oxygen tension in animal tissues, *Rev. Sci. Instrum.* 13:524 (1942).
4. A. Rémond, Ph.W. Davies and D.W. Bronk, Influence of the vascular bed on the pattern of oxygen tension in the cerebral cortex, *Fed. Proc.* 5(1):86 (1946).
5. A. Rémond, Aspects physiopathologiques de l'oxygène cortical, *Rev. Neurol.* 80:579 (1948).
6. E. Roseman, C.W. Goodwin and W.S. McCulloch, Rapid changes in cerebral oxygen tension induced by altering the oxygenation and circulation of the blood, *J. Neurophysiol.* 9:33 (1946).
7. D. Jamieson and H.A.S. van den Brenk, Comparison of oxygen tensions in normal tissues and yoshida sarcoma of the rat breathing air or oxygen at 4 atmospheres, *Brit. J. Cancer* 17:70 (1963).
8. D.W. Lübbers, Oxygen delivery and microcirculation in the brain, *in:* "Microcirculation in Circulatory Disorders," H. Manabe, B.W. Zweifach, K. Messmer, eds., Springer-Verlag, Tokyo-Berlin-Heidelberg-New York-London-Paris (1988).
9. H. Baumgärtl and D.W. Lübbers, Microcoaxial needle sensor for polarographic measurement of local O_2 pressure in the cellular range of living tissue. Its construction and properties, *in:* "Polarographic Oxygen Sensors," Gnaiger/Forstner, eds., Springer-Verlag, Berlin-Heidelberg (1983).
10. D.W. Lübbers, Kritische Sauerstoffversorgung und Mikrozirkulation, *Marburger Universitätsbund*, Jahrbuch (1966/67).
11. J. Manil, R.H. Bourgain, M. v. Waeyenberge, F. Colin, E. Blockeel, B. De Mey, J. Coremans and R. Paternoster, Properties of the spontaneous fluctuations in cortical oxygen pressure, *Adv. Exp. Med. Biol.* 169:231 (1984).
12. H. Baumgärtl, W. Reschke and D.W. Lübbers (1965), quoted by D.W. Lübbers, Microcirculation and hypoxia, *in:* "Neurohumoral and Metabolic Aspects of Injury," A.G.B. Kovach, H.B. Stoner, J.J. Spitzer, eds., Plenum Publishing Corporation, New York (1973)
13. H. Baumgärtl, W. Reschke and D.W. Lübbers (1966), quoted by D.W. Lübbers, Microcirculation and oxygen supply of the brain, *Acta Cardiol. Suppl.* XIX:209 (1974).
14. T.J. Sick, P.L. Lutz, J.C. LaManna and M. Rosenthal, Comparative brain oxygenation and mitochondrial redox activity in turtles and rats, *J. Appl. Physiol.* 53(6):1354 (1982).
15. W.C. Seyde and D.E. Longnecker, Cerebral oxygen tension in rats during deliberate hypotension with sodium nitroprusside, 2-chloroadenosine, or deep isoflurane anesthesia, *Anesthesiology* 64:480 (1986).
16. T.B. Aleksandrova, G.S. Kilibaeva, T.V. Ryasina, I.T. Demchenko, Y.E. Moskalenko and I.M. Rodionov, Distribution of partial pressure of oxygen in the brain of spontaneously hypertensive rats, Translated from *Byulleten' Éksperimental 'noi Biologii i Meditsiny* 103(1):15, Plenum Publishing Corporation (1987).
17. H.A. Crockard, L. Symon, N.M. Branston, J. Juhasz and A. Wahid, Measurements of oxygen tension in the cerebral cortex of baboons, *J. Neurol. Sci.* 27:17 (1975).
18. P. Nair, W.J. Whalen and D. Buerk, PO_2 of cat cerebral cortex: response to breathing N_2 and 100% O_2, *Microvas. Res.* 9:158 (1975).
19. R.H. Smith, E.J. Guilbeau and D.D. Reneau, The oxygen tension field within a discrete volume of cerebral cortex, *Microvas. Res.* 13:233 (1977).
20. M. Fennema, J.N. Wessel, N.S. Faithfull and W. Erdmann, Tissue oxygen tension in the cerebral cortex of the rabbit, *in:* Oxygen Transport to Tissue XI, Adv. Exp. Med. Biol. 248:451 (1988), K. Rakusan, G.P. Biro, Th.K. Goldstick, Z. Turek, eds., Plenum Press, New York-London (1988).
21. Z.-C. Feng, E.L. Roberts, Th.J. Sick and M. Rosenthal, Depth profile of local oxygen tension and blood flow in rat cerebral cortex, white matter and hippocampus, *Brain Res.* 445:280 (1988).

CRITICAL O_2 DELIVERY IN RAT BRAIN

Robert Schlichtig,[1,2] Jill Herrick,[2] and Edwin M. Nemoto[1]

[1] Department of Anesthesiology and Critical Care Medicine, University
   of Pittsburgh, Pittsburgh, PA
[2] Veterans Affairs Medical Center, University Drive, Pittsburgh, PA
   15240

INTRODUCTION

As O_2 delivery (DO_2) of whole body,[1,2] intestine,[3,4] liver,[5] or skeletal muscle[6] is progressively decreased in anesthetized animals, O_2 consumption (VO_2) is initially maintained constant via increased O_2 extraction by the tissues (O_2 supply independence). However, below a critical threshold DO_2 value (DO_2c), VO_2 of these organs decreases in proportion to DO_2 (O_2 supply dependence). More importantly, dysoxia (i.e. O_2 demand that exceeds O_2 supply)[7] appears to commence at the onset of liver O_2 supply dependence, as reflected by the simultaneous decrease in VO_2 and increase in hepatic mitochondrial reduction.[5] Accordingly, it tentatively appears that dysoxia may be identified, in liver at least, by the DO_2c inflection of a biphasic VO_2-DO_2 relation.

Not all organs manifest a biphasic VO_2-DO_2 relationship, i.e. clearly identifiable O_2 supply independent and O_2 supply dependent regions, during all conditions. For example, kidney VO_2 decreases in direct proportion to DO_2 during progressive flow stagnation, throughout the physiologic range, presumably reflecting decreasing tubular energy demand to reclaim NaCl as DO_2 and glomerular filtration simultaneously decrease.[8] This kidney relation between VO_2 and DO_2 most likely represents "O_2 demand dependence," wherein VO_2 is primarily determined by O_2 demand rather than by O_2 supply. Dysoxia therefore cannot likely be identified in kidney simply by observing the response of VO_2 to DO_2 reduction during flow stagnation.

The goal of the present investigation was to determine the characteristics of the VO_2-DO_2 relationship of the brain in rats lightly anesthesthetized with N_2O anesthesia. We wished to determine whether the relationship is characterized by O_2 supply independence, as in liver, or O_2 demand dependence, as in kidney.

METHODS

Seventeen Wistar rats were mechanically ventilated on 1.0% halothane/ 70%

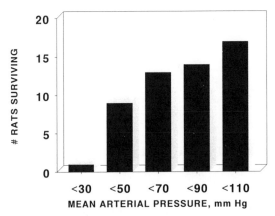

Figure 1. Number of rats surviving phlebotomy at various blood pressures

N₂O/ 29% O₂ during insertion of femoral artery and vein catheters, a 25 µm platinum microelectrode and 28 ga needle into the superior sagittal sinus for H_2 clearance cerebral blood flow (CBF) measurement (T 1/2) and cerebral venous blood sampling. Following instrumentation, they were ventilated with 70% N_2O/30% O_2. The rats were subjected to stepwise, progressive, hemorrhagic arterial hypotension in 20 mm Hg increments. Brain DO_2 was calculated as CBF x CaO_2, and Brain VO_2 was calculated as CBF x (CaO_2 - CvO_2). Brain O_2 extraction ratio was calculated as VO_2/DO_2. Rats were killed when blood pressure varied by more than 10 mm Hg during CBF measurement, and these values were not included in the analysis.

RESULTS

Figure 1 shows the number of rats surviving at various blood pressures. Only one rat survived to a blood pressure of less than 30 mm Hg, and 15 survived to a blood pressure less than 50.

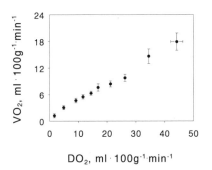

Figure 2. Response of brain VO₂ to DO₂ reduction. Values represent mean ± SE.

576

Figure 2 shows the relation between VO_2 and DO_2 of pooled data. The response of VO_2 to DO_2 reduction appeared linear, as previously noted in kidney,[8] rather than biphasic, as in liver and intestine. [4]

Figure 3 shows the relation between O_2 extraction ratio and DO_2. There appeared to be no evidence of O_2 regulation, i.e. no increase in O_2 extraction ratio, above a DO_2 value of approximately 20 ml · $100g^{-1}$ · min^{-1}. Below the DO_2 value of 20 ml · $100g^{-1}$ · min^{-1}, O_2 extraction ratio increased progressively, achieving a maximum

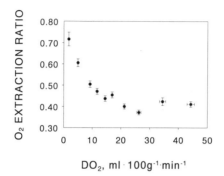

Figure 3. Response of O_2 extraction ratio to DO_2 reduction. Values represent mean ± SE.

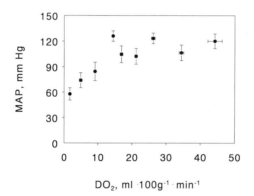

Figure 4. Mean arterial pressure (MAP) during DO_2 reduction.

value of about 70%, i.e. close to critical O_2 extraction ratio of whole body, liver, and intestine. [8]

Figure 4 shows the relation between MAP and DO_2. DO_2 varied very widely above a MAP of 90 mm Hg.

DISCUSSION

We did not observe a biphasic relation between VO_2 and DO_2 of the brain in this investigation. We believe that our observations are consistent with variable O_2

demand, that occurred as a consequence of incomplete anesthesia, such that brain O_2 demand was therefore permitted to vary with the level of consciousness and degree of immobilization stress.[9] DO_2 presumably rose to meet increased O_2 demand, when present, but remained normal in those rats wherein O_2 demand was normal.

Consistent with our hypothesis that the linear VO_2-DO_2 relation represented O_2 demand dependence, rather than O_2 supply dependence, are several observations. First, O_2 extraction ratio did not increase as DO_2 decreased between 20 and 50 ml $100g^{-1} \cdot min^{-1}$ (figure 3), even though brain is normally capable of increasing O_2 extraction ratio to very high fractions when needed. Second, the highest values of O_2 extraction ratio achieved in this investigation were only about as high as critical O_2 extraction ratio achieved in other organs.[2-5] In other words, it is unlikely that true O_2 supply dependence was achieved in this investigation. Finally, DO_2 varied very widely within the range of normal blood pressure, suggesting responsiveness to variable O_2 demand.

We conclude that the response of brain VO_2 to DO_2 reduction is not biphasic when O_2 demand is permitted to vary, and that additional parameters such as mitochondrial redox state are needed to identify brain dysoxia in awake and semi-awake conditions.

REFERENCES

1. S.M. Cain. Peripheral oxygen uptake and delivery in health and disease. Clin. Chest Med. 4: 139-148 (1983).
2. S.A. Bowles, R. Schlichtig, H.A. Klions, D.J. Kramer. Arteriovenous pH and PCO_2 detects critical O_2 delivery during progressive hemorrhage in dogs. Journal of Critical Care 7: 95-105 (1992).
3. D.P. Nelson, C.E. King, S.L. Dodd, P.T. Schumacker, S.M. Cain. Systemic and intestinal limits of O_2 extraction in the dog. J. Appl. Physiol. 63: 387-394, 1987.
4. R. Schlichtig, D.J. Kramer, M.R. Pinsky. Flow redistribution during progressive hemorrhage is a determinant of critical O_2 delivery. J. Appl. Physiol. 70: 169-178 (1991).
5. R. Schlichtig, H.A. Klions, D.J. Kramer, E.M. Nemoto. Hepatic dysoxia commences during O_2 supply dependence. J. Appl. Physiol. 72: 1499-1505 (1992).
6. D.L. Bredle, R.W. Samsel, P.T. Schumacker, S.M. Cain. Critical O_2 delivery to skeletal muscle at high and low PO_2 in endotoxemic dogs. J. Appl. Physiol. 66: 2553-2558 (1989).
7. R.J. Connett, C.R. Honig, T.E.J. Gayeski, G.A. Brooks. Defining hypoxia: a systems view of VO_2, glycolysis, energetics, and intracellular PO_2. J. Appl. Physiol. 68: 833-842 (1990).
8. R. Schlichtig, D.J. Kramer, J. R. Boston, M.R. Pinsky. Renal O_2 consumption during progressive hemorrhage. J. Appl. Physiol. 70: 1957-1962 (1991).
9. C. Carlsson, M. Hagerdal, A.E. Kaasik, B.K. Siesjo. A catecholamine-mediated increase in cerebral oxygen uptake during immobilization stress in rats. Brain Res. 119: 223-231 (1977).

CHANGES IN OXYGENATION STATES OF RAT BRAIN TISSUES DURING
GLUTAMATE-RELATED EPILEPTIC SEIZURES - NEAR-INFRARED STUDY

Miwa Yanagida and Mamoru Tamura

Biophysics Division, Research Institute for
Electronic Science, Hokkaido University, Sapporo
JAPAN

INTRODUCTION

Glutamic acid functions as excitatory neurotransmitter in mammalian central nervous systems. Hippocampus is characterized as most glutaminergic rich area in the cerebrum, which plays key role for many neural activities. Several naturally occuring epilepsy is related to the disorder of glutaminergic nervous systems. Kainic acid and N-methyl-D-aspartic acid (NMDA) are well known agonists which bind different subclass of glutaminergic receptors. These agonists, therefore, have potent neurotoxicity, of which example is that kainic acid-induced seizure is a good model for naturally occuring epilepsy. During the seizure, the marked increases in oxygen consumption and blood-flow are well-recognized and the latter overcomes the former, resulting the increase in hemoglobin oxygenation state. The redox behavior of intracellular space, mitochondria, is, however, not well characterized yet. Recently, the marked and transient reduction of cytochrome oxidase was demonstrated during bicucul-

Oxygen Transport to Tissue XV, Edited by P. Vaupel
et al., Plenum Press, New York, 1994

lin-induced seizue (1), where near-infrared spectrophotometry was used for simultaneous monitoring the hemoglobin oxygenation state and redox state of mitochondria. The redox state of copper not heme moeity of cytochrome oxidase was measured selectively by this method (2). In this paper using near-infrared photometry, we will report the changes of oxygenation states of brain tissure of rat during glutamate-agonists induced epileptic seizure.

EXPERIMENTAL PROCEDURES

Male Wister rats weighing 180-240g were used in the present study. Animals were anesthetized with urethane (1.0g/kg body weight) and ventilated artificially through trachea cannula. Both femoral artery and vein were cannulated, through which gas analysis of arterial and venous bloods were performed. Drugs were administered intravenously through the catheter. Arterial blood prssure was also monitored continuously. Near-infrared spectrophotometer used was that described previously using four-wavelengths algorithm (2).

RESULT

Fig.1-A shows the typical traces of the redox change of cytochrome oxidase during seizure, where we measured the redox state of copper in the cytochrome oxidase. Oxyhemoglobin content was also shown in the figure. Before administration of drugs, rat was breathed with 100% oxygen in a short period, which gave the fully oxygenated state of hemoglobin and fully oxidized cytochrome oxidase. By 100% oxygen respiration, hemoglobin was more oxygenated but cytochrome oxidase remaind unchanged. Administration of kainic acid caused the transient increase in oxyhemoglobin content, due to the transient increase in blood pressure. Cytochrome oxidase was not oxidized during the transient period of increased oxygenation

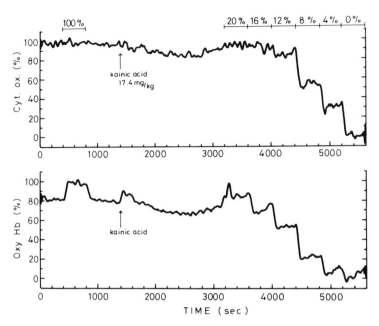

Fig.1-A. Effect of kainic acid-infusion on the redox state of
cytochrome oxidase (Top) and oxygenation state of hemoglobin
in the rat brain.   The percent shown in the top is the FiO_2.

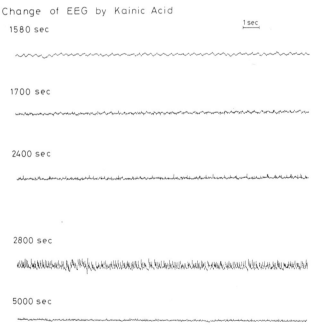

Fig.1-B.   EEG traces before and after the kainic acid-infusion.

state of hemoglobin. Then, cytochrome oxidase was reduced to original level within 3min. The change of hemoglobin oxygenation state nearly paralleled the change of redox state of cytochrome oxidase. After the recovery of initial level, rat was subjected to gradual hypoxia by decreasing oxygen concentration of inspired gas in step-wise fashion. By nitrogen-respiration, hemoglobin was fully deoxygenated and reduction of copper was assumed to be completed. This gave the full scale of reduction of copper signal. The changes in EEG during and after the administration of kainic acid are shown in Fig.1-B. The numbers in seconds correspond those of abscessia of Fig.1-A. At 1700sec, the rapid and excitatory spikes appeared, which became more significant with time, cf. 2400 and 2800sec. The large spikes in 2800sec lasted more than 30min. By lowering oxygen concentration in the inspired gas, 4% oxygen-respiration at 500sec, gave the hypoxic condition, where about 70% of cytochrome oxidase was in the reduced state and hemoglobin was almost fully deoxygenated. The EEG-spikes at this stage were markedly smaller than that at air-respiration of 2800sec. This was due to energy-depletion by hypoxia, since re-ventilation with air showed the similar EEG spikes of 2800sec.

NMDA showed only transient increase in hemoglobin oxygenation (Fig.2-A). Gradual reduction of cytochrome oxidase was not observed after the administration. Deoxygenation of hemoglobin was also not observed. The response in EEG was different from that of kainic acid (Fig.2-B), where the relatively slow and suppresed EEG (2600sec) appeared after the excitatory EEG (1800sec).

MK801, known as the antagonist for NMDA, blocked almost completely the effect of NMDA in both oxygenation state of brain tissue (Fig.3-A) and EEG (Fig.3-B).

Since seizure accompanies the marked increase in oxygen consumption, which may affect the relationship between the intracellular oxygen concentration at mitochondrial space and intracelluar space, such as capillary and venous system. Fig.4 summarizes the relationship between the redox state of cytochrome oxidase and hemoglobin oxygenation state under the various conditions. The experimental points deviated from the straight line with 45 . This is due to the large differ-

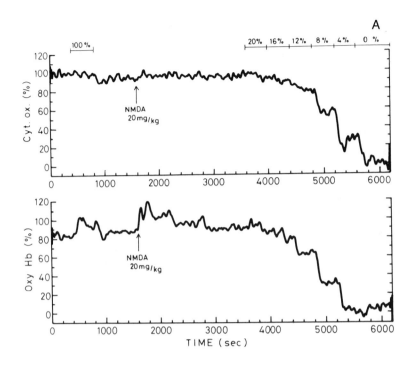

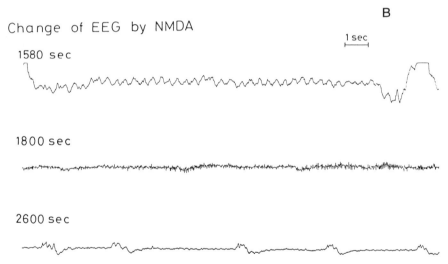

Fig.2. A: Effect of NMDA on the redox state of cytochrome oxidase and hemoglobin oxygenation state of rat brain. B: EEG.

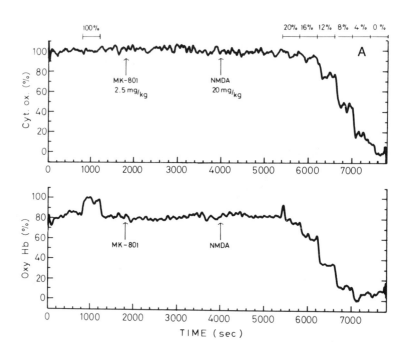

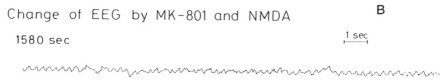

Change of EEG by MK-801 and NMDA

B

1580 sec

1 sec

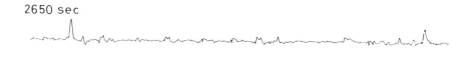

2650 sec

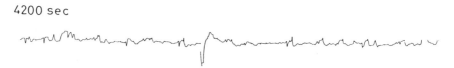

4200 sec

Fig.3. Effect of MK801-infusion.

ences of the oxygen affinity between these chromophores ;
i.e., the oxygen concentration giving half maximal reduction
of copper of cytochrome oxidase in mitochondria is 7×10^{-8}M,
where as that of hemoglobin, 2×10^{-5}M.   No significant differences in the curves were obtained with the rats under the
various experimental conditions examined in this study.

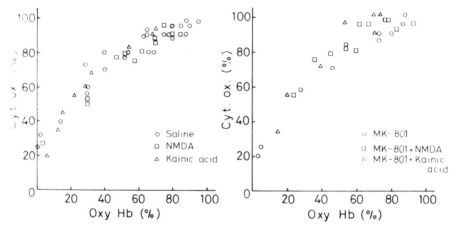

Fig.4. The relationship between percent oxidation of cytochrome oxidase and percent oxygenation of hemoglobin in the
rat brain.

DISCUSSION

Unlike the chemically induced seizures by bicuculline
and pentyren tetrazolium (1), glutamate agonist-induced
seizure showed the relatively small changes in both EEG and
cerebral oxygenation state (Fig.1-3).   The observed gradual
reduction of cytochrome oxidase with kainic acid was possibly
due to the vasoconstriction of low PCO_2, rather than the
lowered cardiac output.   As observed in biochemical binding
study, the effect of NMDA and kainic acid gave the different
behaviors in EEG and oxygenation state of cerebral tissue.
MK801 was also demonstrated as antagonist for NMDA in vivo.

The oxygen gradient between capillary and intracelluar space was not affected by seizures (Fig.4), though the oxygen consumption rate differed more than 5-times among the experimental conditons.

REFERENCES

1. Y.Hoshi and M.Tamura, *Brain Reserch* (in press)
2. O.Hazeki and M.Tamura, *Adv.Exp.Med.Biol.* 248 <u>63</u> (1989)

LEVELS OF DOPAMINE AND ITS METABOLITES IN THE EXTRACELLULAR MEDIUM OF THE STRIATUM OF NEWBORN PIGLETS DURING GRADED HYPOXIA

Anna Pastuszko, Nasser S.Lajevardi, Chao-Ching Huang, Outi Tammela, Maria Delivoria-Papadopoulos and David F.Wilson

Departments Pediatrics and of Biochemistry and Biophysics School of Medicine, University of Pennsylvania, Philadelphia, PA 19104, USA

INTRODUCTION

Neuronal injury resulting from ischemic/hypoxic episodes is thought to be mediated in part by a variety of monoamines and amino acid neurotransmitters. The contribution of the cytotoxicity of the excitatory amino acids (aspartate, glutamate) to ischemic/hypoxic injury has been well documented. More recently, several studies have provided evidence for a role of catecholamines in mediation of postischemic damage. Phebus et al (1986), Globus et al (1988), Kavano et al (1988), Slivka et al (1988), Vulto et al (1988), Damsma et al (1990), Obrenovitch et al (1990), Baker et al (1991) and others have demonstrated that dopamine is released in the striatum during ischemic/hypoxic episodes. Globus and colleagues (1987) suggested that dopamine release may contribute to the selective striatal vulnerability to ischemia. They reported that lesion of substantia nigra protects against development of striatal injury when animals are exposed to ischemia/hypoxia . This protective effect was related by the authors to inhibition of extracellular release of dopamine during ischemic/hypoxic episode. Additionally, Weinberger et al (1985) showed that, in gerbils, depletion of catecholamines by pretreatment with α-methyl-ρ-tyrosine greatly decreased the damage to nerve terminals induced by ischemia.

Accumulation of extracellular monoamines in ischemic regions of the brain region has been also proposed as a possible mechanism of postischemic hypoperfusion (Melamed et al, 1980) and a vasoconstrictor action of dopamine in the striatum has been suggested (Lindvall et al, 1981; Lavyne et al 1977).

The effect of hypoxia/ischemia on metabolism of dopamine in immature brain is much less well documented. Gordon et al (1990), using *in vivo* microdialysis, demonstrated that brief periods of moderate hypoxia markedly disrupted striatal catecholamine metabolism in the immature rodent brain. The authors, in agreement with Silverstein and Johnson (1984), reported that hypoxic exposure suppressed the striatal level of major dopamine catabolites, DOPAC and homovanillic acid.

In the present study, we have investigated the effect of graded low and high flow hypoxia on the extracellular levels of dopamine and its major catabolites in striatum of newborn piglets. It was observed that both high and low flow hypoxia caused an increase in the extracellular level of dopamine and a decrease in its major catabolic products- DOPAC and homovanillic acid. The extent of the increase in dopamine in extracellular medium was dependent on the degree to which the oxygen pressure in the cortex was decreased and the relationship between oxygen pressure and dopamine levels were the same in the two models. The alterations in the extracellular level of the catabolites were also similar in both hypoxic conditions except that recovery required much longer times after hypocapnic hypoxia (low flow hypoxia or ischemia) than after hypoxic hypoxia (high flow hypoxia).

MATERIALS AND METHODS

Animal preparation: Newborn piglets, age 2-4 days, were used throughout this study. These animals have been chosen because the level of development of the brain of the piglet is approximately equal to that of a term newborn. Anesthesia was induced by halotane (4% mixed with 100% O2) and 1% lidocaine was used as a local anesthetic. In all animals, tracheotomy was performed and the femoral artery and vein were cannulated. Fentanyl (30 μ g/kg) was injected intravenously at approximately one hour intervals throughout the experiment. The head of the piglet was fixed in a Kopf stereotaxic frame and the scalp reflected to expose the skull. A hole 1.2 cm in diameter was made in the skull over the parietal hemisphere and the dura removed. A cranial window for measuring cortical oxygen pressure was placed in the hole and the surface of the brain under window was superfused with Ringer solution. A small hole was also drilled in the skull and a microdialysis probe was implanted into the striatum. After surgery, the animals were paralyzed with tubocurarine and mechanically ventilated with 22% O_2 and 78% N_2O. The control rate of respiration was 25/minute. The arterial blood pressure and end-tidal CO_2 were continuously monitored.

Models of hypoxia: Graded hypoxia of the brain was induced by two methods: 1) increasing the ventilatory rate (decreasing systemic $PaCO_2$) and 2) decreasing FiO_2.

In first model, animals were subjected to stepwise increases in the ventilatory rate from 25 to 65, 80, and 95/min at constant respiratory volume, holding the rate constant at each level for 15 min. The ventilatory rate was then returned to the control value and the animal allowed to recover for a period of 30 min. To measure effect of mild hyperventilation, the animals were subjected to a single period of increased ventilatory rate (up to 65/min) where they were maintained for 20 min and then the ventilatory rate returned to the control value and maintained for an additional 30 min.

Hypoxic-hypoxia was induced by stepwise reduction of the percent of oxygen in the inspired gas from 22% (control) to 14%, 11% and 9%. Each value of FiO_2 was maintained constant for 18 min before being changed to the next value. At the end of the treatment, the FiO_2 was returned to 22% and recovery followed for 30 minutes. A more mild, single step, treatment of hypoxia was also performed by decreasing the percent oxygen in the inspired gas from the control (22%) to 14% for 18 min and than returning it to the control value.

Measurements of tissue oxygen pressure using the oxygen dependent quenching of phosphorescence: The phosphorescent oxygen probe (the Pd complex of meso tetra-(4-carboxyphenyl) porphine) was infused into the blood as a complex with bovine serum albumin dissolved in physiological saline at pH 7.4. The lifetime of the phosphorescence was measured and used to calculate the oxygen pressure as previously described (Wilson et al, 1988; Vanderkooi et al, 1989; Pawlowski and Wilson, 1992).

Microdialysis measurements: An unbuffered Ringer solution was pumped through the microdialysis probe at 3.5 µl/min. The dialysate samples were collected at 3 min intervals following a 1.5 hr stabilization period and were immediately analysed using a BAS Liquid Chromatography System. 10 µl of dialysate was directly injected into the microbore column and level of dopamine, DOPAC and HVA were measured by electrochemical detection as described early (Pastuszko et al, 1992).

Statistical analysis: The average of 6 samples immediately before the hypoxia was defined as control (100%). All other values are expressed as the % of control ± SEM. The statistical significance of the experimental values was determined using one way analysis of variance (ANOVA) with repeated measures and multiple range analysis for the means using 95% confidence intervals.

RESULTS

The effects of graded hyperventilation (hypocapnic hypoxia) and hypoxic hypoxia on physiological parameters of newborn piglets are shown in table 1. It can be seen that as the rate of ventilation increase, $PaCO_2$ decreased from

Table 1. The physiological data during graded hypoxic hypoxia and graded hypocapnic hypoxia.

	MAP (Torr)	pH	$PaCO_2$ (Torr)	PaO_2 (Torr)
Graded hypoxic hypoxia				
Baseline	93 ± 12	7.39 ± 0.03	40 ± 3	104 ± 19
Hypoxia (14% FiO_2)	97 ± 19	7.37 ± 0.05	39 ± 2	47 ± 13
Hypoxia (11% FiO_2)	94 ± 23	7.35 ± 0.06	37 ± 4	32 ± 4
Hypoxia (9% FiO_2)	82 ± 28	7.25 ± 0.08	33 ± 7	21 ± 4
Normoxia	94 ± 20	7.05 ± 0.02	35 ± 5	108 ± 11
Graded hypocapnic hypoxia				
Baseline	78 ± 9	7.40 ± 0.01	40 ± 3	94 ± 27
Hypocapnia (rate 65 cpm)	68 ± 7	7.59 ± 0.06	20 ± 1	124 ± 14
Hypocapnia (rate 80 cpm)	55 ± 12	7.70 ± 0.06	14 ± 1	112 ± 12
Hypocapnia (rate 95 cpm)	54 ± 11	7.70 ± 0.05	11 ± 1	109 ± 22
Normocapnia	85 ± 18	7.40 ± 0.02	31 ± 4	98 ± 21

The data are expressed as means ± SEM for 9 piglets and 6 piglets in the graded hypoxic hypoxia and graded hypocapnic hypoxia studies, respectively.

approx. 40 Torr to 20, 14 and 11 Torr and arterial pH increased from 7.4 (control) to 7.59, 7.7 and 7.7, respectively. After return of the ventilatory rate to control values, the pH quickly returned to the control value (7.4). Measurements of the oxygen pressure in the cortex of the brain showed that it decreased parallel to $PaCO_2$ from a control value of 35-40 Torr to 27, 20 and 17 Torr, respectively. In the hypoxic hypoxia model, $PaCO_2$ did not change significantly, but PaO_2 decreased from approx. 100 Torr to 47, 32 and 21 Torr. Cortical oxygen pressure decreased stepwise, in these conditions, from approx. 35 Torr (control) to 27, 17 and 4 Torr. The arterial pH also decreased from about 7.4 to 7.37, 7.35 and 7.25, respectively; after 30 min recovery the pH was 7.05, much below control value.

During mild hypoxic hypoxia (tissue PO_2 decreased to about 25 Torr) the changes in pH were not significant, whereas in hypocapnic hypoxia the same decrease in tissue oxygen pressure was accompanied by an increase in pH to 7.58 (Table 2).

Table 2. The physiological data during mild hypoxic hypoxia and mild hypocapnic hypoxia.

	MAP (Torr)	pH	$PaCO_2$ (Torr)	PaO_2 (Torr)
Mild hypoxic hypoxia				
Baseline	93 ± 15	7.39 ± 0.05	38 ± 3	108 ± 26
Hypoxia (14% FiO$_2$)	92 ± 16	7.37 ± 0.03	39 ± 2	40 ± 17
Normoxia	88 ± 15	7.35 ± 0.02	38 ± 4	96 ± 19
Mild hypocapnic hypoxia				
Baseline	91 ± 6	7.40 ± 0.01	40 ± 3	96 ± 16
Hypocapnia (rate 65 cpm)	69 ± 10	7.58 ± 0.06	21 ± 2	118 ± 12
Normocapnia	95 ± 5	7.40 ± 0.03	36 ± 4	112 ± 10

The data are expressed as means ± SEM for 8 piglets and 5 piglets in mild hypoxic hypoxia and mild hypocapnic hypoxia studies, respectively. FiO_2 is the percent of oxygen in the inspired gas; cpm is the ventilatory rate in cycles per minute. MAP = mean arterial blood pressure.

The effects of mild and graded hypoxic hypoxia and hyperventilation on extracellular level of dopamine and its major metabolites DOPAC and HVA in the striatum are shown in Tables 3 and 4. The control values were 10.4 ± 1.2.pmole/ml for dopamine, 1991 ± 336 pmole/ml for DOPAC and 1655 ± 302 pmole/ml for HVA. In both models of mild hypoxia, decrease in the cortical oxygen pressure to about 25 Torr resulted in similar changes in the extracellular level of dopamine, DOPAC and HVA. The extracellular level of dopamine increase by 50-80%, whereas the levels of DOPAC and HVA decrease by 20-25% and 10-15%, respectively.

During graded hypoxic hypoxia and hypocapnic hypoxia, release of dopamine and decrease in the level of DOPAC and HVA were dependent on the decrease of oxygen pressure. When oxygen decreased to about 17 Torr, the level of dopamine in extracellular medium rose by about 150-200%, while the levels of DOPAC and HVVA decreased by 25 - 35% and 10 - 25%, respectively. During the 30 minutes recovery period, the extracellular level of dopamine returned to control values in both models. The extracellular levels of DOAPC and HVA, on the other hand, returned to control values during 30 minutes of

Table 3. The cortical oxygen pressure and extracellular level of dopamine and its metabolites in the striatum in mild hypoxic hypoxia and mild hypocapnic hypoxia.

	Cortical O_2 (Torr)	DA	DOPAC (% of baseline)	HVA
Mild hypoxic hypoxia				
Baseline	32 ± 3	100	100	100
Hypoxia (14% FiO_2)	22 ± 3	186 ± 24[a]	82 ± 3[a]	92 ± 5
Normoxia	30 ± 3	107 ± 4	99 ± 5	99 ± 8
Mild hypocapnic hypoxia				
Baseline	40 ± 3	100	100	100
Hypocapnia (65 cpm)	27 ± 8	150 ± 24[a]	75 ± 11[a]	95 ±
Normocapnia	35 ± 6	24		
		109 ± 11	91 ± 7	89 ± 8

The extracellular levels of DA, DOPAC and HVA are expressed as % of baseline. The values are given as the mean ± SEM for 8 piglets and 5 piglets for mild hypoxic hypoxia and mild hypocapnic hypoxia, respectively. The superscript a indicates values significantly different from baseline as determined by one way analysis of variance, followed by Wilcoxon signed-rank test. [a] $p<0.05$. FiO_2 is the percent of oxygen in the inspired gas, cpm is the ventilation rate in cycles per minute.

Table 4. The cortical oxygen pressure and extracellular levels of dopamine, DOPAC and HVA in the striatum during graded hypoxic hypoxia and graded hypocapnic hypoxia.

	Cortical O_2 (Torr)	DA	DOPAC (% of baseline)	HVA
Graded hypoxic hypoxia				
Baseline	35 ± 2	100	100	100
Hypoxia (14% FiO_2)	26 ± 4	166 ± 10[a]	93 ± 4[a]	98 ± 5
Hypoxia (11% FiO_2)	17 ± 4	296 ± 59[a]	74 ± 6[b]	91 ± 6
Hypoxia (9% FiO_2)	4 ± 2	629 ± 124[a]	44 ± 6[b]	68 ± 8[b]
Normoxemia	33 ± 7	143 ± 14	88 ± 5[a]	80 ± 15[a]
Graded hypocapnic hypoxia				
Baseline	40 ± 3	100	100	100
Hypocapnia (rate 65 cpm)	27 ± 9	170 ± 30[a]	98 ± 12	105 ± 8
Hypocapnia (rate 80 cpm)	20 ± 6	200 ± 38[b]	75 ± 8[b]	78 ± 10[a]
Hypocapnia (rate 95 cpm)	17 ± 6	250 ± 88[b]	65 ± 6[b]	75 ± 8[a]
Normocapnia	30 ± 10	120 ± 23	55 ± 5[b]	62 ± 9[b]

The extracellular levels of DA, DOPAC and HVA are expressed as % of baseline. The values are given as the mean ± SEM for the 9 and 6 piglets in graded hypoxic hypoxia and graded hypocapnic hypoxia, respectively. The letters, a and b, indicate values significantly different from baseline as determined by one way analysis of variance, followed by Wilcoxon signed-rank test. [a] $p < 0.05$, [b] $p < 0.01$.

recovery after hypoxic hypoxia conditions but after graded hyperventilation remained below baseline even after 60 min of recovery.

DISCUSSION

In the perinatal period, infants with various clinical disorders are commonly exposed to brief, as well as prolonged, periods of hypoxia. Exposure of the immature brain to moderate hypoxia may cause permanent changes in synaptic function and have a significant impact on future neuronal development (Ihle et al, 1985; Lun et al 1986; Hedner and Lundberg, 1979; 1980). It has been suggested that moderate hypoxia in early postnatal rats produced long lasting changes in dopamine metabolism and dopamine related behavior. In our study, we investigated the effects of hypoxic conditions on metabolism of dopamine in striatum of newborn piglets. Controlled, graded levels of hypoxic insult to the brain of animals was generated by hyperventilation or alteration FiO_2. Hyperventilation is a physiological mechanism for decreasing $PaCO_2$ which results in increasing pulmonary blood flow. Thus, hyperventilation has been used clinically to improve lung function in cases with pulmonary hypoperfusion or to treat brain edema induced by perinatal asphyxia.

In both models of brain hypoxia, decreases in oxygen pressure in the cortex were accompanied by marked increases in the extracellular level of dopamine and decreases in the level of the major catabolites of dopamine, DOPAC and HVA. During mild hypoxic conditions the extent of alteration in the extracellular levels of dopamine, DOPAC, and HVA in both pathological models was dependent on the extent of decrease in the oxygen pressure in the tissue. Two different mechanism for the increase extracellular dopamine due to hypoxia have been proposed: Increase in exocytotic release due to neuronal depolarization and/or; inhibition of reuptake of dopamine. When the ventilatory rate or FiO_2 was returned to control values, the extracellular dopamine levels returned to normal values, consistent with reinstatement of the reuptake systems as the oxygen pressure return to baseline. The decrease in extracellular level of DOPAC and HVA during hypoxic hypoxia and hyperventilation are consistent with inhibition of monoamine oxidase. The mechanism of this inhibition, however, remains to be establish. Following an episode of hypoxic hypoxia, the levels of DOPAC and HVA returned to baseline values within about 30 minutes whereas recovery from graded hyperventilation required 1-2 hours. Thus, full recovery of dopamine catabolism required much longer times after hyperventilation than after hypoxic hypoxia. Our data indicate that factor(s) in addition to oxygen contribute to long term alteration in dopamine catabolism by episodes of hyperventilation.

One of the major differences between the two hypoxic models is the change in pH: hypoxic hypoxia caused a decrease in pH whereas in hypocapnic hypoxia there was an increase in pH. The decrease of pH during hypoxic hypoxia is primarily due to accumulation of lactate. It was observed that during graded hypoxic hypoxia the level of blood lactate increase from approximately 2 mM (control) to 2.6 mM (FiO_2 = 14), 4.2 mM (FiO_2 = 11), 9.6 mM (FiO_2 = 9) and 10.5 mM after 30 min recovery. Several studies have suggested that accumulation of lactate can contribute to the damage to brain by ischemic/hypoxic insult (Ginsberg et al, 1980; Kalimo et al, 1981; Pulsinelli et al, 1982; Rehncrona et al, 1981; Siemkowicz and Hansen, 1978; Welsh et al, 1983). Schurr et al (1988), however, concluded from their experiments that lactic acid at concentrations of up to 20 mM has little or no detrimental effect on hypoxic neuronal tissue as manifested by electrophysiological measurements. Rather, it appeared from studies of these authors that lactate in 10 mM concentration is beneficial to neuronal tissue during hypoxia.

The mechanism of this beneficial role of lactate needs further evaluation. White and Clark (1990), Boakye et al (1991) and White et al (1989) reported that in isolated cortical synaptosomes treated to mimic ischemia, addition of lactate decreased uptake of calcium and release of acetylcholine. These authors suggested that lactate may suppress calcium uptake under ischemic/hypoxic conditions, thereby protecting against cell death by calcium overload .

Hypocapnic hypoxia caused long term alterations in catabolism of dopamine, whereas after hypoxic hypoxia level of DOPAC and HVA returned quickly to control values. It is possible that lactate accumulated during hypoxic hypoxia may have aided the rapid recovery observed in this model.

Physiologically important observations from this study include:

1. Even small changes in oxygen pressure result in alterations in dopamine metabolism in brain of newborn piglets;
2. Alterations in dopamine metabolism may persist for hours after even brief hypoxic episodes.
3. Hypocapnic hypoxia causes much longer lasting alterations in catecholamine metabolism than does hypoxic hypoxia.

Acknowledgment. This work was supported in part by grants NS-31465 and NS-10939.

REFERENCES

Baker, A.J., Zornow, M.H., Scheller, M.S., Yaksh, T.L., Skilling, S.R., Smullin, D.H., Larson, A.A., and Kuczenski, R., 1991, Changes in extracellular concentration of glutamate, aspartate, glycine, dopamine, serotonin and dopamine metabolites after transient global ischemia in the rabbit brain, J. Neurochem. 57: 1370.

Boakye, P., White, E.J., and Clark, J.B., 1991, Protection of ischemic synaptosomes from calcium overload by addition of exogenous lactate, J. Neurochem. 57: 88.

Damsma, G., Boisvert, D.P., Mudrick, L.A., Wenkstern, D., and Fibiger, H.C., 1990, Effects of transient forebrain ischemia and pargyline on extracellular concentrations of dopamine, serotonin and their metabolites in the rat striatum as determined by in vivo microdialysis, J. Neurochem. 54; 801.

Ginsberg, M.D., Welsh, F.A., and Budd, W.W., 1980, Deleterious effect of glucose pretreatment on recovery from diffuse cerebral ischemia in the cat. I. Local cerebral blood flow and glucose utilization, Stroke,11: 347.

Globus, M.Y-T., Ginsberg, M.D., Dietrich, W.D., Busto, R., and Scheinberg, P., 1987, Substantia nigra lesion protects against ischemic damage in the striatum, Neurosci. Letters, 80: 251.

Globus, M.Y-T., Busto, R., Dietrich, W.D., Martinez, E., Valdes, I., and Ginsberg, M.D., 1988, Effect of ischemia on the in vivo release of striatal dopamine, glutamate and γ-aminobutyric acid studied by intracerebral microdialysis, J. Neurochem. 51: 1455.

Gordon, K., Statman, D., Johnston, M.V., Robinson, T.E., Becker, J.B., and Silverstein, F.S., 1990, Transient hypoxia alters striatal catecholamine metabolism in immaturate brain : An in vivo microdialysis study, J. Neurochem. 54: 605.

Hedner, T., and Lunborg, P., 1979, Regional changes in monoamines synthesis in the developing brain during hypoxia, Acta Physiol. Scand. 106: 139.

Hedner, T., and Lundborg, P., 1980, Catecholamine metabolism in neonatal rat brain during asphyxia and recovery, Acta Physiol. Scand. 109: 169.

Ihle, W., Gross, J., and Moller, R., 1985, Effect of chronic postnatal hypoxia on dopamine uptake by synaptosomes from striatum of adult rats, Biomed. Biochem. Acta, 44: 433.

Kalimo, H., Rehncrona, S., Soderfeldt, B., Olsson,Y., and Siesjo, B.K., 1981, Brain lactic acidosis and ischemic cell damage. 2. Histopathology, J. Cereb. Blood Flow Metab., 1: 313.

Kawano, T., Tsutsumi, K., Miyake, H., and Mori, K., 1988, Striatal dopamine in acute cerebral ischemia of stroke resistant rats, Stroke, 19: 1540.

Lavyne, M.H., Koltun, W.A., Clement, J.A., Rosene, D.L., Pickren, K.S., Zervas, N.T., and Wurtman, R.J., 1977, Decrease in neostriatal blood flow after D-amphetamine administration or electrical stimulation of the substantia nigra, Brain Res. 135: 76.

Lindvall, O., Ingvar, M., Stenevi, U., 1981, Effects of methamphetamine on blood flow in the caudate-putamen after lesions of the nigrostriatal dopaminergic bundle in the rat, Brain Res. 211: 211.

Lun. A., Gross, J., Beyer, M., Fischer, H.D., Wustmann, C., Schmidt, J., and Hecht, K., 1986, The vulnerable period of perinatal hypoxia with regard to dopamine release and behavior in adult rats, Biomed. Biochem. Acta, 45: 619.

Melamed, E., Moskowitz, M.A., and Wurtman, R.J., 1980, Involvement of monoamines in the pathogenesis of cerebral ischemia, In: Bes, A., Geraud, G., eds. Cerebral Circulation and Neurotransmitters, Amsterdam, Excerpta Medica, 173.

Obrenovitch, T.P., Sarna, G.S., Matsumoto, T., and Symon, L., 1990, Extracellular striatal dopamine and its metabolites during transient cerebral ischemia, J. Neurochem., 54: 1526.

Pastuszko, A., Lajevardi, N., Chen, J., Tammela, O., Wilson, D.F., and Delivoria-Papadopoulos, M., 1992, The effects of graded levels of tissue oxygen pressure on dopamine metabolism in the striatum of newborn piglets, J. Neurochem.,in press.

Pawlowski, M., and Wilson, D.F.,1992, Monitoring of the oxygen pressure in the blood of live animals using the oxygen dependent quenching of phosphorescence, Adv. Exptl. Med. Biol. in press.

Phebus, L.A., Perry, K.W., Clemens, J.A., and Fuller, R.W., 1986, Brain anoxia releases striatal dopamine in rats, Life Sci. 38: 2447.

Pulsinelli, W.A., Waldman, S., Rawlinson, D., and Plum, F., 1982, Moderate hyperglycemia auguments ischemic brain damage: a neuropathologic study in the rat, Neurology, 32:1239.

Rehncrona, S., Rosen, I., and Siesjo, B.K., 1981, Brain lactic acidosis and ischemic cell damage. 1.Biochemistry and neurophysiology, J. Cereb. Blood Flow Metab., 1: 313.

Schurr, A., Dong, W-Q, Reid, K.H., West, C.A., and Rigor, B.M., 1988, Lactic acidosis and recovery of neuronal function following cerebral hypoxia in vitro, Brain Research, 438: 311.

Siemkowicz, E., and Hansen, A.J., 1978, Clinical restitution following cerebral ischemia and hypo-, normo-, and hyperglycemic rats, Acta Neurol. Scand., 58: 1.

Siverstein, F.S., and Johnson, M.V.,1984, Effects of hypoxia-ischemia on monoamine metabolism in the immature brain, Ann. Neurol. 15: 342.

Slivka, A., Brannan, T.T., Weinberger, J., Knott, P.J., and Cohen, G., 1988, Increase in extracellular dopamine in the striatum during cerebral ischemia: A study utilizing cerebral microdialysis, J. Neurochem. 50: 1714.

Vanderkooi, J.M., Maniara, G., Green, T.J., and Wilson,D.F., 1987, An optical method for measurement of dioxygen concentration based upon quenching of phosphorescence, J. Biol. Chem., 262: 5476.

Vulto, A.G., Sharp,T., Ungerstedt, U., and Versteeg, D.H.G., 1988, Rapid postmortem increase in extracellular dopamine in the rat brain as assessed by brain microdialysis, J. Neurochem., 51: 746.

Weinberger, J., Nieves-Rosa., and Cohen, G., 1985, Nerve terminal damage in cerebral ischemia: protective effect of alpha-methyl-para-tyrosine, Stroke, 16: 864.

Welsh, F.S., Sims, R.E., and McKee, A.E., 1983, Effect of glucose on recovery of energy metabolism following hypoxia-oligemia in mouse brain: dose dependent and carbohydrate specificity, J. Cereb. Blood Flow Metab., 3: 486.

White, E.J., and Clark,J.B., 1990,Involvement of lactic acidosis in anoxia-induced perturbations of synaptosomal function, J. Neurochem., 55: 321.

White,E.J., Juchniewicz, H.J., and Clark,J.B., 1989, Effects of lactic acidosis on the function of cerebral cortical synaptosomes, J. Neurochem., 52: 154.

Wilson, D.F., Rumsey, W.L., Green,T.J., and Vanderkooi, J.M., 1988, The oxygen dependence of mitochondrial oxidative phosphorylation measured by a new optical method for measuring oxygen concentration, J. Biol. Chem. 263: 2712.

THE INFLUENCE OF PROFOUND HYPOTHERMIA AND REWARMING ON PRIMATE CEREBRAL OXYGEN METABOLISM

P. W. McCormick,[1] J. M. Zabramski,[2]
J. McCormick,[2] J. Kurbat[2]

[1]Department of Neurosurgery
St. Vincent's Hospital
Toledo, OH

[2]Division of Neurosurgery
Barrow Neurological Institute
Phoenix, AZ

INTRODUCTION

The repair and reconstruction of human blood vessels have great potential for altering the natural history of patients at risk for cerebral infarction.[1,2,5] The greater a patient's potential benefit from surgical intervention, however, the greater is the risk of surgical morbidity.[3,4] The central problem is that oxygen delivery to the brain must be compromised before the vessel can be repaired, and the available collateral blood supply is poor in sicker patients.

Cooling the central nervous system (CNS) before cerebral oxygen delivery is interrupted protects against ischemic injury.[6] Cooling the CNS to temperatures below 20° C has regained popularity as a surgical adjunct.[7,11] At these lower temperatures cerebral oxygen demand is reduced, thereby decreasing the likelihood of injury if oxygen delivery ceases temporarily.

The relationship between cerebral oxygen extraction and brain temperatures below 20° C has not been evaluated scientifically in humans or subhuman primates. Furthermore, how rewarming the brain from very cold temperatures influences cerebral metabolism has yet to be studied. This report describes the influence of brain temperatures between 2° and 20° C on cerebral oxygen extraction in subhuman primates during both cooling and rewarming.

METHODOLOGY

Three adult baboons (25 kg) were anesthetized with intravenous pentobarbital and xylazine. They were intubated and an arterial and jugular bulb catheter were placed.

Femoral-femoral bypass was used to allow extracorporeal oxygenation and cooling of the animal's blood. Brain parenchymal temperature was measured using a customized thermocouple placed in the right frontal gray matter. Brain temperature was lowered from 20° C to 2° C and subsequently rewarmed. Arterial and cerebral mixed venous blood were sampled simultaneously. Arterial blood was taken from the femoral artery, and cerebral mixed venous blood was taken by slow aspiration from the right jugular bulb catheter. The sampled blood was analyzed immediately on a co-oximeter for arterial and cerebral venous oxygen saturation. The lactic acid content of each sample was also measured. Global cerebral oxygen extraction was calculated as the arterial-venous oxygen content difference. Global cerebral lactate production was calculated as the venous-arterial lactate difference. These values were normalized to a baseline normothermic, anesthetized value.

Cooling to less than 15° C damages circulating plasma proteins and formed blood elements. Consequently, the baboons underwent partial exchange-transfusion to store whole blood for use in the rewarming process. The blood was exchanged-transfused during cooling with a dextran saline solution on a volume for volume basis.

After being rewarmed, the baboons were sacrificed by lethal injection of potassium chloride.

RESULTS

No technical difficulties in cooling the animals were encountered. Rewarming rates were variable. Brain temperature lagged behind core body temperature as measured by an esophageal thermometer during cooling and rewarming. After rewarming all three animals had a clinically obvious coagulopathy despite efforts to preserve and recirculate fresh whole blood.

During cooling, cerebral oxygen extraction dropped progressively below 20° C. Brain parenchymal temperature and cerebral oxygen extraction were positively correlated (Fig. 1). Although cerebral temperatures as low as 2° C were reached, measurable cerebral oxygen extraction continued. This finding indicates that a "critical temperature" below which cerebral oxygen metabolism ceased cannot be achieved clinically in baboons.

Rewarming led to increases in cerebral oxygen extraction. There was a weak positive correlation between brain parenchymal temperature and oxygen extraction (Fig. 2). At a given temperature in the 2-20° C range, oxygen extraction was greater during rewarming than cooling (Fig. 3). On one occasion, cerebral lactate production occurred in all three animals during cooling but was common during rewarming in all the animals (Fig. 4).

CONCLUSION

Cerebral ischemic injury is ameliorated by hypothermia.[6,7,8,9] The proposed mechanism is that cerebral oxygen consumption is lowered by hypothermia. The brain can therefore tolerate reduced oxygen delivery transiently. This mechanism has recently been challenged, but there is no doubt that cerebral oxygen consumption decreases with temperature (Fig. 1).[12,13] In some animal models, a brain temperature of 20° C is associated with an 80% drop in cerebral oxygen extraction and a marked increase in the half-life of high energy phosphates.[8,9]

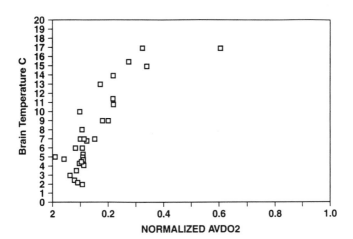

Figure 1. Normalized cerebral arterial-venous oxygen difference as a function of cerebral parenchymal temperature during cooling.

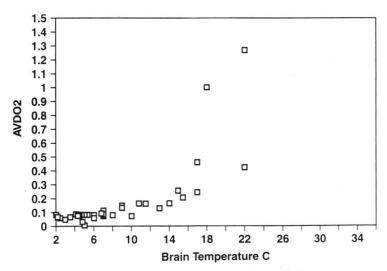

Figure 2. Cerebral arterial-venous oxygen difference as a function of brain parenchymal temperature during warming.

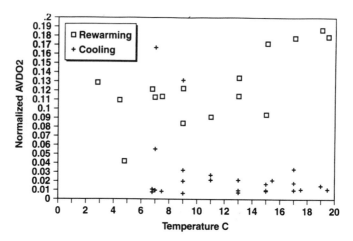

Figure 3. Normalized cerebral arterial-venous oxygen difference as a function of brain temperature during rewarming and cooling. Note that oxygen extraction is greater at any given temperature during rewarming.

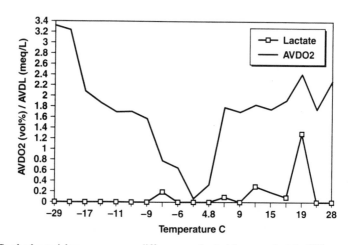

Figure 4. Cerebral arterial-venous oxygen difference and arterial-venous lactate difference as a function of brain temperature in one animal. Cerebral lactate production occurred predominantly during rewarming in all animals.

An important point suggested by the above work and emphasized by this report is that a so-called "critical temperature," below which cerebral oxygen metabolism stops, does not exist at clinically obtainable temperatures (i.e., brain temperature of 2° C). Because significant (30% of anesthetized, normothermic baseline) cerebral oxygen extraction continues at the clinically obtainable brain temperatures of 15-18° C, cessation of cerebral oxygen delivery will cause an oxygen availability consumption mismatch is if lasts long enough. This mismatch will cause anaerobic metabolism and lactic acidosis will ensue.

The predictable limitations of cerebral hypothermic protection are suggested by the availability-consumption mismatch paradigm. No matter how far cerebral temperature is lowered, in the clinical realm, hypoxic protection will be time dependent. We have previously outlined these theoretical consequences of a "residual oxyhemoglobin reserve" in nonperfused cerebral tissue.[10]

Another important issue in clinical hypothermic cerebral ischemic protection is cerebral rewarming. This portion of the equation has not yet been addressed adequately. The data presented here indicate that cerebral oxygen utilization is much less influenced by temperature during rewarming than during cooling. Furthermore, at any given brain temperature, oxygen consumption is significantly greater during rewarming than during cooling.

The accentuated cerebral oxygen metabolism during rewarming creates a tremendous opportunity for a mismatch between oxygen delivery and utilization. Indeed, multiple episodes of cerebral lactic acid production were documented during the rewarming phase.

Our laboratory investigations on the metabolic demands of cerebral oxygen during rewarming are preliminary and ongoing. Nevertheless, it is plausible that re-establishment of ionic gradients across cellular and organelle membranes in neuronal and glial cells accounts for increased oxygen utilization during rewarming. These gradients, which are necessary for normal function, are energy dependent and deteriorate rapidly when cerebral oxygen delivery is low.

As minimally invasive technologies for measuring human cerebral oxygen metabolism become more available, it should be possible to sustain cerebral hypothermic protection for a longer period by using multiple episodes of transient circulatory arrest under hypothermic conditions. This procedure will maintain aerobic respiration and preserve cellular ionic hemostasis.

REFERENCES

1. North American Symptomatic Carotid Endarterectomy Trial Collaborators, Beneficial effect of carotid endarterectomy in symptomatic patients with high-grade carotid stenosis, *N Engl J Med* 325:445 (1991).
2. P.W. McCormick, F. Tomecek, J. McKinney, J.I. Ausman, Disabling cerebral transient ischemic attacks, *J Neurosurg* 75:891 (1991).
3. R.M. Sundt, Jr., B.A. Sandok, J.P. Whisnant, Carotid endarterectomy, Complications on preoperative assessment of risk, *Mayo Clin Proc* 50:301 (1975).
4. F.B. Meyer, T.M. Sundt, Jr., D.G. Piepgras, et al., Emergency carotid endarterectomy for patients with acute carotid occlusion and profound neurologic deficits, *Ann Surg* 203:82 (1986).

5. P. W. McCormick, R.F. Spetzler, J.D. Bailes, J.M. Zabramski, J.L. Frey, Thrombo-endarterectomy of the symptomatic occluded internal carotid artery, *J Neurosurg* 76:752 (1992).

6. J. O'Conner, T. Wilding, P. Farmer, J. Sher, M. Ergin, R. Griepp, The protective effect of profound hypothermia on the canine nervous system during one hour of circulatory arrest, *Ann Thorac Surg* 41:255 (1986),

7. R.F. Spetzler, M. Hadley, D. Rigamonti, L. Carter, P. Raudzens, S. Shedd, E. Wikinson, Aneurysms of the basilar artery treated with circulatory arrest, hypothermia, and barbiturate cerebral protection, *J Neurosurg* 68:868 (1988).

8. J. Tanaka, K. Shiki, T. Asou, H. Yasui, K. Tokunaga, Cerebral autoregulation during deep hypothermic nonpulsatile cardiopulmonary bypass with selective cerebral perfusion in dogs, *J Thorac Cardiovasc Surg* 95:124 (1988).

9. R. Stocker, N. Herschkowitz, E. Bossi, M. Stoller, T. Cross, W. Ave, J. Seelig, Cerebral metabolic studies in situ by 31 P-nuclear magnetic resonance after hypothermic circulatory arrest, *Pediatr Res* 20:867 (1986).

10. P.W. McCormick, M.C. Stewart, G.D. Lewis, J.M. Zabramski, Optical Imaging of Brain Function and Metabolism, Plenum Press, London (1992).

11. P.W. McCormick, G. Balakrishnan, M. Stewart, G. Lewis, J.I. Ausman, Cerebral oxygen metabolism measured during hypothermic circulatory arrest: A case report, *J Neurosurg Anesthesiol* 3:302 (1991).

12. T. Suno, J.C. Drummond, P.M. Patel, M.R. Grafe, J.C. Watson, D.J. Cole, A comparison of the cerebral protective effects of isoflurane and mild hypothermia in a model of incomplete forebrain ischemia in the rat, *Anesthesiology* 76:161 (1992).

13. M.M. Todd, D.S. Warner, A comfortable hypothesis reevaluated, *Anesthesiology* 76:161 (1992).

NON-INVASIVE CEREBRAL OXYGEN MONITORING AND INTRACELLULAR REDOX

STATE DURING SURFACTANT ADMINISTRATION

Hubert Fahnenstich and Stephan Schmidt*

Department of Neonatology
and Department of Gynecology and Obstetrics*
University of Bonn
Adenauerallee 119, 5300 BONN, FRG

INTRODUCTION

By introducing surfactant replacement therapy in clinical routine, the spectrum of treating respiratory distress syndrome in infants (IRDS) could be dramatically improved (Segerer and Obladen, 1990). However, there are still a lot of open questions regarding its action on oxygen supply to the brain, cerebral hemodynamics and intracellular redox state.

Some studies are done according to changes of blood flow and blood flow velocities (Vidyasagar and Shimada, 1987) while giving surfactant. Results remain partly controversial (McCord et al., 1988; Jorch et al., 1989). We focused on changes in oxygen monitoring with a new technique called near infrared spectroscopy (NIRS) (Jöbsis, 1977), which was recently introduced in clinical research (Brazy et al., 1985, Schmidt et al., 1989).

The aim of this study was to monitor cerebral changes in oxy- and deoxyhemoglobin and in the intracellular redox state during and after surfactant application in premature infants suffering form IRDS. In addition, we looked for similarities and differences in oxygen monitoring between transcutaneous pO_2 and NIRS.

PATIENTS AND METHODS

14 premature infants suffering from IRDS were examined. All of those received surfactant supplementation for the first time in a dose of 100 mg/kg body weight. FiO2 was up 0.6 and chest x-ray showed severe hyaline membrane disease. Gestational ages ranged from 25 to 33 weeks (mean 28) and birth weight from 680 g to 1400 g (mean 950 g).
A bovine lung surfactant preparation was used (Alveofact[R]).

All infants were continuously monitored using combined

transcutaneous oxy- and capnometry, pulsoxymetry, heart rate and respiration rate. For the near infrared monitoring we used a prototype from Radiometer[R], Copenhagen. Blood pressure and blood gas analyses were drawn sporadically.

NIRS was applied in the transmission mode that means light enters the infant's head in the temporal region at one side and is collected at the opposite side. Light is generated by laser diodes in 4 different wavelengths of 775, 805, 845 and 904 nm. Fiber optics conduct the light from the generating side of the instrument to the head and back from the head to a photomultiplier. Depending on intracerebral absorbance of light, the connected personal computer calculates changes in oxy-, deoxyhemoglobin and oxidized cytochrome (Rea et al., 1985). Parameters are displayed on the screen and by a plotter, respectively. Values were given in an arbitrary scale expressed as $mmolxl^{-1}xcm$ and then could be converted into absolute quantities expressed as $mmolxl^{-1}$ or $mmolx100g^{-1}$ brain weight (Delpy et al., 1988).

RESULTS

Data from 11 out of 14 patients could be evaluated for all monitored parameters. In the other cases movement artefacts or a low signal to noise ratio in the NIRS examination made an evaluation impossible.

Figure 1 shows an example with typical traces in an infant with severe IRDS. Transcutaneous pO2 and intracerebral oxyhemoglobin react very similar: Immediately after surfactant instillation both parameters decrease, reaching a lower limit and afterwards rise to a high limit. The difference of both traces is revealed in a time delay of oxyhemoglobin in comparison to the transcutaneous signal. In spite of early FiO2 reduction in some patients pO2 reached absolute transcutaneous values above 100 mmHg, although the ventilator settings for oxygen were reduced as transcutaneous pO2 went above 70 mmHg.

In most patients oxidized cytochrome showed no changes. However in three infants slight variations could be found (Fig. 2): An initial decrease as well as a subsequent increase afterwards, according to changes of oxyhemoglobin and transcutaneous pO_2. Corresponding characteristic features of all those patients were high oxygen demand with an FiO_2 0,8 to 1.0 and birthweights below 1 kg. Chest x-ray showed a grade IV hyaline membrane disease.

Just after deconnecting the infant from the ventilator and by surfactant application cutaneous pCO_2 increased in nearly every patient. Not all traces returned to the former pCO_2 levels and remained on a slight higher level; the highest differences were about 10 mmHg. In regard to systolic and diastolic pressure, mean arterial blood pressure and heart rate, respectively, no changes could be detected.

DISCUSSION

Intratracheally surfactant application has a profound influence on oxy- and deoxyhemoglobin in brain. An initial rise in deoxyhemoglobin is a consequence of the bolus application. The air passages were obstructed by the fluid for a period up to three minutes. Although the clinical relevance is not known, the bolus instillation should be avoided. The procedure of

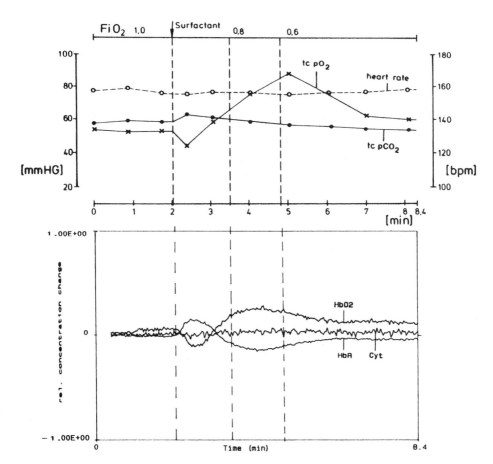

Figure 1. Continuously monitored parameters during surfactant replacement therapy: Oxyhemoglobin (HbO$_2$), deoxyhemoglobin (HbR), cytochrome a/a$_3$ (Cyt), transcutaneous pO$_2$ and pCO$_2$ (tc pO$_2$, tc pCO$_2$) and heart rate.

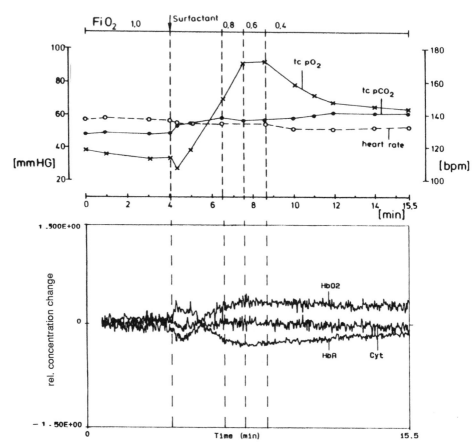

Figure 2. The cytochrome a/a_3 trace decreases just after applying surfactant and returns about 90 seconds later to the base line.

applying surfactant could be replaced by a continuous instillation through double-lumen tubes.

Increasing oxyhemoglobin in brain tissue is of benefit for neonates in a hypoxic condition, but may be harmful to the retina, especially for premature babies. As graphically demonstrated (Fig. 1 and 2), in some cases oxyhemoglobin remained on a higher level than before surfactant application. Therefore the question arises, whether it is possible that surfactant supplementation therapy could be a factor in the retinopathia of prematurity?

As the last step in the oxidative energy metabolism the oxidized cytochrome a/a3 reflects the intracellular redoxstate. In most cases no changes could be seen in the cytochrome signal after surfactant replacement. This reflects the high affinity of the enzyme to oxygen, not only in vitro (Oshino et al., 1974) but also in vivo (Jöbsis, 1972).

However, a few children showed a little decrease after surfactant instillation and also later, correlating with the oxyhemoglobin increase. We speculate that there is a difference in the affinity to oxygen between in vitro and in vivo and that the intracranial oxygen tension of these patients is at the threshold, where the intracellular redox-state is altered.

There are still some open and controversial questions according to the method of near infrared spectroscopy, mostly focused on the cytochrome signal, while the oxy- and deoxyhemoglobin is recognized as valid (Pryds et al., 1990). The good correlations between transcutaneous pO_2 measurements and the NIRS support these results.

Because of some assumptions and limitations to calculate absolute quantities (Delpy et al., 1988), we prefer to give the values as relative changes expressed as $mmol \times l^{-1} \times cm$ in this paper.

REFERENCES

Brazy JE, Lewis DV, Mitnick MH, Jöbsis vander Vliet FF: Noninvasive monitoring of cerebral oxygenation in preterm infants: preliminary observations. Pediatrics 75:217-225 (1985).

Delpy, DT, Cope M, van der Zee P, Arridge S, Wray S, Wray J: Estimation of optical pathlength through tissue from direct time of flight measurement. Phys Med Biol 33:1433-1442 (1988).

Jöbsis FF: Oxidative metabolism at low PO_2. Fed Proc 31:1404-1413 (1972).

Jöbsis FF: Noninvasive, infrared monitoring of cerebral and myocardial oxygen sufficiency and circulatory parameters. Science 198:1264-1267 (1977).

Jöbsis-Vandervliet FF: Near infrared monitoring of cerebral cytochrome c oxidase: Past and present (and future ?), in: Fetal and neonatal physiological measurements, HN Lafeber, ed., pp. 41-55, Excerpta Medica, Amsterdam (1991).

Jorch G, Rabe H, Garge M, Michel E, Gortner L: Acute and protracted effects of intratracheal surfactant application on internal carotid blood flow velocity, blood pressure and carbon dioxide tension in very low birth weight infants. Eur J Pediatr 148:770-773 (1989).

McCord B, Halliday HL, McClure G, Reid MC: Changes in pulmonary and cerebral blood flow after surfactant treatment for severe respiratory distress syndrome, in: Surfactant replacement therapy, ed. B Lachmann, pp. 195-200, Springer, Berlin (1988).

Oshino N, Sugano T, Oshino R, Chance B: Mitochondrial function under
    hypoxic conditions: The steady states of cytochrome a + a_3 and
    their relation to mitochondrial energy states. Biochem Biophys Acta
    368:298-310 (1974).
Pryds O, Greisen G, Skov LL, Friis-Hansen B: Carbon dioxide related changes
    in cerebral blood flow in mechanically ventilated preterm neonates.
    Comparison of near infrared spectrophotometry and [133]Xenon
    Clearance. Pediatr Res 27:445-449 (1990).
Rea PA, Crowe J, Wickramasinghe Y, Rolfe P: Non-invasive optical methods
    for the study of cerebral metabolism in the human newborn: a
    technique for the future? J Med Eng Technol 9:160-169 (1985).
Schmidt S, Lenz A, Eilers H, Helledie N, Krebs D: Laser spectrophotometry
    in the fetus. J Perinat Med 17: 57-62 (1989).
Segerer H, Obladen M: Surfactant substitution treatment of neonatal
    respiratory distress syndrome. Pediatric Rev Commun 5:67-82 (1990).
Vidyagasar D, Shimada S: Pulmonary surfactant replacement in
    respiratory distress syndrome. Clin Perinatol 14:991-1015 (1987).

RESOLUTION OF NEAR INFRARED
TIME-OF-FLIGHT BRAIN OXYGENATION IMAGING

David A. Benaron and David K. Stevenson

Medical Spectroscopy and Imaging Laboratory Section
Neonatal and Developmental Medicine Laboratory
Stanford University School of Medicine
Stanford, California, U.S.A. 94305

INTRODUCTION

Near-infrared spectroscopy (NIRS) is an emerging technique for continuous, noninvasive bedside monitoring of tissue structure, oxygenation, and blood flow. It relies upon the relationship that variations in the concentration of light-absorbing oxygen-carrying pigments produce proportional changes in the way these proteins absorb light, and that such variations in concentration, as well as variations in tissue structure, affect the path of light through tissue. NIRS has already been shown to be a nonionizing, relatively safe form of radiation that functions well as a medical probe, [1-13] with red and near-infrared light passing easily through structures such as the skull,[2,3] penetrating deeply into many tissues,[4-6] and well tolerated in large doses.[7] Thus, variations in light absorbance and scattering at different wavelengths can be used to deduce concentration of physiologic intermediates of deep tissues such as the brain, provided that the distance light has traveled though the tissue between emission and detection is known, and to deduce tissue structure, provided that the path of the light through the tissue is known.

Recent advances in the ability to produce and measure near-infrared (NIR) light passing through tissue has led to an explosion in the number of such medical NIR applications under development. In our laboratory, we have been using a picosecond time-of-flight and absorbance (TOFA) near-infrared multi-wavelength spectro-photometer[14] to study the potential of such optical-based imaging and quantitation. We have imaged the interior of scattering bodies, both inanimate model systems[14] as well as mammals,[14,15] and have produced images of whole animals in which major organs are visible. In humans, we are using a similar approach to locate and define intracranial bleeding in critically ill infants.[15] We have measured the resolving power of such a system to be 1-2 mm in premature neonatal brain, and better than this in adult breast.[16] Lastly, we are investigating approaches to measure cerebral blood volume, cerebral blood flow, and arterial and venous saturation, parameters useful in the detection and treatment of diseases related to problems in the delivery of oxygen to tissue.

In this report, we discuss several active areas of our research, and present data from ongoing experiments. We address measurement issues and imaging issues separately, though a combination of imaging and quantitation approaches will ultimately yield additional information by allowing regional problems to be identified spatially.

QUANTITATION

Basis for Quantitation of Oxygenation

As with all forms of optical oximetry, quantitative measurement of pigments such as hemoglobin *in vitro* using NIRS is based upon the principle that changes in the absorbance of light (ΔA) are related to changes in concentration (ΔC) by Beer's Law ($A = \varepsilon CL$), where L is the distance light has traveled through the medium (called the optical path length) and ε is a constant called the extinction coefficient.[8,17,18] *In vivo*, however, Beer's Law is inaccurate due to additional light losses caused by light scattering, though it may serve as a starting point. Temporal variations in absorbance, caused by changes in the optical spectrum of certain proteins as the partial pressure of oxygen varies,[19] have been used to estimate changes in oxygenation in the extremities,[11-13,17,20,21]

Oxygen Transport to Tissue XV, Edited by P. Vaupel
et al., Plenum Press, New York, 1994

heart,[22] and brain,[1,23,24] as well as to measure local blood volume and flow.[25-27] Estimates can be quantitative when the distance light travels through the tissue is known.[9,28]

Oxygen-sensitive NIRS differs from pulse oximetry in that NIRS can be used to independently measure oxygenation in the arteries, veins, and small blood vessels via hemoglobin spectroscopy, or to measure oxygen sufficiency within the cell via cytosolic and/or mitochondrial cytochrome spectroscopy, or both. Sensitivity to oxygen-carrying pigments gives NIRS techniques the potential to measure hemoglobin oxygen saturation ($HbO_2\%$), cellular and mitochondrial cytochrome aa3 oxygenation state ($CytO_2$), cerebral blood flow (CBF), and cerebral blood volume (CBV). Therefore, NIRS holds promise as early warning and monitoring systems for impending and existing hypoxic injuries.[9,25,26,29-32]

In theory, NIRS techniques such as niroscopy[1] and regional cerebral spectroscopy[23] allow quantitation of changes in concentration of nearly any substance in the body that absorbs light, though current work has focussed upon oxygen carrying pigments, glucose, lipids, and cholesterol. Widespread clinical use has been delayed, however, because conversion of the optical signals into quantitative measurements has been problematic.

Optical Path Length - The Third Variable

In the past, quantitative NIRS has been based upon assumptions that the distance light travels through tissue, called the optical path length (L), is constant among subjects and independent of the wavelength of light used. Concentration, or changes in concentration, could then be determined from measurements at several wavelengths by solving multiple equations for multiple unknowns. A constant optical path length cancels out in ratios of concentrations, such as when calculating percentage hemoglobin saturation via pulse oximetry.[18] Other NIRS methods use a predicted value for L, estimated *a priori* from either animal models[5] or the geometry of the emitter and detector.[33] Errors in either that estimated value of L, or errors regarding the stability of L, can result in inaccurate estimates of absolute pigment concentration.

In order to assess the magnitude and variability in optical path length *in vivo*, we studied transcranial optical path length in 34 infants, aged 1 day to 3 years, using phase-modulated spectroscopy at 754 nm and 816 nm.[10] Optical transcranial path lengths (mean ± SE) were 8.58 ± 0.88 cm, 11.13 ± 0.85 cm, and 11.34 ± 0.93 cm at 754 nm, and 8.76 ± 0.90 cm, 11.20 ± 0.79 cm, and 11.13 ± 0.91 cm at 816 nm, using emitter-detector separations of 1.8, 2.5, and 3.0 cm, respectively. Optical path length decreased as emitter-detector separation, head circumference, or age decreased. Significantly, the ratio of two path lengths at different wavelengths of the light (a measure of wavelength independence), was within 20% of unity for only two-thirds of infants, and ranged from 0.5 to 3.2 in the remaining patients, confirming that path is not independent of wavelength.[15] We could not account for all variability in optical path length using the parameters we recorded, nor by the error of measurement. Our observations raise questions about the accuracy of quantitative NIRS methods based upon assumed or estimated optical path lengths, and suggest 1) NIRS instrument configuration, patient age, and head size, and wavelength each influence optical path length, 2) that accurate quantitative measurements in clinical use may require concurrent measurement of both absorbance and optical path length at each wavelength, and 3) that the current difficulty of performing quantitative NIRS measurements may be related to uncorrected path errors in the method currently used to determine concentration.

Variability in optical path length may give rise to considerable error in the calculation of cerebral oxygenation in some infants if both absorbance and path length are not contemporaneously measured at each wavelength. Substituting a two-fold difference between optical paths at different wavelengths (a range observed in about 10% of the infants studied) into equations for the determination of saturation from optical measurements could result in an over- or under- estimate of the relative concentration of one of the hemoglobin pigments by two-fold. With an estimated venous blood hemoglobin saturation of 66%, a two-fold error could change measured saturation to as low as 50% or as high as 80%. As the lower and upper limit saturations require different clinical responses, use of pigment concentration determinations using algorithms based upon assumed optical path lengths may be of limited value.

Possible sources of such variability in optical tissue path length include the known variations in the optical characteristics among the brains of different infants,[34] the local gross topological irregularity of the convoluted brain surface, and the changes in path length that occur during changes in pigment concentration. Delpy *et al.* describe a characteristic differential path length factor (DPF), a relatively constant ratio between the measured optical path length and emitter-detector separation for a given tissue, reported as 3.85 ± 0.57 (mean ± S.D.) for the brain of living infants,[35] and 4.39 ± 0.28 for the brain of post-mortem infants.[8] Thus, cranial DPF for living infants is expected to be between 2.73 and 4.99 for 95% of all living infants tested, and similar to the DPF's we measured (4.81 at 1.8 cm, 4.47 at 2.5 cm, and 3.75 at 3.0 cm). Delpy and colleagues report that variability in DPF decreases as emitter-detector spacing increases, particularly once over 5 cm,[36] presumably reflecting a lessening of the influence of local irregularities in brain structure at the larger emitter-detector separations. However, persistent variability in DPF was found even at wide emitter-detector separations. Therefore, the behavior of light in tissue with regard to path length is complex and remains difficult to predict. Use of standardized algorithms using predicted or estimated optical path lengths in order to quantitatively solve for hemoglobin oxygen saturation and cytochrome oxygenation is likely to result in limited accuracy due to the presence of outliers, unless optical path length is measured, not estimated, at each wavelength.

Patterson[37] and others[38,39] have analyzed the effects of scattering from tissue upon light, and found the behavior to be complex. Their theoretical calculations predict that the length of the paths traveled by light in tissue will exceed the separation between the emitter and detector, even if the tissue is very thin, a prediction confirmed in this study.

Other studies support the view that L is not constant. Optical path length varies with pigment concentration, which has been used to monitor oxygenation changes in piglets,[9] and spatially with variations in tissue structure, which has been used to form images of phantoms and tissue.[14,15,36,40] At the microscopic level, low-coherence interferometry,[41-43] the measurement of interference patterns between two reflected light signals caused by inequalities in optical paths due to scattering, has been used to image retinal structures down to 2 μm in tissues 2 mm thick.[44] Photon path has also been shown to vary with tissue state, such as with changes in hemoglobin concentration with changing tissue oxygenation. Falling oxygen levels cause more deoxygenated hemoglobin to form, increasing absorption at some wavelengths. At those wavelengths, far-traveling photons have a greater chance of encountering the additional deoxygenated hemoglobin than do the short-traveling photons. Thus, a rise in absorption increases the probability that highly scattered photons will become absorbed far more than it increases that probability for the minimally-scattering photons, and the average photon path will decrease. There is also theoretical support for the wavelength dependence of optical path length.[45] Thus, optical path length cannot be considered a constant.

Concurrent Measurement of Absorbance and Path Length

While quantitative NIRS has been an elusive goal when optical path length is assumed but not measured, the combination of path length and absorbance measurements has allowed quantitation of central cerebral venous saturation changes in the brain of infants undergoing cardiac arrest during open heart cardiac surgery.[9,28] This provides further evidence that there is value in measuring, and not estimating, optical path length at each NIRS wavelength used.

Application of such technology to patient care may facilitate the quantitative measurement of oxygenation in organs not currently accessible to study, potentially allowing early-warning of impending or existing ischemic-hypoxic injury, and thus holds exciting clinical potential.[46] Once problems related to quantitation have been solved, possible clinical forms for such a device include an ultrasound-like probe that would yield noninvasive saturation images for such tests as noninvasive brain oximetry, noninvasive heart catheterizations producing images of ventricular and muscle wall oxygenation, and maternal transabdominal fetal saturation monitors. Currently, several groups are now introducing real-time continuous path measurements to their absorbance measurements. The goals of such measurements, as defined during the Workshop on Near-Infrared Spectroscopy held by the National Institutes of Health[47] are listed in Table I.

IMAGING

Basis for Imaging

Images of the interior of living bodies can be formed using x-ray tomography,[48] magnetic resonance,[49] ultrasound,[50] positron-emission,[51] thermal-emission,[52] electrical impedance,[53] and other probes. Each of these methods has drawbacks that limit use as a continuous, noninvasive, nondestructive monitor for living organ-

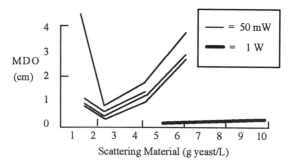

Figure I. Relationship of minimum detectable object size (MDO) and amount of scattering, plotted at different threshold limits from 1-50%. Detection is worst with average path (50% threshold) and low peak power (50 mW), and best at 1% threshold and high power (1 W). Neonatal brain is approximated by 10 g/L yeast, while breast is equivalent to 5 g/L yeast.

isms.[14] Light-based tissue imaging is possible because variations in absorption and scattering over space and time influence photon travel though tissue. For example, tumors frequently differ from neighboring tissues by attenuating light to a greater degree, possibly due to the presence of a plentiful supply of blood vessels and high concentrations of mitochondria.[7,11-13] Such, spatial variations in absorbance have been used to form transillumination "shadowgrams" of tumors,[11-13] to detect cerebral bleeding,[54] and to reconstruct steady-state tomographs of two-dimensional structure.[55,56]

However, optical imaging of tissue has been difficult to achieve because light is strongly scattered by tissue, producing a wide range in the paths taken by, and the time required for, photons to traverse the tissue. As opposed to conventional radiological methods in which photon travel is linear, scattering produces highly irregular photon paths that degrade image quality, much as detail is lost with distance in a fog. Scattering is also the major attenuator of transmitted photon intensity in tissue.[57] The average photon travels less than 100 μm into tissue before scattering,[58] and multiple scattering events occur for virtually all photons propagating through tissue[58-60] Simple models for this diffusive behavior resemble molecular diffusion equations, while more accurate treatments consider that light scattering has a forward-weighted anisotropy.[58]

Path-Resolved Approaches

The potential use of light as a noninvasive imaging tool for visualizing oxygenation or structure within scattering systems such as the brain has led to a search for methods that are fast and of good resolving power. Time-resolved optical methods, in which photon transit time affects the image, were first suggested in 1971,[61] and fall broadly into two categories: either all photons are imaged, and the image is mathematically reconstructed from delays experienced by a group of photons as they travel between emitter and detector, or the "ballistic" photons (those passing through tissue without scattering[58]) are imaged, and thus photon path is linear and conventional radiological analysis applies. Reconstruction approaches have yielded images using both real and ideal data, but are computation-intensive and slow,[62,63] while the rarity of unscattered photons in tissue precludes true ballistic imaging.

Ballistic photon imaging is made possible by the collection of minimally-scattering "snake" photons, which are orders of magnitude more common than ballistic photons,[40] and has been used to image phantom objects through chicken breast several millimeters thick and other scattering media,[40,64,65] to collect light through portions of a fish body,[66] and to improve optical localization of the bony portions of fingers.[67] The advantages of the ballistic approach are that images are easily generated by integrating the linearly-traveling photons over time, that increases in absorption improve resolution,[67] and that the photons respond to the vast array of standard optics techniques developed for other linear-traveling photon systems.[68]

We have focussed upon the time-resolved technique of time-constraint,[14,18] which measures only a constant, early fraction of detected photons. In theory, the further light travels through tissue, the more likely that the light has diffused randomly and contains little spatial information. Thus, optical variation of the tissue directly between the emitter and detector disproportionately affect the intensity and transit time of these early-arriving photons, and changes in this transit time can be used as an imaging variable. The model for such photon behavior in the simplest forms has been standard diffusion equations, such as for heat transfer, while at the more complex level considers that light does not diffuse randomly though tissue, but rather has a forward-weighted anisotropy.[58]

Table II. Effect of Various Factors on Resolution

Increased Factor	Effect upon Resolution
Media scattering (μ_s)	Varies
Media absorbance (μ_a)	Varies
Object size (r_o)	Enhances
Object contrast ($\Delta\mu$) Enhances	
Obj. acentricity ($\Delta_{eo} - \Delta_{od}$)	Degrades
Emit-detect separation (r_{ed})	Degrades
No. of emitters/detectors (n_{ed})	Enhances
Pulses counted (n_p) Enhances	
Laser power (I_p)	Enhances
Pulse width (t_p)	Degrades
Pixel size (r_{pix})	Degrades
Threshold percent ($t_\%$)	Varies

Imaging is divided into two functions: 1) detection (e.g., whether an object is present or not, which is relevant to detection of strokes, intraventricular hemorrhages, and tumors), and 2) localization (e.g., the ability to localize one or more structures to the appropriate boxels, which is relevant to image construction). We constructed a picosecond time-constrained time-of-flight and absorbance (tc-TOFA) spectrophotometer[14] to study such optical-based detection and localization.

Object Detection

We defined a detection algorithm to determine the minimal detectable object (MDO), the smallest object identified as being present with 95% confidence. In a model system in which the relative photon transit delay (y) caused by different diameter objects (x), the MDO is defined by the following formula:

$$MDO = \bar{x} - \frac{\bar{y} - t\,\hat{\sigma}A^{\frac{1}{2}}}{\hat{\beta}\,(1-\varepsilon)}, \text{ with } A = \frac{1-\varepsilon}{n} + \frac{\bar{y}^2}{\hat{\beta}^2\,SSE_x}, \varepsilon = \frac{t\,\hat{\sigma}^2}{\hat{\beta}^2\,SSE_x}, \text{ and } \sigma^2 = \frac{SSE_x}{n-2},$$

where β is the slope of a linear regression in the form of $y = \beta x + \alpha$, barred values are group means, hatted values are estimates, SSE_x is the sum of squared errors between estimated and actual values, and t is the t-statistic for a two-tailed 95% confidence interval for n samples and n-2 degrees of freedom. A smaller MDO implies improved resolution. By varying scattering instead of object size as the x variable, the maximum amount of scattering that allows detection of a given sized object is also determinable using this equation. Results of one such determination, based upon detecting 100% absorptive objects submerged centrally in a 100 mm cube containing yeast in water (a model for neonatal brain) are shown (Fig. 2). The fraction of photons imaged varies from 1% to 50%. Based upon these model data, time-constraint appears to allow detection of solid, 100% absorbing objects as small as 1-2 mm in diameter in neonatal brain, and less than this in adult breast tissue, and the approach offers superior resolution to pure ballistic or all-photon approaches. Since this study, algorithm changes have improved resolution to less than 1-2 mm for neonatal brain. Some types of brain bleeding should be clearly detectable in vivo, and imaging of such events should be possible at this level. Living tissue contains many light absorbers, and image resolution should be enhanced during times of increased tissue absorbance.[66] In addition, resolution is affected by multiple other factors (Table II).

In critically ill infants, illnesses producing maldistributions of heme in the brain are being studied.[15] After human studies approval and parental informed consent obtained, we studied infants with intraventricular hemorrhage (bleeding in the brain), measuring at multiple skull locations, to see if presence of bleeding can be identified. Using a comparison of path and absorbance on one side of the head versus the other, superficial bleeding (subdural hematomas, cephalohematomas) can be easily identified, and some instances of intraventricular bleed are detectable as well.

Object Localization

We first tested two-dimensional imaging capability using inanimate objects (e.g., a soft-sided lunch box)[15] and organic matter (e.g., an olive suspended in blood).[14] In both cases, image resolution was encouraging. Three-dimensional reconstruction was then demonstrated using a milk-filled acrylic cube measuring 50 mm on a side, in which plastic Helvetica numerals, "O" and "I", were attached. Using an automated mechanical stage, the cube was moved between the emitter and detector, until a series of collections had been obtained over the entire face of one side of the cube. Three such measurements were made, using three faces of the cube, mutually orthogonal to one another. A fourth plane of measurement was also performed at an angle offset 45 degrees from each of the previous planes of measurement. A three-dimensional reconstruction was performed by constructing a three-dimensional matrix by computer. For each cell in this three dimensional matrix, the value was determined by the product of the threshold delays from each of the planar images at the point that the emitter-detector axis would have passed through each of the planar images. False color was assigned and the images were recorded on film. In planar reconstruction at the level of the "I", an image of the "I" was clearly visible while the "O" was not (not shown).

Three-dimensional reconstructions were then applied to animals.[15] First, an expired rat pup was suspended in blood and imaged in an anterior-posterior planar fashion. Images were generated from calculated threshold times, assigned gray-scale values, and captured on film. An image of total absorbance without time resolution was unrevealing, showing only greater delays in the thicker portions of the body, whereas the TOFA threshold image reveals major organs: heart, liver, spleen/pancreas, and intestinal gas. The locations of these organs and gas patterns correlate with x-ray and autopsy findings. Images from rodents have also been obtained by other groups using different optical methods.[69]

Next, human infant heads were imaged.[15] There were significant lateralized, regional differences in absorbance for infants with superficial hematomas (subdural or bony). The findings were less apparent with deep intracranial (intraventricular) bleeding, but still often detectable in small infants (< 1 kg). Our results demonstrate that time-constrained TOFA allows imaging in scattering media such as intact animals, and supports the power of path-sensitive over absorbance-sensitive approaches to tissue imaging.

Comparison of Current Time-Resolved Imaging Approaches

Both time-resolved and frequency-resolved techniques have been shown to be useful path-sensitive approaches in image reconstruction and in subsurface object detection, and both approaches yield theoretically equivalent data related by Fourier-transform.[70] In the frequency domain, Chance et al. pioneered multi-frequency phase-modulated spectrophotometry,[54] in which phase shifts related to the average delays experienced by photons traveling through tissue are measured as a function of modulation frequency. Sevick[71] has shown that such an approach allows detection of subsurface structure and control over depth of focus. An interesting variation is that of Gratton et al., who use phased arrays as a probe, similar to the approach used in ultrasound.[72-74]

Other laboratories, including ours, have focused on time-resolved approaches. Using images reconstructed mathematically from time-of-flight curves taken at multiple locations, Delpy et al. have been able to demonstrate two- and three-point structure resolution, and recently reduce computation time to less than twenty minutes under carefully controlled starting conditions.[75-77] There are also strong parallels with impedance imaging techniques.[77] We have favored time-domain approaches as a path length is determined for each detected photon, rather than the ensemble averages determined by frequency-domain approaches. However, it remains unclear at this time which method will prove superior in the future, and it is likely that each will have strong points that will support use under certain clinical conditions.

GOAL: COMBINATION OF IMAGING AND MEASUREMENT

At present, the medical tools for the evaluation of neurologic function are inadequate for the early detection of brain injury caused by a lack of oxygen, and therefore identification of the nature and timing of these injuries is likely to lead to health-saving and life-saving intervention. Quantitative optical measurement of deep-tissue oxygenation, first proposed by Jöbsis,[1] is possible if the distribution of path lengths is known. The combination of a quantitative measurement with a spatial localization will be central to the development of a noninvasive, continuous imaging monitor based upon NIR technology. Algorithms are being considered to allow simultaneous imaging and calculation of tissue oxygenation in three-dimensions. Fields in which such a tool may be presently sufficiently developed to be of use include:

Fetal Monitoring

A fetus in the womb presents a monitoring dilemma. On one hand, access is difficult and attempts to obtain information about the fetus can result in injury from the monitoring process itself (e.g., hemorrhage after blood drawing, infection or premature birth after amniotic fluid sampling). On the other hand, infants are born with neurologic disease, due in part to deficiencies in oxygen delivery to portions of the brain during some phase of development or labor. A superior monitoring technique could potentially reduce the frequency of such injuries. The exact timing of fetal neurologic injury remains unclear, as no direct method exists to measure sufficiency of oxygen delivery to the fetus. Identification of the nature and timing of these injuries could lead to life-saving intervention and the development of tools to avoid such injuries, if possible. Current methods of evaluating a fetus include listening with a stethoscope and external electronic heart rate monitoring,[78] but these are unreliable.[79] Some fetuses exhibit a normal heart rate while undergoing severe injury, while others have abnormal heart rate patterns leading to an emergency surgical delivery, when the infant was actually experiencing no actual difficulty. The result is a 25% rate of surgical delivery in the United States, without a significant decline in the rate of infants born with neurologic injury.[80] What is needed is a better tool for assessing fetal oxygen delivery, and an optical tool may fill this need by providing both oxygenation measurement and metabolic evaluation.

Pulse Gated Imaging

Measuring system spatial variation in absorbance that occurs with systolic arterial pulsations may allow quantitative imaging of arterial, and perhaps venous, saturation, similar to the manner as performed in pulse oximetry only now as an image. Such a tool would be valuable as a fetal monitor, but also useful for intensive care, emergency room, and anesthetic management.

Neonatal Cerebral Monitoring

During the perinatal/neonatal period, infants are at high risk for neurologic injury. Currently, in the intensive care environment, decisions are made as to maintenance or reduction of support, which carries the benefit of less iatrogenic injury, versus escalation of support, which carries the benefit of less immediate neurologic injury. In many cases, the ideal situation would be to be able to monitor the delivery of oxygen to the critical organs (heart, brain, kidney) to better assess the correct level of care to provide. Physicians often err on the side of too much support, for fear of doing injury from doing too little. The problem is that too high a level of support often is equally damaging or fatal, particularly in the case of premature or sick infants who must be supported in the most optimal manner in order to produce the best long-term outcome. Currently, there is no tool to evaluate infants at risk for early injury due to oxygenation problems. Although, in the past, it has been unclear how much of NIR absorption occurs at the level of the brain, and how much occurs at the level of the scalp. Studies by McCormick et al.[81] suggest that much of the signal is from the brain, while studies by Kurth et al.[82] support this view by demonstrating that transcranial path length does not change appreciably in piglets after the removal of the skull. Thus, it is likely that the majority of the NIRS signal reflects oxygenation within the brain itself, and use of such a probe may therefore have particular benefit to critically ill newborn infants. Non path-resolved approaches have been used to image body oxygenation,[83] and path resolved approaches should improve upon these images.

CONCLUSIONS

Light-based imaging, though still in its infancy, is rapidly becoming a reality and may become a powerful clinical imaging and measurement tool. We have extended the technique of optical imaging using time-constrained time-of-flight and absorbance analysis, capable of producing whole-body images of animals and objects *in situ*. An advantage of our approach is the simplicity of the calculations, as each pixel is independent of neighboring ones, allowing on-the-fly computation. With such a device, blood flow and oxygenation may be measured in a spatial fashion. Other potential applications include noninvasive diagnosis of blood clots, diagnosis and management of heart dysfunction, imaging of stroke or cerebral hemorrhage, and metabolite monitoring. Spectral discrimination could allow remote identification of tumor or neural tissue by type, of fresh blood clot from old, frozen from untreated tissue in tumors undergoing cryotherapy, or even detailed spectrographic chemical analysis. Light-based imaging may also permit diffusometry,[72] the characterization of tissue and tissue components based upon optical properties. Lastly, development of clinically relevant model systems will allow comparison between, and standardization of, different optical imaging techniques. Ideally, the combination of a quantitative measurement with a spatial localization will be central to the development of a clinical tool based on this technology. It is likely that several clinical conditions could currently benefit from such optical devices, even without further technological breakthroughs, including fetal and neonatal monitoring. As a result, the medical potential of a combined quantitation and imaging NIR tool is believed to be great.

ACKNOWLEDGEMENTS

Supported through NIH RR-00081, the Walter and Idun Berry Fellowship Fund for Human Development and the Zaricor Family Fund at Stanford. Portions of this review have appeared in print earlier.

REFERENCES

1. F.F. Jöbsis, Noninvasive infrared monitoring of cerebral and myocardial oxygen sufficiency and circulatory parameters, *Science* 198:1264-6 (1975).
2. P.W. McCormick, M. Stewart, G. Lewis, M. Dujovny, and J.I. Ausman, Intracerebral penetration of infrared light, J. Neurosurg. 76:315-8 (1992).
3. C.D. Kurth, presented at NIH workshop on near-infrared spectroscopy, D. Hirtz, Chairperson, April 1992.
4. B. Chance, Comparison of time-resolved and -unresolved measurements of deoxyhemoglobin in brain, Proc. Natl. Acad. Sci. 85:4971-5 (1988).

5. D.T. Delpy, M. Cope, P. van der Zee, S.R. Arridge, S. Wray, and J.S. Wyatt, Estimation of optical pathlength through tissue from direct time of flight measurement, *Phys. Med. Biol.* 33:1433-42 (1988).
6. L.O. Svaasand and R. Ellingsen, Optical properties of human brain, *J. Cereb. Blood Flow Metabol.* 3:293-9 (1983).
7. J.C. Hebden and R.A. Kruger, Transillumination imaging performance: a time-of-flight imaging system, *Med. Phys.* 17:351-6 (1990).
8. J.S. Wyatt, et al., Measurement of optical pathlength for cerebral near infrared spectroscopy in newborn infants, *Dev. Neurosci.* 12:140-4 (1990).
9. D.A. Benaron, *et al.*, Non-invasive estimation of cerebral oxygenation and oxygen consumption using phase-shift spectrophotometry, *Proc. IEEE Eng. Med.* Biol. 12,:2004-7 (1990).
10. D.A. Benaron, *et al.*, Optical path length of 754nm and 816nm light emitted into the heads of infants, *Proc. IEEE Eng. Med. Biol.* 12:1117-9 (1990).
11. B. Drexler, J.L. Davis, and G. Schofield, Diaphanography in the diagnosis of breast cancer, *Radiology* 157:41-4 (1985).
12. V. Marshall, D. C. Williams, and K .D. Smith, Diaphanography as a means of detecting breast cancer, *Radiology* 150:339-43 (1984).
13. G.A. Navarro and A.E. Profio, Contrast in diaphanography of the breasts, *Med. Phys.* 15:181-87 (1988).
14. D.A. Benaron, M.A. Lenox, and D.K. Stevenson, Two-D and three-D images of thick tissue using time-constrained time-of-flight and absorbance (tc-TOFA) spectrophotometry, *SPIE* 164:35-45 (1992).
15. D.A. Benaron, unpublished.
16. D.A. Benaron, Noninvasive measurement and imaging of tissue structure and oxygenation using time-of-flight absorbance (TOFA) spectroscopy, *Proc. IEEE Eng. Med. Biol.* 14:2402-4 (1992)
17. G.A. Millikan, The oximeter, an instrument for measuring continuously the oxygen saturation of arterial blood in man, *Rev. Sci. Instrum.* 13:434-44 (1942).
18. D.A. Benaron, W.E. Benitz, R.A. Ariagno, and D.K. Stevenson, Noninvasive methods for estimating in vivo oxygenation, *Clinical Pediatrics* 31:258-73 (1992).
19. These proteins include: hemoglobin, myoglobin, mitochondrial cytochrome aa₃, cytosolic cytochrome oxidase, and other copper- or iron-containing proteins.
20. M. Ferrari, Q. Wei, L. Carraresi, R.A. DeBlasi, and G. Zaccanti, Time-resolved spectroscopy of human forearm, *J. Photochem. Photobiol.*, in press.
21. Y. Kakihana and M. Tamura, Near-infrared optical monitoring of cardiac oxygen sufficiency through thoracic wall without open-chest surgery, *SPIE* 1431:14-20 (1991).
22. C.M. Alexander, L.E. Teller, and J.B. Gross, Principles of pulse oximetry: theoretical and practical considerations, *Anesth. Analg.* 68:368-76 (1989).
23. P.W. McCormick, *et al.*, Noninvasive cerebral optical spectroscopy for monitoring cerebral oxygen delivery and hemodynamics, *Crit. Care. Med.* 19:89-97 (1991).
24. J.E. Brazy, D.V. Lewis, M.G. Mitnick, and F.F. Jöbsis, Monitoring of cerebral oxygenation in the intensive care nursery, *Adv. Exp. Med. Biol.* 191:843-7 (1986).
25. J.S. Wyatt, A.D. Edwards, D. Azzopardi, and E.O.R. Reynolds, Magnetic resonance and near infrared spectroscopy for investigation of perinatal hypoxic-ischaemic brain injury. Arch. Dis. Child. 1989:64:953-63.
26. J.S. Wyatt, *et al.*, Quantitation of cerebral blood volume in human infants by near-infrared spectroscopy, *J. Appl. Physiol.* 68:1086-91 (1990).
27. A.D. Edwards *et al.*, Effects of indomethacin on cerebral haemodynamics in very preterm infants, *Lancet* 335:1491-95 (1990).
28. C.D. Kurth, J.M. Steven, S.C. Nicolson, B. Chance, and M. Delivoria-Papadopoulos, Kinetics of cerebral deoxygenation during deep hypothermic circulatory arrest in neonates, *Anesthesiology*, in press.
29. P.W. McCormick, M. Stewart, M.G. Goetting, and G. Balakrishnan, Regional cerebrovascular oxygen saturation measured by optical spectroscopy in humans, *Stroke* 22:596-602 (1991).
30. J.E. Brazy, D.V. Lewis, M.H. Mitnick, and F.F Jöbsis, Noninvasive monitoring of cerebral oxygenation in newborn infants by near-infrared transillumination, *Pediatrics* 75:217-25 (1985).
31. A.D. Edwards, *et al.*, Cotside measurement of cerebral blood flow in ill preterm infants by near-infrared spectroscopy, *Lancet* ii;770-1 (1988).
32. A.D. Edwards, *et al.*, Effects of indomethacin on cerebral haemodynamics in very preterm infants, *Lancet* 335:1491-5 (1990).
33. D.T. Delpy, *et al.*, Quantitation of pathlength in optical spectroscopy, *Adv. Exp. Med. Biol.* 248:41-6 (1989).
34. B. Chance, Early detection of brain ischemia and hemorrhage by optical methods, *SPIE* 1641:162-9 (1992).
35. P. Van der Zee, et al., Experimentally measured optical pathlengths for the adult head, calf, and forearm and the head of the newborn infant as a function of inter optode spacing. *Adv. Exp. Med. Biol.* (in press).
36. D.T. Delpy. presented at the NIH Workshop NIR Spectroscopy, D. Hirtz, Chairperson, NIH, April 1992.
37. M.S. Patterson, Time resolved reflectance and transmittance for the non-invasive measurement of tissue optical properties, *Appl. Optics* 28:2331-6 (1989).
38. R.F. Bonne, Model for photon migration in turbid biological media, *J. Opt. Soc. Am.* 4:423-32 (1987).
39. P. van der Zee and D.T. Delpy, Computed point spread functions for light in tissue using a measured volume scattering function, *Adv. Exp. Med. Biol.* 1988;222:191-7.
40. L. Wang, P.P. Ho, G. Zhang, and R.R. Alfano, Ballistic 2-D imaging through scattering walls using an ultrafast optical Kerr gate, *Science* 253:769-71 (1991)
41. H.H. Gilgen, R.P. Novak, and R.P. Salathe, *J. Lightwave Tech.*, 7:1225 (1989).
42. A.F. Fercher, K. Mengedoht, and W. Werner, *Opt. Lett.*, 13:186 (1988).
43. R.C. Youngquist, S. Carr, and D.E.N. Davies, *Opt. Lett.*, 12:158 (1987).
44. D. Huang, *et al.*, Optical coherence tomography, *Science* 254: 1178-81 (1991).
45. Essenpreis, *et al.*, Spectral dependence of temporal point spread functions in human tissues, *Appl. Optics*, in press.
46. M. Cope P. van der Zee, M. Essenpreis, S.R. Arridge, D.T. Delpy, Data analysis methods for near infrared spectroscopy of tissue: problems in determining the relative cytochrome aa₃ concentration. *SPIE 1431*:251-62. (1991).
47. NIH Workshop on Near-Infrared Spectroscopy, D. Hirtz, chairperson. National Institute of Neurological Diseases and Stroke, National Institutes of Health, Chevy Chase, Maryland, April 1992.
48. G.N. Hounsfield, Computerized transverse axial scanning (tomography), *Br. J. Radiol.* 46:1016-47 (1973).
49. R. Damadian, M. Goldsmith, and L. Minkoff, *Physiol. Chem. Phys.* 9:97 (1977).
50. J.J. Wild and J.M. Reid, Application of echo-ranging techniques to the determination of structure of biological tissues, *Science* 115:226-30 (1952).
51. G.D. Hutchins *et al.*, A one-dimensional multigated time-of-flight acquisition system, *IEEE Trans. Nucl. Sci.* NS32:835-42 (1985).
52. A.M. Gorbach and E.N. Tsicalov, Visualization of processes in the brain cortex: a new method, *Proc.. IEEE Eng. Med. Biol. Soc.* 12:1245-6 (1990).
53. J.C. Newlee, D.G. Gisser, and D. Isaacson, *Proc. IEEE Trans. Biomed. Eng.* 35, 828 (1988).
54. B. Chance, Early detection of brain ischemia and hemorrhage by optical methods, *SPIE* 1641:162-9 (1992).
55. J.R. Singer, F.A. Grünbaum, P. Kohn, and J.P. Zubelli, Image reconstruction of the interior of bodies that diffuse radiation, *Science* 248:990-3 (1990).
56. R. Araki and I. Nashimoto, Near-infrared imaging in vivo: imaging of Hb oxygenation in living tissues, *SPIE* 1431:321-32 (1991).
57. B.C. Wilson, M.S. Patterson, S.T. Flock, and D.R. Wyman, in: *Photon Migration in Tissue*, B. Chance, Ed. (Plenum, New York, 1989).
58. S.T. Flock, B.C. Wilson, and M.S. Patterson, Total attenuation coefficients and scattering phase functions of tissues and phanton materials at 633nm, *Med. Phys.* 14: 835-41 (1987).
59. M.S. Patterson, B. Chance, and B.C. Wilson, Time-resolved reflectance and transmittance for the noninvasive measurement of tissue optical properties, *Appl. Opt.* 28:2331-6 (1989).

60. K.M. Yoo and R.R. Alfano, Time-resolved coherent and incoherent components of forward light scattering in random media. *Opt. Lett.* 15:320-22 (1990).
61. M.A. Duguay and A.T. Mattick, Ultrahigh speed photography of picosecond light pulses and echoes, *Appl. Opt.* 10: 2162-70 (1971).
62. F. H. Schlereth, J. A. Fossaceca, A. D. Keckler, and R. L. Barbour, Imaging in diffusing media with a neural net formulation: a problem in large scale computation, *SPIE* 1641:46-57 (1992).
63. R.L. Barbour *et al.*, Imaging of diffusing media by a progressive iterative backprojection method using time-domain data, *SPIE* 1641:21-34 (1991).
64. J.C. Hebden, R.A. Kruger, and K.S. Wong, Time resolved imaging through a highly scattering medium, *Appl. Optics* 30:788-94 (1991).
65. K.M. Yoo, F. Liu, and R.R. Alfano, Imaging through a scattering wall using absorption, *Opt. Lett.* 16:1068-70 (1991).
66. L. Wang, Y. Liu, P.P. Ho, and R. R. Alfano, Ballistic imaging of biomedical samples using picosecond optical kerr gate, *SPIE* 1431:97-101 (1991).
67. S. Andersson-Engels, R. Berg, and S. Svanberg, Time-resolved transillumination for medical diagnostics, *Opt. Lett.* 15:1179-81 (1990).
68. R.R. Alfano, paper presented at the Science/Innovation 1992 conference, sponsored by the American Association for the Advancement of Science, San Francisco, CA, July 1992.
69. E. Gratton, personal communication.
70. J. R. Lakowicz, G. Laczko, H. Cherek, E. Gratton, and M. Limkeman, Analysis of fluorescence decay kinetics from variable-frequency phase shift and modulation data, *Biophys. J.* 46:463-77 (1984).
71. E.M. Sevick, presented at the NIH workshop on near-infrared spectroscopy, Chevy Chase, MD, April 1992.
72. B. Chance, presented at the NIH Workshop on Near-Infrared Spectroscopy, Chevy Chase, MD, April 1992.
73. F. Fishkin, E. Gratton, M.J. vandeVen, and W.W. Mantulin, Diffusion of intensity modulated near-infrared light in turbid media, *SPIE* 1431:122-35 (1991).
74. A. Knüttel, J. M. Schmitt, and J. R. Knutsen, *App. Opt.*, in press (1992).
75. S. R. Arridge, P. van der Zee, M. Cope, and D. T. Delpy, Reconstruction methods of infrared absorption imaging, *SPIE* 1431:204-15 (1991).
76. D. T. Delpy, presented at the NIH Workshop on Near-Infrared Spectroscopy, Chevy Chase, MD, April 1992.
77. R.R. Alfano, personal communication.
78. P.J. Placek, K.G. Keppel, S.M. Taffel, and T.L. Liss, Electronic fetal monitoring in relation to cesarean delivery, for live births and stillbirths in the US, 1980, *Public Heal. Rep.* 99:173-83 (1980).
79. K.K. Shy, *et al.*, Effects of electronic fetal-heart-rate monitoring, as compared with periodic auscultation, on the neurologic development of premature infants, *New. Engl. J. Med.* 322:588-93 (1990).
80. D.A. Luthy, *et al*, A randomized trial of electronic fetal monitoring in preterm labor, *Obstet. Gynecol.* 69:687-95 (1987).
81. P.W. McCormick, M. Stewart, G. Lewis, M. Dujovny, and J.L. Ausman, Intercerbral penetration of light, *J. Neurosurg.* 76:315-8 (1992).
82. C.D. Kurth, J.M. Steven, D.A. Benaron, B. Chance, Near-infrared monitoring of the cerebral circulation, *J. Clin. Mon.*, in press.
83. I. Oda, et al., Noninvasive hemoglobin oxygenation monitor and computed tomography by NIR spectrophotometry, *SPIE* 1431:284-93 (1991).

MEASUREMENT OF CHANGES IN CEREBRAL HAEMODYNAMICS DURING INSPIRATION AND EXPIRATION USING NEAR INFRARED SPECTROSCOPY

C.E. Elwell, H. Owen-Reece[*], M. Cope, A.D. Edwards[*], J.S. Wyatt[*], E.O.R. Reynolds[*], D.T. Delpy

Departments of Medical Physics and Paediatrics[*] .
University College London, U.K.

INTRODUCTION

Near infrared spectroscopy (NIRS) has been employed over the last decade to monitor the changes in tissue oxygenation of intact organs (Jobsis 1977, Brazy et al. 1985, 1986, Ferrari et al. 1986a, 1986b, Hampson et al. 1988, Reynolds et al. 1988). Quantification of cerebral blood flow (CBF) and cerebral blood volume (CBV) using this technique has been described in both neonates and adults (Edwards et al. 1988, Wyatt et al. 1990, Elwell et al. 1992). An NIRS instrument is now commercially available (NIRO 500, Hamamatsu, Japan) which is capable of measuring the changes in the concentration of cerebral oxy - and deoxyhaemoglobin ([HbO$_2$] and [Hb]) at a rate of 2 Hz. This has allowed the detailed investigation of the haemodynamic effects of respiratory and cardiac manoeuvres over the period of one breath.

Pulsus paradoxus describes the changes in mean arterial blood pressure (MAP) and cardiac output (CO) seen on inspiration and expiration (Weatherall et al. 1987). The effect is accentuated in patients with increased airways obstruction (e.g. asthma, positive expiratory pressure ventilation). It would be expected that autoregulatory responses to fluctuations in MAP would act to maintain a constant cerebral blood flow so that the cerebral circulation would not be influenced by cardiovascular changes. Current methods of measuring cerebral haemodynamics involving the use of ionising radiation can provide high spatial resolution but are less able to provide information about the temporal changes in [HbO$_2$] and [Hb] over short time periods (<10s).

The purpose of this study was to use NIRS to investigate whether, in healthy adults, the cardiovascular changes known to occur with ventilation against an increased expiratory pressure (IEP), are reflected in the cerebral circulation. The magnitude and nature of the cerebral haemodynamic changes seen with ventilation in 6 healthy adult volunteers are presented, and possible explanations for these observations are discussed.

THEORY

NIRS

The details of NIRS have been discussed fully elsewhere (Cope et al. 1988, Cope 1991). Briefly, the technique depends upon the relative transparency of biological tissue to light in the infrared region allowing the measurement of absorption by the chromophores oxyhaemoglobin (HbO_2) and deoxyhaemoglobin (Hb). A modified Beer-Lambert law which describes optical attenuation in a highly scattering medium (Delpy et al. 1988) can be used to quantify the changes in the concentration of these chromophores. This can be expressed as:

$$Attenuation(OD) = \log\frac{I_o}{I} = \alpha c L B + G \tag{1}$$

where OD represents optical densities, I_0 the incident light intensity, I the detected light intensity, α the absorption coefficient of the chromophore ($mM^{-1}.cm^{-1}$), c the concentration of chromophore (mM), L the physical distance between the points where light enters and leaves the tissue (cm), B a "pathlength factor" which takes into account the scattering of light in the tissue and G a factor related to the geometry of the tissue. If measurements are only made of the *changes* in attenuation, then L, B and G can be assumed to remain constant and *changes* in chromophore concentration can be derived from the expression:

$$\delta c = \frac{\delta OD}{\alpha L B} \tag{2}$$

The absorption coefficients of HbO_2 and Hb have been deduced from lysed blood (Wray et al. 1988). The pathlength factor, B, has been measured in the adult head by time of flight studies to have a mean value of 5.93 ± S.D. 0.42 (van der Zee et al. 1992).

In this paper the term Hb_{diff} will be used to represent the difference between the [HbO_2] and [Hb] signals and the term Hb_{sum} to represent the sum of the two signals.

Physiology

Both heart rate (HR) and stroke volume are subject to changes on inspiration and expiration. These are mediated by neural and mechanical mechanisms. The resulting variations in cardiac output are synchronous with the ventilatory rate.

During inspiration the diaphragm moves downwards and intrathoracic pressure falls. This pressure drop is transmitted via the thin walls of the low-pressure right heart to the whole right sided circulation, whereas the thick walled left ventricle, as a high pressure system, remains largely immune to the change. Venous return to the right side of the heart increases, so the amount of blood pumped onwards into the pulmonary circulation increases.

Thus, while the pressure in the left ventricle changes very little, the pressure in the pulmonary circulation becomes more negative and blood 'pools' in the lungs reducing the blood flow from the lungs into the left heart. This effect is magnified by pulmonary vasodilation. Stroke volume falls, heart rate does not rise fast enough to compensate and cardiac output falls for the duration of the inspiration.

On expiration, the rise in intrathoracic pressure is again transmitted to the right sided circulation. This effect is enhanced when an expiratory resistance is applied. The blood in the pulmonary circulation is "squeezed" out of the lungs into the left heart and the stroke volume increases. The heart rate does not entirely compensate and so the cardiac output rises.

DATA COLLECTION

The subjects for this study comprised six healthy adult males (age range 25-44, median 27) with no known respiratory or cardiovascular disorders.

Instrumentation and Procedure

Near infrared light was carried to and from the NIR spectrometer (NIRO 500, Hamamatsu Photonics KK, Japan) through fibre optic bundles. The optodes were positioned high on the left side of the forehead 4 - 5 cm apart. The exact position of the optodes was dependent upon the level of the hairline in each subject, but did not vary more than ±1 cm (Figure 1). The optodes were held in position with double sided adhesive rings and self adhesive tape, and the head was then wrapped in black cloth to reduce background light. Pulsed laser diodes produced light at four wavelengths (779, 821, 855, 908 nm) and a photomultiplier tube was employed for detection of transmitted light. Data were collected every 0.5 second and the changes in concentration of HbO_2 and Hb were calculated using a previously established algorithm (Wray et al. 1988).

The cuff of a non invasive continuous blood pressure monitor (Finapress 2300, Ohmeda, USA) was placed on the second finger of the left hand which was kept stationary at the level of the heart. The monitor, working in beat to beat mode, recorded both mean arterial pressure (MAP) and the heart rate (HR). A transcutaneous blood gas electrode

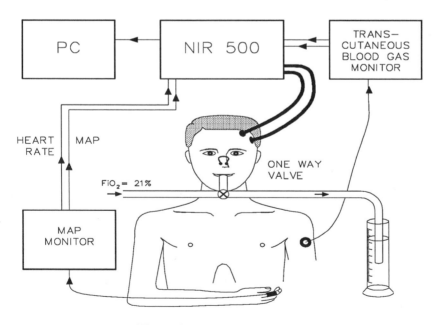

Figure 1 . Experimental Setup.

(Novametrix 850, USA) was placed on a fleshy part of the upper left arm and was used to continuously monitor transcutaneous carbon dioxide tension ($TcPCO_2$). The analogue outputs of both the blood pressure and transcutaneous blood gas monitor were linked directly to the spectrometer for real time display and storage along with the NIRS data.

The breathing circuit comprised a mouthpiece and T piece with a one way valve on the expiratory side and the inspiratory arm left open to room air. The IEP was introduced into the circuit by placing the expiratory line under water in a measuring cylinder at a depth which was varied between 5 and 20 cmH_2O in 5 cm increments.

All subjects wore a noseclip and lay supine. They breathed room air initially against atmospheric pressure to familiarise themselves with the equipment and to provide baseline data. Once comfortable the expiratory arm was placed in the water and the subjects breathed against IEP of 5, 10, 15 and 20 cmH_2O, for approximately 2 minutes at each level. Respiratory rate was not experimentally controlled.

DATA ANALYSIS

Data were smoothed in software by applying a rolling average over three points. Data were inspected and after rejection of obvious artefact, three representative sections during the expiratory period were selected from each level of IEP, in all six subjects. Where possible three consecutive expiratory periods were chosen. Minima and maxima [HbO_2] were defined and the magnitude and direction of the changes in [Hb], [HbO_2], Hb_{sum}, and Hb_{diff}, between these points were calculated. Because of the difference in monitoring sites, a time offset of between 0.5 and 1.5 seconds was present between the MAP and NIRS data. This was accounted for in the calculation by defining the minima and maxima of the MAP trace independently from that of the NIRS data. The magnitude and direction of the changes in MAP and HR were then calculated (measured peak to peak), and in addition, the baseline MAP was calculated by taking the average MAP for the same time period. Δ[HbO_2], Δ[Hb], ΔHb_{sum}, ΔHb_{diff}, ΔMAP, ΔHR and baseline MAP were averaged for each level of IEP for all six subjects. The level of IEP was then correlated with both ΔHb_{sum} and ΔMAP.

RESULTS

Figure 2(a) shows the NIRS, MAP and HR data collected from one subject breathing against an IEP of 20 cmH_2O. The section of data between the two vertical lines is expanded in Figure 2(b) to highlight the changes seen during one breath. All traces commence at the start of expiration.

Table I shows the magnitude and direction of the changes recorded during expiration in the NIRS, MAP and HR data. Assuming a cerebral haemoglobin volume (CHV) of 84 $\mu mol.l^{-1}$ (Sakai et al. 1985) the changes in Hb_{sum} can be expressed as a percentage change in total cerebral haemoglobin volume. Likewise ΔMAP can be expressed as a percentage of the baseline MAP for the equivalent period. These percentage changes are shown in Table II.

The regression of ΔHb_{sum} (y) on the IEP level (x) for all points was $y = 19.6x - 4.1$; $r = 0.96$, and for ΔMAP (y_l) against IEP was $y_l = 1.3x - 8.9$; $r = 0.96$.

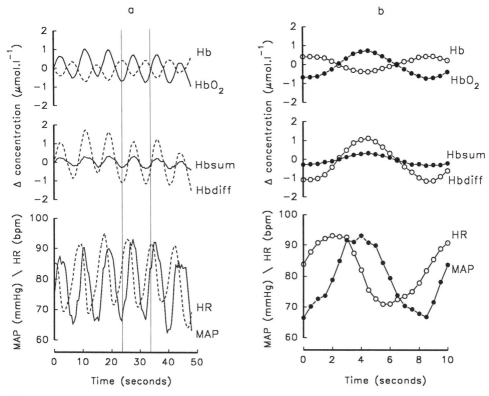

Figure 2 . (a) NIRS, MAP and HR data collected from one subject breathing against an IEP of 20 cmH$_2$O and (b) the same data expanded to show changes during one breath.

Table I . The mean changes in the NIRS, MAP and HR data recorded during expiration at each level of IEP on all subjects (mean ± S.D.).

IEP	Δ[HbO$_2$]	Δ[Hb]	ΔHb$_{sum}$	ΔHb$_{diff}$	ΔMAP	ΔHR
cmH$_2$O	μmol.l^{-1}	μmol.l^{-1}	μmol.l^{-1}	μmol.l^{-1}	mmHg	bpm
0	0.4 ± 0.1	0.0 ± 0.2	0.4 ± 0.2	0.6 ± 0.1	5.8 ± 2.9	3.3 ± 3.1
5	0.7 ± 0.4	-0.4 ± 0.3	0.4 ± 0.2	1.1 ± 0.7	13.7 ± 1.9	9.0 ± 5.3
10	1.0 ± 0.5	-0.5 ± 0.2	0.6 ± 0.4	1.5 ± 0.8	14.1 ± 2.8	12.8 ± 7.2
15	2.0 ± 1.3	-1.0 ± 0.8	1.0 ± 0.7	2.8 ± 2.0	18.9 ± 3.4	15.1 ± 6.3
20	2.3 ± 1.3	-1.1 ± 0.7	1.2 ± 0.7	3.5 ± 2.0	21.1 ± 4.9	17.1 ± 7.7

Table II . Percentage changes in CHV and MAP for each level of IEP (mean ± S.D.)

IEP (cmH$_2$O)	%ΔCHV	%ΔMAP
0	0.5 ± 0.3	6.2 ± 0.3
5	0.4 ± 0.2	14.5 ± 3.6
10	0.7 ± 0.5	15.7 ± 4.3
15	1.2 ± 0.8	19.3 ± 4.3
20	1.5 ± 0.9	21.9 ± 6.7

DISCUSSION

The changes in cerebral haemodynamics measured by NIRS were, on expiration, an *increase* in [HbO$_2$] accompanied by a smaller *decrease* in [Hb]. These changes were reversed on inspiration. The magnitude of these changes showed a strong correlation with the level of IEP.

[HbO$_2$] and [Hb] are calculated from the total absorption of NIR light within a field of view incorporating arterial, venous and capillary compartments. Although the changes in [HbO$_2$] and [Hb] can be separated, the relative contribution of the three compartments to the total signal cannot be measured. It is however possible to make some deductions concerning firstly the changes in cerebral blood volume and flow that occur during ventilation, and secondly which compartments contribute to the Hb$_{sum}$ signal.

Cardiovascular changes associated with expiration must be considered. In the venous circulation there is an increase in central venous pressure and hence intra-cranial pressure while the arterial changes described by pulsus paradoxus include an increase in MAP and cardiac output. It would be expected that these pressure changes would increase cerebral blood volume by a) distending the arterial part of the cerebral circulation and b) impeding venous return and promoting venous distension. However, if the observed increase in Hb$_{sum}$ was solely due to distention of the vessels then [HbO$_2$] and [Hb] would change in parallel. They do not, and if oxygen extraction is constant for this brief period, this can only be interpreted as alteration in CBF.

The decrease in [Hb] can be explained as an increase in CBF which, as well as increasing the delivery of arterial [HbO$_2$], effectively washes deoxygenated blood out of the venous compartment (approximately 30% of which is Hb). Although [HbO$_2$] and [Hb] can be expected to rise due to the increase in mean arterial and central venous pressure, the 'pulse' of increased MAP appears to be associated with a significant increase in CBF which overrides the volume effect, producing a net decrease in [Hb]. This explanation is supported by the correlation of the level of IEP with both Hb$_{sum}$ and MAP changes.

Depending upon the breathing rate of the subject the mean time taken for MAP to go from a minimum to a maximum was four seconds. There are few data documenting the time response of global (i.e. non microcirculatory) homeostatic control mechanisms in the cerebral circulation over such short time periods. Other quantitative non invasive methods of measuring changes in cerebral haemodynamics cannot achieve the temporal resolution necessary to detect the effects of transient changes in MAP and the cardiovascular system.

Laser doppler flowmetry is one technique which can continuously monitor changes in CBF, although absolute quantification of these changes is not yet possible. In a recent publication describing the time course of CBF during rapid hypovolaemic hypotension (Florence et al 1992), oscillations in CBF and MAP during baseline conditions can be seen which appear to be compatible with the respiratory linked changes we have observed, although they are not commented upon in the text.

The changes in Hb_{sum} observed are very small - on average 1% of total blood volume despite the increase in MAP with each level of IEP. These small changes are clearly reproducible and as such indicate the sensitivity of the NIRS technique for monitoring subtle changes in cerebral haemodynamics. It is interesting to note that since the adult skull is effectively a sealed box, the increase in blood volume observed can only be achieved by displacement of an equal volume of cerebrospinal fluid (assuming the tissues to be incompressible). Although there may be errors in both the latter assumption and in the conversion of $\Delta Hbsum$ to change in cerebral blood volume (Wyatt et al. 1990), this NIRS method may allow this parameter to be monitored.

CONCLUSION

We conclude that the increased temporal resolution now available with NIRS systems allows the near continuous monitoring of the cerebral haemodynamic effects of respiratory and cardiac changes during one breath. The data presented indicate that homeostatic mechanisms do not maintain CBF constant over short time periods (<10 seconds). Over these short time periods small respiratory linked changes in cerebral haemodynamics can be observed in the brain.

ACKNOWLEDGEMENTS

The authors are grateful to Matthias Essenpreis for his assistance in the preparation of this manuscript. This work has been supported by grants from the Wellcome Trust, the M.R.C., the S.E.R.C., the Wolfson Foundation and Hamamatsu Photonics KK.

REFERENCES

Brazy, J.E., Lewis, D.V., Mitnick, M.H., Jöbsis, F.F., 1985. Noninvasive monitoring of cerebral oxygenation in preterm infants: preliminary observations. *Pediatrics,* 75:217-225

Brazy, J.E., Lewis, D.V., 1986, Changes in cerebral blood volume and cytochrome aa3 during hypertensive peaks in preterm infants. *Pediatrics,* 108:983-987.

Cope, M., Delpy, D.T., 1988. A system for long term measurement of cerebral blood and tissue oxygenation in newborn infants by near infrared transillumination. *Med. Biol. Eng. & Comp.,* 26, 3:289-294.

Cope, M. 1991. The development of a near infrared spectroscopy system and its application for non invasive monitoring of cerebral blood and tissue oxygenation in the newborn infant. *PhD Thesis, University of London.*

Delpy, D.T., Cope, M., van der Zee, P., Arridge, S.R., Wray, S., Wyatt, J.S., 1988. Estimation of optical pathlength through tissue from direct time of flight measurement. *Phys. Med. & Biol.,* 33, 12:1433-1442.

Edwards, A.D., Wyatt, J.S., Richardson, C.E., Delpy, D.T., Cope, M., Reynolds, E.O.R.,

1988. Cotside measurement of cerebral blood flow in ill newborn infants by near infrared spectroscopy. *Lancet,* ii:770-771.

Elwell, C.E., Cope, M., Edwards, A.D., Wyatt, J.S., Delpy, D.T., Reynolds, E.O.R., 1992. Measurement of cerebral blood flow in adult humans using near infrared spectroscopy - methodology and possible errors. *Adv. Exp. Med. & Biol.* (in press).

Ferrari, M., De Marchis., Giannini. I., Nicola, A., Agostino, R., Nodari, S., Bucci, G., 1986a. Cerebral blood volume and haemoglobin oxygen saturation monitoring in neonatal brain by near infrared spectroscopy. *Adv. Exp. Med. & Biol.,* 200:203-212

Ferrari, M., Zanette, E., Giannini, I., Sideri, G., Fieschi, C., Carpi, A., 1986b. Effects of carotid compression test on regional cerebral blood volume, haemoglobin oxygen saturation and cytochrome-c-oxidase redox level in cerebrovascular patients. *Adv. Exp. Med. & Biol.,* 200:213-222.

Florence, G., Seylaz, J., 1992. Rapid autoregulation of cerebral blood flow: a laser-doppler flowmetry study. *J. Cereb. Blood Flow Metab.* 12(4):674-680

Hampson, N.B., Piantadosi, C.A., 1988. Near infrared monitoring of human skeletal muscle oxygenation during forearm ischemia. *J. Appl. Physiol.* 64 (6):2449-57.

Jöbsis, F.F. 1977. Noninvasive, infrared monitoring of cerebral and myocardial oxygen sufficiency and circulatory parameters, *Science,* 198:1264-1267.

Reynolds, E.O.R., Wyatt, J.S., Azzopardi, D., Delpy, D.T., Cady, E.B., Cope, M., Wray, S., 1988. New non-invasive methods for assessing brain oxygenation and haemodynamics. *Brit. Med. Bull.,* 44, 4:1052-1075.

Sakai, F., Nakazawa, K., Tazaki, Y., Ishii, K., Hidetada, H., Igarashi, H., Kanda, T., 1985. Regional cerebral blood volume and haematocrit measured in normal human volunteers by single-photon emission computed tomography. *J. Cereb. Blood Flow Metab,* 5:207-213.

van der Zee, P., Cope, M., Arridge, S.R., Essenpreis, M., Potter, L.A., Edwards, A.D., Wyatt, J.S., McCormick, D.C., Roth, S.C., Reynolds, E.O.R., Delpy, D.T., 1992. Experimentally measured optical pathlengths for the adult head, calf and forearm and the head of the newborn infant as a function of interoptode spacing. *Adv. Exp. Med. & Biol.* (in press)

Weatherall, D.J., Ledingham, J.G.G., Warrel, D.A., 1987. *Oxford Textbook of Medicine,* 2nd Edition, Oxford University Press, II:13.308

Wray, S., Cope, M., Delpy, D.T., Wyatt, J.S., Reynolds, E.O.R., 1988. Characterisation of the near infrared absorption spectra of cytochrome aa$_3$ and haemoglobin for the non invasive monitoring of cerebral oxygenation. *Biochim. Biophys. Acta,* 933:184-192.

Wyatt, J.S., Cope, M., Delpy, D.T., Richardson, C.E., Edwards, A.D., Wray, S.C., Reynolds, E.O.R., 1990. Quantitation of cerebral blood volume in newborn infants by near infrared spectroscopy. *J. Appl. Physiol.* 68, 3:1086-1091.

626

INCREASED CAPILLARY SEGMENT LENGTH IN CEREBRAL CORTICAL MICROVESSELS OF RATS EXPOSED TO 3 WEEKS OF HYPOBARIC HYPOXIA

Joseph C. LaManna[1], Boris R. Cordisco[1], Derek E. Knuese[2] and Antal G. Hudetz[2]

[1]Departments of Neurology, Physiology/Biophysics, and Neuroscience Case Western Reserve University, Cleveland, OH 44106, U.S.A.; and
[2]Department of Physiology, Medical College of Wisconsin, Milwaukee WI 53226, U.S.A.

INTRODUCTION

The common mammalian physiological response to moderate hypoxia, such as experienced with exposure to altitude up to about 5000m, initially includes increased ventilation and increased cerebral blood flow, followed by elevated hemoglobin concentration (Dempsey and Forster, 1982). We have previously shown that rats follow this usual pattern (Shockley and LaManna, 1988; LaManna et al., 1984; LaManna et al., 1989; LaManna et al., 1992; LaManna, in press). Rats adapt to moderate hypoxia by increased ventilation, increased blood hemoglobin and failure to gain weight (LaManna et al., 1992). For the brain, the most dramatic response to continued hypoxia was an increase in capillary density, resulting in decreased intercapillary distance achieved through angiogenesis that allows brain tissue oxygen diffusion flux to remain adequate. This structural plasticity is accompanied by functional changes as indicated by the increased glucose transporter density observed in the hypoxic adapted rat brain (Harik et al., 1991). The purpose of this present study was to begin to characterize any changes in the geometry of the microvascular capillary network resulting from hypoxic induced angiogenesis.

METHODS

Wistar rats (3 - 6 months of age) were kept in 2 hypobaric chambers, housed 3 to a cage, 1 cage per chamber, maintained at 380 torr (0.5 ATM) continuously for up to 3 weeks, except for 1 hour per day to feed and water and change the bedding. Littermate controls were kept in similar cages outside the chambers but in the same room.

Oxygen Transport to Tissue XV, Edited by P. Vaupel
et al., Plenum Press, New York, 1994

At the end of 3 weeks, control and hypoxic rats were anesthetized with ether in a bell jar until unresponsive to tail or foot pinch. The chest cavity was then quickly opened. A small incision was made in the apex of the left ventricle. A 16-gauge animal feeding tube was introduced through this incision into the aorta. The rats were then perfused through the aorta with a normal saline solution that contained 1 unit/ml heparin and 0.1% lidocaine at normal pressure. The descending aorta was clamped and the brain perfusion-fixed with 10% formalin. A syringe was used to perfuse the brain with 7% gelatin containing carbon black (30g india ink to 500ml gelatin) at 40 °C for 1-2 minutes. The rat head was then removed, immersed in fixative and kept overnight at 4 °C. The next day the brain was removed from the skull and stored in fixative.

The brains were transferred into phosphate buffer and cut serially into 500 micron coronal sections at room temperature using a vibratome. All sections were cleared in a series of glycerol-saline solutions from 50, 75, 90, and 100% over a period of about 8 weeks. Within the anterior cerebral cortex, 5 regions of interest were identified from a stereotaxic atlas (Palkovits and Brownstein, 1988) as frontal motor (FMC); frontopolar (FPC1 and FPC2); frontal sensory (FSC); parietal motor (PMC); and parietal sensory (PSC). Two sections per region of interest were selected from both the control and the hypoxic brains for measurement.

Within these regions of interest capillary segment length was measured from branch point to branch point using a PC-based image analysis system developed at the Medical College of Wisconsin. Sections were laid on a microscope slide and a cover slip was placed on the top. The carbon- black filled vascular network inside the cleared tissue section was imaged using a video microscope using transillumination and a long working distance (8mm) objective lens of 40X (NA = 0.5). The spatial course of each capillary segment was traced in the video image by moving a superimposed video

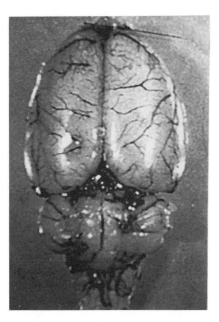

Figure 1. Surface view of control rat brain perfused with carbon black.

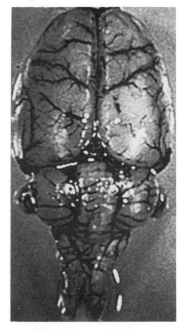

Figure 2. Surface view of a 3 week hypoxic rat brain perfused with carbon black.

cursor along the vessel as controlled by a mouse in the X and Y dimensions. The Z coordinate (i.e., depth below the surface of the sample) along the course of each vessel was assessed by optical sectioning, that is, by adjusting the elevation of the microscope stage to focus on the vessel section currently being traced. As a result, all X, Y, and Z coordinates along the segments were stored by the computer, and the true three-dimensional length of each segment was calculated from the coordinates following calibration with a stage micrometer.

Vessel tracing was started at the depth of the cortex about halfway between the cortical surface and the underlying white matter. For each region of interest, the measurement was limited to a coronal sectional area of 0.5 mm^2 centered around the starting point. From there, vessel segments were traced in all directions at random. Only segments with clearly identified terminating branch points were traced. At least 111 and as many as 280 segments were measured in each section.

Segment length data were compiled into frequency distribution histograms which were found to be similar and lognormal for all regions of interest in the control brain. This was less evident for certain regions of the hypoxic brain for which a shift from short to long lengths was suggested. Because the distributions were not normal, comparisons between the mean capillary segment lengths of the normal and hypoxic brains were made by the Mann-Whitney test for significance ($p < .05$).

RESULTS

The gross appearance of a control rat brain perfused with carbon black gelatin is shown in Figure 1, that of an hypoxic brain is shown in Figure 2. The hypoxic brain clearly has more carbon black filled vessels even in this low magnification, surface view. The brains of hypoxic adapted rats were always distinguishable from control brains by direct visual inspection.

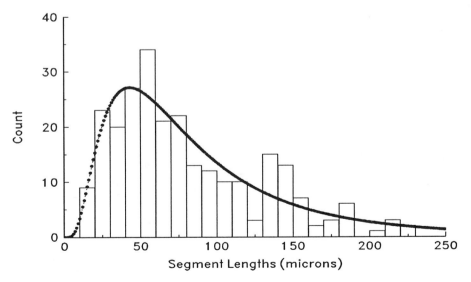

Figure 3. Cerebral cortical capillary segment length distribution. Histogram and log normal curve ($r^2 = 0.85$) from the frontopolar region of a normoxic control rat.

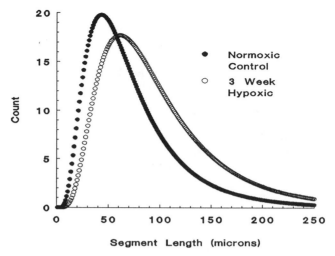

Figure 4. Comparison of log normal curves fit to the capillary segment length distribution of the frontopolar-2 region of a normoxic and a 3 week hypoxic rat brain

The distribution of capillary segment lengths from the frontopolar cortex (FPC1) of a control, normoxic rat is shown in the histogram of Figure 3. The distribution can be described as log normal and fit to the curve shown ($r^2 = 0.85$). The peak frequency was at a segment length of 43 ± 3 (s.e.m.) microns.

Figure 4 is a plot of the fitted log normal curves for frontopolar regions (FPC2) of a normoxic and 3 week hypoxic rat brains. The graph demonstrates a right shift and

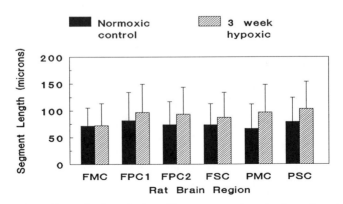

Figure 5. Mean ($\pm$ s.d.) cerebral cortical capillary segment lengths from 6 rat brain regions.

broadening in the distribution of capillary segment lengths. The peak frequency was shifted from 43 ± 2 microns in the normoxic curve ($r^2 = 0.92$), to 61 ± 2 microns in the hypoxic curve ($r^2 = 0.92$).

Except for the frontal motor cortex, there was a significant increase in the mean capillary segment length and a right shift of the histogram in the microvascular networks of the hypoxic brains compared to the normoxic brains (Figure 5; note that the error bars are standard deviation). The increases were 18% and 26% in the 2 frontopolar regions, 19% in the frontal sensory cortex, and 46% and 30% in the parietal motor and sensory cortical regions (Table I).

DISCUSSION

Chronic exposure of rats to moderate hypoxia for 3 weeks stimulates angiogenesis (LaManna et al., 1992). The increased capillary density results in decreased intercapillary distances and allows, with elevated hemoglobin concentration, cerebral blood flow to return to baseline normoxic rates. To begin to characterize the structural changes in microvessel distribution, segment lengths were measured in control and 3 week hypoxic rats. The distribution of segment lengths was log normal with mean segment lengths between 67 and 82 microns (Figure 5) in the six brain regions studied. This distributional shape is reminiscent of the distribution of capillary transit times observed in hemodilution transients (Eke et al., 1979; Tomita et al., 1983; Shockley and LaManna, 1988).

Chronic exposure to simulated altitude resulted in more capillaries, and the new capillaries shifted the distribution to longer segment lengths (Figure 4). Mean segment lengths increased to 72 to 103 microns (Figure 5). The observed increases in capillary segment length were a bit less than the previously reported increases in cortical capillary density (Table I). Consistent with the capillary segment length data, the frontal motor cortex was the least affected by hypoxia, compared to other frontal and parietal regions, as judged by capillary density changes (LaManna et al., 1992).

Table I

Brain Region	Increase in Mean Capillary Segment Length (%)	Increase in Capillary Density (%)[*]
FMC	1	46
FPC1	18	76
FPC2	26	
FSC	19	54
PMC	46	65
PSC	30	68

[*] From LaManna, et al., 1992.

It cannot be known from these results if the increased lengths were due to new, longer segments or elongation of existing capillaries. In addition, it is not known if this finding is generalized to the entire brain, or is limited to those areas of the cerebral cortex that we studied. Finally, it must be considered that the large increase in glucose transport observed in the rats exposed to 3 weeks of hypoxia (Harik et al., 1991) may result in physiological compensations independent of oxygen delivery requirements.

REFERENCES

Dempsey, J.A. and Forster, H.V., 1982, Mediation of ventilatory adaptations, Physiol. Rev., 62: 262-346.

Eke, A., Hutiray, G., and Kovach, A.G.B., 1979, Induced hemodilution detected by reflectometry for measuring microregional blood flow and blood volume in cat brain cortex, Am. J. Physiol., 236: H759-H768.

Harik, S.I., Behmand, R.A., and LaManna, J.C., 1991, Chronic hypobaric hypoxia increases the density of cerebral capillaries and their glucose transporter protein, J. Cereb. Blood Flow Metab., 11 (Suppl): S496.(Abstract)

LaManna, J.C., (in press), Rat brain adaptation to chronic hypobaric hypoxia, in: "Oxygen Transport to Tissue XIV (Advances in Experimental Medicine and Biology, v.)," W. Erdmann and D. Bruley, eds., Plenum Press, New York.

LaManna, J.C., Light, A.I., Peretsman, S.J., and Rosenthal, M., 1984, Oxygen insufficiency during hypoxic hypoxia in rat brain cortex, Br. Res., 293: 313-318.

LaManna, J.C., McCracken, K.A., and Strohl, K.P., 1989, Changes in regional cerebral blood flow and sucrose space after 3-4 weeks of hypobaric hypoxia (0.5 ATM), in: "Oxygen Transport to Tissue XI (Advances in Experimental Medicine and Biology, v. 248)," K. Rakusan, G.P. Biro, T.K. Goldstick, and Z. Turek, eds., pp. 471-477, Plenum Publishing Corp, New York.

LaManna, J.C., Vendel, L.M., and Farrell, R.M., 1992, Brain adaptation to chronic hypobaric hypoxia in rats, J. Appl. Physiol., 72: 2238-2243.

Palkovits, M. and Brownstein, M.J., 1988, "Maps and Guide to Microdissection of the Rat Brain," Elsevier, New York.

Shockley, R.P. and LaManna, J.C., 1988, Determination of rat cerebral cortical blood volume changes by capillary mean transit time analysis during hypoxia, hypercapnia, and hyperventilation, Br. Res., 454: 170-178.

Tomita, M., Gotoh, F., Amano, T., Tanahashi, N., Kobari, M., Shinohara, T., and Mihara, B., 1983, Transfer function through regional cerebral cortex evaluated by a photoelectric method, Am. J. Physiol., 245: H385-H398.

RYTHROCYTE FLOW HETEROGENEITY

N THE CEREBROCORTICAL CAPILLARY NETWORK

Antal G. Hudetz [12], Gabriella Fehér [3], Derek E. Knuese [1], and John P. Kampine [2]

[1]Department of Physiology
[2]Department of Anesthesiology
Medical College of Wisconsin
Milwaukee, WI 53226
[3]Experimental Research Department
Semmelweis Medical University
Budapest, Hungary H-1082

NTRODUCTION

A remarkable characteristic of the cerebrocortical microcirculation is the fast flow f erythrocytes through narrow, tortuous capillaries. In the absence of capillary ecruitment (Göbel et al, 1990) the high flow velocity may represent a functional eserve for oxygen supply to cerebral tissue. In addition, significant spatial variability of rythrocyte flow exists in the cortex (Hudetz et al, 1992). During reduced perfusion ressure, the "flow reserve" could be utilized by the partial redistribution of flow from ie normally well perfused capillaries to poorly perfused capillaries. Such a edistribution of cerebrocortical capillary flow from "functionally superperfused" to ormally perfused capillaries was suggested by Lübbers and Leniger-Follert (1978) based n their measurements of microflow in the cerebral cortex by hydrogen clearance. The ossibility of microflow redistribution was suggested in several physiological states, in articular, during acute changes in blood pressure (Leniger-Follert and Lübbers, 1975). lthough the latter observations were carried out in very small tissue volumes (min. '.05mm^3) the proposed hypothesis has not been directly tested in individual capillaries) date.

The objective of the present work was to determine if redistribution of red lood cell flow in cerebrocortical capillaries may play a role in the maintenance of erfusion of the microcirculation. We first studied if heterogeneity of erythrocyte flow elocity or of erythrocyte flux is maintained in individual cortical capillaries during cute decreases of cerebral perfusion pressure by various maneuvers. We then

xygen Transport to Tissue XV, Edited by P. Vaupel
t al., Plenum Press, New York, 1994

investigated whether heterogeneity of capillary flow velocity reflected preferential flow pathways in the network. To this end, arterio-venous flow pathways in a cortical capillary network were reconstructed. The distribution of red cell velocity, cell flux and transit time along the pathways were determined and compared.

METHODS

Microcirculation of the superficial parietal cerebral cortex was studied using a closed cranial window technique in the rat. Sprague-Dawley rats of 250 to 350 gram were anesthetized by 50mg/kg sodium-pentobarbital. Body temperature was controlled at 37 ± 1 °C. Both femoral arteries and one of the femoral veins were cannulated for blood pressure measurement, blood withdrawal and for the injection of drugs, fluorescent cells and dyes, respectively. The head was placed in a stereotaxic apparatus and a burr hole of approximately 3mm in diameter was created in the right parietal bone, about 3mm from the midline and 5mm from the bregma. The dura was opened. A cranial window containing three ports was mounted onto the parietal bone of the rat following craniotomy. The window space was perfused with heated (37 °C), oxygenated (6% O_2, 6% CO_2, 88% N_2) artificial cerebrospinal fluid. Both perfusion rate and pressure in the window were controlled independently. During the experiment, the animals' lungs were artificially ventilated with 25 to 30% O_2 in N_2. End-tidal CO_2 was maintained between 35 and 40mmHg.

Capillary circulation within the parietal cerebral cortex to a depth of about 70μm was visualized using epifluorescence. Erythrocytes labeled with fluorescein-iso-thiocyanate (FITC) (Hudetz et al, 1992) were injected intravenously to achieve a final labeled cell fraction of about 0.02% in the circulation. The movement of labeled cells in a selected capillary network in each animal was video-recorded for periods of 1 to 2 minutes.

The experimental protocols included (a) stepwise lowering of the mean arterial pressure and (b) stepwise elevation of the local extravascular (intracranial) pressure. Hypotension was induced by controlled hemorrhage through the femoral arterial line in steps of 20mmHg to a minimum of 40mmHg. Intracranial pressure was increased by elevating the hydrostatic pressure in the window by raising the height of the CSF reservoir connected to the outflow port of the cranial window. Control ICP was set to 5mmHg, and it was elevated in steps of 10mmHg to 75mmHg. Video recording of the microcirculation was repeated at each perfusion pressure level, about 10 minutes after reaching steady state conditions.

The velocity of labeled cells was measured over one minute periods in each capillary segment from the video recordings using the dual window digital cross correlation technique (Hudetz et al, 1992). In some cases cell velocity was also measured frame by frame, using a computer assisted image tracking system. The flux of fluorescent erythrocytes in several capillaries was determined by automated cell counting (Knuese et al, 1992). Flow paths of red blood cells through the capillary network were reconstructed using a three-dimensional microvascular network mapping system (Hudetz and DeVito, 1992) which also included the routines for image tracking. For three-dimensional network reconstruction, small amounts of FITC-labeled gamma-globulin was also injected intravenously in selected experiments. The microcirculation was then video-recorded during slow scanning of the focal plane (optical sectioning). Blood vessels were traced from several video images, always selecting the one recorded at the best focus of the vessel segment currently traced. To obtain true spatial vessel lengths, the depth of the optical section was decoded by the computer by counting the video frames recorded on the tape.

RESULTS

At normal cerebral perfusion pressure, the mean velocity of labeled red blood cells in cortical capillaries was 1.47±0.58 (SD) mm/s. Most of the dispersion of data was due to the heterogeneity of velocity within individual capillary networks. The coefficient of variation of velocity was between 0.38 and 0.59 within each of five individual networks. The differences in velocity of individual capillaries appeared to be stationary, at least, over the one minute period of observation. Thus, within this time frame, the range of velocity values reflected mainly spatial rather than temporal heterogeneity.

When cerebral perfusion pressure (CPP) was decreased by either systemic hypotension or intracranial pressure elevation, mean capillary erythrocyte velocity was well maintained when CPP was above 70mmHg. Below 70 mmHg, a fall in cell velocity

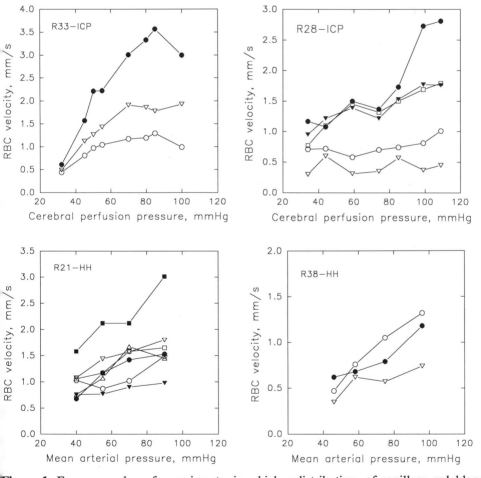

Figure 1. Four examples of experiments in which redistribution of capillary red blood cell flow velocity was observed. Cerebral perfusion pressure was decreased either by elevating the local intracranial pressure (top two panels) or by hemorrhage (bottom two panels).

with decreasing CPP was apparent in several capillaries, and was characterized by decrease rate of about 14% per 10mmHg.

Not all capillaries behaved uniformly, however, during pressure reduction. In small fraction of vessels, red cell velocity began to decrease at the first or second CP level below control. In most of these vessels, cell velocity continued to decline wit further decreases of CPP, while the velocity of other capillaries was well maintained Figure 1 illustrates this finding in four experiments.

The same finding is corroborated by the analysis of data points from a experiments combined. Figure 2 summarizes all velocity measurements from th intracranial pressure experiments. The data suggest the preferential loss of high velocit values with decreasing perfusion pressure. The range of velocity was reduced from 3.25mm/s (CPP=120-70mmHg) to 1.54mm/s (CPP=40-20mmHg). This is indicated b a decrease in range and skewness of the data. With CPP between 70 and 120 the rang and skewness were 3.25 and 4.6, while at a CPP of 20 to 40 they were 1.54mm/s an 2.0, respectively. Thus the data suggest that larger reductions of velocity may hav occurred in capillaries with initially high flow velocity than in those with initially lo velocity.

In some of the experiments, the flux of labeled erythrocytes in the capillarie was also determined. Figure 3 depicts the results of paired measurements of red ce velocity and red cell flux in a capillary network. Changes in red cell flux with perfusio pressure correlated linearly with changes in cell velocity in the same capillaries. A finit intercept on the velocity axis suggested zero red cell flux at an erythrocyte velocity c about 0.5mm/s.

Next we attempted to investigate if the heterogeneity of erythrocyte velocit reflected heterogeneous perfusion of arterio-venous capillary flow pathways. The clarit of the microscopic image of one of the experiments (R28) allowed us to reconstruct th capillary network in sufficient detail to answer this question for that particular network Mean diameter and length of vessel segments in the network were $4.5\pm1.1\mu m$ (SD) an $61\pm44\mu m$ (SD), respectively. Five different capillary flow paths connecting a $6\mu m$ arteriole and a $9\mu m$ venule were positively identified (Figure 3). The length of flo paths ranged from 152 to $374\mu m$. The mean cell velocity of capillary segments in serie

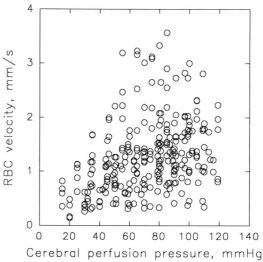

Figure 2. Red blood cell velocity data from seven experiments with intracranial pressure elevation. Note the change in the distribution of high velocity values with decreasing perfusion pressure.

long the flow paths varied from 1.2 to 1.6mm/s from path to path. Transit time of abeled erythrocytes was also heterogeneous (107 to 301ms) and correlated significantly vith path length (r=0.88, n=9) (Figure 4). In contrast, erythrocyte flux, measured at bout midway along each A-V path, was the same (within 5%) in all five paths.

DISCUSSION

The present study revealed significant heterogeneity of erythrocyte flow velocity nd of erythrocyte flux in the cerebrocortical microcirculation. Heterogeneity of capillary low is of interest because it may decrease the efficiency of transport of O_2 and other olutes to/from tissue. Renkin (1969) showed that changes in heterogeneity of capillary erfusion may alter the net capillary exchange at constant overall tissue blood flow. This

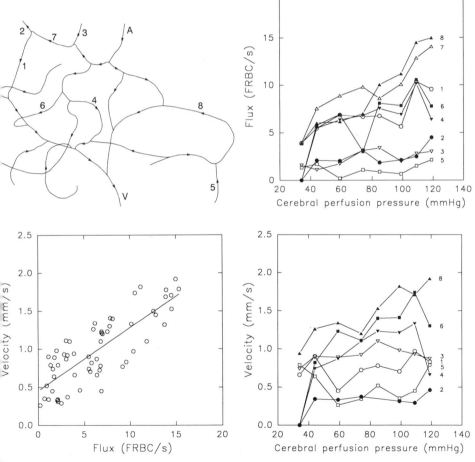

Figure 3. Reconstruction of a cerebrocortical capillary network (top left) and the dependence of red blood cell velocity and red blood cell flux on cerebral perfusion pressure altered by the elevation of intracranial pressure (right). Note the significant correlation (r=0.81) between erythrocyte velocity and flux (bottom left).

637

is particularly important for cerebral tissue, which has no cellular oxygen reserves and apparently has no capacity to recruit capillary blood flow (Göbel et al, 1990). One may then ask why flow heterogeneity is present in the cerebral microcirculation. Our data suggest that when cerebral perfusion pressure is decreased, the heterogeneity of capillary red blood cell velocity and flux is reduced by a shift in velocity distribution from high to low flow vessels. Thus, flow heterogeneity at normal physiological conditions may indicate the presence of a functional "flow reserve" in the capillary network.

Using locally generated hydrogen clearance to measure blood flow in micro-volumes of cerebral tissue, Lübbers found that changes in microflow did not parallel the change in regional flow at all sites of the brain cortex during electrical stimulation of the tissue (Lübbers and Leniger-Follert, 1978). As an explanation, the hypothesis of "functionally superfused" capillaries in addition to "flow-adapted" capillaries in the cerebral cortex was forwarded. According to this hypothesis, superfused capillaries would function as a reserve to allow redistribution of flow to the flow-adapted capillaries with relatively little change in overall flow in times of increased metabolic demand. Furthermore, when microflow was studied during changes in arterial blood pressure, autoregulation was partial: at certain measuring sites microflow followed the changes in arterial pressure (Leniger-Follert and Lübbers, 1975). Our present results are in agreement with these findings and together they support the concept of "flow reserve" in the cortical microcirculation.

If redistribution of capillary erythrocyte flow during reduced perfusion pressure proves to be a consistent phenomenon, than the important question will be whether it is the consequence of passive rheological factors or there are physiological control mechanisms involved. The greater decrease in velocity in capillaries with high initial flow could, in principal, be explained by the recruitment of parallel capillaries. However, no signs of capillary recruitment in our experiments were observed. Partial de-recruitment of high flow (thoroughfare) capillary channels in hypotensive states may theoretically occur via the contraction of precapillary sphincters whose existence, however, is questionable, especially in the cerebral microcirculation. Alternatively,

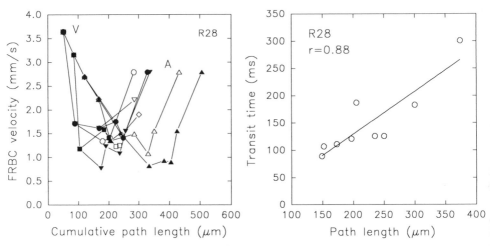

Figure 4. Left: Longitudinal variation of erythrocyte velocity in capillary segments along five major flow paths between the same arteriole and venule in the microvascular network depicted in Figure 3. Right: Red cell transit time and flow path length are correlated in the network. Three additional flow paths from unidentified arteriolar source(s) but converging on the same venule were included in the figure.

precapillary arterioles may modulate the distribution of flow rate in the capillary network by changing the pressure gradient across the capillary bed (Lindbom and Arfors, 1985). Lipowsky (1986) studied, by computer simulation, the effect of reduced perfusion pressure on flow distribution in the mesenteric microvascular network. He described that "Those vessels which bridge more rapidly flowing vessels, analogous to rungs on a ladder, tend toward greater reductions in flow as DeltaP is reduced." Since this simulation did not include physiological control mechanisms, it provides a plausible explanation for flow redistribution by the operation of rheological factors alone.

In other organs, such as striated muscle, capillary flow heterogeneity, as measured by the coefficient of variation of red cell velocities of capillary segments, appeared to be independent of the mean flow velocity (Duling and Damon, 1987). The fractional distribution of red cell flux was also unaffected by vasodilation (Damon and Duling, 1986).

These findings do not exclude the possibility of capillary flow redistribution during reduced perfusion pressure. In our work, changes in heterogeneity of capillary flow were characterized by calculating the range or standard deviation of data which measure the "absolute" heterogeneity, as opposed to the relative or "true" heterogeneity, the latter being measured by the coefficient of variation of data (Duling and Damon, 1987). A change in shape of a distribution, however, may not be reflected by a change in the coefficient of variation. Furthermore, since the statistical distribution of velocity data in Figure 2 was skewed, the coefficient of variation was not used to characterize the dispersion of these data.

Tyml and Mikulash (1986) found an increase in spatial heterogeneity of red cell velocity in skeletal muscle microcirculation during reduced flow. The increase in heterogeneity appeared to be the result of random flow stoppages throughout the capillary network. The same phenomenon was studied in a computer model of the skeletal muscle microcirculation and yielded similar results (Hudetz, 1991). In the cerebral microcirculation, however, flow redistribution was found during moderate reductions in perfusion pressure and flow stoppages occurred only when perfusion pressure was reduced to very low levels. Several factors, including differences in capillary architecture and the distinctly high flow velocity of erythrocytes in cerebral capillaries may be responsible for the lack of increase in flow heterogeneity during moderate decreases in perfusion pressure.

Erythrocyte flux is proportional to both red cell velocity and tube hematocrit and therefore, is a more accurate index of tissue perfusion and conductive oxygen transport than flow velocity. For this reason, red cell flux was determined together with red cell velocity in some of our experiments. A good correlation (r=0.81) between red cell velocity and red cell flux of individual capillary segments was obtained, which supported the use of velocity as an index of flow. However, the slope of the regression between cell velocity and flux suggested that cell flux was more sensitive to variations in perfusion pressure than cell velocity. The linear regression model predicted zero red cell flux at a cell velocity of 0.5mm/s. There may be several explanations to this finding. Erythrocyte perfusion may stop at a critical low velocity due to rheological reasons including aggregation or plugging of capillaries by various blood cells. The critical velocity of 0.5mm/s appears to be fairly high for capillary plugging to occur in the microvascular bed. However, the narrow size of cerebral capillaries may be important from this point of view. Yamakawa et al (1987) observed plugging of cerebral capillaries by leukocytes in severe hemorrhagic shock; the length of time of flow stagnation in each capillary was increased with decreasing arterial pressure. The probability of capillary plugging as a function of cell velocity was not evaluated. Another possible explanation may be the preferential flow of red blood cells at bifurcations. As shown by Schmid-

Schoenbein et al (1980) red cells will fail to enter capillary branches whose flow velocity is below a critical value. Thus, it is conceivable that equalization of the distribution of capillary flow velocity during reductions of perfusion pressure may play a fortuitous protective role by helping to maintain flow velocity and cell flux in the network.

Since the cerebral microvascular bed contains several capillary anastomoses, the question arises whether heterogeneity of erythrocyte velocity measured in individual capillary segments may reflect heterogeneous perfusion of arterio-venous capillary flow pathways. Therefore, we have made a first attempt to determine the distribution of path lengths and red cell transit times along reconstructed arterio-venous pathways in the cerebral capillary network. The obtained correlation between transit time flow path length suggested that mean flow velocity along the paths was more evenly distributed than either the path length or the transit time. If one assumes a nearly equal capillary diameter along each path, then the velocity would be expected to be lower along the long flow paths, and higher along the short flow paths. This does not appear to be the case in the studied cerebral network. A simple explanation would be if capillary diameters along the longer paths were larger than those along the shorter paths (Sarelius, 1986). From the limited number of data (five A-V flow paths) we cannot deduce a significant correlation between length and diameter, however, the data collected so far are consistent with this hypothesis. Several other factors may play a role equalizing flow velocity along the A-V paths. These include local irregularities in capillary cross section (Secomb, 1987), hemodynamic conditions at bifurcations and confluences (Ellis et al, 1989; Wells et al, 1992) and variations in tube hematocrit. In the cerebral microcirculation, a further important factor may be the richly anastomosing pattern of the capillary network.

At normal cerebral perfusion pressure, red cell fluxes measured along different arterio-venous flow paths were quite similar, despite the widely different path lengths and transit times along the same paths. This observation suggests that red cell flow along the arteriovenous capillary pathways may be more stable than velocity or flux in randomly selected capillary segments. We hypothesize that the observed hypotensive flow redistribution may, in a yet undefined manner, help to maintain a balanced perfusion of flow pathways across the entire capillary network. In order to test this hypothesis, systematic measurements of red blood cell flux along reconstructed A-V flow paths will be necessary.

SUMMARY

The heterogeneity of erythrocyte flow velocity and erythrocyte flux and their dependence on decreased cerebral perfusion pressure were studied in the rat cerebral cortex using intravital video microscopy. With decreased perfusion pressure, both mean and range of erythrocyte flow velocity of individual capillaries was reduced. Both cell velocity and cell flux decreased more in high flow capillaries than in low flow capillaries. The results are compatible with the hypothesis that redistribution of capillary flow during hypotension may help to maintain the perfusion of arterio-venous capillary flow pathways. Although the data are preliminary, they represent the first direct measurements of capillary flow path length and transit time in the capillary network of the cerebral cortex.

ACKNOWLEDGEMENT

This work was supported by the grants BCS-9001425 from the National Science Foundation and 90-0095 from the Medical College of Wisconsin.

REFERENCES

Damon, D.H, and Duling, B.R., 1986, Measurement of the distribution of capillary erythrocyte flow in striated muscle microcirculation, in: "Microvascular Networks: Experimental and Theoretical Studies," A.S. Popel, P.C. Johnson, eds., Karger, Basel.

Duling, B.R., and Damon, D.H., 1987, An examination of the measurement of flow heterogeneity in striated muscle, Circ. Res. 60:1.

Ellis, C.G., Tyml, K., and Strang, B.K., 1989, Variation in axial velocity profile of red cells passing through a single capillary, Adv. Exp. Med. Biol. 248:543.

Göbel, U., Theilen, H., and Kuschinsky, W., 1990, Congruence of total and perfused capillary network in rat brains, Circ. Res. 66:271.

Hudetz, A.G., 1989, Critical dependence of network resistance on functional capillary density: percolation phenomenon in the microcirculation, FASEB J. 3:A1406.

Hudetz, A.G., and DeVito, T., 1992, Three-dimensional network mapping of the cerebrocortical microcirculation, FASEB J. 6:A2075.

Hudetz, A.G., Weigle, C.G.M., Fenoy, F.J., and Roman, R., 1992, Use of fluorescently labeled erythrocytes and digital cross-correlation for the measurement of flow velocity in the cerebrocortical microcirculation, Microvasc. Res. 43:334.

Knuese, D., Hudetz, A.G., and Fehér, G., 1992, Automated measurement of fluorescently labeled erythrocyte flux in cerebrocortical capillaries, FASEB J. 6:A2077.

Leniger-Follert, E., and Lübbers, D.W., 1975, Interdependence of capillary flow and regional blood flow in the brain, in: "Cerebral Circulation and Metabolism," T.W. Langfitt et al, eds., Springer, New York.

Lindbom, L., and Arfors, K.-E., 1980, Non-homogeneous blood flow distribution in the rabbit tenuissimus muscle: differential control of total blood flow and capillary perfusion, Acta Physiol. Scand. 122:225.

Lipowsky, H.H., 1986, Network hemodynamics and the shear rate dependency of blood viscosity, in: "Microvascular Networks: Experimental and Theoretical Studies," A.S. Popel, P.C. Johnson, eds., Karger, Basel.

Little, J. R., Cook, A., Cook, S. A., and MacIntyre, W. J., 1981, Microcirculatory obstruction in focal cerebral ischemia: albumin and erythrocyte transit, Stroke 12:218.

Lübbers, D.W., and Leniger-Follert, E., 1978, Capillary flow in the brain cortex during changes in oxygen supply and state of activation, Ciba Foundation Symposium 56:21.

Renkin, E.M., 1969, Exchange of substances through capillary walls, in: "Ciba Foundation Symposium on Circulatory and Respiratory Mass Transport," G.E.W. Wolstenhome, J. Knight, eds., J. and A. Churchill, Ltd., London.

Schmid-Schoenbein, G.W., Skalak, R., Usami, S., and Chien, S., 1980, Cell distribution in capillary networks, Microvasc. Res. 19:18.

Secomb, T.W., 1987, Flow dependent rheological properties of blood in capillaries, Microvasc. Res. 34:46.

Tomita, M., Gotoh, F., Amano, T., Tanahashi, N., Kobari, M., Shinohara, T., and Mihara, B., 1983, Transfer function through regional cerebral cortex evaluated by photoelectric method, Am. J. Physiol. 245:H385.

Tyml, K., and Mikulash, K., 1988, Evidence for increased perfusion heterogeneity in skeletal muscle during reduced flow, Microvasc. Res. 35:316.

Wells, S.M., Potter, R.F., Sainani, D.R., and C.G. Ellis, 1992, Red blood cell flow at converging capillary bifurcations, FASEB J. 6:A2088.

Yamakawa, T., Yamaguchi, S., Niimi, H., and Sugiyama, I., 1987, White blood cell plugging and blood flow maldistribution in the capillary network of cat cerebral cortex in acute hemorrhagic hypotension: an intravital microscopic study, Circulat. Shock 22:323.

LIGHT INTENSITY ATTENUATION IN THE RAT BRAIN TISSUE ASSESSED BY TELEVISION PHOTOMETRY

András Eke, Cornélia Ikrényi, and Enikő Sárváry

Experimental Neuropathology, Department of Pathology, University of
Alabama at Birmingham, Birmingham, AL 35294, U.S.A. and
Experimental Research Department, 2nd Institute of Physiology
Semmelweis University of Medicine, Budapest, Hungary 1082 *

INTRODUCTION

Methods for non-destructive spectrophotometric assessment of brain metabolism, oxygenation, blood flow and microcirculation *in vivo* has become increasingly important to researchers in the last three decades. The high spatial and temporal resolution offered by the optical approach, its non-destructive nature has also attracted considerable interest to the rapidly growing field of optical imaging of brain function and metabolism[1]. The use of near infrared (NIR) light has opened the perspective for non-invasive monitoring of cerebral oxygenation[2] and time-resolved NIR-spectroscopy by direct measurement of the optical pathlength of photons made absolute measurement possible[3,4] and also proved to be an excellent tool to study photon migration in the brain tissue. Most of the surface fluoro-reflectometric methods work in the shorter wavelength range where it remains still difficult to analyze light penetration into the brain tissue since attenuation of light occurs over much shorter distances than that time-resolved spectroscopy can currently handle with adequate resolution[4]. A direct determination of the catchment volume of these measurements at the very site of photometric detection assumes a direct measurement of light attenuation profile in the tissue and becomes important when proper interpretation of *in vivo* data[5,6,7,8,9] or calculation of absolute values from these data is needed. These questions have gained increasing importance during the methodological development of multiparametric imaging of microregional circulation in the brain cortex[9,10]. The primary objective of the present study, therefore, was to approach these problems experimentally by assessing light attenuation kinetics *ex vivo* in the brain within the visible wavelength range (589 nm) by measuring signal contribution from different depth of rat brain samples, among them, the cortical region of the brain where reflectometric measurement is usually

---

*Current address of authors.

Oxygen Transport to Tissue XV, Edited by P. Vaupel
et al., Plenum Press, New York, 1994

done *in vivo*. The *ex vivo* measurements were carried out under illumination and detection geometry identical to the one used *in vivo*.

METHODS

Samples for the photometric measurements were taken from the brain of Wistar rats of 400-410 g bodyweight under 1-1.2 % Halothane inhalation anesthesia. Rinsing of the brain by heparinized saline by arterial infusion via a catheter introduced into the abdominal aorta was performed during euthanasia by exanguination. This procedure effectively

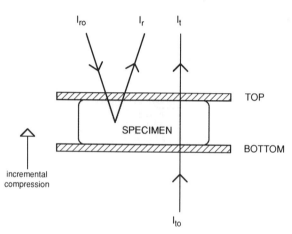

Figure. 1. Schematics of the photometric arrangement. A chamber with transparent glass top and bottom holds a sample of brain tissue, which can be compressed by precision movement of the bottom against the top while measurements of photometric parameters indicated are carried out by a quantitative video photometer (Figure 2).

Symbols:
I_{ro} = Incident intensity of light under epiillumination
I_r = Backscattered intensity of light under epiillumination
I_{to} = Incident intensity of light under transillumination
I_t = Transmitted intensity of light under transillumination

eliminates the erythrocytes from the brain tissue as has been verified by histology. The brain was then carefully removed from the cranium and frozen by immersion in liquid nitrogen and stored in closed plastic bags until the measurement, when they were allowed to thaw at room temperature. Samples from different areas of the brain including the temporoparietal region of the cortex and underlying white matter have been taken. The photometric arrangement is shown in Figure 1. The trans- and epiillumination time-unresolved photometric system consisted of a newvicon camera focused onto the surface of

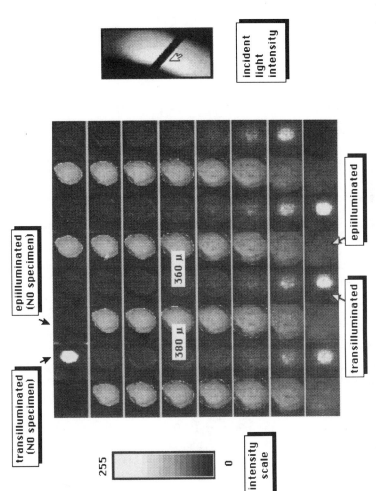

Figure 2. Collage of 8 bit digitized images of a rat brain sample (cortical gray matter) obtained in epi- and transillumination mode of photometric detection during incremental compression of the specimen from a thickness of 600 micra to 20 micra. Images are presented in 256 level intensity scale shown on the left. Incident epiillumination intensity (*Iro*) was determined by digitizing at the arrow on the image of the annular epiilluminator as seen by the television camera while being focused on a marker on the surface of a mirror (shown on the insert to the right). Note the lowering backscattered and rising transmitted intensity as sample thickness is being decreased.

the tissue sample placed in a special chamber with its transparent bottom advanced to any given position within the range of 1000 - 20 micra against its transparent top by a Narishige micromanipulator. The tissue specimen was transilluminated by a small tungsten light bulb from beneath and epiilluminated by an annular fiber optic epiilluminator placed

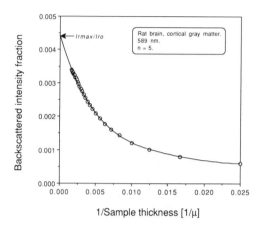

Figure 3. Method of extrapolating to *Irmax/Iro*, the fraction of incident energy backscattered from a sample of infinite thickness. The mean of 5 measurements is shown. The backscattered intensities measured at different degree of sample compression were fitted by a fifth order polynomial of the following form:

$$y = 4.4^{-3} - 0.7x + 60.6x^2 - 2731.5\ x^3 + 60470x^4 - 500660x^5 \qquad r^2 = 1.0$$

Its zero intercept converts to the value of *Irmax*, the intensity backscattered from a tissue layer of infinite thickness.

around the macro lens assembly of the video camera. Digitized video images of the tissue sample under epi- and transillumination applied intermittently were taken by an 8 bit video board at every stage of incremental tissue compression from typically 600 micra to 20 micra in steps of 20 micra (Figure 2). The image files were analyzed by a Macintosh II computer system with a public domain image processing program "NIH-Image". Original sample thickness was adjusted in the range of 1000 - 600 micra. Backscattered and transmitted light intensities at 589 nm were measured from these tissue samples compressed to an increasingly smaller thickness along the axis of the photometric measurement. Data from measurements of backscattered intensities obtained in samples of cortical gray matter are reported.

RESULTS

Light attenuation profiles in the brain cortex - beyond the actual range of sample thickness - was determined by plotting the ratio of the backscattered intensity *(Ir)* and the incident epiillumination intensity *(Iro)* against the reciprocal of sample thickness *(1/d)* (Figure 3). This function was fitted by a fifth order polynomial, whose zero intercept yields the fraction of incident intensity backscattered from a sample of infinite thickness.

The "effective" depth from which contribution still occurs to the reflectance signal *in vivo* was determined from the normalized backscattered intensity profile shown in Figure 4, which is in fact the polynomial function shown in Figure 3 normalized by its zero intercept, *Irmax/Iro*. Data for five samples of cortical gray matter are shown of which two samples yielded very similar profiles showing up as one in the figure (second curve from the top). The contribution of superficial layers of the cortex to the measured reflectance is much greater than that of deeper layers. In the given samples of cortical gray matter, the depth of tissue volume from which 90% of the total backscattered photons get re-emitted and detected varied between 800 and 2000 micra. At the level of 63% of the total backscattered energy this value is between 300 - 700 micra (Figure 4).

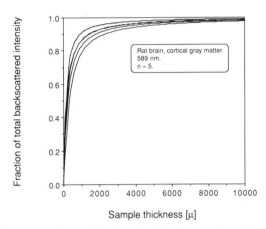

Figure 4. Light attenuation profile determined in five samples of rat cerebrocortical gray matter. Data are normalized to the total backscattered (reflectance) signal that could be measured from a tissue volume of infinite thickness. Catchment volume under the actual reflectometric arrangement can be readily determined at any level detector sensitivity.

DISCUSSION

Propagation of light into tissue, the effect of scattering, absorption and tissue structure has been studied by a number of investigators employing one or more of the following approaches: theoretical[12,13,14,15,16], computer modeling/simulation[4,14,17], *in vivo* measurements (time-resolved and -unresolved)[3,4,5,6,18,19,20] and *ex vivo* measurements in tissue samples[7,8,11,20,21,22], tissue models or turbid media[3,4,22,23]. Our method provides means for an *ex vivo* assessment of light attenuation in tissue under conditions of epiillumination photometry in a detection geometry that is identical to that employed *in vivo*. It can determine the catchment volume at any given wavelength and detection geometry for surface photometric methods utilizing epiillumination and reflection measurement. This parameter is needed for quantitation and interpretation of photometric data in terms of relative signal contribution from superficial as opposed to deeper tissue layers, *etc*. This method can be used for any soft tissue, like liver, kidney, mucous membrane *etc*. Measurement of tissue fluorescence can also be added. Backscattering and absorption can be separately determined, which can further enhance the interpretation of light attenuation kinetics in the samples. The method may be used to match the performance of artificial brain models[3,4] to characteristics of the brain tissue and is to be used to determine the catchment volume of the reflectometric method for multiparametric assessment of the cerebrocortical microcirculation[9,10,24].

An adaptation of the method of Groenhuis *et al*[23] to the circumstances of *in vivo* reflectometry of the brain cortex can further enhance our approach by bridging between the *in vivo* reflectance data[9,10,24], *in vivo* measures of scattering and absorption characteristics of the tissue[23] and similar data provided by our tissue compression method. Eggert and Blazek[11] reported a very concise set of relative levels of reflection, absorption and scattering, coefficients of scattering and absorption, and penetration depth for human brain samples in the spectral range of 200 - 900 nm. They calculated the penetration depth from measured reflectance and transmittance according to Beer's law as the depth at which the total optical power is reduced to 37%. At 590 nm they found it around 800 micra, which is comparable to our value of 300 - 700 micra obtained for the rat brain (see Figure 4).

It is well established that with large size scatterers (size equal to or larger than the wavelength of light), there is a strong forward scattering. This forward scattered light will tend to be attenuated by the absorbers within the tissue (and *in vivo* by haemoglobin) before it is scattered back towards the tissue surface. The small subcellular size scatterers of size below that of the wavelength of light, on the other hand exhibit an almost isotropic scattering distribution. The total scattering effect at any angle is determined by the particle size distribution and the overall scattering coefficient which itself depends upon both the scattering efficiency and the number of scatterers per unit volume. In the tissues, there are a large number of small particles, and although their scattering efficiency is low, their high number combined with an isotropic scattering distribution means that their contribution to the backscattered signal is dominant. It is recognized that the compression of the sample displaces and/or distorts large size scatterers more than subcellular scatterers, and should thus alter forward scattering more than backward scattering. However, because compression leaves the ratio of their numbers in the sample and the dominance of backscattering unaffected, the measured light attenuation profile cannot be considered significantly distorted by the process of sample compression.

ACKNOWLEDGMENTS

This work has been jointly supported by grants-in-aid of the Department of Pathology, University of Alabama at Birmingham and National Science Foundation Grant No. 2040 (Hungary). The help with the pertinent theoretical background by D.T. Delpy, and discussion by B. Chance on the significance of the results is greatly appreciated.

REFERENCES

1. B. Chance, A. Villinger, U. Dirnagl, K.M. Einhäupl, Optical imaging of brain function and metabolism, J Neurol. 239:359 (1992).
2. F.F. Jöbsis, Non invasive, infrared monitoring of cerebral and myocardial oxygen sufficiency and circulatory parameters, Science. 198:1264 (1977).
3. B. Chance, J.S. Leigh, H. Miyake *et al*, Comparison of time-resolved and -unresolved

measurements of deoxyhemoglobin in the brain, Proc Natl Acad Sci USA. 85:4971 (1988).

4. D.T. Delpy, M. Cope, P. van der Zee et al, Estimation of optical pathlength through tissue from direct time of flight measurement, Phys Med Biol. 33(12):1433 (1988).

5. B. Chance, V. Legallis, B. Schoener, Combined fluorometer and double-beam spectrophotometer for reflectance measurements, Rev Scient Instr. 34(12):1307 (1963).

6. F.F. Jöbsis, M. O'Connor, A. Vitale, H. Vreman, Intracellular redox changes in functioning cerebral cortex. I. Metabolic effect of epileptiform activity, J Neurophysiol. 34:735 (1977).

7. D.M. Benson and J.A. Knopp, Effect of tissue absorption and microscope optical parameters on the depth of penetration for fluorescence and reflectance measurements of tissue samples, Photochem and Photobiol. 39(4):495 (1984).

8. E. Dóra, Further studies on reflectometric monitoring of cerebral microcirculation. Importance of lactate anions in coupling between cerebral blood flow and metabolism, Acta Physiol Hung. 66(2):199 (1985).

9. A. Eke, Gy. Hutiray, A.G.B. Kovách, Induced hemodilution detected by reflectometry for measuring microregional blood flow and blood volume in cat brain cortex, Am J Physiol. 236(5):H759-H768 (1979).

10. A. Eke, Reflectometric imaging of local tissue hematocrit in the cat brain cortex, in: "Cerebral Hyperemia and Ischemia: From the Standpoint of Cerebral Blood Volume" M. Tomita, T. Sawada, H. Naritomi and W.D. Heiss, eds., Elsevier Science Publishers (1988).

11. H.R. Eggert and V. Blazek, Optical properties of human brain tissue, meninges, and brain tumors in the spectral range of 200 to 900 nm, Neurosurgery. 21(4):459 (1987).

12. P. Kubelka, New contributions to the optics of intensely light-scattering materials. Part I, J Opt Soc Am. 38(5):448 (1947).

13. V. Twersky, Multiple scattering of waves and optical phenomena, J Opt Soc Am. 52:145 (1962).

14. R.A.J. Groenhuis, H.A. Ferwerda, and J.J. Ten Bosch, Scattering and absorption of turbid materials determined from reflection measurements. 1:Theory, Appl Optics 22(16):2456 (1983).

15. W.L. Butler, Absorption spectroscopy in vivo: Theory and application, Ann Rev Plant Physiol. 15:451 (1964).

16. J. Langerholc, Beam broadening in dense scattering media, Appl Optics. 21(9):1593 (1982).

17. G.H. Weiss, R. Nossal and R. F. Bonner, Statisctics of penetration depth of photons re-emitted from irradiated tissue, J Mod Optics. 36(3):349 (1989).

18. P.W. McCormick, M. Steward, G. Lewis et al, Intracerebral penetration of infrared light, J Neurosurg. 76:315 (1992).

19. A.P. Bruckner, Picosecond light scattering measurements of cataract microstructure, Appl Optics. 17(19):3177 (1978).

20. J.G. Fujimoto, S. De Silvestri, and E.P. Ippen, Femtosecond optical ranging in biological systems, Optics Letters. 11(3):150 (1986).

21. S.L. Jacques, C.A. Alter, and S.A. Prahl, Angular dependence of HeNe laser light scattering by human dermis, Lasers in the Life Sciences. 1(4):309 (1987).

22. S.T. Flock, B.C. Wilson and M.S. Patterson, Total attenuation coefficients and scattering phase functions of tissues and phantom materials at 633 nm, Med Phys. 14(5):835 (1987).

23. R.A.J. Groenhuis, J.J. Ten Bosch, and H.A. Ferwerda, Scattering and absorption of turbid materials determined from reflection measurements. 2:Measuring method and calibration, Appl Optics 22(16):2463 (1983).
24. A. Eke, Instrumentation and technology for multiparametric mapping of intra-parenchymal circulation in the brain cortex, Adv Exp Med Biol. 317:671 (1992).

QUANTITATIVE MULTICOMPONENT SPECTRAL ANALYSIS USING NEURAL NETWORKS

Chii-Wann Lin[1] and Joseph C. LaManna[2]

[1]Department of Biomedical Engineering
[2]Departments of Neurology, Physiology/Biophysics, and Neurosciences
Case Western Reserve University, School of Medicine
Cleveland, Ohio 44106, U.S.A.

INTRODUCTION

Recent developments in dye chemistry and modern optics have made simultaneous measurement of multiple intracellular ion species possible[1]. Analysis of optical spectra from intact tissues is complicated because of the presence of multiple components. Quantitative descriptions of these components are required to apply these techniques to analytical chemistry and cellular physiology. Ratio methods[2] have been applied to many areas of quantitative optical signal measurement because the quantitative data is independent of dye concentration, path length and light source intensity. However, it is known that the ratio method can give erroneous results[3] without special attention to the choice of the optimal wavelengths for these methods. Full spectra carry all the information needed for qualitative and quantitative analysis. Methods like principal component regression (PCR) and partial least-squares (PLS), which have been used for full spectra calibration in most chemometrics literature[4,5], or multicomponent stripping for image applications [6,7,8] need heavy computation times to perform their optimization processes.

It has been shown that a simple linear neuron model with Hebbian-type synaptic modification can perform a principal components analysis[9] and preserve the topological characteristic of the input pattern[10]. An artificial neural network (ANN) model has advantages over PCR and PLS in some aspects[5] as a method for multicomponent analysis. The quantitative application of ANN with spectral recognition and prediction combining the concepts of association memory and principal components analyzer has been reported[11]. The proof for the optimal convergence without local minima has been derived[11,12,13,14]. With merely linear independent patterns, the storage matrix will have crosstalk problems with the encoded information. Under such nonideal conditions, the generalized delta rule (GDR) has been used to deal with non-orthogonal input patterns[15]. Due to the similarity of the learning objective function to the one in multiple linear regression, this learning process will produce a least squares solution with significant components when the input patterns are not linearly independent. This feature detection or extraction property of self-organized behavior using local rules, like Hebb's rule, has been used to explain, e.g., the possible mechanism of opponent color processing[16] in the visual cortex.

In contrast to other uses of ANN for spectral recognition[17,18], we used the networks to distinguish the similarity between spectra with continuous output not just as a classifier with a discrete index. Thus, instead of teaching each discrete pattern, only a few teaching patterns are required and the ANN interpolates intermediate values. This decreases teaching time and increases analysis speed, making real-time applications possible. In this paper, we demonstrate the feasibility of a quantitative application with feature detection of a self-organized neural network using two-component spectra of the pH sensitive dye, (carboxyseminaphthorhodafluor -1, SNARF-1; Molecular Probes, INC., Eugene, Oregon, U.S.A.), generated from microspectrofluorometric data. This is an extended application of our previous work with neural network for quantitative spectral measurement with the absorption dye, Neutral Red (NR)[11].

SNARF-1 has been used biologically for intracellular pH measurement because it requires only a single excitation source but gives out two distinct longer wavelength emissions[19,20,21,22], one characteristic of the acid form of the dye (590 nm) and the other characteristic of the basic form of the dye (640 nm). The ratio of these two peaks follows the Henderson-Hasselbalch equation, is proportional to the solution pH and is independent of dye concentration or path length[2]. This ratio calculation method has been applied to the measurement of intracellular pH in the in vitro hippocampal brain slice[23] and in vivo in brain cortex using NR[24].

SNARF-1 is loaded into cells by means of the membrane permeant ester form (SNARF-1 AM) along the concentration gradient. The dye is then hydrolyzed by intracellular esterases to release the free fluorophore which, because of its higher ionic charge, is retained by the cells. SNARF-1 is good for physiological pH range measurement because of its pK value (7.5) and its long wavelength fluorescent emission (> 550 nm). The leakage of the dye, photobleaching caused by excessive exposure, and nonuniform dye distributions (due to compartmentalization or esterase activity) can lead to errors for pH measurement. Ratio calculation of overlapped spectrum by peak positions, in theory, can have measurement outcomes independent of the excitation intensity, path length and indicator concentration. To use full spectra of fluorescence, this ANN model was first developed as a learning device, from a set of training spectra, then used as a one pass calculation for evaluating unknown spectra due to pH changes.

THE NEURAL NETWORK MODEL

A three-layered, feed-forward artificial neural network (ANN) model, consisting of an input layer, a hidden layer and an output layer with $N_i = 25$, $N_j = 25$ and $N_k = 8$ nodes, shown in figure 1 was developed in C language on an PC. All the nodes (neurons) exhibit real, continuous-valued activities and are bounded in between 0 and 1 to represent the firing frequency of neural activities. The teaching patterns (P^n) are normalized using the Euclidean vector norm method. Nodes in the input layer acted as a buffer for the external input and their output, o_{Ni}, was directly equal to the input values, i.e. $o_{Ni}=p^n$. Output activities of the hidden and output nodes were transformed by the value of linear summation of their inputs (i) multiplied by the synaptic strengths (w), $o=f(iw)$ by a sigmoidal function. The sigmoidal function not only gives nonlinear properties to each node to simulate the response of real neurons, but also increases the dynamic range of response. The nondecreasing, differentiable properties of this function will also prevent output saturation and stay in maximum response around the operating point as illustrated in figure 2. With the backpropagation method for weight modification, these characteristics of sigmoidal function actually help to guarantee convergence of the networks. The convergence criterion is determined by the value of the objective function between the expected patterns (T) and

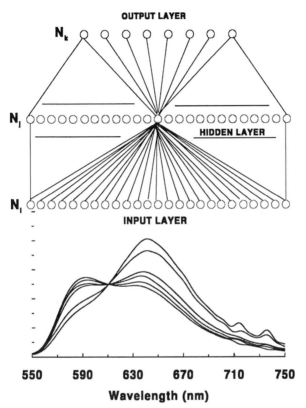

Figure 1. Artificial neural network (ANN) model for quantitative spectra measurement. Normalized fluorescent emission spectra (550nm to 750 nm) from SNARF-1 are fed into the input layer (N_i = 25; for sufficient resolution). A connection weight matrix is used to represent the connection strength between the layers (hidden units, N_j = 25 and output units N_k = 8). The teaching spectra with known pH values were assigned with binary number between 0 and 255 as the expected pattern of the output layer. The actual output of each feedforward cycle is compared to this expected pattern to calculate the error, then the weight matrix is modified with a backpropagation method. This learning process converges until the error is smaller than a preset limit. The real time evaluation of similar untrained spectra can be achieved with these trained weight matrices, which have multicomponent information encoded.

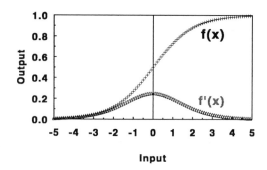

Figure 2. A sigmoidal function f(x) and its first derivative f'(x) is shown to demostrate the nondecreasing, differentiable properties and its nonsaturating output. With backpropogation method, the first derivative function acts as a noise filter to limit the maximum response range around zero.

the actual output activities of the output layer (O), $\Sigma_p \Sigma_j (t_{pj} - o_{pj})^2/2$,which is set to 0.01 times the number of the output nodes in the simulation. The expected patterns of the output layer were assigned by binary coding of known pH spectra to a value between 0 and 255. The weight modification is done according to the GDR following presentation of pattern p, as $\Delta_p w_{ji} = \eta * \Psi_{pj} * i_{pi}$, where η is a small positive constant for learning rate, $\Psi_{pj} = (t_{pj} - o_{pj})f'_j(i*w)$ for the output layer and $\Psi_{pj} = f'_j(i*w) \Sigma_k \Psi_{pk} * w_{kj}$ for the hidden layer. If the learning rate is small enough, the update of the weight matrix can be performed after presentation of all patterns.

To allow distinguishing states for each training patterns (spectra), at least n nodes in the output layer are required for 2^n patterns. As the number of output nodes is increased beyond the minimum necessary, the resolution is more and more improved. For example, if one output node is allowed, then we can only train two spectra, pH 4 for 0 and pH 9 for 1. If eight output nodes are allowed, then we can distinguish 256 different spectra with pH 4 and pH 9 set corresponding to the activity values of 0 and 255 with the expected patterns of (0 0 0 0 0 0 0 0) and (1 1 1 1 1 1 1 1). For the 5 pH unit range, this provides a theoretical resolution of about 0.02 pH units. For training spectral pH units apart, this resolution improves to better than 0.005 pH units. The prediction of the pH of an unknown spectrum uses the preset number of output nodes to interpret the output activities with a binary weighted method. For example, for an output layer of eight nodes, the output activity of each individual node is $0 < o_i < 1$ (i= 0..7,), the interpreted value will be $2^7 * o_7 + ... + 2^0 * o_0$. Therefore, the interpreted value of output activities will be a value between 0 and 255 in this case. More extensive mathematical analysis of this model has been presented previously[11].

SIMULATION RESULTS

By minimizing the objective function of this model, $\Sigma_p \Sigma_j (t_{pj} - o_{pj})^2/2$, which is similar to the objective function of multiple linear regression function, the weight matrix will evolve toward the significant components by using GDR. This is identical to the method

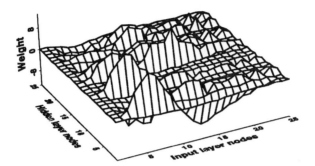

Figure 3. Connection weight matrix between input and hidden layer will store information of the two principle components in SNARF-1 spectra after trained with pH 6.62 and pH 7.72. The two peak positions correspond to the acid (590 nm) and basic (640 nm) components. The information in this weight matrix can be further enhanced by training with more extreme samples, like pH 5 and pH 9.

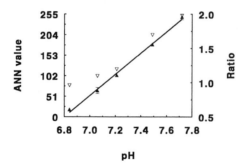

Figure 4. Calibration curve for the interpretation of artificial neural networks output activities. The data points (filled triangular) are values getting from training patterns with known pH value. The ratio calculation (open triangular)of these samples are plotted to show the linearity of ANN model. This calibration curve is then applied to the value generate from unknown pH spectra to estimate the sample pH.

used to find the eigen vectors in linear algebra. Using normalized spectra generated from microspectrofluorometry of SNARF-1 having different pH to train the network with 25 nodes to cover the visible range from 550 nm to 750 nm, we can reach a convergent state where the two principal components of SNARF-1 are identified and stored in the weight matrix of the input to hidden layer as shown in figure 3. The geometric appearance of this weight matrix shows that two inverse peaks are present in the connection weights from each hidden node to all the input nodes. The network can distinguish two states by adjusting the weight matrix toward either positive or negative. The two peak positions correspond to the acid and basic forms of SNARF-1 at about 590 nm and 640 nm respectively.

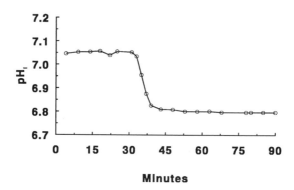

Figure 5. Intracellular pH measurement by SNARF-1 AM with quantitative output of artificial neural networks. Hippocampal slice is exposed to 100% N_2 in HEPES-ACSF. The fluorescent emission spectra are taken, then fed to the trained networks for estimation of pH changes during anoxia.

With the convergent weight matrix from a network trained with the spectra of pH 6.62 and pH 7.72, unknown spectra of intermediate pH values can be predicted by the output activities of the hidden and output layers. After the principal components have been identified by the learning procedure, the subsequent prediction of unknown spectra can be considered as the inner product of the input vector with convergent weight matrix.

By looking at the output activities of the output layer using a binary weighted method after convergence, a calibration curve can be constructed from a limited number of teaching spectra with known pH values. Simulation with different numbers of teaching spectra gives the average activity value at each specific pH. These values are then plotted vs pH to give a calibration curve. The calibration curve constructed from the fluorescent ratio (I636/I591) determined by a standard multiple linear regression method is plotted for purposes of comparison. As shown in figure 4, this new method maps the input spectra to the output activities of the output nodes linearly from pH 6.8 to pH 7.8 while the calibration curve from ratio calculation starts to deviate from linear at about pH 7.2.

In hippocampal brain slices in vitro, anoxia results in an intracellular acidification. Fluorescent spectra generated from microspectrophotometry with nonrecovering anoxic response of a hippocampal brain slice are used to demonstrate the feasibility of this model for quantitative measurement (figure 5). A convergent weight matrix from the learning phase of the simulation is used to give the projected output value corresponding to its input spectrum in one step of the process. Mathematically, this convergent weight matrix multiplied by the input vectors yields the index of similarity. This activity output value can then be transformed to pH value by applying the calibration curve derived above.

DISCUSSION

The quantitative application of the ANN model for spectral measurement has been reported with absorption dye (NR)[11]. The general structure of this method can also be adopted for fluorescent spectral measurement using SNARF-1. A simple, local interactive learning rule, like GDR, can identify the eigenvectors (principal components) of the incoming information and encode them in the weight matrix (synaptic junction), after a successful learning procedure as suggested by Oja[9]. This convergent weight matrix can then be used to predict similar untrained patterns with the output activities showing the correlation between input and teaching patterns. Unlike the "wild guess" which occassionaly occurs in conventional methods, this model tends to follow the interpolation of trained patterns by using full spectral characteristics. Extrapolation of unknown similar spectra can also be exploded provided that expected patterns are not assigned to extreme numbers.

By considering that information is carried by frequency coding instead of an all or none single pulse in the central nervous system and the limited resources neurons can provide for activation, we used 0 and 1 for the notation of silent and maximum firing frequency in our model. At the input layer, this is coded by the Euclidean vector norm to normalize the input pattern to values between 0 and 1. After this layer, coding is done by a sigmoidal function which transforms the input of each node to an output between 0 and 1. As pointed out in the previous section, this function is important in the sense of dynamic range and noise quenching for the behavior of networks. Real time application of the trained networks is straight forward as a feed forward model. Dynamic modification of the trained weight matrix can be incorporated into the model to fulfill the variation of samples.

In conclusion, this model (figure 1) has been shown to be capable of quantitative measurement for spectral recognition and prediction in both absorption and fluorescent spectra. It also presents a new method for spectrophotometric measurement where quantitative information depends on the general characteristics of spectra. This model might be generalized for application to multisensory data fusion and pattern-oriented sensory information processing.

REFERENCES

1. G.T. Rijkers, L.B. Justement, A.W. Griffioen, and J.C. Cambier, Improved method for measuring intracellular Ca^{++} with Fluo-3, *Cytometry* **11**: 923-927 (1990)
2. V.W. Macdonald, J.H. Keizer, F.F. Jöbsis, Spectrophotometric measurements of metabolically induced pH changed in frog skeletal muscle, *Arch. Biochem.* **184**: 423-430 (1977)
3. U. Heinrich, J. Hoffmann, and D.W. Lübbers, Quantitative evaluation of optical reflection spectra of blood-free perfused guinea pig brain using a nonlinear multicomponent analysis, *Pflügers Arch.* **409**: 152-157 (1987)
4. E.V. Thomas, And D.M. Haaland, Comparison of multivariate calibration methods for quantitative spectra analysis, *Anal. Chem.* **62**:1091-1099 (1990)
5. P.J. Gemperline, J.R. Long, and V.G. Gregoriou, Nonlinear multivariate calibration using principal components regression and artificial neural networks, *Anal. Chem.* **63**:2313-2323 (1991)

6. S. Kawata, K. Sasaki, and S. Minami, Component analysis of spatial and spectral patterns in multispectral images. I. basis, *J. Opt. Soc.Am. A* **4**: 2101-2106 (1987)
7. S. Kawata, K. Sasaki, and S. Minami, Component analysis of spatial and spectral patterns in multispectral images. II. Entropy minimization, *J. Opt. Soc.Am. A* **6**: 73-79 (1989)
8. M. Nakamura, Y. Suzuki, and S. Kobayashi, A method for recovering physiological components from dynamic radionuclide images using the maximum entropy principle: a numerical investigation, *IEEE trans. Biomed. Eng.* **36**: 906-917 (1989)
9. E. Oja, A simplified neuron model as a principal component analyzer, *J. Math. Biol.* **15**: 267-273 (1982)
10. T. Kohonen, Self-organized formation of topological correct feature maps. *Biol. Cybern.* **43**: 59-69 (1982)
11. C.W. Lin, J.C. LaManna, and Y.Takefuji, Quantitative measurement of two-component pH-sensitive colorimetric spectra using multilayer neural networks, *Biol. Cybern.* (in press)
12. T. Kohonen, An adapative associative memoryprinciple, *IEEE Comput.* **23**: 444-445 (1974)
13. P. Baldi, and K. Hornik, Neural networks and principal component analysis: learning from examples without local minima, *Neural Networks* **2**: 53-58 (1989)
14 T.D. Sanger, Optimal unsupervised learning in a single-layer linear feedforward neural network, *Neural Networks*, **2**: 459-473 (1989)
15. D.E. Rumelhart, and J.L McClelland, "The PDP Research Group: Parallel Distributed Processing", MIT Press, Cambridge (1988)
16. J. Rubner, and K.Schulten, Development of feature detector by self-organization, *Biol. Cybern.* **62**: 193-199 (1990)
17. B.J. Wythoff, S.P. Levine, and S.A. Tomellini, Spectral peak verification and recognition using a multilayered neural network, *Anal. Chem.* **62**: 2702-2709 (1990)
18. B. Meyer, T. Hansen, D. Nute, P. Albersheim, A. Darvili, W. York, and J. Sellers, Identification of the 1H-NMR spectra of complex oligosaccharides with artificial neural networks, *Science* **251**: 542-544
19. J.E. Whitaker, R.P. Haugland, and F.G. Prendergast, Spectral and Photophysical studies of Benzo[c]xanthene dyes: dual emission pH sensors, *Anal. Biochem.* **194**: 330-344 (1991)
20. O.Seksek, N. Henry-Toulmé, F. Sureau, and J. Bolard, SNARF-1 as an intracellular pH indicator in laser microspectrofluorometry: a critical assessment, *Anal. Biochem.* **193**: 49-54 (1991)
21. K.J. Buckler, and R.D. Vaughan-Jones, Application of a new pH-sensitive fluoroprobe (carboxy-SNARF-1) for intracellular pH measurement in small, isolated cells, *Pflügers Arch.* **417**: 234-239 (1990)
22. S. Bassnett, L. Reinisch, and D.C. Beebe, Intracellular pH measurement using single excitation-dual emission fluorescence ratios, *Am. J. Physiol.* **258**: C171-C178 (1990)
23. J.C. LaManna, and K.A. McCracken, The use of neutral red as an intracellular pH indicator in rat brain cortex in vivo. *Analyt. Biochem.* **142**: 117-125 (1984)
24. T.J. Sick, T.S. Whittingham, J.C. LaManna, Determination of intracellular pH in the in vitro hippocampal slice preparation by transillumination spectrophotometry of neutral red. *J. Neurosci. M.* **27**: 25-34

SKELETAL MUSCLE AND OTHER TISSUES

MORPHOMETRY OF THE SIZE OF THE CAPILLARY-TO-FIBER INTERFACE IN MUSCLES

Odile Mathieu-Costello

Department of Medicine, 0623
University of California, San Diego
La Jolla, CA 92093-0623

INTRODUCTION

Capillary-to-fiber (C/F) perimeter ratio in transverse sections is an index of capillary surface per fiber surface, i.e. it allows one to incorporate the increased surface area due to capillary tortuosity and branching into the estimate of a muscle potential for O_2 transfer. This is important considering the role of the capillary-to-fiber interface in determining O_2 flux rates in red muscles (Gayeski and Honig, 1986; Groebe and Thews, 1990). A greater capillary surface per fiber surface can allow adequate flux rates to be maintained at a lower PO_2 at the red cell surface, or higher fluxes to be achieved at a similar red cell PO_2 (rev. Honig et al, 1991).

We derived stereological equations which show how C/F perimeter ratio in transverse sections is related to other aspects of muscle capillarity (e.g. capillary-to-fiber number ratio, capillary number per fiber cross-sectional area, capillary length per fiber volume, etc.), fiber size and capillary diameter (Mathieu-Costello et al, 1991). Knowing these relationships is useful to determine the effect of each variable on the size of the C/F interface, and also to calculate C/F perimeter ratio from other estimates of muscle capillarity such as capillary number, length, surface or volume density. It also permits to study the effect of fiber shortening, i.e. changes in sarcomere length within the physiological range on C/F perimeter ratio. We showed that it is a unique feature of C/F perimeter ratio to account for capillary geometry and fiber size and yet itself vary little with sarcomere length. This permits direct comparisons of the potential for blood-tissue exchange between muscles of different fiber size or examined at different sarcomere length (Mathieu-Costello et al, 1991).

In this study, we compared calculated values of C/F perimeter ratio using different morphometric variables with direct estimates by intersection-counting in muscle transverse sections and summarized data on the effect of light (LM) and transmission electron microscopy (TEM) resolution on this estimation. Our purpose was to determine how close estimates of C/F perimeter ratio were obtained via different methods in muscles with different capillary geometry or with large differences in capillary density and fiber size.

MATERIAL AND METHODS

Thirty six perfusion-fixed muscle samples from a total of eighteen animals were used. They included the flight muscles of hummingbirds (_Selaphorus rufus_; body mass M_b, 3-4g) and bats (_Eptesicus fuscus_; M_b, 15-16g), the red muscle of tunas (_Katsuwomus pelamis_; Mb, 1.5-2kg), hindlimb muscles of bats and soleus muscle of rats (M_b, 342-745g). We chose those samples because of their differences in capillary density or geometry and fiber size. Fiber cross-sectional area varied 10-fold, from $201 \pm 14 \ \mu m^2$ in hummingbird flight muscle to $1,988 \pm 127 \ \mu m^2$ in rat M. soleus, and capillary density ranged from $1301 \pm 129 \ mm^{-2}$ in rat M. soleus to $8,001 \pm 782 \ mm^{-2}$ in hummingbird flight muscle (Table 1).

Table 1
Group mean values of fiber cross-sectional area and capillary numerical density, i.e. capillary number per fiber cross-sectional area, at 2.1 μm sarcomere length in each muscle*

	Fiber cross-sectional area μm^2	Capillary density mm^{-2}
Hummingbird flight muscle (n = 7)	201 ± 14	8,001 ± 782
Bat pectoralis (n = 6) hindlimb (n = 6)	318 ± 10 447 ± 35	6,394 ± 380 2,865 ± 238
Tuna red muscle (n = 8)	475 ± 25	3,391 ± 197
Rat soleus muscle (n = 9)	1,988 ± 127	1,301 ± 129

*From Mathieu-Costello et al, 1992b (hummingbird) and 1992c (bat); calculated from Mathieu-Costello 1987 (rat) and 1992a (tuna).

Tissue Preparation and Sectioning

Muscle preparation, sampling, processing for electron microscopy and the morphometric analysis of capillary density and geometry, fiber size and ultrastructure have been reported elsewhere (Mathieu-Costello, 1987; Mathieu-Costello et al 1992a-c). Briefly, the tissues were fixed by vascular perfusion _in situ_. The entire vasculature was perfused with saline (11.06 g NaCl/L, 350 mosm, 20,000 U heparin/L) via a cannula inserted directly into the left ventricle with the right atrium cut open to secure outflow. Perfusion fixation followed with glutaraldehyde fixative (6.25% solution in 0.1 M sodium cacodylate buffer; total osmolarity of the fixative 1,100 mosm; pH 7.4) at a non pulsatile pressure of 80-100 mmHg (bat and rat), 150-170 mmHg (hummingbird) and 80-90 mmHg (tuna). Samples were taken from pectoralis and supracoracoideus muscles of hummingbird (Mathieu-Costello et al 1992b), pectoralis and hindlimb muscles of bats (Mathieu-Costello et al, 1992c), red muscle of tuna (Mathieu-Costello et al, 1992a) and rat M. soleus (Mathieu-Costello, 1987) and processed for electron microscopy using standard procedures.

One micrometer thick sections were cut on a LKB Ultrotome III and stained with 0.1% aqueous toluidine blue solution. From each muscle sample, four to eight blocks were cut into four transverse and four longitudinal sections following a procedure described elsewhere in detail (Mathieu-Costello, 1987). Briefly, a minimum of three sections were taken either parallel to the muscle fiber axis at consecutive angles a approximately 1° apart (longitudinal sections) or perpendicular to the fiber axis at consecutive angles approximately 5° apart (transverse sections). Sarcomere length was measured on each longitudinal section (average of 10 measurements of groups of consecutive sarcomeres systematically sampled over the entire area of each section) examined at magnification 630x. A section was considered to be longitudinal when changing a in either direction produced fiber sections with a greater sarcomere length. It was considered transverse when changing a gave sections with a smaller A-band spacing. Ultrathin transverse sections (50-70 nm) were contrasted with uranyl acetate and bismuth subnitrate (Riva, 1974) and examined with a Zeiss 10 electron microscope.

Morphometry

Capillary-to-fiber perimeter ratio in transverse sections, $B_B(0)$, was calculated by each of two methods.

1. $B_B(0)$ is the product of capillary length per fiber volume, $J_V(c,f)$, capillary perimeter, $\pi \cdot \bar{d}(c)$, and the ratio of fiber cross-sectional area, $\bar{a}(f)$, and fiber cross-sectional perimeter, $\bar{b}(f)$, based on the equation (Mathieu-Costello et al 1991) :

$$B_B(0) = [J_V(c,f) \cdot \pi \cdot \bar{d}(c) \ / \ c'(K',0)] \cdot [\bar{a}(f) \ / \bar{b}(f)] \qquad (1)$$

where $c'(K',0)$ is an anisotropy coefficient relating capillary perimeter per fiber cross-sectional area and capillary surface per volume of fiber. $J_V(c,f)$ is the product of capillary density in transverse sections (i.e. capillary number per fiber cross-sectional area) and the $c(K,0)$ anisotropy coefficient (Mathieu et al 1983):

$$J_V(c,f) = c(K,0) \cdot Q_A(0) \qquad (2)$$

Except for muscles with a large degree of capillary tortuosity [$c(K,0)$ coefficient (Eq. 2) > 1.53], the value of $c'(K',0)$ is 1. The maximal value of $c'(K',0)$ is 1.27 [for $c(K,0) = 2$; see Mathieu-Costello et al, 1991].

2. $B_B(0)$ is also the product of capillary surface per fiber volume, $S_V(c,f)$, and the ratio of fiber cross-sectional area, $\bar{a}(f)$, and perimeter, $\bar{b}(f)$, based on the equation (Mathieu-Costello et al, 1992c).

$$B_B(0) = [S_V(c,f) \ / \ c'(K',0)] \cdot [\bar{a}(f) \ / \bar{b}(f)] \qquad (3)$$

663

Eq. 3 is obtained from Eq. 1 by replacing the product of capillary cross-sectional perimeter $[\pi \cdot \bar{d}(c)]$ and capillary length per fiber volume, $J_V(c,f)$, by the quantity it represents, i.e. capillary surface per fiber volume, $S_V(c,f)$.

We calculated $B_B(0)$ via Eq. 1 and 3 in each muscle using values for anisotropy coefficient, $c'(K',0)$, fiber cross-sectional area, $\bar{a}(f)$, fiber cross-sectional perimeter, $\bar{b}(f)$, and capillary length per fiber volume, $J_V(c,f)$, in the same samples reported elsewhere (Mathieu-Costello et al 1992a-c). In Eq. 3, we used the estimates of capillary surface per fiber volume, $S_V(c,f)$, measured by intersection-counting on vertical (i.e. longitudinal) sections with a cycloid grid using the method developed by Baddeley et al (1986). The measurements were done on the same longitudinal sections used to estimate capillary length per fiber volume, $J_V(c,f)$, and the orientation coefficients $c(K,0)$ and $c'(K',0)$. Estimates of $S_V(c,f)$ in hummingbird and bat flight muscles, bat hindlimb and rat M. soleus have been reported elsewhere (Mathieu-Costello et al 1992b,c). In tuna red muscle, we measured a total of 25-35 fields selected by systematic random sampling in each sample. They were measured at magnification 400x with a O(6x6) cycloid (Cruz-Orive, University of Bern, Switzerland) eyepiece test system.

Calculated values of $B_B(0)$ via Eqs. 1 and 3 were compared with direct estimates by intersection-counting using the equation

$$B_B(0) = l_c/l_f \tag{4}$$

where l_c and l_f are the intersections of test lines with the boundary of capillaries and fibers, respectively in transverse sections. We also summarize data on the effect of light (LM) and electron microscopy (EM) resolution on the estimate of $B_B(0)$ by intersection-counting in hummingbird flight muscle and rat M. soleus. All measurements of $B_B(0)$ by intersection-counting in transverse sections used in this paper are from Mathieu-Costello et al (1992a-c). They were obtained using both the horizontal and vertical lines of a square grid superimposed on pictures taken from the same transverse sections used to estimate capillary density, fiber size and capillary diameter. LM measurement were done with either a l00-point square grid eyepiece at magnification 1,000x (tuna red muscle and rat M. soleus) or a 144-point square grid on micrographs projected at a final magnification of 2,060x (hummingbird flight muscle). EM measurements were done with a 144-point square grid on micrographs projected at a final magnification of 15,000x (bat pectoralis), 12,000x (hummingbird flight muscle and bat hindlimb) and 9,000x (rat M. soleus). We examined totals of 15 ± 0 (EM) and 22 ± 2 (LM) micrographs per sample in hummingbird flight muscle, 16 ± 0 in bat pectoralis (EM), 39 ± 0 in bat hindlimb (EM), 76 ± 2 (EM) and 75 ± 1 (LM) in rat M. soleus, and 63 ± 4 (LM) in tuna red muscle.

Statistical Analysis

Data are expressed as mean ± SE. Estimates of $B_B(0)$ in the same samples using different methods were compared by paired t-test. Differences were taken as significant for $P < 0.05$.

RESULTS AND DISCUSSION

Capillary-to-fiber perimeter ratio was approximately two-fold greater in hummingbird (0.39 ± 0.02) and bat flight muscles (0.46 ± 0.02) than in rat soleus muscle (0.23 ± 0.03), and it was 0.30 ± 0.01 and 0.27 ± 0.02 in tuna red muscle and bat hindlimb, respectively (all direct estimates by intersection counting). There was no significant difference between light (LM) and transmission electron microscopy (TEM) estimates of C/F perimeter ratio by intersection-counting in transverse sections of either hummingbird flight muscle or rat M. soleus (Fig.1).

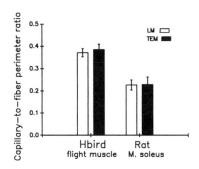

Fig. 1   Histogram of capillary-to-fiber perimeter ratio in muscle transverse sections, $B_B(0)$, measured by intersection-counting by light (LM) and transmission electron microscopy (TEM) in hummingbird flight muscle (n = 7) and rat M. soleus (n = 9). Values are group mean ± SE.

Capillary surface per fiber volume ranged from 47.2 ± 3.3 to 74.7 ± 3.8 (group mean 57.6 ± 3.4) mm^2/mm^3 in tuna red muscle. Calculated values of C/F perimeter ratio via Eq. 3 were highly correlated with direct estimates by intersection-counting (r = 0.84; n = 36), and the two estimates were not significantly different from each other in any muscle (Fig. 2). Similarly, calculated values of C/F perimeter ratio via Eq. 1 were very close and not significantly different from those obtained by direct measurement by intersection-counting in hummingbird and bat flight muscle. However, in other muscles (bat hindlimb, rat soleus and tuna red muscle) there was a significant difference of 10 - 17% between the two estimates of C/F perimeter ratio (Fig. 2). The difference was not in the same direction in all muscles, indicating that it was not the result of a bias in the calculated estimates. Instead, it could be due to the cumulative effect of the small imprecision of the estimate of each variable used to calculate C/F perimeter ratio (a larger number of variables is used in the calculation of $B_B(0)$ via capillary length density and diameter (Eq. 1) than via capillary surface density (Eq. 3).

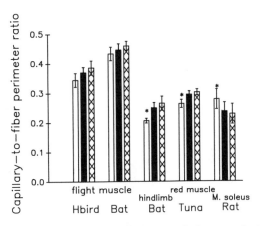

Fig. 2 Histogram of capillary-to-fiber perimeter ratio in muscle transverse section, $B_B(0)$, measured by intersection-counting (cross-hatched bars) and calculated via Eq. 1 (open bars) and Eq. 3 (solid bars) in each muscle. Values are group means ± SE. * Significantly different ($P<0.05$) after calculation via Eq. 1 compared with intersection-counting measurements in transverse sections.

Capillary surface per fiber surface is the product of C/F perimeter ratio and the $c'(K',0)$ anisotropy coefficient (Mathieu-Costello et al, 1991). It is also the product of capillary surface per fiber volume and the ratio of fiber cross-sectional area and cross-sectional perimeter (see Eq. 3). The value of the capillary anisotropy coefficient $c'(K',0)$ was 1 in almost all samples, indicating that C/F perimeter ratio was a direct estimate of capillary-to-fiber surface ratio in those muscles (Mathieu-Costello et al, 1992a-c).

Capillary-to-fiber perimeter ratio was greater in hummingbird and bat flight muscle than in other muscles (Fig. 2). The examination of capillary surface per fiber surface $S_s(c,f)$ relative to the volume of mitochondria in the muscle fibers showed that $S_s(c,f)$ at a given mitochondrial volume per unit length of fiber was two times greater in bat and hummingbird flight muscle than in rat M. soleus (Mathieu-Costello et al 1992b,c). In bat hindlimb it was intermediate between those in flight muscle and rat M. soleus (Mathieu-Costello et al 1992c) and it was similar in rat M. soleus and tuna red muscle (Mathieu-Costello et al 1992a). The finding of a greater capillary surface per fiber surface in the flight muscles suggests a greater capacity for O_2 fluxes, consistent with the suggestion of an important role of the capillary-to-fiber interface in blood-tissue O_2 kinetics (Honig et al 1991). It is also consistent with measurements of O_2 uptake/ml of mitochondria in flying hummingbirds that are about twice as high as those in locomotory muscles of mammals running at $\dot{V}O_2$max (Suarez et al, 1991).

SUMMARY

Capillary-to-fiber perimeter ratio is a morphometric estimate of muscle capillarity in transverse sections which accounts for the three-dimensional arrangement of the capillary network. We compared different methods for estimating capillary-to-fiber perimeter ratio in muscles with large differences in fiber size and capillary density or geometry (hummingbird and bat flight muscle, bat hindlimb, tuna red muscle and rat M. soleus). There was no significant difference between light and electron microscopy estimates of capillary-to-fiber perimeter ratio by direct intersection-counting in transverse sections. Calculated values via capillary surface per fiber volume and fiber cross-sectional area/perimeter were not significantly different from those obtained by direct intersection-counting in muscle transverse sections in any muscle. A closer estimate of capillary-to-fiber perimeter ratio to that obtained by direct intersection-counting in transverse sections was calculated via capillary surface density than capillary length per fiber volume and capillary diameter, possibly because of the greater number of variables used to calculate capillary-to-fiber perimeter ratio via capillary length density and diameter. A greater capillary-to-fiber perimeter ratio was found in hummingbird and bat flight muscle than in the other muscles, consistent with an important role of the capillary-to-fiber interface in determining O_2 flux rates and measurements of mitochondrial respiratory rates in flying hummingbird that are about two times greater than those in locomotory muscles of mammals running at $\dot{V}O_2$max.

ACKNOWLEDGEMENTS

We are very grateful to Mr. Peter Agey for technical assistance. The work was supported by Grant 5P01 HL-17731 from the National Institute of Health.

REFERENCES

Baddeley, A.J., Gundersen, H.J.G., and Cruz-Orive, L.M., 1986, Estimation of surface area from vertical sections. J. Microscopy, 142:259-276.

Gayeski, T.E.J., and Honig, C.R., 1986, O_2 gradients from sarcolemma to cell interior in red muscle at maximal $\dot{V}O_2$. Am. J. Physiol., 251:H789-H799.

Groebe, K., and Thews, G., 1990, Role of geometry and anisotropic diffusion for modelling PO_2 profiles in working red muscle. Resp. Physiol., 79:255-278.

Honig, C.R., Gayeski, T.E.J., Groebe, K., 1991, Myoglobin and Oxygen Gradients. In: "The Lung: Scientific Foundations", edited by R.G. Crystal, J.B. West, P.J. Barnes, N.S. Cherniack and E.R. Weibel, Raven Press, New York, pp. 1489-1495.

Mathieu, O., Cruz-Orive, L.M., Hoppeler, H., and Weibel, E.R., 1983, Estimating length density and quantifying anisotropy in skeletal muscle capillaries. J. Microscopy, 131:131-146.

Mathieu-Costello, O., 1987, Capillary tortuosity and degree of contraction or extension of skeletal muscles. Microvasc. Res., 33:98-117.

Mathieu-Costello, O., Agey, P.J., Logemann, R.B., Brill, R.W., and Hochachka, P.W., 1992a, Capillary-fiber geometrical relationships in tuna red muscle. Can. J. Zool., 70:1218-1229.

Mathieu-Costello, O., Ellis, C.G., Potter, R.F., MacDonald, I.C., and Groom, A.C., 1991, Muscle capillary-to-fiber perimeter ratio: morphometry. Am. J. Physiol., 261:H1617-H1625.

Mathieu-Costello, O., Suarez, R.K., and Hochachka, P.W., 1992b, Capillary-to-fiber geometry and mitochondrial density in hummingbird flight muscle. Resp. Physiol., 89:113-132.

Mathieu-Costello, O., Szewczak, J.M., Logemann, R.B., and Agey P.J., 1992c, Geometry of blood-tissue exchange in bat flight muscle compared with bat hindlimb and rat soleus muscle. Am. J. Physiol., 262:R955-R965.

Riva, A., 1974, A simple and rapid staining method for enhancing the contrast of tissues previously treated with uranyl acetate. J. Microsc. (Paris), 19:105-108.

Suarez, R.K., Lighton, J.R.B., Brown, G.S., and Mathieu-Costello, O., 1991, Mitochondrial respiration in hummingbird flight muscles. Proc. Natl. Acad. Sci. USA, 88:4870-4873.

CAPILLARY PROLIFERATION RELATED TO FIBRE TYPES IN HYPERTROPHIED AGING RAT M. PLANTARIS

H. Degens, Z. Turek, L.J.C. Hoofd and
R.A. Binkhorst

Department of Physiology
University of Nijmegen
The Netherlands

INTRODUCTION

Most studies on ageing describe an age-related muscle fibre atrophy and an increase in the percentage of type I (oxidative) and IIa (oxidative glycolytic) fibres and a decrease in the percentage of IIb (glycolytic) fibres (Kovanen, 1989). Compensatory hypertrophy is characterised by enlargement of existing fibres and an increased percentage of type I fibres (Riedy et al., 1985). Since muscle fibre type and size are correlated with the capillary supply to a fibre (Egginton and Ross, 1989), changes in muscle capillary supply might accompany changes in fibre type composition and fibre cross-sectional areas. Absence of capillary proliferation with hypertrophy would result in increased diffusion distances from the capillary to the interior of fibres, which might impede the delivery of oxygen to the interior of fibres. However, little is known about capillarisation in ageing rat muscles not to mention capillarisation in hypertrophied ageing muscle. Therefore, in the present study we investigated the capillarisation in muscles at various ages and, in particular, we wanted to elucidate whether compensatory hypertrophy in ageing muscle was accompanied by capillary proliferation. This was done by the extended method of Capillary Domains as developed by Hoofd et al. (1985; Egginton and Ross, 1989).

METHODS

Female Wistar rats were used. Functional overload resulting in hypertrophy of the m. plantaris (Table 1) was obtained by denervation of synergists (Binkhorst, 1969). Six weeks later the overloaded (O) muscles and muscles of control (C) rats were excised. At that time the rats were 5, 13 and 25 months old. Their body weights are given in table 1. On transverse sections of the muscles, cut at -25 ^{0}C, the fibres were classified

Oxygen Transport to Tissue XV, Edited by P. Vaupel
et al., Plenum Press, New York, 1994

as type I or II based on ATP-ase activity, with type II fibres subclassified into IIa (oxidative) and IIb (glycolytic) based on SDH activity. Capillaries were depicted by the combined staining for alkaline phosphatase and dipeptidyl peptidase IV (Batra et al., 1989). On photomicrographs of the sections the fibre type composition was assessed. Using a digitising tablet, fibre outlines were read into the computer as contour coordinates and capillary locations as coordinates of capillary centres. Fibre cross-sectional areas (FCSA in μm^2) were derived from complete fibre contours on these photographs. The capillary density (CD) was defined as the number of capillaries per square millimetre of tissue. Capillary domains were constructed, defined as the area bounded by lines perpendicular to the midpoint of lines equidistant from adjacent capillaries (Hoofd et al., 1985). From overlapping of domains and muscle fibres the local capillary-to-fibre ratio (LCFR) for each fibre was derived. The LCFR for a fibre was defined as the sum of fractions of each domain area overlapping the fibre. As one domain is the region geometrically supplied by one capillary, the LCFR can be interpreted as the number of capillaries geometrically supplying a fibre (Egginton et al., 1988). The correlation coefficients and slopes of the regression lines between local capillary-to-fibre ratio and fibre cross-sectional area for each fibre type separately, were calculated for each group. The slope of the regression line gives an indication for the capillary supply per fibre cross-sectional area for each individual fibre type. This was also done for all fibres pooled in each group to determine changes in capillary supply per fibre cross-sectional area irrespective of fibre type, thereby circumventing fibre type specific effects.

ANOVA was applied to test for age and overload effects. When an age effect was found a Bonferroni corrected t-test was applied to test for differences between groups (Wallenstein et al., 1980). The correlation coefficients for the relation between local capillary-to-fibre ratio and fibre cross-sectional area were tested for significance with a t test as was also done to detect differences in slopes of regression lines between groups or fibre types. Differences were considered significant at P < 0.05.

Table 1. Body weight (BW), muscle weight (MW), and capillary density (CD) of control (C) and overloaded (O) rat plantaris muscle of different age.

		5 MONTHS	13 MONTHS	25 MONTHS
C:	BW (g)	225 ± 5 (20)	303 ± 7 (20)	307 ± 8.1 (17)
	MW (mg)	329 ± 12 (19)	348 ± 14 (20)	357 ± 13 (16)
	CD (mm^{-2})	882 ± 32 (15)	755 ± 45 (20)	652 ± 24 (16)
O:	BW (g)	215 ± 3 (18)	285 ± 6 (19)	296 ± 11 (15)
	MW (mg)	434 ± 13 (16)	446 ± 16 (18)	456 ± 19 (15)
	CD (mm^{-2})	802 ± 41 (15)	657 ± 32 (19)	548 ± 30 (15)

Values are mean ± SEM; number of animals in parentheses.

RESULTS

In order to limit the number of data only the data of the deep region (more oxidative) of the m. plantaris are given. The data of the superficial (more glycolytic) region show a similar pattern. Table 1 shows the data for body and muscle weight, and capillary density. The P values as obtained by the ANOVA for fibre type related variables are given in table 2. For age effects no general direction could be given (no arrows for age effects in table 2), as the effects of age were not always similar. Table 3 shows the percentage of fibre types, cross-sectional areas and local capillary-to-fibre ratio. Table 3 also shows the characteristics of the regressions between local capillary-to-fibre ratio and fibre cross-sectional areas.

Table 2. P values as obtained by ANOVA for age and overload effects on fibre type related variables in the deep region of rat m. plantaris.

	Age			Overload		
	I	IIa	IIb	I	IIa	IIb
%	NS	P < 0.001	P = 0.005	P < 0.001↑	NS	P < 0.001↓
FCSA	P < 0.001	P < 0.001	P = 0.003	P < 0.001↑	P < 0.001↑	P < 0.001↑
LCFR	P = 0.03	P < 0.001	P = 0.001	P < 0.001↑	P < 0.001↑	NS
Slope	P < 0.001	P < 0.001	P < 0.001	P < 0.001 ↓	P < 0.001 ↓	NS

The direction of the arrows indicates the direction of the overload effect; %: number percentage of the respective fibre types; FCSA: fibre cross-sectional area in μm^2; LCFR: local capillary-to-fibre ratio; Slope:slope of the regression line forced through the origin.

Local capillary-to-fibre ratio and fibre cross-sectional area. The correlation coefficients between local capillary-to-fibre ratio and fibre cross-sectional area for each fibre type separately and all fibres pooled for each group are given in table 3 and were all significant (P < 0.015). In most cases the slope of type I fibres was largest and the slope of IIb fibres smallest with those of IIa fibres in between. Figure 1 illustrates this.

Age. No age effects on muscle weight were found. The percentage of type IIa fibres was lower in muscles of 5 months old rats, than in those of other age, while for the percentage of type IIb fibres the opposite was found. The cross-sectional areas of fibres of each type were smaller in muscles of 5 than in those of 13 months old rats. Only the cross-sectional area of IIb fibres was significantly larger in muscles of 13 than in those of 25 months old rats. The capillary density decreased with increasing age (P < 0.001). The local capillary-to-fibre ratio of each fibre type was significantly lower in muscles of 25 months old rats than in those of younger rats. However, for type I fibres no significant difference between muscles of 25 and 5 months old rats was found. It appeared that the slope of the regression lines between local capillary-to-fibre ratio and fibre cross-sectional area decreased with increasing age for each fibre type in both control and overloaded muscles.

Overload. An almost 30% increase in muscle weight as a result of the overload was obtained in each age group (P < 0.001). This was reflected in increased cross-sectional areas of fibres of each type. The percentage of type I fibres was increased with overload at all ages, whereas the percentage of IIb fibres was decreased. Overload resulted in a decreased capillary density (P = 0.001). The hypertrophy was accompanied by an increased local capillary-to-fibre ratio for each fibre type, except for IIb fibres. The slopes of the regression lines between local capillary-to-fibre ratio and fibre cross-sectional area of the overloaded muscles were lower than the slopes of the regression lines of the corresponding control muscles (P < 0.001) except for IIb fibres.

Table 3. Fibre type composition (number percentage), fibre cross-sectional area (FCSA), Local capillary-to-fibre ratio (LCFR) and correlation coefficients (R) and slopes of the regressions between LCFR and FCSA in control and overloaded muscles of different age.

	5 MONTHS CONTROL				13 MONTHS CONTROL				25 MONTHS CONTROL			
	I	IIa	IIb	All	I	IIa	IIb	All	I	IIa	IIb	All
%	15.34 ± 1.24 (15)	51.63 ± 1.48 (15)	33.05 ± 2.04 (15)		16.18 ± 0.89 (20)	59.71 ± 1.70 (20)	24.13 ± 1.80 (20)		17.17 ± 2.10 (18)	56.50 ± 3.16 (18)	26.32 ± 3.07 (18)	
FCSA (µm²)	1279 ± 53 (15)	1613 ± 67 (15)	2360 ± 84 (15)	1755 ± 77 (15)	1471 ± 59 (20)	2129 ± 100 (20)	3121 ± 174 (20)	2192 ± 84 (20)	1688 ± 131 (17)	2061 ± 108 (17)	2601 ± 114 (17)	2088 ± 86 (16)
LCFR	1.263 ± 0.049 (15)	1.523 ± 0.061 (15)	1.828 ± 0.083 (15)	1.557 ± 0.053 (15)	1.271 ± 0.083 (20)	1.669 ± 0.070 (20)	2.021 ± 0.081 (20)	1.664 ± 0.051 (20)	1.050 ± 0.081 (16)	1.437 ± 0.072 (16)	1.594 ± 0.061 (16)	1.410 ± 0.052 (16)
R	0.518 (97)	0.605 (269)	0.497 (140)	0.617 (506)	0.438 (97)	0.530 (355)	0.243 (105)	0.516 (557)	0.698 (141)	0.686 (440)	0.715 (181)	0.713 (762)
Slope	1004 ± 40 (15)	948 ± 37 (15)	774 ± 33 (15)	872 ± 36 (15)	859 ± 45 (20)	800 ± 45 (20)	658 ± 37 (20)	755 ± 44 (20)	728 ± 38 (16)	688 ± 29 (16)	624 ± 30 (16)	671 ± 26 (16)

	5 MONTHS OVERLOADED				13 MONTHS OVERLOADED				25 MONTHS OVERLOADED			
	I	IIa	IIb	All	I	IIa	IIb	All	I	IIa	IIb	All
%	31.79 ± 2.31 (15)	49.11 ± 2.95 (15)	19.10 ± 2.81 (15)		27.16 ± 1.73 (19)	61.04 ± 2.27 (19)	11.79 ± 2.10 (19)		23.29 ± 1.63 (15)	63.18 ± 3.72 (15)	13.60 ± 3.17 (15)	
FCSA (µm²)	2249 ± 159 (15)	2743 ± 182 (15)	3288 ± 164 (14)	2592 ± 156 (14)	3036 ± 145 (19)	3294 ± 132 (19)	3514 ± 168 (14)	3242 ± 116 (19)	3032 ± 186 (15)	3030 ± 153 (15)	3183 ± 262 (10)	3032 ± 121 (15)
LCFR	1.840 ± 0.082 (14)	2.176 ± 0.117 (15)	2.229 ± 0.134 (14)	2.027 ± 0.098 (14)	2.012 ± 0.107 (19)	2.179 ± 0.112 (19)	2.024 ± 0.208 (13)	2.117 ± 0.106 (19)	1.719 ± 0.139 (15)	1.701 ± 0.065 (15)	1.578 ± 0.148 (10)	1.700 ± 0.070 (15)
R	0.661 (125)	0.619 (154)	0.671 (57)	0.654 (336)	0.419 (98)	0.461 (193)	0.524 (42)	0.460 (333)	0.520 (106)	0.595 (261)	0.646 (41)	0.569 (408)
Slope	890 ± 46 (13)	806 ± 47 (14)	713 ± 37 (14)	788 ± 41 (14)	674 ± 42 (19)	670 ± 40 (19)	658 ± 59 (13)	655 ± 37 (19)	576 ± 35 (15)	572 ± 34 (15)	479 ± 21 (10)	560 ± 32 (15)

All: data for the pooled fibres; %: number percentage of the respective fibre types; Slope: slope of the regression line forced through the origin; R: Pearson correlation coefficient, all R values $P < 0.015$ with in parentheses number of fibres; for other data n is number of animals. Values are mean ± SEM.

DISCUSSION

In the present study we investigated whether compensatory hypertrophy in muscles of various ages is accompanied by capillary proliferation. This was determined by a new index to quantify capillarisation, i.e. the local capillary-to-fibre ratio (capillaries geometrically supplying a fibre).

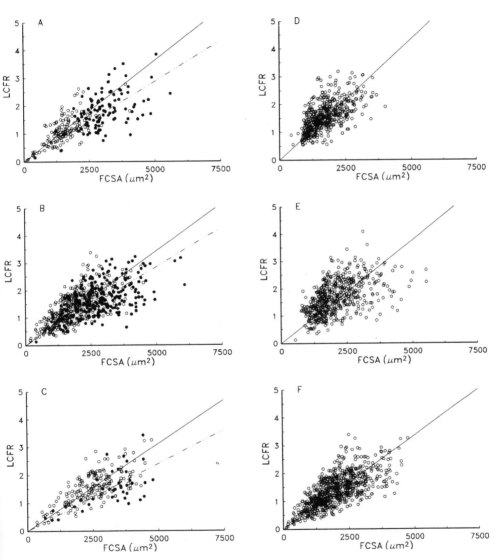

Figure 1. Regressions of local capillary-to-fibre ratio (LCFR) against fibre cross-sectional area (FCSA) in the deep (more oxidative) region of rat m. plantaris. **A:** LCFR of type I fibres in control and overloaded muscles (as an example of 25 months old rats). **B:** idem for IIa fibres and **C:** for IIb fibres. **D.**, **E.**, and **F.** show plots of the pooled fibres in control muscles of 5, 13 and 25 months old rats respectively. ○—— Control; ●——···—— Overloaded.

Local capillary-to-fibre ratio and fibre cross-sectional area

It is stated by Egginton and Ross (1989) that "Direct scaling of local capillary-to-fibre ratio with fibre area suggests that capillarisation is primarily determined by fibre size". This implies, that changes in fibre areas might affect capillarisation. In figure 1 some plots of our material are shown. The steeper the slope of the regression lines is, the better the capillary supply per fibre cross-sectional area is. Implications of several changes in fibre cross-sectional areas and/or local capillary-to-fibre ratio, assuming no changes in fibre number will be described below.

An increase in local capillary-to-fibre ratio always indicates capillary proliferation. On the other hand a decrease indicates capillary loss. If the fibre cross-sectional areas increase, without changes in the local capillary-to-fibre ratio, the slope of the regression line becomes flatter. If the slope remains the same, there must have been capillary proliferation in pace with the increases in fibre size. A slope in between indicates a capillary proliferation lagging behind the increases in fibre areas. A decrease in fibre cross-sectional area without a change in local capillary-to-fibre ratio results in a steeper slope of the regression lines. When this decrease in fibre cross-sectional area is accompanied by a decrease in the local capillary-to-fibre ratio the slope of the regression line can remain similar or become flatter. The former situation indicates a proportional capillary loss and the latter a larger than proportional capillary loss. Thus, in the latter situation the capillary supply per fibre cross-sectional area is reduced.

The steeper slope of the regression lines for oxidative (type I and IIa) fibres than for glycolytic (IIb) fibres indicates a more intense capillary supply for the former than the latter. This is also covered by Egginton and Ross (1989).

Age

The increased fibre cross-sectional areas of each fibre type in muscles of 13 compared with those of 5 months old rats, were not accompanied by increases in local capillary-to-fibre ratio. This resulted in decreased slopes of the regression lines between local capillary-to-fibre ratio and fibre cross-sectional area for each fibre type, except IIb fibres and all fibres pooled. It indicates that the capillary supply per fibre cross-sectional area was lower in muscles of 13 than in those of 5 months old rats. In muscles of 25 months old rats, only the fibre cross-sectional areas of IIb fibres was declined compared with those of 13 months old rats. Between 13 and 25 months the local capillary-to-fibre ratio of each fibre type, as well as all fibres pooled, decreased, indicating loss of capillaries during this period. This loss of capillaries further decreased the slope of the regression lines between local capillary-to-fibre ratio and fibre cross-sectional area for type I and IIa fibres and thus their capillary supply per fibre cross-sectional area. One might argue that an age-related decrease in fibre number might occur. This, however, would result in an increased local capillary-to-fibre ratio and increased slope of the regression line between local capillary-to-fibre ratio and fibre cross-sectional area, when the number of capillaries remains the same, or increases. Thus the results suggest, even more when an age-related decrease in fibre number occurs, that the capillary supply per fibre cross-sectional area decreases with increasing age, while real capillary loss only takes place at advanced age.

Overload

Overloading the plantaris muscle by denervation of synergists results in a compensatory hypertrophy. The fibre cross-sectional areas of each fibre type are increased in overloaded muscles in each age group, indicating that compensatory hypertrophy, due to overload, is not limited by age. Gollnick et al. (1981), using an almost similar model as used in our study, found that the number of fibres in the m. plantaris did not change with compensatory hypertrophy. Hence, the increased local capillary-to-fibre ratio accompanying the increases in fibre cross-sectional areas for each fibre type indicates capillary proliferation. This capillary proliferation lags behind the increases in fibre cross-sectional areas as can be deduced from the lower slopes of the regression lines between local capillary-to-fibre ratio and fibre cross-sectional area for each fibre type in overloaded muscles than in control muscles. However, this conclusion as inferred from these data must be viewed with some caution, as will be pointed out below. The local capillary-to-fibre ratio is primarily determined by fibre cross-sectional area (Egginton and Ross, 1989). The cross-sectional area of type IIb fibres is largest and of type I fibres smallest, with that of type IIa fibres in between. In overloaded muscles the percentage of type I fibres is increased in expense of IIb fibres, which might have been accomplished by transformation of relatively small IIb fibres into IIa fibres, while relatively small IIa fibres have been transformed into type I fibres. This might result in increased mean fibre cross-sectional areas and a concomitant increase in mean local capillary-to-fibre ratio for each fibre type, without changes in the number of capillaries. Therefore, to conclude more firmly to capillary proliferation, the regression between local capillary-to-fibre ratio and fibre cross-sectional area for all fibre types pooled were calculated for each group. It appeared that though the slopes were lower in the overloaded muscles, the local capillary-to-fibre ratio of the pooled fibres was higher in overloaded than in control muscles. This confirms the inference drawn above. As similar results were obtained in each age group it is concluded that capillary proliferation occurs with overload at all ages, though lagging behind the increases in fibre cross-sectional areas.

Capillary fibre density

Similar results as obtained by comparing the slopes of the regression lines between local capillary-to-fibre ratio and fibre cross-sectional area were obtained by comparing the capillary fibre densities (calculated as mean local capillary-to-fibre ratio divided by mean fibre cross-sectional area for each animal separately), for each fibre type in each group. This indicates that the capillary fibre density is comparable to the slope of the regression lines between fibre cross-sectional area and local capillary-to-fibre ratio.

CONCLUSION

With ageing capillary loss occurs. Compensatory hypertrophy is similar in each age group. Concomitant with hypertrophy capillary proliferation was found in each age group, which lagged behind the increase in fibre cross-sectional areas.

REFERENCES

Batra, S., Rakusan, K., and Kuo, C., 1989, Spatial distribution of coronary capillaries: A-V segment staggering. *in*: Oxygen Transport to Tissue-XI. Eds. K. Rakusan, G.P. Biro, T.K. Goldstick, Z. Turek, Plenum Press, New York and London, pp 241-247.

Binkhorst, R.A., 1969, The effect of training on some isometric contraction characteristics of a fast muscle. *Pflügers Arch*. 309:193-202.

Egginton, S., and Ross, H.F., 1989, Influence of muscle phenotype on local capillary supply. *in*: Oxygen Transport to Tissue-XI. Eds. K. Rakusan, G.P. Biro, T.K. Goldstick, Z. Turek, Plenum Press, New York and London, pp 281-291.

Egginton, S., Turek, Z., and Hoofd, L.J.C., 1988, Differing patterns of capillary distribution in fish and mammalian skeletal muscle. *Resp. Physiol.* 74:383-396.

Gollnick, P.D., Timson, B.F., Moore, R.L., and Riedy, M., 1981, Muscular enlargement and number of fibers in skeletal muscles of rats. *J. Appl. Physiol.* 50:936-943.

Hoofd, L., Turek, Z., Kubat, K., Ringnalda, B.E.M., and Kazda, S., 1985, Variability of intercapillary distance estimated on histological sections of rat heart. *in*: Oxygen Transport to Tissue-VII. Eds. F. Kreuzer, S.M. Cain, Z. Turek, T.K. Goldstick, Plenum Press, New York, pp. 239-247.

Kovanen, V., 1989, Effects of ageing and physical training on rat skeletal muscle. An experimental study on the properties of collagen, laminin, and fibre types in muscles serving different functions. *Acta Physiol. Scand.* 135 (S577):7-56.

Riedy, M., Moore R.L., and Gollnick, P.D., 1985, Adaptive response of hypertrophied muscle to endurance training. *J. Appl. Physiol.* 59:127-131.

Wallenstein, S., Zucker, C.L., and Fleiss, J.L., 1980, Some statistical methods useful in circulation research. *Circ. Res.* 47:1-9.

DETERMINATION OF MYOGLOBIN-DIFFUSIVITY
IN INTACT SKELETAL MUSCLE FIBERS
AN IMPROVED MICROSCOPE-PHOTOMETRICAL APPROACH

Thomas Peters, Klaus D. Jürgens,
Gabriele Günther-Jürgens* and Gerolf Gros

Zentrum Physiologie
Medizinische Hochschule Hannover
*Regionales Rechenzentrum für Niedersachsen
Universität Hannover
Hannover, FRG

INTRODUCTION

In concepts of oxygen transport to muscle tissue an important contribution of myoglobin-facilitated oxygen diffusion to the intracellular oxygen transport is frequently assumed (Wittenberg and Wittenberg, 1990). However, there is lack of direct evidence for a corresponding high diffusivity of myoglobin in intact muscle cells. Jürgens et al. (1990) were the first to present a method to measure the intracellular diffusion coefficient of myoglobin in mammalian muscle fibers. It is based on transmission spectroscopy of dissected and superfused rat diaphragms. In geometrically defined microscopic areas of such samples, photooxidation of oxymyoglobin is performed by short UV pulses. The observed absorbance change at 420 nm, which is subsequently recorded with a computer equipped microscope photometer (Fig.1), is the consequence of the translational myoglobin diffusion along the fiber axes. Metmyoglobin diffuses out of the photometric field while oxymyoglobin enters it simultaneously.

ADVANCEMENTS OF THE METHOD

Consideration of Interfering Absorbance Changes

The absorbance curves recorded at 420 nm are not exclusively due to diffusion kinetics of myoglobin but are superimposed by changes caused for instance by movements of the sample or alterations of cell structures. UV irradiation of the tissue with the used quantum of energy is not free of sideeffects in this respect. Experiments with abdominal muscle layers from the frog, free of myoglobin, show that myoglobin independent absorbance changes caused by UV irradiation are about identical at any wavelength in the spectral range from 380 to 700 nm. To take this into account the method has been improved by a dual wavelength recording technique. The appropriate second wavelength, close to 420 nm, is 473 nm, an isosbestic wavelength for met- and oxymyoglobin, at which the difference spectrum crosses the baseline flatly.

The light from a halogen bulb, which is transmitted through the sample, is passed through a grating monochromator, alternately set to 420 and 473 nm every second by a stepper motor, before it is guided to the photomultiplier tube (Fig.1). The absorbance recorded at 420 nm is corrected by subtracting the result of the simultaneous measurement at 473 nm (Fig.2).

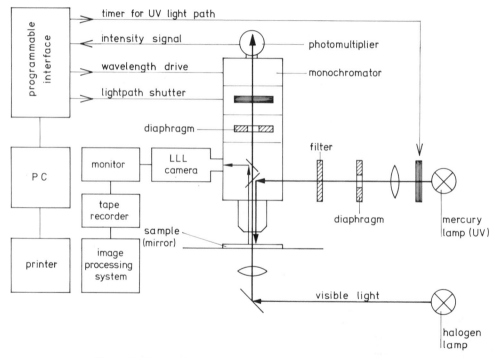

Figure 1. Scheme of the photometrical setup and the imaging system.

Consideration of the Initial Condition

The initial distribution profile of metmyoglobin caused by the UV irradiation is assumed to depend on the irradiance distribution. A super pressure mercury short arc lamp (Osram HBO100W/2) is used as UV source. The emitted radiation of the small discharge arc of this lamp is focussed onto the sample to get an irradiance as high as possible, enabling UV pulses <2 s for sufficient photooxidation of oxymyoglobin. This illumination generates an approximately gaussian distribution of irradiance along the muscle fiber axes. The irradiance of the sample perpendicular to the muscle fiber axes, however, is almost constant over a distance of 215 μm.

For diffusion measurements rectangular irradiated fields, oriented with their longer sides perpendicular to the muscle fiber axes, and rectangular photometric fields, in the middle of the irradiated fields, are chosen by field diaphragms in the ray paths of UV and transmitted light. The width of the irradiated field is varied between 36 and 497 μm for the single recordings, while the height of the photometric fields is set maximally to

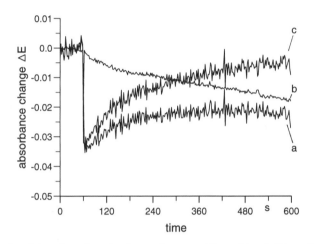

Figure 2. Examples of time dependent absorbance changes at 420 nm (a) and 473 nm (b) as well as the resulting absorbance change difference (E_{420}-E_{473}) (c), observed at $x = 0$.

215 μm, upper and lower boundary congruent with fiber borders. This allows measurements over several parallel fibers. The ensuing distribution of UV intensity in the irradiated field is measured by placing a mirror at the plane of the sample and recording the reflected image with a low light level camera attached to the microscope photometer (Fig.1). The video tape recordings are analyzed with a digital image processing system. The determined profiles (Fig.3) are considered as the initial conditions for the evaluation of the recorded diffusion kinetics, where it is assumed that metmyoglobin concentration is proportional to UV intensity.

Consideration of Metmyoglobin Reduction

The recorded kinetics may be influenced by reduction of metmyoglobin in the sample. Enzymatically catalyzed metmyoglobin reduction has been observed in muscle tissue and isolated myocytes (Al-Shabani and Price, 1977; Taylor and Hochstein, 1982).

Baylor and Pape (1988) have described reduction of injected metmyoglobin in frog muscle fibers as a first order, irreversible reaction with an average rate constant of 0.00027 s^{-1} (22°C). Assuming a) the applicability of the law of Lambert-Beer for our photometrical recordings, b) longitudinal diffusion of myoglobin in the muscle fibers and c) simultaneous reduction of metmyoglobin corresponding to a first order kinetics, the following differential equation holds for the absorbance change E(x,t)

$$dE/dt = D_{Mb} \, d^2E/dx^2 - k_{Mb}E, \tag{1}$$

where D_{Mb} is the diffusion coefficient of myoglobin and k_{Mb} is the reduction rate constant. Diffusion in y- and z-direction is supposed to be negligible.

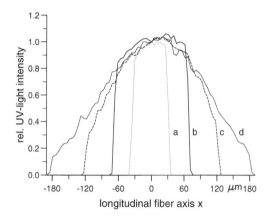

Figure 3. Distribution of light intensity on the exposed sample at different widths of the irradiated field: 72 μm (a), 144 μm (b), 248 μm (c), and 355 μm (d).

Computing Procedure

The differential equation is numerically solved for the respective boundary conditions, as well as the corresponding initial condition given by the UV irradiance profile, with the Crank-Nicolson algorithm on a Cyber 990 at the regional computer center for lower saxony (RRZN) in Hannover, FRG.

The value of D_{Mb} is optimized by a least square fit of the solution of the differential equation to the corrected absorbance curves (program EO4FDF of the NAG library). This has been done for nine different values of k_{Mb}, ranging from 0.0 to 0.005.

RESULTS

Examples of fits, gained by solving the differential equations by the Crank-Nicolson algorithm and optimizing the values of D_{Mb} for the recorded curves with the least square method, are shown in Fig.4. The results of the fittings for several measurements, each consisting of a set of different widths of the irradiated field (varying between 36 and 497 μm) lead for rat diaphragm muscle to a value of D_{Mb} (mean $\pm$ SD, n=26) of (1.2 ± 0.7) 10^{-7} cm^2 s^{-1} and a value of k_{Mb} (mean $\pm$ SD) of 0.0012 ± 0.0011 s^{-1} (20°C). If k_{Mb} was set to zero, D_{Mb} was determined to be (2.7 ± 1.7) 10^{-7} cm^2 s^{-1} (20°C).

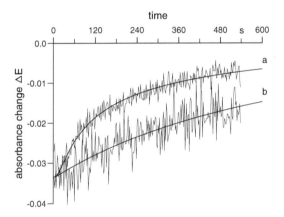

Figure 4. Examples of measured time dependent absorbance change differences $(E_{420}\text{-}E_{473})$ at x=0 and best fits for two different widths of the irradiated field: 144 μm (a) and 355 μm (b).

DISCUSSION

The Advantages of the Improved Method

A single recording of myoglobin diffusion with the described method takes ten minutes or even longer. Long measuring periods make these recordings susceptible to disturbances. Furthermore, UV irradiation can cause sideeffects in the tissue. With the described dual wavelength recording it is possible to take this into account and to correct for artifacts. Necessity of short UV pulses requires focussing the radiation of the UV source onto the sample, which results in inhomogeneous irradiation. In consequence a longitudinal gradient of initial metmyoglobin concentration, especially within broad irradiated fields, has to be considered. This is also achieved by the applied method.

The Values of D_{Mb} and k_{Mb}

Myoglobin diffusivity and metmyoglobin reduction may be different in muscle fibers of various types. According to Metzger et al. (1985) rat diaphragm exhibits a mixture of 40% type I, 27% type IIa and 34% type IIb fibers. Thus, our result represents a mean value of myoglobin diffusivity in intact skeletal muscle fibers. The value of $(1.2 \pm 0.7)\ 10^{-7}\ cm^2\ s^{-1}$ (20°C) found for D_{Mb}, assuming simultaneous metmyoglobin reduction, is in the range of the values, which have been reported by Moll (1968) for layers of rat heart and skeletal muscle homogenates ($D_{Mb} = 1.5\ 10^{-7}\ cm^2\ s^{-1}$ (20°C)) and by Baylor and Pape (1988) for longitudinal diffusion of metmyoglobin in frog muscle fibers ($D_{Mb} = 1.6\ 10^{-7}\ cm^2\ s^{-1}$ (22°C)). It is about three times smaller than the self-diffusion coefficient of myoglobin in an aqueous solution of 18g% (Riveros-Moreno and Wittenberg, 1971), which is often used in mathematical models of O_2 supply to muscle tissue (e.g. Groebe, 1990). It is also somewhat smaller than the preliminary value, which we reported for measurements with the unrefined method (Jürgens et al., 1990).

Comparison of the mean value of k_{Mb} (0.0012 s^{-1}), determined in our investigation, with the value of 0.00027s^{-1} (22°C) reported by Baylor and Pape (1987), suggests that the reduction of metmyoglobin proceeds faster in rat diaphragm muscle fibers than in frog muscle fibers. Although the observation of a slow metmyoglobin reduction in frog muscle fibers, in which myoglobin is normally absent, points to an only modest catalysis of metmyoglobin reduction in such fibers, it seems probable that the reducing system is more active in muscle cells containing myoglobin naturally. Taylor and Hochstein (1982) reported metmyoglobin reduction in isolated myocytes from rat heart ventricle to occur with a reaction rate constant of 0.0023 s^{-1} at 37°C. In comparison to our experimental conditions, higher temperature in their measurements may explain the somewhat faster metmyoglobin reduction in the investigated myocytes than found here. Both literature values, however, range within the standard deviation of our result.

Physiological Significance of D_{Mb}

Disregarding more complex models of intracellular diffusion processes, it is possible to obtain a rough estimate of the contribution of myoglobin-facilitated oxygen diffusion to total O_2 transport in rat diaphragm muscle cells at 20°C under the following assumptions: Intracellular myoglobin diffusivity in all directions is the same as along the fiber axis. Convective transport does not play a role in intracellular O_2 transport. Oxygen half saturation pressure of myoglobin is 0.7 mmHg (Antonini and Brunori, 1971). Highest intracellular oxygen partial pressure is 30 mmHg at the cell boundaries. Myoglobin is completely deoxygenated at the mitochondria. Free oxygen is in chemical equilibrium with myoglobin. Intracellular distribution of myoglobin is uniform and the intracellular concentration is 170 μmol/l, the value which we measured for rat diaphragm. The diffusion coefficient of oxygen in muscle is 0.79 10^{-5} cm^2 s^{-1} (Homer et al., 1984) and oxygen solubility in muscle is 3.93 10^{-5} ml cm^{-3} mmHg^{-1}, corresponding to the value for aqueous 0.155 mM NaCl (Bartels et al., 1959).

For this situation myoglobin facilitated oxygen diffusion is calculated to contribute 5% to total intracellular oxygen flux. If no reduction of metmyoglobin is assumed to occur during our measurements, facilitated oxygen diffusion is calculated to be 10% of free oxygen diffusion. These figures do not give support to concepts, in which myoglobin plays an important role as an intracellular oxygen carrier.

REFERENCES

Al-Shaibani, K.A., and Price, R.J., 1977, Enzymatic reduction of metmyoglobin in fish, *J. Food Sci.* 42:1156.

Antonini, E., and Brunori, M., "Hemoglobin and Myoglobin in their Reactions with Ligands", North-Holland Publishing, Amsterdam (1971) p.222

Bartels, H., Bücherl, E., Hertz, C.W., Rodewald, G., and Schwab, M., "Lungenfunktionsprüfungen, Methoden und Beispiele klinischer Anwendungen", Springer, Berlin (1959) p.408

Baylor, S.M., and Pape, P.C., 1988, Measurement of myoglobin diffusivity in the myoplasm of frog skeletal muscle fibers, *J. Physiol.* 406:247.

Groebe, K., 1988, A versatile model of steady state O_2 supply to tissue. Application to skeletal muscle, *Am. J. Physiol.* 254:H1179.

Homer, L.D., Shelton, J.B., Dorsey, C.H., and Williams, T.J., 1984, Anisotropic diffusion of oxygen in slices of rat muscle, *Am. J. Physiol.* 246:R107

Jürgens, K.D., Peters, T., and Gros, G., 1990, A method to measure the diffusion coefficient of myoglobin in intact skeletal muscle cells, *Adv. Exp. Med. Biol.* 277:137.

Metzger, J.B., Scheidt, K.B., and Fitts, R.H., 1985, Histochemical and physiological characteristics of the rat diaphragm, *J. Appl. Physiol.* 58:1085.

Moll, W., 1968, The diffusion coefficient of myoglobin in muscle homogenate, *Pflügers Arch.* 299:247.

Riveros-Moreno, V., and Wittenberg, J.B., 1972, The self-diffusion coefficients of myoglobin and hemoglobin in concentrated solutions, *J. Biol. Chem.* 247:895.

Taylor, D., and Hochstein, P., 1982, Reduction of metmyoglobin in myocytes, *J. Mol. Cell. Card.* 14:133.

Wittenberg, B.A., and Wittenberg, J.B., 1990, Transport of oxygen in muscle, *Ann. Rev. Physiol.* 51:857.

NONINVASIVE MEASUREMENT OF FOREARM OXYGEN CONSUMPTION DURING EXERCISE BY NEAR INFRARED SPECTROSCOPY

Roberto A. De Blasi[1,2], Immacolata Alviggi[1], Mark Cope[3], Clare Elwell[3], Marco Ferrari[2,4]

[1]Istituto di Anestesiologia e Rianimazione, I Universita' di Roma, Policlinico Umberto I, 00161 Rome, Italy
[2]Laboratorio di Biologia Cellulare, Istituto Superiore di Sanità, 00161 Rome, Italy
[3]Department of Medical Physics and Bioengineering, University College London, London, WCIE 6JA, U.K.
[4]Dipartimento di Scienze e Tecnologie Biomediche e Biometria, Universita' dell'Aquila, 67100 L'Aquila, Italy

INTRODUCTION

The evaluation of the oxygen consumption (VO_2) related to muscle metabolic changes can be a very useful assessment for clinical and physiological interpretations. Local VO_2 can be evaluated by measuring the VO_2 changes on the whole body but this measurement is subject to a large variability and requires the assumption of a constant basal metabolism. Otherwise methods for the measurement of local VO_2 are invasive and difficult to apply in dynamic conditions. A simple and non-invasive technique for the measurement of skeletal muscle VO_2 could find many physiological and clinical applications in the evaluation of muscle metabolism particularly under different workload conditions. Near infrared (NIR) spectroscopy has been developed experimentally and clinically for the non-invasive monitoring of changes in brain and muscle oxygenation (Jobsis-Vander Vliet, 1977). Changes in NIR light propagation across skeletal muscle are affected by scattering and absorption effects due to haemoglobin (Hb) and myoglobin (Mb). Trends in human skeletal muscle deoxygenation have been studied previously during cuff ischaemia at rest and with extreme exercise (Hampson & Piantadosi, 1988; Chance et al., 1988; Chance et al., 1992; De Blasi et al., 1992). Although the NIR spectrum of Mb overlaps that of Hb (De Blasi et al., 1991), recently magnetic resonance spectroscopy has been employed to separate the responses of Mb and Hb to mild and severe deoxygenation (Wang et al., 1990).

Quantitative measurements of muscle VO_2 have been obtained by combining the Hb/Mb absorption changes with the knowledge of the differential pathlength factor (DPF) (Cope et al., 1988). Recently NIR spectroscopy was applied to measure calf VO_2 at rest by evaluating the Hb/Mb desaturation rate in the tissue after inducing a vascular occlusion (Cheatle et al., 1991). During arterial occlusion O_2 extraction is limited only by the O_2 diffusion from the erythrocytes to the cells. Since among tissues skeletal muscle shows the highest variability in energy turnover from the resting state through to maximal activity (Wittenberg & Wittenberg, 1989) it represents an excellent organ to investigate the adequacy of O_2 supply to the extreme metabolic demand. The sustained maximal voluntary contractions represent a standard method widely used to stimulate both slow contracting, highly oxidative (type I), and fast contracting, highly glycolytic (type II), fibers (Hultman et al., 1991).

Previously we evaluated the VO_2 of human forearm at rest (De Blasi et al. 1992) on six subjects by inducing a 10 min vascular occlusion. A notable repeatability was observed when VO_2 was measured consecutively on each subject. Two maximal voluntary contractions were also executed during vascular occlusion in order to verify the increment of VO_2 due to the increase of metabolic demand.

The aim of the present study was to non-invasively study human forearm VO_2 in untrained volunteers comparing the results obtained when two maximal voluntary contractions (MVC) were performed with and without blood flow limitation.

MATERIALS AND METHODS

Six healthy untrained subjects were enrolled in the study (ages 21-39). Verbal consent was obtained from all subjects. A fast scanning spectrophotometer (Model 6500, NIRSystems, Silver Spring, MD) was used for NIR measurements. The procedure for spectral analysis was recently described (De Blasi et al. 1992). Measurements were performed on the right forearm brachio-radial muscle which was the dominant arm in all cases. Two optical fibers (200 cm long and 0.5 cm active diameter) were applied 2.8-3.2 cm apart using a metal support. NIRSystems software was utilized to automatically collect a scan every 5 s. Each subject was submitted to two consecutive protocols. In the first protocol (A) two isometric maximal voluntary contractions (MVC) of 30 s duration were performed 15 and 75 s respectively after the start of vascular occlusion (240-260 mmHg). The occlusion was released after 175 s. In the second protocol (B) two isometric MVC of 30 s length were executed without vascular occlusion at 15 and 75 s respectively. In order to assess the repeatability of the measurements protocols were repeated on different days. The NIR spectral features, expressed as log $(1/T_d)$ (where T_d is diffuse transmittance), were observed after each experiment in order to verify the quality of measurements during the exercise.

Absorption spectra were analyzed according to a modified Lambert-Beer law in order to obtain the quantification of Hb/Mb changes during the study. DPF values were measured separately on the forearm by time-resolved spectroscopy (Ferrari et al., 1992). We found in separate experiments, on 3 out of the 7 subjects, that DPF decreased by less than 10% throughout MVC. Therefore a constant DPF was assumed throughout the protocols. Variations in muscle absorption coefficients were assumed to result only from changes in the concentration of oxy-Hb and deoxy-Hb respectively assuming that changes in saturation were mainly due to Hb.

The Hb saturation changes are expressed as micromoles per liter of tissue (μM/L) assuming a molecular weight of 64000 for Hb. The muscle $\Delta\mu_a$ was split into $\Delta[Hb]$ and $\Delta[HbO_2]$ using a multilinear regression analysis (Cope et al. 1988) of the Hb and HbO_2 spectra between 750 and 900 nm (Wray et al., 1988). VO_2 was measured by calculating the rate of oxy to deoxy-Hb change in muscle in sixty seconds and taking into account the molecular ratio between Hb (fully saturated) and O_2 (1:4) (i.e. $0.5*4*60*d\{\Delta[HbO_2]-\Delta[Hb]\}/dt$).

In protocols A and B VO_2 was calculated by regression analysis of data measured during the first 15-20 s of MVC when the desaturation process was linear. VO_2 was expressed as μM/min per 100 g of tissue using 1.33 g/ml as the density of muscle.

Results were statistically evaluated using a paired t-test. The repeatability of the measurements of the two consecutive MVC performed without vascular occlusion on the 6 subjects was evaluated by a repeatability test (Bland and Altman, 1986). Results were expressed as mean $\pm$ standard error (SEM).

RESULTS

Figure 1 reports the results of protocol A. The first contraction caused a fast Hb/Mb desaturation rate which was completed within 15-20 s. The second contraction did not provoke any further Hb/Mb desaturation. The variance of Hb/Mb maximum desaturation levels measured on the subjects was clearly larger than the variance of the desaturation rate demonstrating an independence between these two variables. The recovery phase (T_R) showed a high variability as well. A compensatory hyperoxia was observed in all cases. A fast Hb/Mb desaturation rate was also found when two consecutive MVC were performed without vascular occlusion (fig.2).

Despite a narrow difference in the Hb/Mb desaturation rate

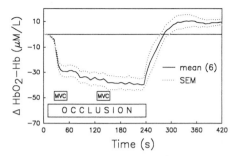

Figure 1. Time course of brachio-radial muscle Hb/Mb desaturation when two MVC were performed during vascular occlusion (protocol A). The first contraction caused a high Hb/Mb desaturation rate which was completed within 15-20 s. The second contraction did not provoke any further Hb/Mb desaturation.

among subjects even in this case the maximum desaturation level and T_R were very different from one subject to another. The second contraction showed a Hb/Mb desaturation rate very similar to the first one. In this case the recovery period was not accompanied by the compensatory hyperoxia.

Table 1 shows the VO_2 results of protocol A and B performed on 6 subjects. No statistically significant difference was found between VO_2 measured during MVC with vascular occlusion and during MVC without occlusion, or between the VO_2 of the two consecutive MVC in protocol B. The VO_2 of the consecutive MVC, performed without vascular occlusion on 6 subjects in different days, were used in the repeatability test (Bland and Altman,

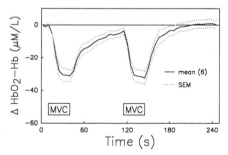

Figure 2. Time course of brachio-radial muscle Hb/Mb desaturation when two MVC were performed without vascular occlusion. A similar Hb/Mb desaturation rate was found in both MVC.

Table 1. Forearm brachio-radial muscle VO_2 ($\mu M/min/100g$) during vascular occlusion with MVC (protocol A) and two MVC without occlusion (protocol B). d_1 and d_2 refer to different days; I and II refer to the first and the second MVC.

	OCCLUSION + MVC Protocol A		REPEATED MVC Protocol B			
N°	d_1	d_2	$d_1(I)$	$d_2(I)$	$d_1(II)$	$d_2(II)$
1	12.8	31.2	13.0	31.8	12.2	31.1
2	29.4	34.5	22.0	36.8	18.7	38.8
3	13.7	20.3	18.9	22.1	20.7	22.9
4	14.2	13.4	11.1	12.7	12.4	17.6
5	28.3	22.2	40.3	22.9	33.2	13.6
6	11.2	15.1	13.6	7.5	20.3	6.7
MEAN SEM	18.3±3.1	22.8 ±3.2	19.8 ±4.0	22.3 ±4.1	19.6 ±2.9	21.8 ±4.4

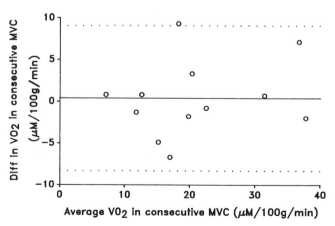

Figure 3. Repeatability test for pairs of consecutive VO_2 measurements during MVC performed without vascular occlusion. Dotted lines represent two standard deviation of differences. There was no correlation between the difference and VO_2 values.

1986). Fig. 3 shows the plot for pairs of consecutive measurements. There does not look to be any relation between the difference and VO_2 values. Only 1 out 12 measurements was an outlier.

DISCUSSION

Skeletal muscle VO_2 at rest and during exercise has been previously evaluated by different methods. These methods can be complex and/or difficult to perform repeatedly so that they are often inconvenient to apply clinically.

Recently the possibility of measuring the DPF by time resolved spectroscopy (Cope et al. 1988) allowed Cheatle et al. (1991) first to quantitate VO_2 at rest on calf muscles of volunteers and patients with peripheral vascular diseases. To the best of our knowledge, the present results constitute the first non invasive measurement of forearm VO_2 during exercise.

The O_2 transport from red cell to mitochondria is caused by the PO_2 gradient from capillary to Mb ($P_{Mb}O_2$) and the conductance (Honig et al., 1992). When blood flow is interrupted, as in protocol A, the Hb/Mb desaturation rate is proportional to VO_2. The relative small difference in the Hb/Mb desaturation rates compared to the desaturation levels in protocol A suggests that the aerobic metabolic activity ceases, on untrained subjects, independently of the desaturation rate (VO_2).

The control of energetic processes in contracting human skeletal muscle during isometric exercise has been recently reviewed (Sahlin, 1991). Hartling et al. (1989), performing consecutive exercise in trained subjects found a mean value much higher than we measured (210.1 ± 56 $\mu MO_2/100ml/min$). This value was obtained by performing repetitive contractions at 90% of maximal work load. However, during repetitive contractions, ATPase activity is associated with high rates of cross-bridge linking of filaments and causes higher O_2 demand compared to a prolonged isometric contraction (Spriet et al., 1987).

During exercise the increase in VO_2 is many-fold greater than that for flow, so as percentage O_2 extraction increases and capillary PO_2 falls markedly (Honig et al., 1992). The observation that desaturation of Hb/Mb occurs during exercise even when blood flow is preserved demonstrates that the homeostatic adjustments are not sufficient to maintain constant the PO_2 near the cells. The rapid and extreme desaturation causes the appearance of an imbalance between supply and demand. The plateau in protocols B indicates that an equilibrium point is reached in 15-20 s of exercise so that no more Hb/Mb desaturation is observed (Fig.3). VO_2 data during MVC measured with and without occlusion were similar, although in subject 5 a major VO_2 variability was observed when MVC was performed on different days, which may be explained by a technical error in the execution of the exercise. The observed VO_2 variability between the protocols could be explained by the difficulty of replicating the same muscle work with and without cuff compression by untrained volunteers. The repeatability of consecutive MVC without vascular occlusion was satisfactory.

The results of this study show that VO_2 values during MVC were very similar both in the presence and absence of blood flow limitation in most of the tested subjects. This suggests that muscle VO_2 might be evaluated accurately without the use of cuff occlusion. The advantage of using this non-invasive technique is that it makes possible the continuous monitoring of muscle metabolic activity during exercise. The good repeatability of measurements allows the application of this method for physiological and clinical purposes.

Acknowledgements
This research was supported in part by C.N.R. contribution N.92.01027.CT04. The financial support of Telethon-Italy to the project is gratefully acknowledged. De Blasi's stay at University College has been supported by CNR n° 12110729.

REFERENCES

Bland, J.M. and Altman, D., 1986, Statistical methods for assessing agreement between two methods of clinical measurement. *The Lancet.* 2:307.

Chance, B., Nioka, S., Kent, J., McCully, K., Fountain, M., Greenfeld, R. & Holtom, G., 1988, Time-resolved spectroscopy of hemoglobin and myoglobin in resting and ischemic muscle. *Analytical Biochem* 174:698.

Chance, B., Dait, M.T., Zhang, C., Hamaoka, T. & Hagerman, F., 1992, Recovery from exercise-induced desaturation in the quadriceps muscles of elite competitive rowers. *Am. J. Physiol.* 262:C766.

Cheatle, T.R., Potter, L.A., Cope, M., Delpy, D.T., Coleridge Smith, P.D. & Scurr, J.H., 1991, Near-infrared spectroscopy in peripheral vascular disease. *Br. J. Surg.* 78:405.

Cope, M., Delpy, D.T., Reynolds, E.O.R., Wray, S., Wyatt, J. & van der Zee, P., 1988, Methods of quantitating cerebral near infrared spectroscopy data. *Adv. Exp. Med. Biol.* 222:183.

De Blasi, R.A., Quaglia, E. & Ferrari, M., 1991, Skeletal muscle oxygenation monitoring by near infrared spectroscopy. *Biochem. Int.* 25:241.

De Blasi, R.A., Cope, M. & Ferrari, M., 1992, Oxygen consumption of human skeletal muscle by near infrared spectroscopy during tourniquet-induced ischemia in maximal voluntary contraction. *Adv. Exp. Med. Biol.* In: Oxygen Transport to

Tissue XIV, Ed. W. Erdman and D.F. Bruley, Plenum Press, New York, 771.

Ferrari, M., Wei, Q., Carraresi, l., De Blasi, R.A. & Zaccanti, G., 1992, Time-resolved spectroscopy of human forearm. *J. Photochem. Photobiol.* (in press)

Hampson, N.B. & Piantadosi, C.A., 1988, Near infrared monitoring of human skeletal muscle oxygenation during forearm ischemia. *J. Appl. Physiol.* 64:2449.

Hartling, O.J., Kelbæk, H., Gjørup, T., Schibye, B., Klausen, K. & Trap-Jensen, K., 1989, Forearm oxygen uptake during maximal forearm dynamic exercise. *Eur. J. Appl. Physiol.* 58:466.

Honig, C.R., Connett, R.J., & Gayeski, T.E.J., 1992, O_2 transport and its interaction with metabolism; a systems view of aerobic capacity. *Med. Sc. in Sports and Exercise* 24:47.

Hultman, E., Greenhaff, P.L., Ren, JM. and Söderlund, K. (1991) Energy metabolism and fatigue during intense muscle contraction. *Biochem. Soc. Trans.* 19:347.

Jobsis-Vander Vliet, F.F., 1977, Non invasive infrared monitoring of cerebral and myocardial oxygen sufficiency and circulatory parameters. *Science.* 198:1264.

Sahlin, K., 1991, Control of energetic processes in contracting human skeletal muscle. *Biochem. Soc. Trans.* 19:353.

Spriet, L.L., Soderlund, K., Bergstrom, M. & Hultman, E., 1987, Energy cost and metabolic regulation during intermittent and continuous tetanic contractions in human skeletal muscle. *Can. J. Physiol. Pharm.* 66:134.

Wang, Z., Noyszewski, E.A. & Leigh, Jr., 1990, In vivo MRS measurement of deoxymyoglobin in human forearms. *Magn. Res. Med.* 14:562.

Wittenberg, B.A. & Wittenberg, J.B. (1989). Transport of oxygen in muscle. *Ann. Rev. of Physiol.* 51:857.

Wray, S., Cope, M., Delpy, D.T., Wyatt, J.S. & Reynolds, E.O.R., 1988, Characterization of the near infrared absorption spectra of cytochrome aa3 and hemoglobin for the non-invasive monitoring of cerebral oxygenation. *Biochem. Bioph. Acta* 933:184.

CONTINUOUS TISSUE OXYGENATION ASSESSMENT

DURING BLOODFLOW ALTERATIONS

IN AN ISOLATED HINDLIMB MODEL OF THE PIG

S.O.P. Hofer,[1] A.J. van der Kleij,[2] P.F. Gründeman,[1] and P.J. Klopper [1]

[1]Department of Surgical Research
[2]Departments of Hyperbaric Medicine and Surgery
 Academic Medical Center, University of Amsterdam, Meibergdreef 9
 1105 AZ Amsterdam, The Netherlands

INTRODUCTION

In clinical practice tissue perfusion is mostly assessed by accumulating "indirect" parameters such as blood pressure, pulse, urine output or capillary refill. It has been pointed out that these "indirect" parameters of tissue perfusion can be normal, when actual tissue perfusion is abnormal.[1-3] It would be preferable, therefore, to determine "direct" parameters. A "direct" parameter reflecting adequate tissue perfusion is assessment of tissue oxygenation.[4,5]

In this study a continuous oxygen tension (PO_2) sensor was used[6] in skeletal muscle in an isolated hindlimb model of the pig. This "direct" sensor was compared with two "indirect" monitors of peripheral perfusion, i.e. transcutaneous oximetry and laser Doppler flowmetry, during periods of arterial flow reduction and intermittent reperfusion. Extracorporeal circulation (ECC) was utilized to induce arterial flow reductions. The pig was used because skin characteristics and blood supply are very similar to those found in man.[7]

The aim of this study was to assess the relationship between skeletal muscle PO_2 (PmO_2), transcutaneous PO_2 ($PtcO_2$), Laser Doppler flowmetry (LDF) and regional bloodflow. The data indicate that PmO_2 reflects bloodflow alterations adquately and its clinical use is advocated.

MATERIALS AND METHODS

Animals & Anaesthesia

Seven female Yorkshire pigs weighing 29 to 34 kg were used. For general anaesthesia a mixture of oxygen (FiO_2 50%) and nitrous oxide was given in combination with Nembutal iv (6-8 mg/kg/hr) on an infuser. Analgesia (Sufenta iv, 15 µg) and muscle relaxation (Pavulon iv, 0.2 mg/kg) were administered as needed. Central and hindlimb temperature were measured with a thermocouple (Ellab instruments, Copenhagen, Denmark). ECG, arterial and venous pressure and pulse rate were registered continuously on a recorder. Respiration was maintained by a volume controlled respirator (UV705, Aga Medical AB, Lidingö, Sweden). To prevent septicaemia all animals received amoxycillin 1 gram after induction of anaesthesia.

Model

In this model the hindlimb of the pig was used. The paw was excluded from the circulation by a tourniquet around the ankle. After laparotomy, the aortic bifurcation and iliac arteries were exposed. Both internal iliac arteries and veins as well as the deep circumflex iliac arteries and veins were ligated to reduce collateral bloodflow. To prevent further collateral flow, skin was dissected circumferentially at the level of the distal thigh, disclosing the underlying muscles. The external iliac artery was bypassed by means of ECC using a conventional roller-pump (Gambro Dreissen, Sweden) in order to vary bloodflow to the isolated hindlimb.

The EC circuit contained rigid polyvinylchloride (PVC) tubing (Baxter Labs., Irvine, USA; 1/4 x 3/32 inch and 3/16 x 1/16 inch, implant tested) including a heat exchanger. The entire EC circuit was insulated to prevent environmental heat exchange and to guarantee regional perfusion at 37°C. The PVC tubing was primed with Hartman's solution (US Pharmacopeia; 150 ml) and debubbled. The ECC drainage cannula (16 Fr) was inserted into the abdominal aorta just distal to the bifurcation and connected to the pump inlet site. The right external iliac artery was cannulated using a 14 Fr catheter and connected to the ECC outlet. Blood pressure at the outlet site of the roller-pump was matched with mean arterial blood pressure and provided the blood flow which was offered to the extremity as 100% perfusion. Blood pressure and blood temperature in the hindlimb were kept at a constant level.

Just prior to cannulation heparin (150 U/kg) was given, followed by hourly doses of 100 U/kg after the first hour to reduce the risk of thrombosis-induced microvascular damage and blood clotting in the ECC. After the first hour blood clotting was assessed every hour by determining the activated coagulation time on site (Hemochron 801, Laméris, Utrecht, The Netherlands).

Monitors of tissue perfusion

I. PmO_2 was measured continuously using a non-heated polarographic Clark type oxygen sensor (Continucath 1000 TM, Biomedical Sensors, Shiley, High Wycombe, England), as described earlier.[6] The distal 5 cm of the 10 cm long flexible polyethylene tubing (outer diameter (OD) 0.55 mm) is the oxygen sensor. Calibration in saline, equilibrated with 5% oxygen, at 38°C was done before implantation and after removal of the oxygen sensor. A temperature measuring probe was inserted into the muscle close to the oxygen sensor. All tissue oxygen tension values were corrected for temperature changes.

II. The transcutaneous PO_2 sensor (TCM 1, Radiometer, Copenhagen, Denmark) polarographically quantitates oxygen diffusing from the skin through its thin polypropylene membrane.[8] The probe contains a thermistor-controlled heating element. Temperature in all experiments was set to 44°C. Prior to application, the system was calibrated to zero and environmental oxygen tension.

III. Dermal blood flow was measured with a 1 mW laser Doppler flowmeter (Periflux PF3, Perimed, Stockholm, Sweden). In this device, laser light scattered from tissue *in vivo* is broadened in line width as a result of the Doppler shift produced by moving red cells in the microcirculation. Light from the helium-neon laser illuminates a 1 mm area of measurement.[9]

Blood sampling

Arterial blood gas analyses were performed in an acid-base analyzer (ABL 2, Radiometer, Copenhagen, Denmark) and corrected for temperature. Hemoglobin and hematocrit were determined every hour.

Study design

Baseline recordings started after one hour of circulatory stabilization. Consecutively 50% arterial flow reduction, reperfusion, 75% arterial flow reduction, reperfusion, 100% arterial flow reduction and reperfusion were induced by means of ECC. Each period of altered circulation lasted for 30 minutes. Blood samples and temperature readings were performed at 1, 5 and 30 minutes after flow alteration. Instrumental monitoring values were recorded continuously.

All results are presented in percentage of baseline values. Baseline values are the values at the end of the stabilization period and are considered to be 100%. Response of PmO_2, $PtcO_2$ and LDF to bloodflow alterations were checked for significance. Each last value before a change in bloodflow was compared with the values 1, 5 and 30 min after this change (see figs 1-3).

Statistical analysis

Results were calculated as means $\pm$ standard error of the mean (SEM). Student's t-test was used to compare means and to test coefficients of correlation and regression. A value of $p \leq 0.05$ was considered statistically significant.

RESULTS

All animals survived the surgical procedure and remained stable during the entire experiment. Mean arterial pressure (82 ± 4 mm Hg) and pulse rate (81 ± 6/min) remained stable in all animals. Arterial blood gases remained constant throughout the experiments (PaO_2 181 ± 5 mm Hg, FiO_2 50%). Hemoglobin and hematocrit showed no significant differences between baseline and final values.

The results caused by subsequent flow alterations on PmO_2, $PtcO_2$ and LDF are presented in figures 1, 2 and 3. PmO_2 and $PtcO_2$ reflected alterations in bloodflow adequately. No significant differences between baseline values and values recorded 30 min after all reperfusion periods were found. There was a good correlation between PmO_2 and bloodflow (r=0.81, p=0.004), $PtcO_2$ and bloodflow (r=0.90, p<0.001) and, PmO_2 and $PtcO_2$ (r=0.92, p<0.001). LDF showed no satisfying response during 50% and 75% flow reductions. During reperfusion following these reductions a significant increase in laser Doppler flow could be noticed at some moments. During 100% flow reduction laser Doppler flow decreased significantly, yet never dropped under 50% of baseline. No correlation could be found between hindlimb temperature and blood flow.

The response times, $T_{50\%}$ and $T_{90\%}$, were assessed. $T_{X\%}$ being the time after which X% of the final value was reached after the start of the change in flow. The results are shown in tables 1 and 2. The intramuscular electrode showed a non-significant drift of $\pm$ 1.5% during the experiments.

Table 1. 50% and 90% response times ($T_{50\%}$, $T_{90\%}$) of skeletal muscle PO_2 (PmO_2) after flow reduction ($\downarrow$) and after flow reestablishment ($\uparrow$).

	PmO_2		
	$\downarrow$	$\uparrow$	(flow: $\downarrow$,$\uparrow$)
$T_{50\%}$	80-90	90-210	(seconds)
$T_{90\%}$	5-8	4-12	(minutes)

Table 2. 50% and 90% response times ($T_{50\%}$, $T_{90\%}$) of transcutaneous PO_2 ($PtcO_2$) after flow reduction ($\downarrow$) and after flow reestablishment ($\uparrow$).

	$PtcO_2$		
	$\downarrow$	$\uparrow$	(flow: $\downarrow$,$\uparrow$)
$T_{50\%}$	30-60	30-240	(seconds)
$T_{90\%}$	3-4	8-9	(minutes)

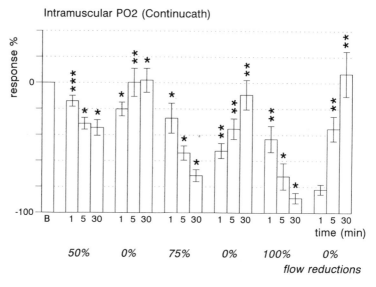

Figure 1. Representation of %-response of PmO_2 to consecutive alterations in bloodflow 1, 5 and 30 minutes after induced bloodflow alteration. All values are means $\pm$ SEM. Significance of each PmO_2 response compared to the final value before the last alteration in bloodflow: * p$\leq$ 0.001, ** p$\leq$ 0.006, *** p$\leq$ 0.02.

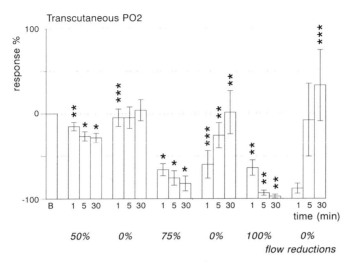

Figure 2. Representation of %-response of PtcO$_2$ to consecutive alterations in bloodflow 1, 5 and 30 minutes after induced bloodflow alteration. All values are means $\pm$ SEM. Significance of each PtcO$_2$ response compared to the final value before the last alteration in bloodflow: * p$\leq$ 0.01, ** p$\leq$ 0.03, *** p$\leq$ 0.05.

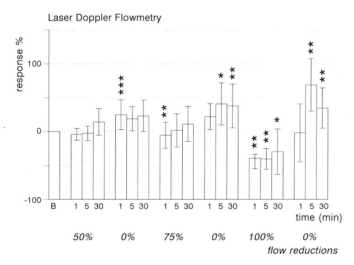

Figure 3. Representation of %-response of LDF to consecutive alterations in bloodflow 1, 5 and 30 minutes after induced bloodflow alteration. All values are means $\pm$ SEM. Significance of each LDF response compared to the final value before the last alteration in bloodflow: Figure 3: * p$\leq$ 0.01, ** p$\leq$ 0.03, *** p$\leq$ 0.05.

DISCUSSION

The purpose of this study was to assess the relationship between skeletal muscle PO_2, transcutaneous PO_2, laser Doppler flowmetry and regional bloodflow during periods of selective bloodflow reduction and subsequent reperfusion.

The main findings were that PmO_2 and $PtcO_2$ correlated well with bloodflow. PmO_2 offered more consistent and stable results compared to the other two methods. $PtcO_2$ responded slightly faster to alterations in bloodflow than PmO_2. PmO_2 and $PtcO_2$ responded faster to flow reductions than to reperfusion. LDF showed poor correlation with bloodflow, even in the no-flow state laser Doppler flow values never dropped under 50% of baseline.

An isolated hindlimb model perfused by ECC was used. Collateral bloodflow reduction was gained by ligation of all arterial and venous vessels distal of the aortic bifurcation and circumferential dissection of skin and muscle at the level of the distal thigh. A no-flow state of the external iliac vein during occlusion of the external iliac artery, as well as a vigorous reactive hyperemia following the arterial occlusion, were considered proof for an insignificant collateral circulation. A similar type of hindlimb isolation has been reported by other authors in canine models.[10,11] Normal perfusion pressure was matched with central blood pressure, providing adequate tissue perfusion.[12,13] Hindlimb perfusion was the only variable parameter in this model and it could be manipulated accurately to assess a relationship between bloodflow and instrumental monitors.

The PO_2 sensor was inserted in the gluteal musculature. Alterations in skeletal muscle oxygenation have shown to be an early indicator of impaired flow.[14-16] The principle of the PO_2 sensor is similar to the tonometric method in which a silastic tube (OD 1.3 mm) is implanted and saline (0.9%) is slowly perfused through the tube to allow tissue gases to equilibrate with the saline in the tube.[17-21] The sealed one-way PO_2 sensor measures PO_2 over a length of 5 cm and has an OD of 0.55 mm. The advantage of this new device over the method in which a silastic tube is implanted is that a) no frequent recalibration is required; b) no leakage occurs; c) it is small; and d) it is easy to handle. For clinical use, calibration can be performed inside the protective cover of the sensor, which is filled with sterile saline. At the end of each experiment the PO_2 sensor was recalibrated and showed a non-significant drift of $\pm$ 1.5%. Baseline values were 42 mm Hg $\pm$ 1.4 mm Hg (Mean $\pm$ SEM) at FiO_2 50%. This agrees with results reported by other authors.[13,14,16,22] Although the sensor may be very small, one has to keep in mind that it is an invasive method, and therefore causes minor tissue damage.

The transcutaneous PO_2 sensor as described by Huch et al[8] was applied to monitor impaired arterial flow. The device was originally developed to measure arterial PO_2 through the heated skin. The heat that enables the technique also interferes with the vasoconstrictive reflexes that occur as a result of the sympathetic response. $PtcO_2$ has, therefore, a non-linear relationship with blood flow until the point is reached where vasoconstriction due to hypoperfusion overcomes vasodilatation due to heat. This perfusion-dependent turning point is not known. From that point on $PtcO_2$ can be expected to be linear to perfusion. In this study, the perfusion-dependent turning point seemed to be between 50% and 75% flow reduction, because $PtcO_2$ showed a 28% decrease to a 50% flow reduction and a 82% decrease to a 75% flow decrease. Very low $PtcO_2$ values probably did not reflect true tissue PO_2. Oxygen-consumption by the tissue and the measuring probe most likely exceeded the amount being delivered to the skin. This problem was faced in the 75% flow reduction. In two animals during a 75% flow reduction $PtcO_2$ reached zero quickly. Absolute $PtcO_2$ values were unreliable in low perfusion conditions. This can be a disadvantage when deciding on a critical point of tissue viability. This is probably the reason for a substantial heterogeneity between minimum $PtcO_2$ readings consistent with spontaneous healing.[23,24] Baseline values in this study were: 74 mm Hg $\pm$ 13.8 mm Hg (Mean $\pm$ SEM), which reflects a large variation. Practical problems consisting of recalibration or relocation of the probe, during the experiment, made the use of the transcutaneous sensor not ideal. Still, $PtcO_2$ measurements have been used successfully under many different circumstances.[25-27]

Laser Doppler flow consists for 80% of a signal which is derived from the thermoregulatory AV-shunts of the skin, not the nutrient capillaries.[28] Clinically severe skin ischemia may exist with adequate laser Doppler flow when microcirculation is unevenly distributed, mainly occurring in AV-anastomoses.[29] Laser Doppler flow reflects moving red blood cells in a small sample volume. In the no-flow state no zero values were recorded. This can be explained by oscillating red blood cells. Other authors reported encouraging results with LDF to detect impaired perfusion under different circumstances.[29-32]

In conclusion, the continuous intramuscular PO_2 sensor was superior to transcutaneous PO_2 measurement and laser Doppler flowmetry in this isolated hind limb model of the pig. Clinical application might well broaden our knowledge of tissue oxygenation during periods of impaired perfusion.

SUMMARY

A continuous intramuscular oxygen tension sensor was compared, with transcutaneous oximetry and laser Doppler flowmetry, during periods of arterial flow alterations in an isolated hindlimb model in the pig. The intramuscular oxygen tension sensor correlated well with bloodflow and was superior to the other two methods.

REFERENCES

1. O. Nelimarkka, L. Halkola, and J. Niinikoski, Effect of graded hemorrhage on renal cortical perfusion in dogs, *Am. J. Surg.* 141:235 (1981).
2. N. Chang, W.H. Goodson III, F. Gottrup, and T.K. Hunt, Direct measurement of wound and tissue oxygen tension in postoperative patients, *Ann. Surg.* 197:470 (1983).
3. A. Gosain, J. Rabkin, J.P. Reymond, J.A. Jensen, T.K. Hunt, and R.A. Upton, Tissue oxygen tension and other indicators of blood loss or organ perfusion during graded hemorrhage, *Surgery* 109:523 (1991).
4. F. Gottrup, R. Firmin, J. Rabkin, B.J. Halliday, and T.K. Hunt, Directly measured tissue oxygen tension and arterial oxygen tension assess tissue perfusion, *Crit. Care Med.* 15:1030 (1987).
5. T.K. Hunt, J. Rabkin, J.A. Jensen, K. Jonsson, K. von Smitten, and W.H. Goodson III, Tissue oximetry: an interim report, *World J. Surg.* 11:126 (1987).
6. S.O.P. Hofer, A.J. van der Kleij, and K.E. Bos, Tissue oxygenation measurement: a directly applied Clark-type electrode in muscle tissue, *Adv. Exp. Med. Biol.* 317:779 (1992).
7. L.K. Bustad and R.O. McClellan, Use of pigs in biomedical research, *Nature* 208:531 (1965).
8. R. Huch, D.W. Lübbers, and A. Huch, Quantitative continuous measurement of partial oxygen pressure on the skin of adults and newborn babies, *Pflugers Arch.* 337:185 (1972).
9. M.D. Stern, In vivo evaluation of microcirculation by coherent light scattering, *Nature* 254:56 (1975).
10. H.J. Granger, A.H. Goodman, and D.N. Granger, Role of resistance and exchange vessels in local microvascular control of skeletal muscle oxygenation in the dog, *Circ. Res.* 38:379 (1976).
11. D.L. Bredle, R.W. Samsel, P.T. Shumacker, and S.M. Cain, Critical O_2 delivery to skeletal muscle at high and low PO_2 in endotoxemic dogs, *J. Appl. Physiol.* 66:2553 (1989).

12. W.P.J. Fontijne, P.H. Mook, H. Schraffordt Koops, J. Oldhoff, and C.R.H. Wildevuur, Improved tissue perfusion during pressure regulated hyperthermic regional isolated perfusion, *Cancer* 55:1455 (1985).

13. W.P.J. Fontijne, P.H. Mook, J.M. Elstrodt, H. Schraffordt Koops, J. Oldhoff, and C.R.H. Wildevuur, Isolated hindlimb perfusion in dogs: the effect of perfusion pressures on the oxygen supply (PtO_2 histogram) to the skeletal muscle, *Surgery* 97:278 (1985).

14. A.J. van der Kleij, D.R. de Koning, G. Beerthuizen, R.J.A. Goris, F. Kreuzer, and H.P. Kimmich, Early detection of hemorrhagic hypovolemia by muscle oxygen pressure assessment: Preliminary report, *Surgery* 93:518 (1983).

15. J.W. Brantigan, E.C. Ziegler, K.M. Hynes, T.Y. Miyazawa, and A.M. Smith, Tissue gases during hypovolemic shock, *J. Appl. Physiol.* 37:117 (1974).

16. J. Niinikoski and L. Halkola, Skeletal muscle PO_2: indicator of peripheral tissue perfusion in hemorrhagic shock, *Adv. Exp. Med. Biol.* 94:585 (1977).

17. T.K. Hunt, A new method of determining tissue oxygen tension, *Lancet* 2:1370 (1964).

18. J. Niinikoski and T.K. Hunt, Measurement of wound oxygen tension with implanted Silastic tube, *Surgery* 71:22 (1972).

19. F. Gottrup, R. Firmin, N. Chang, W.H. Goodson III, and T.K. Hunt, Continuous direct tissue oxygen tension measurement by a new method using an implantable silastic tonometer and oxygen polarography, *Am. J. Surg.* 146:399 (1983).

20. K. Jonsson, J.A. Jensen, W.H. Goodson III, J.M. West, and T.K. Hunt, Assessment of perfusion in postoperative patients using tissue oxygen measurements, *Br. J. Surg.* 74:263 (1987).

21. V.E. Hjortdal, E.J.F. Timmenga, D. Kjolseth, T.B. Henriksen, E.S. Hansen, J.C. Djurhuus, and F. Gottrup, Continuous direct tissue oxygen tension measurement, *Ann. Chir. Gyn.* 80:8 (1991).

22. V.E. Hjortdal, E. Hauge, and E.S. Hansen, Differential effects of venous stasis and arterial insufficiency on tissue oxygenation in myocutaneous island flaps. An experimental study in pigs, *Plast. Reconstr. Surg.* in press (1992).

23. J. Megerman and W.M. Abott, Transcutaneous oxygen tension determination, *in:* "Practical non-invasive vascular diagnosis", R.F. Kempczinski, J.S.T. Yao, eds., Chicago Year Book Medical Publishing (1987).

24. R.G. Karanfilian, T.G. Lynch, V.T. Zirud, F.T. Padberg, Z. Jamil, and R.W. Hobson, The value of laser Doppler velocimetry and transcutaneous oxygen tension determination in predicting healing of ischemic forefoot ulcerations and amputations in diabetic and non-diabetic patients, *J. Vasc. Surg.* 4:511 (1986).

25. T.R.S. Harward, J. Volny, F. Golbrandson, E.F. Bernstein, and A. Fronek, Oxygen inhalation-induced transcutaneous PO_2 changes as a predictor of amputation level, *J. Vasc. Surg.* 2:220 (1985).

26. G.R. Rhodes, Uses of transcutaneous oxygen monitoring in the management of below-knee amputations and skin envelope injuries (SKI), *Am. Surg.* 51:701 (1985).

27. D. Serafin, C.B. Lesesne, R.Y. Mullen, and N.G. Georgiade, Transcutaneous PO_2 monitoring for assessing viability and predicting survival of skin flaps: experimental and clinical correlations, *J. Microsurg.* 2:165 (1981).

28. A. Bollinger and B. Fagrell, "Clinical Capillaroscopy", Hogrefe & Huber Publishers, Lewiston (NY), Toronto (1990).

29. K. Kvernebo and E. Seem, Erythromelalgia - pathophysiological and therapeutic aspects; a preliminary report, *J. Oslo City Hosp.* 37:9 (1987).

30. G.G. Hallock and T.J. Koch, External monitoring of vascularized jejunum transfers using laser Doppler flowmetry, *Ann. Plast. Surg.* 24:213 (1990).

31. F.A. Matsen III, C.R. Wyss, C.L. Robertson, P.A. Öberg, and G.A. Holloway, The relationship of transcutaneous PO_2 and laser Doppler measurements in a human model of local arterial insufficiency, *Surg. Gynecol. Obstet.* 159:418 (1984).

32. M. Walkinshaw, A. Holloway, A. Bulkley, and L.H. Engrav, Clinical evaluation of laser Doppler blood flow measurements in free flaps, *Ann. Plast. Surg.* 18:212 (1987).

THE RELATIONSHIP BETWEEN MIXED VENOUS AND HEPATIC VENOUS O_2 SATURATION IN PATIENTS WITH SEPTIC SHOCK

A. Meier-Hellmann, L. Hannemann, M. Specht, W. Schaffartzik,
C. Spies, K. Reinhart

Department of Anesthesiology and Surgical Intensive Care Medicine
Steglitz Medical Center, Free University of Berlin
Hindenburgdamm 30, D-1000 Berlin 45, Germany

INTRODUCTION

Mixed venous O_2 saturation (SvO_2) is a useful parameter for the monitoring of the relationship between whole body oxygen supply (DO_2) and oxygen consumption (VO_2) in the critically ill patient.[1,2,3] Even under normal conditions, there is considerable difference in O_2 saturations between the different organs. In septic patients there is not only an impairment of convective oxygen transport, but also redistribution of cardiac output (C.O.) among the different organs. Thus, measurements in patients with septic shock yielded 15% lower mean values for hepatic venous ($ShvO_2$) than for mixed venous saturation, but no differences between SvO_2 and $ShvO_2$ were found in patients without septic shock.[4] Because the gastrointestinal tract is a major source for septicemia,[5,6,7] the monitoring of $ShvO_2$ could be useful to detect and prevent tissue hypoxia in this region. Additionally, catecholamines used in the treatment of septic shock may alter the distribution of regional blood flow to the various organs. In patients undergoing cardiac surgery and in patients with sepsis or ARDS, SvO_2 and $ShvO_2$ increased equally after rising C.O. by dopamine and dobutamine[8]. Vasopressors such as epinephrine and norepinephrine are also used in the treatment of septic shock, and newly developed substances, e.g., dopexamine, are being tested in respect to their influence on the splanchnic

Oxygen Transport to Tissue XV, Edited by P. Vaupel
et al., Plenum Press, New York, 1994

perfusion.[9] Whether changes in $ShvO_2$ induced by these catecholamines are adequately reflected by SvO_2 in septic patients is still unknown. It was the aim of this study to investigate how norepinephrine, epinephrine, dopamine and dopexamine affect this relationship between SvO_2 and $ShvO_2$.

PATIENTS AND METHODS

The study was approved by the ethics committee of our hospital. All patients (n = 21) fulfilled the sepsis criteria according to Bone[10] and were mechanically ventilated (Servo 900 C, Siemens AB, Solna, Sweden). The analgesic sedatives fentanly/midazolam were given to all patients based on individual requirements. Besides the established monitoring procedure for patients with septic shock (arterial cannula 20G, Swan-Ganz pulmonary artery catheter), an additional catheter was positioned in the hepatic vein by fluoroscopy via the right internal jugular vein or the right femoral vein.

Cardiac output was determined at each stage in triplicate by thermodilution (Edwards CO computer). Blood samples were drawn in duplicate (arterial, mixed venous, hepatic venous) for blood gas analysis from each patient by slow, synchronous aspiration from the catheters in two heparinized syringes. The samples were immediately stored on ice and analyzed within 15 minutes. A hemoximeter (OSM3 Radiometer, Copenhagen) was used to determine O_2 saturation and hemoglobin concentration, and O_2 partial pressure was measured with a blood gas analyzer (ABL 300 Radiometer, Copenhagen). The blood gas analyzer was calibrated immediately before and after each study. Oxygen transport related variables were determined according to standard formulas.

PROTOCOL

The following conversions of catecholamine infusion were performed:

A: from dobutamine (12.2 ± 2.1 $\mu g/kg/min$) to epinephrine at a dosage establishing the same arterial mean pressure as under dobutamine (mean: 0.21 ± 0.13 $\mu g/kg/min$);

B: from dobutamine (11.4 ± 2.3 $\mu g/kg/min$) to norepinephrine at a dosage establishing the same arterial mean pressure as under dobutamine (mean: 0.25 ± 0.11 μg);

C: from dobutamine (14.2 ± 1.1 $\mu g/kg/min$) to a combination of dobutamine and 4 $\mu g/kg/min$ dopexamine;

D: from norepinephrine (0.25 ± 0.11 $\mu g/kg/min$) to a combination of norepinephrine and 2.8-3.0 $\mu g/kg/min$ dopamine.

The measurements (before and after conversion) were started when the patients were stable (change in C.O. < ±5% with repeated measures) and repeated after 60 min and 120 min. Each subject received only one of the above conversions.

Differences between initial values and values after conversions were tested for statistical significance by Wilcoxon test for independent samples. Calculations including regression analysis were performed with the statistics package SPSS/PC+ (SPSS, Chicago, Il). A p <0.05 was considered to be statistically significant. All results are given as means ± SD.

RESULTS

At baseline all patients were in stable hemodynamic condition with pulmonary capillary wedge pressure (PCWP) between 14 and 17 mmHg, a DO_2 of 755 ± 219 ml/min/m^2, and a VO_2 of 160 ± 40 ml/min/m^2. At baseline, the difference between SvO_2 and $ShvO_2$ was 15 ± 9% with large individual variations (range 1% to 37%).

The correlation coefficient for changes in SvO_2 and $ShvO_2$ induced by catecholamine conversions was r^2 = 0.62 (p<0.001).

Conversion of the catecholamine regimen produced several changes in SvO_2, $ShvO_2$, and the difference between the two (Table 1).

A conversion in catecholamine therapy from dobutamine had no influence on SvO_2 (from 77 ± 4% to 76 ± 2%, n.s.) but caused a decrease of $ShvO_2$ from 64 ± 8% to 54 ± 10%. Thus difference between SvO_2 and $ShvO_2$ increased significantly from 12 ± 5% to 22 ± 9%.

After changing the therapy from dobutamine to norepinephrine, SvO_2 decreased from 75 ± 5% to 69 ± 5%, $ShvO_2$ decreased from 62 ± 13 to 49 ± 13% and the difference between both increased from 13 ± 10 to 19 ± 9%.

Adding 4 μg/kg/min dopexamine to dobutamine caused a slight increase of SvO_2 from 75% ± 5 to 77% ± 3%. No significant change occured in the difference between SvO_2 and $ShvO_2$ after adding dopexamine.

Adding dopamine to norepinephrine, SvO_2 increased from 69 ± 4 to 74 ± 4% (p<0.05), and $ShvO_2$ from 53 ± 13% to 64 ± 10% (p<0.05). The difference between SvO_2 and $ShvO_2$ was diminished from 16 ± 11% to 10 ± 7% after the administration of dopamine. This difference was of borderline significance (p=0.08).

DISCUSSION

The baseline difference between SvO_2 and $ShvO_2$ was 15 ± 9% which is in the same range as that reported by Dahn et al.[11] in patients with septic shock.

Tab 1. Mixed venous O_2 saturation (SvO_2), hepatic venous O_2 saturation ($ShvO_2$) and the difference between SvO_2 and $ShvO_2$ before and after change of catecholamine treatment

Catecholamine conversion	SvO_2 (%)		$ShvO_2$ (%)		SvO_2 - $ShvO_2$	
	before	after	before	after	before	after
A: Dob to Epi	77±4	76±2	64±8	54±10 *	12±5	22±9 *
B: Dob to Nor	75±5	69±5 *	62±13	49±13 *	13±10	19±9 *
C: Dob to Dob and Dpx	75±5	77±3 *	58±12	59±13	17±11	18±13
D: Nor to Nor and Dop	69±4	74±4 *	53±13	64±10 *	16±11	10±7

Dob = dobutamine, Epi = epinephrine, Nor = norepinephrine, Dop = dopamine,
Dpx = dopexamine, * = $p < 0.05$ between before and after

The correlation between changes in SvO_2 and $ShvO_2$ ($r^2 = 0.62$) is similar to that demonstrated by Ruokonen et al.,[8] who concluded that changes in SvO_2 induced by sympathomimetic substances reflect changes in $ShvO_2$. That conclusion is true only if there is no relative change of blood flow in the splanchnic region. In our study, the change from dobutamine to epinephrine did not influence SvO_2, while the observed decline of $ShvO_2$ significantly increased the difference between the two parameters. The conversion in catecholamine therapy from dobutamine to norepinephrine also increased the difference between SvO_2 and $ShvO_2$ significantly. We suspect that the increased difference between SvO_2 and $ShvO_2$ is due to a decrease in splanchnic perfusion mediated by the known effect of epinephrine and norepinephrine on intestinal alpha-adrenergic receptors.[12,13] Another study investigating patients undergoing liver surgery showed a marked decline of $ShvO_2$ after skin incision, and almost no change of SvO_2.[14] The authors hypothesized that this discrepancy is due to a release of endogenous alpha-mimetic catecholamines resulting in a selective impairment of perfusion in the splanchnic area. Therefore the use of alpha-mimetics in the treatment of septic shock to increase DO_2, as recommended by some authors,[15,16] seems questionable because of the possible reduction of splanchnic perfusion. Traditional therapy that attempts to redistribute blood flow to more "vital organs" at the expense of splanchnic perfusion, may be counterproductive in septic shock.

Adding 4 μg/kg/min dopexamine to dobutamine did not change the difference between SvO_2 and $ShvO_2$. This finding corresponds to that of Leier[17] who described a proportional rise of C.O. and splanchnic perfusion for dopexamine in heart failure patients. Additionaly, dopexamine has been shown to preserve blood flow to the gut mucosa in an animal model of endotoxic shock.[18] For this reason dopexamine may be useful as adjunct therapy in septic shock.

The addition of 2.8-3.0 μg/kg/min dopamine to norepinephrine resulted in a relatively greater increase in $ShvO_2$ than in SvO_2. Low-dose dopamine has been demonstrated to improve perfusion of the splanchnic area.[19,20,21] However, our increase in $ShvO_2$ may reflect a decrease in nutritive blood flow at the level of the mucosa at the same time that total blood flow to the splanchnic region is increased. Giraud et al.[22] demonstrated that dopamine increases the perfusion in the superior mesenteric artery but decreases the perfusion of the intestinal mucosa. To differentiate whether changes in the difference between SvO_2 and $ShvO_2$ are caused by redistribution of both flow or microcirculatory alterations, splanchnic perfusion needs to be measured together with $ShvO_2$ to determine VO_2 of the splanchnic region.

Changes in O_2 saturation only reflect a changed ratio of oxygen supply and consumption. $ShvO_2$ is nevertheless clinically relevant even if splanchnic perfusion cannot be measured. An intraoperative $ShvO_2$ below 40% was found to correlate with a postoperative increase in liver transaminases and subsequent liver failure.[23] In 12 % of our patients we observed $ShvO_2$ values below 40% while SvO_2 remained in the normal range ($>70\%$). Both sepsis and the vasopressors which are used to treat septic shock may increase the difference between SvO_2 and $ShvO_2$. Changes in the splanchnic O_2 supply/consumption ratio are unfortunately not always adequately reflected by corresponding changes in SvO_2. Therefore, monitoring $ShvO_2$ may prove helpful in management of patients with severe septic shock.

SUMMARY

It was the purpose of this study to measure the relationship between hepatic venous O_2 saturation ($ShvO_2$) and mixed venous O_2 saturation (SvO_2) in septic patients (n=21) following treatment with various catecholamines (epinephrine, norepinephrine, dopamine, dopexamine). At baseline mean SvO_2 was 74 ± 5 % while mean $ShvO_2$ was 59 ± 12 %. Alpha-mimetic substances such as epinephrine and norepinephrine reduced $ShvO_2$ and increased the difference between SvO_2 and $ShvO_2$. $Beta_2$-mimetic and dopaminergic substances (dopexamine, dopamine) did not change the difference between SvO_2 and $ShvO_2$. These results show that SvO_2 does not necessarily reflect all changes of $ShvO_2$. Monitoring $ShvO_2$ may be helpful in managing septic shock by adding information on adequacy of O_2 supply/consumption ratio in the crucial splanchnic region.

REFERENCES

1. K. Reinhart. Oxygen transport and tissue oxygenation in septic shock. In: Sepsis - An interdisciplinary challenge. Reinhart K, Eyrich K, Springer, Berlin - Heidelberg - New York, (1989)

2. K. Reinhart. Clinical assessment of tissue oxygenation - value of hemodynamic and transport-related variables. In: Tissue Oxygen Utilization. G. Guiterez, J.L. Vincent (Eds) Springer, Berlin - Heidelberg New York, S. 269 - 285 (1990)

3. K. Reinhart, L. Hannemann, M. Specht. The role of O_2 transport-related variables in the assessment of the tissue oxygenation in the clinical setting. In: Yearbook on Intensive Care and Emergency Medicine 1992. Vincent JL (ed.). Springer, Berlin - Heidelberg - New York (1992)

4. M.S. Dahn , M.P. Lange, L. A. Jacobs. Central mixed and splanchnic venous oxygen saturation monitoring. Intens Care Med 14: 373 (1988)

5. E.A. Deitch, R. Berg, R. Specian. Endotoxin promotes the translocation of bacteria from the gut. Arch Surg 122: 185 (1987)

6. P.F. Fink. Gastrointestinal mucosal injury in experimental models of shock, trauma, and sepsis. Crit Care Med, 19:627-641 (1991)

7. J.L. Meakins, J.C. Marshall. The gut as the motor of multiple system organ failure. In: Splanchnic Ischemia and Multiple Organ Failure. Marston A, Bulkley GB, Fiddian Green RG et al. (eds.). St Louis, CV Mosby, pp 339 - 348 (1989)

8. E. Ruokonen, J. Takala, A. Uusaro. Effect of vasoactive treatment on the relationship between mixed venous and regional oxygen saturation. Crit Care Med 19: 1365 - 1369 (1991)

9. L. Hannemann, A. Meier-Hellmann, K. Reinhart. Regional blood flow in sepsis. Clin Int Care 3:28-31 (1992)

10. R. C. Bone, C.J. Fisher, T.P. Clemmer, G.J. Slotman, C.A. Metz, R.A. Balk, the methylprednisolone severe sepsis study group. Sepsis syndrome: a valid clinical identity. Crit Care Med 17: 389 - 393 (1989)

11. M.S. Dahn, M.P. Lange, R.F. Wilson, L.A. Jacobs, R.A. Mitchel. Hepatic blood flow and splanchnic oxygen consumption measurements in clinical sepsis. Surgery 107: 295 - 301 (1989)

12. D.N. Granger, P.D.J. Richardson, P.R. Kvietys, N.A. Mortillaro. Intestinal blood flow. Gastroenterology 78: 837 - 863 (1980)

13. F.D. Reilly, R.S. McCuskey, E. v.Cilento. Hepatic Microvascular Regulatory Mechanisms. I. Adrenergic Mechanisms. Microvascular Research 21, 103-116 (1981)

14. M. Kainuma, Y. Fujiwara, N. Kimura, A. Shitaokoshi, K. Nakashima, Y. Shimado. Monitoring Hepatic Venous Hemoglobin Oxygen Saturation in Patients Undergoing Liver Surgery. Anesthesiology 74:49-52 (1991)

15. P.E. Bollaert, Ph. Bauer, G. Audibert, H. Lambert, A. Larcan. Effects of Epinephrine on Hemodynamics and Oxygen Metabolism in Dopamine-Resistant Septic Shock. Chest 98/4:949-953 (1990)

16. S.J. Mackenzie, F. Kapadia, G.R. Nimmo, I.R. Armstrong, I.S. Grant. Adrenaline in treatment of septic shock: effects on haemodynamics and oxygen transport. Intensive Care Med 17:36-39 (1991)

17. C.V. Leier. Regional blood flow responses to vasodilators and inotropes in congestive heart failure. Am J Cardiol.62: 86E-93E (1988)

18. S.M. Cain, S.E. Curtis. Systemic and regional oxygen uptake and delivery and lactate flux in endotoxic dogs infused with dopexamine. Crit Care Med 19:1552-1560 (1991)

19. D.J. Johnson, J.A. Johannigman, R.D. Branson, K. Davis, J.M. Hurst. The Effect of Low Dose Dopamine on Gut Hemodynamics during PEEP Ventilation for Acute Lung Injury. J Surg Research 50:344-349 (1991)

20. J. Lundberg, D. Lundberg, L. Norgren, E. Ribbe, J. Thörne, O. Werner. Intestinal Hemodynamics during Laparotomy: Effects of Thoracic Epidural Anesthesia and Dopamine in Humans. Anesth Analg 71:9-15 (1990)

21. O. Winsö, B. Biber, J. Martner. Does Dopamine Suppress Stress-Induced Intestinal and Renal Vasoconstriction? Acta Anaesthesiol Scand 29:508-514 (1985)

22. G.D. Giraud, K.L. MacCannell. Decreased nutrient blood flow during dopamine- and epinephrine-induced intestinal vasodilatation. J Pharm Exp Ther 230: 214 - 220 (1984)

23. M. Kainuma, K. Nakashima, I. Sakuma, M. Kawase, T. Komatsu, Y. Shimada, Y. Nimura, T. Nonami. Hepatic Venous Hemoglobin Oxygen Saturation Predicts Liver Dysfunction after Hepatectomy. Anesthesiology 76:379-386 (1991)

OXYGEN SUPPLY AND PLACENTAL OXYGEN METABOLISM

[1]David J. Maguire, [2]Graeme R. Cannell and [1,2]Russell S. Addison

[1]Faculty of Science and Technology, Griffith University, Brisbane, Australia
and [2]Conjoint Internal Medicine Laboratory, Royal Brisbane Hospital
Brisbane, Australia

INTRODUCTION

There have been numerous previous reports of investigations into the relationship between oxygen supply and oxygen metabolism in human tissues and organs and a variety of animal tissues and organs. Those studies have encompassed both *in vivo* and *in vitro* preparations and have included perfusions with whole blood and with artificial perfusion in the presence and absence of synthetic, natural and modified natural oxygen carriers.

A number of investigators have specifically reported the relationship between circulation flow rates and oxygenation status in placentae of humans and of animals. Kunzel and Moll (1972) and Moll and Herberger (1976) studied the transfer of oxygen from maternal blood flow to foetus in guinea pigs. They suggested that there was a linear relationship between flow and oxygen uptake in their system, in which maternal supply was mechanically manipulated in animals into which arterio-spiral shunts had been introduced. Weir and Miller (1985) advocated the use of oxygen transport as an indicator of perfusion viability in the isolated perfused placental lobule. Mendoza et al. (1989) have investigated the relation between intra-uterine growth retardation and maternal oxygen transport.

Most previous studies into placental oxygen disposition have been concerned with the question of maintenance of adequate supply to the foetus (i.e. trans-placental oxygen flux) and have made but scant reference to provision of oxygen to the tissues of the placenta itself. Such approaches neglect the manifest reports on the range and severity of complications observed in infants exposed to placentae which are functionally stressed.

It might be speculated that under certain conditions of temporary oxygen deprivation the foetal tissues might be kept oxygenated at the cost of reduced placental function. Such temporary oxygen deficits may be tolerated in this tissue in spite of its abundant population of mitochondria. It might be necessary to invoke an aerobic/anaerobic switching mechanism in the placenta to accomodate to the altered levels of oxygenation. By contrast, even small long term oxygen deficits would certainly be expected to have major deleterious consequences for placental tissue and therefore also for the developing foetus.

We have previously reported the conditions used in an *in vitro* placental perfusion technique (Addison et al., 1991) and have demonstrated that those conditions maintain adequate (i.e. physiologically appropriate) oxygenation to both the maternal and the foetal tissue compartments in that system.

Using those standard conditions, we have reported a number of investigations into clearance and metabolism of clinically significant steroids (Addison et al., 1991). Results of those studies are summarized in Figure 1. Recently we have begun to investigate the placental disposition of therapeutics used to control maternal blood pressure during pregnancy. It is expected that these compounds will influence placental vasculature, thereby modifying the clearance of test substances. By altering flow of perfusion medium, it is

Oxygen Transport to Tissue XV, Edited by P. Vaupel
et al., Plenum Press, New York, 1994

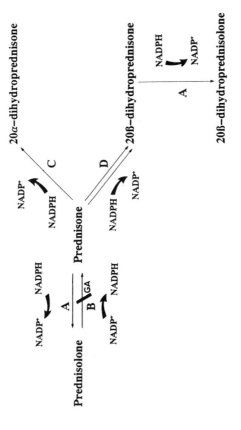

Figure 1. Proposed metabolic pathway for prednisolone in placenta, showing the inhibitory action of glycyrrhetenic acid (GA) and enyme induction by anti-epileptic drugs (double arrows).

A = 11ß–reductase ⎫ 11ß–hydroxysteroid dehydrogenase (11ß–OHSDH)
B = 11ß–oxidase ⎬
C = 20α–hydroxysteroid dehydrogenase
D = 20ß–hydroxysteroid dehydrogenase
GA = Glycyrrhetinic acid

likely that they will also produce general or local alteration to tissue oxygenation and thereby modify placental metabolism of a range of substances.

The present study was initiated in order to define the effect of mechanical restriction of total perfusate flow and the ratio of maternal to foetal circulation flows upon apparent oxygenation status of the perfused placenta.

METHODS

The perfusion system, a modification of the method of Miller et al. (1985) was as described by Addison et al. (1991). The perfusate was tissue culture medium M199, obtained from Sigma Chemical Company, (St.Louis, Mo., U.S.A.) and supplemented with heparin (25IU/ml), gentamicin (100mg/l), glucose (2g/l), sodium bicarbonate (2.9g/l) and dextran (foetal 29g/l: maternal 7.5 g/l). Term human placentae were obtained at caesarian section within 5 min of delivery from healthy women with no significant drug history and transported immediately in cold, oxygenated perfusate to an adjacent laboratory. An artery-vein pair to an intact peripheral lobule was cannulated for foetal circuit perfusion with maternal perfusion being established by insertion of two cannulae approximately 0.8 cm through the decidual plate. The volume of perfusate in the maternal and foetal circuits was 150 and 100 ml respectively. The pH was maintained between 7.35 and 7.45 by the addition of sodium bicarbonate. Tissue temperature was maintained at 37^0C and foetal circuit pressure below 40 mm Hg. Perfusion was maintained in dual recirculating mode while maternal and fetal circulation flow rates were varied over a range of 3 to 25 and 1 to 6 ml/min, respectively. Maternal to foetal circulation flow ratios ranged from 2:1 to 25:1. Perfusate gas analyses were performed as previously described (Addison et al, 1991)

In experiments to investigate the effect of respiratory inhibition, antimycin was added only to the maternal circulation at final maternal perfusate concentrations corresponding to 10mM (after first addition) and 100mM (after second addition). Antimycin was added at 35 and 90 minutes after the start of the perfusion. The inhibitor was allowed to equilibrate for fifteen minutes before sampling perfusate for gas analysis.

RESULTS

In Fig.2a, maternal to foetal oxygen transfer rate is plotted against maternal circuit flow rate. Maximum transfer rate was obtained at a maternal perfusate flow rate of 25 ml/min. When foetal perfusate flow rate was varied over a six-fold range, no changes in transfer rate were observed.

In Fig.2b, oxygen consumption rates and oxygen transfer rates, both expressed as a fraction of the values obtained for the standard conditions we use, are plotted against maternal circuit flow rates. From this plot it is observed that oxygen consumption rate also increased as maternal perfusate flow rate increased but decreased when foetal perfusate flow was restricted.

In Fig.2c, the same parameters are plotted relative to the values obtained for oxygen transfer under those standard conditions, to emphasize the different contributions of oxygen transfer and oxygen consumption to oxygen depletion through the placenta.

In Fig.3, oxygen consumption rates and oxygen transfer rates are plotted against the ratio of maternal to foetal circuit flow rates. At very low flow ratios (corresponding to low values for maternal perfusate flow rate) and high flow ratios (corresponding to low values for foetal perfusate flow rate), oxygen consumption rate was depressed. However, there is no consistent pattern to this relationship.

In an attempt to define the extent of respiratory chain (i.e. oxidative) metabolism occuring in the perfused placenta, antimycin was added to the maternal supply (Fig.4). Each addition of antimycin produced a significant decrease in oxygen consumption rate. There appears to be some recovery from inhibition after each addition of antimycin. Maximal inhibition obtained at the highest concentration of antimycin used was approximately 75% of uninhibited value.

DISCUSSION

From Fig.2a it can be seen that, over the range of perfusate flow conditions used, a

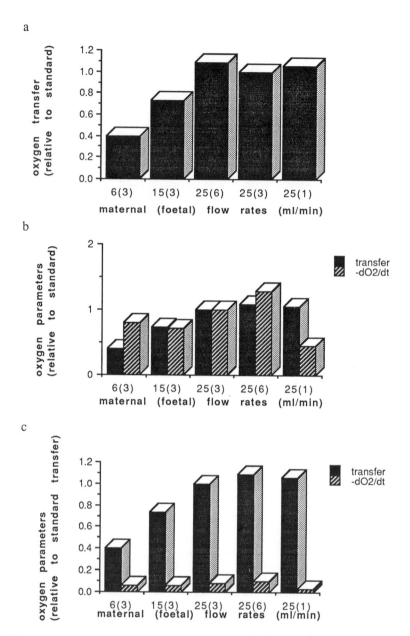

Figure 2 Oxygen parameters plotted against perfusate circulation flow rates; (a) oxygen transfer rate against maternal circuit flow rate, (b) oxygen transfer rate and oxygen consumption rate, both expressed as a fraction of the value obtained for each parameter using "standard" conditions, against maternal (foetal) circuit flow rates and (c) as for (b) but all values expressed relative to values obtained for oxygen transfer using "standard" conditions

maternal circulation flow rate of 25 ml/min gave the maximum rate of oxygen transfer from maternal to foetal compartments. At that flow rate, alterations to foetal circulation flow rate did not appear to significantly affect oxygen transfer. However, from Fig.2b it is apparent that at very low foetal circulation flow rates (1 ml/min), oxygen consumption in the placenta drops by at least 50%, although good transfer of oxygen still occurs. This suggests that, under these conditions, insufficient perfusate flow through the foetal circulation impedes the removal of metabolic end products. This, in turn, leads to depression of normal oxygen metabolism within the placenta. It can also be seen that at low maternal circulation flow rates

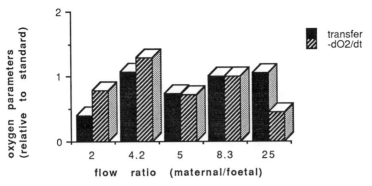

Figure 3. Oxygen parameters plotted against the ratio of maternal circulation flow rates to foetal circulation flow rates.

oxygen consumption rates are also depressed. Under these conditions it is likely that oxygen consumption is limited by the supply of oxygen to the foetal tissue of the placenta. At these low maternal circulation flow rates oxygen-consuming metabolism appears to be maintained at the expense of transfer of oxygen from maternal to foetal compartments (oxygen consumption is comparatively less limited than oxygen transfer).

However, it should not be inferred from Fig.2b that oxygen consumption ever approaches the level of oxygen transfer; the graphical representation used grossly distorts the situation as is apparent when the results are plotted in a more comparative fashion (Fig.2c). It is nevertheless significant that oxygen consumption is not more deeply inhibited under hypoxic conditions, thereby indicating the requirement for some level of oxidative metabolism to be maintained even under conditions of reduced oxygen supply to the foetus. It can be inferred from Fig.3 that flow ratio is probably a secondary, and possibly unimportant, factor in the maintenance of oxygen parameters in this compound tissue.

In vitro perfusion is a technique which has been extensively used to study organ and tissue metabolism in many species. The technique has provided useful information regarding the human placenta, particularly in respect of hormone synthesis and metabolism, and the metabolism and clearance of natural and synthetic compounds to which placentae are exposed. If the information obtained from such studies is to have clinical significance it is important that the conditions which prevail during the perfusion are close to physiological. In this tissue, which is responsible for maintenance of foetal nutrient supply, oxygen is a key compound.

About half the oxygen is depleted from maternal blood during its circulation through the placenta and a significant proportion is used by the tissues of the placenta. Respiratory demands (involving the electron transport pathway) might be expected to account for a large proportion of the oxygen consumed in this tissue. This contribution to oxygen consumption has been calculated on a number of occasions from estimations of lactate production and glucose utilization rates.

It has previously been demonstrated that viable perfusions can be maintained for 6 hours in a dual recirculatin mode with maternal and foetal circulation flow rates of 25 and 3 ml/min, respectively. In the present investigation it was observed that there are two critical factors in maintaining normal placental function, namely adequate maternal and foetal circulation flow rates.. Those prime factors affect the rates of oxygen delivery to the maternal circulation and waste removal from the foetal circulation, respectively. The question of whether flow ratio is an important consideration was also addressed. When this was varied much below the previously established "standard" conditions (corresponding to a reduction in maternal circulation flow rates, oxygenation could not be maintained at a level that would satisfy the demands of an aerobically metabolizing tissue. Under these conditions, however, the tissue may have the capacity to switch to anaerobic metabolism. An equally dramatic response was seen when flow ratios were increased by mechanical reduction of the foetal circulation flow rates; this is probably a response to the accumulation of metabolites in the foetal circulation. It is not known how long these altered metabolic states can be maintained in this tissue in the *in vitro* experiments described here. It is also not yet possible to comment upon whether these situations ever arise *in vivo* nor for how long altered metabolism might be maintained under those conditions.

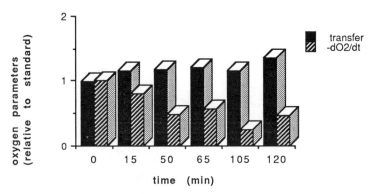

Figure 4. The effect of antimycin upon oxygen parameters expressed as a fraction of the value obtained at zero time, against maternal (foetal) circuit flow rates

In the *in vivo* experiments that Moll and Herberger (1976) conducted on surgically manipulated guinea pigs, only maternal circulation flow rates were able to be altered. The highest (maternal circulation) placental blood flow rates observed in that system were up to 30 ml/min. and placental supply was able to be varied over a wide range of figures up to that value. The linear relationship observed by those workers between maternal circulation flow rates and total placental oxygen uptake is probably of physiological significance. As Moll and Herberger (1976) indicated, at least one previous study has confirmed that variations in foetal growth rates are associated with variations in placental flow rates (Bruce and Abdul-Karim, 1973). From the present study, it might be inferred that reduced foetal circulation flow rates can also limit placental function.

In experiments in which antimycin, a respiratory chain inhibitor, was added to maternal perfusate, a maximal 75% inhibition of oxygen consumption rate occurred. This might indicate that there is a residual component of oxygen consumption that is independent of the respiratory chain. A more likely explanation is that the final concentrations of antimycin achieved in some parts of the placenta were not sufficient to completely inhibit respiration, despite the ten-fold difference between concentrations between the first and second additions of antimycin. The slight but reproducible recovery from inhibition after each addition of antimycin may reflect equilibration of the inhibitor between maternal and foetal compartments. Another possibility is that this recovery reflects only the distribution of antimycin through the maternal tissue and that the residual oxygen consumption observed is due to the foetal tissue alone. For this situation to prevail, it would be necessary to invoke the existence of a perfusion barrier to prevent the passage of antimycin from maternal to foetal circulations. There are no reports of measurements of placental clearance for this compound although from previous studies in our laboratory it appears that clearance across the placenta is reduced by increasing hydrophilicity and increasing size (Maguire et al, in press).

An extension of that hypothesis is that the component of oxygen consumption that was observed to persist at low maternal circulation flow rates may represent only consumption of oxygen by the maternal tissue component of the placenta. Yet a further extension of that hypothesis is that the effect induced by reduced foetal circulation flow rates is manifested by suppression of oxygen consumption only in the foetal tissue component.

CONCLUSIONS

The collection of useful data from an *in vitro* human placental perfusion experiment depends upon the maintenance of tissue in a physiological state. It appears that this tissue has at least two viable states and presumably a range of intermediate oxygenation conditions exist in some regions of this tissue. By mechanically altering flow rates and flow ratios, it has been possible to define a range of conditions over which oxygen metabolism appears to be relatively constant. At flow rates above this range, mechanical damage to tissues is to be expected. Further work will be required to fully define the metabolic consequences of altered flow rates and flow ratios in this organ. Any future investigations will also need to address the question of the existence of separate and independent respiring compartments.

REFERENCES

Addison, R.S., Maguire, D.J., Mortimer, R.H. and Cannell, G.R., 1991, Metabolism of prednisolone by the isolated perfused human placental lobule, J. Steroid Biochem. Molec. Biol. 39:83-90.

Bruce, N.W. and Abdul-Karim, R.W., 1973, Relationship between fetal weight, placental weight and maternal placental circulation in the rabbit at different stages of gestation, J. Reprod. Fertil. 32:15-24.

Kunzell, W. and Moll, W., 1973, Uterine oxygen consumption and blood flow of the pregnant uterus, Z. Gebutsh. Perinat. 178:108-117.

Maguire, D.J., Addison, R.S., Harvey,T.J., Mortimer, R.H. and Cannell,G.R., 1992, A comparison of parameters used to standardize results from *in vitro* perfusions of human placentae, Adv. Exp. Biol. Med. in press.

Mendoza, G.J.B., Brown, E.G., Calem-Grunat, J. Chervenak, F., Karmel, B.Z., Krouskop, R.W., LeBlanc, M.H. and Winslow, R.M., 1989, Intrauterine growth retardation related to maternal erythrocyte oxygen transport, Adv. Exp. Biol. Med. 248:377-386.

Miller, R.K., Weir, O.J., Maulik, K.D. and di Sant'Agnese, P.A., 1985, Human placenta in vitro: characterization during 12 h of dual perfusion, Contrib. Gynecol. Obstet. 13:77-84.

Moll, W. and Herberger, J., 1976, Oxygen uptake of the guinea pig at decreased and increased maternal placental blood flow, Adv. Exp. Biol. Med. 75:705-712.

Weir, P.J. and Miller, R.K., 1985, Oxygen transport as an indicator of perfusion viability in the isolated human placental lobule, Contr. Gynec. Obstet. 13:127-131.

DIMINUTION OF HISTIDINE-INDUCED REOXYGENATION DAMAGE BY GLYCINE IN POSTHYPOXIC RENAL CELLS

G. Gronow,[1] M. Mályusz,[1] W. Niedermayer[2], and N. Klause[2]

[1]Department of Physiology
[2]Clinic of Nephrology
University of Kiel
D-2300 Kiel, Germany

INTRODUCTION

Free oxygen radicals are generated in cells at inner membranes of mitochondria, in the endoplasmatic reticulum, and in the cytosol. Under physiological conditions and at normal oxygen tension, these oxygen species are detoxified by protective enzymes (e.g. superoxide dismutase, SOD, and catalase) as well as by electron accepting scavengers like α-tocopherol or polyalcohols (Chance et al., 1979). In hyperoxia or during reperfusion, however, tissue activities of protective enzymes and/or the capacity of oxygen radical scavanging cell constituents becomes insufficient, and free oxygen radicals oxidize cellular macromolecules and membranes (Baker et al., 1985; Gronow et al., 1989).

Amino acids may modify postanoxic tissue reperfusion injury. Beneficial amino acids like glycine ore alanine have been shown to reduce reperfusion injury in posthypoxic kidney cells (Weinberg et al, 1987; Gronow et al., 1990). The role of histidine remains unclear. On the one hand, histidine in extremely high concentration (about 190 mmol /l) has been sucessfully used as a buffer substance (Fig. 1 A,B) in cardiac and renal preservation fluids (Bretschneider et al., 1988; Kallerhoff et al., 1988). On the other hand, histidine may induce in biological membranes lipid peroxidation by a catalytic formation of hydroxyl radicals (Sundberg et al., 1974; Winkler et al., 1984).

The histidine-mediated oxygen radical pathway (Fig. 1 C) includes the acceptance of one electron at the nucleophilic imidazole ring of histidine, forming an imidazoyl radical. This radical may reduce molecular oxygen a) monovalently to the superoxide anion, and b) divalently, under the catalytic action of iron, to $\cdot$OH, the hydroxyl radical. $\cdot$OH may then extract hydrogen from unsaturated membrane lipids, forming an alkyl radical (I). This may initialize a chain reaction: after diene formation and oxygen binding lipid peroxidation may further destabilize membranes (Fig. 1 D,E) by newly formed alkyl radicals (II).

The question arose as to what extent histidine-mediated lipid peroxydation in reoxygenated renal cells (Klause et al., 1989) may be compensated, at least in part, by the known beneficial effect of glycine in posthypoxic cells (Weinberg et al., 1987; Gronow et al., 1990). We tested in the present experiments in reoxygenated renal tubular cells the effect of histidine, glycine, and of a combination of histidine plus glycine on a) lipid peroxidation, b) maintenance of intracellular potassium, c) ADP-linked control of mitochondrial respiration, and on d) the loss of cellular macromolecules, cytoplasmatic lactate dehydrogenase and mitochondrial glutamate dehydrogenase, into the incubation medium.

Oxygen Transport to Tissue XV, Edited by P. Vaupel
et al., Plenum Press, New York, 1994

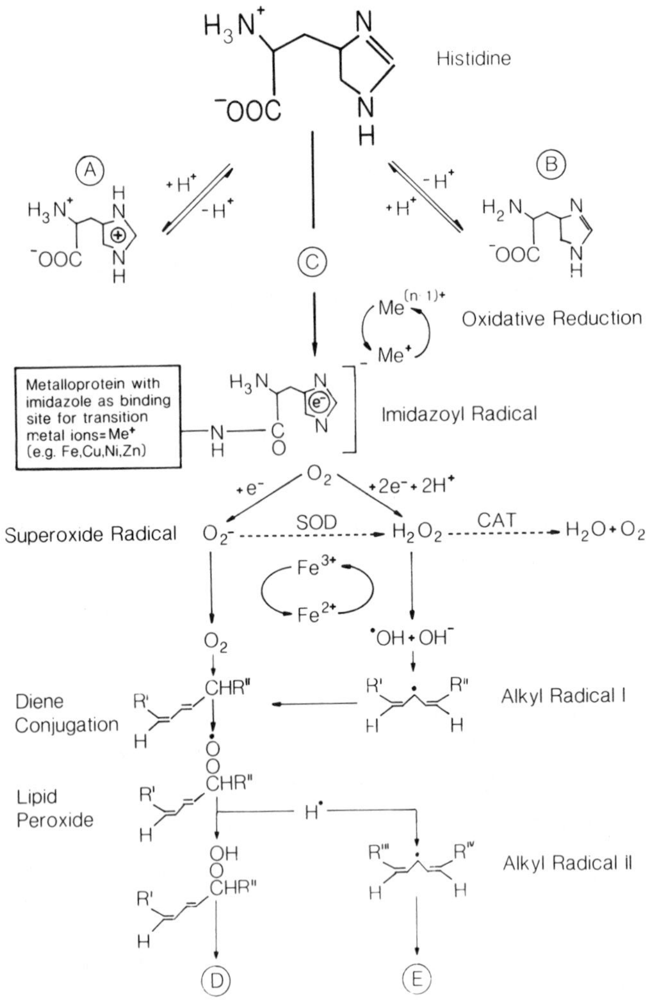

Figure 1. The amino acid histidine may buffer pH in biological material by acceptance (A) or release (B) of H^+. Histidine may also catalyze free oxygen radical formation (C) in the presence of iron: the imidazole ring in histidine transfers one (superoxide radical formation, left chain) or two electrons to molecular oxygen (hydroxyl radical formation, right chain). The strong biological oxidant $\cdot OH$ then extracts hydrogen from unsaturated fatty acids in membranes, forming an alkyl radical (I). This radical reacts as a diene with molecular oxygen to lipid peroxides, destabilizing the membrane (D) and generating a new alkyl radical (II). This radical may oxidize in a chain reaction other membrane lipids (E). SOD = superoxide dismutase, CAT = catalase, Me = transition metal ion.

METHODS

Isolated tubular segments (ITS) from rat renal cortex were prepared by collagenase treatment. Details of this method have been reported elsewhere (Gronow et al., 1984, 1989). ITS were incubated at $37°C$ in a modified Krebs-Ringer-bicarbonate (KRB) medium containing 0.5 g /dl bovine albumine and 10 mmol /l lactate. The tested KRB-media contained amino acid additives (numbers indicate mmol /l) as follows: (A) HIS = 100 histidine + 10 taurine; (B) GLY = 10 glycine + 100 taurine; (C) CONTROL = 110 taurine; (D) HIS + GLY = 100 histidine + 10 glycine. The amino acid derivative taurine exerted no significant effect on parameters under study, it was added to compensate the osmotic differences between individual test media. Osmolality of all test media was maintained konstant at 300 mmosmol /l by the omission of 55 mmol/l NaCl from the basic KRB-medium. Extreme hypoxia (PO_2 for 30 min < 1 mm Hg) was introduced by gassing the surface of the suspension with water saturated 95% N_2 : 5% CO_2. Subsequent 120 min reoxygenation was achieved by gassing with 95% O_2: 5% CO_2. All probes were immediately withdrawn, centrifuged and analyzed for protein, K^+, enzymes, and mitochondrial respiration.

Renal mitochondria were isolated and tested as described by Goldstein (1975). The mitochondrial respiratory control ratio (RCR = state 3 over state 4 respiration) was calculated as the ratio of 0.5 mmol /l ADP-stimulated oxygen consumption (in the presence of 5 mmol /l malate and 5 mmol /l glutamate) over mitochondrial respiration after the ADP-effect had worn off. Tubular and mitochondrial protein was measured colorimetrically by the method of Lowry et al. (1951). Lipid peroxidation was estimated in the supernatant of homogenized and centrifuged ITS (10 min at 600 x g) as thiobarbituric acid-positive material (TBAM) according to the assay of Ohkawa et al. (1979). Intracellular K^+ was extracted from ITS and determined by standard flame photometry. Measurements of enzyme activities in the supernatant of centrifuged ITS (LDH = lactate dehydrogenase, EC 1.1.27; GlDH = glutamate dehydrogenase, EC 1.4.1.3) were performed according to standard procedures and previously described methods (Gronow et al., 1984; 1989). All values are expressed per mg tubular protein and are means ±SD of 14 observations (n= 14). Statistical analysis was employed as paired t-Test. A P-value of 0.05 or less was assumed to indicate a significant difference.

RESULTS and DISCUSSION

Lack of oxygen and metabolic energy reduces transmembraneous ion pumping and in consequence induces cellular swelling as well as the loss of cell constituents (MacKnight and Leaf, 1977; Völkl et al., 1988; Gronow et al., 1990). In the present experiments extreme hypoxia (extracellular PO_2 < 1 mm Hg) was accompanied by a loss of about 30% of intracellular K^+ (Fig.2, left panel). Addition of amino acids had no significant effect on the K^+ loss. In the reoxygenation period, K^+ declined to about 60% of untreated cells (dashed line). Addition of histidine (HIS) to the incubation medium further reduced intracellular K^+-content (open circles), after 120 min reoxygenation K^+ reached one third of its initial value. In contrast, with glycine (GLY) in the incubation medium, intracellular K^+ improved significantly after reoxygenation to about 80% (no HIS added) or about 60% (HIS added) of control values.

In the presence of HIS the observed K^+-loss was accompanied by the appearance of a cytoplasmatic macromolecule in the incubation medium, lactate dehydrogenase (LDH, Fig. 2, right panel), indicating unphysiological membrane permeability in the reoxygenation period. GLY, in contrast, not only suppressed LDH-loss significantly during reoxygenation but also in extreme hypoxia no significant differences could be observed with respect to untreated cells (dashed line). Under control conditions (no GLY or HIS added, open circles) the rate of LDH-loss in hypoxia increased one order of magnitude and returned to values near normal after two hours of reoxygenation. In contrast to the control observations, the LDH-leakage remained in presence of histidine significantly elevated, with HIS as the sole amino acid by 146%, with HIS plus GLY by 76%.

Respiratory control ratio (RCR) was reduced in mitochondria isolated from O_2-deprived and subsequently reoxygenated renal tubular cells. Under control conditions RCR fell by about 48% (Tab. 1). This decrease in RCR was significantly reduced by the addition of glycine to the incubation medium, RCR fell only by 19%. A similar beneficial effect of amino acids on the mitochondrial respiratory control ratio in renal cells has been described for a mixture of 8 amino acids containing glycine (Gronow et al., 1986). In contrast to glycine, histidine (HIS) in the incubation medium intensified the posthypoxic decline in RCR, no significant ADP-stimulated mitochondrial respiration could be observed (RCR = 1.2). The combination of GLY plus HIS improved significantly mitochondrial respiratory control rate (RCR = 1.5). The leakage of a mitochondrial marker enzyme, glutamate dehydrogenase (GlDH), varied in parallel to alterations in mitochondrial respiratory function.

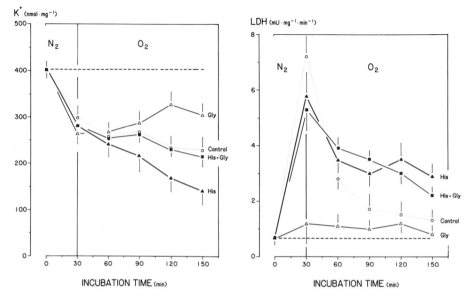

Figure 2. Effect of histidine (His), glycine (Gly), and of a histidine plus glycine combination (His + Gly) on intracellular potassium (K^+) content (left panel), and on loss of cytoplasmatic lactate dehydrogenase (LDH) in isolated tubular segments (ITS) of rat renal cortex. ITS were incubated in Krebs-Ringer-bicarbonate medium (37°C) and reoxygenated (O_2) after extreme hypoxia ($N_2 = PO_2 < 1$ mm Hg). Mean $\pm$ SD, n = 14

An increase in GlDH-loss was accompanied by a decrease in RCR, and vice versa (Fig. 3, left panel). Under control conditions, GlDH-leakage nearly doubled after reoxygenation (open circles). Histidine (HIS) significantly stimulated the loss of GlDH by additional 82%. This posthypoxic increase in GlDH-leakage indicated severe membrane defects in mitochondria and was paralleled by a loss of mitochondrial respiratory control (Tab. 1). In contrast to histidine, glycine reduced the posthypoxic GlDH-leakage to control values (dashed line). In the presence of combined GLY + HIS the GlDH-loss in the reoxygenation period was, similar to the observed loss of LDH, about half the leakage observed with HIS as the sole amino acid. With respect to glycine, however, GlDH-loss remained still significantly elevated.

The formation of lipid peroxidation products, monitored by the release of thiobarbituric acid-positive material (TBAM), declined - as one would expect - without oxygen delivery to zero (Fig. 3, right panel), and incresead in the reoxygenation period to

Table 1. Effect of glycine (GLY) and histidine (HIS) on mitochondrial respiratory control rate (RCR = state 3 / state 4 respiration) in posthypoxic cells of isolated tubular segments of rat kidney cortex. O2K = aerobic control, no amino acids added. Control = posthypoxic cells, taurine added (mean $\pm$ SD, n = 14).

	O2K	HIS	GLY	CONTROL	HIS + GLY
RCR	$4.8 \pm 0.35^*$	$1.2 \pm 0.27^*$	$3.9 \pm 0.31^*$	2.5 ± 0.27	$1.5 \pm 0.25^*$

* significant different (p < 0.05) in comparison to control

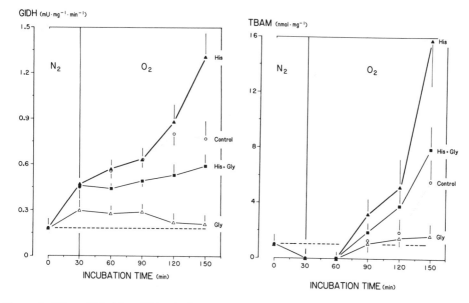

Figure 3. Effect of histidine (His), glycine (Gly), and of a histidine plus glycine combination (His + Gly) on loss of mitochondrial glutamate dehydrogenase (GlDH, left panel), and on the liberation of lipid peroxidation products = thiobarbituric acid-positive material (TBAM, right panel) from of cells of isolated tubular segments (ITS) of rat renal cortex. ITS were incubated in Krebs-Ringer-bicarbonate medium (37°C) and reoxygenated (O₂) after extreme hypoxia (N₂ = PO₂ < 1 mm Hg). Mean ± SD, n = 14

about 5 nmol /mg at control conditions. In the presence of oxygen, histidine (HIS) stimulated the TBAM-liberation with respect to control observations about threefold. Glycine (GLY) suppressed TBAM-release to values of untreated cells (dashed line). The combination of GLY and HIS reduced TBAM-liberation to about half of the value observed with histidine as the sole amino acid.

Generally, histidine effects were small in hypoxia but pronounced in the presence of oxygen, indicating oxygen-mediated cytotoxiciy of histidine. During reoxygenation histidine probably catalyzed the formation of ·OH-radicals (Sundberg et al., 1974; Winkler et al., 1984) which oxidized unsaturated fatty acids in biological membranes (Fig. 1 C). Lipid peroxidation of biological membranes generates thiobarbituric acid-positive material (TBAM), mainly malone dialdehyde (Chance et al., 1979; Gronow et al., 1989). Accordingly, the liberation of TBAM decreased in hypoxia, but increased severalfold in the presence of histidine (Fig. 3). This histidine-stimulated TBAM-liberation was accompanied by a parallel loss of intracellular K^+ and cytoplasmatic LDH (Fig. 2) in the reoxygenation period. The observed loss of mitochondrial GlDH (Fig. 3) and the concomitant reduction of mitochondrial respiratory control rate (Tab. 1) also supported the hypothesis of severe membrane damage in the presence of high concentrations of histidine.

Hearts and kidneys perfused with HTK-solution have been succesfully preserved, probably due to the buffering capacity of histidine (Bretschneider et al., 1988; Kallerhoff et al., 1988). Histidine/HCl accepts a proton at the imidazol ring (Fig. 1 A, pK_a 6.1) as well as it donates a proton from the amino group (Fig. 1 B, pK_a 9.15). However, a formerly applied high concentration of histidine in HTK-solution (about 190 mmol /l) may have also enabled cellular and interstitial deposition of histidine. Thus, with the onset of reperfusion and oxygen supply, histidine might have facilitated membrane fragmentation the catalytic generation of free oxygen radicals. This risk, however, might be minimized during organ transplantation by 3 additional protective mechanisms: 1) low perfusate temperature, 2) flushing the vascular tree after preservation, and 3) by the presence of the hydroxyl radical scavenger mannitol. Mannitol is a component of the HTK-solution and, in fact, supresses the formation of thiobarbituric acid-positive material in reoxygenated renal tubular cells (Gronow et al., 1989).

Glycine, in contrast to histidine, reduced reoxygenation damage in the present experiments. The exact mechanism of protection by glycine in renal cells remains to be clarified (Weinberg et al., 1990). Support of posthypoxic volume regulation by glycine was indicated in the present experiments by an increased K^+-reaccumulation (Fig. 2). These findings are in agreement with earlier observations where glycine reduced cellular swelling by about 50% (Gronow et al, 1990). Reduced cellular swelling also supports the integrity of cellular membranes, thus minimizing the loss of cytoplasmatic LDH (Fig. 1) and of mitochondrial GlDH (Fig. 3). Maintenance of the internal milieu and intactness of cellular membranes would also improve mitochondrial respiratory control (Tab. 1), which, in turn, would provide more metabolic energy for ion pumping, e.g. K^+-reaccumulation (Fig. 2).

Cytotoxicity of histidine in posthypoxic renal cells, however, could not totally be prevented by glycine in the present experiments. It is concluded that the risk of histidine-mediated free oxygen radical formation in cardiac and renal preservation fluids should be reduced by the replacement of histidine with glycine and/or a more physiological buffer substance, e.g. sodium bicarbonate or -lactate.

The technical assistance of R. Bock is gratefully acknowledged

REFERENCES

Bretschneider,H.J., Helmchen,U., and Kehrer,G., 1988, Nierenprotektion, *Klin. Wochenschr.* 66:817.

Baker,G.L., Corry,R.C., and Autor,A.P., 1985, Oxygen free radical induced damage in kidneys subjected to warm ischemia and reperfusion, *Ann. Surg.* 202:628.

Chance,B., Sies,H., and Boveris,A., 1979, Hydroperoxide metabolism in mammalian organs, *Physiol. Rev.* 59:527.

Goldstein,L., Glutamine transport by mitochondria isolated from normal and acidotic rats. *Am. J. Physiol.* 229:1027.

Gronow.G., Klause,N., and Mályusz,M., 1990, Support of hypoxic renal cell volume regulation by glycine, *Adv. Exp. Med. Biol.* 277:705.

Gronow,G., Meya,F., and Weiss, C., 1984, Studies on the ability of renal cells to recover after periods of anoxia, *Adv. Exp. Med. Biol.* 169:589.

Gronow,G., Prechel,P., and Klause,N., 1989, Cytoprotective effect of isotonic mannitol at low oxygen tension, *Adv. Exp. Med. Biol.* 248:755.

Gronow,G., Skrezek,Ch., and Kossmann,H., 1986, Correlation between mitochondrial respiratory dysfunction and Na^+-reabsorption in the reoxygenated rat kidney, *Adv. Exp. Med. Biol.* 200:515.

Kallerhoff,M., Blech,M., Isemer,F.-E., Kehrer,G., Kleinert,H., Langheinrich,M., Helmchen,U., and Bretschneider,H.J., 1988, Metabolic, energetic and structural changes in protected and unprotected kidneys at temperatures of 1°C and 25°C, *Urol. Res.* 16:57.

Klause,N., Beuke,H.P., Mályusz,M., Gronow.G., 1989, Puffersubstanzen bei der Nierenkonservierung. Die Rolle des Histidins und des Glycins, *Urol. Nephrol.* 1:171.

Lowry,O.H., Rosebrough,N.J., Farr,A.L., and Randall,R.J., 1951, Protein measurement with the folin phenol reagent, *J. Biol. Chem.* 193:265.

MacKnight,A.D.C., and Leaf,A., 1977, Regulation of cellular volume, *Physiol. Rev.* 57:510.

Ohkawa,H., Ohishi,N, and Yagi,K., 1979, Assay for lipid peroxides in animal tissues by thiobarbituric acid reaction, *Anal. Biochem.* 95:351.

Sundberg,R.J., and Martin,R.B., 1974, Interactions of histidine and other imidazole derivatives with transition metal ions in chemical & biological systems, *Chemical Rev.* 74:471.

Völkl,H., Paulmichl,M., and Lang,F., 1988, Cell volume regulation in renal cortical cells, *Renal Physiol. Biochem.* 3:158.

Weinberg,J.,M., Abarzua,D.J.A., Rajan,T., 1987, Cytoprotective effect of glycine and gluthathione against hypoxic injury in renal tubules, *J. Clin. Invest.* 80:1446.

Weinberg,J.,M., Venkatchalam,M.,A., Garza-Quintero,M., Roeser,M.,F., and Davis,J.A., 1990, Structural requirements for protection by small amino acids against hypoxic injury in kidney proximal tubules, *FASEB J.* 4:3347.

Winkler,P., Schaur,R.J., and Schauenstein,E., 1984, Selective promotion of ferrous iron-dependent lipid peroxydation in Ehrlich ascites tumor cells by histidine as compared with other amino acids, Biochem. Biophys. Acta 196:220.

THE OXYGEN PERMEABILITY OF CULTURED ENDOTHELIAL CELL MONOLAYERS

C. Y. Liu[1], S. G. Eskin[2], and J. D. Hellums[1]

[1]Department of Chemical Engineering
Rice University, Houston, TX 77251
[2]Department of Internal Medicine
University of Texas Medical School, Houston, TX 77225

INTRODUCTION

The first barrier encountered by oxygen after exiting the lumen of the capillary is the capillary wall endothelium. Prior workers' estimates of the oxygen permeability of the endothelium have differed by orders of magnitude, with some studies suggesting that the endothelial resistance to oxygen transport is of dominant importance (Rasio and Goresky, 1979; Rose and Goresky, 1985; Fletcher and Schubert, 1984). The present study was undertaken to directly measure the oxygen permeability of cultured bovine aortic, and human umbilical vein endothelial cell monolayers.

METHODS

Bovine aortic endothelial cells (passages 8 to 14) and human umbilical vein endothelial cells (passages 1 to 2) were cultured in monolayer on fibronectin-coated Silastic® silicone rubber membranes (Dow Corning) of 0.005" thickness and 4.5 cm² area as previously described (Liu, 1992). The oxygen permeabilities of fully confluent monolayers were measured in a specially designed diffusion cell apparatus.

Figure 1 shows a schematic of the diffusion cell. Shown are the cross section and the top views of the top and bottom sections. The diffusion cell consists of two chambers formed by a lid, a top section, a bottom section, and a base plate. The upper chamber is 95 ml in volume and is perfused with humidified gas. Rotometers maintained the gas flow at 243 std ml/min. The lower chamber is 16.6 ml in volume and is filled with saline (0.9% NaCl). During electrode calibration, saline at known oxygen tension enters and exits the lower chamber via narrow conduits which can be closed off by plastic stopcocks. Vigorous stirring of the saline is accomplished by a magnetic stir bar and a highly precise disc encoder controlled magnetic stirrer. This specially designed stirrer allows for absolute reproducibility in the stirring conditions. Temperature control is maintained by submerging the diffusion cell in a water bath at

Oxygen Transport to Tissue XV, Edited by P. Vaupel
et al., Plenum Press, New York, 1994

37°C. To eliminate temperature and stirring effects on the experimental measurements, the electrode is calibrated under conditions identical to that of the experiments. The oxygen tension in the saline of the bottom chamber was monitored with a miniature Clark-type electrode with a polyethylene membrane (Diamond General Corp. 731).

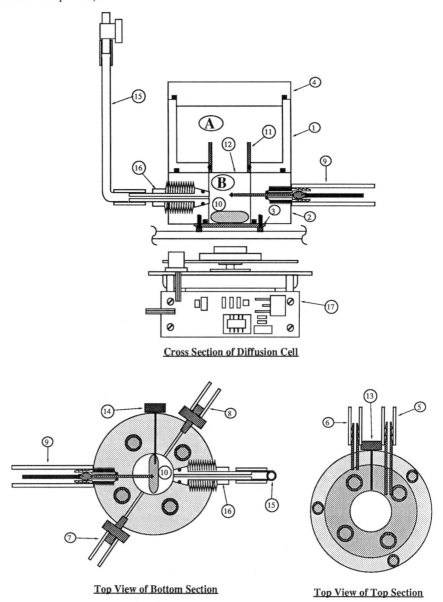

Cross Section of Diffusion Cell

Top View of Bottom Section

Top View of Top Section

Figure 1. Schematic of Diffusion Cell. A)Upper Chamber (gas); B)Lower Chamber (saline); 1)Top Section; 2) Bottom Section; 3)Base Plate; 4)Lid; 5)Upper Chamber Gas Outlet; 6)Upper Chamber Gas Inlet; 7)Lower Chamber Saline Inlet; 8)Lower Chamber Saline Outlet; 9)Clark-Type Electrode; 10)Magnetic Stir Bar; 11)Ring Holding Silastic® Membrane; 12)Silastic Membrane; 13)Thermocouple to Upper Chamber; 14)Thermocouple to Lower Chamber; 15)Glass Tube Manometer; 16)Capillary Fitting to Manometer; 17)Disc Encoder Stirring Apparatus

The pressure in the lower chamber was monitored by a glass tube manometer connected to the lower chamber saline by a stainless steel capillary fitting of 0.08 cm diameter and 6 cm length. In this way, atmospheric pressure can be maintained in the tightly sealed lower chamber by adjusting the level in the manometer to that of the silicone rubber membrane.

When the endothelial monolayers achieved full confluence and total surface coverage of the silicone rubber membranes, they were mounted in the carefully calibrated diffusion cell in one of two configurations (Figure 2). In the first configuration, the monolayer is on the gas (upper chamber) side of the silicone rubber. In the second configuration, the monolayer is on the saline (lower chamber) side of the silicone rubber. Prior to the start of a permeability experiment, the lower chamber of the diffusion cell was filled with degassed saline at very low oxygen tension. Then, the upper chamber was perfused with fully humidified oxygen. The increase in oxygen tension in the saline was recorded by both a strip chart recorder (Houston Instruments Omnigraphic 1000) and a computer data acquisition system (Apple MacIntosh SE with A/D converter). The experiments were repeated on the bare silicone rubber membranes.

The resistances to the flow of oxygen from the upper chamber to the lower chamber of the diffusion cell for either mounting configuration are shown in Figure 2. Note that in the case where the cells are mounted in configuration 1, a thin residual film of media remains on the monolayer throughout the experiment. Figure 3 shows photomicrographs of confluent monolayers of bovine aortic and human umbilical vein endothelial cells.

Integration of the transient oxygen mass balance differential equation yields a relationship between the increase in the lower chamber oxygen tension and the mass transfer coefficients of the resistance layers.

$$-\left(\frac{\alpha V}{A}\right)\ln\left(\frac{P_L(t) - P_U}{P_{L0} - P_U}\right) = Mt \tag{1}$$

where:
α = bunsen solubility coefficient of O_2 in saline
V = volume of lower chamber of diffusion cell
A = area of silicone rubber membrane
P_L = O_2 tension in saline of lower chamber
P_{L0} = initial O_2 tension in saline of lower chamber
P_U = O_2 tension in gas of upper chamber
M = overall mass transfer coefficient
t = time

A plot of the left hand side of equation (1) would be linear with slope M.

The overall mass transfer coefficients for experiments with the endothelial monolayers mounted in configurations 1 and 2 and with the bare silicone rubber membrane, M_1, M_2, and M_0, can be expressed as:

$$M_1 = \left(\frac{1}{k_{gbl}} + \frac{1}{k_{rm}} + \frac{1}{k_{ec}} + \frac{1}{k_s} + \frac{1}{k_{lbl}}\right)^{-1} \tag{2}$$

$$M_2 = \left(\frac{1}{k_{gbl}} + \frac{1}{k_s} + \frac{1}{k_{ec}} + \frac{1}{k_{lbl}}\right)^{-1} \tag{3}$$

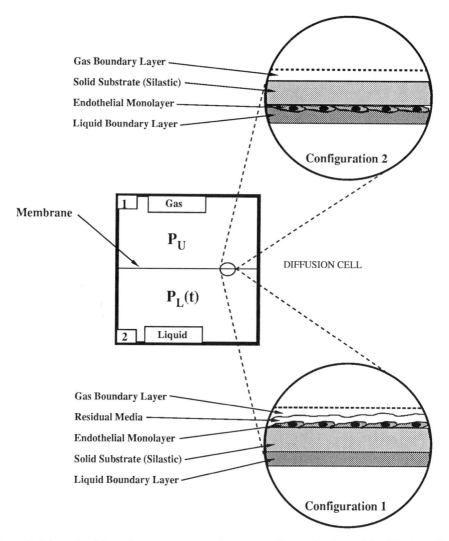

Figure 2. Schematic of the resistances separating the upper and lower chambers of the diffusion cell with the endothelial monolayers mounted in configurations 1 and 2.

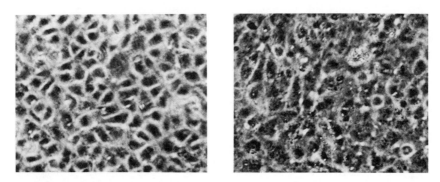

Figure 3. Photomicrographs of confluent bovine aortic endothelial cells (left) and human umbilical vein endothelial cells (right) cultured on Silastic® silicone rubber membranes.

$$M_0 = \left(\frac{1}{k_{gbl}} + \frac{1}{k_s} + \frac{1}{k_{lbl}} \right)^{-1} \tag{4}$$

where: k_{gbl} = mass transfer coefficient of the gas boundary layer
k_{rm} = mass transfer coefficient of the residual media
k_{cc} = mass transfer coefficient of the endothelial monolayer
k_s = mass transfer coefficient of the silicone rubber membrane
k_{lbl} = mass transfer coefficient of the liquid boundary layer

The net mass transfer coefficient of the endothelial monolayer and the residual media film can be obtained from (2) and (4); this represents a lower bound to the mass transfer coefficient of the monolayer alone.

$$k_{ec, lb} = \left(\frac{1}{k_{rm}} + \frac{1}{k_{ec}} \right)^{-1} = \left(\frac{1}{M_1} - \frac{1}{M_0} \right)^{-1} \tag{5}$$

Similarly, the mass transfer coefficient of the endothelial monolayer alone can be determined from (3) and (4).

$$k_{ec} = \left(\frac{1}{M_2} - \frac{1}{M_0} \right)^{-1} \tag{6}$$

RESULTS AND DISCUSSION

As validation of the experimental approach, the oxygen permeability coefficient of silicone rubber, PC_{sil}, was determined using membranes of different thicknesses (Liu, 1992). The permeability coefficient of silicone rubber was determined to be $2.73 \pm 0.07 \times 10^{-13}$ (avg. $\pm$ s.d.) gmol/cm sec mmHg. Since PC_{sil} is a physical property, it should be independent of the combination of thicknesses used in its determination. Indeed, this was clearly shown to be the case. Furthermore, the value of PC_{sil} agrees very well with prior workers measurements (Major et al., 1972; Galletti et al., 1966). The results of these validation experiments with the silicone rubber membranes demonstrates the high accuracy and precision of the diffusion cell apparatus.

Permeability experiments were performed on bovine aortic and human umbilical vein endothelial monolayers mounted in configuration 1. Experiments with the monolayer mounted in configuration 2 were successfully performed only with the human umbilical vein endothelial cells; the bovine cells tended to be sheared off the surface of the silicone rubber by the vigorous stirring of the lower chamber saline. The confluence, surface coverage, and the overall integrity of the monolayers were verified visually by phase contrast microscopy (Nikon Diaphot) both before and after the permeability experiments (Figure 3).

Figure 4 shows the result of a typical experiment, in this case, with bovine aortic endothelial cell monolayers mounted in configuration 1. The left hand side of equation (1) is plotted versus time for both the experiments with and without the monolayer present on the silicone rubber membrane. The lines drawn through the points are the least squares fits. As expected, the plots are linear with time, and the slopes represent M_1 and M_0.

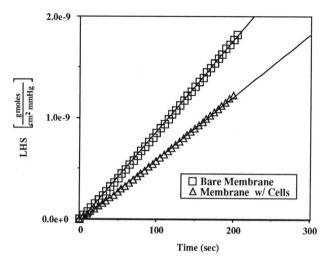

Figure 4. Results of a typical permeability experiment. Here, the left hand side of equation (1) is plotted versus time for experiments with a monolayer of bovine aortic endothelial cells in configuration 1 (triangles) and for a bare silicone rubber membrane (squares). The lines drawn through the points are the least squares fit.

The lower bounds to the mass transfer coefficient for the cultured bovine aortic and human umbilical vein endothelial cell monolayers at 37°C were determined to be $1.99 \pm 0.46 \times 10^{-11}$ (avg.$\pm$s.d., n=16) gmoles/cm^2 sec mmHg and $2.75 \pm 0.73 \times 10^{-11}$ (avg.$\pm$s.d., n=15) gmoles/cm^2 sec mmHg respectively. Lower bounds to the permeability coefficient of the cultured monolayers were obtained by multiplying $k_{cc,lb}$ by the thickness of the monolayer. Electron microscopy of *in vivo* capillaries show the endothelium lining to vary from approximately 2μm at its thickest to less than 0.2μm at its thinnest (Weibel, 1984). Using an average value for thickness of 1μm, the lower bound for the permeability coefficient, PC_{lb}, was determined to be $1.99 \pm 0.46 \times 10^{-15}$ (avg.$\pm$s.d.) gmoles/cm sec mmHg and $2.75 \pm 0.73 \times 10^{-15}$ (avg.$\pm$s.d.) gmoles/cm sec mmHg for the bovine and human cells respectively. Dividing PC_{lb} by the bunsen solubility coefficient of the endothelial cells, α_{cc}, would yield the lower bounds to the effective diffusivity, $D_{cc,lb}$, or permeability in the units of diffusivity for the cell monolayer. Using a value of 1.4×10^{-9} gmoles/cm^3 mmHg for α_{cc} typical for tissue (Altman and Dittmer, 1971), $D_{cc,lb}$ was calculated to be $1.42 \pm 0.33 \times 10^{-6}$ (avg.$\pm$s.d.) cm^2/sec for the bovine cell monolayers and $1.96 \pm 0.52 \times 10^{-6}$ (avg.$\pm$s.d.) cm^2/sec for the human cell monolayers.

By use of configuration 2 (Figure 2) the mass transfer coefficient for the human umbilical vein endothelial cells was measured to be $1.22 \pm 0.45 \times 10^{-10}$ (avg.$\pm$s.d., n=8) gmoles/cm^2 sec mmHg. Again, assuming an average thickness for the monolayers of 1μm, the permeability coefficient, PC, of the human cells was calculated to be $1.22 \pm 0.45 \times 10^{-14}$ (avg.$\pm$s.d.) gmoles/cm sec mmHg. Furthermore, dividing PC by a typical tissue bunsen solubility coefficient of 1.4×10^{-9} gmoles/cm^3 mmHg (Altman and Dittmer, 1971) yields a value of $8.73 \pm 3.21 \times 10^{-6}$ (avg.$\pm$s.d.) cm^2/sec for the effective diffusivity, D_{eff}, for the human umbilical vein endothelial cell monolayers. These results represent the first such oxygen permeability values for the endothelium determined in direct measurements.

The values of D_{cc} determined in this work are compared with prior estimates in Table 1.

728

Table 1. Different Workers' Estimates of the Effective Diffusivity of Oxygen in the Endothelium

Source	Temp., °C	$D_{ec} \times 10^6$, cm^2/sec
Rasio and Goresky, 1979	25	0.03
Rose and Goresky, 1985	37	0.46[1]
Fletcher and Schubert, 1984	32.5	3.00[1]
Groebe and Thews, 1986	37	13
Liu (this work)		avg. ± s.d.
Lower Bound, Bovine Aortic	37	1.42 ± 0.33
Lower Bound, Human Umbilical Vein	37	1.96 ± 0.52
Human Umbilical Vein	37	8.73 ± 3.21

[1]These values were calculated from reported values of the oxygen permeability of the capillary wall. The wall thickness was assumed to be 1μm. Since the capillary wall consists of the extravascular space and the basement membrane in addition to the endothelium, these values can be thought of as lower bounds for that of the endothelium alone.

The most striking comparison between the D_{ec} determined in this work and previous estimates is offered by Rasio and Goresky (1979). Their value, determined in the rete mirabile of the eel, is more than two orders of magnitude smaller than the values of the D_{ec} from human cells from the present work. Clearly the results of Rasio and Goresky (1979) is not applicable to the human endothelium, perhaps due to differences in the tissue of the rete mirabile and its configuration.

Rose and Goresky (1985) determined a value for the "permeability of the capillary wall" from analysis of indicator dilution studies in a canine heart perfusion system. From their analysis, Rose and Goresky (1985) estimated a permeability value of 4.6×10^{-3} cm/sec, and they suggested that a substantial proportion of the resistance is localized to the capillary membrane. Hence, the diffusivity in Table 1 is reported as if the resistance were in the endothelial layer. Another way of looking at the results of Rose and Goresky (1985) is that the resistance to O_2 transport is distributed throughout the extraluminal tissue. Their permeability value corresponds to that of a layer of tissue 19μm in thickness (with a diffusivity equal to that measured in the current work). However, this thickness is on the order of 3 times the distance from the capillary to the middle of the cardiac muscle and is many times the distance from the blood to the sarcolemma (Weibel, 1984; Rose and Goresky, 1985). The indicator dilution analysis certainly gives a measurement that is related to the oxygen permeability of the preparation. However, it does not seem to have directly determined the oxygen permeability of the endothelium.

Fletcher and Schubert (1984) analyzed data on oxygen tension profiles in an isolated feline heart preparation by use of a mathematical model of tissue diffusion. They found the best fit between the model and the experiment was obtained with a capillary wall permeability of 3×10^{-2} cm/sec. They realized that this value of permeability was low and suggested that the model was incomplete. Their value is roughly one third of the value determined in the present work for human umbilical vein endothelial cells.

Compared to the value for D_{ec} of 8.73×10^{-6} cm^2/sec determined in the cultured human cell monolayers, the best previous estimate was provided by Groebe and Thews (1986). They estimated a value of 13×10^{-6} cm^2/sec based on the protein or water content of the endothelium. This value is significantly higher ($p < 0.005$) than the value determined in this work by about 49%. To obtain their value from a correlation of a tissue's oxygen diffusivity and its water content (Vaupel, 1976), Groebe and Thews assumed that the endothelium was 80% water. If a value of 72% is assumed for the water content, then the same correlation would yield a value consistent with the one determined in this work. Therefore, it follows that either D_{ec} is lower than the endothelial percentual water content would suggest, or that Groebe and Thews overestimated the water content of the endothelium.

All the prior workers discussed here except Groebe and Thews (1986) have neglected the intraluminal resistance to oxygen transport in analysis of their experimental results. The intraluminal resistance has been shown to be of the same order as the extraluminal resistance (Hellums, 1977; Baxley and Hellums, 1983). Taking the intraluminal resistance into account would yield a capillary wall permeability closer to that of the present work.

Intuitively, there is nothing about the physical composition of the endothelium that suggests that it should have an effective oxygen diffusivity many times lower than other tissues. The value for D_{ec} of the human umbilical vein endothelial cell monolayers in this work was determined from direct measurements of the oxygen mass transfer coefficient, and it falls in the range expected for tissue. The experimental system used was thoroughly tested with thin silicone rubber membranes, a material whose oxygen permeability is well established. This lends confidence to the results of this work, which leads to the conclusion that prior workers have overestimated the resistance to oxygen transport of the endothelium, except for Groebe and Thews (1986), whose estimate for D_{ec} is slightly higher than the value determined here. The endothelial resistance to oxygen transport is not of dominant importance in determining oxygen transport to tissue.

REFERENCES

Altman, P. L., and Diller, D. S., 1971, "Biological Handbooks: Respiration and Circulation," Federation of American Societies for Experimental Biology, Bethesda, MD.

Baxley, P. T., and Hellums, J. D., 1983, A simple model for simulation of oxygen transport in the microcirculation, *Annals of Biomed. Eng.*, 11:401.

Fletcher, J. E., and Schubert, R. W., 1984, Capillary wall permeability effects in perfused capillary/tissue structures, *in:*"Adv. Exp. Med. and Biol., Vol. 180," D. Bruley, H. I. Bicher, and D. Reneau, eds., Plenum Press, New York and London.

Galletti, P. M., Snider, M. T., and Silbert-Aiden, D., 1966, Gas permeability of plastic membranes for artificial lungs, *Med. Res. Eng.* 2nd Quarter 1966:20.

Groebe, K. and Thews, G., 1986, Theoretical analysis of oxygen supply to contracted skeletal muscle, *in:*"Adv. Exp. Med. and Biol., Vol 200," I. S. Longmuir, ed., Plenum Press, New York and London.

Hellums, J. D., 1977, The resistance to oxygen transport in the capillaries relative to that in the surrounding tissue, *Microvas. Res.* 13:131.

Liu, C. Y., 1992, "A Study on the Resistances to Oxygen Transport in the Microcirculation," Ph.D. thesis, Rice University, Houston.

Major, C. J., and Kammermeyer, K., 1962, Gas permeability of plastics, *Modern Plastics* 39(no.11):135.

Rasio, E. A., and Goresky, C. A., 1979, Capillary limitation of oxygen distribution in the isolated rete mirabile of the eel (anguilla anguilla), *Circ. Res.* 44:498.

Rose, C. P., and Goresky, C. A., 1985, Limitation of oxygen uptake in the canine coronary circulation, *Circ. Res.* 56:57.

Vaupel, P., 1976, Effect of percentual water content in tissues and liquids on the diffusion coefficients of O_2, CO_2, N_2, and H_2, *Pflugers Arch.* 361:201.

Weibel, E. R., 1984, "The Pathway for Oxygen," Harvard University Press, Cambridge MA, and London.

TRANSCUTANEOUS OXYGEN PARTIAL PRESSURE AND DOPPLER ANKLE PRESSURE DURING UPPER AND LOWER BODY EXERCISE IN PATIENTS WITH PERIPHERAL ARTERIAL OCCLUSIVE DISEASE

Yuefei Liu, Jürgen M. Steinacker, Martin Stauch

Abt. Sport- und Leistungsmedizin
Universität Ulm
7900 Ulm, Germany

INTRODUCTION

Transcutaneous measurement of oxygen partial pressure (tcpO$_2$) with heated Clark-elektrodes can represent both the arterial oxygen partial pressure and the blood flow at the site where the tcpO$_2$ is measured[1-4]. The blood flow dependency of tcpO$_2$ has to be considered if changes in arterial pO$_2$ should be monitored. This application is of special value during heavy exercise, where often arterial blood sampling is impossible. On the other hand, changes in local blood flow can be observed by measurements of tcpO$_2$. In this case, skin blood flow is used as an indicator of regional blood flow[5], especially in the limbs of patients with peripheral arterial occlusive disease (PAOD)[6]. At rest, this approach has been proved as clinically valuable for objective graduation of PAOD[7].

In PAOD, the blood supply of the lower extremities is often limited only during exercise, so measurements during exercise will enhance the possibility to detect PAOD. Therefore, the walking distance in a treadmill stress test (TT) is usually in accordance with the severity of the PAOD [8], but it depends on the cooperation of a patient.

To obtain objective results of the functional reserve of a diseased leg in PAOD, Doppler ankle pressure (DAP)[9] was introduced. This method is sensitive at rest, but complicated during exercise, because it is difficult, to find the same site of measurement after exercise, the inflation of the cuff itself disturbs blood flow, and the method is not continuous. There could be an advantage of tcpO$_2$ during exercise, because the method is noninvasive, simple and continuous.

In this study tcpO$_2$ should be examined during exercise on the chest, which should represent changes in paO$_2$, and on the calf, which should represent local leg blood flow, in patients and controls during exercise. Exercise was performed mainly by the tigh muscles in supine cycle ergometer exercise (CE), the legs were not stressed during upper body exercise with a special rowing ergometer (RE)[10,11]. The relation between tcpO$_2$ and DAP should be examined and compared with walking distance. It should be also possible to determine, in which conditions the measurement of tcpO$_2$ may be useful during exercise.

Oxygen Transport to Tissue XV, Edited by P. Vaupel
et al., Plenum Press, New York, 1994

METHODS

Patients: 30 men, 40-70 years of age (58±8), were devided into two groups:
Control group: 10 men, without PAOD, confirmed by angiography or DAP.

PAOD group: 20 men, with chronic stable intermittent claudication without rest pain. PAOD was diagnosed by the angiography and DAP. All the patients had at least illiac arterial lesions, some combined with femoral or popliteal arterial lesions.

In all patients significant heart or lung failure as well as diabetes mellitus was excluded. There were no differences in age, blood pressure and smoking habits between the two groups. All the patients gave informed consent to take part in this study.

Stress Test

TT, CE and RE were performed by all patients in random order on different days. TT was performed at a speed of 3 km/h and slope of 12% on the treadmill as long as possible. The distance the subjects could walk was defined as walking distance. For the control group the subjects should walk over 1000 m.

The CE was a multiple stage test in supine position, beginning with 25 Watts, increasing by 25 Watts, each stage lasted 3 minutes followed by an 1 min break, ended by exhaustion or strong pain on the legs.

For the RE a modified rowing ergometer was used. Instead of a sliding seat a fixed seat was used, so that the subjects could exercise in a sitting position without moving the lower body. The protocol was the same as that of CE.

Table 1. Comparison of the maximum performance between the control group and the PAOD group during TT, CE, and RE.

	n	TT	CE	RE
control	10	> 1000 m	125±33 W	111±24 W
PAOD	20	161(62-504) m	72±31 W	102±28 W
P		<0.01	<0.01	NS

TT = treadmill test; CE = cycle-ergometry; RE = rowing-ergometry; m = walking distance in meters, the numbers in the bracket are the minimum and maximum value; P = significance level; NS = no significance.

Measurements

DAP was measured with a 8MHz continuous wave ultrasound Doppler at the ankle, DAP was taken at rest, at the end of each stage and 1', 3', 5' after the stress test in CE and RE.

Transcutaneous pO_2 was monitored continuously with heated Clark-type electrodes at 45°C, which were fixed on chest (central) and calf (peripheral) during CE and RE.

During CE and RE, heart rate, blood pressure from the upper arms was measured and blood samples for capillary pO_2 were taken at the same time with DAP. Leg pain or other complaints of the subjects were recorded.

RESULTS

Physical Performance in TT, CE and RE

Maximum performance during the different forms of exercises is shown in Table 1. In the controls, maximum performance was higher than that of the PAOD group except for RE. The performance of PAOD in CE was significantly lower than that in RE (P<0.01), while the performance of controls in CE was lightly higher than that in RE (NS).

Blood Pressure and Doppler Ankle Pressure

There was no significant difference of systolic and diastolic blood pressure between patients and controls in CE and RE.

DAP is reported in Table 2. At rest, DAP was lower in CE than in RE. During CE and RE, DAP of the control group increased (P<0.01). In the PAOD group DAP decreased remarkably during CE (P<0.01), while it remained relatively constant in RE.

Table 2. Comparison of the Doppler ankle pressure (mmHg) between control- and PAOD-group and between the CE and RE

	n	CE		RE	
		before	end	before	end
control	10	136±30	165±35	170±33	213±53
PAOD	20	85±37	44±42	113±30	101±44
P		<0.01	<0.01	<0.01	<0.01

CE = cycle-ergometry; RE = rowing-ergometry; before = before exercise;
end = at the end of exercise; P = significance level.

Table 3. Comparison of the peripheral $tcPO_2$ between control group and PAOD group during CE and RE

	n	CE		RE	
		before	end	before	end
control	10	58±9	73±12	69±9	82±9
PAOD	20	50±9	22±22	64±14	60±4
P		<0.05	<0.01	NS	<0.05

CE = cycle-ergometry; RE = rowing-ergometry; before = before exercise;
end = at the end of exercise; P = significance level; NS = no significance.

Central and Peripheral $tcpO_2$

Central $tcpO_2$ (obtained from the chest) increased during CE and RE (P<0.05). There was no significant difference between the two groups before and during exercise. Changes of capillary pO_2 were similar to that of central $tcpO_2$ with a significant correlation (r=0.81, P<0.01, Figure 1).

At rest, peripheral $tcpO_2$ (measured on calf) was lower in CE than in RE (Table 3). In the controls, peripheral $tcpO_2$ increased during CE and RE, while in the PAOD group peripheral $tcpO_2$ clearly decreased in CE, but remained relatively unchanged in RE (Figure 2, Figure 3).

Relationship Between Peripheral $tcpO_2$, DAP and Performance

The peripheral $tcpO_2$ correlated nonlinearly with the DAP during CE ($r^2= 0.64$, P<0.01). If the DAP was greater than 21 mmHg, a hyperbolic relationship between the peripheral $tcpO_2$ and the DAP ($tcpO_2 = 69-1496/DAP$) could be met (Figure 4). The correlations between $tcpO_2$, DAP and performance are shown in Table 4.

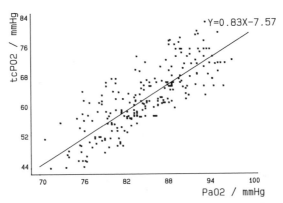

Figure 1. Transcutaneous oxygen partial pressure ($tcpO_2$) on the chest (central) correlated linearly with capillary blood oxygen partial pressure (PaO_2) during rowing- and cycle-ergometry (r=0.81, P<0.01).

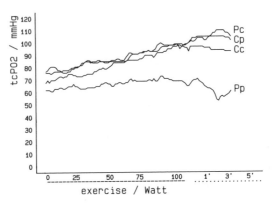

Figure 2. Typical registration of $tcpO_2$ measured on the chest (central) and calf (peripheral) of a control without PAOD (Cc,Cp) and a patient with PAOD (Pc,Pp) during RE. Peripheral $tcpO_2$ remained constant in the patient, while it increased in the control.

DISCUSSION

This study was based on previous reports about the relationship between $tcpO_2$, paO_2 and skin blood flow[2,3]. Lübbers postulated that $tcpO_2$ depends on capillary blood flow and reaches paO_2 at high flows which are attained by heating of the electrode. $tcpO_2$ is also influenced by skin structure, O_2-consumption of the electrode, and O_2-diffusion through the membrane of the electrode. This model was confirmed in several studies for the arm and the leg in normal subjects during rest.

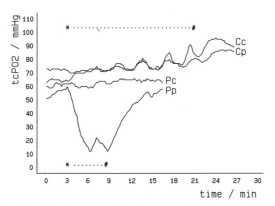

Figure 3. Typical registration of $tcpO_2$ measured on chest (central) and calf (peripheral) of a control without PAOD (Cc,Cp) and a patient with PAOD (Pc,Pp) during CE. The peripheral $tcpO_2$ decreased in the patient. * Start of exercise; # end of exercise.

Steinacker and Spittelmeister[3] reported for the arm a hyperbolic relationship between $tcpO_2$, cutaneous blood flow and perfusion pressure at rest. Wyss et al.[12,13] found a similar relation between $tcpO_2$ and the arteriovenous pressure gradient in the leg and we found similar results in patients with scleroderma[14]. This was confirmed by Gardner et al.[15] for patients with PAOD during rest, and they observed that there was a curvilinear relationship between foot $tcpO_2$ and ankle systolic pressure, but they found a linear relationship during recovery from an exercise test.

In this study, we found a strong hyperbolic relationship between $tcpO_2$ and Doppler ankle pressure in patients with PAOD during exercise. It is interesting, that we calculated

Table 4. Correlation coefficients between walking distance and maximal performance on the CE (Pmax) with the peripheral $tcpO_2$ and DAP at rest (rest) and at the end point of exercise (end).

	walking distance		Pmax CE	
	rest	end	rest	end
peripheral $tcpO_2$	0,23	0,62*	0,13	0,56*
DAP	0,45*	0,68*	0,29	0,49*

*: $p < 0,05$

nearly the same DAP-intercept in our patients during exercise (defined at zero $tcpO_2$) as Wyss et al. found for normals at rest (21 to 22 mmHg). The intercept seems smaller for the arm (5 mmHg)[3], which finding underlines, that $tcpO_2$ can only be interpreted, when the measurement conditions are known.

Our analysis describes why at rest DAP but not peripheral $tcpO_2$ in patients with PAOD was already significantly lower than in control subjects. Since the selected patients had no pain at rest, there was enough blood supply to the lower extremities at rest, and certainly, the $tcpO_2$ remained normal. The decreased $tcpO_2$ before CE may be considered to result from the supine position of the body[16]. During exercise DAP of the PAOD-group decreased further and at the same time the peripheral $tcpO_2$ decreased also significantly. Moreover, the $tcpO_2$ measured on the chest increased identically with the capillary pO_2 during exercise. This relationship between the two parameters means that in normal range of cutaneous blood supply changes in blood flow do not result in a remarkable change of the peripheral $tcpO_2$, therefore, the PAOD patients without rest pain had normal $tcpO_2$, but DAP may be decreased. During exercise, when blood supply is much more disturbed, further decreases of perfusion pressure are accompanied by a big decrease of peripheral $tcpO_2$. In other words, in critical ischemia during exercise, in which condition DAP is much more difficult to obtain, the change of peripheral $tcpO_2$ is more sensitive than that of the DAP due to the hyperbolic relationship of both parameters.

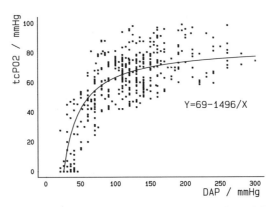

Figure 4. The nonlinear relationship between the $tcpO_2$ measured on calfs (peripheral) and Doppler ankle pressure (DAP) in patients with PAOD during cycle-ergometry (For DAP $\geq$ 21 mmHg, $tcpO_2$ = 69-1496/DAP; r^2=0.64, P<0.01)

Like walking distance or DAP, peripheral $tcpO_2$ can also differentiate patients with PAOD from subjects without PAOD. Furthermore, peripheral $tcpO_2$ correlated with walking distance and DAP (Table 4). Therefore, peripheral $tcpO_2$ can be comparable to these classical parameters that can be used in assessing severity of PAOD. Because the transcutaneous measurement of pO_2 is an objective, continuous method, and it is also noninvasive and easy to carry out[17], the $tcpO_2$ during exercise can be very useful in appreciating the functional reserve of blood supply to the lower extremities.

CONCLUSION

From this study it can be concluded that during exercise a strong hyperbolic relationship exists between $tcpO_2$ and Doppler ankle pressure in patients with PAOD, as it was established for normals and patients during rest. With decreasing leg blood flow peripheral $tcpO_2$ reaches zero at a Doppler ankle pressure of about 21 mmHg due to the oxygen consumption of the electrode and the skin. In patients with PAOD the functional reserve of blood supply to lower extremities can be tested by lower body exercise and measurement of peripheral $tcpO_2$ and Doppler ankle pressure.

REFERENCES

1. R. Huch, D.W. Lübbers, A. Huch, The transcutaneous measurement of oxygen and carbon dioxide tension for the determination of arterial blood gas values with control of local perfusion and peripheral perfusion pressure, Theoretical analysis and practical application, in: "Oxygen measurement in biology and medicine," J.P. Payne, D.W. Hill, ed., London and Boston (1975).
2. D.W. Lübbers, Theoretical basis of the transcutaneous blood gas measurements, Crit Care Med. 9:721-733 (1981).
3. J.M. Steinacker, W. Spittelmeister, Dependence of transcutaneous O_2 partial pressure on cutaneous blood flow, J Appl Physiol. 64:21-25 (1988).
4. J.M. Steinacker, W. Spittelmeister, R. Wodick, Examinations on the blood flow dependence of tcPO₂ using the model of the "circulatory hyperbola". in: "Continuous transcutaneous monitoring," A. Huch, R. Huch, G. Rooth, ed., Plenum Publishing Corp, New York (1987).
5. K.K. Tremper, K. Waxman, W.C. Shoemaker, Effects of hypoxia and shock on transcutaneous PO_2 values in dogs, Crit Care Med. 7: 526-539 (1979).
6. S. Ohgi, K. Ito, T. Mori, Quantitative evaluation of the skin circulation in ischemic legs by transcutaneous measurement of oxygen tension, Angiology. 32:833-839 (1981).
7. G.M. Andreozzi, S. Signorelli, G. Butto, C. Scrofani, R. Leotta, L.D. Pino, M. Rerrara, S. Monaco, Oxygen transcutaneous tensiometry ($tcpO_2$) for microcirculatory evaluation of peripheral arterial disease, CV World Report 3: 37-39 (1990).
8. S. Cross, D. Kneafsy, F. Given, The treadmill in peripheral vascular disease, Ir Med J. 80:404-406 (1987).
9. M.R. Marinelli, K.W. Beach, M.J. Glass, J.F. Primozich, D.E. Strandness, Noninvasive testing vs clinical evaluation of arterial disease, JAMA. 241: 2031-2034 (1979).
10. Y.F. Liu, J.M. Steinacker, A. Stange, K. Röcker, M. Stauch, Exercise testing on a modified rowing ergometry compared to bicycle ergometry in patients with peripheral vascular occlusive disease, Int J Sports Med. 12:130 (1991).
11. J.M. Steinacker, C. Hübner, K Röcker, A. Berger, M. Stauch, Modified rowing ergometry in upper body exercise testing compared to supine bicycle ergometry in surgical patients. Med Si Sports Exerc 23:(Suppl)S4 (1991).
12. C.R. Wyss, F.A. Matsen III, R. King, C.W. Simmons, E.M. Burgess, Dependence of transcutaneous oxygen tension on local arteriovenous pressure gradient in normal subjects, Clin Sci. 60:499-506 (1981).
13. C.R. Wyss, C. Robertson, S.J. Love, R.M. Harrington, F.A. Matsen III, Relationship between transcutaneous oxygen tension, ankle blood pressure, and clinical outcome of vascular surgery in diabetic and nondiabetic patients, Surgery. 101: 56-62 (1987).
14. J.M. Steinacker, F. Nobbe, Transcutaneous pO₂ for therapy control in mixed connective tissue disease and scleroderma, in: "Clinical oxygen pressure measurement II," A.M. Ehrly, J. Hauss, R. Huch, ed., Springer-Verlag, Berlin (1985).
15. A.W. Gardner, J.S. Skinner, D.W. Cantwell, L.K. Smith, E.B. Diethrich, Relationship between foot transcutaneous oxygen tension and ankle systolic blood pressure at rest and following exercise, Angiology. 42:481-490 (1991).
16. C.J. Hauser, P. Appel, W.C. Shoemaker, Pathophysiologic classification of peripheral vascular disease by positional changes in regional transcutaneous oxygen tension, Surgery. 95: 689-693 (1984).
17. K. Linge, D.H. Roberts, G.S.E. Dows, Indirect measurement of skin blood flow and transcutaneous oxygen tension in patients with peripheral vascular disease, Clin Physiol Meas. 8: 293-302 (1987).

O_2 CONSUMPTION VS. O_2 SUPPLY

THE RELEVANCE OF MEASURING O_2 SUPPLY AND O_2 CONSUMPTION FOR ASSESSMENT OF REGIONAL TISSUE OXYGENATION

A. Meier-Hellmann, L. Hannemann, W. Schaffartzik, M. Specht, C. Spies, K. Reinhart

Department of Anesthesiology and Surgical Intensive Care Medicine
Steglitz Medical Center, Free University of Berlin
Hindenburgdamm 30, D-1000 Berlin 45, Germany

INTRODUCTION

Tissue hypoxia is considered to be a relevant factor in the pathogenesis of sequential organ failure (multiple organ failure, MOF), the main cause of death in patients with septic shock and/or ARDS.[1] In these disorders, not only the global O_2 transport to tissue but also the distribution of cardiac output (C.O.) among organ systems and the microcirculatory nutritive blood flow are disturbed.[2] The therapeutic approach is to keep O_2 supply above the normal level ($DO_2 > 600$ ml/min/m^2) to compensate for a deficit in O_2 extraction. It has been recommended to increase DO_2 until no further rise in O_2 consumption (VO_2) occurs.[3,4] It has been shown that hyperdynamic patients with increased DO_2 levels have a significantly lower mortality, compared to normodynamic patients.[5] Other authors[6,7] demonstrated that VO_2 rose after increase of DO_2 in patients with septic shock. This was considered as evidence of tissue hypoxia. Bihari et al.[8] showed that patients with tissue hypoxia determined by a positive O_2 flux test all died whereas patients with a negative O_2 flux test all survived. A negative O_2 flux test is therefore considered to be an indicator of adequate tissue oxygenation.

However, it remains questionable whether the global O_2 transport parameters are sensitive enough to reflect tissue oxygenation at the organ level, e.g. the splanchnic region. In animal models, intestinal O_2 uptake was decreased in endotoxemic conditions despite adequate oxygen supply.[9] The pHi is considered to be a sensitive marker for hypoxia of the gastric mucosa.[10,11] It has been demonstrated that critically ill patients had an increased mortality if pHi values were < 7.35 on admission to the ICU when compared to another group with initial pHi values > 7.35, in whom DO_2 was raised whenever pHi fell below normal levels.[12]

We investigated whether gastric mucosal oxygenation is adequate in patients with hyperdynamic septic shock and markedly increased DO_2, and if not, whether a further increase of DO_2 by volume substitution is an efficient therapeutic approach.

PATIENTS AND METHODS

The study was approved by the ethics committee of our hospital. We studied 10 patients who fulfilled the criteria of septic shock (plausible focus or positive hemoculture, temperature > 38.5°C or < 35°C, systolic arterial hypotension < 90 mm Hg and permanent need for volume substitution without source of hemorrhage, leukocytosis > 12.0 G/l or < 4.0 G/l, thrombocytopenia > 30%/24h without source of hemorrhage, tachypnea, disorientation). All patients were mechanically ventilated and a pulmonary artery catheter was placed in each patient.

Initially all patients received volume substitution by colloidal solutions (hydroxyethylstarch) (HES 10%) for hemodynamic stabilization until the left-ventricular filling pressure was in the upper normal range (14-17 mm Hg). All patients also required dobutamine (average dosage: 11.0 ± 5.4 ug/kg/min) to achieve a mean arterial pressure $\geq$ 70 mm Hg and DO_2 above the norm.

Following hemodynamic stabilization, the global O_2 transport parameters and the pHi (Trip'TGS catheter, Tonometrics Inc.) were determined. If pHi was < 7.35 under the above mentioned therapy more volume was added to increase C.O. and DO_2, and measurements were repeated after 2 hours had elapsed.

Hemodynamic and O_2 transport parameters and pHi were determined according to the following formulas:

DO_2 = C.O. x CaO_2 x 10
VO_2 = C.O. x (CaO_2-CvO_2) x 10
CaO_2 = (Hb x 1.36 x SaO_2) + (PaO_2 x 0.0031)
CvO_2 = (Hb x 1.36 x SvO_2) + (PvO_2 x 0.0031)

DO_2 : O_2 supply, VO_2 : O_2 consumption, C.O. : cardiac output, CaO_2: arterial O_2 content, CvO_2: mixed venous O_2 content, Hb: hemoglobin, 1.36 : O_2 carrier capacity (ml O_2/g Hb), 0.0031: O_2 dissolved in 100 ml blood per mm Hg PaO_2.

$$pHi = 6.1 + \log_{10} \frac{<\text{art. bicarbonate concentration}>}{F \times PCO_2 \text{ of NaCl sol. in the tonometer}}$$

pHi: pH value of the gastric mucosa, F: time-dependent equilibration factor for saline solution in the gastric tube. All patients were treated with the H_2 receptor antagonist Ranitidin to reduce $[H^+]$ because a high gastric acidity could lead to an underestimation of pHi.

Statistics: paired t-test (SPSS/PC+, SPSS), values as means ± SD, level of significance: $p < 0.05$.

RESULTS

At baseline, DO_2 was 717 ± 187 ml/min/m^2 (min: 445, max: 980 ml/min/m^2), VO_2 was 155 ± 31 ml/min/m^2 and pHi was 7.20 ± 0.05 (min: 7.11, max: 7.29, Tab.1).

The patients received on average 1246 ± 594 ml HES 10% (min: 500, max: 2750 ml). Pulmonary capillary wedge pressure (PCWP) increased from 14 ± 2 mmHg (min: 10, max: 17 mm Hg) to 17 ± 1 mmHg (min: 15, max: 20 mm Hg) after volume substitution.

Do_2 increased to 852 ± 254 ml/min/m^2 (min: 534, max: 1355 ml/min/m^2) whereas VO_2 did not change significantly (Tab.1). At the same time pHi increased significantly to 7.25 ± 0.05 (Table 1).

DISCUSSION

Our results show that additional volume infusion in hyperdynamic septic shock patients further increased DO_2 and improved pHi but did not increase VO_2. These findings suggest a regional tissue hypoxia despite a negative O_2 flux test. The pHi values < 7.35 in all patients despite a mean initial DO_2 of 717 ± 187 ml/min/m^2 are further evidence of this tissue hypoxia in the splanchnic region.

An increase in DO_2 by volume substitution significantly raised the pHi. The fact that tissue oxygenation could be improved by application of colloidal volume, even when cardiac filling pressures were in the upper normal range underlines the importance of adequate volume treatment in septic shock.[13,14]

Gutierrez et al.[12] demonstrated significantly better survival rates in patients whose global O_2 transport was increased whenever the pHi fell (below 7,35 or by more than 0,10 units from the previous measurements) compared to patients who were treated according to a standard regimen. In our study 5 of the 10 patients

Tab 1. Oxygen supply (DO$_2$), oxygen consumption (VO$_2$) and pH of gastric mucosa (pHi) before and after volume substitution.

Patient No.	DO$_2$ (ml/min/m^2) before/after volume		VO$_2$ (ml/min/m^2) before/after volume		pHi before/after volume		
1.	445	611	138	142	7.20	7.23	
2.	512	534	108	106	7.22	7.26	
3.	603	728	185	176	7.22	7.28	
4.	613	698	163	158	7.24	7.27	
5.	632	802	148	144	7.22	7.27	
6.	698	706	105	117	7.29	7.34	
7.	876	948	191	179	7.19	7.25	
8.	878	1042	157	171	7.14	7.18	
9.	934	1096	168	172	7.18	7.26	
10.	980	1355	187	238	7.11	7.18	
mean	717	852 *	155	160	7.20	7.25	*
±SD	187	254	31	37	0.05	0.05	

SD = standard deviation, * = $p < 0.05$ before vs. after

subsequently died. The pHi prior to volume substitution was the same in surviving patients and in those who later died of septic shock. However, following volume substitution, surviving patients had a significantly higher mean pHi at 7.29 ± 0.36 than non-survivors (7.19 ± 0.88). This is in agreement with results reported by Gutierrez et al.,[15] who found a significantly lower pHi in non-survivors than in survivors. These findings strongly suggest a tissue hypoxia in the splanchnic region and demonstrate the importance of pHi.

We conclude that the measurement of pHi in patients with hyperdynamic septic shock may be a useful parameter for the detection of and a guide to the treatment of regional tissue hypoxia. Adequate volume infusion for preventing tissue hypoxia is an important first step in the hemodynamic support of sepsis. The increase of pHi in our study after volume treatment suggests an improvement of tissue oxygenation in the splanchnic region, at a time when the whole body VO$_2$ was not a sensitive enough measure to detect these changes.

SUMMARY

Septic shock and ARDS are associated with disturbed tissue oxygenation. It has been suggested to increase O_2 supply (DO_2) above the normal level (> 600 ml/min/m^2) to compensate for the tissue hypoxia. The lack of a rise in O_2 consumption (VO_2) after increases of DO_2 has been presumed to indicate adequate tissue oxygenation (negative O_2 flux test). We were interested in whether a negative O_2 flux test precludes an improvement of regional tissue oxygenation. The pH value of the gastric mucosa (pHi) is considered to be a sensitive marker for hypoxia in the splanchnic region. We measured pHi as well as DO_2 and VO_2 in 10 patients with hyperdynamic septic shock to assess the effect of volume substitution on tissue oxygenation. The initial therapeutic approach (volume substitution and catecholamines) led to a DO_2 of 717 ± 187 ml/min/m^2. However, all patients had pHi values < 7.35 indicating regional tissue hypoxia. An additional increase of DO_2 by colloidal volume substitution caused a significant rise of pHi from 7.20 ± 0.05 to 7.25 ± 0.05 but did not change VO_2. We conclude that a negative O_2 flux test does not rule out regional tissue hypoxia, and second, an increase in DO_2 may improve tissue oxygenation without measurable changes in VO_2. Furthermore, adequate volume substitution is an important step in the treatment of septic shock to increase total body blood flow and more specifically regional blood flow.

REFERENCES

1. W.J. Sibbald, A. Bersten, F.S. Rutledge. The role of tissue hypoxia in multiple organ failure. In: Reinhart K, Eyrich K (Hrsg.) Clinical Aspects of O_2 Transport and Tissue Oxygenation. Springer, Berlin - Heidelberg - New York, S. 102-114 (1989)

2. K. Reinhart. Oxygen Transport and Tissue Oxygenation in Sepsis and Septic Shock. In: Reinhart K, Eyrich K (Hrsg.) Sepsis - An Interdisciplinary Challenge. Springer, Berlin - Heidelberg - New York, S. 125-139 (1989)

3. S.M. Cain, S. Curtis. Experimental models of pathologic oxygen supply dependency. Crit Care Med 19: 603-612 (1991)

4. P. Schumacker, S. Cain. The concept of a critical oxygen delivery. Intensive Care Med 13: 223-229 (1987)

5. J.D. Edwards, G.C.S. Brown, P. Nightingale, R.M. Slater, E.B. Faragher. Use of survivors' cardiorespiratory values as therapeutic goals in septic shock. Crit Care Med 17:1098-1103 (1989)

6. W.C. Shoemaker, P.L. Appel, H.B. Kram, K. Waxman, T.S. Lee. Prospective trial of supranormal values of survivors as therapeutic goals in high-risk surgical patients. Chest 94:1176-1186 (1988)

7. W.C. Shoemaker, P.L. Appel, R. Bland. Use of physiological monitoring to predict outcome and to assist in clinical decisions in critically ill postoperative patients. Am J Surg 146:43-50 (1983)

8. D. Bihari, M. Smithies, A. Gimson, J. Tinker. The effects of vasodilation with prostacyclin on oxygen delivery and uptake in critically ill patients. N Eng J Med 317:397-403 (1987)

9. S.M. Cain, S.E. Curtis. Systemic and regional oxygen uptake and delivery and lactate flux in endotoxic dogs infused with dopexamine. Crit Care Med 19:1552-1560 (1991)

10. J.B. Antonsson, C.C. Boyle, K.L. Kruithoff. Validity of tonometric measures of gut intramural pH during endotoxemia and mesenteric occlusion in pigs. Am J Physiol 259:G519-523 (1990)

11. R.G. Fiddian-Green, S. Baker. Predictive value of the stomach wall pH for complications after cardiac operations. Crit Care Med 15:153-156 (1987)

12. G. Gutierrez, F. Paliazas, G. Doglio, N. Wainsztein, A. Gallesio, J. Pacin, A. Dubin, E. Schiavi, M. Jorge, J. Pusajo, F. Klein, E. San Roman, B. Dorfman, J. Shottlender, R. Giniger. Gastric intramucosal pH as a therapeutic index of tissue oxygenation in critically ill patients. Lancet; 339: 195-199 (1992)

13. M.T. Haupt, E.M. Gilbert, R.W. Carlson. Fluid loading increases oxygen consumption in septic patients with lactic acidosis. Am Rev Respir Dis 131:912-916 (1985)

14. E.M. Gilbert, M.T. Haupt, R.Y. Mandanas, A.J. Huaringa, R.W. Carlson. The effect of fluid loading, blood transfusion, and catecholamine infusion on oxygen delivery and consumption in patients with sepsis. Am Rev Respir Dis; 134:873-878 (1986)

15. G. Gutierrez, H. Bismar, D.R. Dantzker, N. Silva. Comparison of gastric intramucosal pH with measures of oxygen transport and consumption in critically ill patients. Crit Care Med 20:451-457 (1992)

INVESTIGATION OF THE HUMAN OXYGEN TRANSPORT SYSTEM DURING CONDITIONS OF REST AND INCREASED OXYGEN CONSUMPTION BY MEANS OF FRACTIONATION EFFECTS OF OXYGEN ISOTOPES

K.-D.Schuster, H.Heller, and M.Könen

Institute of Physiology, University of Bonn
5300 Bonn 1, FRG

INTRODUCTION

From the fact that oxygen uptake reaches a maximal level due to exhausting exercise the question arises which of the various pathways of the oxygen transport system approaches a borderline of oxygen transporting capacity so as to prevent a further increase of oxygen consumption. This question has been of long-standing interest and it is still a matter of debate in spite of numerous studies. Interestingly, measuring fractionation effects of isotopic oxygen molecules may provide additional information on this field. It has been shown for the situation of rest that the oxygen molecule $^{16}O_2$ is transported 0.9% more rapidly from inspiratory gas to tissue than its isotopic species $^{16}O^{18}O$, leading to an overall fractionation effect of respiration (Schuster and Pflug, 1989). This is due to the fact that the pathways of diffusion and metabolism, which constitute lower resistances to the lighter molecule, slightly lessen the overall resistance for $^{16}O_2$. From the paper cited above and subsequent investigations it has been concluded that oxygen transport to tissue at rest is far more limited by convective processes and metabolism than by diffusion. The aim of this study is to investigate the way in which these relations are changed under conditions of increased oxygen consumption so as to obtain further data for assessing the various pathways of the oxygen transport system.

METHODS

Experimental Protocol

Experiments were performed on healthy humans at rest and various levels of exercise between 50 and 250 W. Subjects sat on a bicycle ergometer breathing environmental air. Each level of performance was maintained for at least 5 to 10 min. A reco-

Oxygen Transport to Tissue XV, Edited by P. Vaupel
et al., Plenum Press, New York, 1994

very phase of more than an hour's duration was introduced after each working phase. During steady state conditions, the subject expired about 40 l into a bag. End-expiratory and mixed-expiratory partial pressures of oxygen and carbon dioxide as well as volume expired during sampling period and also sampling time were measured. From these data, inspiratory oxygen flow $\dot{V}_I O_2$, expiratory oxygen flow $\dot{V}_E O_2$, and oxygen consumption, $\dot{V} O_2$, were calculated.

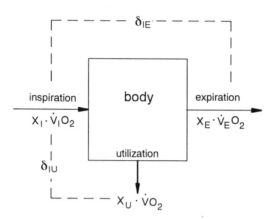

Figure 1. Model of $^{16}O^{18}O$ input and outputs of the body. $\dot{V}_I O_2$, $\dot{V}_E O_2$, $\dot{V} O_2$: inspiratory flow, expiratory flow, and consumption of $^{16}O_2$. X:$[^{16}O^{18}O]/[\,^{16}O_2]$, δ_{IE}: fractionation measured between inspiratory and expiratory gas, δ_{IU}: overall fractionation. I, E, U: indices for inspiration, expiration, utilization.

Quantifying Fractionation Effects

In the model shown in fig.1, the whole body is reduced to only one compartment. Assuming steady state conditions, the flow of $^{16}O^{18}O$ from inspiratory air (I) to expiratory gas (E) and into the sink of mitochondrial utilization (U) can be described by

$$X_U \cdot \dot{V} O_2 = X_I \cdot \dot{V}_I O_2 - X_E \cdot \dot{V}_E O_2 \tag{1}$$

where X is the isotopic ratio $[^{16}O^{18}O]/[\,^{16}O_2]$ of the gas species indicated and $\dot{V} O_2$, $\dot{V}_I O_2$, and $\dot{V}_E O_2$ are utilization, inspiratory flow and expiratory flow of $^{16}O_2$ respectively. If the overall resistance of oxygen transport and metabolism through the body is different for $^{16}O^{18}O$ and for $^{16}O_2$, a fractionation effect occurs leading to different isotopic ratios X_I, X_E and X_U. The percentage deviation of isotopic abundance between inspiratory and expiratory gas has been measured as

$$\delta_{IE} = \frac{X_I - X_E}{X_I} \cdot 100\ \% \tag{2}$$

which depends mainly on the ventilatory rate.

The percentage deviation of isotopic abundance between inspiratory oxygen and oxygen utilized is analogously defined:

$$\delta_{IU} = \frac{X_I - X_U}{X_I} \cdot 100 \ \%. \tag{3}$$

Since it is impossible to measure X_U, δ_{IU} cannot be determined directly from eq. (3). However, inserting eq.(3) into eq. (1) yields after some simple transformations

$$\delta_{IU} = - \delta_{IE} \cdot \frac{\dot{V}_E O_2}{\dot{V} O_2} \tag{4}$$

which has been applied to quantify the overall fractionation effect.

Analysis of Oxygen Isotope Ratios

$^{16}O^{18}O/^{16}O_2$ ratios of expiratory gas sampled in a bag were determined with a respiratory mass spectrometer which had been adapted to analyse isotopic composition in respiratory gas (Schuster et al., 1979). $^{16}O_2$ and $^{16}O^{18}O$ partial pressures were simultaneously measured on mass peaks 32 and 34 respectively. To avoid side effects and drift errors, a reference technique was applied similar to that of Schuster (1985). Briefly, dry sample gas was compared with a reference gas of natural isotopic composition composed of the same main components N_2, $^{16}O_2$, CO_2, and Ar. A comparison was made by measuring successively sample and reference for about 5 min continuously.

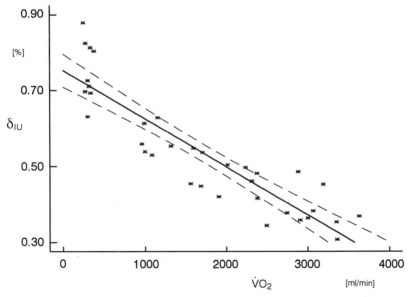

Figure 2. Regression line with 95 % confidence limits of overall fractionation effect δ_{IU} on oxygen consumption $\dot{V}O_2$.

RESULTS

6 healthy subjects were studied, three of them were capable of achieving and sustaining steady-state conditions at all performances including the highest working level (250 W). Experiments at 250 W were performed separately from all others, on a different day, measuring resting values again. Since the regression lines of overall fractionation effect δ_{IU} on oxygen consumption $\dot{V}O_2$ are not significantly different when comparing data of the transition rest-250 W with all other data, all results were summarized in fig.2. It shows δ_{IU} as a function of $\dot{V}O_2$ for all levels of activity studied. At rest, δ_{IU} amounted to 0.74 ± 0.08 %. This value denotes that uptake, subsequent transport and utilization of oxygen occurs with a relatively higher rate of 0.74 % for $^{16}O_2$ than for $^{16}O^{18}O$ under stationary resting conditions. δ_{IU} steadily decreased with increasing oxygen consumption up to the highest rate of 3600 ml/min yielding the regression line

$$\delta_{IU} \, [\%] = 0.74 - 1.3 \cdot 10^{-4} \cdot \dot{V}O_2 \; [\text{ml/min}]. \tag{5}$$

The coefficient of correlation and number of measurements are -0.90 and 35 respectively.

DISCUSSION

Comparison with Data from Literature

Two previous publications are known dealing with fractionation effects of oxygen isotopes during ergometer work, that of Pflug (1975) and that of Heller and Schuster (1990). The latter paper presents first results at an early stage of this investigation and can therefore be omitted from further discussion. The former paper measures also the overall fractionation effect. 8 humans were studied at rest and loadings of 100 W and 200 W of cycling work. Although the methods of isotope analysis and of determining the overall fractionation effect were different from those of this paper, very similar results were obtained. Mean values and standard deviations given in [%] for the situations of rest, 100 W and 200 W, amount to 0.86 ± 0.18, 0.71 ± 0.16 and 0.5 ± 0.13, calculated from the data provided by Pflug (1975). The respective numbers of the present investigation are 0.74 ± 0.08, 0.48 ± 0.06 and 0.40 ± 0.06. Although Pflug's values are slightly higher, the tendency to decrease with increasing work load is equal so that both papers confirm each other in this main point.

Linkage between Fractionation Effects and the Oxygen Transport System

For steady-state conditions, the path of oxygen from inspiratory air to tissues including utilization can be considered as an overall resistance across which the oxygen flow is driven by the total oxygen partial pressure gradient which is equal to the oxygen partial pressure of inspiratory gas. In this model, a δ_{IU}-value unequal to zero means that the overall resistance of the oxygen transport system is different for $^{16}O^{18}O$ and for $^{16}O_2$. δ_{IU} as defined according to eq. (4) can also be defined in terms of resistances as

$$\delta_{IU} = \frac{R_O{}^* - R_O}{R_O} \cdot 100 \; [\%] \tag{6}$$

where R_O^* and R_O denote the overall resistances for $^{16}O^{18}O$ and $^{16}O_2$ transport respectively. The overall resistance of oxygen transport can be considered as consisting of a cascade of resistances in series whereby these resistances may refer to the various pathways of oxygen diffusion, convection and utilization. For each single pathway, a δ-parameter can be defined similarly to eq.(6).

Fig.3 shows fractionation parameters δ on a linear scale expected according to Graham's law (Schuster and Pflug, 1989) or measured (Feldman et al., 1959) for characteristic processes of oxygen transport together with the overall effect, δ_{IU}, of this study. A δ-value of a single process contributes to the overall effect according to its resistance relative to the overall resistance of the oxygen transport system. For example, an overall δ-value of a highly diffusion limited transport system is expected to approach the δ-value of diffusion which has been calculated to be 3% (Schuster and Pflug, 1989).

Interpretation of the Results

At rest, the δ_{IU}-value is located between the δ-parameters of convection and utilization but far away from that of diffusion (fig.3). This reflects the relationships of the resistances of these 3 processes. The convective resistance of ventilation and blood flow amount to more than 50% of the overall resistance, the resistance of utilization to about 25% and that of pulmonary and tissue diffusion to 20% or less (Otis, 1987). The δ_{IU}-values decrease with increasing oxygen consumption thus moving still closer to the δ-value of convection (fig.3). This suggests that resistances of low fractionating processes such as ventilation and blood flow become even more dominant, whereas on the contrary a limitation of oxygen transport due to diffusion does not increase further up to oxygen consumption rates of 3600 ml/min. The end-expiratory oxygen partial pressures remained close to 100 mmHg during the lower performances, but they increased at the highest level of work load. This implies that hyperventilation occurred indicating that the resistance of ventilation decreased relatively. Therefore a limitation of oxygen transport brought about by convective processes as suggested by decreasing δ_{IU} can be mainly attributed to the blood flow pathway.

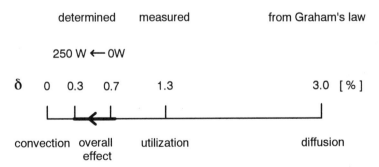

Figure 3. Fractionation parameters δ on a linear scale expected from Graham's law or measured (Feldman et al., 1959) for characteristic processes of oxygen transport. Bar on the scale: overall effect δ_{IU} determined in the present paper for loadings between 0 and 250 W.

The factors that limit oxygen transport during conditions of increased oxygen consumption have been a subject of long-standing debate, and each stage in the transport system has been supposed to be a candidate for site of limitation (Kaijser, 1970, Dempsey et al., 1984, Cerretelli and di Prampero, 1987, Hoppeler et al., 1990, Piiper, 1990, Manier et al., 1991, Piiper and Haab, 1991). It is currently proposed that the limits to whole body oxygen transport are multifactorial but that the greatest role as a limiting factor is played by the resistance of circulating blood (di Prampero and Ferretti, 1990). This is in line with the result of the present paper.

SUMMARY

The aim of the study was to assess various pathways of the oxygen transport system at rest and ergometer work by the utility of information derivable from different behaviour of the isotopic oxygen molecules $^{16}O_2$ and $^{16}O^{18}O$ during transport. 6 healthy humans were studied at rest and at different levels of ergometer work, ranging from 50 to 250 W. Isotope analysis was performed by applying a reference technique. Samples of inspiratory and expiratory gas, taken during steady state conditions, were analysed by a respiratory mass spectrometer on their $^{16}O^{18}O/^{16}O_2$ ratios by comparing them with a reference gas of appropriate composition. Ventilatory minute volume, oxygen consumption and end-expiratory oxygen partial pressure were also measured. At rest, the δ_{IU}-value quantifying the isotope effect of the overall oxygen transport amounted to 0.74 ± 0.08 %. During ergometer work, the fractionation factor steadily decreased with increasing oxygen consumption, yielding the regression line δ_{IU} [%] = 0.74 $-1.3 \cdot 10^{-4} \cdot \dot{V}O_2$, where $\dot{V}O_2$ is oxygen consumption given in ml/min. With respect to oxygen transport from inspiratory gas to tissue, this result suggests: convective processes of oxygen transport become more limiting with increasing oxygen consumption, whereas diffusion does not become a major limiting step up to oxygen consumption rates of 3600 ml/min, otherwise a reverse relationship between fractionation factor and oxygen consumption should have been found.

REFERENCES

Cerretelli,P., and di Prampero,P.E., 1987, Gas exchange in exercise, in:"Handbook of Physiology", Sect.3 The Respiratory System, Vol.IV, Gas Exchange, Chapter 16, p.297-339, Fishman,A.P., Farhi,L.E., Tenney,S.M., and Geiger,S.R., eds., American Physiological Society, Bethesda.

Dempsey,J.A.,Hanson,P.G.,and Henderson,K.S., 1984, Exercise-induced arterial hypoxaemia in healthy human subjects at sea level,J.Physiol. 355:161-175.

Feldman,D.E.,Yost jr.,H.T., and Benson,B.B.,1959, Oxygen isotope fractionation in reactions catalyzed by enzymes,Science, 129:146-147.

Heller,H., and Schuster,K.-D.,1990, Investigation of oxygen transport to tissue during rest and ergometer work by using oxygen isotopes, Pflügers Arch. 415, suppl.1, R67.

Hoppeler,H.,1990, The different relationship of VO_2max to muscle mitochondria in humans and quadrupedal animals, Respir.Physiol. 80:137-146.

Kaijser,L.,1970, Limiting factors for aerobic muscle performance, Acta Physiol. Scand.,Suppl. 346:5-96.

Manier,G.,Moinard,J.,Téchoueyres,P.,Varène,N.,and Guénard,H.,1991, Pulmonary diffusion limitation after prolonged strenuous exercise, Respir.Physiol. 83:143-154.

Otis,A.B.,1987, An overview of gas exchange, in: "Handbook of Physiology", Sect.3 The Respiratory System, Vol.IV, Gas Exchange, Chapter 1, p.1-11, Fishman,A.P., Farhi, L.E., Tenney,S.M., and Geiger,S.R., eds., American Physiological Society, Bethesda.

Pflug,K.P.,1975, Über den Mechanismus der Sauerstoffisotopen-Fraktionierung bei der Respiration des Menschen, Inaugural-Dissertation: 1-76, Technische Hochschule, Aachen.

Piiper,J.,1990,Unequal distribution of blood flow in exercising muscle of the dog, Respir. Physiol. 80:129-136.

Piiper,J., and Haab,P.,1991, Oxygen supply and uptake in tissue models with unequal distribution of blood flow and shunt, Respir.Physiol. 84:261-271.

di Prampero,P.E., and Ferretti,G.,1990, Factors limiting maximal oxygen consumption in humans, Respir.Physiol. 80:113-128.

Schuster,K.-D., Pflug,K.P., Förstel,H., and Pichotka,J.P., 1979, Adaptation of respiratory mass spectrometer to continuous recording of abundance ratios of stable oxygen isotopes, in: "Recent developments in mass spectrometry in biochemistry and medicine", 2:451-462, A.Frigerio, ed., Plenum Publishing Corp., New York.

Schuster,K.-D.,1985, Kinetics of pulmonary CO_2 transfer studied by using labeled carbon dioxide $C^{16}O^{18}O$, Respir.Physiol. 60:21-37.

Schuster, K.-D., and Pflug, K.P., 1989, The overall fractionation effect of isotopic oxygen molecules during oxygen transport and utilization in humans, Adv.Exp.Med.Biol., 248: 151-156.

DEPENDENCY OF OVERALL FRACTIONATION EFFECT OF RESPIRATION ON HEMOGLOBIN CONCENTRATION WITHIN BLOOD AT REST

H.Heller[1], K.-D.Schuster[1], and B.O. Göbel[2]

[1]Institute of Physiology, University of Bonn
[2]Medizinische Universitäts-Poliklinik Bonn
5300 Bonn 1, FRG

INTRODUCTION

In some of the pathways of respiration the oxygen molecule $^{16}O_2$ is preferentially transported to its heavier, stable isotopic species $^{16}O^{18}O$ owing to different molecular weights. Therefore a change in isotopic composition of oxygen occurs during these pathways, so that they exert a fractionation effect on oxygen transported. According to Graham's law and using the values for solubility constants of $^{16}O_2$ and $^{16}O^{18}O$ ($\beta(^{16}O_2)$ and $\beta(^{16}O^{18}O)$) as estimated by Klots and Benson (1963), it can be calculated that the diffusion rate constant should be greater for $^{16}O_2$ than for $^{16}O^{18}O$ by 3% . Feldman et al. (1959) found for reactions of the respiratory chain that $^{16}O_2$ is metabolized 1.3 % more rapidly than $^{16}O^{18}O$. Therefore O_2-diffusion and O_2-utilization are considered to be fractionating pathways unlike the convective processes ventilation and blood flow which are known to be non-fractionating (fractionation effect: 0 %). This means that respiration consists of a series of fractionating and non-fractionating processes. Moreover, those pathways which are limiting O_2-transport will contribute most to overall fractionation effect of the entire oxygen transport system. Consequently, isotopic analyses of oxygen could help to differentiate between limitations of oxygen transport caused by different pathways of respiration. These limiting pathways can be detected by comparing $^{16}O^{18}O/^{16}O_2$ ratios within oxygen before and after entire oxygen transport under varying conditions.

Previous investigations on humans have demonstrated that at rest respiration exhibits an overall fractionation effect on oxygen in which $^{16}O_2$ is transported with a 0.9 % or 0.72 % higher rate than $^{16}O^{18}O$ (Schuster and Pflug, 1989; Heller and Schuster , 1990). From above-given fractionation effects of O_2-diffusion and O_2-utilization it has been concluded that at rest oxygen transport to tissues is mostly limited by convective processes and metabolism. In order to split overall fractionation effect into contributing fractionating and non-fractionating processes, the aim of the present study is to look at the dependency of overall fractionation effect on varying hemoglobin concentrations within blood at rest. This could be important for investigating the influence of blood flow as a convective process on the entire oxygen transport system.

METHODS

Experiments were carried out on 6 patients suffering from various degrees of anemia of a variety of etiologies, and on 6 healthy humans. The test subjects breathed room air at rest in a sitting position. After a short period of breathing to attain steady state conditions, the person expired up to 40 l into a bag. Respiratory and circulatory conditions were quantified by measuring volume expired into the bag with a spirometer, period of expiration with a watch, alveolar and expiratory partial pressures of oxygen and carbon dioxide with a respiratory mass spectrometer (Varian MAT, Type M3), and heart frequency with a pulse oximeter (Dynavit Conditronic 30). Furthermore blood pictures of patients and those of healthy test subjects were obtained.

Samples from room air and expiratory gas mixture were analysed with the same respiratory mass spectrometer to determine $^{16}O^{18}O/^{16}O_2$ ratios by comparing with a reference gas of appropriate gas composition. With the aid of this method which is similar to that described by Schuster et al. (1979), isotopic analysis of $^{16}O^{18}O/^{16}O_2$ ratios can be performed directly and continuously on expired gas without combustion of oxygen to CO_2, a method which was applied in previous investigations in order to facilitate isotopic analysis of oxygen (Schuster and Pflug, 1989).

The fractionation effect between inspired (I) and expired gas (E) is given as δ_{IE}-value . With the abbreviation $X = (^{16}O^{18}O/^{16}O_2)$, δ_{IE} is defined as

$$\delta_{IE} = \frac{X_I - X_E}{X_I} 100 \quad (\%) \tag{1}.$$

According to Schuster and Pflug (1989), the overall fractionation effect of respiration δ_{IU} can be derived from eq.(1) as

$$\delta_{IU} = -\frac{\dot{V}EO_2}{\dot{V}O_2} \delta_{IE} \quad (\%) \tag{2},$$

where $\dot{V}EO_2/\dot{V}O_2$ is the ratio of expiratory oxygen flow to oxygen uptake, i.e. δ_{IU} is defined as the deviation of $^{16}O^{18}O$-abundance between inspired and utilized (U) oxygen.

To assess between day variations in accuracy of isotopic analysis, all measurements of fractionation effects were accompanied by determinations of $^{16}O^{18}O/^{16}O_2$ ratios between room air and a $^{16}O^{18}O$-enriched standard gas mixture of known isotopic composition.

RESULTS

The values of hemoglobin concentration within blood (Hb), and fractionation effects between inspired and expired gas (δ_{IE}) are listed in columns 5 and 6 of table 1. To characterize respiratory and circulatory conditions alveolar partial pressures of O_2 (PAO_2) and CO_2 ($PACO_2$) are given in columns 2 and 3, and hematocrit (HKT) in column 4 respectively. Following Könen et al. (1991), values of overall fractionation effect of respiration (δ_{IU}) are normalized referring to a constant $PAO_2 = 100$ mmHg ($\delta_{IU}{}^n$) in order to be able to disregard variations in ventilatory conditions. δ_{IU}- and $\delta_{IU}{}^n$-values are shown in columns 7 and 8 of the same table.

The relationship between normalized $\delta_{IU}{}^n$-values and hemoglobin concentration within blood is plotted in figure 1. As can be seen from table 1 and figure 1, $\delta_{IU}{}^n$ rises from 0.57 % to 0.78 % with respect to an increase in hemoglobin content from 6.6 to 17.6 g/100 ml. This increase in $\delta_{IU}{}^n$-values can be described in terms of a linear rela-

Table 1. Fractionation effects of stable, isotopic oxygen molecules during respiration due to varying levels of hemoglobin content in blood.

Subject	PAO_2 (mmHg)	$PACO_2$ (mmHg)	HKT	Hb (g/100ml)	δ_{IE} (%)	δ_{IU} (%)	$\delta_{IU}{}^n$ (%)
A	113	35	0.20	6.6	-0.15	0.67	0.57
B	112	28	0.22	7.6	-0.12	0.55	0.46
C	121	22	0.24	8.5	-0.08	0.59	0.43
D	113	32	0.24	7.9	-0.13	0.64	0.54
E	115	31	0.26	9.2	-0.13	0.68	0.56
F	117	27	0.30	10.3	-0.10	0.57	0.44
G	116	31	0.46	15.1	-0.15	0.81	0.68
H	104	37	0.45	15.2	-0.27	0.83	0.80
I	113	29	0.42	14.2	-0.15	0.68	0.58
J	82	47	0.54	17.6	-0.39	0.64	0.78
K	111	32	0.51	16.2	-0.16	0.73	0.64
L	107	35	0.46	14.8	-0.18	0.70	0.64

$\delta_{IE}, \delta_{IU}, \delta_{IU}{}^n$: differences in ${}^{16}O^{18}O$-abundances between inspired and expired oxygen, inspired and utilized oxygen, and between inspired and utilized oxygen according to a normalization of δ_{IU}-values referring to a constant $PAO_2 = 100$ mmHg. $PAO_2, PACO_2, HKT, Hb$: alveolar partial pressures of O_2 and CO_2, hematocrit, and hemoglobin concentration within blood, respectively.

tionship to Hb-values. The slope of regression line amounts to 0.024 (%100ml/g) and its intercept is 0.303 % . The correlation coefficient of n = 12 independent measurements is calculated to be r = 0.79 , and is therefore different from zero (Sachs, 1974; P < 0.01). This means that, disregarding varying ventilatory conditions, overall fractionation effect depends on hemoglobin concentration within blood in terms of

$$\delta_{IU}{}^n = 0.303 + 0.024[Hb] \quad (\%) \tag{3},$$

where [Hb] is given in g/100 ml.

Of course, similar to eq. (3), a linear relationship between $\delta_{IU}{}^n$ and hematocrit can also be obtained. No significant relationship becomes apparent between $\delta_{IU}{}^n$ and the parameters PAO_2, and $PACO_2$, and between $\delta_{IU}{}^n$ and heart frequency respectively.

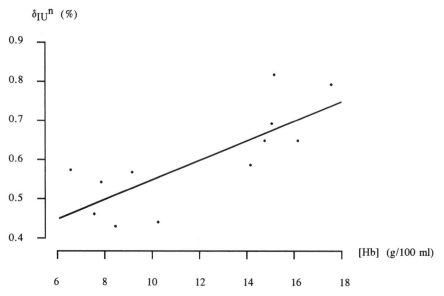

Figure 1. Linear relationship between normalized values of overall fractionation effect of respiration $\delta_{IU}{}^n$ and hemoglobin concentration within blood [Hb]: $r = 0.79$, $n = 12$.

DISCUSSION

Resistance model of respiration

First eq. (2) is based on the assumption that oxygen transport has to overcome only a single resistance placed between inspiratory gas and tissues. This single-resistance model can be enlarged by splitting the one fractionation effect of entire respiration into fractionation effects of the included pathways ventilation (δ_V), O_2-diffusion within lungs (δ_{DL}), blood flow (δ_B), O_2-diffusion within tissues (δ_{DT}), and O_2-utilization (δ_U) respectively. Each of these pathways exerts its own resistance on oxygen transport (R_V, R_{DL}, R_B, R_{DT}, R_U). Since total resistance of entire respiration (R_{IU}) is additively connected to these resistances as

$$R_{IU} = R_V + R_{DL} + R_B + R_{DT} + R_U \tag{4},$$

overall fractionation effect of respiration can be added from the fractionation effects of each pathway. In case of steady state conditions one can deduce from eq. (4) that

$$\delta_{IU} = \frac{R_V}{R_{IU}} \delta_V + \frac{R_{DL}}{R_{IU}} \delta_{DL} + \frac{R_B}{R_{IU}} \delta_B + \frac{R_{DT}}{R_{IU}} \delta_{DT} + \frac{R_U}{R_{IU}} \delta_U \tag{5},$$

where fractionation effects are weighted by the ratio of resistance according to each pathway to total resistance of respiration. Ventilation and blood flow are known to be non-fractionating, convective processes so that δ_V or δ_B are equal to zero. Therefore eq.

758

(5) can be reduced to

$$\delta_{IU} = \frac{R_{DL}}{R_{IU}} \delta_{DL} + \frac{R_{DT}}{R_{IU}} \delta_{DT} + \frac{R_U}{R_{IU}} \delta_U \qquad (6).$$

On first glance at this equation, δ_{IU} seems to be independent of δ_V or δ_B. But in the case of a limitation of oxygen transport by convective processes, R_V and R_B will increase. With eq. (4) and assuming R_{IU} to be constant under conditions of rest, for healthy test subjects as well as for anemic patients, one or more of the remaining resistances have to be diminished. This means that one or more of the remaining fractionation effects δ_{DL}, δ_{DT}, and δ_U will be weighted to a lower extent and δ_{IU} decreases.

As above mentioned δ_{IU}-values were normalized referring to a constant $PAO_2 = 100$ mmHg, the influence of varying resistance of ventilation was excluded, so that R_V can be considered to be constant. This suggests that a drop in δ_{IU}^n-values is caused mostly by a rise in R_B when hemoglobin concentration within blood decreases. From Ohm's law and Fick's principle it can be derived that R_B is indeed in inverse proportion to [Hb] as

$$R_B \sim \frac{1}{SO_2 \, [Hb] \, \dot{Q}} \qquad (7),$$

where SO_2 is the oxygen saturation within blood and $\dot{Q}$ is the cardiac output.

Interpretation of data

In chronic anemia and with regard to Fick's principle, two different mechanisms are known to compensate reduced O_2-carrying capacity of anemic blood: increased cardiac output and enhanced oxygen release from blood to tissues, leading to a rise in difference of O_2-concentration in arterial and venous blood ($avDO_2$). The latter mechanism would be synonymous with an increase in R_B, because, applying Ohm's law again, the more $avDO_2$ or partial pressure difference of oxygen (PO_{2B}) rose the greater the resistance of blood flow had to increase:

$$R_B \sim PO_{2B} \qquad (8).$$

Since heart frequency observed in patients (96.6 min^{-1}) was significantly greater than heart frequency of healthy test subjects (84,7 min^{-1}) (Sachs,1974; $P < 0.025$), an enlarged cardiac output can be assumed. But nevertheless δ_{IU}^n is diminished in anemic patients. With regard to eq. (7) and eq. (8), the question arises as to which size in severity of anemia a drop in hemoglobin concentration can be compensated by which size of increase in cardiac output. From the increased heart frequency and decrease of δ_{IU}^n-values in anemic patients one can conclude that either the rise in cardiac output was not sufficient to compensate anemia or both mechanisms contributed to compensation leading altogether to an increase in blood flow resistance (see eq. (7) and (8)).

From the clinician's point of view anemia is not associated with dyspnea, tachycardia, and other cardiovascular symptoms until hemoglobin concentration declines 7 to 8 g/100 ml (Begemann, 1986; Rossi, 1991; Simon, 1991). Above this range of hemoglobin content within blood, regulatory mechanisms and effects of chronic anemia such as a rise in levels of 2,3-diphosphoglycerat (2,3-DPG) content of red blood cells, decrease in viscosity of anemic blood and redistribution of blood flow to oxygen-dependent tissues, respectively should be able to avoid anemic symptoms. Below the range of 7 to

8 g/100 ml these mechanisms are not considered to be able to compensate reduction in O_2-carrying capacity of anemic blood, and cardiac output therefore has to increase.

All $\delta_{IU}{}^n$-values of anemic patients are lower than those of healthy test subjects. This suggests that in anemia oxygen transport to tissues is limited by perfusion, despite redistribution of blood flow, rise in 2,3-DPG content of red blood cells, and an increase in cardiac output, respectively. This limitation starts to influence entire oxygen transport above a hemoglobin concentration of 8 g/100 ml. A correlation coefficient amounting to 0.79 points to a high mean variation of $\delta_{IU}{}^n$-values estimated, which suggests that with respect to eq. (5) there are still remaining regulatory mechanisms influencing δ_{IU} and these may differ from person to person.

SUMMARY

In this study it was investigated in which way varying hemoglobin concentrations within blood influence overall fractionation effect of respiration, meaning a change in composition of isotopic oxygen molecules $^{16}O_2$ and $^{16}O^{18}O$ within oxygen transported during entire respiration. Since overall fractionation effect of respiration is known to consist of different fractionating and non-fractionating processes, measuring it under condition of anemia could be useful in relating changes in isotopic compositions of oxygen to limitations of entire oxygen transport caused by one or more of these processes. Experiments were performed on 6 patients suffering from various degrees of anemia of a variety of etiologies and on 6 healthy humans. All test subjects breathed air at rest. Samples from inspiratory and expiratory gas were taken in order to analyse $^{16}O^{18}O/^{16}O_2$ ratios with the aid of respiratory mass spectrometry. Values of overall fractionation effect decreased with respect to a drop in hemoglobin concentration from 17.6 to 6.6 g/100 ml in terms of a linear relationship (r=0.79) provided that values of overall fractionation effect were normalized so as to exclude the influence of varying ventilatory conditions. It could be shown that at a value of hemoglobin content of 6.6 g/100 ml, $^{16}O_2$ was transported in preference to $^{16}O^{18}O$ with a 0.57 % higher rate compared to a value of 0.78 % obtained at a hemoglobin concentration of 17.6 g/100 ml. From these results together with a resistance model of respiration it is concluded: In anemic patients oxygen transport to tissues is more limited by perfusion than in healthy subjects. In contrast to the clinician's point of view, this limitation starts to influence entire oxygen transport above a hemoglobin concentration of 8 g/100 ml. But the low correlation coefficient points out that there are still remaining processes within respiration despite ventilation and perfusion which influence overall fractionation effect.

REFERENCES

Begemann, H., 1986, Anämien, in:" Klinische Hämatologie", pp.216-218, Begemann,H. und Rastetter,J.,eds., Thieme, Stuttgart, New York.

Feldman,D.E., Yost,jr.,H.T., and Benson,B.B.,1959, Oxygen isotope fractionation in reactions catalyzed by enzymes, Science,129:146-147.

Heller,H., and Schuster,K.-D., 1990, Investigation of oxygen transport to tissues during rest and ergometer work by using oxygen isotopes, Pflügers Arch.,415,suppl.1:R67.

Klots,C.E., and Benson,B.B., 1963, Isotope effect in the solution of oxygen and nitrogen in distilled water, J.Chem.Phys., 38:890-892.

Könen,M., Heller,H., and Schuster,K.-D., 1991, Influence of ventilation on transport of isotopic oxygen molecules to tissues at rest, Pflügers Arch. 419, suppl.1:R117.

Rossi,E.C., 1991, Pathophysiology of anemia, in:"Principles of transfusion medicine", pp.91-93, Rossi,E.C., Simon,T.L., and Moss,G.S., eds., Williams & Wilkins, Baltimore, Hong Kong, London, Munich, San Franciscio, Sydney, Tokyo.

Sachs,L., 1974,"Angewandte Statistik", p.212, p.329, Springer, Berlin.

Schuster,K.-D., Pflug,K.P., Förstel,H., and Pichotka,J.P., 1979, Adaptation of respiratory mass spectrometer to continuous recording of abundance ratios of stable oxygen isotopes, in:"Recent developments in mass spectrometry in biochemistry and medicine", 2:451-462, A.Frigerio, ed., Plenum Publishing Corp., New York.

Schuster,K.-D., and Pflug,K.P.,1989, The overall fractionation effect of isotopic oxygen molecules during oxygen transport and utilization in humans, Adv.Exp.Med.Biol.,248: 151-156.

Simon,T.L., 1991, Red cell transfusion, in:"Principles of transfusion medicine", pp.95-98, Rossi,E.C.,Simon,T.L., and Moss,G.S., eds., Williams & Wilkins, Baltimore, Hong Kong, London, Munich,San Franciscio, Sydney, Tokyo.

MEASURED AND PREDICTED VALUES OF OXYGEN CONSUMPTION DURING ISOFLURANE ANESTHESIA IN MAN

Luigi S. Brandi [1], Francesco Giunta [2], Marco Oleggini [3], Tommaso Mazzanti [3], and Nicoletta Fossati [3]

[1] Researcher in Anesthesiology and Intensive Care
[2] Associate Professor in Anesthesiology and Intensive Care
[3] Staff Anesthesiologist
Department of Anesthesiology and Intensive Care, University of Pisa, Italy

INTRODUCTION

Continuous oxygen consumption monitoring during inhalation anesthesia can be done by metabolic gas exchange measurements (indirect calorimetry). This method requires meticulous attention to technique, and many factors limit its usefulness in daily clinical practice. During inhalation anesthesia, the major limiting factor is the presence of exhaled anesthetic agents [1]. Different systems and solutions have been proposed to obtain accurate and precise measurement of oxygen consumption during inhalation anesthesia [2]. However, these systems are complex in use and dear (*e.g.,* mass spectrometry) to be taken in account in daily clinical practice. With the recent progress in the development of closed circuit anesthesia systems, it has become possible to practice inhalation anesthesia together with on line registration of oxygen consumption [3]. This measurement has been improving our ability to study various pathophysiological problems during anesthesia and operation [3]. In a totally closed circuit system the rate of oxygen delivery is determined by the rate of oxygen consumption by the patient. The system measures the end-expiratory anesthetic circuit volume and oxygen concentration and adjusts the oxygen flow to maintain a constant circuit volume. According to a simple physical principle (conservation of mass), the rate of mass flowing into a system (patient) normally must equal the rate of mass flowing from the system

Oxygen Transport to Tissue XV, Edited by P. Vaupel
et al., Plenum Press, New York, 1994

(patient). If these rates are not equal, then the difference between the two must be accounted by either accumulation or reaction. For oxygen, the difference between the inhaled mass flow and exhaled mass flow, represents oxygen consumption.

At basal conditions (basal metabolic rate) oxygen consumption in mammals of all size, from mice to elephants, is estimated according to Brody and Kleiber's equations. In humans, the values of oxygen consumption estimated by these equations are similar to the values measured by indirect calorimetry in normal subjects at rest [4,5].

Data regarding oxygen consumption during anesthesia are still contradictory. Anesthesia is said to decrease whole-body oxygen consumption, but the magnitude of this effect is still in doubt. In animal models, whole-body oxygen consumption during anesthesia is as high as or higher than the basal metabolic rate [6]. Theye and Michenfelder observe in dogs that the decrease in whole-body oxygen consumption with anesthetic agents (*e.g.*, halotane, enflurane, and isoflurane) is a summation of events in individual organs in which an anesthetic-induced change in function resulted in a change in metabolic requirements [7]. In man, even with different measurement techniques, general anesthesia is associated with a decrease in whole-body oxygen consumption by 7 to 40% of the measured or estimated basal values [7,8,9,10,11,12,13,14,15,16]. Recently, the intraoperative decrease in oxygen consumption has been attributed to inadequate oxygen delivery than to decreased metabolic demand [17], and the intraoperative oxygen debt has been correlated with the incidence of postoperative organ failure [18].

The aims of this study were: 1) to compare, during isoflurane anesthesia, the oxygen consumption as measured by the totally closed circuit system with the theoretical values as estimated by the Brody and Kleiber's equations 2) to test the hypothesis that reduced intraoperative oxygen consumption might not reflect inadequate tissue oxygenation.

PATIENTS AND METHODS

Sixty-four patients (37 males, 27 females; ASA I-II) who underwent major elective abdominal surgery (time course between 60-480 minutes) were selected for the study. Before the enrollment into the study, a complete medical and laboratory work-up was carried out to exclude the presence of significant cardiovascular, respiratory, renal or endocrine disease. Their mean age was 57.8 ± 16 years (range 19-85), body weight was 69 ± 13 kg. Morphine (0.1 mg/kg) and atropine (0.01 mg/kg) were given by intramuscular injection one hour before surgery. Anesthesia was induced with fentanyl (3 μg/kg), thiopental (4 mg/kg), pancuronium bromide (0.1 mg/kg). After endotracheal intubation with a cuffed tube, the lungs of patients were artificially ventilated, and anesthesia was maintained with isoflurane (end tidal 0.5-0.8 %), and $N_2O:O_2$ mixture (40:60). During the intraoperative period patients received a fix amount (5 ml/kg/h) of saline intravenously and blood or colloid when required. No complications were observed during the anesthesia. Throughout the study, core temperature, heart rate, and arterial pressure were measured continuously. The end-tidal carbon dioxide concentration was maintained at 4.0-4.5 %

In five of these patients, oxygen consumption was also measured by the Fick principle, using the thermodilution technique, every 30 minutes throughout the intraoperative period. Each of these patients was monitored using a 7 Fr, flow-directed thermistor-tip catheter, and an indwelling radial artery catheter. Cardiac output was determined by standard thermodilution technique and cardiac computer. Injections of 10 mL of a room-temperature (21 to 24 °C) solution of 5% dextrose in water were used. Injection times were always < 4 sec, thus eliminating possible effects of varying injection rates on calculations. The value of cardiac output used for the calculation of oxygen consumption, was the average of three serial measurements obtained within 2 to 3 mins, providing that the intermeasurement variance was < 10%. If variance was >10%, two additional measurements were made, and high and low values rejected. Immediately after cardiac output measurement, arterial and mixed venous blood samples were obtained simultaneously from the catheter in the radial and from the distal port of the pulmonary artery catheter. Blood gases were measured immediately by an automated blood gas laboratory (IL System 1312 Instrumentation Laboratory, Lexington, Ma, USA). Hemoglobin concentration and oxyhemoglobin saturation were measured directly using a cooximeter (IL 282 Instrumentation Laboratory). From these values we derived values for arterial and mixed venous oxygen content (CaO_2 and CvO_2) and $C(a-v)O_2$ as follows:

$$CaO_2 = (1.39 * Hgb * SaO_2) + 0.0031 * PaO_2$$

$$CvO_2 = (1.39 * Hgb * SvO_2) + 0.0031 * PvO_2$$

$$C(a-v)O_2 = CaO_2 - CvO_2$$

in which Hgb (g/dL) is the hemoglobin concentration, SaO_2 and SvO_2 (%) the arterial and mixed venous oxygen saturation, and PaO_2 PvO_2 (torr) the arterial and mixed venous oxygen tension, respectively, 1.39 is the amount of oxygen/g Hgb, and $(0.0031) * (PO_2)$ is the amount of oxygen dissolved in plasma. Oxygen consumption (VO_2) was measured as:

$$VO_2 = CO * (CaO_2 - CvO_2)$$

Using the totally closed circuit system, oxygen consumption was measured continuously. At the onset of cardiac output measurement, five minutes of consecutive measurements of oxygen consumption were averaged and used for the comparison with the thermodilution technique.

In other ten patients, arterial blood samples were obtained at timed-intervals (time 0, 30, 60, 90, 120, 150, End) for determination of blood glucose, lactate, pyruvate, and alanine concentrations. Their mean age was 58 ± 6 years, body weight was 72.6 ± 11 kg. In two and in one of these patients we did not obtain the measures of pyruvate and alanine, respectively.

In all cases the anesthetic equipment consisted of a totally closed circuit anesthesia ventilator (Physioflex, Physio BV Medical System, Hoksteen, The Netherlands). In this system the gas is moved unidirectionally around by a blower at about 70 L/min. In the system four membrane chambers are integrated for ventilation. Besides end-expiratory feed back control of inhalation anesthetics, and inspiratory closed loop control of oxygen, the system offers on-line registration of oxygen consumption, flow, volume and respiratory pressures as well as a capnogram [3]. For each patient, the total intraoperative oxygen consumption was expressed as the mean of the measures obtained every minute by the totally closed circuit system during surgical procedure. The theoretical intraoperative values of oxygen consumption were also estimated according to the Brody and Kleiber's equations ($VO_2 = 10.15 * kg^{0.73}$, and $VO_2 = 10 * [0.3BW + 3]$, respectively). For substrates determination, arterial blood was drawn into chilled tubes containing 1 N perchloric acid, and immediately centrifugated.The deproteinized supernatants were stored at -20 °C until analysis. Glucose, lactate, pyruvate, and alanine were all assayed by enzymatic methods by an automated spectrophotometric method (ERIS Analyzer 6170, Eppendorf Gratebau, Hamburg, Germany).

All data are expressed as Mean $\pm$ SD. Paired t test analysis was used to compare mean group values. Analysis of variance (ANOVA) with repeated measures over time was used as appropriate. Linear regression was calculated with standard methods. A $p < 0.05$ was considered statistically significant.

RESULTS

Under the condition of this study, oxygen consumption measured by using the totally closed circuit system was 144 ± 28 mL/min. When oxygen consumption was estimated using Brody and Kleiber's equations, the corresponding values were 223 ± 30 mL/min and 237 ± 38 mL/min, respectively ($p < 0.001$). Therefore, during isoflurane anesthesia the measured oxygen consumption was 34 ± 9 % (range 10-49 %) lower than the values estimated by the traditional equations (Fig. 1). A linear relationship was observed between oxygen consumption estimated by the Brody's equation and oxygen consumption measured by the totally closed circuit system during isoflurane anesthesia (Fig. 2). There was a progressive deviation of measured oxygen consumption from oxygen consumption estimated by the Brody's formula for patients with increasing body weight.

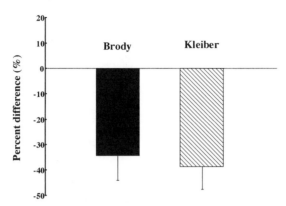

Figure 1. Percent differences between oxygen consumption as measured by the totally closed circuit system and by the Brody and Kleiber's equations in 64 patients during isoflurane anesthesia.

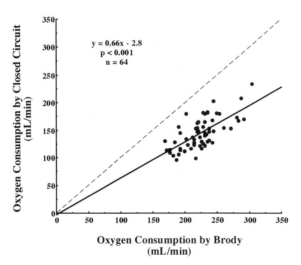

Figure 2. Relation between oxygen consumption as measured by the Brody's equation and the totally closed circuit system in 64 patients during isoflurane anesthesia. The *dotted line* is the identity line.

In five patients, mean oxygen consumption measured by the Fick method was 73.9 ± 13 mL/min/m² (1.8 ± 0.42 mL/min/kg), while mean oxygen consumption measured by the totally closed circuit system was 68.4 ± 8 mL/min/m² (1.69 ± 0.18 mL/min/kg). The mean difference between the two methods was 5.6 ± 16 mL/min/m² (0.14 ± 0.41 mL/min/kg) (0.1> p < 0.05) (Fig. 3).

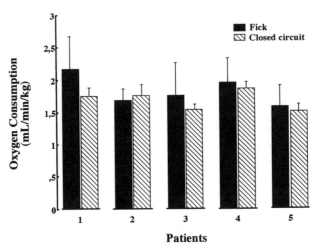

Figure 3. Mean values of oxygen consumption as measured by the totally closed circuit system and by the Fick method in five patients during isoflurane anesthesia.

Arterial substrate concentrations, plasma glucose levels, and lactate/pyruvate ratio are shown in Table I. A progressive increase of arterial lactate (p < 0.001), pyruvate (p < 0.01), and glucose (p < 0.01) was observed during the study. No significant variation was observed in alanine. There was a strong significant relationship between lactate and pyruvate (R² = 0.88, p < 0.001). Therefore, the lactate/pyruvate ratio did not change during the time-course of the study (p NS). Besides, significant relationships between lactate, pyruvate, and glucose (R² = 0.54, p < 0.001, and R² = 0.37, p < 0.01, respectively) and between lactate and alanine (R² = 0.45, p < 0.001), were observed. In these patients, oxygen consumption measured by the totally closed circuit system did not significantly change over time (131.1 ± 21.9 mL/min at baseline, and 132.6 ± 22.7 mL/min at the end of the study, p NS). Again, these values of oxygen consumption were 57 ± 7 % (range 45-74 %) of the theoretical values estimated from Brody's equation (p < 0.001). For all measurements, no significant relationship was observed neither between absolute values of arterial lactate and intraoperative oxygen consumption, nor between the respective time-related absolute or percent variations (Fig 4). Mean intraoperative reduction in body temperature was 1.6 ± 0.8 °C (range 0.6-3.2 °C).

Table 1. Arterial substrates concentrations, plasma glucose levels, and lactate/pyruvate ratio in ten patients during isoflurane anesthesia [1]

Time (Min)	Lactate (mmol/L)	Pyruvate (μmol/L)	Alanine (μmol/L)	Glucose (mmol/L)	L/P
0	1.04 ± 0.5	67 ± 29	314 ± 74	8.7 ± 1.1	19 ± 1.0
30	1.09 ± 0.6	71 ± 21	309 ± 77	9.8 ± 1.6	16 ± 0.5
60	1.29 ± 0.7	99 ± 74	318 ± 74	10.6 ± 2.1	16 ± 0.5
90	1.45 ± 0.9	107 ± 81	322 ± 91	10.7 ± 1.8	16 ± 0.4
120	1.73 ± 1.2	134 ± 102	345 ± 117	11.5 ± 2.3	17 ± 0.5
150	1.84 ± 1.2	149 ± 106	349 ± 119	12.2 ± 2.5	16 ± 0.4
End	2.18 ± 1.6	169 ± 133	363 ± 147	12.6 ± 2.3	17 ± 0.6

[1] *Time 0* is immediately after induction of anesthesia; *Time End* is after skin closure. LP, lactate/pyruvate ratio.

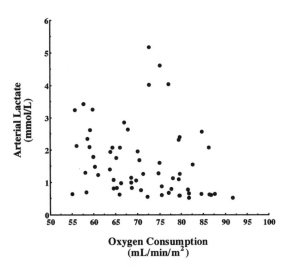

Figure 4. Relation between oxygen consumption as measured by the totally closed circuit system and lactate levels (n = 70) during isoflurane anesthesia in ten patients.

DISCUSSION

At present time, the new developments in totally closed circuit anesthesia and ventilation offer one line registration of oxygen consumption and avoid the intraoperative use of other invasive, non invasive and expensive techniques. First, our data show that during isoflurane anesthesia, oxygen consumption measured by a totally closed circuit system is 35 % lower than the expected value calculated according to the Brody and Kleiber's equations. This reduction in oxygen consumption cannot be explained solely by the reduction in body temperature occurring during anesthesia. It is known that 1 °C decrease in body temperature induces a 5-7 % decrease in oxygen consumption [19]. In our patients we observed a mean decrease of 1.6 °C in body temperature that corresponds to a mean decrease in oxygen consumption of about 7-10 %. Besides, mechanical ventilation and neuromuscular blockade also contribute to the decrease in oxygen consumption during anesthesia, probably by decreasing the work and hence the oxygen consumption of the respiratory muscles. In normal subjects the oxygen cost of breathing amounts to 0.5-1 mL of oxygen consumed by the respiratory muscles per litre of minute ventilation [20,21]. If this assumption is correct, in our patients, the oxygen cost of breathing was about 7 mL/min of oxygen. Mechanical ventilation, therefore, contributed a mere 3-4 % of the overall decrease in oxygen consumption during anesthesia. Therefore, the effect of the hypothermia and muscle paralysis cannot explain all the decrease in oxygen consumption observed in our patients during inhalation anesthesia. Experimental studies in animals [7] pointed out that anesthetic agents (e.g., isoflurane) cause a decrease in whole-body oxygen consumption that represents a summation of events in individual organs in which an anesthetic-induced change in function results in a change in metabolic requirements. While decreased oxygen consumption during operation in man has been previously recognized [8,9,10,11,12,13,14,15], it has usually been attributed to decreased metabolic demand caused by anesthetic agents and hypothermia. But, a recent study suggests that the reduced oxygen consumption during operations may reflect inadequate tissue oxygenation [17]. These Authors observed a strong relationship between the mean intraoperative oxygen consumption and lactate concentrations, suggesting a condition of oxygen deficit and anaerobic metabolism. More recently, Shoemaker and co-workers [18] reported that the intraoperative decrease in oxygen consumption and the calculated oxygen debt correlated with the development of postoperative complications and organs failure. In our subgroup of ten patients, we found no relationship between intraoperative oxygen consumption and lactate concentrations. Possibly, our patients' group cannot be compared with the Waxman's group, which included critically ill surgical patients with severe preoperative complications and with (35%) hepatic dysfunction, a well known condition that can influence significantly lactate metabolism [22]. In Waxman's study, intraoperative lactate levels were fivefold higher than preoperative levels, while in our study intraoperative lactate levels were only doubled at the end of the study, compared with the basal (time 0) levels. Possibly, an oxygen deficit could be present in our group of patients, as the lactate/pyruvate ratio was higher than normal [23] but did not change significantly over time. Blood lactate levels are thought to primarily reflect the imbalance between oxygen demand and oxygen supply. However, the involved metabolic process can be complex, as increased lactate production by aerobic pathways can occurs. Moreover, lactate levels can be influenced not only by an increased production through the anaerobic glycolitic pathway, but also by an alteration in the clearance mechanisms (by skeletal muscle, liver, and myocardium) [24] that could contribute to the maintenance of higher blood lactate levels. Anesthetic agents can interfere with lactate metabolism by altering blood flow to the liver [25], which is the most important organ in lactate clearance.

Second, we observed a significant increase in plasma glucose, lactate and pyruvate over time during the intraoperative period. The hyperglycemia we observed in our patients is the consequence of an altered glucose metabolism caused by isoflurane anesthesia [26]. It is known that isoflurane anesthesia decreases insulin mediated glucose utilization at peripheral tissues [26,27]. Besides, isoflurane anesthesia induces an increase in hepatic glucose, lactate, and pyruvate production, through an increase in plasma epinephrine, a well-known activator of glicogenolisys and glycolisys [27]. On the basis of such data it appears likely that the release of cathecolamines is a contributory factor which may in part explain some of the changes in lactate and pyruvate observed in the present series during isoflurane anesthesia. This is supported by the observation that the intravenous administration of epinephrine in normal human subjects is associated with an increase in lactate and pyruvate [28]. The increase in lactate levels due to epinephrine administration is due to two factors. One is an increase in anaerobic glucose metabolism with an excess of lactate production. The other is an increase in aerobic glucose metabolism with an increase in pyruvate and a proportionate increase in lactate. Therefore, the increased intraoperative lactate levels obseved in our patients could be explained not only by a condition of oxygen debt, but also by different mechanisms that involve either production or utilization.

We conclude that Brody and Kleiber's equations do not reflect the actual oxygen consumption during isoflurane anesthesia, and that lactate concentrations do not correlate with measured intraoperative oxygen consumption. Therefore, in this study, whole body oxygen consumption markedly decreased during anesthesia most likely because of decreased tissue metabolic requirements. It is important to underline that the significance of intraoperative lactate determination may be misinterpreted, especially when used for assessing the imbalance between oxygen demand and oxygen supply during isoflurane anesthesia.

REFERENCES

1. S.J. Aukburg , R.T. Geer, H. Wollman, G.R. Neufeld, Errors in measurements of oxygen uptake due to anesthetic gases, Anesthesiology. 62:54 (1984).

2. K.L. Svensson, H.G.Sonander, O. Stenquist, Validation of a system for measurement of metabolic gas exchange during anesthesia with controlled ventilation in an oxygen consumption lung model, Brit J Anaesth. 64:311 (1990).

3. A.P. K. Verkaaik, V. Erdman, Respiratory diagnostic possibilities during closed circuit anesthesia., Acta Anaesth Belgica. 41:178 (1990).

4. L.S. Brandi, M. Oleggini, S. Lachi, M. Frediani, S. Bevilacqua, F. Mosca, E. Ferrannini, Energy metabolism of surgical patients in the early postoperative period; a reappraisal, Crit Care Med. 16:18 (1988).

5. L.S. Brandi, A. De Vitis, T. Mazzanti, F. Giunta: Il consumo ed il trasporto di ossigeno in terapia intensiva ed in anestesia, in: "Anestesia a bassi flussi e a circuito chiuso", F. Giunta, ed., Piccin Editore, Padova (1991).

6. M. Mikat, J. Peters, M. Zindler, J. Ardnt, Whole body oxygen consumption in awake, sleeping, and anesthetized dogs, Anesthesiology. 60:220 (1984).

7. R.A. Theye, J.D. Michenflender, Whole-body and organ VO_2 changes with enflurane, isoflurane, and halotane, Brit J Anaesth. 47:813 (1975).

8. J.F. Nunn, R.L. Matthews R.A., Gaseous exchange during halotane anaesthesia: the steady respiratory state, Brit J Anaesth. 31:330 (1959).

9. R.A. Theye: Thiopental and oxygen consumption, Anesth Analg; 49:69 (1970).

10. R.A. Theye, G.R.Tuohy; Consideration in the determination of oxygen uptake and ventilatory performance during methoxyfluorane anesthesia in man, Anesth Analg. 43:306 (1978).

11. R. Calverley, T.Y. Smith, C.W. Jones, C. Pry-Roberts, E.I. Eger, Ventilatory and cardiovascular effect of enflurane anesthesia during spontaneous ventilation in man, Anesth Analg. 57:610 (1978).

12. E.I. Eger, T.Y. Smith, R.K. Stoelting, D.J. Cullen, L.B. Kadis, C.E. Whitcher, Cardiovascular effects of halotane in man, Anesthesiology. 32:396 (1970).

13. W.C. Stevens, T.H. Cromwell, M.J. Halsey, E.I Eger, T.F. Shakespeare, S.H. Boniemar, The cardiovascular effects of a new inhalation anesthetic, Forane in human volunteers at constant arterial carbon dioxide tension, Anesthesiology; 35:8 (1971).

14. S. Gregoretti, S. Gelman, A. Dimick, E.L Bradley, Hemodynamic changes and oxygen consumption in burned patients during enflurane or isoflurane anesthesia, Anesth Analg. 69:431 (1989).

15. J.P. Viale G.J. Annat, S.M. Tissot, J.P. Hoen, E.M. Butin, O.J. Bertrand, J.P. Motin, Mass spectrometric measurements of oxygen uptake during epidural analgesia combined with general anesthesia, Anesth Analg. 70:89 (1990).

16. D. Benhamou, J.M. Desmonts, La consommation d'oxygen per et postanesthesique, Ann Fr Anest Reanim. 3:205 (1984).

17. K. Waxman, L.S. Nolan, W.C. Shoemaker: Sequential perioperative lactate determination. Physiological and clinical implication, Crit Care Med. 10:96 (1982).

18. W.C. Shoemaker, P.L. Apple, H.B. Kram, Tissue oxygen debt as a determinant of lethal and non lethal postoperative organ failure, Crit Care Med. 16:418 (1988).

19. A. Holdcroft, "Body temperature control in anaesthesia, surgery and intensive care", Ballier Tindall,London (1980).

20. K.J. Christensen, A.P. Andersen, S. Jorgensen, Energy expenditure on breathing during anaesthesia; Acta Anaesth Scand. 29:280 (1980).

21. J.F. Nunn: "Applied respiratory physiology", Butterworth, London (1987).

22. P.L. Almenoff, J. Levy, M.H. Weil, N.B. Goldberg, D. Vega, E.C Rackow, Prolongation of the half-life of lactate after maximal exercise in patients with hepatic dysfunction, Crit Care Med. 17:870 (1989).

23. B.A. Mizock, Controversies in lactic acidosis. Implications in critically ill patients, JAMA. 258:497 (1987).

24. S.E. Buchatler,M.R. Crain, R. Kreisberg, Regulation of lactate metabolism in vivo, Diabet Metab Rev. 5:379 (1989).

25. S. Gelman, K.C. Flower, L.R. Smith, regional blood flow during isoflurane and halotane anesthesia, Anesth Analg. 63:557 (1984).

26. M. Diltoer, F. Camu, Glucose homoeostasis and insulin secretion during isoflurane anesthesia in humans, Anesthesiology. 68:880 (1988).

27. F.F. Horber, S. Krayer, J Miles, P. Cryer, K. Rehder, M.W. Haymond, Isoflurane and whole body leucine glucose, and fatty acid metabolism in dogs, Anesthesiology. 73:82 (1990).

28. Green NM, Effects of epinephrine on lactate, pyruvate, and excess lactate production in normal human subjects, J Lab Clin Med. 58:682 (1961).

COMBINED EPIDURAL AND GENERAL ANESTHESIA PREVENTS EXCESSIVE OXYGEN CONSUMPTION POSTOPERATIVELY

Wolfgang Heinrichs und Norbert Weiler

Department of Anesthesiology
Johannes Gutenberg-University, Medical School
Langenbeckstr. 1, D-W-6500 Mainz

INTRODUCTION

In the postoperative period patients are at risk of excessive oxygen consumption (VO_2). However, patients suffering from cardiovascular disease may be unable to increase their oxygen transport capacity sufficiently and may be especially vulnerable to tissue hypoxia as part of the reaction to intraoperative stress. During the last 10 years contradictory results concerning the benefits of a combined epidural and light general anesthesia have been published. Some of the results indicate that postoperative catabolism may be depressed and that the neuroendocrine response to stress may be inhibited by such a combined technique[1,2]. We studied the effect of a combined epidural and light general anesthesia on VO_2 in the early postoperative period.

METHODS

Three groups of patients were studied: Group I included 10 patients scheduled for major urological procedures of at least 3 hours duration who received a combined epidural and light general anesthesia. Group II contained 17 patients with procedures comparable to group I but who received a standard general anesthesia with isoflurane, N_2O and fentanyl. In addition 13 patients undergoing minor urological procedures of less than 2 hours duration and undergoing standard general anesthesia were included in the study as a control group (Group III). All patients gave informed consent. Preoperative management was the same in the 3 groups. Assessment of perioperative risk was performed according to the ASA-classification. There was no difference between Groups I and II. Group III contained more patients who were classified into ASA grades 1 and 2. Muscle relaxation was performed with vecuronium in all patients. In Group I patients, an epidural catheter was placed preoperatively at L3/L4 interspace and tested for correct positionning using 4 ml of 2% mepivacaine with epinephrine 1:200,000.

After induction of anesthesia epidural block was established with 0.5% bupivacaine for intraoperative analgesia and 0.25% bupivacaine for postoperative pain relief. The initial dosage was determined (according to Bromage's method) to reach a sensory level of T6. Two thirds of the initial dosage was then given at further 90 minutes intervals. End-tidal isoflurane concentrations ranged between 0.3 and 0.6Vol% in this group. In Groups II and III, end-tidal isoflurane concentrations of 1.0 to 1.5 were applied. Postoperative analgesia was achieved in these groups using repeated iv doses of 7.5 mg piritramide.

Oxygen consumption was measured in the recovery room using the Deltatrac^R (Datex) metabolic monitor. Measurements were performed with a canopy room air dilution technique. Arterial oxygen saturation of the patients was monitored continuously using pulse oximetry. Patients who were unable to breath room air in the early postoperative period were not enter into the study. Data acquisition was started within 10 minutes of extubation and continued for at least 60 minutes until a steady state of oxygen consumption was reached. We recorded the average VO_2 during the initial 5 minutes of the measurement period and during another 5-minute period after the steady state was reached (45-60 min after extubation).

RESULTS

Patients in the 3 groups were comparable in age, height and body weight (table 1). Duration of procedures in group I and II ranged between 4 and 7 hours. Group I and II were further comparable in terms of intraabdominal procedures, intraoperative blood loss, fluid replacement, and fall in body temperature during the operation.

Table 1. Patient Data

Group	I	II	III
Age (Years)	59 (16)	47 (16)	53 (16)
Height (cm)	173 (4)	172 (8)	173 (10)
Weight (kg)	76 (8)	76 (15)	77 (14)

Standard deviation in brackets

Figures 1-3 show the typical course of oxygen consumption and carbon dioxide production (VCO_2)in patients of Groups I, II and III. The readings in the Group I patient are stable throughout the observation period. Oxygen consumption is in the physiological range. In contrast, in the Group II patient during the early postoperative periode, largely increased values of oxygen consumption and carbon dioxide production are found. The increased values of VO_2 and VCO_2 return to normal within 30 minutes. In the Group III patient VO_2 and VCO_2 values are within the normal range throughout the whole measuring period.

In Figure 4 mean values and standard deviations of oxygen consumption are given for all patients in relation to their body weight. Group II patients showed a markedly increased VO_2 within the first 5 minutes of the measurement period. Compared to Groups I and III the differences were highly significant. 45-60 minutes later, during the steady state the excessively high values of VO_2 had disappeared and no further difference could be found between the 3 groups.

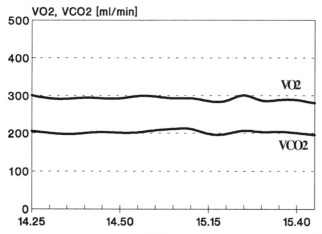

Figure 1. Typical course of oxygen consumption (VO$_2$) and carbon dioxide production (VCO$_2$) in a patient of Group I.

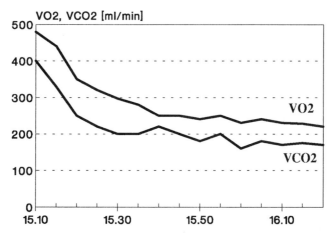

Figure 2. Typical course of oxygen consumption (VO$_2$) and carbon dioxide production (VCO$_2$) in a patient of Group II.

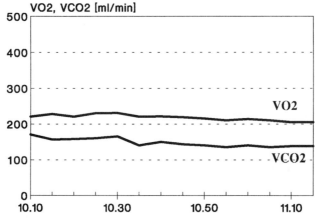

Figure 3. Typical course of oxygen consumption (VO$_2$) and carbon dioxide production (VCO$_2$) in a patient of Group III.

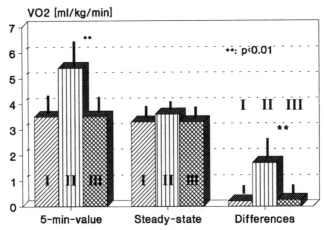

Fig. 4. Mean values and standard deviations of oxygen consumption during the initial measurement periode (5-min-value) and steady state.

DISCUSSION

During the past 10 years several studies have compared combined epidural and light general anesthesia with conventional anesthesiological techniques. The results of these studies are controversial. Authors who found the combination doubtful suggested that cardiovascular instability may arise from the synergy of epidural sympathetic block on the one hand and with cardiovascular depression due to general anesthesia on the other hand[3,4,5,6,7,8]. In contrast, those who came out in support of a combined epidural and general anesthesia found a faster return to normal in gut function, a satisfactory postoperative analgesia, a lower stress response, and a reduction in overall postoperative complications[1,2]. The latter factors may have contributed to the reduction in oxygen consumption in our Group I patients.

Our results demonstrate that a combined technique of general and epidural anesthesia prevents excessive oxygen consumption postoperatively. Patients suffering from cardiovascular disease who may not be able to increase their oxygen transport capacity sufficiently (therefore developing tissue hypoxia postoperatively) may benefit from the addition of an epidural block. The risk and costs of this epidural anesthesia are almost certainly outweighed by an improvement in overall patient safety.

REFERENCES

1. J.B. Dahl, J. Rosenberg, W.E. Dirkes, T. Mogensen, H. Kehlet, Prevention of postoperative pain by balanced analgesia, Brit J Anaesth. 64:518 (1990).
2. M.P. Yeager, D.D. Glass, R.K. Neff, T. Brink-Johnsen, Epidural Anesthesia and analgesia in high-risk surgical patients, Anesthesiology 66:729 (1987).
3. J.F. Baron, M. Bertrand, E. Barre, G. Godet, O. Mundler, P. Coriat, P. Viars, Combined epidural and general anesthesia versus general anesthesia for abdominal aortic surgery, Anesthesiology 75:611 (1991).
4. H. Lessire, M. Pfisterer, M.L. Schweppe-Hartenauer, C. Puchstein, Hämodynamische Auswirkungen der Kombination von Allgemein- und Peridualanaesthesie während der Narkoseeinleitung bei geriatrischen Patienten, Anaesthesist 40:375 (1991).

5. K. Reinhart, U. Foehring, T. Kersting, M. Schäfer, D. Bredle, A. Hirner, K. Eyrich, Effects of thoracic epidural anesthesia on systemic hemodynamic function and systemic oxygen supply-demand relationship, Anesth Analg 69:360 (1989).

6. W. Seeling, F.W. Ahnefeld, H. Heinrich, G. Rosenberg, D. Spilker, Aortofemoraler Bifurkationsbypass - Der Einfluß des Anaesthesieverfahrens (NLA, thorakale kontinuierliche Katheterperidualanaesthesie) auf Kreislauf, Atmung und Stoffwechsel. Hämodynamische Veränderungen durch Peridualanaesthesie und Narkoseeinleitung, Anaesthesist 34:217 (1985).

7. W. Seeling, F.W. Ahnefeld, H. Hamann, H. Heinrich, S. Hutschenreiter, G. Rosenberg, D. Spilker, J. Vollmar, Aortofemoraler Bifurkationsbypass - Der Einfluß des Anaesthesieverfahrens (NLA, thorakale kontinuierliche Katheterperidualanaesthesie) auf Kreislauf, Atmung und Stoffwechsel. Intraoperatives Kreislaufverhalten, Anaesthesist 34:417 (1985).

8. P.M.C. Wright, J.P.H. Fee, Cardiovascular Support during combined extradural and general Anaesthesia, Brit J Anaesth 68:585 (1992).

INCREASED OXYGEN AFFINITY CONTRIBUTES TO TISSUE HYPOXIA IN CRITICALLY ILL PATIENTS WITH LOW OXYGEN DELIVERY

Reiner Dauberschmidt,[1] Heinz Mrochen,[1] Werner Kuckelt,[2] Ullrich Hieronymi,[1] and Manfred Meyer[1]

[1]Clinic of Anaesthesiology and Intensive Care Medicine, Department of Functional Evaluation in Critical Care Medicine, Friedrichshain Hospital D-O-1017 Berlin

[2]Department of Anaesthesiology and Intensive Care Medicine, Central Hospital "Links der Weser", D-W-2800 Bremen, Germany

INTRODUCTION

The acute organ system failure (OSF) is a serious complication in intensive care patients, in the postoperative period as well as after trauma and resuscitation, respectively[1]. In most intensive care patients the oxygen demand is high, especially in septic conditions[2]. The development of a cumulative oxygen consumption deficit is one of the causes of an OSF[3]. The role of a changed oxygen affinity for the development of such an oxygen consumption deficit in critically ill patients is not clear.

From experimental investigations and some clinical studies, in accordance with theoretical concepts, it was concluded that a shift of the blood oxygen dissociation curve to the right (decrease of P_{50}) might be advantageous for the oxygen transport to tissue at normoxia and mild hypoxia, respectively, but disadvantageous for oxygen uptake in cases of severe hypoxia [4,5,6,7,8].

In a first clinical study we could show that in patients with extremely low oxygen delivery an increase of the oxygen affinity (lowering of P_{50}) substantially contributes to tissue hypoxia even though there is a sufficient arterial oxygenation[9].

The aim of this study was to assess whether or not changes in oxygen affinity are responsible for a tissue hypoxia in patients at high risk of an OSF and if so, in which way those changes take effect.

MATERIAL AND METHODS

39 critically ill patients were included into the study. 15 patients survived and 24 died. An oxygen delivery index ($\dot{D}O_2$) not higher than 350 ml/min$\cdot$m² was defined as "considerably low $\dot{D}O_2$". In 9 patients of the 24 nonsurvivors a $\dot{D}O_2 \leq 350$ ml/min $\cdot$ m² was measured at least once during the investigational period. On this base the measurements were grouped according to the following criteria:

- Group 1: 83 measuring points with $\dot{D}O_2 > 350$ ml/min$\cdot$m² in 24 nonsurvivors
- Group 2: 71 measuring points with $\dot{D}O_2 > 350$ ml/min$\cdot$m² in 15 survivors
- Group 3: 19 measuring points with $\dot{D}O_2 \leq 350$ ml/min$\cdot$m² in 9 nonsurvivors

Increases of lactate concentration in blood were used as indicator for tissue hypoxia. All patients had indwelling catheters in a peripheral artery (femoral or radial artery, respectively) and in the pulmonary artery. Blood samples were taken simultaneously from both catheters for measurement of blood gases, acid base status, hemoglobin concentration and lactate concentration. At the same time the respiratory gases were analyzed and the expiratory minute volume was registered.

For the measurements the following equipment was used:

- Arterial and mixed venous blood gases (PaO_2, $P\bar{v}O_2$, $PaCO_2$, $P\bar{v}CO_2$) and acid base status: ABL-1 (Radiometer Copenhagen)
- Arterial and mixed venous oxygen saturation, and hemoglobin concentration (SaO_2, $S\bar{v}O_2$, Hb): IL 282 (Instrumentation Laboratory)
- Lactate concentration: Determination with Lactate Monotest (Boehringer Mannheim) at $25°C$ and 365 nm
- Inspiratory and expiratory oxygen fraction (F_IO_2, F_EO_2): OM11 (Beckman Instruments)
- Expiratory carbon dioxide fraction (F_ECO_2): LB2 (Beckman Instruments)
- Oxygen content (CaO_2, $C\bar{v}O_2$), cardiac index (C.I.), oxygen consumption index ($\dot{V}O_2$), oxygen delivery index ($\dot{D}O_2$), and oxygen affinity (P_{50}) were calculated according to standard formulae.

The distribution of data was characterized by the median value ($\tilde{x}$), 10th and 90th percentiles, respectively. Statistical analyses were performed using the Kolmogorov-Smirnov test for homogeneity and the Median test. The relationship between the measured parameters was characterized by linear and exponential regression analysis, respectively. Statistical significance was accepted when $p < 0.01$.

RESULTS

Blood gases and values of the acid base equilibrium were similar in nonsurvivors and in survivors[9]. No significant differences were found. The arterial oxygenation was sufficient in all patients[9]. The oxygen affinity was not statistically significant different in the 3 investigated groups, but the lactate concentration differed (Table 1.). The highest lactate concentrations were measured in patients with extremely low oxygen delivery (group 3).

With regard to the relationships between the parameters the following can be shown:
- In groups 1 and 2, respectively, the oxygen affinity correlates with the oxygen extraction in some degree. A correlation between lactate and the oxygen transport parameters was not seen (Table 2.).
- In group 3, a correlation of P_{50} as well as of lactate with the oxygen extraction can be found. Between P_{50} and lactate there exists a highly significant linear correlation ($r = 0.809$; $p < 0.001$, Figure 1.). This correlation is also observed if from the 9 non-surviving patients only those measuring points were taken where the oxygen delivery first falls below 350 ml/min • m². The same is true for the last measuring points with $\dot{D}O_2 \leq 350$ ml/min • m² (Table 3.; Figures 2. and 3.).

Table 1. Oxygen affinity (P_{50}) and lactate concentration in groups 1, 2 and 3

Group	n	P_{50} (mm Hg)			Lactate (mmol/l)		
		10th Perc.	$\tilde{x}$	90th Perc.	10th Perc.	$\tilde{x}$	90th Perc.
1	83	25,1	27,1	30,2	1,20	1,98	3,97
2	71	26,2	28,4	30,1	0,84	1,53	2,30
3	19	21,8	25,7	29,7	1,60	6,10*	9,50

* $p < 0.001$ in comparison to groups 1 and 2, respectively.

Table 2. Groups 1 and 2: Relationships of some oxygen transport parameters with P_{50} and lactate, respectively

Parameter	Group 1[1]		Group 2[2]	
	P_{50}	Lactate	P_{50}	Lactate
$\dot{V}O_2$	0.208	- 0.086	0.016	- 0.153
$\dot{D}O_2$	- 0.142	- 0.132	- 0.171	- 0.102
$a\bar{v}DO_2/CaO_2$	0.358**	0.048	0.190	0.037
C.I.	0.144	- 0.165	- 0.207	- 0.134
$P\bar{v}O_2$	0.154	0.015	0.349**	- 0.096
Lactate	- 0.076		0.174	

[1]Group 1: 83 measuring points; [2]group 2: 71 measuring points; ** $p < 0.01$;

- In group 3, no significant correlations were observed between P_{50} and cardiac index or between P_{50} and oxygen delivery, respectively (Table 3.).

The relationship between P_{50} and lactate seems to be rather exponential than linear which is furthermore suggested by a plot of the measuring values (Figure 1.). These figure show that drastic increases of lactate concentration as an expression of marked tissue hypoxia will be measured just if P_{50} falls below the reference area of 26 to 28 mm Hg.

If only the first and the last measuring points were taken into account, respectively, showing a $\dot{D}O_2 \leq 350$ ml/min•m² in the 9 nonsurvivors, a quite similar exponential curve is to be seen (Figures 2. and 3.). But these results have to be confirmed by further examinations.

DISCUSSION AND CONCLUSIONS

An increase of oxygen affinity has been found in different situations in intensive care medicine, as in critically ill patients[10], in patients with barbiturate intoxications[11], with CO-intoxication[8,12], with burns[13], with respiratory or metabolic alkalosis[8], with sepsis[14], with pancreatitis[15], or after transfusion of large volumes of bank blood[14,16,17]. However, only Sheldon[16] has demonstrated a relationship between changes of oxygen affinity and lactate production in patients after massive transfusion.

The presented results show that in patients with sufficient arterial oxygenation but extremely low oxygen delivery an increase of the oxygen affinity may be harmful as it

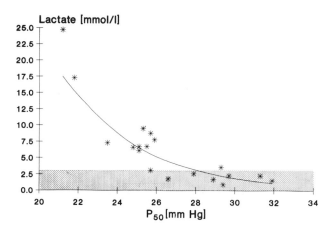

Figure 1. Group 3: Exponential correlation between P_{50} and lactate in nine nonsurviving patients with a $\dot{D}O_2 \leq 350$ ml/min · m² (19 measuring points).

Lactate concentrations above 3.0 mmol/l (above the marked area) are defined as pathologically.

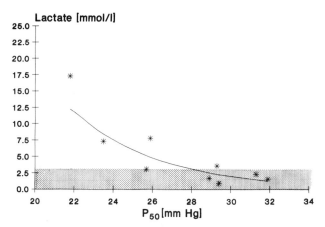

Figure 2. Group 3: Exponential correlation between P_{50} and lactate of the first measurement with a $\dot{D}O_2 \leq 350$ ml/min · m² during the investigational period.

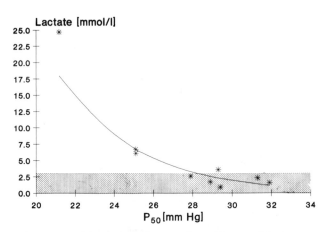

Figure 3. Group 3: Exponential correlation between P_{50} and lactate of the last measurement with a $\dot{D}O_2 \leq 350$ ml/min $\cdot$ m^2 during the investigational period.

Table 3. Group 3: Relationship of some oxygen transport parameters with P_{50} and lactate, respectively (19 measurements in 9 patients)

Parameter	All Measuring Points (n = 19)		1st Measurement[1] (n = 9)		Last Measurement[1] (n = 9)	
	P_{50}	Lactate	P_{50}	Lactate	P_{50}	Lactate
$\dot{V}O_2$	- 0.206	- 0.241	- 0.254	0.487	- 0.165	0.147
$\dot{D}O_2$	0.369	- 0.435	0.459	- 0.206	0.506	- 0.518
$a\bar{v}DO_2/CaO_2$	- 0.476	0.658**	- 0.423	0.331	- 0.631	0.741
C.I.	0.279	- 0.377	0.304	- 0.298	0.271	- 0.347
$P\bar{v}O_2$	0.665**	- 0.601**	0.651	- 0.533	0.658	- 0.637
Lactate	- 0.809***		- 0.830**		- 0.858**	

[1] see text for explanation; ** p < 0.01; *** p < 0.001

worsens the disproportion between a high oxygen demand of the tissue and a restricted ability to deliver the needed oxygen by limitation of the release of oxygen. An increase in blood flow cannot meet the demand, and the venous-capillary oxygen tension difference may fall to critical levels. A drastic increase in lactate concentration in blood is a sensible indicator, pointing to a tissue hypoxia of higher degree.

On the other hand, variations in oxygen affinity in case of a P_{50} above the reference level of about 26 mm Hg seem to have none or only minor influence on the development of a tissue hypoxia.

These results show that in critically ill patients with extremely low oxygen delivery a decrease of P_{50} to values below the reference area additionally limits the oxygen supply to tissues. Changes in oxygen affinity, therefore, may become an extra factor contributing essentially to the development of a tissue hypoxia.

REFERENCES

1. W.A. Knaus, E.A. Draper, D.P. Wagner, and J.E. Zimmerman, Prognosis in acute organ system failure, *Ann. Surg.* 202: 685 (1985)

2. R.W. Samsel and P.T. Schumacker, Oxygen delivery to tissues, *Europ. Respir. J.* 4: 1258 (1991)

3. W.C. Shoemaker, P.L. Appel, and H.B. Kram, Tissue oxygen debt as a determinant of lethal and non-lethal postoperative organ failure, *Crit. Care Med.* 11: 640 (1983)

4. M.J. Sold, Is there an optimal P_{50} of haemoglobin?, *Anaesthesia* 37: 640 (1982)

5. D.C. Willford, E.P. Hill, and W.Y. Moores, Theoretical analysis of optimal P_{50}, *J. Appl. Physiol.: Respirat. Environ. Exercise Physiol.* 52: 1043 (1982)

6. Z. Turek, F. Kreuzer, M. Turek-Maischeider, and B.E.M. Tingnalda, Blood O_2 content, cardiac output, and flow to organs at several levels of oxygenation in rats with a left-shifted blood oxygen dissociation curve, *Pflügers Arch.* 376: 201 (1978)

7. R.C. Koehler, R.J. Traystman, and M.D. Jones, Influence of reduced oxyhemoglobin affinity on cerebrovascular response to hypoxic hypoxia, *Am. J. Physiol.* 251: H756 (1986)

8. W. Hess, Die Sauerstoffaffinität des Hämoglobins - Ihre Bedeutung unter physiologischen und pathophysiologischen Bedingungen, *Anaesthesist* 36: 455 (1987)

9. R. Dauberschmidt, U. Hieronymi und W. Kuckelt, Sauerstoffbereitstellung und Sauerstoffverbrauch bei kritisch kranken Patienten: Sind Änderungen der Sauerstoffaffinität Ursache für eine Gewebehypoxie?, *Anaesthesiol. Notfallm. Schmerzther.* 28: in press (1983)

10. J.A. Myberg, R.K. Webb, and L.I.G. Worthley, The P_{50} is reduced in critically ill patients, *Intens. Care Med.* 17: 355 (1991)

11. M. Meyer, R. Dauberschmidt, and H. Gaida, On changes in the oxygen affinity of haemoglobin in patients with barbiturate intoxication, *in* "Oxygen Measurement in Biology and Medicine", J.P. Payne and D.W. Hill, eds., Butterworths, London (1975)

12. A. Zwart, G. Kwant, B. Oeseburg, and W.G. Zijlstra, Human whole blood oxygen affinity, effect of carbon monoxide, *J. Appl. Physiol.: Respirat. Environ. Exercise Physiol.* 57: 14 (1984)

13. N. Nishimura and M. Fukuda, P_{50} in burn injury, *Crit. Care Med.* 10: 384 (1982)

14. H.B. Hechtman, G.R. Grindlinger, A.M. Vegas, J. Many, and C.R. Valeri, Importance of oxygen transport in clinical medicine, *Crit. Care Med.* 7: 419 (1979)

15. A.G. Greenberg, L. Terlizzi, and G.W. Peskin, Oxyhemoglobin affinity in acute pancreatitis, *J. Surg. Res.* 22: 561 (1977)

16. G.F. Sheldon, Diphosphoglycerate in massive transfusion and erythroporesis, *Crit. Care Med.* 7: 407 (1979)

17. R. Weisel, R. Dennic, J. Mauny, R. Valeri, and H. Hechtman, Adverse effects of transfusion therapy during abdominal aortic aneurysectomy, *Surgery* 83: 682 (1978)

PROTECTIVE REGULATION OF OXYGEN UPTAKE AS A RESULT OF REDUCED OXYGEN EXTRACTION DURING CHRONIC INFLAMMATION

D.K. Harrison[1], N.C. Abbot[1,3], F.M.T. Carnochan[2], J. Swanson Beck[3], P.B. James[4] and P.T. McCollum[2]

Vascular Laboratory, Departments of Medical Physics[1] and Surgery[2] Department of Pathology[3] and Department of Epidemiology and Public Health[4], Ninewells Hospital and Medical School, Dundee DD1 9SY, Scotland

INTRODUCTION

Previous studies of chronic inflammation using the tuberculin reaction in human skin as a model have demonstrated large increases in blood flow within the lesion (Beck and Spence, 1986). This occurs in response to the increase in oxygen consumption presented by the infiltration of cells, mainly T-lymphocytes and macrophages (Gibbs et al., 1984). Despite this increase in flow, transcutaneous pO_2 ($tcpO_2$) values remain low at the centre of the reaction (Abbot et al., 1990a). Extracellular pH falls (Harrison et al., 1986), but transcutaneous pCO_2 measurements rise during the course of the tuberculin reaction (Abbot et al., 1990a), indicated that the tissue acidosis was purely respiratory in origin. Thus, despite a large observed increase in O_2 uptake rate (Abbot et al., 1990b) and low tissue pO_2, demand does not appear to exceed the rate of oxygen delivery to the cells.

Whilst protective, pO_2-dependent regulation of local O_2 uptake rate has been demonstrated in the cells of a number of organs (Harrison et al., 1990; Hoeper, 1991) including skin (Albrecht et al., 1988), this paper examines the possibility that the oxygen consumption of infiltrating cells may be similarly regulated.

Our conclusions are based on results from two series of experiments, one of which is reported in detail (Harrison et al., 1992) and the other in preliminary form (Abbot et al., 1990b) elsewhere, but neither of which set out initially to answer the question raised in this paper.

METHODS

Hyperbaric Oxygen Experiments

Measurements of $tcpO_2$ and local oxygen consumption rates were carried out prior to (0h) and at 24h, 48h, 72h and 96h following injection of the antigen (0.1ml, 10 TU, purified protein derivative, Glaxo, Greenford, UK) in 13 normal volunteers (10 men and 3 women; mean age 35 +/- 10.9, sd). The measurements were performed at the site of injection under conditions of breathing pure oxygen at 1 atmosphere absolute (1ATA) and subsequently pure oxygen at 2 atmospheres absolute (2ATA) in a monoplace hyperbaric chamber (Hyox Systems, Aberdeen, UK).

The oxygen consumption rate (VO_2) was estimated, after raising the $tcpO_2$ to at least 200mmHg by means of the subject breathing 100% oxygen from the initial rate of fall of $tcpO_2$, $d(pO_2)/dt$, in the forearm skin during suprasystolic cuff occlusion of the brachial artery. The method, as applied to the tuberculin reaction in skin, is described elsewhere (Abbot et al, 1990b).

The subjects were classified at 48h into two groups according to the intensity of their reactions (Abbot et al, 1992):

Weak positive reactions with induration less than 10mm diameter (5 subjects) and

Strong positive reactions with induration greater than 10mm and exhibiting "central relative slowing" (Beck et al., 1989; see also Harrison et al., 1993)

Tissue Spectrophotometry Experiments

Lightguide spectrophotometric measurements were carried out using a Photal MCPD-1000 instrument (Otsuka Electronics Co., Osaka, Japan) in the visible range (500-620nm) in order to measure haemoglobin oxygenation (SO_2) during the tuberculin reaction (Harrison et al., 1992). The method used for estimation of SO_2 is also summarised elsewhere in this volume (Hickman et al., 1993).

The experiments were carried out according to the above protocol in 18 normal subjects (11 males and 7 females; mean age 38 +/- 10.3, sd) but only under normobaric conditions, breathing room air (except for VO_2 measurements which were necessarily carried out with the subjects breathing 100% oxygen). No differentiation was made in these experiments between weak and strong reactors.

The laser Doppler (LD) and SO_2 measurements were used to estimate local relative oxygen extraction (O_2 Ext). This was done by calculating the product of the laser Doppler concentration of moving blood cells (CMBC) and the degree of oxygen desaturation of haemoglobin (Harrison et al., 1992). The saturation of arterial blood was taken as 97%, thus:

$$O_2 \text{ Ext} = CMBC \times (97 - SO_2).$$

The experimental protocols were all approved by the Tayside Committee on Medical Ethics.

The levels of significance during the course of the reaction for both the hyperbaric and spectrophotometry experiments were tested statistically using Student's t test for paired values.

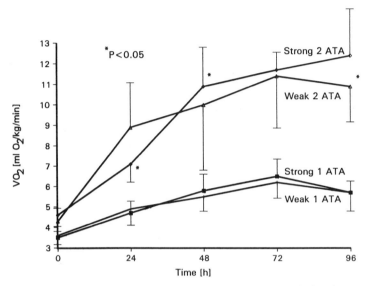

Figure 1. Changes (Mean +/- SEM) in VO_2 measured at 1 and 2ATA during the course of the tuberculin reaction in strong and weak reactors.

RESULTS

Hyperbaric Oxygen Experiments

Significant increases in LD flux and VO_2, but decreases in $tcpO_2$ (all at p < .001) were observed at all stages of the reaction and under all conditions compared with 0h. However, the most interesting findings are shown in figure 1. In all cases, including control skin (0h), VO_2 was raised when breathing oxygen at 2ATA compared with 1ATA. The difference became greater during the development of the reaction and was statistically significant (p < 0.05) for strong reactors at 24 and 48h and weak reactors at 96h.

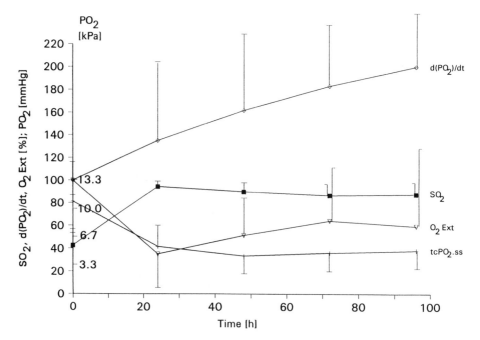

Figure 2. Changes (Mean +/- SEM) in tcpO$_2$, relative intramicrovascular oxygen extraction rate (O$_2$ Ext), haemoglobin saturation (SO$_2$) and relative tissue oxygen uptake rate, d(pO$_2$)/dt (Harrison et al., 1992; by permission).

Tissue Spectrophotometry Experiments

The results of the spectrophotometric measurements are summarised in figure 2. It can be seen that, similarly to results from the hyperbaric experiments, VO$_2$ (here expressed in terms of d(pO$_2$)/dt) demonstrated a large increase compared with control (p < .01 at 24h and < .001 at all other stages). However, SO$_2$ increased compared with control (p < .001 at all stages) but tcpO$_2$ decreased (p < .001 at all stages). Not shown in the figure are the LD flux values which were significantly increased (p < .001) throughout the reaction. Despite this increase in perfusion, oxygen extraction (O$_2$ Ext) decreased (p < .001 at 24h and p < .05 at 72h and 96h).

DISCUSSION

Results from the experiments involving hyperbaric oxygen demonstrated significant increases in tcpO$_2$ between measurements at 1ATA and 2ATA in both weak and strong reactors at all stages of the reaction. The changes in oxygen uptake rate, compared with control, were statistically significant at 24h and 48h (strong reactors) and 96h (weak reactors). A small (not statistically significant) increase in oxygen consumption was observed between 1ATA and 2ATA in normal skin. This may be due to local changes in the diffusion gradient between the source of oxygen (the dermal capillaries) and the electrode induced by the greatly increased pO_2. However, the difference between the estimated oxygen consumption at 1ATA and 2ATA increased significantly in both weak and strong reactors as the tuberculin reaction progressed, indicating a real increase in oxygen consumption as a result of breathing hyperbaric oxygen at 2ATA.

Spectrophotometric measurements during the tuberculin reaction under normobaric conditions demonstrated the presence of increased intracapillary haemoglobin oxygenation. This implies an increase in oxygen availability within the capillary circulation as a consequence the markedly increased volume perfusion (Harrison et al., 1992). It is thus unlikely that the low $tcpO_2$ values arose from an inadequate blood flow within the lesion. The experiments demonstrated, as in the hyperbaric oxygen experiments, that oxygen consumption in skin increases significantly during the course of the tuberculin reaction. However, this series demonstrated a simultaneous decrease in oxygen extraction.

Histological and immunocytochemical studies of the tuberculin reaction have demonstrated the presence of oedema (which causes an increase in intercapillary distance) and an exudate of inflammatory cells, protein rich fluid and cellular debris (e.g. fibrin) in the interstitial fluid of the dermis (Turk, 1980; Poulter et al., 1982; Gibbs et al., 1984; 1991). Such exudates probably form sites of resistance for the diffusion of oxygen from the capillaries to the indigenous and infiltrating cells both in terms of increased diffusion distances and decreased oxygen permeability.

The discrepancies between intracapillary oxygenation and $tcpO_2$ on the one hand, and oxygen consumption and extraction on the other, provide physiological evidence for such an increased resistance for the diffusion of oxygen during the course of the tuberculin reaction.

Elsewhere in this volume, Harrison et al. (1993) have demonstrated that the phenomenon of "central relative slowing" previously reported by Beck et al., 1989 (regions of low perfusion at the centre of strong reactions surrounded by areas of higher flow) may also be present throughout the area of erythema. These local heterogeneities in flow, possibly induced by increases in interstitial pressure due to oedema (Beck et al., 1989) may also contribute to the occurrence of areas of local hypoxia.

Protective regulation of oxygen consumption as a result of hypoxia has been observed in many organs (Hoeper, 1991). In particular, measurements of VO_2 and tissue pO_2 in skeletal muscle (Harrison et al., 1990) indicated a significant reduction of VO_2 in the absence of anoxia (less than 5% of tissue pO_2 values were below 5mmHg). It would therefore appear that local protective regulation of VO_2 occurs before, and can indeed prevent, cellular anoxia ($pO_2 < 0.1$mmHg). The low $tcpO_2$

levels in the tuberculin reaction, coupled with the presence of a diffusional resistance and possible localised areas of impaired perfusion (Harrison et al., 1993), may indicate the presence of hypoxic regions which could be sufficient to trigger such a protective limitation of VO_2.

The raising of the intracapillary pO_2 by hyperbaric oxygen increases the diffusion gradient from blood to tissue and appears to be sufficient to overcome the diffusional resistance. This reduces or eliminates the tissue hypoxia permitting the affected cells to resume a normal metabolic rate. The fact that this mechanism appears to apply to the infiltrating as well as the indigenous cells is in agreement with the mechanism for regulation first proposed by Kessler et al., 1981. The cells to be first affected by hypoxia are always those lying between the venous ends of capillaries (the "lethal corner"). In their model, however, (see Hoeper, 1991) the mitochondrial enzyme monoamine oxidase B (MAO B) triggers a signal chain acting along the capillary endothelial cells (Kessler et al., 1984) which can also regulate the consumption of oxygen in cells nearer the arterial end of the capillaries. The effect of this mechanism is to ensure that even those cells at the lethal corner do not become anoxic.

CONCLUSIONS

Tissue hypoxia during the tuberculin reaction is probably due to impaired diffusion of oxygen together with a maldistribution of capillary blood flow. Furthermore, the resultant hypoxia when the subject is in a normoxic environment may bring into effect a local protective relative reduction in oxygen uptake rate. When the diffusional resistance is overcome by raising the local pO_2 gradient under hyperbaric conditions, the necessity for the protective down-regulation is reduced, and the cellular O_2 uptake rate increases.

ACKNOWLEDGEMENTS

The authors are grateful to the Scottish Home and Health Department and the University of Dundee Research Initiatives Fund for financial support for this work, to Dr Dick Lerski, Director, Department of Medical Physics for his continuing support, and of course to the volunteer subjects for their patience and cooperation. The monoplace hyperbaric chamber was kindly lent by Hyox Sytems Ltd., Aberdeen, Scotland.

REFERENCES

Abbot, N.C., Spence, V.A., Beck, J.S., Carnochan, F.M.T., Gibbs, J.H. and Lowe J.G., 1990a, Assessment of the respiratory metabolism in the skin from transcutaneous measurements of

PO$_2$ and PCO$_2$: potential for non-invasive monitoring of response to tuberculin skin testing, *Tubercle* 71:15.

Abbot, N.C., Beck, J.S., Carnochan, F.M., Spence, V.A. and James, P.B., 1990b, Estimating skin respiration from transcutaneous PO$_2$/PCO$_2$ at 1 and 2 atm abs on normal and inflamed skin, *J. Hyperbar. Med.* 5:91.

Abbot, N.C., Swanson Beck J., Carnochan, F.M., Lowe, J.G. and Gibbs, J.H., 1992, Circulatory adaptation to the increased metabolism in skin at the site of the tuberculin reaction, *Int. J. Microcirc: Clin. Exp.* in press.

Albrecht, H.P., Frank, K.H., Duemmler, W. and Kessler, M., 1988, Intracapillary haemoglobin oxygenation and local O$_2$ uptake rate of human skin, *Pflueg. Arch. ges. Physiol.* 412:R36.

Beck, J.S. and Spence V.A., 1986, Patterns of blood flow in the microcirculation of the skin during the course of the tuberculin reaction in normal human subjects, *Immunology* 58:209.

Beck, J.S., Gibbs, J.H., Potts, R.C., Kardjito, T., Grange, J.M., Jawad, E.S. and Spence, V.A., 1989, Histometric studies on biopsies of tuberculin skin test showing evidence of ischaemia and necrosis, *J. Pathol.* 159:317.

Gibbs, J.H., Ferguson, J., Brown, R.A., Kenicer, K.J.A., Potts, R.C., Coghill, G. and Beck J.S., 1984, Histometric study of the localisation of lymphocyte subsets and accessory cells in human Mantoux reactions, *J. Clin. Pathol.* 37:1227.

Gibbs, J.H., Grange, J.M., Beck, J.S., Jawad, E., Potts, R.C., Bothamley, G.H. and Kardito, T., 1991, Early delayed hypersensitivity responses in tuberculin skin tests after heavy occupational exposure to tuberculosis, *J. Clin. Pathol.* 44:919.

Harrison, D.K., Spepnce, V.A., Beck, J.S., Lowe, J.G. and Walker, W.F., 1986, pH changes in the dermis during the course of the tuberculin skin test, *Immunology* 59:497.

Harrison, D.K., Kessler, M. and Knauf, S.K., 1990, Regulation of capillary blood flow and oxygen supply in skeletal muscle in dogs during hypoxaemia, *J. Physiol. (Lond.)* 420:431.

Harrison, D.K., Evans, S.D., Abbot, N.C., Swanson Beck, J. and McCollum, P.T., 1992, Spectrophotometric measurements of haemoglobin saturation and concentration in skin during the tuberculin reaction in normal human subjects, *Clin. Phys. and Physiol. Meas.* 13:in press.

Harrison, D.K., Abbot, N.C., Swanson Beck, J. and McCollum, P.T., 1993, Laser Doppler perfusion imaging compared with lightguide laser Doppler flowmetry, dynamic thermographic imaging and tissue spectrophotometry for investigating blood flow in human skin, *Adv. Exp. Med Biol.* this volume.

Hickman, P., Harrison, D.K., Evans, S.D., Belch, J. and McCollum, P.T., 1993, Use of lightguide reflectance spectrophotometry in the assessment of peripheral arterial disease, *Adv. Exp. Med Biol.* this volume.

Hoeper, J., 1991, "Influence of Local Oxygen Deficiency on Function and Integrity of Liver, Kidney and Heart," Gustav Fischer, Stuttgart.

Kessler, M., Hoeper, J., Luebbers, D.W. and Ji, S., 1981, Local factors affecting regulation of microflow, O$_2$ uptake and energy metabolism, *Adv Physiol. Sci.* 25:155.

Kessler, M., Hoeper, J., Harrison, D.K., Skolasinska, K., Kloevekorn, W.P., Sebening, F., Volkholz, H.J., Beier, I., Kernbach, C., Rettig, V. and Richter, H., 1984, Tissue oxygen supply under normal and pathological conditions, Adv. Exp. Med. Biol., 169:69.

Poulter, L.W., Seymour, G.J., Duke, O., Janossy, G. and Panayi, G., 1982, Immunohistological analysis of delayed-type hypersensitivity in man, *Cell. Immunol.* 74:358.

Turk, J.L., 1980, "Delayed Hypersensitivity," *Research Monographs in Immunology 3rd Ed*, Vol 1, Elsevier/North Holland, Amsterdam.

METHODS AND MODELING

MEASUREMENTS OF INTRACELLULAR CONCENTRATIONS OF OXYGEN: EXPERIMENTAL RESULTS AND CONCEPTUAL IMPLICATIONS OF AN OBSERVED GRADIENT BETWEEN INTRACELLULAR AND EXTRACELLULAR CONCENTRATIONS OF OXYGEN

Harold M. Swartz

Dartmouth Medical School
Hanover, NH 03755, U.S.A.

INTRODUCTION

The intracellular concentration of oxygen ($[O_2]$) is the pertinent parameter for most physiological, pathophysiological, and therapeutic considerations, but it seldom is measured directly. This paradox is explained by a combination of a lack of awareness and a lack of methodology. The literature is quite mixed in regard to the occurrence of significant gradients between the intracellular and extracellular compartments. Everyone agrees, of course, that there must be some gradient because oxygen enters from the outside of the cell and is consumed inside the cell, principally by the mitochondria. The disagreements are in regard to the size of the gradient, with arguments being made on theoretical grounds that there should or should not be a significant gradient. There also are some experimental reports of indirect measures of intracellular oxygen concentrations and these, like the theoretical reports, have quite variable conclusions with reports of both no significant gradients and relatively large gradients (1-11).

Recently, experimental limitations on the study of oxygen gradients have become reduced by the development of new methods. We have used the technique of Electron Paramagnetic Resonance (EPR or, equivalently, Electron Spin Resonance, ESR) Oximetry (12,13) to make selective measurements of intracellular $[O_2]$ in several mammalian cell lines and compared these with measurements of extracellular $[O_2]$ (14-16). We also have calculated the gradients expected, assuming the free diffusion of oxygen into and through cells (14). The overall conclusion from our studies is that there can be quite significant gradients between the intracellular and extracellular compartments. In this paper the results of some of these experiments are summarized and the implications of the findings are considered in some detail.

METHODS

EPR oximetry is based on the fact that under appropriate conditions, the shape and other parameters of EPR spectra are very sensitive to the $[O_2]$, with resolution of less than 0.1 micromolar concentrations being feasible (17). In order to increase experimental reliability, we used several different methods to obtain selective oxygen-dependent EPR spectra from the intra- and extracellular compartments. The $[O_2]$ were measured in suspensions of four different mammalian cell lines (CHO, mouse thymus-bone marrow, myoblasts, and tumor macrophage cells) at 37°C. In some experiments the rate of respiration of the cells was enhanced by the addition of an uncoupler of oxidative phosphorylation, carbonyl cyanide M-chlorophenylhydrazone (CCCP) . Calculations of the expected gradients of oxygen were made with a model based on simple diffusion of oxygen, with the consumption of oxygen occurring inside the cell in shells which simulated the location of mitochondria.

Suspensions of cells were placed in gas permeable tubes and placed in an EPR spectrometer for measurements at 37°C with a stream of gas with the desired composition flowing around the gas permeable tube. Several different methods were used to measure [O_2] in the intracellular and extracellular compartments.

In most experiments the intracellular compartment was studied selectively by using a combination of an oxygen sensitive neutral nitroxide that freely permeated into cells and a paramagnetic broadening agent whose negative charge prevented it from crossing the membranes of viable cells; this is illustrated in Figure 1. As a consequence the paramagnetic broadening agent made the spectra of the extracellular compartment too broad to affect the measurements of the spectra of the neutral nitroxides which were inside viable cells.

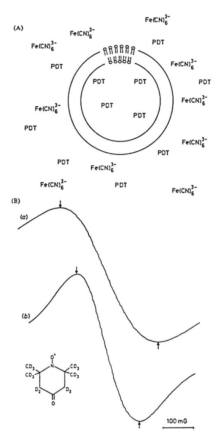

Fig. 1. Method of measuring intracellular oxygen. (A) Schematic representation of cell, nitroxides (PDT) and broadening agents (ferricyanide). The broadening agent effectively eliminates the EPR spectra of extracellular nitroxides. (B) EPR spectra used to measure intracellular oxygen: spectra of 0.10 mM PDT (chemical formula shown) in the presence (a) and absence (b) of air. The peak-to-peak linewidths are measured as shown by the small arrows. The difference, ΔW_0, changes linearly with oxygen concentration. Calibrations are made in the media in which the oxygen concentration is measured (reproduced from J. Chem. Soc. with permission) (18).

Initially [O_2] in the extracellular compartment was measured in separate experiments in which an aliquot of cells did not have the broadening agent added and, instead of a neutral nitroxide, a positively charged nitroxide was used (14). The charged nitroxide did not cross the cell membrane and, therefore, measured the [O_2] in the extracellular compartment. Care was taken to keep all other conditions the same so as to assure the validity of the comparisons of the two measurements. Experiments were conducted in the presence and absence of an uncoupler of oxidative phosphorylation in order to stimulate respiration. The differences between the two compartments then could be compared with cells having different rates of respiration (the rates of respiration were measured directly in aliquots of cells with the various concentrations of the uncoupler).

Because of a concern that the use of two different experiments to measure intracellular and extracellular [O_2] might have led to an experimental artifact, other methods were developed which permitted the simultaneous measurement of [O_2] in both compartments (15,16). These methods used the same method to measure intracellular [O_2], but provided means to protect the nitroxide used for the measurements of extracellular [O_2] from the broadening agent. In one set of experiments the amount of broadening agent was reduced moderately and a negatively charged nitroxide was used for the measurements of extracellular [O_2] (15). Its spectrum therefore was not broadened unacceptably by the negatively charged broadening agent. Both the neutral and the charged nitroxide could be observed simultaneously by the use of appropriate isotopes of nitrogen, which resulted in clearly separated EPR spectra. This approach was used in both CHO cells and a mouse tumor macrophage cell line. The cells were studied with and without an uncoupler of oxidative phosphorylation.

In another set of experiments the nitroxide used for the measurement of [O_2] in the extracellular compartment was enclosed in a liposome (16). The membrane of the latter was freely permeable to oxygen but not to the broadening agent. These measurements were made in a cell line, mouse myoblasts, with a relatively high rate of respiration and, therefore, there was no need to stimulate respiration.

RESULTS

Figures 2 and 3 indicate that with the initial methodology that was employed, in which [O_2] in the two compartments was measured separately, there was no measurable gradient without respiratory stimulation but there was a very significant gradient with increased rates of respiration. Because the same methodology produced results in which the two compartments were approximately equal in the absence of respiratory stimulation, and then no longer were equal with respiratory stimulation it is less plausible that the observations of gradients were due to experimental artifacts.

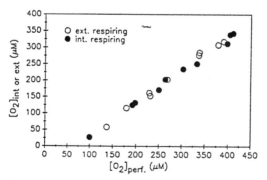

Fig. 2. Measurement of intracellular and extracellular O_2 in CHO cells. Suspensions containing 10^8 cells/ml were labelled with 15^N PDT and drawn into Teflon tubing. Spectra were recorded at different [O_2] in the perfusing gas; ΔW was measured and converted into an extracellular or intracellular oxygen concentration by using appropriate calibration curves. The figure shows that there is no difference between the extracellular and intracellular [O_2] of unstimulated CHO cells (reproduced with permission from J. Cell. Physiol.) (14).

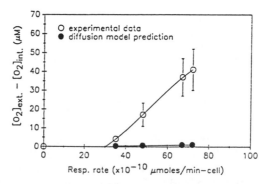

Fig. 3. Difference in extracellular and intracellular oxygen concentration as a function of cellular respiration rate. Cells were perfused at a constant oxygen concentration of 365 μM and respiration rates were stimulated by the addition of CCCP. For each concentration of CCCP, $[O_2]_{ext}$ and $[O_2]_{int}$ were measured, and the difference was plotted vs. respiration rate. Respiration rate vs. [CCCP] was determined in separate experiments (reproduced with permission from J. Cell. Physiol.) (14).

Table 1 summarizes the results of another set of experiments with CHO cells in which the measurements of intracellular and extracellular $[O_2]$ were made simultaneously, using a negatively charged nitroxide to measure the extracellular $[O_2]$. With this improved technique a small but significant gradient could be observed in cells without respiratory stimulation and a larger difference was found with respiratory stimulation. These results are consistent with those in Figures 2 and 3. The improved resolution of the "simultaneous" method apparently made it possible to resolve the small gradient in unstimulated cells.

Table 2 summarizes the results of similar experiments in another cell line, tumor macrophages. Again there were detectable differences between the two compartments. The rates of respiration and the gradients were similar in both cell lines.

Table 1. Differences in $[O_2]_i$ and $[O_2]_e$ in CHO Cells at Various Perfused $[O_2]$ (reproduced with permission from Biochim. Biophys. Acta) (15).

Perfused $[O_2]$ (μM)	Average $[O_2]_e$ (μM)	Average $\Delta[O_2]_{e-i} \pm$ s.e.m. (No. of exp.)
Unstimulated CHO cells		
200	139	4.5 ± 3.8 (6)
150	94	12.3 ± 5.3 (6)
100	47	9.2 ± 2.4 (6)
50	10	3.7 ± 0.6 (6)
CHO cells stimulated by 5 μM CCCP		
200	103	38.0 ± 13.0 (2)
150	62	44.0 ± 5.5 (2)
100	26	18.5 ± 9.5 (2)

Table 2.   Differences in $[O_2]_i$ and $[O_2]_e$ in M5076 Tumor Cells at Various Perfused $[O_2]$ (reproduced with permission from Biochim. Biophys. Acta) (15).

Perfused $[O_2]$ (μM)	Average $[O_2]_e$ (μM)	Average $[O_2]_{e-i}$ ± s.e.m. (No. of exp.)
Unstimulated M5076 tumor cells		
200	137	12.3 ± 4.4 (12)
150	95	15.5 ± 3.1 (12)
100	53	15.1 ± 3.0 (12)
50	14	9.5 ± 3.0 (11)
M5076 tumor cells stimulated by 1 μM CCCP		
200	90	26.6 ± 3.9 (7)
150	48	26.3 ± 5.5 (7)
100	20	12.1 ± 2.8 (7)

Figure 4 summarizes the results of experiments with another cell line, myoblasts. In these experiments the extracellular $[O_2]$ was measured by the use of liposome encapsulated charged nitroxides. The rates of respiration of these cells were higher than those of the other two cell lines.

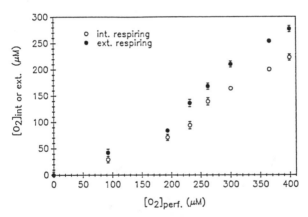

Fig. 4. Extracellular and intracellular oxygen concentrations obtained using a nitroxide encapsulated in liposomes to measure $[O_2]_{ext}$ while simultaneously measuring $[O_2]_{int}$. Samples of respiring cells were perfused with different concentrations of oxygen, ΔW measured, and the ΔW's converted to extracellular and intracellular oxygen concentrations using calibrations from experiments with cells with know $[O_2]$. The resulting $[O_2]_{ext}$ and $[O_2]_{int}$ values are plotted vs the $[O_2]$ in the perfusing gas (reproduced with permission from Magnetic Resonance in Med.) (16).

DISCUSSION

These results presented here with three different cell lines, using several different experimental approaches, all indicate that significant gradients in $[O_2]$ can occur between the extracellular and intracellular compartments. Preliminary results from additional experiments which are not described here, using other cell lines and other variations of the EPR methods, gave similar results. While experimental artifact cannot be absolutely excluded, we have not been able to find a plausible experimental reason that indicates that these results are likely to be incorrect.

The possibility of experimental artifact is considered because the finding of gradients of this magnitude would seem to have rather far reaching implications on the structure and function of cells. This is because calculations based on generally accepted assumptions of the properties of cells and oxygen lead to the conclusion that such a gradient should not have occurred. The results of such a calculation are shown in Figure 3. The solid points in this figure are the gradient that would be expected to occur with the measured rate of consumption of oxygen in cells of the same dimension as the CHO cells, assuming that molecular oxygen diffuses in cytoplasm at the same rate as in water and that it passes freely through the cell membrane. The results of the experimental determinations of intracellular $[O_2]$ therefore imply that the common assumptions about the diffusion of oxygen in cells may be incorrect.

There are several possible explanations for the observed discrepancy between the expected and observed gradients of $[O_2]$. The possibility of experimental artifact has been mentioned already and it was suggested that this is unlikely. The calculations of the differences expected on the basis of diffusion might be incorrect but the method that we used is based on standard, widely used methods. We directly tested the assumption that the diffusion of oxygen in cytoplasm differs greatly from diffusion in water but found that the rates were the same within experimental error (14). The exclusion of these possibilities leaves several interesting alternatives which seem to have significant implications for the organization of cells.

One logical possibility is that within the cell, oxygen is not fully available to interact with the paramagnetic probes that were used in these experiments. Because the effects of oxygen on EPR spectra are based on simple collisions, this would require some type of binding of oxygen within the cell. It seems likely that if this occurs it would have been noted previously because this would require large amounts of such a binding molecule and there are few molecules other than polymers with active surfaces and heme containing proteins that are known to bind oxygen avidly.

Another possibility is that there is a mechanism for pumping out oxygen once it enters cells. This seems unlikely because if the calculations of the expected rate of diffusion are correct, this would require a tremendously active pump to establish such a gradient. It should be noted, however, that the opposite effect - increasing $[O_2]$ above surrounding tissues has been observed in the retina of fish and this does appear to be based on active transport of $[O_2]$ (19-21).

Perhaps the most plausible explanation is that there is a barrier to the free diffusion of oxygen into the cell. On the basis of the experimental results this barrier would seem to have to be at the cell membrane, because the methods used in this study measured the average $[O_2]$ throughout the cell, so a barrier at the mitochondria, for example, would not have resulted in the observed gradient. There are a few reports that are consistent with such a possibility. Measurements of the partition coefficient of model membranes suggest that under some circumstances oxygen can be much less soluble in membranes than in aqueous solutions (22-25). This occurs when the membrane is quite rigid; in the fluid state membranes usually have $[O_2]$ 4-6 fold greater than the surrounding aqueous medium. The presence of ß-mercaptoethylamine has been reported to inhibit oxygen transport in phospholipid membranes (26). Some proteins in membrane also can fairly rigorously exclude oxygen (27,28). If the membrane is a barrier to the free diffusion of oxygen, then it must be organized in ways that have not been recognized previously and further, there are likely to be physiological and pathological states that are associated with changes in this type of organization.

Subczynski et al. recently reconsidered the question of whether the cell membrane could be an effective barrier to oxygen (29). They concluded, on the basis of their experimental results with CHO cells, that it was unlikely that the cell membrane could be an effective barrier to oxygen. Their approach, however, was based on a steady state technique which measured a parameter related to the $[O_2]$ and therefore required that their probes for $[O_2]$ were located specifically and that these locations included all possible plausible sites where oxygen could be highly excluded. Therefore while they have made a very comprehensive attempt to resolve this question, it is not clear that their results are conclusive.

Another experimental question that appears to have implications for the interpretation of the results summarized here, is whether the oxygen dependency of cytochrome oxidase is similar in isolated mitochondria and intact cells. Dean and coworkers found a significant difference (1-5) while more recent results by Robiolio, et al. found no significant difference at the low [O_2] they used in their studies (8). This latter finding implies that oxygen freely moves across the membranes. There are at least two possible explanations that could account for both sets of results. The most probable explanation is that the two systems and experimental procedures are sufficiently different that they are not really comparable. A less likely but more interesting explanation is that cells have a mechanism for allowing low concentrations of oxygen into cells while tending to restrict higher concentrations of oxygen. This would make sense from a teleological point of view because cells need only low levels of oxygen in order to carry out aerobic metabolism but higher concentrations of oxygen are potentially quite toxic. A possible mechanism for allowing low concentrations of oxygen to enter cells while controlling the occurrence of higher levels would be to have a barrier to the free diffusion of oxygen that has a pore-like structure or function in it, which becomes more restrictive with increased [O_2].

CONCLUSIONS

Regardless of our ability to explain the basis for the experimental results, our results, which have been summarized here indicate that:

1. It is necessary, under some circumstances, to measure intracellular oxygen concentrations directly to obtain values that are pertinent for the processes being investigated.

2. The experimental findings, together with calculations of gradients expected on the basis of free diffusion of oxygen into cells, indicate that under some circumstances, free diffusion of oxygen into cells does not occur.

3. Cells appear to have a heretofore unrecognized mechanism that affects the entrance or availability of oxygen in the intracellular compartment.

ACKNOWLEDGEMENTS

This research was supported by a grant from the National Institutes of Health GM34250 and used the facilities of the Illinois EPR Research Center which is supported by NIH Grant RR01811.

REFERENCES

1. D.P. Jones, T.Y. Aw, and F.G. Kennedy, 1983, Isolated hepatocytes as a model for the study of cellular hypoxia, *In* : Isolation, Characterization and Use of Hepatocytes. R.A. Harris and N.W. Cornell, eds., Elsevier Sciences Publishing, Co., New York, .

2. D.P. Jones and H.S. Mason, 1978, Gradients of O_2 concentration in hepatocytes, *J. Biol. Chem.* 253:4874.

3. D.P. Jones, 1984, Effect of mitochondrial clustering on O_2 supply in hepatocytes, *Am. J. Physiol.* 247:C83.

4. D.P. Jones and F.G. Kennedy, 1982, Intracellular oxygen supply during hypoxia, *Am. Physiol. Soc.* 243:C247.

5. D.P. Jones and F.G. Kennedy, 1982, Intracellular O_2 gradients in cardiac myocytes. Lack of a role for myoglobin in facilitation of intracellular O_2 diffusion, *Biochim. Biophys. Res. Comm.* 105:419.

6. B.A. Wittenberg and J.B. Wittenberg, 1985, Oxygen pressure gradients in isolated cardiac myocytes, *J. Biol. Chem.* 260:6548.

7. C.R. Honig, T.E.J. Gayeski, W. Federspiel, A. Clark, Jr., and P. Clark, 1984, Muscle O_2 gradients from hemoglobin to cytochrome: new concepts, new complexities, *Adv. Exp. Med. Biol.* 169:23.

8. M. Robiolio, W.L. Rumsey, and D.F. Wilson, 1989, Oxygen diffusion and mitochondrial respiration in neuroblastoma cells, *Am. Physiol. Soc.* 256:C1207.

9. I.R. Katz, J.B. Wittenberg, B.A. Wittenberg, 1984, Monoamine oxidase an intracellular probe of oxygen pressure in isolated cardiac myocytes, *J. of Biol. Chem.* 259:7504.

10. M. Tamura, N. Oshino, B. Chance, and I.A. Silver, 1978, Optical measurements of intracellular oxygen concentration of rat heart in vitro, *Arch. of Biochem. and Biophys.* 191:8.
11. J.J.P. Fengler and R.E. Durand, 1990, Respiration-induced oxygen gradients in cultured mammalian cells, *Int. J. Radiat. Biol.*, 58:133.
12. S. Belkin, R.J. Mehlhorn, and L. Packer, 1988, Electron spin resonance oxymetry, *Methods in Enzymol*, 167:670.
13. H.M. Swartz and M.A. Pals, 1989, Measurement of intracellular oxygen, *In*: Handbook of Biomedicine of Free Radicals and Antioxidants, J. Miquel, H. Weber, and A. Quintanilha, eds., CRC Press Inc., Boca Raton, FL.
14. J. Glockner, H.M. Swartz, and M. Pals, 1989, Oxygen gradients in CHO cells: measurement and characterization by electron spin resonance, *J. Cell. Physiol.*, 140:505.
15. H. Hu, G. Sosnovsky, and H.M. Swartz, 1992, Development of EPR method for simultaneous measurement of intra- and extra-cellular $[O_2]$ in viable cells, *Biochim. Biophys. Acta*, 1112:161.
16. J.F. Glockner, S.W. Norby, and H.M. Swartz, 1992, Simultaneous measurement of intracellular and extracellular oxygen concentrations using a nitroxide-liposome system, *Magnetic Reson. in Med.*, 29:12-18.
17. W. Froncisz, C.-S. Lai, and J.S. Hyde, 1985, Spin-label oximetry: Kinetic study of cell respiration using a rapid-passage T_1-sensitive electron spin resonance display, *Proc. Natl. Acad. Sci. USA*, 87:411.
18. H.M. Swartz, 1987, Use of nitroxides to measure redox metabolism in cells and tissues, *J. Chem. Soc.* 83:191.
19. J.B. Wittenberg and B.A. Wittenberg, 1961, Active transport of oxygen and the eye of fish, *Biol. Bull.*, 121:379.
20. M.B. Fairbanks, J.R. Hoffert, and P.O. Fromm, 1974, Short circuiting the ocular oxygen concentrating mechanism in the teleost Salmo gairdneri using carbonic anhydrase inhibitors. *J. Gen. Physiol.* 64:263.
21. M.B. Fairbanks, J.R. Hoffert, and P.O. Fromm, 1969, The dependence of the oxygen-concentrating mechanism of the teleost eye (Salmo gairdneri) on the enzyme carbonic anhydrase, *J. Gen. Physiol.* 54:203.
22. Subczynski, W.K. and J.S. Hyde, 1984, Diffusion of oxygen in water and hydrocarbons using an electron spin resonance spin-label technique. *Biophys. J.* 45:743.
23. W.K. Subczynski, J.S. Hyde, and A. Kusumi, 1989, Oxygen permeability of phosphatidylcholine-cholesterol membranes. *Proc. Natl. Acad. Sci. USA*, 86:4474.
24. W.K. Subczynski, J.S. Hyde, and A. Kusumi, 1991, Effect of alkyl chain unsaturation and cholesterol intercalation on oxygen transport in membranes: a pulse ESR spin labeling study. *Biochem.* 30:8578.
25. W.K. Subczynski, E. Markowska, and J. Sielewiesiuk, 1991, Effect of polar carotenoids on the oxygen diffusion-concentration product in lipid bilayers. An ESR spin label study. *Biochim. Biophys. Acta*, 1068:68.
26. A. Vachon, V. Roman, C. Lecomte, G. Folcher, M. Fatome, P. Braquet, and F. Berleur, 1987, A radioprotector: cysteamine, inhibits oxygen transport in lipidic membranes, *Int. J. Radiat. Biol.*, 52:847.
27. W.K. Subczynski, G.E. Renk, R.K. Crouch, J.S. Hyde, and A. Kusumi, 1992, Oxygen diffusion-concentration product in rhodopsin as observed by a pulse ESR spin labeling method, *Biophys. J.*, In press.
28. C. Altenbach, T. Marti, H.G. Khorana, and W.L. Hubbell, 1990, Transmembrane protein structure: Spin labeling of bacteriorhodopsin mutants, *Science*, 248:1088.
29. W.K. Subczynski, L.E. Hopwood, and J.S. Hyde, 1992, Is the mammalian cell plasma membrane a barrier to oxygen transport?, *J. Gen. Physiol.*, 100:69.

DETECTION OF ABSORBERS IN A DYNAMIC SYSTEM USING NIR PHASE MODULATED DEVICE (PMD)

K. A. Kang, L. He, and B. Chance

Johnson Foundation, D501 Richards Bldg. , Department of
Biochemistry and Biophysics, University of Pennsylvania
Philadelphia, PA 19104-6089, USA

INTRODUCTION

The application of Near Infra Red (NIR) Spectroscopy to the biological system analysis has progressed rapidly during the past decade. This method has a great advantage for the biological system application because measurements can be performed non-invasively and the health risk caused by applying this light source is almost none. This method has been used for the analysis of a homogeneous steady state and slow dynamic biological systems. The theoretical derivation of phase shift in a homogeneous semi-infinite medium was derived by Patterson and Chance (1990). Sevick and Chance (1991) has developed an algorithm using Phase Modulated Spectroscopy (PMS) of dual wave lengths (754 and 816 nm) for measuring hemoglobin oxygen saturation. Smith and Chance (1992) measured brain oxygen saturation using dual wave lengths of PMS and time resolved spectroscopy (TRS). Haida and Chance (1992) developed a method for obtaining the ratio of oxy- and deoxy-hemoglobin absorption coefficients by using dual wavelengths measurements at two different separations between the source and the detector.

The basic theoretical principle of PMD in a homogeneous scattering medium is measuring transport delay between two points (a source and a detector) in terms of the phase delay of modulated wave. The concept of the phase modulated photon wave is analogous to a infinitely long string (figure 1), sinusoidally moving at a velocity of V_w, except that the light intensity of NIR spectroscopy decreases exponentially with the distance from the source. Assuming a point of this string is marked specifically when the point passes the source position, then it will take the time, τ_d, for this point to get to the detector which is separated with the distance of ρ. In other word, when this mark passes the source, the position of the string at the detector should be the one which has passed the source point the time of τ_d ago. If the two string waves passing through the source and the detector are superimposed at a certain time, there would be a phase difference of θ, between these two points.

Therefore, the transport delay may also be expressed as phase delay, θ (in radian), between the source and the detector as follows.

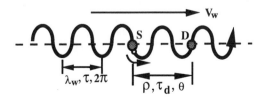

Figure 1. Basic principle of Phase Modulation Device (PMD). S and D denotes the source and the detector, respectively.

Oxygen Transport to Tissue XV, Edited by P. Vaupel
et al., Plenum Press, New York, 1994

$$\theta(\rho)=2\pi\frac{\rho}{\lambda_w} \quad = 2\pi\frac{\tau_d}{\tau} = 2\pi \ f \ \frac{\rho}{V_w}$$

(1)

where λ_w is the wave length, τ is the period of the sinusoidal wave, and f is the frequency of the wave.

When Eq. (1) is expressed for the velocity of the wave, V_w,

$$V_w = 2\pi \ f\frac{\rho}{\theta(\rho)}$$

(2)

For the system which has no boundary, the phase shift, $\theta(r)|_{inf}$, can be expressed as

$$\theta(\rho)|_{inf} = -\rho\sqrt{\frac{\mu_a}{D}}\sqrt{1+(\frac{2\pi f}{\mu_a C_n})^2} \ \sin\frac{\phi}{2}$$

(3)

where $\phi = \tan^{-1}(\frac{2\pi f}{\mu_a C_n})$,

(4)

μ_a and μ_s' are the absorption and the effective scattering coefficient, respectively, D is the diffusion coefficient, $D=1/[3(\mu_a +\mu_s')]$, C_n is light velocity in the scattering media, which is c/n (c is the light velocity in vacuum and n is the refractive index of the medium), and the subscript 'inf' denotes infinite space domain.

For a semi-infinite system (Patterson and Chance, 1990), the phase shift, $\theta(r)|_{sinf}$, is

$$\theta(\rho)|_{sinf} =-\psi \sin\frac{\phi}{2} -\tan^{-1}\frac{-\psi \sin\frac{\phi}{2}}{1+\psi \cos\frac{\phi}{2}}$$

(5)

where $\psi = \rho\sqrt{\frac{\mu_a}{D}}\sqrt{1+(\frac{2\pi f}{\mu_a C_n})^2}$,

(6)

and the subscript, 'sinf', denotes semi-infinite domain. Therefore, with knowing the absorption and the scattering coefficients, wave length, λ_w, may be computed by using the relationship,

$$\lambda_w = \rho \ \frac{2\pi}{\theta(\rho)} \ .$$

(7)

Therefore, for an infinite domain,

$$\lambda_w|_{inf} =\frac{2\pi}{\sqrt{\frac{\mu_a}{D}}\sqrt{1+(\frac{2\pi f}{\mu_a C_n})^2} \ \sin\frac{\phi}{2}}$$

(8)

and for a semi-infinite domain,

$$\lambda_w|_{sinf} =\frac{2\pi \ \rho}{\psi \sin\frac{\phi}{2}+\tan^{-1}\frac{-\psi \sin\frac{\phi}{2}}{1+\psi \cos\frac{\phi}{2}}} \ .$$

(9)

The followings are the approximated wave lengths for special cases in an infinite medium.

If $2\pi f << \mu_a C_n$, $\lambda_w|_{inf} = \frac{2 \ C_n}{f} \ \sqrt{\mu_a \ D} \ .$

(10)

For the case of $2\pi f << \mu_a C_n$ and $\mu_s' >> \mu_a$, $\lambda_w|_{inf} =\frac{2 \ C_n}{\sqrt{3} \ f} \sqrt{\frac{\mu_a}{\mu_s'}} \ .$

(11)

808

$$\text{If } 2\pi f = \mu_a C_n, \quad \lambda_w|_{inf} = \frac{2\pi}{4\sqrt{2}\,\sin\frac{\pi}{8}}\sqrt{\frac{D}{\mu_a}}\,. \tag{12}$$

For the case of $2\pi f = \mu_a C_n$ and $\mu_s' \gg \mu_a$, $\quad \lambda_w|_{inf} \cong \dfrac{8}{\sqrt{\mu_a\,\mu_s'}}\,.$ \hfill (13)

$$\text{If } 2\pi f \gg \mu_a C_n, \quad \lambda_w|_{inf} = \frac{\sqrt{2\pi\,C_n}}{\sin\frac{\pi}{4}}\sqrt{\frac{D}{f}}\,. \tag{14}$$

For the case of $2\pi f \gg \mu_a C_n$ and $\mu_s' \gg \mu_a$, $\quad \lambda_w|_{inf} \cong \dfrac{2\sqrt{C_n}}{\sqrt{\mu_s'\,f}}\,.$ \hfill (15)

For typical measurements in biological media, in the range of USA FDA safety regulation of laser power, the separation, ρ, is usually much smaller than the wave length, For example, for the infinite medium with $\mu_a = 0.05$ cm^{-1} and $\mu_s' = 10.0$ cm^{-1}, the wave length is, approximately, 10.3 cm. Therefore, a phase shift greater than 360^0 is very rare.

In a heterogeneous medium, a wave propagating in three dimensions is distorted by the localized absorbers or scatterers, therefore, the phase shift measured at positions near to an absorber is different from the medium without it. Whether the phase shift increases or decreases depends on the position, the volume, and the relative optical properties of the absorber or the scatterer to the media, Therefore, by analyzing the change in phase shift, the localized heterogeneity may be detected. When a localized absorber changes its volume in time the phase shift also changes in time. By quantifying the change in phase, the amount of change in absorber volume can be measured. In this paper it is demonstrated that the change in absorber volume as fast as 1 Hz can be detected by PMD.

THEORETICAL PREDICTION OF PHASE: SIMULATION RESULTS AND DISCUSSION

The governing equation for the photon fluence rate, $P(x,y,z,t)$, in an isotropic scattering medium can be expressed as a simple diffusion equation with constant consumption rate, μ_a (Patterson, 1990).

$$\frac{1}{C_n}\frac{\partial P}{\partial t} - D\,\nabla^2 P + \mu_a P = S(x,y,z,t) \tag{16}$$

where x, y, z is the spatial location in x, y, z direction (cm), respectively, t is the time (ps), and $S(x,y,z,t)$ is a source term. In order to see the possibilities of detecting the absorber changing its volume as fast as 1 Hz, by PMD, two computer simulations of a closed system were performed. The system simulated was a cube which has the dimension of 12 cm x 12 cm x 12 cm [figure 2 (a)]. For this simulated system, absorbing boundaries were chosen;

$$P(x=0.0, y, z, t) = P(x=12, y, z, t) = 0.0 \tag{17-a}$$

$$P(x, y=0.0, z, t) = P(x, y=12, z, t) = 0.0 \tag{17-b}$$

$$P(x, y, z=0.0, t) = P(x, y, z=12, t) = 0.0 \tag{17-c}$$

At the source, sinusoidally modulated intensity was placed;

$$P(x=6.0, y=4.0, z=0.0, t) = 1000{,}000\,(3.0 + \sin(2\pi f\,t)) \tag{17-d}$$

The position of the detector was at x=6.0, y=8.0, z=0.0.

Parameters used for the simulation were $\mu_a = 0.05$ (cm^{-1}), $\mu_s' = 10.0$ (cm^{-1}), $C_n = 3.0/1.33 \times 10^{10}$ (cm/s), and f = 200 (MHz). The numerical method used for the computation was a probabilistic numerical technique, the Bruley-Williford-Kang (B-W-K) technique [Williford, 1974; Bruley, (in press)]. This technique uses a transient density function at each nodal point. As a result, heterogeneous and non-isotropic problems can be solved by using proper density functions for different regions in three dimensions. The computation is done by the Cray Y-MP at the Pittsburgh Super Computing Center, Pennsylvania, USA.

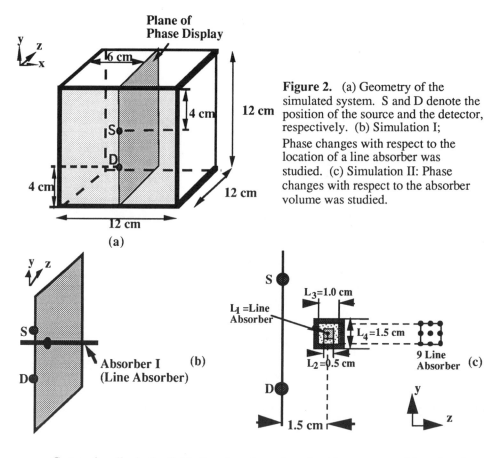

Figure 2. (a) Geometry of the simulated system. S and D denote the position of the source and the detector, respectively. (b) Simulation I; Phase changes with respect to the location of a line absorber was studied. (c) Simulation II: Phase changes with respect to the absorber volume was studied.

Conventionally, in the field of engineering, when there is a transport delay, the phase shift should be expressed in negative terms [see equations (3) and (4)]. However, in this paper, to follow previous researchers in NIR fields the delayed phase shift is expressed as positive value.

Simulation I: Phase Change with respect to the Position of a Line Absorber

This simulation was performed to study the effect of a location of the line absorber to the phase change. With the position of a perfect line absorber of the length 12 cm [x=0~12 cm, y, z; figure 2 (b)], phase changes with respect to its position in y and z direction were simulated. Figure 3 shows the three dimensional display of phase computed at the detector with the function of various positions of the line absorber in a simulated system. The simulation results showed that the phase detected at the detector, compared to the control

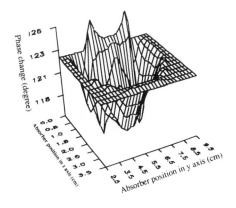

Figure 3. Phase change with respect to the line absorber position [see figure 2 (b) for the simulation system].

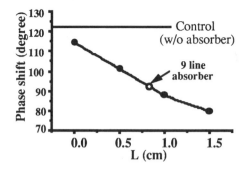

Figure 4. Phase change with change in absorber volume [see figure 3 (c) for the simulated system].

value (i.e. phase shift without absorber) increases rapidly close to the surface (approximately 0.5 cm) where the source and the detector were located. The phase change was maximized when the absorber was located very close to the source or the detector However, as the absorber moved away from the surface of the source and detector, the mean phase decreases rapidly and becomes minimized at approximately, z=2 cm, and then increased slowly back to the control value. At the plane, z=3.5 cm, the absorber location was too far to effect the mean phase shift. Sevick and Chance (in press) has studied on pathlength change with respect to the position of a black sphere. As in their study the simulation result showed that when the absorber is located near to the surface of the source and the detector, the phase increased because the absorber cuts the shorter paths between the source and the detector and, as a result, the mean phase shift (or the mean pathlength), becomes longer. From the gradient of the phase change it can also be shown that the photon density is not evenly distributed. Instead, the density of the near field photon is much denser and the change in phase could be more sensitive around the area close to the plane where the sources and detectors are located.

Simulation II: Phase Change with respect to the Volume of Absorber

The second simulation was design to see if there was any the phase change while an absorber changes its volume. In order to avoid the inconsistency of an increase or decrease of phase, the center of the absorber was fixed at 1.5 cm from the plane, z=0.0, which is far enough from the distance of phase increase as shown in the first simulation. For this simulation, five different absorber volumes were studied: (1) a line absorber ($L_1 = 0.0$ cm), (2) the edge length of the parallelpiped, $L_2=0.5$ cm, (3) the edge length, $L_3=1.0$ cm, (4) the edge length, $L_4=1.5$ cm, and (5) nine line absorbers in a cross sectional area of 1.0 cm^3 [figure 2 (c)], simulating a capillary bundle.

Figure 4 illustrates the simulation result of the phase change with the function of the volume of the absorber. When the center of different absorbers (x=1~12, y=7, and z=1.5 cm) located at the same position as the edge length (L) of the parallelepiped cross section were increased, the phase shift decreased. The absorber centered at 1.5 cm from the surface, z=0.0 cm, cut longer pathlengths. When the volume of the absorber increased the larger portion of long paths between the source and the detector disappeared. In other words, the volume of an absorber affected the mean phase shift by changing the degree of distortion. Therefore, the phase shift for a smaller object will be different from larger one although the center of the absorber location remains at the same position. As a result, when there is a change in the volume of an absorber in time, phase will also be changing in time. For example, if an absorber changes its cross section edge length from 0.5 cm to 1.0 cm, the phase shift changes from 100° to 90° (figure 4). If the absorber is a bundle of capillaries, and the volume of the capillaries expands, the phase changes from that of the bundle of line absorbers to 1 cm^3 cross sectional area filled with the expanded capillaries.

EXPERIMENTAL STUDY: RESULTS AND DISCUSSION

The experimental model studied was a cylinder of 13.5 cm diameter and 14.0 cm height, with an absorber in it [figure 5 (a)]. This cylinder had multiple ports around the wall for the fixture of light guides. For the experiment, two ports separated by 5.5 cm was used with the rest closed. The absorber used were: (1) A black absorber of diameter, 1.5 cm [figure 5 (b)] and (2) A bundle of silicone capillaries. The black absorber was designed in

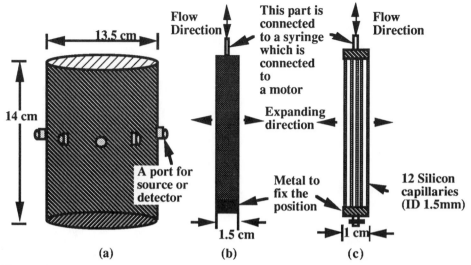

Figure 5. Schematic diagram of the experimental system. A black absorber (b) and a capillary bundle (c; 12 capillaries, ID of a capillary was 1.5 mm) which pulsated at a constant rate were located in a cylinder (a) filled with 0.25 % intralipid.

such a way that when there was a volume increase by injecting the liquid into it, the diameter of the absorber increased without longitudinal expansion in order to avoid multi-dimensional effect which might complicate the analysis of experimental result. The capillary model was composed of 12 capillaries evenly distributed in a 1 cm diameter circle and filled with 0.003 % indocyanine green in 0.25 % of intralipid solution [figure 5 (c)]. During the experiment absorbers were located in the cylinder filled with 0.25 % intralipid (donated by Kabi Pharmacia, Clayton, NC) and centered between the source and the detector. Both absorbers had metal ending on the bottom, which stabilized the position of the absorber during pulsation. Upper ends of absorbers were connected to a syringe, which was connected to a motor. During experiments the motor pushed or pulled the syringe at a constant RPM to pump a pre-determined amount of liquid in and out of the absorbers. For the experiment, the source and the detector were separated by 5.5 cm. Dual wavelength, 754 and 816 nm, NIR PMD (NIM Inc., Philadelphia, PA) was used to measure the phase change in terms of pathlength and recorded on a chart recorder.

Experiment I: Volume Change of the Black Absorber

Chance (1989) has studied dynamic change of hemoglobin oxygenation/deoxygenation during pathological condition of the brain by using the continuous wave and the time resolved spectroscopy. Studies on patients during cardiac bypass surgery and carotid artery occlusion for endarterectomy using PMD have been performed by Chance and his coworkers (Personal communication). In this study the experiments were designed to see if PMD could be used for the measurement in absorber volume or concentration change as fast as 1 Hz.

The first experiment was designed to see following variables,

(1) Location of the pulsating black absorber: For this experiment pulsation rate and the absorber expansion volume were constant at 7 RPM and 10 ml (diameter change, 0.4 cm), respectively. As can be seen in the figure 6 (a), as the center of the absorber moved far away from the source and detector the change in pathlength decreased, which could be expected from the simulation result (see figure 3). When the absorber was located at 1.5 cm from the rim of the cylinder, the pathlength of the wavelength, 816 nm, increased due to the cut on short pathlengths,

(2) Volume of black absorber: For this experiment, the absorber location was at 2.0 cm from the rim of the container and pulsation rate was 7 RPM. As the change in the absorber diameter increased due to the larger pumping volume, the pathlength changes increased rapidly [figure 6 (b)]. This was due to the increase of long path elimination due to the absorber volume expansion.

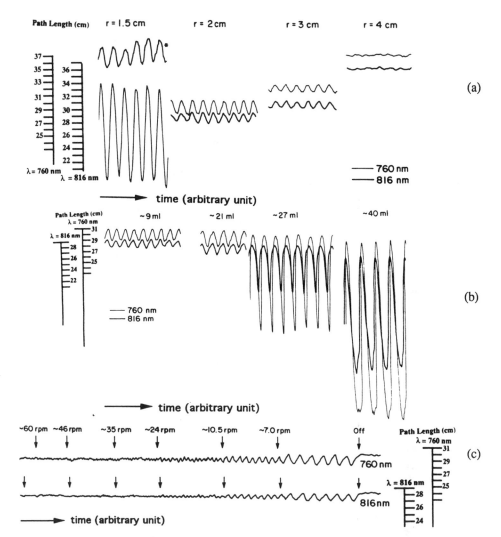

Figure 6. Phase (or pathlength) at various experimental conditions. Changes in (a) the location, (b) the pulsating volume, and (c) the pulsating frequency of black absorber. The medium in the cylinder was 0.25 % intralipid and the separation between the source and the detector was 5.5 cm.

(3) Pulsation rate: As can be seen figure 6 (c), when the pulsation rate increased the pathlength change measured decreased slowly, It was found that this phenomena was not due to the actual phase shift but due to the signal damping effect due to the slow machine time constant. For this experiment, a time constant of 2 second was used. When longer time constant than 2 second was used the signal almost disappeared at the moter speed less than 60 RPM.

Experiment II: Capillary Pulsation

For a second experiment, in order to simulate blood vessel pulsation, the capillary bundle [see figure 5 (c)] was used. The location of the capillary center was at 2.0 cm from the rim of the intralipid container. 6 ml of 0.003 % indocyanin green in 0.25 % intralipid solution was pulsated into 12 silicon capillaries at a predetermined rate. From the result, it can be shown the pulsation was clearly recorded without difficulties. As in the case of the black absorber, due to the machine time constant (2 seconds) the signal becomes reduced when the motor pumping rate increased. However, when the time domain signal at 60 RPM

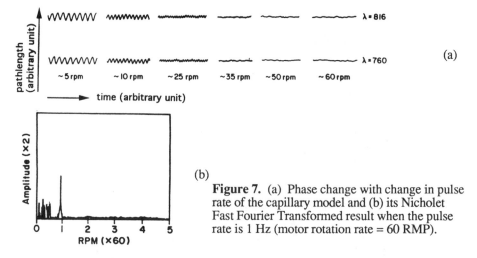

Figure 7. (a) Phase change with change in pulse rate of the capillary model and (b) its Nicholet Fast Fourier Transformed result when the pulse rate is 1 Hz (motor rotation rate = 60 RMP).

was transferred to frequency domain using Nicholet Fast Fourier Transformer, a clear peak appeared at 1 Hz.

CONCLUSION AND FUTURE APPLICATION

From the simulation and the experiments, it is concluded that PMD can be used for the detection of fast dynamic changes of absorber (~ 1 Hz). When the change is periodical the detectability can be improved by converting the time domain signal to frequency domain by using Fast Fourier Transformer.

This method could be applied to measuring the change of blood flow (or hemoglobin concentration) in time under certain physiological conditions, for example, in the determination of change in tissue arterial oxygen saturation.

ACKNOWLEDGMENT

This work was partially supported by NIH grant HL 44125.

REFERENCES

Bruley, D.F., "Modeling O2 Transport: Development of Methods and Current State", Proc. 1992 ISOTT, (in Press).

Chance, B., Smith, D.S., Nioka, S., Miyake, H., Holton, G., and Maris, M., "Photon migration in muscle and brain", 121-135, in Photon Migration in Tissue (Chance, B., ed.), Plenum, 1989.

Haida, M. and Chance, B., "A method to estimate the ratio of absorption coefficients of two wave lengths using phase modulated near infrared light spectroscopy", Proc. 1992 ISOTT, (in Press),

Patterson, M.S., Chance, B., and Wilson, B.C., "Time resolved reflectance and transmittance for the non-invasive measurement of tissue optical properties", Applied Optics, **28** (12), 2331-2336, 1989.

Patterson, M.S., Moulton, J.D., and Wilson, B.C., Chance, B., "Application of time-resolved light scattering measurements to photodynamic therapy dosimetry", Proc. SPIE, **1203**, 62-75, 1990.

Sevick, E.M., Wang, N.G., and Chance, B., Time dependent photon migration imaging, Proc. SPIE, **1599**, (in press).

Sevick, E.M., Chance, B., Leigh, J., Nioka, S., and Maris, M., "Quantitation of time-and frequency-resolved optical spectra for the determination of tissue oxygenation", Analytical Biochemistry, **195**, 330-351, 1991.

Smith, D.S., Levy, W.J., Carter, S., Wang, N.W., Haida, M., Chance, B., "Brain vascular hemoglobin saturation and light scattering in a population of normal volunteers", Abstract for Joint Anglo-American Neuro-Anesthesiology Mtg., London, 1992.

Williford, Jr., C., Bruley, D., and Artique, R., "Probabilistic Modelling of Oxygen Transport in Brain Tissue", NeuroResearch, **2**, 153-170, 1974.

NEAR-INFRARED OPTICAL IMAGING OF TISSUE PHANTOMS WITH MEASUREMENT IN THE CHANGE OF OPTICAL PATH LENGTHS

Eva M. Sevick[*], Christina L. Burch[*], and Britton Chance[†]

[*]Department of Chemical Engineering, Vanderbilt University
Nashville, TN 37235 USA
[†]Department of Biophysics and Biochemistry
University of Pennsylvania
Philadelphia, PA 19104 USA

INTRODUCTION

The possibility to non-invasively image hypoxic tissue volumes based upon oxy- and deoxy-hemoglobin absorbance exists with the development of near-infrared (NIR) biomedical optical imaging. However, image reconstruction presents problems for biomedical optical imaging since the direct correlation between incident and detected light is destroyed by multiple scattering. Using pulsed time measurements, Hebden and Kruger[1,2] and Andersson-Engels, et al.[3] have attempted to minimize the loss of correlation in their optical images by monitoring the intensity of scattered light that has travelled short distances within various "time-of-flight" windows between 37 and 320 picoseconds in duration. Upon integrating I(t) over time windows bounded by varying T_1 and T_2,

$$I^* = \int_{T_1}^{T_2} I(t)\, dt \qquad (1)$$

they reported I* images of 5 mm diam. absorbers located at varying depths within three to four centimeter thick tissue phantoms. These measurements were conducted using single source/single detector transillumination scanning measurements. In each of their studies, greater resolution was achieved upon using "time-of-flight" windows of smaller duration, as low as 37 picoseconds.

More recently, using multi-detector frequency domain techniques in reflectance geometries, Sevick, et al.[4] have demonstrated two-dimensional images of phase-shift, θ, providing the detection of a 3 mm perfect absorber located 1.2 cm deep within a tissue phantom. Phase-shift images created in the presence and absence of the absorber at 30 to 100 MHz modulation frequencies showed not only could "images" of the obscured object be formed from $\Delta\theta$ ($\theta_{presence} - \theta_{absence}$), but that the $\Delta\theta$ image was dependent upon modulation frequency: (i) at low modulation frequencies, the absorber was detected by negative values of $\Delta\theta$, (ii) at high modulation frequencies, by positive values of $\Delta\theta$, (iii) and at intermediate frequencies, the absorber was detected by $\Delta\theta = 0$. At a constant frequency, the presence of the absorber caused θ to decrease when it was located far and caused θ to increase when it was located close to the source and detector. Subsequent studies employing Monte Carlo simulations and single source/single detector measurements confirmed that the modulation frequency at which $\Delta\theta = 0$ (termed the zero-phase-shift frequency) is a unique function of the absorber z-position in x-y reflectance measurements[5]. Each of these studies indicate that the depth of tissue interrogated may be "focused" upon by simply changing the modulation frequency using reflectance measurements.

Since the frequency-domain parameter of θ is related to the mean "time-of-flight" ($<t>$) or optical path length ($<L>$)[6], we hypothesize that similar results should be obtained upon evaluating the time-resolved intensity using the following relationship:

$$<L> = c\frac{\int_{T_1}^{T_2} I(t)\,t\,dt}{\int_{T_1}^{T_2} I(t)\,dt} \qquad (2)$$

where c is the speed of light in the medium.

In this case, one might expect that there exists a unique time window, bounded by T_1 and T_2, for which the presence of an absorber at depth z causes no change in $<L>$. Thus, as in the frequency-domain measurements, the depth of tissue interrogated in time-domain studies may be "focused" upon simply by varying the time-window.

The objective of this study was, therefore, to demonstrate the detectability and the localization of an absorber located at varying z depths from values of $\Delta<L>$ ($<L>_{presence}$ - $<L>_{absence}$) as a function of: (i) time-window duration, Δt; (ii) upper "time-of-flight" bound, T_2; and (iii) lower "time-of-flight" bound, T_1. In the following, values of $\Delta<L>$ obtained from Monte Carlo simulation of photon migration are presented for a reflectance geometry with a perfect absorber located at varying positions along the midplane between the source and detector. The results and their implications for three dimensional localization of tissue optical heterogeneities are examined in light of a simple model for reflectance photon migration imaging. Future work to quantitate the x,y,z position and geometry from x,y reflectance measurements as well as future approaches to characterize the optical properties of tissue heterogeneities (such as hypoxic tissue zones) are also discussed.

MODEL FOR REFLECTANCE PHOTON MIGRATION IMAGING

The physical basis of reflectance photon migration imaging (PMI) has been described elsewhere[5,7], but is briefly reiterated here. Consider the transport of photons from a single point source to a point detector located a distance ρ in reflectance geometry on the surface of a scattering medium such as tissue. Photons emitted at the source and ultimately received at the detector have travelled a distribution of optical path lengths. The optical path length travelled by a migrating photon correlates with the probable penetration depth into the tissue. For example, photons which travel the longest optical path length have the greatest probability for penetrating deeply into the medium; and photons which travel the shortest optical path length migrate close to the

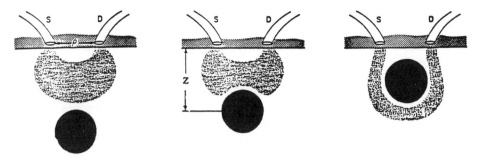

Figure 1 Physical basis of PMI. Reproduced from reference (6).

surface. In addition, the greater the separation between a source and detector, the longer optical path lengths and the greater the penetration depth. The volume of space that is significantly sampled by all photons migrating between the source and detector is defined as the "photon sampling volume" or PSV. Located far from the PSV, the presence of a light absorbing tissue volume does not significantly affect the distribution of optical path lengths of photons travelling within the PSV (Figure 1a). However if an absorbing volume is positioned close to the PSV, as shown schematically in Figure 1b, photons which have travelled the greatest penetration and are associated with the longest optical path length, are eliminated from the photon migration process. Thus the presence of the absorber effectively shortens the distribution of optical path lengths and decreases its mean, $<L>$. If the absorber position is moved closer to the surface (Figure 1c), detected photons may travel with increasing numbers and probabilities "around" as compared to "in front of" the absorber. In this case, the presence of the absorber effectively lengthens the distribution of optical path lengths and $<L>$. Furthermore, there should exist an intermediate position in which the numbers and probabilities for photon transport "around" and "in front of" the absorber are comparable, resulting in no net change in $<L>$. Thus, this physical model of PMI predicts: the presence of an absorber should initially cause (i) a decrease and (ii) a subsequent increase in $<L>$.

In the physical model described above, it is the interaction between the PSV and the light absorbing volume at varying positions that is the basis for increased and decreased $<L>$. However, in order to probe the depth of an absorbing volume at one position, one may varying the size of the PSV upon evaluating $<L>$ of photons which travel "time-of-flights" bounded by T_1 and T_2. Upon increasing T_2, photons which travel long "time-of-flights" and greater penetration depths are considered in the $<L>$ measurements. Upon increasing T_1, photons which travel short "time-of-flights" and shallow depths are excluded from the $<L>$ measurements.

From this qualitative model of time-domain PMI, several predictions regarding the relationships between $\Delta<L>$, T_1, T_2 and absorber position can be made:

(i) Regardless of Δt, T_1, and T_2, the approach of a perfect absorber midplane between a single source/detector in reflectance geometry will cause a decrease and subsequent increase in $<L>$.

(ii) The presence of the absorber will be detected from $\Delta<L>$ at distances farther from the source and detector when greater "time-of-flights" are considered.

(iii) For a given absorber position, the $\Delta<L>$ due to its presence will be positive when photons with long "time-of-flights" are considered, and negative when short "time-of-flights" are considered. At some intermediate window, termed the "zero path length change window" (ZPW), there will be no change in $\Delta<L>$ due to the presence of the absorber.

(iv) The ZPW is a unique function of the z- position and dimensions of the absorber. As the absorber positions are located at increasing depth, the ZPW must be associated with longer "time-of-flights."

MONTE CARLO SIMULATIONS OF I(t)

In order to examine the hypothesis, variance reduction Monte Carlo techniques similar to those used by Wilson and Adam[8] were employed to generate I(t). Specifically, 10^7 photons were injected one scattering length ($l^* = 1/(1-g)\mu_s$, where $(1-g)\mu_s$ is the isotropic scattering coefficient) into the phantom. Successive isotropic steps were taken, each of length, $L = -\ln(R)/(\mu_a + (1-g)\mu_s)$, where R is a uniformly distributed random number[9] between 0 and 1 and μ_a is the absorption coefficient. The time duration of the step was computed from $t = L/c$, where c is 3.0×10^{10} cm/sec $\div$ n, where n ($=1.4$) is the refractive index of the medium. At each step, the photon lost a fraction, $\mu_a/(\mu_a + (1-g)\mu_s)$, of its weight, which was initially set to one. In the simulated phantom containing the absorber, the photon migration was stopped if the photon migrated into the volume simulating the perfect absorber. Otherwise, the photon migration continued until the photon either (i) encountered a detector or (ii) migrated out of the phantom undetected. If the photon was detected at a 2 mm-diam. detector, then simulation parameters of total elapsed time, final photon weight, and the location and photon weight at each time step were recorded. The latter data enabled mapping of the PSV.

Unfortunately, three dimensional Monte Carlo simulations did not provide adequate time-resolved statistics at detector positions at significant distances away from the source (> 1 cm) in the presence of the absorber. For this reason, two dimensional simulations were conducted using the parameters listed in Figure 2. CPU time for the launching of 10^7 photons on a 486 50 MHz IBM machine took approximately 6 hours. Since these simulations were conducted in two-dimensional space with values of c, $(1-g)\mu_s$, and μ_a for three-dimensional photon migration, the

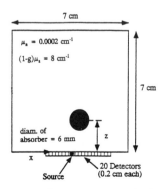

Figure 2 Schematic for 2-D Monte Carlo simulations.

effective speed of the photon in 2-D space can be considered to be $\sqrt{3/2}$ greater than in 3-D. All "time-of-flights" reported herein are therefore $\sqrt{3/2}$ greater than one would expect experimentally.

In order to investigate the effect of absorber position upon $\Delta <L>$ as a function of Δt, T_1, and T_2, two dimensional Monte Carlo simulations for the following conditions were conducted: (i) in the absence of the absorber, and (ii) in its presence with the centroid positioned from z = 0.34 cm to z = 3.1 cm in 14 increments. Values of $\Delta <L>$ (= $<L>_{presence}$ - $<L>_{absence}$) were computed for each simulation from simulated I(t) and equation (2) at varying T_1 and T_2. Only those photons arriving at a detector 2 cm away from the source are considered herein.

RESULTS AND DISCUSSION

$\Delta <L>$ due to the presence of the absorber at varying positions Figure 3 illustrates the computed values of $\Delta <L>$ versus absorber position for three different time-windows of 975 picoseconds duration. Consistent with the physical model of PMI described above, $\Delta <L>$ was zero when the absorber is located far (>3.0 cm for T_2 = 975 picoseconds) from the source and detector plane and the photon migration was unaffected by its presence. However, as the absorber moved closer, photons which travelled the longest optical path lengths were extinguished from the migration process, resulting in a optical path shortening (or a negative value of $\Delta <L>$). As the absorber became located closer, photons began to travel "around" the absorber, reversing the $\Delta <L>$ trend to a point at which the presence of the absorber caused no change ($\Delta <L>$ = 0). Further approach of the absorber resulted in the elimination of photons which travelled the shortest optical path lengths, causing optical path lengthening (or a positive value of $\Delta <L>$). In addition, Figure 3 shows that the absorber was detected by nonzero $\Delta <L>$ values at greater z distances away from the source and detector when T_2 was lengthened from 975 picoseconds to 1462 and 1950 picoseconds. Again, this is consistent with the model of PMI which predicts that the absorber will be detected at greater z depths when greater "time-of-flights" are considered.

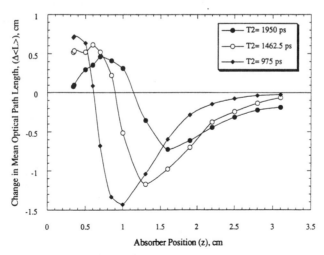

Figure 3 $\Delta <L>$ versus absorber position as a function of T_2.

$\Delta <L>$ **due to the presence of the absorber at varying "time-of-flight" windows.** Figures 4 and 5 similarly show $\Delta <L>$ versus absorber position for various time-windows in which (a) $T_1 = 19.5$ picoseconds and T_2 was varied between 975 and 1462 picoseconds and (b) $T_2 = 1462$ picoseconds and T_1 was varied between 19.5 and 585 picoseconds. Figure 4 also illustrates that absorber detection from non-zero values of $\Delta <L>$ occurred at deeper absorber positions at greater "time-of-flights" or increased T_2. Multi-frequency plots of $\Delta\theta$ versus z^5 are analogous to that shown in Figure 4.

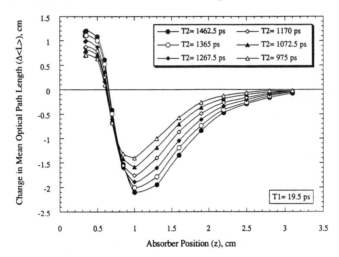

Figure 4 $\Delta <L>$ versus absorber position as a function of T_2.

Figure 5 is also consistent with the PMI model, showing little change in the absorber detectability at deep absorber positions with varying T_2. However, the absorber position associated with $\Delta <L> = 0$ and with photon transport with equal numbers and probabilities "around" as "in front of" the absorber, was extremely sensitive to changing T_1. Comparison of Figures 4 and 5 show that the absorber position associated with $\Delta <L> = 0$ dramatically changed with T_1, but changed little with T_2. It is important to note that in frequency-domain measurements, changing modulation frequency is comparable to changing T_1^5. Thus, time-domain measurements may provide more sensitive localization information than possible in the frequency-domain.

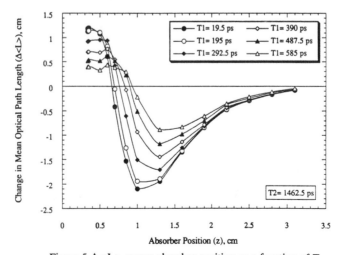

Figure 5 $\Delta <L>$ versus absorber position as a function of T_1.

"Time-of-flight" windows at which $\Delta <L> = 0$ Figure 5 suggests that time-window at which $\Delta <L> = 0$, or the ZPW, provides information regarding the z- position and dimensions of the absorber. Thus upon "tuning" Δt, T_1 and T_2 to find the ZPW, localization information may be obtained. This is similar to the previously proposed frequency-domain imaging[5] in which the modulation frequency is "tuned" until $\Delta \theta = 0$ for identification of absorber position. Multi-pixel frequency-domain "images" obtained by scanning at multiple frequencies demonstrate this behavior[5]. In the time-domain measurements, scanning can be accomplished by interrogating photon migration (i) within a time window of constant Δt at increasing T_1 or (ii) in various time-window durations, Δt at constant T_1 and increasing T_2. Again, time-domain scanning employing increasing T_1 is analogous to multi-frequency scans in which the modulation frequency is increased.

Figure 6 illustrates $\Delta <L>$ due to the presence of an absorber at $z = 7$ mm as monitored in various sized time-windows, Δt, as a function of T_2. There are several points to note from Figure 6: (i) Regardless of Δt, at relatively small T_2, the presence of the absorber resulted in path shortening (negative $\Delta <L>$) and at relatively large T_2, caused optical path lengthening (positive $\Delta <L>$). This is consistent with the results shown in Figure 4. (ii) At increasing Δt, the PSV associated with the photon migration increased, causing the absorber to be placed relatively less deep. Thus, path lengthening occurred at $\Delta t = 1365$ picoseconds. At $\Delta t = 780$ picoseconds, predominate path shortening occurred. (iii) The values of T_2 associated with the ZPW (at $\Delta <L> = 0$) increased with Δt. In the case of an arbitrarily placed absorber

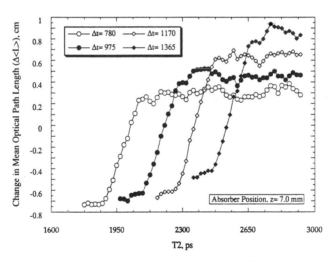

Figure 6 $\Delta <L>$ versus T_2 as a function of Δt.

probed with photons travelling a wide Δt time-window, photons travelling the upper "time-of-flight" limit, T_2 must penetrate greater depths and photons travelling the lower "time-of-flight" limit, T_1, must penetrate more shallow depths for photon transport to occur "in front of" and "around" the absorber with equal numbers and probabilities. Indeed, Figure 7 shows that the T_1 associated with $\Delta <L> = 0$ decreases with time-window duration, Δt. In addition, T_1 associated with $\Delta <L> = 0$ increases as the depth of the absorber increases. Each of these trends are consistent with the PMI model described in Figure 1.

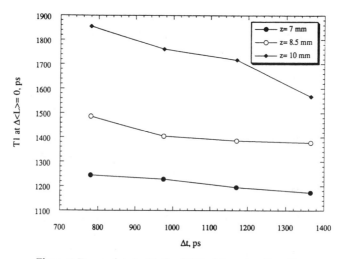

Figure 7 T_1 associated with the ZPW of time duration Δt.

SUMMARY

Using 2-D Monte Carlo simulations, we have demonstrated that values of $\Delta <L>$ at varying Δt, T_1 and T_2 can contain significant information concerning the presence and location of a light absorbing volume in scattering media such as tissue. Specifically, we have illustrated that relationships exist between ZPW measured in x,y reflectance geometries and the absorber x,y,z position. These relationships are predictable yet can be expected to furthermore vary with (i) absorber z-dimensions, (ii) the optical properties of the surrounding media, and (iii) the source/detector separation, ρ. In addition, while we have reported absorber positions located within 1 cm of tissue thickness for ρ = 2 cm, One can expect interrogation of absorbers located at greater tissue thicknesses with greater ρ^4. Most importantly, it is noteworthy that there exists greater opportunity to monitor specific population of photons in time-domain PMI than in frequency-domain PMI. Therefore, time-domain localization may be more sensitive than in the frequency-domain. From comparison to PMI, Figure 8 illustrates the values of ΔI^* computed from equation (1) versus absorber position for the same values T_1 and T_2 as in Figure 3. Upon inspection of Figures 3

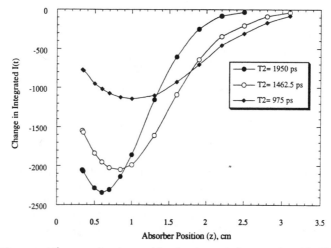

Figure 8 ΔI^* versus absorber position for time- windows employed in Figure 3

and 8, one can see that it is easier to infer the relationship between the PSV and the absorber position from $\Delta<L>$ than from ΔI^*. As a consequence, the measurement of $\Delta<L>$ may enable creation of an inverse localization algorithm for photon migration imaging.

In order to elucidate such a complete imaging algorithm, further study of PMI is warranted: (i) studies using multiple wavelengths to demonstrate the potentials of $\Delta<L>^\lambda$ ($= <L>^{\lambda 1} - <L>^{\lambda 2}$) imaging for elimination of the biomedically unfeasible "absence" condition required in these current PMI studies[4,5]; (ii) studies employing imperfect absorbers and differential scatterers to uncover potential algorithms for characterization of optical properties of tissue heterogeneities, hypoxic tissue volumes, exogenously-duped tissues, etc.; and (iii) studies employing phantoms of varying optical properties to ascertain the limitations of optical imaging all must be conducted in order to uncover an algorithm for detection, localization, and characterization of tissue heterogeneities using PMI.

ACKNOWLEDGEMENTS

This work was supported by NIM, Inc., Hamamatsu Photonics, Inc. and the Whittaker Foundation (EMS).

REFERENCES

1. J.C. Hebden and R.A. Kruger, Transillumination imaging performance: spatial resolution simulation studies, *Med. Phys.* 17:41 (1990).
2. J.C. Hebden, R.A. Kruger, and K.S. Wong, Time resolved imaging through a highly scattering medium, *Appl. Optics.* 30:788 (1991).
3. S. Andersson-Engels, R. Berg, S. Svanberg, and O. Jarlman, Time-resolved illumination for medical diagnostics, *Opt. Lett.* 15:1179 (1990).
4. E.M. Sevick, J.R. Lakowicz, H. Szmacinski, K. Nowaczyk, and M.L. Johnson, Frequency-domain imaging of absorbers obscured by scattering, *J.Photochem. and Photobiol.* 16:169-185, 1992.
5. E.M. Sevick, J.K. Frisoli, C.L. Burch, and J.R. Lakowicz, Localization of absorbers in scattering media using frequency domain measurements of time-dependent photon migration, *in press*.
6. E.M. Sevick, B. Chance, J. Leigh, S. Nioka, and M. Maris, Quantitation of time- and frequency-resolved optical spectra for the determination of tissue oxygenation, *Anal. Biochem.* 195:330 (1991).
7. B.C. Wilson, E.M. Sevick, M.S. Patterson, and B. Chance, Time-dependent optical spectroscopy and imaging for biomedical applications, *Proc. IEEE* 80: 918 (1992).
8. B.C. Wilson and G. Adam, A Monte Carlo model for the absorption and flux distributions of light in tissue, *Med. Phys.* 10:324 (1983).
9. W.H. Press, B.P. Flannery, S.A. Teulkolsky, and W.T. Vetterling, "Numerical Recipes," Cambridge University Press, New York (1989).
10. M.S. Patterson, B. Chance, and B.C. Wilson, Time-resolved reflectance and transmittance for the non-invasive measurement of tissue optical properties, *Appl. Opt.* 28:2331 (1989).

NIRS IN THE TEMPORAL REGION - STRONG INFLUENCE OF EXTERNAL CAROTID ARTERY

DNF Harris[1], FM Cowans[2], DA Wertheim[2]

Departments of Anaesthesia[1], Paediatrics[2], Royal Postgraduate Medical School, London, England. W12 0NN

INTRODUCTION

NIRS in transmission mode has been shown to provide useful information on intra cerebral oxygenation in neonates[1,2], and is beginning to be applied to adults using reflectance oximetry[3,4]. The relative contribution of intra- and extra- cranial blood pools to the NIRS signal is not known, but initial results during selective carotid injection suggested a greater extra-cranial component than theoretical data had suggested. This study investigates the response of NIRS using temporal and frontal optodes to a change in external carotid flow (teeth clenching) and in internal carotid flow (rise in CO_2) using Doppler measurement of blood velocity.

METHODS

6 normal volunteers, aged 26-44, were studied. 4 were male, 2 female.

NIRS

Absorption of NIR by the oxidised and reduced fractions of Haemoglobin (HbO, HbR) was measured at 6 wavelengths from 779-991nm (NIR 1000, Hamamatsu Photonics UK). The transmitting optode was placed over the thinnest part of the temporal bone, taking care to avoid the insertion of temporalis, and the receiving optode attached 5 cm apart, high on the frontal bone. The optodes were secured with adhesive tape and covered with a light-tight bandage. Data was collected every 2 seconds (10K photons).

Teeth Clenching

After 2 minutes at rest, subjects clenched their teeth as hard as they could for 30 seconds. 30 minutes later the test was repeated (in a preliminary study blood velocity returned to baseline 12 minutes after release of clenching). Subjects were instructed to

Oxygen Transport to Tissue XV, Edited by P. Vaupel
et al., Plenum Press, New York, 1994

breathe at the same rate and depth throughout, with no breath holding. A further 30 minutes rest was given before the hypercapnic tests.

CO₂

Subjects took deep slow regular breaths, with End tidal CO_2 ($EtCO_2$) and FIO_2 measured throughout. After 2 min on room air, subjects breathed 100% oxygen for 5 minutes. At end expiration the fresh gas was stopped, and subjects rebreathed from the closed circuit until the $EtCO_2$ had risen 3 kPa. After 20 minutes rest the test was repeated. FIO_2 never fell below 0.5, and SaO_2 remained at 100% in all subjects.

Doppler

External Carotid Artery velocity (ECV) was measured in the neck (Vingmed CFM 700). Care was taken to ensure no movement of the probe during clenching, and minimal increase in jugular venous signal during hypercapnia. Middle Cerebral Artery velocity (MCAV) was measured transcranially using the standard technique[5].

RESULTS

Teeth Clenching

HbR increased sharply (0.45 +/- 0.02 mmol.cm) and HbO fell (-0.39 ± 0.08 mmol.cm) during clenching (see fig. 1); on release HbR fell quickly to near baseline (+0.03 at 1 minute), while HbO rose above baseline (0.13 +/- 0.07) and was slower to return (1.5-4 minutes). During clenching Hb Diff (HbO-HbR) fell by 0.95 +/- 0.16 mmol.cm. For each subject the change in Hb Diff on the second test was within 8% of the first. There was no change in the Cytochrome signal during the test. ECV did not change during clenching, but increased sharply on release (30 +/- 10%), returning slowly to baseline (6 ± 4 min). MCAV was unchanged.

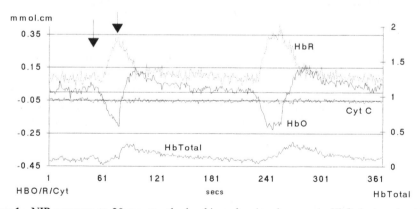

Figure 1. NIR response to 30 sec. teeeth clenching, showing decrease in HbO during clenching, with hyperaemic rebound after. Arrows show start and end of clenching. Cytochrome signal is stable throughout.

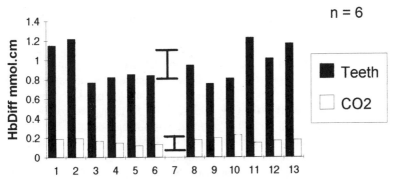

Figure 2. HbDiff response of 6 subjects to teeth clenching and to hypercapnia (2 tests for each subject). The bars indicates +/- 1 S.D.

CO$_2$

On breathing 100% Oxygen HbO increased (0.08 +/- 0.03) and HbR decreased (0.07 +/- 0.02) to produce an increase in Hb Diff of 0.15 +/- 0.008 mmol.cm, for a 2.8 +/- 0.2% increase in SaO$_2$. At maximum EtCO$_2$ (increase of 3.0 +/- 0.02 kPa) HbO increased (0.1 +/- 0.03) and HbR decreased further (0.07 +/- 0.02), for an increase in Hb Diff of 0.18 +/- 0.03 mmol.cm) (see figure 2). There was no change in MCAV or ECV with O$_2$. MCAV increased 70 +/- 8% at max. EtCO$_2$, while ECV rose slightly (10 +/- 3%).

The change in HbDiff with teeth clenching was much greater than for hypercapnia (0.95 +/- 0.16 v. 0.18 +/- 0.03 mmol.cm, p < 0.05).

DISCUSSION

With NIRS, the accepted theory suggests that mean depth of penetration of the signal increases in proportion to the interoptode spacing, as the scattering of the infra-red beam becomes random within a short distance of the surface. According to Monte Carlo modelling, at 5 cm separation the majority of the signal should have passed through the intracranial tissues, and the contribution of skin, subcutaneous and bony tissues should be

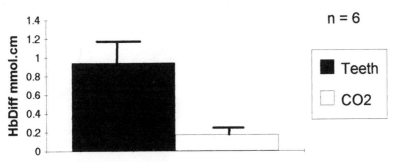

Figure 3.   Difference in HbDiff response to Teeth Clenching and Hypercapnia (mean of 6 subjects)

small. Indeed McCormick[6] has suggested that even at 3 cm optode separation changes in intra-cerebral oxygenation tissue can be measured.

Hypercapnia produced an increase in intracranial flow, with only a small increase in extra-cranial flow, and could be used as a marker of a change in intracranial oxygen delivery: teeth clenching produced a classical hyperaemic response in extracranial tissues, with no change in intracranial flow. The change in oxygenation measured by NIRS during teeth clenching was 5 times that for CO_2, although the % change in arterial velocity for teeth clenching was half that of CO_2. Optode positioning and stability is critical for accurate NIRS measurements;, and contraction of temporalis could have produced movement of the optodes, although this usually affects all signals in the same direction. No movement was visible, and the stability of the amplified cytochrome signal suggests that none occurred. The temporalis muscle was between the optodes, and blood flow / 100g would be higher than for non-muscular areas, especially during hyperaemia; however the muscle is less than 5 mm thick and mainly tendinous at this point. As hypercapnia and teeth clenching are different stimuli, these results cannot show what proportion of the signal comes from the 2 carotid territories, but they suggest that the contamination from tissues supplied by the external carotid artery may be much greater than has been thought.

Other optode positions away from temporalis over less well perfused tissues might show a smaller signal from external carotid territory. It is difficult to produce an isolated uniform change in external carotid flow, but testing with heat and cold would be more similar physiologically to hypercapnia and may prove useful.

REFERENCES

1. A.D. Edwards, J.S. Wyatt, C. Richardson et al, Cotside Measurements of cerebral blood flow in ill newborn infants by near infrared spectroscopy, Lancet Oct 1: 770 (1988).
2. J.E. Brazy, M.D. Lewis, M.H. Mitnick et al, Noninvasive monitoring of cerebral oxygenation in preterm infants: preliminary observations, Pediatrics 75 : 217 (1985).
3. N.B. Hampson, E.M. Camporesi, B.W. Stolp et al, Cerebral Oxygen availability by NIR spectroscopy during transient hypoxia in humans, J. Appl. Physiol. 69(3) : 907 (1990).
4. M. Ferrari, E. Zanette, G. Sideri et al, Effects of carotid compression, as assessed by near infrared spectroscopy, upon cerebral blood volume and haemoglobin oxygen saturation, J.R.S.M. 80 : 83 (1987).
5. R. Aaslid, K-F. Lindegaard, W. Sorteberg etal, Cerebral autoregulation dynamics in humans, Stroke 20 : 45 (1988).
6. P.W. McCormick, M. Stewart, G. Lewis et al, Intracerebral penetration of infra-red light, J. Neurosurg. 76: 315 (1992)

A METHOD TO ESTIMATE THE RATIO OF ABSORPTION COEFFICIENTS OF TWO WAVELENGTHS USING PHASE MODULATED NEAR INFRARED LIGHT SPECTROSCOPY

Munetaka Haida and Britton Chance

Johnson Research Foundation, D501 Richards Bldg., Department of Biochemistry and Biophysics, School of Medicine, University of Pennsylvania, Philadelphia, PA 19104-6089, USA

INTRODUCTION

Near infrared (NIR) spectroscopy provides a very useful tool to monitor the oxygen saturation of living biological tissue non-invasively (1-3). Since the biological tissue has a very high effective scattering factor ($\mu s'$), the light travels a relatively long path length making it difficult to compute the absorption coefficient (μa) by usual methods. Phase Modulation Spectroscopy (PMS) is one method to measure the optical path length, and estimate the μ_a from a highly scattering media. By measuring the ratio of the μa's of two different light wavelengths, we can determine the hemoglobin (Hb) oxygen saturation within the tissue (4). A technique using two modulated frequencies at two wavelength has been reported by Sevick et al. (4). This method requires a more complicated system for determining the ratio of μ_a. In this report, we present an improved method for obtaining the ratio of the absorption coefficients using a single frequency PMS system.

THEORY

The photon density response in a homogeneous media can be estimated by the diffusion equation of photons by Ishimaru (5)

$$\frac{1}{c_n}\frac{\partial}{\partial t}\phi(r,t) - D\nabla^2\phi(r,t) + \mu_a\phi(r,t) = S(r,t) , \qquad [1]$$

where S(r, t) is the input light function. D is the photon diffusion constant defined as $D=1/[3(\mu_a+(1-g)\mu_s)]$, g is the directional cosine and μ_s is the scattering coefficient, $(1-g)\mu_s$ is the effective scattering factor (μ_s') and c_n is the light velocity in the tissue ($c_n=c/n$; n is the refractive index of tissues), respectively. In this paper, the absorption coefficients are based upon Napierian log expression.

A response function to the input of light impulse, $S(r,t) = \delta(t) \bullet \delta(r-r_s)$, in the semi-infinite boundary conditions and a reflectance configuration, R(ρ,t) has been obtained by Patterson et al. (6)

Oxygen Transport to Tissue XV, Edited by P. Vaupel
et al., Plenum Press, New York, 1994

$$R(\rho,t) = (4\pi Dc_n)^{-\frac{3}{2}} z_0 t^{-\frac{5}{2}} \exp(-\mu_a c_n t)\exp(-\frac{\rho^2+z_0^2}{4\pi Dc_n t}) \,, \qquad [2]$$

where ρ is the distance between the light source and detector and z_0 is the mean free path length of the media ($z_0=1/(1-g)\mu_s$).

For the PMS, the amplitude of the input signal $S(r,t)$ in equation (1) is modulated with a frequency f ($S(r,t) = A\sin(2\pi ft) + A$). The response function at the detector position separated from the source by a distance, ρ(cm), is a convolution of equation (1) with the input function $S(r,t)$. In the frequency domain, the convolution of two functions is the multiplication of their Fourier transformed functions. The Fourier transformed function of equation (2) has been obtained by Patterson et al (7). A Fourier transformation of the $A\sin(2\pi ft)$ is a delta function at frequency f. Multiplication with the Fourier transformed equation (2) has a component of frequency f as shown in equation (3). Equation (3) represents the phase components of the system response, when it is stimulated by the amplitude modulated input light.

$$\theta(\rho,f) = -\Psi\sin\frac{\Theta}{2} - \tan^{-1}\frac{-\Psi\sin\dfrac{\Theta}{2}}{1+\Psi\cos\dfrac{\Theta}{2}}, \qquad [3]$$

where,

$$\Psi = \sqrt{3(1-g)\mu_s}\sqrt{(\mu_a c_n)^2 + (2\pi f)^2 c_n^{-1}}\,\rho,$$

$$\Theta = \tan^{-1}(\frac{2\pi f}{\mu_a c_n}).$$

It is easy to show using Figure 1 that the second term of the equation (3) is equal to $\frac{\Theta}{2} - \delta$. The value of δ depends on the separation ρ, but it is negligibly small at large Ψ. The following relation will always hold, $\frac{\Theta}{2} < \frac{\pi}{4}$ and $\sin\frac{\Theta}{2} < 0.707 < \cos\frac{\Theta}{2}$.

The phase angle θ of the photon density wave, therefore, will change linearly with the ρ, and we can define a wave number, k, as follows,

$$k = \sqrt{3(1-g)\mu_s}\sqrt{(\mu_a c_n)^2 + (2\pi f)^2 c_n^{-1}}\,\sin(\frac{\Theta}{2}) \qquad [4]$$

From equation (4), we can obtain the wavelength, $\lambda=2\pi/k$, and phase velocity, $v=\lambda f=2\pi f/k$, of the photon density wave in terms of the separation, ρ. The phase delay (θ) due to tissue at separation, ρ, can be expressed as follows,

$$\theta = k\rho + \frac{\Theta}{2} - \delta, \qquad [5]$$

where δ is a negligibly small term (Figure 1).

For two different light wave lengths, λ_1 and λ_2, it can be expected that the relations $\mu a^{\lambda_1} \neq \mu a^{\lambda_2}$ and $\mu s^{\lambda_1} = \mu s^{\lambda_2}$ hold. When we measure two phase delays of two wave lengths $\theta_1^{\lambda_1}, \theta_1^{\lambda_2}$ and $\theta_2^{\lambda_1}$ and $\theta_2^{\lambda_2}$, at two different separations, ρ_1 and ρ_2, it is easy to eliminate the $\frac{\Theta}{2} - \delta$ and μ_s' term from equation (4) and (5) by simple calculation.

830

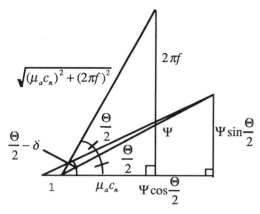

Figure 1. A schematic explanation of equation (3), whose second term is equal to $\frac{\Theta}{2} - \delta$. In the case of large Ψ, δ is close to zero.

$$r_\theta = \frac{(\theta_1^{\lambda_1} - \theta_2^{\lambda_1})}{(\theta_1^{\lambda_2} - \theta_2^{\lambda_2})} = \frac{\sin(\frac{\omega\tau^{\lambda_2}}{2r})}{\sin(\frac{\omega\tau^{\lambda_2}}{2})} \sqrt[4]{\frac{r^2 + (\omega\tau^{\lambda_2})^2}{1 + (\omega\tau^{\lambda_2})^2}} , \qquad [6]$$

where $\omega = 2\pi f$, $\tau^{\lambda_2} = \dfrac{1}{\mu_a^{\lambda_2} c_n}$ and $r = \dfrac{\mu_a^{\lambda_1}}{\mu_a^{\lambda_2}}$.

Equation (6) has only two unknown values $\mu a^{\lambda 1}$ and $\mu a^{\lambda 2}$, or their ratio (r) = $\mu a^{\lambda 1}/\mu a^{\lambda 2}$. In case of $\omega\tau < 1$, this equation is simplified as follows,

$$r = \frac{1}{r_\theta^2}. \qquad [7]$$

Figure 2 shows the relationship between the calculated value of $\dfrac{1}{r_\theta^2}$ and ratio of μa using equation (6) in the case of $\mu a\lambda 2 = 0.06$ (cm-1) at f=200MHz, which shows that the equation (7) holds in r>0.6 region.

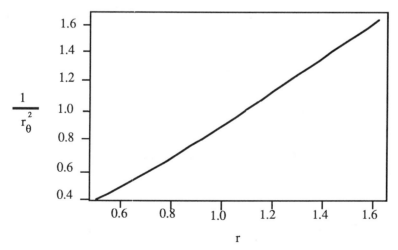

Figure 2. The relationship between $1/r_\theta^2$ vs. r, at $\mu a = 0.06$ (cm-1) and f=200 MHz.

MATERIAL AND METHOD

We made an experiment to prove the validity of the above algorithm using Intralipid solutions and India ink as the absorber.

We made the Time Resolved Spectroscopy (TRS) measurements and PMS measurements on 1% Intralipid solution (Kabi Pharmatica Inc., NC, U.S.A.) and Black India Ink (Faber-Castell, No 4416, NJ, U.S.A.). For the TRS measurements, we used a semiconductor laser source ($\lambda = 830$ nm, HAMAMATSU, PLP, Hamamatsu, Japan), a time correlated single photon counting system (TENNELEC, Time Correlated Single Photon Counting System, USA) and a multichannel plate-photo multiplier tube detector (HAMAMATSU, R1712-U, Hamamatsu, Japan). For PMS measurements, a phase modulated spectroscopy system ($\lambda =754$ nm and 816 nm, the modulation frequency is 200 MHz, NIM Corp., PMD-3000b, PA, USA) was used. The Intralipid was diluted to 1 % (w/w) solution by distilled water. The fiber diameters were 250 µm (single mode fiber) for the source and 3 mm for the detector in the TRS measurements, and 5 mm for the source and 6 mm for the detector in the PMS, respectively. The container size was 17.5 x 28.0 x12.0 (cm³), the inside wall of which was painted black. The amount of Intralipid solution was 5000 ml. The fibers were fixed in the Intralipid solution in a reflectance configuration. The separation of the source and detector fiber was 4 cm for the TRS measurements, and 2.5 cm and 3 cm for the PMS,respectively. The absorption coefficient of the solution was changed by adding a small amount of the India ink into the solution. The TRS and PMS measurements were made alternatively on the same concentration of the India ink. The India ink was added up to the concentration of 37.5 (µg/ml). We determined the absolute value of the absorption coefficients, μ_a^{780}, by the TRS measurements. The obtained experimental time resolved curves were de-convoluted using an instrument function which was obtained at the time of the experiment to get a true response function of the system. The response function of each concentration of the India ink was fitted by equation (2) using the least mean square method to

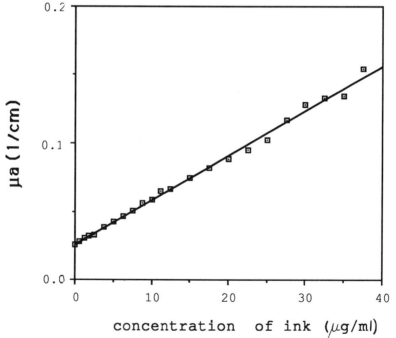

Figure 3. The concentration of India ink(µg/ml) vs. the absorption coefficient μ_a^{780}, measured by TRS method. The regression line is expressed as
$y = 3.254 \times 10^{-3} x + 2.58 \times 10^{-2}$, $r^2 = 0.996$.

get the parameter μ_a^{780}. We measured the phase shifts in the solutions using the dual wave length system ($\lambda_1=756$ nm and $\lambda_2=816$ nm) at the two different separations (2.5 cm and 3 cm), and calculated r_θ, by using equation (6).

RESULT AND DISCUSSIONS

Figure 3 shows the relationship between the concentration of the India ink and the obtained absorption coefficient, μ_a^{780}. The μ_a^{780} linearly increased with the concentration of the India ink as obtained by was expected. The intercept of the regression line gives the μ_a^{780} of the Intralipid solution, which may include the absorption of water molecules, and of oil droplets (the Intralipid particle) and some effects of the loss of photons from boundaries. Since the boundary effects should mainly affect the light with longer path lengths and results in a higher absorption coefficient, the effects may be seen in the solution with lower absorption coefficients, which may result in a non-linear dependence on the concentration of the ink. The good linear dependence of the results shown in Figure 3 indicates that we can neglect such effects of the boundary in these experiments.

Figure 4 shows the relationship between the calculated ratio of the absorption coefficients of two wave lengths, r, ($r=\dfrac{\mu_a^{754}}{\mu_a^{816}}$), using equation (6) and (7) and the absorption coefficient of the solution, μ_a^{780}. Since the absorption coefficients of India ink should be the same for the three wave lengths (754,780 and 816) which we used, the ratio r will tend to approach 1 at higher concentrations of India ink. Equation (7) holds at the theoretical region $\mu a^{\lambda 2}>0.06$ (cm^{-1}) and at f=200MHz. This is also seen in Figure 4, which shows that equation (7) is working as well.

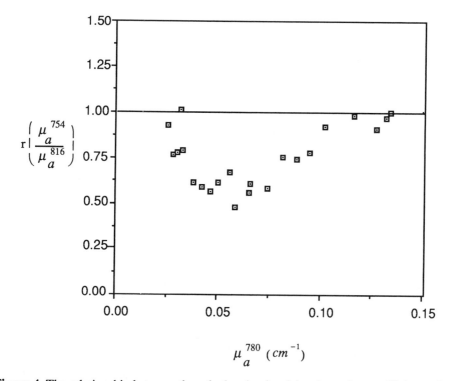

Figure 4. The relationship between the calculated ratio of the absorption coefficients of two wave lengths, r, ($r=\dfrac{\mu_a^{754}}{\mu_a^{816}}$).

Table 1. comparison of the three methods to measure the ratio of μ_a's.

methods	Number of wavelengths	Number of Modulation Frequencies	Number of Separation	Restrictions	Advantages	Disadvantages
2 wave length	two	one	one	applicable region of the object is restricted	Simple	Less accurate, can not eliminate blood volume effects
2 wave lengths and 2 frequencies	two	two	one	$2\pi f \gg \mu_a C$		expensive
2 wave lengths and 2 separation	two	one	two	$\mu_a C \gg 2\pi f$		Limited to the relatively Homomgeneous regions

Compared with currently used other methods, this method has several advantages (Table I): (a) It can eliminate the problems related to instability of the machine, because the processes of subtraction and division eliminate unstable factors such as machine drift. (b) It can use the phase, or phase related values other than the true path length value, which means we can measure the ratio without any calibration of the machine. Larger changes in separation yields higher accuracy of the results. However it is well known that the altering the separation will change the detecting region of the objects (8), which restricts the choice of the range of separation. There should be an optimum combination of separations, which depends on the size and the absorption coefficients of the objects to be measured.

CONCLUSIONS

Equation (7) indicates that the ratio of two phase angle difference at two different separations obtained by two different light wavelengths provides a good estimate of the ratio of μ_a at these wavelength, which can ultimately be used to monitor the oxygen saturation within tissue non-invasively.

ABSTRACT

Near infrared spectroscopy provides a very useful tool to monitor the oxygen saturation of the living tissue non-invasively. We can calculate the hemoglobin oxygen saturation within the tissue, using the ratio of the absorption coefficient (μ_a) at two different wave lengths of light. Biological tissue has a very high effective scattering factor (μ_s'), which elongates an optical path length and makes it difficult to compute the μ_a by the conventional method using continuous light. Phase Modulated Spectroscopy (PMS) measures the path length which is a complex function of the μ_a and μ_s'. To get the ratio of the μ_a, we have to eliminate the effects of the μ_s' from the obtained value by the PMS method. In this report, we present a theory and an experimental result which show that the inverse of the squared ratio of two phase angle differences at two different separations obtained by two different light wavelengths provides a good estimate of the ratio at these wavelength.

ACKNOLEDGEMENT

This work was partially supported by NIH grant 44125.

REFERENCES

1. Chance, B., M.T., Dait, C., Zhang, T., Hamaoka, and F., Hagerman, (1992) *Am, J. Physiol.* **262;** C766-C775.
2. Chance B. (1992) *Clin. J. Sport Med.* **2,** 132-138.
3. Morris, J. B., S., Carter, N., Guerrero, B., Chance (1992), *Circ Shock*, **37;** 39.
4. Sevick, E, B. Chance, J. Leigh, S. Nioka, and M. Maris(1991), *Analy Biochem,* **195**; 330-351,
5. Ishimaru, A (1978) Wave Propagation and Scattering in Random Media, pp175-188, Academic Press, Sandiego.
6. Patterson, M.S., B. Chance, and B. C. Wilson(1989), Appl. Opt. **28;** 2331-2336.
7. Patterson, M.S., J.D. Moulton, B.C. Wilson and B.Chance (1990) *Proc SPIE-Int Soc. Opt. Eng* **1203**; 62-75.
8. Cui, W., C., Kumar, B., Chance (1991) *Proc SPIE-Int Soc. Opt. Eng* **1431**; 180-191.

NIRS IN ADULTS - EFFECTS OF INCREASING OPTODE SEPARATION

D.N.F. Harris[1], F.M. Cowans[2], D.A. Wertheim[2], and S. Hamid[1]

Departments of Anaesthesia[1], Paediatrics[2], Royal Postgraduate Medical School, London, England. W12 0NN

INTRODUCTION

Since its development by Jobsis[1] Near Infra-red Spectroscopy (NIRS) nas been used to study cerebral oxygenation non-invasively in both neonates[,2,3] and more recently in adults[4,5]. The penetration of NIRS is said to be a function of the interoptode distance, and Monte Carlo modelling has been used to demonstrate the calculated light path, showing that the majority of the light passes through the intra-cranial tissues above about 4 cm separation, with increasing contamination from surface tissues as the distance is reduced. McCormick[6] has shown data indicating that there was a significant internal carotid signal with the optodes only 2.8 cm apart, but initial results at this hospital during selective carotid arterial clamping suggested that the relative contribution of the extra-cranial tissues may have been greater than was thought. This study investigates the effect of increasing the optode separation on the amount of internal carotid territory seen by NIRS using hypercarbia to increase internal carotid flow, with Doppler measurement of velocity in Internal and External carotid arteries.

METHODS

Following informed consent, 12 normal volunteers, aged 26-44, were studied: 8 were male, 6 female.

NIRS

Absorption of NIR by the oxidised and reduced fractions of Haemoglobin (HbO, HbR) was measured at 6 wavelengths from 779-991nm (NIR 1000, Hamamatsu Photonics UK). The optodes were placed high on the frontal bone, with the transmitting optode lateral to the sagittal sinus and the receiving optode 3 cm apart. . The optodes were secured with adhesive tape and covered with a light-tight bandage. Aqueous gel was used to improve optical coupling. After a CO_2 challenge the lateral optode was moved further apart in 1 cm steps and the CO_2 challenge repeated, until the count rate limit was reached (usually 7 or 8 cm). HbO, HbR, HbDiff and HbTotal were recorded every 2 seconds (10K photons/sample).

NIR data was normalised for the optode separation to account for the increase in path length and absorption.

CO_2

Subjects took deep slow regular breaths, with End tidal CO_2 (EtCO$_2$), SaO$_2$ and FIO$_2$ measured throughout. After 2 min on room air, subjects breathed 100% oxygen for 5 minutes from a mask and reservoir bag. At end expiration the fresh gas was stopped, and subjects rebreathed from the closed circuit until the EtCO$_2$ had risen 3 kPa; the mask was removed, and blood velocity and EtCo$_2$ allowed to return to normal (c. 3 min). After 20 minutes rest the test was repeated at the new optode spacing. During rebreathing FIO$_2$ remained above 0.5 and SaO$_2$ remained at 100% in all subjects.

Doppler

Middle Cerebral Artery velocity (MCAV) was measured transcranially using the standard technique[7], and External Carotid Artery velocity (ECV) was measured in the neck (Vingmed CFM 700).

RESULTS

Fig. 1 shows a typical study. Change in HbO and HbR are approximately the same magnitude and opposite direction on breathing Oxygen. With CO_2 the change in CO_2 is slightly greater, indicating a small rise in measured Total blood volume. End tidal CO_2 is only recorded by the NIR 1000 every 2 seconds, and under-reads the true value slightly during O_2. Continuous analog measurements were used for the EtCO$_2$ data.

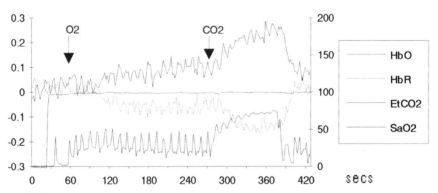

Figure 1 NIR response to O_2 and CO_2 in 1 subject. Left scale is for HbO, HbR in mmol.cm; right scale is SaO$_2$ % and EtCO$_2$ x 10.

HbO and HbR data from NIRS were normalised for the distance between optodes to account for the increase in path length and thus absorption. With 100% O_2 increase in HbDiff was not significantly different between 5, 6 and 7 cm optode separation (see fig. 2); increase in SaO$_2$ was the same (mean 2.9, 2.7, 2.8 %).

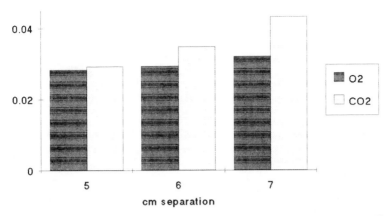

Figure 2. Change in HbDiff during O_2 and CO_2 at 5, 6 and 7 cm separation normalised for the increase in optical path length.

At each distance HbDiff during hypercapnia increased, and was significantly increased from 5 - 7 cm ($p < 0.05$). The increase in CO_2 was the same at each distance (3.0, 3.1, 3.1). Fig. 3 shows the increase in normalised HbDiff for 1 subject between 3 and 7 cm.

Doppler

MCAV rose 69 +/- 11% for a 3 kPa rise in $EtCO_2$; ECV increased 11 +/- 3.5%. There was no change in MCAV or ECV during 100% O_2.

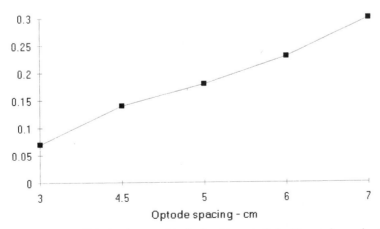

Figure 3. Increase in HbDiff during hypercarbia for 1 subject studied with optode spacing from 3 - 7 cm, showing a progressive increase. HbDiff (mmol.cm) is normalised for the increased separation.

DISCUSSION

Changes in SaO_2 should affect intra- and extra-cranial tissues equally, in proportion to their blood supply. With an increase in optode separation, the change in HbO, HbR and HbDiff should increase due to the increase in light path, foloowing the Beer-Lambert law. The constant increase in HbDiff on breathing oxygen when normalised for the optode separation suggests that the compensation was correct for the increase in the volume of tissue being studied.

Hypercapnia increases intenal carotid flow, producing a doubling of flow for a 3 - 4 kPa increase. External Carotid flow is relatively unaltered (Δ MCAV = 6x Δ ECV), and a CO_2 challenge can be used as a predominantly intra-cranial increase in flow.. The increase in HbDiff with increasing separation during hypercapnia, even after normalisation, suggests that the proportion of intra-cranial tissue in the optical field had increased. The count rate decreases as optode separation increases, so for the same signal-to-noise ratio the sample interval must be increased. With the photon counting technique of the NIR 1000 a sample time of 1-2 seconds is possible at 5 cm, and about 5 seconds at 7 cm. As no plateau was reached in the HbDiff response, it is possible that the intra/extra-cranial tissue ratio could be increased further, at the cost of noisier signals or slower sample times.

This study suggests that at 5 cm separation the proportion of extra-cranial tissue being seen may be higher than has been supposed, and that wider optode separation may improve the selectivity of NIRS for detecting purely intra-cranial events.

REFERENCES

1. F.F. Jobsis, Nonivasive, infrared monitoring of cerebral and myocardial oxygen sufficiency and circulatory parameters, Science 198 : 1264 (1977).
2. A.D. Edwards, J.S. Wyatt, C. Richardson et al, Cotside Measurements of cerebral blood flow in ill newborn infants by near infrared spectroscopy, Lancet Oct 1: 770 (1988).
3. J.E. Brazy, M.D. Lewis, M.H. Mitnick et al, Noninvasive monitoring of cerebral oxygenation in preterm infants: preliminary observations, Pediatrics 75 : 217 (1985).
4. N.B. Hampson, E.M. Camporesi, B.W. Stolp et al, Cerebral Oxygen availability by NIR spectroscopy during transient hypoxia in humans, J. Appl. Physiol. 69(3) : 907 (1990).
5. M. Ferrari, E. Zanette, G. Sideri et al, Effects of carotid compression, as assessed by near infrared spectroscopy, upon cerebral blood volume and haemoglobin oxygen saturation, J.R.S.M. 80 : 83 (1987).
6. P.W. McCormick, M. Stewart, G. Lewis et al, Intracerebral penetration of infra-red light, J. Neurosurg. 76: 315 (1992)
7. R. Aaslid, K-F. Lindegaard, W. Sorteberg et al, Cerebral autoregulation dynamics in humans, Stroke 20 : 45 (1988).

COMPARISON OF CLARK ELECTRODE AND OPTODE FOR MEASUREMENT OF TISSUE OXYGEN TENSION

Harriet Williams Hopf, and Thomas K. Hunt*

Departments of Anesthesia and Surgery*
University of California, San Francisco
San Francisco, CA 94143-0522

INTRODUCTION

Measurement of subcutaneous tissue oxygen tension (PsqO$_2$) depends on the subcutaneous placement of a length of Silastic (Dow-Corning, Midland, MI) tubing (tonometer). Silastic is freely permeable to oxygen, but not to water, and the oxygen tension of saline placed within the tonometer equilibrates quickly with that of the surrounding tissue (Figure 1). Originally, Niinikoski and Hunt[1] allowed the PO$_2$ within the saline to equilibrate and then removed saline from the tonometer for analysis of oxygen tension. Employing a modified Clark electrode, Hunt and colleagues[2] then developed a technique for continuous monitoring of PsqO$_2$. The method was developed as a research tool for examining the effects of local oxygen tension on wound healing and resistance to infection.

The level of PsqO$_2$ in postoperative patients predicts the risk of wound infection more accurately than other risk factors (unpublished data). The amount of collagen deposition in subcutaneously implanted expanded polytetrafluoroethylene (ePTFE) tubes is directly proportional to PsqO$_2$ in surgical patients[3].

These observations make routine monitoring of PsqO$_2$ desirable in patients at risk for postoperative wound complications. Moreover, continuous monitoring of PsqO$_2$ in patients in the intensive care unit may prove valuable as a measure of tissue oxygen delivery. PsqO$_2$ is the most sensitive measure of volume status[4], decreasing long before any change in blood pressure, heart rate, or cardiac output. Decreases in perfusion of bowel and bone occur at about the same time as decreases in PsqO2 in response to hemorrhage[5]. PsqO$_2$ decreases in response to epinephrine infusion[6], cigarette smoking[7], hemodialysis[8], and hypothermia (Sheffield et al, unpublished data), and increases in response to local heat[9]. PsqO$_2$ monitoring may lead to a decrease in wound complications in subcutaneous tissue, bowel, and bone, and allow more optimal management of septic or hypovolemic patients.

Several features make routine clinical monitoring impractical with the modified Clark electrode that we use. The current modification requires constant attention during measurements and recalibration every few hours in a 37°C water bath. Calibration must be manually corrected for subcutaneous temperature. Moreover, the expense of the electrodes requires re-use, leading to concerns about infection control.

Optical electrode ("optode") technology offers some significant advantages. The optode contains a dye which fluoresces in response to light of a certain frequency. The amount of fluorescent light emitted is inversely proportional to oxygen tension, and temperature-dependent.

Inner-Space Medical provided us with an optode which they modified for use in the

Oxygen Transport to Tissue XV, Edited by P. Vaupel
et al., Plenum Press, New York, 1994

Silastic tonometer. The probe contains a thermocouple at the tip which allows for temperature correction. Incident light of the appropriate frequency is carried to the probe tip by a fiberoptic cable, which also carries the fluorescent light back to the measuring device. The probe is easily calibrated in ambient room air, and monitor software calculates PO_2 up to every 2 seconds. Because of slow bleaching of the dye by the incident light, calibration is required every 72 hours in vitro. In vivo, we have measured $PsqO_2$ continuously for up to 24 hours without the need for recalibration. The optode, unlike the Clark electrode, does not consume oxygen, which improves the accuracy of measurements. Data may be downloaded to a computer for storage and analysis.

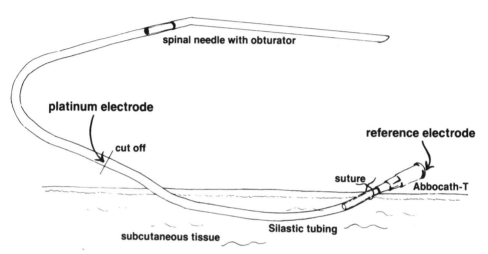

Figure 1. Schematic diagram of the subcutaneous oxygen tonometer. The oxygen probe is inserted through the catheter hub.

Under controlled conditions, the optode and Clark electrode measure PO_2 accurately in vitro over a broad range of values of PO_2 and temperature. In vitro accuracy (in a water bath at 37°C) is ±3 mm Hg for the range 0-100 mm Hg, and ±5% for the range 100-360 mm Hg. Temperature sensitivity is 0.25% per degree centigrade (accuracy data provided by InnerSpace Medical).

Because of its practical advantages for clinical applications, we wished to replace the modified Clark electrode with the optode for $PsqO_2$ measurement. In vitro data, however, are not adequate to prove comparability of the two techniques in vivo. Therefore, we evaluated the comparability of the two methods for measurement of $PsqO_2$ in both rabbits and human volunteers.

METHODS

Calibration

The Clark electrode was calibrated within a Silastic tonometer in a 37°C water bath bubbled with room air (PO_2 set to 150 mm Hg). The silver-silver chloride reference electrode was placed through a stopcock connected by a Luer hub to the Silastic tubing. The tubing was then flushed with saline through the stopcock. The platinum electrode was placed in the open distal end of the Silastic tubing, and then a small amount more saline flushed through the system to ensure an adequate salt bridge between the two electrodes. After a 2 hour warm-up period, the calibration was set to 150 mm Hg. Prior to placing the electrodes within the subcutaneously implanted tonometer, a thermocouple probe was inserted to measure subcutaneous temperature, and the calibration adjusted for the difference from 37°C. A dedicated tissue oximeter measured current flow, which is proportional to oxygen tension in the voltage range used (-0.68 V)[10].

The optode system was allowed to warm-up for at least 2 hours, because lamp output changes when the temperature of the monitor and lamp changes. The machine reaches a fairly constant temperature after one hour. Background activity was measured by connecting the fiberoptic cable to a light-insensitive probe. The dye-containing probe was then connected to the fiberoptic cable and placed in room air. The fluorescent output was measured by the monitor for 24 seconds (12 light flashes), and the calibration set at 150 mm Hg. Using the Stern-Volmer equation (which includes temperature), the monitor software calculates PO_2 relative to the calibrated PO_2 every 2 seconds.

Animal Studies

Approval was obtained from the Committee on Animal Research at the University of California, San Francisco. Rabbits (n = 3) were anesthetized with IM injection of acepromazine and ketamine. A modified 19 gauge spinal needle was used to place 2 tonometers, each consisting of a Luer-hubbed 15 cm segment of Silastic tubing (internal diameter, 0.8 mm; external diameter, 1.0 mm), 1-2 cm apart in the subcutaneous tissue 5-10 cm lateral to the spine. The Clark electrode and optode require different Luer-hubbed connectors, and thus it was impossible to interchange the probes from site to site. The Clark electrode was placed in the tonometer as described above. The optode was placed through the Luer-hubbed connector into the Silastic tube. Saline was then flushed through the probe and tonometer to eliminate air bubbles. After 20-40 minutes of equilibration, a baseline value was recorded for each animal breathing room air (FiO_2 0.21). FiO_2 was then varied (range: 0.21 to 1.0). Values were not recorded until $PsqO_2$ was stable, about 20-30 minutes after each change in FiO_2. No fluid was given to the rabbits, so tissue perfusion, and thus $PsqO_2$, decreased during the several hours of measurement.

Human Volunteers

Approval was obtained from the Committee on Human Research at the University of California, San Francisco. Under local anesthesia with 1% Lidocaine, 2 tonometers were placed subcutaneously, 1-2 cm apart, in the lateral upper arm. All studies were performed 12-18 hours after placement of the tonometers. Measurement of $PsqO_2$ was performed as described above. After a baseline value was obtained with the volunteers (n = 4) breathing room air, 50% oxygen was administered by face mask for 20-30 minutes and a stable value recorded. The measurements were repeated in each volunteer.

Analysis of Data

Limits of agreement (95% confidence intervals) were calculated to evaluate the comparability of measurements using the method of Bland and Altman[11,12]. Absolute values of error increase with increasing PO_2, and thus logarithmic transformation of the data was performed to create a more normal distribution for statistical analysis. Correlation coefficients were also calculated for the two methods of measurement.

RESULTS

Animal Studies

A total of 52 data points were collected in 3 rabbits. Values ranged from 40-176 mm

Hg. The 95% confidence interval for limits of agreement by the optode was 21% below to 28% above the Clark electrode value (Fig. 2). The correlation (Fig. 3) between values measured by Clark electrode vs. optode was significant ($r^2 = 0.929$, p = 0.0001).

In one rabbit, a third tonometer was placed which allowed simultaneous measurement of $PsqO_2$ using a single Clark electrode and 2 optodes. The placement was not over the rib cage, as with the other two, but more ventrally over the abdomen. The PO_2 values for the Clark electrode and the optode in the adjacent tonometer remained very close throughout the experiment. The PO_2 in the third tonometer was slightly higher at FiO_2 0.21, and 70 mm Hg higher at FiO_2 1.0. When the optodes were switched, PO_2 remained the same within each tonometer. This implies that it was local differences in perfusion rather than calibration or other differences between the two optodes which resulted in most of the discrepancy.

Human Volunteers

A total of 22 data points were collected in 4 volunteers. Values ranged from 62-138 mm Hg. The 95% confidence interval for limits of agreement by the optode was 23% below to 24% above the Clark electrode value (Fig. 4). The correlation (Fig. 5) between values measured by Clark electrode vs. optode was significant ($r^2 = 0.721$, p = 0.001).

DISCUSSION

For values from 40-176 mm Hg, the Clark electrode and optode agree within about 25%. $PsqO_2$ values measured in humans (patients and volunteers) and animals range from

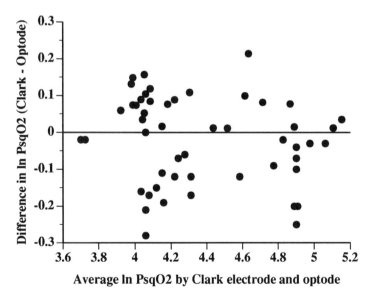

Figure 2. In rabbits, the 95% confidence interval for agreement by the optode was 23% below to 24% above the Clark electrode value.

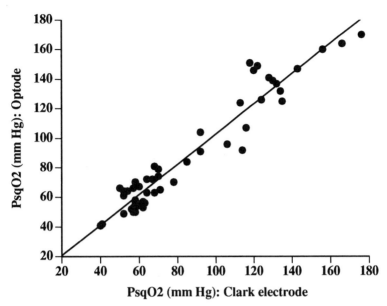

Figure 3. Correlation between $PsqO_2$ values measured by Clark electrode vs. optode ($r^2 = 0.929$).

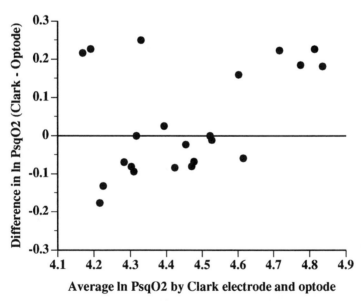

Figure 4. In humans, the 95% confidence interval for agreement by the optode was 21% below to 28% above the Clark electrode value.

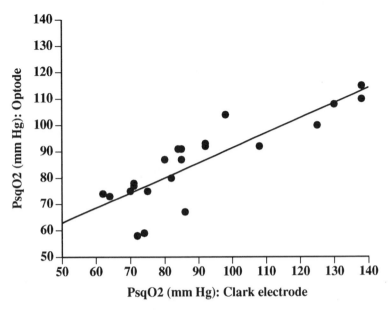

Figure 5. Correlation between $PsqO_2$ values measured by Clark electrode vs. optode ($r^2 = 0.721$).

20-200 mm Hg, with most falling between 35-140 mm Hg. The range measured in this study includes this clinically useful range.

Unfortunately, because the two probes require incompatible Luer-hubbed connectors, it was impossible to measure $PsqO_2$ at exactly the same site. Our experience using 2 optodes in one animal implies that much of the variability between measurements results from local variability in perfusion rather than an intrinsic difference between the techniques. This is supported by in vitro studies with known concentrations of gases which show that both the Clark electrode and optode accurately measure oxygen tension.

The next largest contribution to variability in measurements between the two methods likely results from inaccuracies in Clark electrode calibration and changes in the calibration during a measurement. We routinely and frequently checked the calibration, and the Clark electrode required recalibration more often than the optode. Despite the fact that the Clark electrode consumes oxygen and can be difficult to calibrate, there does not appear to be a bias in the values obtained by either measurement. Optode values are distributed equally above and below Clark electrode values, which implies a random error rather than a consistent bias.

This study demonstrates that the optode can replace the Clark electrode for measurement of oxygen tension within a Silastic tonometer without loss of prior data. The optode has a number of advantages over the Clark electrode which make the change in measuring technique desirable. Both techniques can be used for intermittent monitoring, but the optode requires less operator intervention and is more reliable, with only infrequent loss of data or the need to repeat a measurement because of technical problems. The optode makes continuous monitoring of $PsqO_2$ in critically ill patients feasible. Continuous monitoring is not feasible with the current Clark electrode design.

SUMMARY

Measurement of $PsqO_2$ has proven clinically valuable. The optode is more stable and reliable than the Clark electrode, does not consume oxygen, measures temperature, and is relatively simple to use. The good correlation between values obtained by the Clark electrode and the optode in this study demonstrate that the optode may replace the Clark electrode without loss of prior data.

ACKNOWLEDGEMENTS

This study was supported by NIH GM 27345 and InnerSpace Medical (Irvine, CA).

REFERENCES

1. J. Niinikoski and T.K. Hunt, Measurement of wound oxygen with implanted Silastic tube, *Surgery* 71:22 (1972).

2. N. Chang, W.H. Goodson, F. Gottrup, and T.K. Hunt, Direct measurement of wound and tissue oxygen tension in postoperative patients, *Ann Surg* 197:470 (1983).

3. K. Jonsson, J.A. Jensen, W.H. Goodson, H. Scheuenstuhl, J. West, H.W. Hopf, and T.K. Hunt, Tissue oxygenation, anemia and perfusion in relation to wound healing in surgical patients, *Ann Surg* 214:605 (1991).

4. K. Jonsson, J.A. Jensen, W.H. Goodson, J.M. West, and T.K. Hunt, Assessment of perfusion in postoperative patients using tissue oxygen measurements, *Br J Surg* 74:263 (1987).

5. A. Gosain, J. Rabkin, J.P. Reymond, J.A. Jensen, T.K. Hunt, and R.A. Upton, Tissue oxygen tension and other indicators of blood loss or organ perfusion during graded hemorrhage, *Surgery* 109:523 (1991).

6. J.A. Jensen, K. Jonsson, W.H. Goodson, T.K. Hunt, and M.F. Roizen, Epinephrine lowers subcutaneous oxygen tension, *Curr Surg* 42:472 (1985).

7. J.A.Jensen, W.H. Goodson, H.W. Hopf, and T.K. Hunt, Cigarette smoking decreases tissue oxygen, *Arch Surg* 126:1131 (1991).

8. J.A. Jensen, W.H. Goodson, R. Omachi, S.M. Lindenfeld, and T.K. Hunt, Subcutaneous tissue oxygen falls during hemodialysis, *Surgery* 101:416 (1987).

9. J.M. Rabkin and T.K. Hunt, Local heat increases blood flow and oxygen tension in wounds, *Arch Surg* 122:221 (1987).

10. F. Gottrup, R. Firmin, N. Chang, W.H. Goodson, and T.K. Hunt, Continuous direct tissue oxygen tension measurement by a new method using an implantable Silastic tonometer and oxygen polarography *Am J Surg* 146:399 (1983).

11. D.G. Altman and J.M. Bland, Measurement in Medicine: the analysis of method comparison studies, *The Statistician* 32:307 (1983).

12. J.M. Bland and D.G. Altman, Statistical methods for assessing agreement between two methods of clinical measurement, *The Lancet* i:307 (1986).

PHOTOMETRIC DETERMINATION OF THE O_2 STATUS OF HUMAN BLOOD USING THE OXYSTAT SYSTEM: cO_2 (mL/dL), sO_2 (%), cHb (g/dL)

R. Zander and W. Lang

Inst. of Physiology and Pathophysiology, Mainz University, Mainz (FRG)

INTRODUCTION

The O_2 status of arterial human blood (Zander, 1990) can be completely described by a set of four parameters: cO_2 (mL/dL), sO_2 (%), cHb (g/dL) and pO_2 (mm Hg).

The usefulness of this concept is the fact that all types of hypoxemia can be clearly differentiated, e. g. hypoxic ($pO_2\downarrow$, $sO_2\downarrow$), toxemic ($sO_2\downarrow$) or anemic (cHb$\downarrow$).

However, there is no simple analytic device available for measuring all of the four parameters simultaneously. For example, blood gas analyzers or pulse oxymeters can only measure pO_2 or psO_2 (partial saturation) and calculate the other or vice versa, or multiwavelength oxymeters can measure cHb and sO_2, and calculate only chemically bound cO_2 by ignoring pO_2.

In contrast, the Oxystat system (Zander et al., 1978) calculates sO_2, and measures total cHb and total cO_2 directly, the last being a parameter which is most sensitive to any change of oxygen in blood, irrespective what may have been the cause. Its value is decreased for all types of hypoxemia.

The Oxystat system is based on photometric tests for oxygen and for hemoglobin which have been rationalized in form of disposable cuvettes with a special dosing system for blood (Hb and O_2 cuvette) and a battery-operated mini-photometer for measuring absorbance. It has been developed for rapid clinical use, and represents a powerful diagnostic tool for all hypoxemic situations in blood. To make sure reliable diagnostic values, quality control solutions, both for oxygen and for hemoglobin, are available.

THE OXYSTAT SYSTEM

The Oxystat system is a direct application of a rationalized photometric procedure in determination of oxygen and of hemoglobin in blood and consists of the following units:

The Oxystat Cuvette

The Oxystat cuvette is a disposable cuvette and can be used as an operational unit of a photometric cell and a dosing system at the same time. It is filled with 1 mL of a specific reagent which for oxygen is called: the O_2 Cuvette (aqueous alkaline solution of catechol and an iron(II)-salt under nitrogen), and for hemoglobin: the Hb Cuvette (aqueous alkaline Triton X-100 solution). On top of the light transparent part of the cuvette, there is a dosing system. (Figure 1.)

This is a capillary that fills with blood (about 20 µL), and a plunger which communicates with a part of the capillary, and by pushing down exactly measures 10 µL for reaction. The excess of blood in the capillary works in the case of oxygen measurement as a seal against air, and the blood can be introduced anaerobically into the cuvette.

The Oxystat Photometer

This is a small pocket-sized and battery-operated mini-photometer for measuring absorbance, and programmed to indicate cO_2, sO_2 and cHb on a display. (Figure 2.) A filter is used with a maximum of light transmission around 615 nm and a half-bandwidth of about 10 nm.

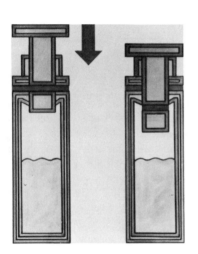

Figure 1. Principle of the Oxystat Cuvette.

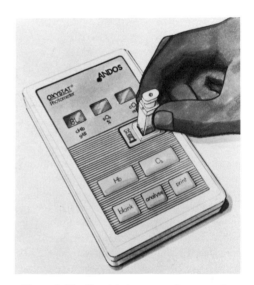

Figure 2. The Oxystat photometer demonstrating the different functions on the display.

The Oxystat Measurement

By using the Oxystat System, direct measurement of the total oxygen concentration and total hemoglobin concentration in blood can be easily performed, because photometry is very simplified:

- application of a drop of blood into the capillary of the dosing system
- absorbance blank
- displacement of the plunger

- shaking and after 90 s absorbance measurement of the endproduct.

Taking into account physically dissolved oxygen of approximately 0.3 mL/dL in the physiological range and using Hüfner's theoretical factor of 1.39 mL/g, O_2 saturation (sO_2) with respect to total hemoglobin is calculated. For a complete analysis, only 30-40 µL (1-2 drops) of blood are required, so that puncturing of arteries normally is unnecessary, and it can be taken from the hyperemized earlobe. At least after 3 minutes, the following values for the O_2 status are indicated on the display of the photometer:

- total O_2 content (cO_2, mL/dL)

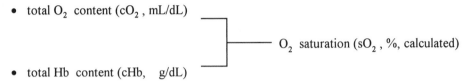

O_2 saturation (sO_2, %, calculated)

- total Hb content (cHb, g/dL)

QUALITY CONTROL AND ACCURACY

A crystalline standard, available both for the O_2 and the Hb cuvette, allows gravimetric calibration (Wolf, 1991; Zander, 1991). For quality control of the Oxystat system, control solutions for oxygen (aqueous KJO_3 solutions: 20 and 10 mL/dL) and for hemoglobin (chlorohemin in alkaline Triton X-100 solution: 15 and 7.5 g/dL) can be obtained in the normal and in the half normal range. Treating these solutions in the same way as blood, all necessary steps in the procedure including both the Oxystat cuvette and the Oxystat photometer can be simulated and checked. By application of the Oxystat system, all relevant data for the O_2 status can be determined with an accuracy and reliability of 3 %.

CONCLUSIONS

Knowledge of the actual O_2 concentration in blood is the most sensitive parameter of the O_2 status because any oxygen deficiency can be immediately noticed. Therefore, the Oxystat system can be recommended as a powerful diagnostic tool for clinical practice, because

- all necessary data (cO_2, sO_2, cHb) for the O_2 status can be obtained within 3 minutes from only 30-40 µL of blood
- can be used anywhere at any time
- can be calibrated by control solutions
- can recognize all hypoxemic situations, even hypoxia in the lungs, e. g. by repeating the actual O_2 measurement after breathing pure oxygen.

REFERENCES

Wolf, H.U.,1991, Calibration and quality control of methods and equipment for the determination of hemoglobin concentration,
in: "The Oxygen Status of Arterial Blood," R. Zander and F. Mertzlufft, eds., Karger, Basel.
Zander, R., 1990, The oxygen status of arterial human blood,
Scand J Clin Lab Invest. 50 (Suppl. 203): 187.

Zander, R., 1991, Calibration and quality control of equipment used for measuring O_2 concentration,
in: "The Oxygen Status of Arterial Blood," R. Zander and F. Mertzlufft, eds., Karger, Basel.

Zander, R., Lang, W., and Wolf, H.U.,1978, A new method for measuring the oxygen content in microliter
samples of gases and liquids: The oxygen cuvette,
in: "Oxygen Transport to Tissue III," Plenum Press, Corp., New York.

LASER DOPPLER PERFUSION IMAGING COMPARED WITH LIGHTGUIDE LASER DOPPLER FLOWMETRY, DYNAMIC THERMOGRAPHIC IMAGING AND TISSUE SPECTROPHOTOMETRY FOR INVESTIGATING BLOOD FLOW IN HUMAN SKIN

D.K. Harrison[1], N.C. Abbot[1,2], J. Swanson Beck[2]
and P.T. McCollum[3]

Vascular Laboratory, Departments of Medical Physics[1] and Surgery[2]
and Department of Pathology[3]
Ninewells Hospital and Medical School
Dundee, DD1 9SY, Scotland

INTRODUCTION

Lightguide laser Doppler flowmetry (LDF_c) is widely used both in micro-circulatory research and in clinical blood flow studies (for a review, see Shepherd and Oberg, 1990). Despite the inability to measure blood flow in absolute terms with the method (flux values are quoted in volts), physiological challenges can be used in order to test local and sympathetic control of the microvascular flow (Khan et al., 1991).

A further limitation of the method arises from the fact that, due to the anatomy of the microvasculature (Braverman et al., 1990) or physiological function (Harrison et al., 1988), tissue perfusion is heterogeneous. Since the catchment volume of the LDF_c probe is of the order of $1mm^3$, flux measurements only millimetres apart may give completely different values

In order to overcome this problem, laser Doppler imaging (LDI) has very recently been introduced into the field of laser Doppler flowmetry. The advantage claimed for LDI is that a more representative sample of microvascular perfusion can be obtained than with conventional LDF_c. Two such imaging devices have been reported, one by Essex and Byrne, 1991, and one by Wardell et al., 1991; 1992. The instrument described by Wardell et al. is now commercially available (Lisca Laser Doppler Perfusion Imager, Lisca development, Linkoping, Sweden) and was loaned to us for evaluation by Moor Instruments Ltd, Axminster, UK.

Oxygen Transport to Tissue XV, Edited by P. Vaupel
et al., Plenum Press, New York, 1994

In order to evaluate the device, it was applied to imaging flux changes induced in human skin during the tuberculin reaction. LDF_c, thermography and lightguide spectrophotometry have been used previously in our laboratory to study the changes in blood flow and oxygen supply which occur during the course of this reaction (Beck and Spence, 1986; Abbot et al., 1992; Harrison et al., 1992). Although, generally, LDF_c is raised throughout the reaction, in particularly intense reactions it can be considerably lower at the centre than at adjacent peripheral sites. This phenomenon is called "central relative slowing" (CRS) (Beck et al., 1989; Abbot et al., 1992). The aim of these experiments, therefore, was to investigate whether LDI might enable CRS - and other relative changes in flow patterns - to be mapped on a more regional basis within the tuberculin reaction.

METHODS

Laser Doppler Imager

The LDI comprises a 2mW helium-neon laser, the beam of which is directed at the tissue via an optical scanner. This consists of two mirrors controlled by two stepping motors: measurements are made sequentially at 4096 points. The back-scattered light is detected by a photo diode at a distance of about 20cm from the skin surface. An area of some 12 x 12cm can be scanned. In the "Step 2" mode, each colour-coded pixel of the image represents the flux recorded from $1mm^2$ areas of skin, the centres of which are 2mm apart. Software allows statistical analysis and display of profiles within the area scanned

Dynamic Thermographic Imaging

The dynamic thermographic imaging technique (DTI), developed in our laboratory, is described elsewhere (Wilson and Spence, 1989). An Agema System 800 (Agema Infrared Systems Ltd, Leighton Buzzard, UK) was used to record images at 1s intervals following cooling of the skin in the area under investigation using a specially constructed cooling element. The parameter used for assessment of flow here was the temperature 100s after the cold challenge.

Tissue Spectrophotometry

A Photal MCPD-100 (Otsuka Electronics Co., Osaka, Japan) spectrophotometer was used in the visible range (500-620nm) to measure relative haemoglobin concentration in terms of the haemoglobin index (HBI) and absolute haemoglobin oxygenation (SO_2) in the skin according to the 6 wavelength analysis technique described by Harrison et al., 1992 (see also Hickman et al., 1993 in this volume).

Experimental Protocol

Measurements were carried out in 6 normal subjects at control sites and 48h after injection of 0.1ml (10TU) purified protein derivative (Glaxo, Greenford, UK), a time at which blood flow changes are usually maximal. A flexible probe holder and reflective stickers were used to ensure accurate location of the spectrophotometer and LDF_c (Perimed PF2B) lightguides. Corresponding values were measured at 10mm intervals from the centre of the reaction to distances of 40mm. Discrete measurements were recorded (LDF_c and tissue spectrophotometry) or read from images (LDI and DTI) and compared by means of linear regression analysis.

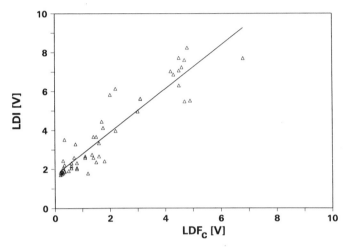

Figure 1. Relation between flux measured by LDI and LDF_c

RESULTS

Significant linear correlations ($p < .001$) were found between flux values obtained from LDI and LDF_c (Fig.1: $r=0.93$, $n=53$), LDI and DTI (Fig.2: $r=0.79$, $n=30$) and LDI and HBI (Fig.3: $r=0.88$, $n=53$) at identical locations. A roughly linear relation between haemoglobin saturation and both LDF_c and LDI can be observed up to flux values of about 2.8V and 4.5V (Fig.4). A plateau is reached above these values at which haemoglobin is 90-97% saturated.

A degree of spatial heterogeneity could be detected in normal skin (mean flux $1.92 \pm 0.26V$, i.e. $\pm 13.5\%$) but during the tuberculin reaction flux differences of up to 5V between adjacent pixels could be identified with LDI (mean flux $5.29 \pm 1.65V$, i.e. $\pm 31.2\%$). Such localised heterogeneities could not be detected with DTI.

Pseudo 3-dimensional representation of images obtained by LDI (Fig.5) enable an even clearer representation of spatial heterogeneity. Such images revealed local areas of relatively low flux surrounded by regions of higher perfusion. Such "crater" effects could also be seen in less intense reactions.

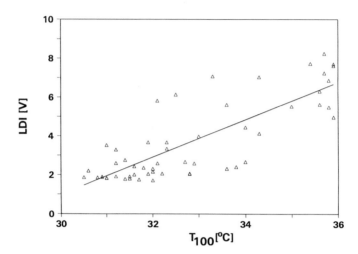

Figure 2. Relation between LDI flux and T_{100}

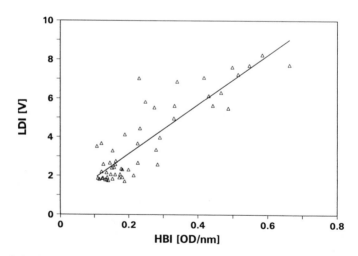

Figure 3. Relation between LDI flux and relative haemoglobin concentration assessed in terms of HBI

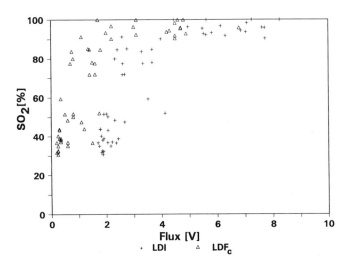

Figure 4. Relation between haemoglobin oxygenation (SO$_2$) and LDF$_c$ and LDI flux values

DISCUSSION

Good correlation was obtained between LDI and LDF$_c$. The scatter is most probably due to biological variations between the time of making the LDI and LDF$_c$ measurements, and the necessity to locate accurately the LDF$_c$ measurement site on the LDI image. The difference in absolute terms arises from being unable to measure absolute values using laser Doppler flowmetry (see Shepherd and Oberg, 1990). Also, two entirely different instruments - and indeed technologies - were being compared. However, *changes* in LDI and LDF$_c$ flux values were proportional over a very wide range within the tuberculin reaction.

Linear correlations were also obtained between LDI and the other two indicators of perfusion, i.e. DTI and HBI. The relationships between tissue haemoglobin saturation and the two laser Doppler fluxes were similar. The right-shifted LDI values in Fig.4 reflect the differences between absolute values seen in Fig.1. The relation between SO$_2$ and LDF$_c$ during the course of the tuberculin reaction and the implication with regard to cellular oxygen supply is discussed elsewhere in this volume (Harrison et al., 1993).

The initial question was whether central relative slowing may be present over an area too small (a diameter less than 10 mm) to be detected by our established LDF$_c$ technique. In fact, LDI revealed that relative slowing may not only be restricted to the centre of the lesion, but could also occur elsewhere within the area of erythema (Fig.5). This may be due to localised oedema possibly occuring in pockets not necessarily corresponding to the visible centre of the lesion. The resulting increased interstitial pressure may then alter flow patterns in a non-homogeneous manner.

A further feature revealed by LDI is the remarkable spatial variation of flux values between areas only 2mm away from each other. In some cases these differences were as great as 5V. Such very large, local differences in flow values during the tuberculin reaction may play an important regulatory role in a similar way to that demonstrated in skeletal muscle (Harrison et al., 1988) and perhaps reflects local demands for oxygen or the build-up of metabolites.

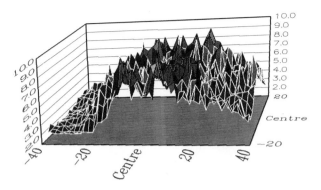

Figure 5. Pseudo-3d perspective of a tuberculin reaction at 48h. A "crater" surrounded by regions of high perfusion is marked.

LDI enables rapid, non-invasive, detailed analysis of blood flow patterns in skin and correlates well with other methods for measuring skin perfusion. Its use to examine heterogeneity of microvascular blood flow patterns may lead to further understanding of the local mechanisms for regulation of oxygen supply to tissue.

ACKNOWLEDGEMENTS

The authors are grateful to Drs. David Boggett and Nick Barnett (Moor Instruments Ltd) for making the LDI available. Funding for this work was provided by the Scottish Home and Health Department (Grant No. K/MRS/50/C1534) and the University of Dundee Research Initiatives Fund. The authors are also grateful for the support of Dr Dick Lerski, Director, Department of Medical Physics, for his support of the project.

REFERENCES

Abbot, N.C., Swanson Beck J., Carnochan, F.M., Lowe, J.G. and Gibbs, J.H., 1992, Circulatory adaptation to the increased metabolism in skin at the site of the tuberculin reaction, *Int. J. Microcirc: Clin. Exp.* in press.

Beck, J.S. and Spence V.A., 1986, Patterns of blood flow in the microcirculation of the skin during the course of the tuberculin reaction in normal human subjects, *Immunology* 58:209.

Beck, J.S., Gibbs J.H., Potts, R.C., Kardjito, T., Grange, J.M., Jawad E.S. and Spence, V.A., 1989, Histometric studies on biopsies of tuberculin skin test showing evidence of ischaemia and necrosis, *J. Pathol.* 159:317.

Braverman, I.M., Keh, A. and Goldminz, D., 1990, Correlation of laser Doppler wave patterns with underlying microvascular anatomy, *J. Invest. Dermatol.* 95:283.

Essex, T.J.H. and Byrne, P.O., 1991, A laser Doppler scanner for imaging blood flow in skin, *J. Biomed. Eng.* 13:189.

Harrison, D.K., Birkenhake, S., Knauf, S.K, Hagen, N., Beier, I. and Kessler, M., 1988, The role of high flow capillary channels in the oxygen supply to skeletal muscle, *Adv. Exp. Med. Biol.* 222:623.

Harrison, D.K., Evans, S.D., Abbot, N.C., Swanson Beck, J. and McCollum, P.T., 1992, Spectrophotometric measurements of haemoglobin saturation and concentration in skin during the tuberculin reaction in normal human subjects, *Clin. Phys. and Physiol. Meas.* in press.

Harrison, D.K., Abbot, N.C., Carnochan, F., Swanson Beck, J., James, P.B. and McCollum, P.T., 1993, Protective regulation of oxygen uptake as a result of reduced oxygen extraction during chronic inflammation, *Adv. Exp. Med. Biol.* this volume.

Hickman P., Harrison, D.K., Evans, S.D., Belch, J. and McCollum, P.T., 1993, Use of lightguide reflectance spectrophotometry in the assessment of peripheral arterial disease, *Adv. Exp. Med. Biol.* this volume.

Khan, F., Spence, V.A., Wilson, S.B. and Abbot, N.C., 1991, Quantification of sympathetic vascular responses in skin by laser Doppler flowmetry, *Int. J. Microcirc: Clin. Exp.* 10:145.

Shepherd, A.P. and Oberg, P.A., 1990, "Laser Doppler Flowmetry," Kluwer Academic Publishers, Boston.

Wardell, K., Jakobsson, A. and Nilsson, G., 1991, Laser imager maps microvascular flow, *Diagnost. Imaging Int.* March/April:44.

Wardell, K., Jakobsson, A. and Nilsson, G., 1992, Laser Doppler perfusion imaging by dynamic light scattering, *IEEE Trans. BME,* in press.

Wilson, S.B. and Spence, V.A., 1989, Dynamic thermographic imaging method for quantifying dermal perfusion: potential and limitations, *Med. Biol. Eng. Comput.* 27:496.

QUANTITATION OF ABSOLUTE CONCENTRATION CHANGE IN SCATTERING MEDIA BY THE TIME-RESOLVED MICROSCOPIC BEER-LAMBERT LAW

M.Oda[*], Y.Yamashita[*], G.Nishimura and M.Tamura

Biophysics Division, Research Institute for Electronic Science
Hokkaido University, Sapporo 060, Japan
[*]Central Research Laboratory, Hamamatsu Photonics K.K.
Hamakita Research Park, 5000 Hirakuchi, Hamakita, Shizuoka
434, Japan

INTRODUCTION

In a scattering media like living tissue, there have been two lines of critical argument concerning the effect of optical absorption on the distribution of the optical pathlength. One is that the optical pathlength is constant when the absorption changes, though it differs markedly from the physical pathlength, such as the thickness of the tissue because of considerable scattering. The other is that the distribution of the pathlength depends on the absorption (1,2). Previously, we have shown the validity of the Beer-Lambert law in rat heads (3) and thigh muscles (4). The requirement of the Beer-Lambert law is the independence of the attenuation of incident light by absorption from that by scattering. This was confirmed by measuring the time of flight of picosecond length light pulses in several rat tissues (5) as well as model systems (6). Equation(1), which was derived from our time-resolved study on the Beer-Lambert law, shows that light intensity along the non-linear path taken by photons through scattering media is exponentially attenuated by absorption. Monte Carlo simulation also confirmed this (7). The present paper expands equation(1) into time-resolved multiwavelength photometry for determination of the absolute concentration of absorber coexisting in scattering media, by which the optical pathlength was directly estimated.

EXPERIMENTAL PROCEEDURE

The experimental set up is illustrated in Fig.1. Picosecond light pulses (<10ps FWHM, 30Hz repetition, 690 to 710nm wavelength range) were generated by a tunable picosecond dye laser (Quantel PTL10) which was pumped by a Q-switched mode-locked Nd:YAG laser (Quantel YAG 501-30). The energy of the light pulses was 0.3mJ/pulse. A streak camera (Hamamatsu C2830) was employed for time-resolved measurements. The model system consisted of a phantom containing 3% yeast suspension and hemoglobin (Fig.1(b)). In the animal experiments, the rats (200-300g) anesthetized by pentobarbital sodium (50mg/kg) were connected to the artificial respiration system (60stroke/min.,10ml/stroke/kg). The substitution of blood with perfluorotributylamin emulsion (FC-43, Green Cross Corp., Japan) was used to reduce hemoglobin concentration, hematocrit, in the rat head.

ANALYSIS

Our time-resolved Beer-Lambert equation in scattering media at a certain wavelength can be written as:

$$A_\lambda(t) = \log\{I_{0\lambda}(t)/I_\lambda(t)\} = E_\lambda Cvt \qquad (1)$$

$A_\lambda(t)$: absorbance at time t

$I_{0\lambda}(t), I_\lambda(t)$: the intensity of transmitted or reflected light at time t without absorption and with absorption

E_λ: the extinction coefficient at a given wavelength

C: concentration of absorber

v: velocity of light in the medium

t: time

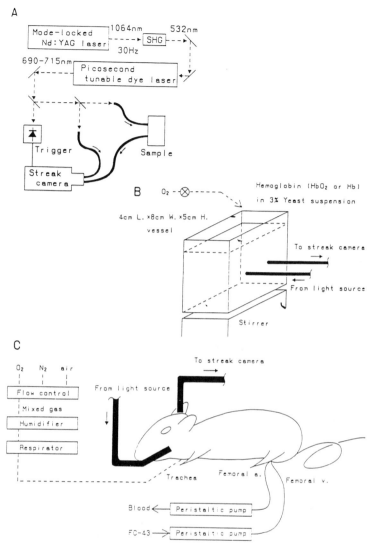

Fig. 1 (A) Block diagram of the experimental setup for time of flight measurements. A 3mm diameter fiber bundle was used for light input and a 1.1mm diameter single fiber for light detection. (B) A phantom of the model system measurement. The detection fiber was set 3cm away from the input fiber. The suspension was purged with O_2 gas to keep the hemoglobin at oxyform, The vessel was then sealed to deoxygenate because of cousumption of oxygen by yeast. (C) Experimental setup for animal study. The input fiber was inserted into the mouth of each rat, and the detection fiber was placed on the top of head connected with the parietal region.

Here, the temporal profile of $I_{0\lambda}(t)$, $I_{0\lambda}$, shows the probability distribution in highly scattering and no absorbing system as a function of time taken by photons travelled through it. With dual-wavelength photometry at $\lambda 1$ and $\lambda 2$, we assume equation(2).

$$I_{0\lambda 1}(t) = I_{0\lambda 2}(t) \tag{2}$$

Then we obtain equation(3) from equation(1).

$$A_{\lambda 2-\lambda 1}(t) = \log\{ I_{\lambda 1}(t)/I_{\lambda 2}(t)\} = (E_{\lambda 2}-E_{\lambda 1})Cvt \tag{3}$$

$A_{\lambda 2-\lambda 1}(t)$: absorbance difference between $\lambda 2$ and $\lambda 1$ at time t

Then equation(4) is obtained, where the slope of equation(3), $A_{\lambda 2-\lambda 1}(t)$ is proportional to the product of the extinction coefficient, concentration and light velocity.

$$\Delta Abs._{\lambda 2-\lambda 1} = A_{\lambda 2-\lambda 1}/t = [\log\{I_{\lambda 1}(t)/I_{\lambda 2}(t)\}]/t = (E_{\lambda 2}-E_{\lambda 1})Cv \tag{4}$$

In the hemoglobin system of equation(4), absolute concentrations can be calculated by solving simultaneos equations for given wavelengths by use of extinction coefficients of oxy- and deoxyhemoglobin (equation(5)).

$$\Delta Abs._{\lambda 2-\lambda 1}/v = (E_{\lambda 2}^{oxy}-E_{\lambda 1}^{oxy})C^{oxy} + (E_{\lambda 2}^{deoxy}-E_{\lambda 1}^{deoxy})C^{deoxy} \tag{5}$$

RESULT

Phantom Experiment

For deconvolution of the traces of time of flight measurement, the profile of input light pulse, h(t), is shown in Fig.2 with 70 ps of FWHM. Fig.3-(A) shows profiles of time of flight at 710 and 690nm of the model phantom containing 0.12mM deoxy-hemoglobin. By deconvoluting the results of Fig.3-(A) using h(t), we obtained Fig.3-(B) where the rising phase after the pulse was well improved. The difference of both temporal profiles at each time gave a straight line in a logarithmic scale as was expected from equation(3). The absolute absorbance differences per 1cm at 690 minus 710nm were plotted against the concentrations of oxy- and deoxyhemoglobin in Fig.4, where the slope of Fig.3-(B) was divided by

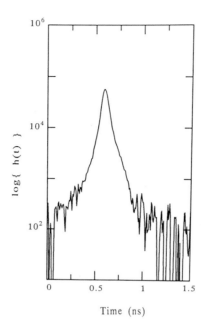

Time (ns)

Fig. 2　Input light pulse profile, h(t), was obtained from measurement of the input pulse using our experimental system. This was used as a system response function when deconvolution was performed.

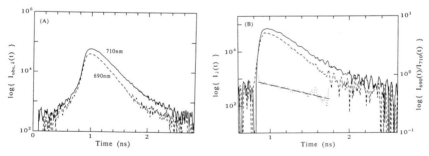

Fig. 3　(A) Measured profile I(t) of the phantom at 710 (solid line) and 690nm (broken line) where the Hb concentration was 0.12mM.　(B) Profiles of $I_{710}(t)$ (solid line) and $I_{690}(t)$ (broken line) after deconvolution ; dotted line was the calculated $\log\{ I_{690}(t)/I_{710}(t) \}$ and solid straight line matched best according to equation(3).

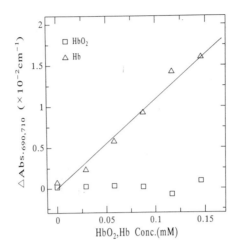

Fig. 4　Plots of ΔAbs 690-710 at different concentrations of Hb and HbO$_2$ in the phantom.　The velocity of light was 0.023cm/ps in water.

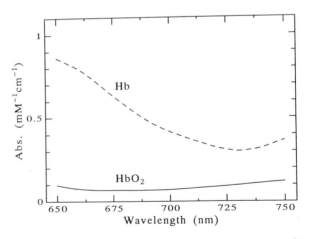

Fig. 5 Absorbance spectrum of the hemoglobin solution.

0.023cm/ps. The absorbance difference at 690-710nm remained zero with increasing oxyhemoglobin whereas it increased linearly with increasing deoxyhemoglobin. This is due to the fact that the absorbance difference at 690 minus 710nm is nearly zero for oxyhemoglobin (cf. Fig.5). The slope of deoxyhemoglobin gave a difference extinction coefficient at 690-710nm. The value was $0.122mM^{-1}cm^{-1}$, identical to that of pure solution, (cf, extinction coefficients at 690 and 710nm are 0.49 and $0.37mM^{-1}cm^{-1}$ and the difference, $0.12mM^{-1}cm^{-1}$, see Fig.4).

Rat head in vivo

Fig.6 shows the temporal profiles of the transmitted light pulse through the rat head measured at 690 and 710nm of the original traces (A) and deconvoluted traces (B). The logarithmic plot of absorption difference against time gave the straight line as was observed with the phantom system of Fig.3. The slopes of the straight line in Fig.6-(B) were divided by 0.022cm/ps and then plotted against various wavelengths where 710nm was used as common reference. The results are given in Fig.7. The spectra thus obtained were the time-resolved absolute absorption spectra of the rat head. The spectrum of 5% hematocrit gave an almost flat base-line, showing a negligible contribution to the absorption due to cytochrome oxidase in the brain tissue as was observed previously (3). Since absorption spectra of oxyhemoglobin and cytochromes are almost flat in this wavelength region, the spectra obtained at various FiO_2 can be regarded as those of deoxyhemoglobin. Indeed, the overall profiles of the spectra resembled that of Fig.4 of deoxyhemoglobin solution, except for the zero absorption at 710nm.

Determination of the Absolute Concentration of Deoxyhemoglobin and SO_2 in the Rat Head

In Fig.7, the concentration of deoxyhemoglobin can be simply estimated from equation(5), where $(E_{\lambda 2}^{oxy}-E_{\lambda 1}^{oxy})C^{oxy}$ is zero. Therefore equation(6) stands at

$$C^{Hb} = \Delta Abs_{\lambda 2-\lambda 1} / E^{Hb}_{\lambda 2-\lambda 1} \qquad (6)$$

where $\lambda 1$ and $\lambda 2$ are appropriate combinations of dual-wavelength pairs. Since the absorbance difference is largest at the pair 690 and 710nm under our experimental conditions, the absolute concentrations of deoxyhemoglobin were calculated using the corresponding extinction

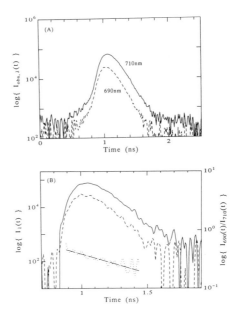

Fig. 6   Profiles of the time of flight in the rat head at 710 and 690nm when the rat breathed 10% FiO_2 : (A) Original traces. (B) Deconvoluted traces.

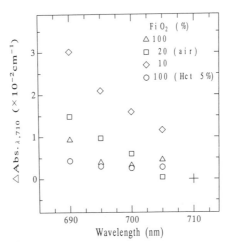

Fig. 7   Plots of $\Delta Abs_{\lambda,710}$ at various wavelengths when FiO_2 was changed. Substituted blood with FC-43 was also used. The velocity of light was 0.022cm/ps in 20% albumin solution.

coefficient, and are plotted against FiO_2 in Fig.8.   The relatively large deviations shown are possibly due to the uncontrolled respiration of the rats resulting from factors such as fluctuations in blood pressure.   The absolute deoxyhemoglobin concentration observed in the rat head during breathing of nomal air was about 0.13mM.   The mean total hemoglobin concentration in the rat head, which had been previously determined by time-resolved photometry, was 0.32mM (5).   Next the figures for oxygen saturation SO_2 were then also obtained and plotted in Fig.8.   During breathing of nomal air, the SO_2 level was 60%. This figure is close to the value found at the jugular vein (6).   All of the figures from data obtained on SO_2 closely approximated those datermined directly by gas analysis (5).

DISCUSSION

The animal as well as the phantom experiments demonstrated that our time-resolved Beer-Lambert Equations of equation(1) and equation(3) are valid for use in scattering media and living tissue, where $I_{0\lambda}(t)$ is not necessary for determination of the absolute concentration.   The critical assumption of equation(2) employed here can be supported by the result of 5% hematocrit in Fig.7, where the flat base line showed a constancy of $I_{0\lambda}(t)$.   Equation(3) offers a great advantage for use in the living tissues, since in general we cannot obtain $I_{0\lambda}(t)$ of equation(1) in circulatory blood systems.   In the rat head, we   can obtain the absolute concentrations of deoxyhemoglobin, and SO_2 values, with reasonable results where total hemoglobin concentration was determined separately by the use of equation(1) of single wavelength photometry (5).   Present three-wavelengths and four-wavelengths methods, however, did not directly give the SO_2 since we could not obtain the oxyhemoglobin concentration because of the flat absorption in this region.   There is no doubt that when using other wavelength pairs having the absorption difference of oxyhemoglobin,   equation(5)   will give the absolute concentration of oxyhemoglobin, and therefore absolute SO_2.   Thus equation(1), which is based on the independence of the distribution of pathlength from absorption, plays an indispensable role for quantification of absorber in living tissue.   Equation(1), however, conflicts with the concept that distribution of pathlength depends on absorption (1,2).

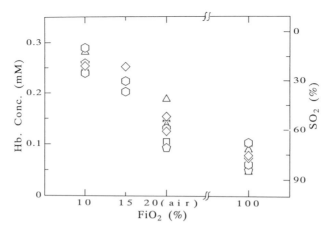

Fig. 8   Relationship between the calculated deoxyhemoglobin concentration in the rat head and FiO_2 by equation(7).   Data were those from five rats (200-300g). 0.32mM of the total hemoglobin concentration in the rat brain was used to calculate the value of SO_2 (6).

REFERENCES

(1) B.Chance, J.S.Leigh, H.Miyake, D.S.Smith, S.Nioka, R.Greenfeld, M.Finander, K.Kaufman, W.Lery, M.Yong, P.Cohn, H.Yoshioka, and R.Boretsky *Proc. Natl. Acad. Sci. U.S.A.* 85 4971-4975(1988)

(2) D.T.Delpy, M.Cope, P.vander Zee, S.Arridge, S.Wray, and J.Wyatt *Physics in Medicine and Biology* 33 1433-1442(1988)

(3) O.Hazeki and M.Tamura *J.Appl.Physiol.* 64 796-802(1988)

(4) M.Seiyama, O.Hazeki and M.Tamura *J.Biochem.* 103 419-424(1988)

(5) Y.Nomura and M.Tamura *J.Biochem.* 109 455-461(1991)

(6) Y.Nomura, O.Hazeki and M.Tamura *Adv.Exp.Med.Biol.* 248 77-80(1989)

(7) A.Hasegawa, Y.Yamada, M.Tamura and Y.Nomura Vol.30 No.31 *Applied Optics* 4515-4520(1990)

MONITORING OF TISSUE OXYGENATION VIA PARAMETERS OF ERYTHRO-POETIC ACTIVITY

Johann Gross,[1] Burkhard Göldner,[2] Olaf Sowade,[2],
Gudrun Fleischak[2] and Ria Krüger[2]

[1]Institute of Pathological and Clinical Biochemistry
[2]Pediatric Clinic
Medical School (Charité), Humboldt University
Berlin, 1040

INTRODUCTION

Monitoring of hypoxia of infants with cyanotic heart disease (CHD) is a basic requirement for the treatment of the disease and prevention of late consequences. Blood gas analysis and determination of hemoglobin concentration (Hb) or hematocrit (Hk) are used as parameters for the assessment of tissue oxygenation in chronically hypoxic infants. Whereas blood gas parameters assess the acute situation, Hb or Hk give informations about the long-term adaptational changes. Both the level of Hb/Hk and O_2-status do not answer the question of compensation of hypoxemia.

The assessment of the status of compensation of hypoxemia seems to be very important with regard to the time of corrective surgery. An inverse association between cognitive function and the length of hypoxemic exposure was described[1].

The formation of red blood cells (rbc) depends on the relation of oxygen delivery and oxygen consumption and therefore it is conceivable that rbc could indicate real tissue hypoxia. A useful parameter to evaluate the formation of rbc is the determination of the percentage of low density cells by the erythrocyte density test[2] (EDT).

In the postnatal period, there are dramatic changes of the metabolic needs and in consequence of the oxygen transport capacity. In children with cyanotic heart disease an overlapping of adaptational effects of hypoxia and effects of the ontogenetic programme occurs in the first months of life in order to meet the needs for growth and development.

The aim of the present study was to compare the behaviour of paO_2, Hk, reticulocytes (reti) and EDT of healthy infants and infants with CHD in order to evaluate EDT as a criterion relevant for the severity of hypoxia.

Oxygen Transport to Tissue XV, Edited by P. Vaupel
et al., Plenum Press, New York, 1994

PATIENTS AND METHODS

Study 1 (table 1) was carried out as longitudinal study in 10 term infants (birth weight 2680-3640 g) and in 23 patients of congenital CHD (birth weight 2570-4720 g). The CHD infants included 16 cases with transpositions of great arteries, 2 cases M. Ebstein, 3 cases with hypoplastic right heart syndrome, 1 case of M. Fallot and 1 case of valvular pulmonal stenosis. The longitudinal study was carried out in the first 5 months of life. Based on the periods of erythropoetic activity the following timing for taking the blood samples was used: day 1 and 2 (for the assessment of prenatal conditions), day 2 and 4 (for the assessment of birth), day 7-9 (for the assessment of decreasing erythropoetic activity after birth), day 25-31 (for the assessment of the minimum of erythropoetic activity in the first trimenon) and day 50-60 and day 130-160 (for the assessment of recovery from the erythropoetic depression).

Study 2 (table 2-3) was carried out as a cross-sectional study in 40 infants of CHD (birth weight 2210-3960) and 42 infants of acyanotic heart desease (AHD, birth weight 2520-4020 g). In general these subjects were studied on two or more occasions. The diagnoses of the CHD infants were similar to study 1, the diagnoses of the AHD infants included 22 cases with ventricle septum defect, 6 cases with pulmonal stenosis, 9 cases of aortic isthmus stenosis, 5 cases of atrium septum defect. All determinations from patients with blood transfusion up to day 12 after transfusion were excluded from the calculations. In the first 5 months of life 13 infants with CHD died: 5 infants between day 1-7, 4 infants between day 29-150 and 4 infants older than 150 days. The study was approved by the Hospital's Ethical Committee.

For all investigations capillary blood was used, the determinations were carried out 2 h after taking the blood sample. Hk was measured by centrifugation method, reticulocyte count by counting after brilliant cresyl blue staining. EDT was carried out as previously described[2]. In principle, Hk-tubes were filled with 5 ul of phthalic esther, density 1.088 kg/l, and 10 ul blood suspended in about 50 ul BSG (phosphate buffered saline glucose, osmolarity 310 mosmol/l). After centrifugation in a hematocrit centrifuge (10 min, 18000 g) the length of the cell column above and below phthalic ester was measured and the percentage of low density cells (% ldc = fraction of cells with a density equal or lower 1.088 kg/l) was calculated. Haematological indices were determined using a H1 (Instrumentation laboratory) or Coulter Counter Model S 880 (Coulter Electronics). Blood gas measurements were performed on a AVL 995 Automatic Blood Gas Analyser.

In order to get statistically relevant data in study 2, the values from the following periods were combined: day 1-7, day 8-28, day 29-150 and beyond day 150. Statistical difference was tested by the U-test of Mann and Whitney.

RESULTS

1. Longitudinal Study on the Behaviour of Hk, Reti and EDT during the First 5 Months of Life

Infants with CHD show, in comparison to controls, in-

creased Hk and EDT values as adaptational changes. There is
no decrease of the Hk-value at the age of 30 days, the time
of trimenon reduction in control infants. In CHD infants the
reticulocyte counts show decreased values in the first 4 days
of life and clearly increased values on day 30 and 60. The
EDT values (% low density cells) tend to increase as early as
in the first week of life, values become statistically significant beyond day 30.

Table 1. Hematocrit, reticulocyte count and EDT in control (C)
(n = 6-10) and infants with CHD (n = 8-17) during the first 5
months of life

Day of life	Hk		Reti (%)		EDT (%ldc)	
	C	CHD	C	CHD	C	CHD
1-2	0.51	0.55	4.3	2.8*	6.9	7.7
	(0.09)	(0.11)	(0.7)	(1.8)	(1.0)	(1.0)
3-4	0.53	0.56*	2.9	2.2*	6.6	7.4
	(0.07)	(0.06)	(0.8)	(1.6)	(0.8)	(2.1)
7-9	0.48	0.54*	1.4	2.1	6.5	7.5
	(0.07)	(0.07)	(0.7)	(1.7)	(0.8)	(2.1)
25-31	0.32	0.51*	0.5	1.7*	4.9	10.0*
	(0.04)	(0.10)	(0.2)	(1.0)	(0.7)	(3.1)
50-60	0.34	0.54*	0.9	1.8*	7.3	10.0*
	(0.04)	(0.10)	(0.4)	(1.3)	(1.3)	(3.3)
130-150	0.36	0.62*	1.0	1.0	4.4	14.0*
	(0.04)	(0.07)	(0.2)	(0.6)	(0.5)	(10.6)

* p < 0.05 between C and CHD infants; mean and (SD)

2. Cross Sectional Study on the Diagnostic Relevance of EDT

The EDT was selected because of the early reaction in
response to chronic hypoxia and its simplicity. Because of
the overlapping of ontogenetic changes and changes caused by
hypoxia it is reasonable to analyse the differences in relation to the erythropoetic periods after birth.
Table 2 indicates the level of paO_2 in controls, infants
with AHD and infants with CHD. As expected, infants with AHD
show paO_2 values in the range of 7 kPa, the CHD in the range
of 4 kPa. There are no changes during the first 5 months of
life. The EDT values clearly differ in the different groups:
infants with CHD show increased values in each period compared to the AHD infants.
The dependency of EDT values on the paO_2 in all AHD and
CHD infants showed that relatively high EDT values occur in
infants with paO_2 lower than 4.1 kPa paO_2 only, but, surpri-
singly "normal" EDT values do also occur frequently here (not
shown). In order to analyse the behaviour of EDT in dependence on the paO_2 the group of CHD infants was divided into
infants with a paO_2 > 4.1 kPa and paO_2 < 4.1 kPa (table 3).
The EDT values show remarkable differences: relatively low

Table 2. paO_2 and EDT in control, AHD and CHD infants in different periods after birth

Age days	Control (n=6-10)	AHD (n=17-97)	CHD (n=61-182)
paO_2 1-7	8.4[1]	6.9	3.9*
	(0.8)	(1.4)	(1.1)
8-28	10.4	7.0	4.0*
	(1.0)	(1.9)	(0.9)
29-150	10.4	7.3	4.2*
	(1.0)	(1.7)	(1.0)
> 150	10.4	7.5	4.0*
	(1.0)	(1.3)	(0.7)
EDT 1-7	6.7[3]	1.1[2]	4.5*
	(1.0)	(1.0-1.5)	(3.1-10.1)
8-28	5.4	1.4	4.1*
	(0.7)	(1.0-3.4)	(1.5-8.0)
29-150	4.4	1.8	8.1*
	(1.0)	(1.0-3.0)	(2.0-21.7)
> 150	4.4	1.6	15.0*
	(0.5)	(0.5-2.5)	(3.2-47.6)

[1] x+/-s; [2] mean (25th-75th percentile); [3] data from study 1
* p < 0.01

levels in the CHD > 4.1 kPa infants and extremly high values in infants with CHD < 4.1 kPa.

In order to analyse the predictive value of EDT in the CHD infants with a paO_2 < than 4.1 kPa two groups were analysed: survivers and nonsurvivers (table 3). The paO_2 values of survivors and nonsurvivors are similar. In contrast, the EDT values clearly differ in both groups in all periods investigated: nonsurvivors show significantly higher values than survivors.

DISCUSSION

Hypoxia of infants with CHD is compensated by the formation of rbc and an increase in P_{50} in order to increase the transport capacity and the supply of oxygen[3]. With increasing Hk the viscosity of blood rises, which, in turn, may impair oxygen delivery to the tissue. Because of the overlapping of ontogenetic and adaptational changes in CHD infants it is important to relate hematological parameters to the periods of erythropoetic activity in the postnatal period. In previous studies we distinguished a period of relatively high erythropoetic activity (day 1-3), a period of low erythropoetic activity (day 8-28) and a period of recovery (beyond day 29)[4].

The density of rbc, measured by the EDT, is mainly a

function of MCHC. The continuous increase in EDT in infants with CHD may be interpreted as production of cells with decreased Hb concentration or as an expression of an increased fraction of newly formed rbc. The low Hb concentration could

Table 3. paO$_2$ (kPa) and EDT % ldc in AHD and CHD infants in different periods after birth

Age (days)	CHD		CHD < 4.1 kPa	
	>4,1kPa (n=23-90)	<4,1kPa (n=38-92)	S (n=16-36)	NS (n=22-62)
paO$_2$ 1-7	4.7 (0.9)	3.4 (0.8)	3.2 (0.8)	3.5 (0.4)
8-28	5.0 (0.6)	3.4 (0.5)	3.5 (0.5)	3.3 (0.4)
29-150	5.0 (0.8)	3.4 (0.6)	3.6 (0.4)	3.3 (0.6)
> 150	4.7 (0.6)	3.5 (0.5)	3.7 (0.4)	3.3 (0.4)
EDT 1-7	4.3 (2.4-6.6)	4.7 (3.3-13.6)	3.4 (3.1-4.7)	13.7* (11.0-19.0)
8-28	1.5 (0.9-3.1)	6.0* (3.9-9.8)	4.6 (3.5-7.9)	13.9* (10.1-19.0)
29-150	2.0 (1.4-4.3)	20.5* (9.0-32.0)	7.3 (2.2-10.6)	27.8* (19.2-38.0)
> 150	2.1 (1.1-4.4)	24.7* (9.4-54.1)	11.5 (3.6-41.8)	45.3* (27.3-58.9)

[1]x+/-s; [2]mean (25th percentile); * p < 0.01; S survivors, NS nonsurvivors

result from disturbances in the haem or the globin synthesis due to disturbances in iron metabolism or protein synthesis[5,6,7].

It is interesting to note that relatively high EDT values are observed below paO$_2$ < 4 kPa only, in addition "normal" EDT values were found. The density of rbc seems to be determined not only by arterial paO$_2$, but also by other factors. A possible reason for low EDT values in infants with CHD and a paO$_2$ < 4.1 kPa is that their hypoxemia is compensated[1,6]. This conclusion is in agreement with observation on serum immunoreactive erythropoetin level[1]. The differences observed in survivors and nonsurvivors also point to the status of compensation of hypoxia. Beside the compensatory changes an oxygen debt may still remain which could cause irreversible tissue damage resulting in long-term consequences or fatal outcome.

In the present study nonsurvivors had significantly higher EDT values than survivors. The severity of tissue injury may be reflected by the magnitude of the increase in EDT value as an expression of the production of rbc with a low Hb concentration. Because protein synthesis could be a limiting reaction in hypoxia, it is conceivable that a decompensated hypoxia is expressed in a decreased Hb concentration[5].

The diagnostic values of EDT carried out between day 26-30 of life seem to be extremely valuable for the prediction of the outcome: diagnostic sensitivity 100 %, diagnostic specificity 96 %, predictive value of the positive test 89 % and predictive value of the negative test 100 %. Because of the low number of patients investigated further studies are necessary before the test could be introduced into clinical practive.

REFERENCES

1. P.Haga, P.M. Cotes, J.A. Till, B.D. Minty and E. Shinebourne, Serum Immunoreactive Erythropietin in Children With Cyanotic and Acyanotic Congenital Heart Disease, Blood 70:822 (1987).
2. J.Gross, A. Lun, G. Fleischak and R. Krüger, The erythrocyte density test (EDT) - a useful screening test for the diagnosis of hypoxia in newborns and infants, in "Perinatal hypoxia", St. Trojan and J. Gross, ed., Universitas Carolina-Pragensis (1989).
3. S.S.Gidding an J. A. Stockman, Erythropoietin in cyanotic heart disease, Am. Heart J. 116:128 (1988).
4. J.Gross, E.L. Grauel und D. Mücke, Erythropoese und Erythrozyt im 1. Trimenon, Dtsch. Ges.wesen 26:678 (1973).
5. M.H.Rosove , J.K. Perloff, W.G. Hocking, J.S. Child, M.M. Canobbio and D.J. Skorton, Chronic hypoxaemia and decompensated erythrocytosis in cyanotic congenital heart disease, The Lancet, August 9:313 (1986).
6. M.R.Ryndal, D.F. Teitel, W.A. Lutin, G.K. Clemons and P.R. Dallman, Serum erythropoietin levels in patients with congenital heart disease, J. Pediatr. 110:538 (1987).
7. S.K.Jindal, B. Gupta, D. Mohanty, K.C. Das, P.S. Bidway and P.L. Wahi, Study of erythropoiesis, erythropoietin and haematological adjustments in congenital cyanotic heart disease. Indian J. Med. Res. 67:1019 (1978).

CARDIAC OUTPUT AND REGIONAL BLOOD FLOW MEASUREMENT WITH NONRADIOACTIVE MICROSPHERES BY X–RAY FLUORESCENCE SPECTROMETRY IN RATS

Ichiro Kuwahira[1], Hidezo Mori[2], Yoshihiro Moue[1], Yoshiro Shinozaki[2], Yasuyo Ohta[1], Hajime Yamabayashi[1], Haruka Okino[2], Norberto C. Gonzalez[3], Norbert Heisler[4], and Johannes Piiper[4]

[1]Department of Medicine and [2]Department of Physiology, Tokai University School of Medicine, Isehara, Kanagawa 259–11, Japan, [3]Department of Physiology, University of Kansas Medical Center, Kansas City, Kansas 66160–7401, USA and [4]Abteilung Physiologie, Max–Planck–Institut für experimentelle Medizin, 3400 Göttingen, FRG

INTRODUCTION

Since its introduction (Rudolph and Heymann, 1967) a number of studies have employed the radioactive microsphere method to evaluate changes in cardiac output, regional blood flow, and distribution of pulmonary blood flow under various experimental conditions. Unfortunately, the storage, handling, processing and disposing of radioactive materials requires many precautions and restrictions. Recently, an X–ray fluorescence system and the technique of labeling microspheres with stable heavy elements were developed and used to assess the coronary, hepatic and renal blood flow of large animals (Morita et al., 1990; Mori et al., 1992; Sakamoto et al., 1992). However, this method has not been applied to the measurement of blood flow in small animals such as rats. Rats are one of the most commonly used experimental animals, since entire organs can be easily analyzed because of their relatively small size.

The purpose of the present study was to investigate whether nonradioactive microspheres, labelled with stable heavy elements and detected by X–ray fluorescence spectrometry, can be applied to the measurement of cardiac output, regional blood flow, and distribution of pulmonary blood flow in rats.

METHODS

Nonradioactive microspheres (Sekisui Plastic Co., Ltd. Japan) are made of inert plastic labelled with different types of stable heavy elements as described in detail previously (Mori et al., 1992). In the present study, microspheres labelled with bromine (Br) or zirconium (Zr) were used. Mean diameter was 15 μm, and specific gravity was 1.34 for Br and 1.36 for Zr. Microspheres were suspended in normal saline and 0.05–0.1% SDS (sodium dodecyl sulfate). In every experiment, the microsphere suspensions were shaken well, and mixed mechanically in a syringe prior to and during infusion to prevent aggregation of spheres.

Oxygen Transport to Tissue XV, Edited by P. Vaupel
et al., Plenum Press, New York, 1994

The X-ray fluorescence activity of stable heavy elements was measured by a wavelength dispersive spectrometer (PW 1480, PHILIPS Co., Ltd.). Specifications of this X-ray fluorescence spectrometer have been described in detail previously (Mori et al., 1992). In brief, when the microspheres are irradiated by the primary X-ray beam, the elements absorb energy, and certain electrons are pushed into a higher orbit. Then, the electrons fall back to the lower orbit and give off measurable energy. This energy level of the X-ray fluorescence is characteristic for each element. Therefore, it is possible to quantify the X-ray fluorescence of several differently labelled microspheres in a mixture. Eight sets of nonradioactive microspheres, which are now commercially available, can be quantified by this spectrometry.

Two sets of experiments were carried out in the present study. A total of 14 male Sprague-Dawley rats weighing 356±18g were used. The rats were anesthetized with halothane, tracheostomized and mechanically ventilated. In the first set of experiments, we evaluated the accuracy and reproducibility of the flow measurement in the systemic circulation. A PE-50 catheter was advanced approximately 40 mm through the right common carotid artery into the left ventricle for microsphere infusion. Blood pressure was recorded while the catheter was inserted. Correct position of the catheter tip into the left ventricle was verified at the end of every experiment, when the animals were sacrificed. Another PE-50 catheter was inserted 10-20 mm into the middle caudal artery for withdrawal of the reference blood sample. In order to assess the accuracy of the flow measurement, microspheres labelled with Br and labelled with Zr, 400,000 spheres of each type (total 1.0 ml of suspensions), were simultaneously infused into the left ventricle of 5 rats. In order to evaluate the reproducibility, microspheres labelled with Br and Zr, 400,000 spheres of each type (0.5 ml each), were infused separately, at intervals of 30 minutes, into the left ventricle of 3 additional rats. The procedures for microsphere infusion and reference blood sample withdrawal have been described before (Kuwahira et al, 1992 a,b). Briefly, the reference blood sample was withdrawn from the middle caudal artery at a rate of 0.7 ml/min; 10 sec later, 0.5 ml(Br or Zr) or 1.0 ml(Br and Zr) of microsphere suspensions was infused and then flushed in with 0.5 ml of warm saline at a rate of 0.7 ml/min. Withdrawal of the reference sample continued for 30 sec after the saline flush was finished. Blood pressure and heart rate were recorded from the middle caudal artery immediately before and after microsphere infusion in order to evaluate changes in systemic hemodynamics following microsphere infusion. At the end of the experiment, the rats were sacrificed by an overdose of sodium pentobarbital and dissected for sampling organs and tissues. Brain, heart, diaphragm, liver, spleen, pancreas, stomach, small and large intestine with mesentery, kidneys, reproductive organs, hindlimb muscles, abdominal muscles, intercostal muscles, skin and fat were removed. These organs and the reference blood sample were weighed, placed in vials and dissolved in 2N-KOH solution. The remaining organs and tissues were also dissolved in order to calculate the total injected activity of infused microspheres (see below). The vials were then centrifuged, and the microspheres were aspirated and trapped on filter paper. The X-ray fluorescence activity of each element was measured by the spectrometer. Cardiac output and regional blood flow were calculated from the following equation:

$$\frac{\text{cardiac output}}{\text{total injected activity}} = \frac{\text{organ blood flow}}{\text{activity in organ}} = \frac{\text{reference sample withdrawal rate}}{\text{activity in reference blood sample}}$$

Fractional distribution of cardiac output (% of cardiac output) was calculated as:

$$\frac{\text{activity in organ}}{\text{total injected activity}} \times 100$$

The data of fractional distribution to investigated organs was compared with that measured with radioactive microspheres in our previous experiments (Kuwahira et al., 1992b).

In the second set of experiments, we evaluated the accuracy and reproducibility of the flow measurement in the pulmonary circulation. A PE-50 catheter was advanced approximately 95 mm through the left femoral vein into the inferior vena cava, 10 mm below the right atrium, for microsphere infusion. A no. 3.5 French umbilical vessel catheter (Argyle), angled to 90° over the distal 10 mm and curved slightly at the tip, was advanced approximately 35 mm through the right external jugular vein into the right ventricle for monitoring right ventricular pressure and heart rate (Stinger et al., 1981). Catheter position was indicated by recording the pressure contours. Correct position of both catheter tips was verified at the end of every experiment. In order to assess the accuracy of the flow measurement, microspheres labelled with Br and those labelled with Zr, 100,000 spheres of each type (total 1.0 ml of suspensions), were simultaneously infused into the inferior vena cava of 3 rats. In order to evaluate the reproducibility, microspheres labelled with Br and Zr, 100,000 spheres of each type (0.5 ml each), were infused separately, at intervals of 30 minutes, into the inferior vena cava of 3 additional rats. The microsphere suspensions were infused and then flushed in with 0.5 ml of warm saline at a rate of 0.7 ml/min. Right ventricular pressure and heart rate were recorded immediately before and after microsphere infusion. The rats were sacrificed at the end of the experiments. The lung was removed and cut into 9 samples. The procedures for dissolving tissues and measuring the activity of each element were identical to those described above. The total injected activity of infused microspheres was calculated by adding up the activities of 9 samples. In this second set of experiments, the reference blood sample was not withdrawn so that fractional distribution of total pulmonary blood flow (% of total pulmonary blood flow) was reported.

All results are presented as means±SE. A paired t test was used to compare data of arterial blood pressure, right ventricular pressure and heart rate before and after microsphere infusion. A P value of less than 0.05 was considered to indicate a statistically significant difference. Correlation and linear regression analyses were applied to the dual flow data: organ blood flows (ml/min/100g tissue) and fractional pulmonary blood flows (% of total pulmonary blood flow), calculated using the two microspheres, respectively.

RESULTS AND DISCUSSION

In the first set of experiments, microspheres labelled with Br and Zr were infused simultaneously into the left ventricle of 5 rats. Micropshere infusion caused no serious effects on central hemodynamics. Mean arterial blood pressure and heart rate did not change significantly (Table 1). MS indicates microspheres.

Table 1. Changes in central hemodynamics following microsphere infusion into the left ventricle.

	Before MS	After MS	
Mean arterial blood pressure	99± 8	101± 9	mmHg
Heart rate	303±17	312±20	/min

Comparison of cardiac output determined with the two microspheres infused simultaneously showed that cardiac output obtained with either microsphere was essentially equal (Table 2).

Table 2. Comparison of cardiac output determined with the two microspheres.

	Br–MS	Zr–MS	
Cardiac output	153±20	152±21	ml/min/kg

Figure 1 shows the results of correlation and linear regression analyses of regional blood flows in ml/min/100g tissue measured with the two microspheres. The results indicate that the blood flows obtained with either microsphere were essentially equal. There was a high correlation between the regional blood flows calculated with either microsphere. The linear regression equation calculated from least square fit of 170 blood flow data points (34 data points for each animal) was:

$$y = 1.00x - 0.93 \ (r = 0.99, \ Sy.x = 3.9)$$

where y is the regional blood flow calculated from the distribution of Zr microspheres and x is the value of blood flow calculated from the distribution of Br microspheres; r is the correlation coefficient, and Sy.x is the standard deviation from regression. The fact that equal blood flows were obtained with two indicators infused simultaneously indicates the accuracy of the present methods, including mixing and distribution of microspheres in the circulation as well as quantification of different elements.

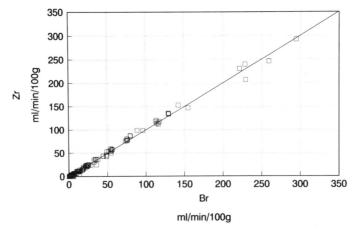

Figure 1. The results of correlation and linear regression analyses of regional blood flows in ml/min/100g tissue calculated using the two microspheres infused simultaneously showed good correlation and regression coefficients: y = 1.00x − 0.93 (n = 170, r = 0.99, Sy.x = 3.9).

In 3 additional rats, microspheres labelled with Br and Zr were infused into the left ventricle at 30 minutes intervals. Figure 2 shows the results of correlation and linear regression analyses of regional blood flows in ml/min/100g tissue measured with the two microspheres. The results indicate that the reproducibility of the flow measurement was high. There was a high correlation between the regional blood flows calculated with either microsphere. The linear regression equation calculated from least square fit of 102 blood flow data points (34 data points for each animal) was:

$$y = 0.99x - 0.45 \ (r = 0.98, \ Sy.x = 10.1)$$

where y, x, r and Sy.x have the same meaning as in the above equation. The results indicate that blood flows obtained within 30 minutes intervals in steady-state conditions were essentially equal.

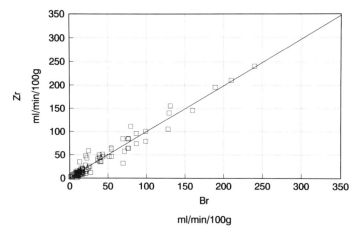

Figure 2. The results of correlation and linear regression analyses of regional blood flows in ml/min/100g tissue calculated using the two microspheres infused separately showed good correlation and regression coefficients: y = 0.99x − 0.45(n =102, r = 0.98, Sy.x = 10.1).

In the second set of experiments, microspheres labelled with Br and Zr were infused simultaneously into the inferior vena cava of 3 rats. Microsphere infusion caused no serious effects on pulmonary hemodynamics. Table 3 shows changes in mean right ventricular pressure and heart rate following microsphere infusion. There were no significant changes in these variables.

Table 3. Changes in pulmonary hemodynamics following microsphere infusion into the inferior vena cava.

	Before MS	After MS	
Mean right ventricular pressure	15.7±0.2	15.5±0.3	mmHg
Heart rate	328±28	324±26	/min

Figure 3 shows the results of correlation and linear regression analyses of fractional pulmonary blood flows (% of total pulmonary blood flow) determined with the two microspheres. The results indicate the accuracy of the pulmonary blood flow measurement. There was a high correlation between the fractional pulmonary blood flows calculated with either microsphere. The linear regression equation calculated from least square fit of 27 data points (9 data points for each lung) was:

$$y = 1.02x - 0.16 \ (r = 0.97, Sy.x = 0.74)$$

where y is the fractional pulmonary blood flow determined with Zr microspheres and x is the value determined with Br microspheres.

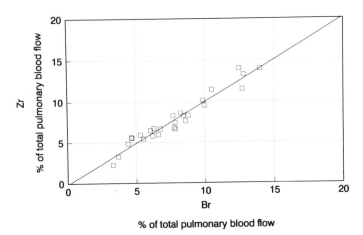

Figure 3. The results of correlation and linear regression analyses of fractional pulmonary blood flow (% of total pulmonary blood flow) determined with the two microspheres infused simultaneously showed good correlation and regression coefficients: y = 1.02x − 0.16 (n = 27, r = 0.97, Sy.x = 0.74).

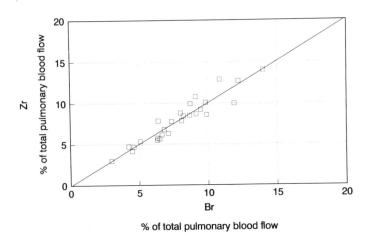

Figure 4. The results of correlation and linear regression analyses of fractional pulmonary blood flows (% of total pulmonary blood flow) determined with the two microspheres infused separately showed good correlation and regression coefficients: y = 1.01x − 0.07 (n = 27, r = 0.95, Sy.x = 0.90).

In 3 additional rats, microspheres labelled with Br and Zr were infused into the inferior vena cava at 30 minutes intervals. Figure 4 shows the results of correlation and linear regression analyses of fractional pulmonary blood flows (% of total pulmonary blood flow) determined with the two microspheres. The results indicate that the reproducibility of the pulmonary blood flow measurement was high. There was a high correlation between the fractional pulmonary blood flows calculated with either microsphere. The linear regression equation calculated from least square fit of 27 data points (9 data points for each lung) was:

$$y = 1.01x - 0.07 \ (r = 0.95, \ Sy.x = 0.90)$$

where y and x have the same meaning as in the above equation.

In order to evaluate the accuracy of the blood flow measurement in the present study, the data of fractional distribution to investigated organs was compared with that measured by us using radioactive microspheres in rats (Kuwahira et al., 1992b). Table 4 shows the results of comparison of fractional distribution between nonradioactive and radioactive microspheres. The data obtained in the present study was consistent with that measured with radioactive microspheres.

Table 4. Comparison of fractional distribution of cardiac output between nonradioactive and radioactive microspheres.

	Nonradioactive	Radioactive
Brain	1.9±0.3	1.5±0.2
Heart	6.9±1.4	5.0[*]
Diaphragm	0.3±0.1	0.6±0.1
Liver	4.4±0.9	2.6±0.8
Spleen	0.6±0.1	1.3±0.2
Pancreas	2.7±0.4	2.6±0.5
Stomach	2.7±0.3	2.2±0.4
Intestines	16.3±1.8	18.0±1.5
Splanchnic	26.7±2.9	26.8±1.9
Portal	22.3±2.4	24.1±2.3
Kidneys	11.0±1.7	16.0±1.6
Reproductive organs	2.6±0.5	2.3±0.2
Hindlimb muscles	4.4±1.6	5.8±0.7
Abdominal muscles	1.2±0.3	1.5±0.2
Intercostal muscles	2.9±0.3	2.8±0.3
Skin	8.7±1.2	8.6±0.9
Fat	0.5±0.1	0.8±0.2

Fractional distribution is presented in percentage of cardiac output.
Fractional distribution determined with radioactive microspheres
was obtained in our previous experiments except heart.
* Literature data (Baker et al., 1979)

In summary, we applied nonradioactive microspheres, labelled with stable heavy elements and detected by X-ray fluorescence spectrometry, to the measurement of cardiac output, regional blood flow, and distribution of pulmonary blood flow in anesthetized rats. Microsphere infusion caused no significant changes in central and pulmonary hemodynamics. The accuracy of the measurement was tested by comparing blood flows obtained with the simultaneous infusions of microspheres labelled with Br and Zr. The reproducibility of the method was tested by comparing the data of blood flows in consecutive determinations in the same animal. The results demonstrated the accuracy and reproducibility of both systemic and pulmonary blood flow measurements. Fractional distribution of cardiac output was consistent with that measured with radioactive microspheres in our previous experiments. It is concluded that the present method with nonradioactive microspheres can be applied to the measurement of cardiac output, regional blood flow, and distribution of pulmonary blood flow in rats.

ACKNOWLEDGMENTS

This study was supported by a Grant–in–Aid for Scientific Research from the Ministry of Education, Science, and Culture of Japan No. 03770443, and Tokai University School of Medicine Research Aid.

REFERENCES

Baker, H.J., Lindsey, J.R., and Weisbroth, S.H., 1979, "The Laboratory Rat", Academic Press, New York.

Kuwahira, I., Gonzalez, N.C., Heisler, N., and Piiper, J., 1992a, Regional blood flow in conscious resting rats determined by microsphere distribution, *J. Appl. Physiol.* (in press).

Kuwahira, I., Gonzalez, N.C., Heisler, N., and Piiper, J., 1992b, Changes in regional blood flow distribution and oxygen supply during hypoxia in conscious rats, *J. Appl. Physiol.* (in press).

Mori, H., Haruyama, S., Shinozaki, Y., Okino, H., Iida, A., Takanashi, R., Sakuma, I., Husseini, W.K., Payne, B., and Hoffman, J.I.E., 1992, New nonradioactive microspheres and more sensitive X–ray fluorescence to measure regional blood flow, *Am. J. Physiol.* (submitted).

Morita, Y., Payne, B., Aldea, G.S., McWatters, C., Husseini, W., Mori, H., Hoffman, J.I.E., and Kaufman, L., 1990, Local blood flow measured by fluorescence excitation of nonradioactive microspheres, *Am. J. Physiol.* 258 (*Heart Circ. Physiol.* 27): H1573–H1584.

Rudolph, A.M., and Heymann, M.A., 1967, The circulation of the fetus in utero: methods for studying distribution of blood flow, cardiac output and organ blood flow, *Circ. Res.* 21:163–184.

Sakamoto, H., Tanaka, Y., Mitomi, T., Shinozaki, Y., Haruyama, S., and Mori, H., 1992, Nonradioactive microspheres and X–ray fluorescence to measure regional blood flow in chronic animal experiments, *FASEB Journal* 6: A1473.

Stinger, R.B., Iacopino, V.J., Alter, I., Fitzpatrick, T.M., Rose, J.C., and Kot, P.A., 1981, Catheterization of the pulmonary artery in the closed–chest rat, *J. Appl. Physiol.: Respirat. Environ. Exercise Physiol.* 51: 1047–1050.

USE OF LIGHTGUIDE REFLECTANCE SPECTROPHOTOMETRY IN THE ASSESSMENT OF PERIPHERAL ARTERIAL DISEASE.

P. Hickman[1], D.K. Harrison[1], S.D. Evans[1], J.J.F. Belch[2] and P.T. McCollum[1]

[1]Vascular Laboratory and
[2]Department of Medicine
   Ninewells Hospital and Medical School
   Ninewells
   Dundee, DD2 1SY
   Scotland

INTRODUCTION

Peripheral vascular disease (PVD) is a major cause of morbidity in the Western World. Its most common manifestation is intermittent claudication which is a symptom of cramp-like muscle pain. It is brought on by walking, relieved by rest and reproduced by further exercise and it may affect the calf, thigh or buttock muscle groups depending on the site and severity of the disease. Approximately 5% of men over 50 years of age suffer from intermittent claudication[1]. It is caused by an inadequate blood flow through the muscle during exercise, although the exact pathophysiological mechanism responsible for the symptom is still unknown[2].

Although angiography can provide structural information, essential for the management of claudicants, the clinical presentation often bears little relationship to the apparent morphology[3]. This is because the haemodynamic significance of any given arterial stenosis or occlusion depends on the combined effects of the occlusive disease and the ability of the alternative collateral pathways to compensate[4]. An assessment of haemodynamics in the affected extremity is therefore essential. Despite the efforts of many vascular laboratories, however, the assessment of claudication remains controversial[5]. Arterial pressure measurement has, in general, been accepted as the most appropriate method of assessment[6]. Although it is a useful screening test, it is not ideal. It is relatively insensitive in that changes in the ankle-brachial ratio (AB ratio) of as much as 0.15 may not be significant[7]. Arterial calcification, which is relatively common in diabetics, makes Doppler-derived pressure measurement unreliable, resulting in spuriously high AB ratios because the vessels are incompressible[8]. There is a poor correlation between the the AB ratio and the measured walking distance of claudicants by treadmill testing[5]. We have recently adopted the technique of lightguide remittance spectrophotometry (LRS) for measurement of the relative haemoglobin concentration (HBI) and absolute haemoglobin oxygen saturation (SO_2) in the skin[9]. LRS has recently been investigated in our laboratory for the assessment of PVD for use in patients with non-compliant arteries and to seek a test which more accurately reflects disease severity. In order to assess the value of LRS as a non-invasive test in patients with PVD we compared the results obtained with LRS against Doppler-derived pressure measurements before and after a standard exercise test in patients with compliant arteries.

MATERIALS AND METHODS

Spectrophotometer

A Photal MCPD-1000 (Otsuka Electronics, Osaka) lightguide spectrophotometer, employing a Y configuration lightguide was used for this investigation. Light from a 150 Watt Xenon lamp was used to illuminate the skin or cuvette via the transmitting fibres and the back-scattered light was transmitted via the receiving fibres to the photometer. The light then passed to a diffraction grating which splits the light into its spectral components in the wavelength range 300 to 1100 nm before falling on the photodiode array of the detector. The signal from the detector was then amplified and digitalised and then transferred to a personal computer for processing. Prior to the clinical investigations, a number of *in vitro* and *in vivo* experiments were carried out to calibrate the system.

In a series of *in vitro* experiments using our instrument we identified 5 isosbestic points (wavelengths of constant absorption, independent of oxygenation) in the wavelength range 500 to 620 nm for haemoglobin. Isosbestic points were also identified in the volar forearm skin of volunteers during cuff occlusions. Using these isosbestic points, a method was developed for the measurement of HBI. This can be calculated from the addition of the gradients of the extinction spectrum between the isosbestic points (see Fig.1.). The HBI may be calculated from the following equation :-

$$HBI = 100 \times [((E_{527.1}-E_{500})/27.1) + ((E_{548.5}-E_{527.1})/21.4)$$
$$+ ((E_{548.5}-E_{571.8})/23.3) + ((E_{571.8}-E_{585.4})/13.6)]\%.$$

where E_x is the extinction at wavelength X and may be calculated from absorption (A_x) according to :-

$$E_x = -\log(1-A_x).$$

Extinction is expressed in units of optical density and, according to the Lambert-Beer law, is directly proportional to the concentration of the absorbing medium. A series of *in vitro* cuvette experiments were performed measuring the HBI of known concentrations of haemoglobin ([Hb]) in a suspension of barium sulphate (acting as a scattering medium). A curvilinear relationship was demonstrated between HBI and [Hb] but at concentrations found physiologically in the skin this proved linear ($r^2 = 0.94$)[9].

A six point method was developed for measurement of the oxygenation index (OXI) (see Fig.2). The parameter OXI is calculated from the gradients of the extinction spectra from the point where the spectra differ most between oxygen and deoxygenated haemoglobin to the nearest isosbestic points and is then normalised for HBI according to the below equation :-

$$OXI = 100/HBI \times [((E_{571.8}-E_{560.1})/11.7) + ((E_{560.1}-E_{548.5})/11.6)]\%.$$

where E_x is the extinction at wavelength x.

OXI was measured against a series of known haemoglobin oxygen saturations (SO_2) *in vitro* in a series of tonometer experiments. A linear relationship between the OXI and the SO_2 was demonstrated in these experiments ($r^2 = 0.97$). In a series of experiments using 6 minute cuff occlusions of the forearm in healthy volunteers we were both able to validate this and also to define 0% haemoglobin oxygen saturation *in vivo*.

Subjects

8 healthy normal volunteers and 13 patients with proven PVD were recruited. The healthy volunteers were aged from 25 to 40 years, of either sex and had a resting AB ratio of greater than 0.95. The patients were aged 45 to 75, of either sex and had a resting AB ratio of less than 0.95 and a proven occlusion of either the aorto-iliac segment or femoro-popliteal segment on angiography. There were thus 3 groups : i)

normal volunteers (n = 8); ii) patients with an aorto-iliac occlusion (n = 5); iii) patients with a femoro-popliteal occlusion.

All subjects were rested supine for at least 15 minutes and then the AB ratio, together with the HBI and SO_2 were measured on the dorsum of the foot. Each subject then underwent a standard exercise test of one minute on a treadmill (10° slope at 3.5 km/hr). The above parameters were then measured at one minute intervals for 5 minutes following exercise.

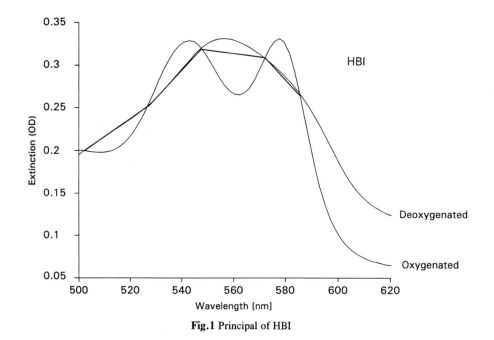

Fig.1 Principal of HBI

RESULTS

Group (i) showed a rise in AB ratio following exercise; group (iii) exhibited a fall in AB ratio with a gradual recovery whilst group (ii) showed a more profound fall in AB ratio with a more prolonged recovery (see Fig.3.).

Group (i) showed a slight but not significant fall in SO_2 after exercise; group (ii) showed a significant fall in SO_2 ($p < 0.01$) and group (iii) showed a highly significant fall in SO_2 (p<0.001) (see Fig.4.). There was also a statistically significant fall in HBI in patients in group (ii), although there was no significant fall in the other two groups (see Fig.5.). There was an excellent correlation between the $t_{1/2}$ recovery time for SO_2 and ankle pressures in all subjects (r =0.91, p,0.001) (see Fig.6.).

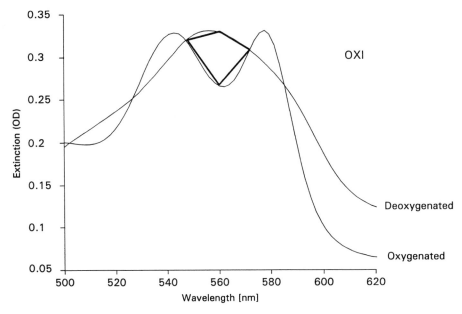

Fig.2. Principal of OXI

DISCUSSION

The ankle pressure of a claudicant falls during exercise[10]. The blood pressure distal to either an arterial stenosis or occlusion falls during exercise in claudicants. This is a direct result of shunting of blood to the area of lowest resistance, namely the exercising muscle, and the high vascular resistance across an arterial stenosis or the collateral arteries bypassing an occlusion[4]. Pathophysiological considerations suggest that exercise muscle blood flows at comparable work loads must always be reduced in claudicants compared to normal subjects and this has been verified by ^{133}Xe xenon

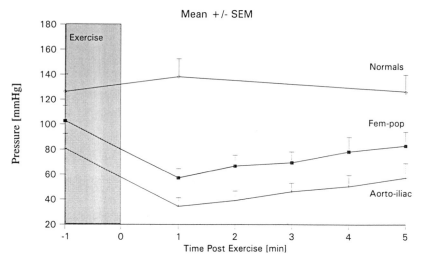

Fig.3 Change in pressure following exercise

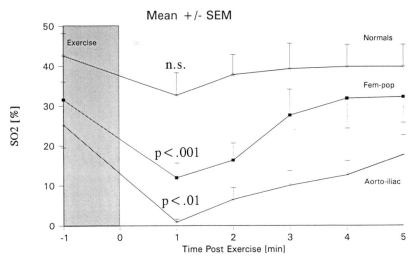

Fig.4 Mean SO$_2$ following exercise

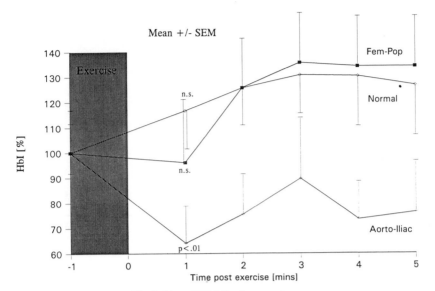

Fig.5 Mean HBI following exercise

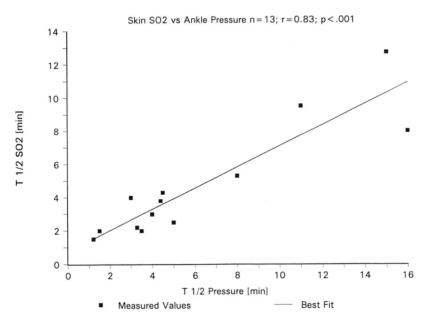

Fig.6 Regression of recovery half times

clearance studies[11]. One would also expect muscle oxygenation to fall if consumption outstrips delivery. Intramuscular oxygen tension has been shown to rise with exercise in normal subjects but to fall in patients with PVD[12]. As the ankle pressure of claudicants falls after exercise one would expect skin perfusion also to fall and there to be a corresponding fall in the SO_2 in the skin. This work has confirmed this. The changes in the skin of normals were not statistically significant but one could speculate that decreases in SO_2 in the skin may be due to shunting of blood from the skin to exercising muscle. The only significant changes in HBI were in patients with aorto-iliac disease who have reduced arterial inflow. We speculate that HBI represents the balance between the arterial inflow and the muscle pump pumping blood away from the capillary beds.

CONCLUSIONS

This preliminary data suggests that LRS may provide a very good and non-invasive method of assessing patients with non-compliant arteries and warrants further extensive study.

REFERENCES

1. J. Dormandy, M. Mahir, G. Ascady et al. Fate of the patient with chronic leg ischaemia. *J. Cardiovasc. Surg.* 30: 314 (1989).
2. E. Lorentsen. Blood pressure and flow in the calf in relation to claudication distance. *Scand. J. Clin. Lab. Investig.* 31:141 (1973).
3. B.L. Thiele, Strandness D.E. Accuracy of angiographic quantification of peripheral atherosclerosis. *Progress in cardiovascular disease.* 26: 223 (1983).
4. E. Strandness, J.W. Bell. An evaluation of the haemodynamic response of the claudicating extremity to exercise. *Surg. Gynae. Obstet.* 119: 1237 (1964).
5. D. Wilkinson, P. Vowden, A. Parkin et al. A reliable and readily available method of measuring limb blood flow in intermittent claudication. *Br. J. Surg.* 74: 516 (1987).
6. A.R. Baker, D.S. Macpherson, D.H. Evans et al. Pressure measurements in arterial surgery. *Eur. J. Vasc. Surg.* 1: 273. (1987).
7. J.D. Baker, P.A.C. DeEtte. Variability of Doppler ankle pressures with arterial disease: An evaluation of ankle index and brachial ankle pressure gradient. *Surgery.* 89: 134 (1980).
8. W.F. Walker, V.A. Spence, P.T. McCollum. Systolic pressure measurements in the ischaemic lower limb. *Hospital Update.* 12: 349. (1986).
9. D.K. Harrison, S.D. Evans, N.C. Abbott et al. Spectrophotometric measurement of haemoglobin saturation and concentration in skin during tuberculin reaction in normal subjects. *Clin. Phys. and Physiol. Meas.* 13: (in Press) (1992).
10. S.A. Carter. Indirect systolic pressures and and pulse waves in arterial occlusive disease of the lower extremities. *Circulation.* 37: 624 (1968).
11. K.H. Tonnensen. Muscle blood flow during exercise in intermittent claudication: Validation of the [133]xenon clearance technique: Clinical use by comparison to plethysmography and walking distance. *Circulation.* 37: 402 (1968).
12. E.J. Jussaila, J. Nijnikoski. Effect of vascular reconstructions on tissue gas tensions in the calf muscles of patients with occlusive arterial disease. *Ann. Chir. Gynaecol.* 70: 56 (1981).

MODELLING ERYTHROCYTES AS POINT-LIKE
O$_2$ SOURCES IN A KROGHIAN CYLINDER MODEL

Louis Hoofd, Cees Bos, and Zdenek Turek

Department of Physiology
University of Nijmegen
The Netherlands

INTRODUCTION

In modelling O$_2$ transport to tissue, the capillary is often considered as a uniform oxygen source. Nevertheless, almost all the oxygen is supplied from the hemoglobin packed in single erythrocytes. Few literature models handle this particulate nature of blood O$_2$ supply, and even fewer consider the consequences in a tissue pO$_2$ model. Then, these particulate models are often too complicated or too laborious to be applied on large portions of tissue or on many tissue cases, as is needed for correct judgement of tissue oxygenation, e.g., as pO$_2$ histograms. For a recent overview, see Popel (1989). Here, the simplest way of representing O$_2$ sources, the point-like source, is worked out for handling erythrocytic O$_2$ supply, and the consequences for tissue O$_2$ considered referring to the simple basic configuration of the Krogh/Kety cylinder model.

METHODS

The model layout is a tissue cylinder, of radius R and length L, with a centrally located capillary, of radius r_c, in where erythrocytes are represented by point-like oxygen sources located on the axis of the cylinder. For simplicity, it is assumed here that these sources are evenly distributed, with and identical spacing Δz, and stay so while moving along the axis, with velocity v. Consequently, radial symmetry is assumed in the model.

Mathematical treatment

The model coordinates are the cylindrical coordinates $\vec{r} = (r,z)$, radial and axial respectively, and there are N erythrocytes, the ith one located at $\vec{r}_i = (0, \{i-\frac{1}{2}\}\Delta z)$, where $\Delta z = L/N$. The situation is considered independent of time by the "flash photograph" technique: every instant when this configuration is reached, so in evenly spaced time intervals $\Delta t = \Delta z/v$. Then, from dimensional analysis it is concluded that the resulting differential equations may approximately be handled as in steady state; including myoglobin-facilitated diffusion, it is described by:

$$\mathcal{P} \nabla^2 p + D_{Mb} \nabla^2 (c_{Mb} s) = M \tag{1}$$

where $\mathcal{P}$, p, M are O_2 permeability, O_2 pressure and tissue O_2 consumption respectively, D_{Mb}, c_{Mb}, s are myoglobin (Mb) diffusion coefficient, total Mb concentration and Mb oxygen saturation respectively. The solution of eq.1 is written here as:

$$p + p_F s = C_p + \frac{M}{4\mathcal{P}} \{ \Phi(\vec{r}) + \sum_{i=1}^{N} \frac{V_i}{\pi |\vec{r} - \vec{r_i}|} \} \tag{2}$$

where $p_F = D_{Mb} c_{Mb}/\mathcal{P}$ is facilitation pressure, C_p is a constant, $\Phi(\vec{r})$ is a homogeneous solution of eq.1, and V_i is the O_2 supply volume of the ith source - as can be deduced from analyzing the radial flux around $\vec{r} = \vec{r_i}$. The "background function" $\Phi(\vec{r})$ must be constructed so that it fulfils the boundary conditions, which read:
- there is no O_2 flux across the cylinder borders, at $r = R$ and $z = 0,L$;
- p must match erythrocytic O_2 pressure p_i for each erythrocyte.

Since - because of the geometry - the axial gradients are unimportant, the first condition can be approximately met by assuming equal supply volumes $V_i = \pi R^2 \Delta z$ for each source. For the second condition, at first p_i must be derived from the incoming arteriolar O_2 pressure p_1. The total O_2 concentration c_i of the ith erythrocyte is:

$$c_i = c_{Hm} s_i + \alpha_e p_i \tag{3}$$

where c_{Hm} is oxygen binding capacity (heme concentration), s_i is the hemoglobin (Hb) oxygen saturation and α_e the erythrocytic O_2 solubility; for simplicity, c_i, s_i and p_i are assumed homogeneous throughout the erythrocyte. In between the "flashes", when the erythrocyte moves on from $z = z_i$ to $z = z_{i+1}$, it releases from its volume V_e an O_2 amount of $V_e \Delta c_i = M V_i \Delta t$ to the surrounding tissue so that:

$$c_{i+1} = c_i - \frac{\pi M R^2 \Delta z^2}{v V_e} \tag{4}$$

From eqs.3,4, the consecutive c_i's and p_i's can be calculated when assuming chemical equilibrium between p_i and s_i via the O_2 dissociation curve. Correction for plasma pO_2 can be made by replacing α_e by $\{V_e \alpha_e + (\pi r_c^2 \Delta z - V_e)\alpha_p\}/V_e$, where α_p is plasma O_2 solubility. For matching p_i to tissue p, the following reasoning is followed:
- any kind of source confined in a small region resembles a point source when "looked at from far away" from the source;
- sources evenly distributed over a sphere look exactly the same as a point source located in the sphere centre, when seen from outside the sphere;
- so, for the tissue, the erythrocyte resembles a sphere evenly filled with O_2 sources;
- consequently, tissue p is matched to p_i at this sphere radius $r = r_e$, where $V_e = {}^4/_3 \pi r_e^3$ (sphere volume of radius r_e) - actually, at $\vec{r} = (r_e, z_i)$.

A homogeneous solution $\Phi(\vec{r})$ of eq.1 now can be constructed so that it matches these boundary conditions:

$$\Phi(r,z) = r^2 - R^2\ln(z + \sqrt{r^2 + z^2}) - R^2\ln\{L - z + \sqrt{r^2 + (L-z)^2}\} + \sum_{n=1}^{N} C_n F_n(r,z) \qquad (5)$$

where C_n are coefficients to be solved and $F_n(r,z)$ are polynomials in r,z with z^n as highest order:

$$
\begin{aligned}
F_1(r,z) &= z \\
F_2(r,z) &= z^2 - \tfrac{1}{2}r^2 \\
F_3(r,z) &= z^3 - \tfrac{3}{2}zr^2 \\
F_4(r,z) &= z^4 - 3z^2r^2 + \tfrac{3}{8}r^4 \\
F_5(r,z) &= z^5 - 5z^3r^2 + \tfrac{15}{8}zr^4
\end{aligned}
$$

...

Actually, it turned out sufficient to limit the summation to these five terms.

Input data

Two situations were considered here:
- Rat heart muscle, data according to Hoofd et al. (1990);
- Dog gracilis muscle, data according to Groebe (1990).

Table 1. Summary of data used in the calculations.

DIMENSIONAL DATA

	R	r_c	L	Δz	V_e	r_e
	μm	μm	μm	μm	$fL = \mu m^3$	μm
Rat	10.0	2.4	500	8-16	66	2.5
Dog	22.6	2.3	912	9-18	66	2.5

TISSUE DATA

	$\wp$	M	p_F	$p_{50\ Mb}$	c_{Mb}
	$mol \cdot m^{-1} \cdot mmHg^{-1} \cdot s^{-1}$	$mol \cdot m^{-3} \cdot s^{-1}$	mm Hg	mm Hg	$mol \cdot m^{-3}$
Rat	$2.35\ 10^{-12}$	0.665	14.0	5.3	0.25
Dog	$1.09\ 10^{-12}$	0.0991	39.6	5.3	0.54

BLOOD DATA

	α_e	c_{Hm}	$p_{50\ Hb}$	n_{Hill}	p_1 (begin)	p_N (end)
	$mol \cdot m^{-3} \cdot mmHg^{-1}$	$mol \cdot m^{-3}$	mm Hg		mm Hg	mm Hg
Rat	$1.57\ 10^{-3}$	21.4	37.0	2.7	100	39.0
Dog	$1.56\ 10^{-3}$	20.3	26.4	2.65	60	23.4

The resulting data are summarized in table 1. For Hb saturation, the Hill equation was applied: $p = p^n/(p^n+p_{50}^n)$; Mb saturation curve is hyperbolic: $p = p/(p+p_{50})$. For easier comparison with literature, pressures are denoted here in mm Hg (1 kPa = 7.5 mm Hg).

As shown in table 1, different values of erythrocyte spacing Δz were considered. In order to appreciate the influence of this spacing per se, the resulting different hematocrit (Hct) was compensated for by adapting the blood velocity v, so that the end-capillary pressure (p_N) remained the same for each situation; in fact, v is calculated from the table data. In the same way, a comparison was made with a Krogh/Kety situation (extended to account for facilitated diffusion by replacing p by $p+p_Fs$ as in eq.2) which in fact now is close to the limit case for $\Delta z \to 0$.

RESULTS

The calculated tissue pO_2's are presented graphically, below, pO_2 on the vertical axis against location (r,z) in the tissue cylinder. Most interesting would be the differences with the Krogh/Kety calculations; in order to quantify such differences, the reasoning below was followed:
- at a location far away from the capillary, the series of single sources will look like a continuous source line;
- at this location, also the Krogh equation can be applied;
- the capillary pO_2, p_c, in the Krogh equation can be chosen so that the calculated tissue pO_2 is the same;
- the difference between this p_c and the actual erythrocytic pO_2, p_i, is called *Extraction Pressure* (EP). This is equivalent to the term *Capillary Barrier* (CB) also used in the literature.

EP (CB) can be calculated for each individual erythrocyte in the array. In all calculations, however, EP turned out to be almost constant over the capillary length. So, for each individual situation a mean value of EP can be presented.

Rat heart

In figure 1, pO_2 profiles are shown for the rat heart case, Krogh/Kety situation (A) and point-source solution for three different hematocrit values (Hct; B, C, D). Note that, because a Krogh cylinder is very much longer than wide, the scale of the r and z axes is different. Whereas in panel A the whole profile along the z axis is smooth, in the particulate case there are up to strong oscillations, extending further from the capillary into the tissue when Hct is lower. These oscillations in the axial direction can be quite large, at the capillary level (r = r_c) up to an amplitude of 29.3 mm Hg [3.91 kPa] in case D. They fade out quickly when receding from the capillary; at the border (r = R) it is 2.9 mm Hg [0.4 kPa] in case D. Then, gradients in the radial direction, along r, will be very different when starting off from an erythrocyte or in between: drop of 29.9 mm Hg [3.99 kPa] against 3.6 mm Hg [0.48 kPa] from r_c to R in case D. Anyhow, as is in the Krogh case A, the steepest gradients are around the capillary. Profiles are much flatter in the outer region, e.g., 2.7 mm Hg [9.36 kPa] from 6 to 10 μm in the Krogh case A and 3.6 - 4.6 mm Hg [0.48 - 0.61 kPa] in case D. Also, the steepening perierythrocytic gradients cause tissue pO_2 levels on the whole to decrease with increasing spacing.

Dog gracilis

In figure 2, pO_2 profiles are shown for the dog gracilis case, also Krogh/Kety situ-

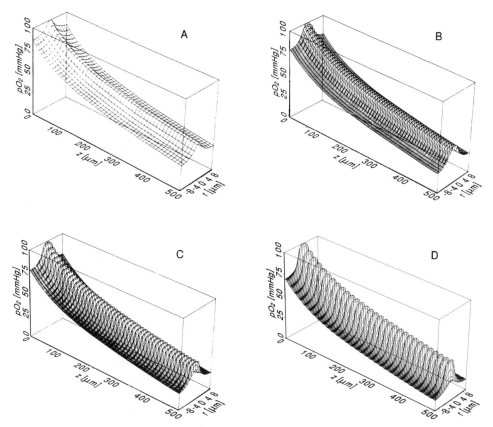

Figure 1. Calculated pO_2 profiles for rat heart case, Krogh situation (**A**), Hct=45.2% (**B**), Hct=33.9% (**C**) and Hct=22.6 (**D**).

ation (**A**) and point-source solution for three different hematocrit values (Hct; **B**, **C**, **D**). The same features appear as discussed above for figure 1, though in case **B** the axial oscillations are so closely spaced that they are hardly visible. Again for case **D**, the axial oscillation amplitude is 44.2 mm Hg [5.89 kPa] at $r = r_c$ decreasing to 0.2 mm Hg [0.03 kPa] at $r = R$ - note that R is over twice as large as with the rat heart! Also, the combination of data (large R, low M, large p_F and low p_i) leads to more flat radial gradients particularly at the end of the cylinder. Also, the axial gradient in pO_2 is very flat, yielding most p's below 10 mm Hg [1.33 kPa]. In cases **A** and **B** p remains positive, in case **C** there is a small portion of anoxic tissue; in case **D** this would be so large that the calculation end the end portion of the cylinder is no longer valid - though not easily seen from the figure, at $z = 912$ μm p drops below zero already closely around the erythrocyte. In other words: Hct is too low here to maintain adequate O_2 supply to all the surrounding tissue.

Extraction Pressures

The smooth, Krogh/Kety-like profiles mostly approached when receding from the capillary allow comparison with such calculations, as pointed out above and quantified in terms of Extraction Pressure EP. A value of EP can be calculated for each individual erythrocyte, but turned out to be almost the same along the z axis, for each p_i, in any particular situation. So, an average value can be provided. The largest standard devia-

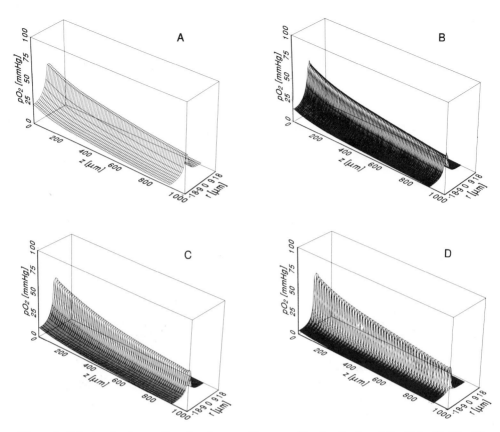

Figure 2. Calculated pO$_2$ profiles for dog gracilis case, Krogh situation (**A**), Hct=44.4% (**B**), Hct=33.3% (**C**) and Hct=22.2% (**D**).

Table 2. Hematocrit values (Hct) and resulting Extraction Pressures (EP) for the cases considered.

	Rat heart			Dog gracilis	
Hct	EP (or CB)		Hct	EP (or CB)	
%	mm Hg	kPa	%	mm Hg	kPa
45.2	5.7	0.76	44.4	8.9	1.19
33.9	8.6	1.15	33.3	14.7	1.96
22.6	16.9	2.25	22.2	29.6	3.95

tion (SD) in the average value was 3.0 mm Hg [0.4 kPa] (dog, case **D**).

The data of the different hematocrits used and of the resulting Extraction Pressures are shown in table 2. Obviously, EP strongly depends on Hct. Note, that a lower Hct was compensated for by an increased flow so as to keep O$_2$ delivering capacity of the capillary the same (resulting in the same capillary end pressure). Nevertheless, there is quite an extra drop in tissue pO$_2$ caused by the wider spacing of the sources. Note, that in the dog gracilis Hct=22% case EP is even larger than the end-capillary pressure. So, the Krogh simulation would start from a negative p_c which is obviously meaningless. This concords with the conclusion above, that the treatment is no longer valid in the end portion of the cylinder of figure 2 panel **D**.

DISCUSSION

In modelling tissue O_2 distribution, there are two steps that cannot be brought together, or not yet. Firstly, there is a quite complicated situation in and around each particular erythrocyte in the flowing capillary blood, which must be solved in order to find out how O_2 is distributed into the surrounding tissue. Secondly, a realistic tissue model must encompass quite a large tissue portion, with several capillaries (Hoofd et al., 1989; Hoofd and Turek, 1992). For a complete model, this means solving a vast number of complicated situations even before starting tissue O_2 distribution. So, in practice, either the small-scale or the large-scale situation was handled. There is few literature handling "in-between" cases, e.g., Groebe (1990) handles 4 capillaries and a somewhat simplified solution for the erythrocyte environment. His figure 2 nicely shows pO_2 peaks around the erythrocytes, similar to those in our figure 2.

Tsai and Intaglietta (1989) investigated a similar layout as used here, diffusion from single sources into a surrounding tissue cylinder. They numerically solved a set of equations including (cylindrical) erythrocyte shape and time dependence. Their results also showed the steep drops in pO_2 around the erythrocytes and the oscillatory phenomena along the array of them. They also pointed out, that tissue pO_2 significantly depended on the actual hematocrit value while keeping the product of hematocrit and flow, e.g., the oxygen delivery, the same; just as is found here. In their figure 3, a moving front of pO_2 around the moving erythrocytes is shown, which indeed looks like a steady moving profile, allowing "flash photography" as applied above.

The concept of EP or CB was used in earlier publications of our group to account for the pericapillary pO_2 drop, assuming to compensate for the particulate nature of blood and for possible other O_2 barriers so that the capillary could be handled as a uniform source as seen from the tissue - at least, the distant tissue. However, there were no general data or theories that could predict values for the cases considered.

It was for the latter, that the point-like source treatment was developed, as laid down above. Though surely a crude treatment, it gives some idea of how large EP will be in any situation one wishes to consider (for any set of capillary and tissue data as laid out in table 1). The mathematics is simple and the only somewhat more complicated part is to match the coefficients C_n of eq.5 to the actual capillary pO_2 profile. Even that might be obsolete, when EP turns out to be almost independent of pO_2; then, e.g., a constant or linear axial profile might be assumed.

It must be stressed, however, that the model is a large simplification. Nothing is modelled about what is happening in the capillary itself, neither in the erythrocyte nor in the plasma. No heterogeneity in erythrocyte spacing was considered. These are small-scale features, so they might have only limited effect on the outcomes of EP. Possibly more of a problem is, that all supply volumes V_i were taken the same. However, from tissue models allowing V_i to vary along the capillary axis, it is deduced that these variations are very limited indeed (Hoofd et al., 1990), for parallel capillaries.

Once values found for EP, it can be implemented very easily in tissue O_2 models. Instead of approaching actual erythrocyte pressure p_i, the tissue approaches p_i-EP_i. Then, pO_2 around the capillary will not be modelled correctly - because of the oscillations in pO_2 there - but this is only for a small portion of tissue. The actual oscillatory phenomenon will be smaller because there is a time damping too - the erythrocyte is not always present at that location but passes by quite quickly so that the actual pO_2 around the capillary might never rise to the steady-state model value here.

A remark on the two types of tissue data considered here; there are obvious differences between the two cases. The rat heart pO_2 came out higher, and the dog gracilis pO_2 profiles flatter, both in z- and in r- direction. This is due to some obvious differences in the data sets used for the two cases (see table 1). Once, the dog gracilis data have an arteriolar pO_2 of 60 mm Hg, against 100 mm Hg for the rat heart. Then, the cylinder radius is much larger, 22.6 μm against 10 μm respectively, so that the steep gradients, mainly extending over a few μm, are less important in the dog gracilis case. Finally, the facilitation pressure p_F is much higher in the dog gracilis data, 39.6 mm Hg against 14 mm Hg, so that a lesser pressure drop Δp is needed for the same driving force drop $\Delta(p+p_F s)$ - see eq.2. Although the calculations here cannot be considered as a tissue O_2 modelling effort, it emphasizes the importance of the input data for the model.

CONCLUSIONS

Tissue pO_2 models, including the Krogh/Kety model, can be extended including a pericapillary Extraction Pressure (EP; or Capillary Barrier CB) to account for delivery phenomena in the blood;

Representation of erythrocytes as point-like sources can be used for an estimate of the importance and magnitude of this EP (CB).

REFERENCES

Groebe, K., 1990, A versatile model of steady state O_2 supply to tissue; application to skeletal muscle, *Biophys. J.* 57: 485-498.

Hoofd, L., Olders, J., and Turek, Z., 1990, Oxygen pressures calculated in a tissue volume with parallel capillaries, *in*: "Oxygen Transport to Tissue - XII", J. Piiper, T.K. Goldstick, and M. Meyer, eds., Plenum Press, New York & London, pp.21-29.

Hoofd, L., and Turek, Z., 1992, Oxygen pressure histograms calculated in a block of rat heart tissue, *in*: "Oxygen Transport to Tissue - XIV", W. Erdmann et al., eds., Plenum Press, New York & London, pp.561-566.

Hoofd, L., Turek, Z., and Olders, J., 1989, Calculation of oxygen pressures and fluxes in a flat plane perpendicular to any capillary distribution, *in*: "Oxygen Transport to Tissue - XI", K. Rakusan, G. Biro, T.K. Goldstick, and Z. Turek, eds., Plenum Press, New York & London, pp.187-196.

Popel, A.S., 1989, Theory of oxygen transport to tissue, *Crit. Rev. Biomed. Engn.* 17: 257-321.

Tsai, A.G., and Intaglietta, M., 1989, Local tissue oxygenation during constant red blood cell flux: a discrete analysis of velocity and hematocrit changes, *Microvasc. Res.* 37: 308-322.

THE MICROVASCULAR UNIT SIZE FOR FRACTAL FLOW HETEROGENEITY RELEVANT FOR OXYGEN TRANSPORT

J.H.G.M. van Beek, J.P.F. Barends and N. Westerhof

The Laboratory for Physiology
Free University
1081 BT Amsterdam
The Netherlands

INTRODUCTION

Blood flow is heterogeneously distributed in the myocardium. The width of this distribution depends on the spatial resolution of the flow measurement. Flow heterogeneity has been described by a fractal relation: the relative dispersion (standard deviation/mean) of the measured flow distribution increases with the spatial resolution of the measurement via a power law (Bassingthwaighte et al., 1989). The dependence of the dispersion of the flow distribution on spatial resolution has also been explained with a fractal vascular network model (Van Beek et al., 1989). Both types of fractal model imply that the heterogeneous flow is not distributed randomly, but that flow shows spatial correlation over large distances.

Neither of the two fractal models does incorporate a limit in spatial resolution below which the dispersion of flow does not increase any further. Indeed, unequal flow distribution has even been measured in adjacent capillaries in skeletal muscle (Tyml and Ellis, 1989). Measures of flow heterogeneity, such as the relative dispersion, may continue to increase with spatial resolution down to the capillary level. It would be useful to define a functional microvascular unit size for which the flow distribution can be reported instead of reporting a complete, but also more complicated fractal description. Heterogeneity in flow results in heterogeneity in oxygen supply that will be counteracted by oxygen diffusion among adjacent regions. In this paper, the functional microvascular unit is taken small enough to allow diffusion to compensate for the effect of internal flow heterogeneity in the unit on the oxygen tension distribution in the tissue. We will try to define the functional microvascular unit size by model calculations of oxygen transport in heterogeneously perfused tissue.

Oxygen Transport to Tissue XV, Edited by P. Vaupel
et al., Plenum Press, New York, 1994

MODEL DESCRIPTION

Oxygen transport model

We model oxygen transport in a slab of tissue extending from x=0 to x=L, representing an isolated perfused organ, where x is the linear spatial coordinate. Oxygen diffusion among adjacent regions and across both surfaces of the slab is taken into account, see Fig. 1. The oxygen transport equation has been developed previously (Van Beek et al., 1992), and is similar to the equation used by Popel and Gross (1979). The one-dimensional form of this equation for the steady state is:

$$\alpha\lambda D\frac{d^2P}{dx^2} - 2\rho F\alpha(P-P_a)=\rho\dot{V}_{O_2}. \tag{1}$$

In this equation α is the O_2 solubility, λ is the ratio of O_2 solubility in tissue to the O_2 solubility in the perfusate, D is the diffusion coefficient, ρ is tissue density, F is flow per unit tissue mass and $\dot{V}_{O_2}$ is the O_2 consumption per unit tissue mass. The oxygen tension P represents the local oxygen tension averaged in a capillary exchange region, and P_a is the arterial oxygen tension. The rationale for Eq. 1 has been discussed before (Van Beek et al., 1992).

The change of oxygen tension between regions in perfused tissue can be characterized by the space constant ξ^{-1} (Van Beek et al., 1992)

$$\xi^{-1}=\sqrt{\lambda D/(2\rho F)}. \tag{2}$$

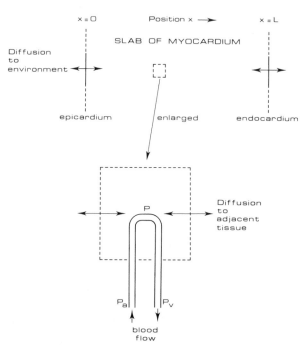

Figure 1. Model for oxygen transport in slab of cardiac tissue. Oxygen is delivered by the perfusate and diffuses among adjacent vascular exchange regions and across the slab's surfaces. P, average tissue O_2 tension. P_a and P_v, arterial and venous O_2 tension. Oxygen consumption is uniform.

To calculate the oxygen tension profile in tissue with heterogeneous perfusion flow F a finite difference form of Eq. 1 is applied:

$$D\frac{P_{i+1}-2P_i+P_{i-1}}{(\Delta x)^2} + \frac{2\rho F_i}{\lambda}(P_a-P_i) = \frac{\rho \dot{V}_{O_2}}{\lambda \alpha} . \qquad (3)$$

Subscript i (i=1 through N) indicates the value at discrete points in the center of N segments of width Δx into which the slab has been divided along the x-axis. The equations for i=1 and i=N are the same but in these special cases oxygen tensions P_0 and P_{N+1} are used which are oxygen tensions in virtual segments outside the slab. This technique of using fictitious oxygen tensions outside the region of interest to introduce the boundary conditions is discussed by Crank (1975). To obtain a reasonable value for the fictitious value P_0 a second order polynomial in x is constructed through P_2, P_1 and P_{epi}, the oxygen tension at x=0. Extrapolation of the polynomial to the position at half a segment width to the left of x=0, outside the slab, defines the value of P_0. The system of N linear equations containing N unknown oxygen tension values is solved using the Crout reduction for tridiagonal linear systems algorithm (Burden and Faires, 1989) programmed in TURBO C (Borland, Scotts Valley CA, USA) on a personal computer. The P_{O2} tensions were calculated at N = 4096 grid points in the slab.

Strategy to determine functional flow unit size

The functional microvascular unit size was assessed supposing fractal perfusion heterogeneity in tissue. To this end a heterogeneous flow distribution was generated in the slab, using the fractal vascular network model (Van Beek et al., 1989) which has been shown to describe the myocardial flow distribution well. According to this model one half of the slab receives a fraction γ of the total flow, while the other half of the slab receives the remaining fraction 1-γ. The flow within these halves of the slab is again distributed according to the same law in sub-halves of the half, and this pattern is recursively repeated. The standard deviations of the flow distributions thus obtained for various spatial resolutions fit experimental data on the distribution of myocardial flow, with γ about 0.45 (Van Beek et al., 1989). Examples of calculated flow distributions are shown in Fig. 2. We assume a homogeneous distribution of oxygen consumption. The resulting mismatch of local flow and oxygen consumption results in a heterogeneous distribution of oxygen tension.

The fractal flow distribution is calculated for 12 recursions of the process of repetitive asymmetric distribution among two halves, resulting in separate flow values for all segments in the slab. The flow can be averaged in a chosen number of adjacent segments. We call the size of the region over which the heterogeneous flow is averaged the spatial resolution of the flow distribution. The obtained flow distribution supplies the values for F_i in Eq. 3. The oxygen tension profile is calculated for various spatial resolutions of the flow distribution. The oxygen tension for the heterogeneous flow distribution is subtracted from the oxygen tension for homogeneous flow (see Fig. 2, right) at the 4096 grid points to assess the effect of heterogeneous flow on the oxygen tension distribution. The average and the standard deviation of these differences are then determined as a function of the spatial resolution of the heterogeneous flow distribution. We will see that there is a critical spatial resolution beyond which greater resolution does not lead to significant changes in the calculated oxygen tension distribution.

Parameter values

Parameter values for tissue perfused with saline solution were taken from experiments in arrested isolated guinea pig hearts at 37 °C (Loiselle, 1989; Van Beek et al., 1992). Flow is 2.8 ml/g_{ww}/min (ww indicates wet weight), oxygen consumption 15 μl/g_{ww}/min, diffusion coefficient 1.5×10^{-5} cm^2/s, oxygen solubility in Krebs-Henseleit solution 0.03 μl/ml/mmHg, tissue density is 1.06 g/ml, and the tissue-to-perfusate partition coefficient is 0.85. Amounts of oxygen are expressed as the volume of dry gas at 0 °C and 760 mmHg pressure (1 mol = 22414 ml). The tissue oxygen tensions at the boundaries are

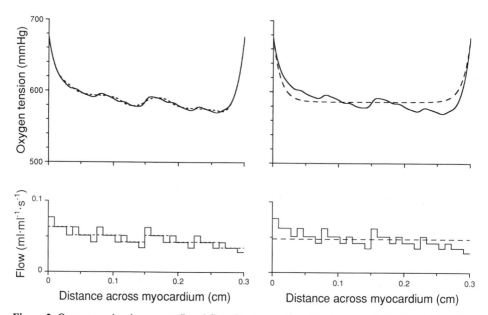

Figure 2. Oxygen tension (upper panel) and flow (lower panel) profiles in the wall of saline-perfused arrested heart. *Left* Fractal heterogeneous perfusion at two spatial resolutions, with $\gamma = 0.45$ (see text). The dotted line is for spatial resolution 375 μm, the solid line for resolution 94 μm. *Right* Heterogeneous and homogeneous perfusion compared. The dashed line is for homogeneous flow, the solid line for heterogeneous flow at resolution 94 μm.

equal to environmental oxygen tensions in the fluid touching the boundaries (Van Beek et al., 1992), and were set equal to arterial oxygen tension, 677 mmHg, for the calculations. The arterial and surface oxygen tensions do influence the level of the calculated profile, but not the analysis of SD.

For blood-perfused tissue, parameters were chosen to resemble those of in vivo canine myocardium: flow 0.8 ml/g_{ww}/min, oxygen consumption 100 μl/g_{ww}/min, effective oxygen solubility 4.16 μl/ml/mmHg (linearized slope of blood oxygen dissociation curve), and tissue-to-blood partition coefficient 0.00613 for conditions where myoglobin is completely oxygenated.

RESULTS

We model the saline-perfused arrested heart, though of limited physiological relevance, because the transport model has been tested and found to apply in this situation (cf. Van Beek et al., 1992). In Fig. 2 (left) the calculated oxygen tension profiles are shown for two spatial resolutions of the flow, 375 and 94 µm. The finer flow heterogeneity on increasing the spatial resolution leads to relatively small deviations (up to 4 mmHg) from the oxygen tension profile calculated for a resolution of 375 µm. In some places P_{O2} increases at higher spatial resolution of flow, in others it decreases, keeping the net effect on the oxygen tension distribution small. Comparing the steep discontinuous profile for the heterogeneous flow with the smooth profiles for oxygen tension shows that diffusion has a filtering effect.

The average and standard deviation of the differences in oxygen tension between homogeneous and heterogeneous flow are computed for a number of chosen spatial resolutions. This was done for two conditions: with and without diffusion of oxygen (see Fig. 3). Changes with spatial resolution are apparent at coarse resolutions. Below a certain threshold additional flow heterogeneity does only lead to negligible changes in SD when compensated by diffusion, but changes continue when there is no diffusion. It is found that below a spatial resolution of 500 µm the increase in standard deviation of the oxygen tension differences is limited to 1 % in the saline-perfused heart with normal diffusion.

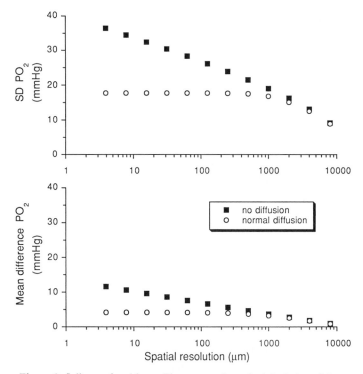

Figure 3. Saline-perfused heart. The mean and standard deviation of the differences for the calculated O_2 tension between heterogeneous and homogeneous flow, as a function of spatial resolution of flow measurement (see text). The width of the slab was taken large, 1.6 cm, to reduce the influence of the slab's surface. The oxygen tension is on average lower for heterogeneous than for homogeneous flow.

This spatial resolution depends on flow and diffusion coefficient but not on oxygen consumption. The 1 % level was chosen to define the functional microvascular unit because there is a rather steep change in standard deviation with coarser spatial resolution: the 5 % level is at a spatial resolution of about 1000 μm.

The standard deviations and averages of the differences in oxygen tension between heterogeneous and homogeneous flow for blood-perfused cardiac tissue are given in Fig. 4. In this case a spatial resolution of 100 μm constitutes the threshold below which the standard deviation increases by 1 % only. The threshold for saline-perfused tissue is much larger than for blood-perfused tissue because of the higher relative importance of diffusion resulting from the low oxygen carrying capacity of saline solution compared to blood. The threshold spatial resolution increases by one order of magnitude for an increase in diffusion coeffient by two orders of magnitude (Van Beek, 1992). The plateau of the standard deviation below the resolution threshold is only modestly influenced by order of magnitude changes in diffusion coefficient: a two orders of magnitude increase in diffusion coefficient leads to a decrease in SD plateau by one third.

The space constant ξ^{-1}, Eq. 2, for the oxygen tension profile in saline-perfused tissue is 114 μm for the conditions studied here. Thus the derived linear dimension of the microvascular unit is four-to-five times the space constant. The same is true for blood perfusion. The space constant increases with the square root of the diffusion coefficient. The dependence on flow and partition coefficient is also given by Eq. 2. It should be noted that the space constant does not change with oxygen consumption.

DISCUSSION

There is marked flow heterogeneity in the myocardium (cf. Bassingthwaighte et al., 1989) and skeletal muscle. Even at levels as small as the capillary bifurcations in skeletal muscle flow distributes asymmetrically (Tyml and Ellis, 1989) with roughly 45 % of the flow entering one capillary and 55 % of the flow entering the other capillary at the bifurcation. Despite the completely different spatial scale, this is in striking correspondence with the fractal flow distribution model that describes microsphere measurements of heterogeneous myocardial flow as a function of spatial resolution: if a tissue block of arbitrary size is divided in two halves roughly 45 % of the flow goes to one half, and 55 % to the other (Van Beek et al., 1989).

The fact that flow is heterogeneously distributed at all scales may be thought of as a fractal property (Bassingthwaighte and Van Beek, 1988; Bassingthwaighte et al., 1989). It would be convenient to report flow heterogeneity for one scale that is relevant for transport. An attempt was made previously to define this microvascular unit size by postulating that fractal models for the relation between relative dispersion (= standard deviation/mean) of flow and spatial resolution for individual animals may be extrapolated to one common interindividual small unit size (Bassingthwaighte et al., 1990). Analysis of data from sheep and baboons resulted in microvascular unit sizes of 50-75 μg. The relative dispersion of flow at this unit size was about 100 % for the fractal power law model, much larger than the relative dispersion of 50 % derived from the fractal vascular network model for this unit size (Bassingthwaighte et al., 1990).

Our present model analysis for conditions in blood-perfused heart results in a flow unit size of order $(100 \text{ μm})^3$, which corresponds with a mass of about 1 μg. This unit size

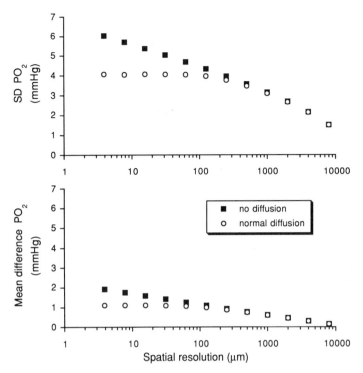

Figure 4. Blood-perfused heart. The mean and the standard deviation of the differences for the calculated O_2 tension between heterogeneous and homogeneous flow as a function of spatial resolution of flow measurement. The width of the slab was 1.6 cm for this calculation. The oxygen tension is on average lower for heterogeneous than for homogeneous flow.

is probably slightly overestimated because of the one-dimensional analysis of the three-dimensional real situation. The two different estimates of the microvascular unit size to report flow heterogeneity are based on very different rationales. The postulate of a common point of convergence (Bassingthwaighte et al., 1990) requires extrapolation over four orders of magnitude, and is not yet corroborated by high resolution flow measurements. However, Bassingthwaighte's hypothesis remains attractive because it recognizes that it is the flow heterogeneity at small scales that is of importance to transport. One common degree of heterogeneity for all individuals at the common unit size does allow differences in heterogeneity at larger scales to exist because the units with high flow may either be randomly dispersed or may tend to cluster, resulting in different fractal dimensions (Van Beek et al., 1989). A third definition of microvascular unit size is anatomical in nature: the unit is the volume of tissue supplied with blood by one terminal arteriole. In dog myocardium such arterioles are located at about 1 mm intervals, suggesting a unit size of 1000 µg (Bassingthwaighte et al., 1974). We have to conclude that the microvascular flow unit size depends on the definition chosen, which may have an anatomical basis, may be based on extrapolation of fractal laws or, as in this study, may be based on the oxygen transport properties of tissue. The present analysis based on oxygen transport suggests that reporting the flow heterogeneity at 1 to 10 µg resolution allows accurate calculation of the oxygen tension distribution in blood-perfused heart.

SUMMARY

In this study we used a computer model for oxygen transport in heterogeneously perfused tissue to define the microvascular unit size of relevance to oxygen transport. Flow within this unit is presumably heterogeneous, but this internal heterogeneity is by definition of negligible importance for the oxygen tension distribution. In saline-perfused heart the linear dimension of the thus defined unit is 500 μm, in blood-perfused heart it is 100 μm.

REFERENCES

Bassingthwaighte, J.B., King, R.B., and Roger, S.A., 1989, Fractal nature of regional myocardial flow heterogeneity, *Circ. Res.* 65:578.

Bassingthwaighte, J.B., and Van Beek, J.H.G.M., 1988, Lightning and the heart: fractal behavior in cardiac function, *Proc. IEEE* 76:693.

Bassingthwaighte, J.B., Van Beek, J.H.G.M., and King, R.B., 1990, Fractal branchings: the basis of myocardial flow heterogeneities? *Ann. N.Y. Acad. Sci.* 591: 392.

Bassingthwaighte, J.B., Yipintsoi, T., and Harvey, R.B., 1974, Microvasculature of the dog left ventricular myocardium, *Microvasc. Res.* 7:229.

Burden, R.L., and Faires J.D., 1989, "Numerical Analysis (Fourth Edition)," PWS-KENT Publishing Company, Boston.

Crank, J., 1975, "The Mathematics of Diffusion (Second Edition)," Clarendon Press, Oxford.

Loiselle, D.S., 1989, Exchange of oxygen across the epicardial surface distorts estimates of myocardial oxygen consumption, *J.Gen.Physiol.* 86:105.

Popel, A.S., and Gross, J.F., 1979, Analysis of oxygen diffusion from arteriolar networks, *Am.J.Physiol.* 237:H681.

Tyml, K., and Ellis, C.G., 1989, Localized heterogeneity of red cell velocity in skeletal muscle at rest and after contraction, *Adv.Exp.Med.Biol.* 248:735.

Van Beek, J.H.G.M., 1992, Fractal models of heterogeneity in organ blood flow, *in*: "Modelling of oxygen transport from environment to cell," S. Egginton and H. Ross, eds., Cambridge University Press, Cambridge.

Van Beek, J.H.G.M., Loiselle, D.S., and Westerhof, N., 1992, Calculation of oxygen diffusion across the surface of isolated perfused hearts, *Am.J.Physiol.* 263 *(Heart Circ. Physiol.* 32), in press.

Van Beek, J.H.G.M., Roger, S.A. and Bassingthwaighte, J.B., 1989, Regional myocardial flow heterogeneity explained with fractal networks, *Am.J.Physiol.* 257 *(Heart Circ. Physiol.* 26):H1670.

TERMINOLOGY AND DEFINITIONS IN RESPIRATORY PHYSIOLOGY

WHY A CONSENSUS MEETING ON TERMINOLOGY AND DEFINITION IN RESPIRATORY PHYSIOLOGY?

The International Society on Oxygen Transport to Tissue (ISOTT) was founded in 1973 to facilitate the exchange of information among those scientists interested in aspects of the transport and/or utilization of oxygen in tissues. Its members encompass virtually all disciplines, extending from various areas of clinical medicine such as anesthesiology, critical care or internal medicine and other disciplines through the basic biomedical sciences of physiology, biochemistry and radiobiology to most branches of biophysics and engineering.

In the past, exchange of scientific information in the field of oxygen transport to tissue has often been made difficult due to a Babel-like confusion of terminology, definitions and symbols. In order to overcome this dilemma, a special round table discussion was planned for the 1992 ISOTT Meeting, recalling the previous proposal of R. Zander and P. Vaupel (Adv. Exp. Med. Biol. 191: 965, 1985). To "catalyze" a standardized nomenclature, the Organizing Committee took every effort to provide all participants with the necessary information by distributing recently published recommendations of R. Zander and F. Mertzlufft (Scand. J. Clin. Lab. Invest. 50, Suppl. 203: 177, 1990, and "The Oxygen Status of Arterial Blood", Basel-Munich-London-New York: Karger, 1991) which have been based on already established terminology (IFCC and IUPAC: J. Clin. Chem. Clin. Biochem. 18: 829, 1980; IUPS: J. Appl. Physiol. 34: 549, 1973)

ISOTT members were invited to submit their written proposals in advance. In addition, two major opinion leaders (O. Siggard-Andersen, J.W. Severinghaus) were invited to contribute with their expertise. In order to provide a sound platform for the round table discussion, the ISOTT Organizing Committee has pre-evaluated all submitted suggestions and, on the ground of this evaluation, only major topics have been chosen for the final discussion.

On the following pages, the résumé of this discussion and additional vota are presented. It is hoped that this information may help to find our way out of Babel and to minimize confusion of terminology, definitions and symbols in the future.

For the editors

Peter Vaupel

TENTATIVE RECOMMENDATION ON TERMINOLOGY AND DEFINITIONS IN RESPIRATORY PHYSIOLOGY: RÉSUMÉ OF THE ISOTT CONSENSUS SESSION 1992

Rolf Zander and Fritz Mertzlufft

Institute of Physiology and Pathophysiology
Johannes Gutenberg-University Mainz, D-6500 Mainz, and
Clinic of Anaesthesiology and Intensive Care Medicine
University of Homburg, D-6650 Homburg-Saar, Germany

GENERAL REMARKS ON SYMBOLS

1. The use of small letters for the symbols "p" (partial pressure), "s" (saturation) and "c" (concentration) (e.g. pO_2, sO_2, cO_2) follows recommendations of the IFCC and IUPAC [4]. This supports the use of contemporary word processing systems and mostly eliminates the need to use subscripts (except for chemical valencies: e.g. O_2, CO_2, H_2CO_3 etc.). The potential risk of misinterpretations and double meanings is reduced also (e.g. "cO_2" [oxygen concentration] v.s. "CO_2" [carbon dioxide] and "sO_2" [oxygen saturation] v.s. "SO_2" [sulfur dioxide]).

2. The symbol shall include the site of measurement or description, e.g. paO_2 (arterial O_2 partial pressure), $s\bar{v}O_2$ (mixed venous oxygen saturation), or $avDO_2$ (arterio-venous oxygen difference). This removes in an intelligible manner the confusion of symbols (e.g. paO_2: PaO_2, p_aO_2, Pa_{O_2}, P_{aO_2} etc.). One wishes to question the rationale of a statement such as "writing S_{aO_2}, $S_{O_2}(a)$, $S_{O_2}(ab)$ or the like, is a matter of taste" [10], because perfect confusion may be the result, here concerning the arterial O_2 saturation (saO_2).

3. It is a convention in chemistry to refer to radicals or compounds containing oxygen with the term "oxi" rather than "oxy" (e.g. carbon monoxide (CO), carbon dioxide (CO_2), oxidized Hb (MetHb) etc.). On the other hand, methods and terms referring to molecular oxygen (oxygenium) should be written with "y" and not with "i" (e.g. oxymetry, pulse oxymetry, oxygenation, Hb with reversibly bound O_2 (Oxy-Hb, O_2Hb) and deoxygenated Hb (Deoxy-Hb, Hb), etc.).

4. Even if a new in vivo method differs considerably from the established in vitro method (e.g. in vivo (transcutaneously) measurement of arterial O_2 saturation or O_2 partial pressure) this does not justify the use of different notations or symbols. Use of the symbol $ptcO_2$ should be avoided for transcutaneously determined "paO_2": If the method is able to measure the arterial pO_2 then the symbol paO_2 should be used. If this is not the case, however, i.e. if indeed the cutaneous pO_2 is determined, then the symbol $pctO_2$ is appropriate. The use of Sp_{O_2} [2,7] or S_{pO_2} [5] or $S_{O_2}(po)$ [10] for arterial O_2 saturation, measured by pulse oxymetry, could erroneously suggest the measurement of an essentially different quantity [10].

5. The number of symbols employed for a given measured value should be kept as small as possible. For this reason the suggestions of Payne and Severinghaus [5] should not be followed, since a total of six different symbols is recommended for the O_2 saturation. Consequences are a worldwide confusion: within only one article [2] arterial oxygen saturation is referred to as Sp_{O_2} (pulse oxymeter reading), FSa_{O_2} (functional saturation), Sa_{O_2} (fractional saturation), O_2Hb % (fractional saturation). Within the same volume of a journal [2,7] Sa_{O_2} is used for fractional oxygen saturation [2] as well as for functional oxygen saturation [7]. Obviously, the notation "fraction" becomes more and more attractive: Besides the widely accepted "fraction" in respiratory physiology (e.g. FIO_2, inspired oxygen fraction), the oxyhemoglobin fraction F_{HbO_2} was proposed [10] for the $So_2(frac)$ [5] or the fractional saturation Sa_{O_2} [2]. But, on the other hand, the symbol F was then introduced as FSa_{O_2} for the functional (not the fractional) saturation and used besides the common FIO_2 [2], the inspired oxygen fraction.

6. Symbols used for any notations should be as simple as possible. Neither the use of NSo_2 to describe the noninvasive technique [1] for the measurement of oxygen saturation, nor that of Sp_{O_2} [2] for pulse oxymetry should be accepted.

7. The symbol for a measured value must be independent of the method (cf. comment 5), and certainly independent of the manufacturer. Recent recommendations to the contrary, e.g. to use the symbol $S_{hp}O_2$ for the value given by an oxymeter from Hewlett Packard [5], or that of Barker et al [2] to use the symbol Sx_{O_2} for the value given by an Oximetrix system, are unacceptable.

In conclusion the following is proposed:

- that no new definitions resulting from the limitations of a method be introduced,
- that symbols and methods are not combined per se, and
- that definitions and symbols be disassociated from any commercial use.

SPECIAL REMARKS ON SYMBOLS AND DEFINITIONS

The special symbols concerning the parameters of oxygen are summarized in Table I. Relevant definitions dealing with oxygen transport by human blood are given in Table II.

TABLE I. Symbols

Term	Unit	Symbol	Specifcation/Comment
O_2 partial pressure	mmHg, kPa	pO_2	pAO_2 alveolar paO_2 arterial blood pcO_2 capillary blood pvO_2 venous blood $p\overline{v}O_2$ mixed venous blood $pctO_2$ skin (cutaneous) ptO_2 tissue
O_2 saturation	%*	sO_2	saO_2 arterial blood svO_2 venous blood $s\overline{v}O_2$ mixed venous blood
Partial O_2 saturation	%*	psO_2	$psaO_2$ arterial blood $psvO_2$ venous blood $ps\overline{v}O_2$ mixed venous blood
Hemoglobin concentration (Synonym: Hb content)	g/L, g/dL, mmol/L	cHb	
O_2 concentration (Synonym: O_2 content)	mL/dL, vol%, % (v/v), L/L	cO_2	caO_2 arterial blood cvO_2 venous blood $c\overline{v}O_2$ mixed venous blood
Oxy-Hb concentration (Synonym: Oxy-Hb fraction)	%*	cO_2Hb	Identical to sO_2
Carboxy-Hb concentration (Synonym: Carboxy-Hb fraction)	%*	$cCOHb$	
Met-Hb concentration (Synonym: Met-Hb fraction)	%*	$cMetHb$	
O_2 solubility (Synonym: O_2 solubility coefficient)	mL/mL/atm, mL/dL/mmHg	αO_2	
Arterio-venous O_2 difference	mmHg, %*, mL/dL	$avDO_2$	The term $avDO_2$ can only be applied to a given organ, whereas $a\overline{v}DO_2$ can also refer to the whole organism.
Alveolo-arterial O_2 difference	mmHg	$AaDO_2$	
O_2 uptake	mL/min	$\dot{V}O_2$	
O_2 transport (Synonym: O_2 transport capacity; O_2 supply; O_2 availability)	mL/min	$\dot{T}O_2$	
O_2 consumption	mL/min	$\dot{Q}O_2$	Identical to $\dot{V}O_2$ when used in conjunction with $a\overline{v}DO_2$ under steady state conditions. Use of $avDO_2$ gives the O_2 consumption of an organ.

* can also be expressed as a fraction (without units)

TABLE II. Definitions

Terms	Definitions	Comments
O_2 partial pressure	The pressure exerted by O_2 in a mixture (e.g. CO_2, N_2, H_2O, etc.) of gases (e.g. alveolar gas, air), in a liquid (e.g. blood, cerebrospinal fluid) or in tissue.	In the case of blood the O_2 partial pressure describes the pressure of both the physically dissolved and chemically bound oxygen.
Normoxia	Normal oxygen partial pressure at a defined location and under defined conditions.	Normoxia in the arterial blood of a patient presumes knowledge of the normal value in relation to the age, sex, relative body weight and barometric pressure.
Hypoxia	Decreased O_2 partial pressure (compared to normoxia).	The term hypoxia will continue to be used generally to describe an oxygen deficit. Greater specifity in terminology is to be preferred, however (e.g. arterial hypoxia, tissue hypoxia, etc.).
Hyperoxia	Increased O_2 partial pressure (compared to normoxia).	An increase in the inhaled oxygen concentration (normobaric) and/or the total pressure in a pressure chamber (hyperbaric) employed therapeutically.
O_2 saturation	1. The concentration (content) of O_2 bound to hemoglobin in relation to the O_2 binding capacity (the theoretical maximum for Hb-bound O_2 expressed as a fraction or as a percentage: $sO_2 = (cO_2 -$ physically dissolved $O_2)/O_2$ capacity.	The result of measuring the O_2 content (after deducting physically dissolved O_2) in relation to the O_2 capacity.
	2. Oxyhemoglobin as a proportion of the total hemoglobin, expressed as a fraction or as a percentage, Total Hb = O_2Hb + Hb + COHb + MetHb etc.: $sO_2 = cO_2Hb/(cO_2Hb + cHb + cCOHb + cMetHb)$.	The result of photometric determination with equipment using $4-7$ wavelengths (Oxymeter). Not recommended [5]: Oxyhemoglobin saturation (HbO_2) or fractional saturation (So_2(frac)).
Partial O_2 saturation	The concentration of oxyhemoglobin as a fraction or percentage of the sum of the concentrations of Deoxy-Hb (Hb) plus Oxy-Hb (O_2Hb) alone: $psO_2 = cO_2Hb/(cO_2Hb + cHb)$.	1. The result of photometric determination using only 2 wavelengths. 2. Obtained by calculation from the pO_2 and the O_2 binding curve under defined conditions (pH, pCO_2, temp., etc.). The term "partial" is used to emphasize that only a portion of the Hb (O_2Hb + Hb) is taken into account resulting in limited diagnostic relevance. The term "available Hb" for the sum of Hb + O_2Hb (i.e. the Hb available for O_2 transport) is unacceptable since the conditions of measurement are not defined: Depending upon the exposure time and magnitude of the pO_2 and the MetHb reductase activitiy, COHb and MetHb are converted into "available" Hb (in vivo and in vitro). The recommendation of Payne and Severinghaus [5] to saturate with a "minimum volume of oxygen" to prevent removal of COHb and MetHb is not practicable.

TABLE II. Definitions, continued

Oxygenation	Reversible cooperative binding of oxygen to the bivalent iron of hemoglobin, whereby deoxygenated hemoglobin is converted to oxygenated hemoglobin. The splitting off of O_2 is referred to as deoxygenation.	Not recommended [5]: In vivo (So_2) or functional O_2 saturation (So_2(func)), or pulse oxymeter saturation (SpO_2). Oxygenation must be distinguished from oxidation, in which an increase in the valency of iron takes place (hemiglobin formation from hemoglobin). The term "reduced Hb" [5] for deoxygenated hemoglobin should be avoided since iron is also present in divalent form (Fe^{++}) in the case of O_2Hb [8]. The general use of the term "oxygenation" in the sense of "oxygen enrichment" should be avoided or specified.
Hypoxygenation	Decrease in O_2 saturation at a defined location and under defined conditions.	
Hb concentration (Hb content) Total Hb concentration (cHb)	1. Concentration of hemoglobin in blood (e.g. g/dL).	The result of the photometric determination of Hb in blood.
	2. Sum of all Hb derivatives in blood (THb = total Hb): THb = cHHb + cO_2Hb + cCOHb + cMetHb.	The result of the spectrophotometric determination in a multi-wavelength oxymeter.
Hemoglobin derivatives:		
Hemoglobin (Hb, HHb)	Deoxy-Hb (Hb without O_2).	
Oxyhemoglobin (O_2Hb)	Oxy-Hb (Hb with bound O_2).	The term "oxidized Hb" should be eliminated.
Carboxyhemoglobin (COHb)	Hemoglobin with reversibly bound carbon monoxide (CO).	CO is bound with a high affinity but reversibly.
Methemoglobin (MetHb, Hb^+, Hi)	Hemoglobin in an oxidized state, also known as hemiglobin, that is unavailable for O_2 transport.	
Sulfhemoglobin (SHb, SulfHb)	Hemoglobin with bound sulphur (H_2S action on hemoglobin).	
Cyanohemiglobin (HiCN)	Hemiglobin with bound cyanide (HCN action on hemiglobin).	Only occurs in vitro.
OxyHb concentration (cO_2Hb)	Proportion of O_2Hb in blood in relation to total Hb; expressed as a fraction (without dimensions) or as a percentage (%). Identical to O_2 saturation (sO_2).	The definition by Siggaard-Andersen [6] of cO_2Hb as the "HbO_2 fraction" in relation to $cHb + cHbO_2$ (rather than to total Hb) should be rejected since the fractions of COHb, MetHb and SulfHb are related to the total Hb. The concentrations (fractions) of all Hb derivatives should be related to total Hb merely for practical reasons.
CarboxyHb concentration (cCOHb)	see cO_2Hb	
MetHb concentration (cMetHb, cHi)	see cO_2Hb	
SulfHb concentration (cSulfHb, cSHb)	see cO_2Hb	

TABLE II. Definitions, continued

O$_2$ concentration (Synonym: O$_2$ content)	The sum of the amounts of chemically bound and physically dissolved oxygen in blood.	
Normoxemia	The normal O$_2$ concentration in a blood sample under defined conditions.	
Hypoxemia	Reduced O$_2$ concentration compared to normoxemia.	The decrease in cO$_2$ is accompanied by:
Hypoxic hypoxemia	Hypoxemia as a result of hypoxia (decreased pO$_2$).	- decreased pO$_2$ and sO$_2$ with normal cHb,
Toxemic (toxic) hypoxemia	Hypoxemia as a result of a decrease in O$_2$ binding ability of Hb (e.g. by formation of COHb or MetHb)(decreased sO$_2$).	- decreased sO$_2$ with normal pO$_2$ and cHb,
Anemic hypoxemia	Hypoxemia as a result of anemia (decreased cHb).	- decreased cHb with normal pO$_2$ and sO$_2$.
Hyperoxemia	Increased O$_2$ concentration compared with normoxemia.	
O$_2$ solubility of the blood	Proportionality between O$_2$ partial pressure and the concentration of physically dissolved oxygen in blood; usually described by the O$_2$ solubility coeffcient.	The most widespread is the Bunsen solubility coeffcient (mL O$_2$ /mL/atm).
Hüfner Number (Synonym: Hüfner factor)	The maximum amount of oxygen that can be bound by 1 g of hemoglobin.	On the basis of a molecular weight of 64458 and the fact that 1 mol Hb can bind a maximum of 4 mol O$_2$ the theoretical value is 1.39 mL O$_2$/g. The fact that in practically all individuals about 3 % of the total Hb exists as COHb, MetHb or SHb should not be expressed as an "in vivo Hüfner number", but as an appropriate reduction in the O$_2$ saturation of the blood (sO$_2$ = 97 %).
O$_2$ capacity	The maximum amount of oxygen that can be bound by Hb in a defined blood volume; expressed as O$_2$ concentration (e.g. mL O$_2$/dl.). The O$_2$ capacity is the product of cHb and the Hüfner number.	The O$_2$ capacity is essentially a theoretical value since no experimental method is available that allows complete saturation of the total Hb with O$_2$. Traces of COHb and MetHb will always remain which, although not interfering with the determination of the O$_2$ capacity, will be included in the measurement of Hb (as total Hb). Not to be confused with the "O$_2$ transport capacity" (see definition).
O$_2$ binding curve (Synonym: O$_2$ dissociation curve)	Graphical relationship (S- shaped) between the O$_2$ saturation of hemoglobin (chemically bound O$_2$) and the O$_2$ partial pressure of the blood: sO$_2$(%) as a function of pO$_2$ (mmHg), or psO$_2$ (%) as a function of pO$_2$ (mmHg).	At a pO$_2$ of over 150 mmHg, a maximum sO$_2$ can be reached of only up to 98 %, a psO$_2$ of 100 %, resp.
O$_2$ content curve (Synonym: O$_2$ concentration curve)	Graphical relationship (S-shaped) between the O$_2$ content (chemically bound plus physically dissolved O$_2$) and O$_2$ partial pressure of the blood: cO$_2$ (mL/dL) as a function of pO$_2$ (mmHg).	At a pO$_2$ of over 150 mmHg, the O$_2$ content curve shows a linear increase whose slope is dependent upon the O$_2$ solubility.

TABLE II. Definitions, continued

Half-saturation pressure (p50, p0.5)	The O_2 partial pressure that leads to 50 % saturation of hemoglobin ($sO_2 = 50\%$ or 0.5).	The p50 (p0.5) provides an approximate indicator of the status of the O_2 binding curve in the form of sO_2 (%) as a function of pO_2 (mmHg) or, in the presence of significant concentrations of COHb or MetHb, as psO_2 (%) as a function of pO_2 (mmHg).
Arterio-venous O_2 difference	The difference between arterial and venous ($avDO_2$) or mixed venous ($a\bar{v}DO_2$) oxygen, expressed in units of partial pressure (pO_2), saturation (sO_2) or concentration (cO_2) (mmHg, %, mL/dl.).	The greatest predictive value is provided by the $avDO_2$ in concentration units; this is the only parameter that yields information on the O_2 consumption of an organism or organ (taking into account the blood flow).
Alveolo-arterial O_2 difference	The difference between the alveolar and arterial O_2 partial pressures.	
O_2 uptake	The amount of O_2 taken up per unit time via the respiration (mL O_2 /min), given by the product of the ventilation and the difference between the concentrations of inhaled and exhaled O_2 : $\dot{V}O_2 = \dot{V} \cdot (FIO_2 - FEO_2)$.	Under steady state conditions identical to the O_2 consumption of the organism.
O_2 transport (Synonyms: O_2 transport capacity; O_2 supply; O_2 availability)	The amount of oxygen supplied to the organism via the blood flow per unit time (mL O_2 /min), given by the product of the cardiac output and the arterial O_2 concentration: $\dot{T}O_2 = C.O. \cdot caO_2$.	Not recommended: O_2 delivery (DO_2).
O_2 consumption	The amount of oxygen consumed by the whole organism per unit time (mL O_2 /min), given by the product of the cardiac output and the arterio-mixed venous O_2 difference: $\dot{Q}O_2 = C.O. \cdot a\bar{v}DO_2$.	Under steady state conditions identical to the O_2 uptake.

REFERENCES

1. Barker SJ, Tremper KK, Gamel DM. A clinical comparison of transcutaneous pO_2 and pulse oximetry in the operating room. Anesth Analg 1986; 65: 805.
2. Barker SJ, Tremper KK, Hyatt J. Effects of methemoglobinemia on pulse oximetry and mixed venous oximetry. Anesthesiology 1989; 70: 112.
3. International Union of Physiolological Sciences. Glossary on respiration and gas exchange. J Appl Physiol 1973; 34: 549.
4. International Federation of Clinical Chemistry and International Union of Pure and Applied Chemistry. Physico-chemical quantities and units in clinical chemistry. J Clin Chem Clin Biochem 1980; 18: 829.
5. Payne JP, Severinghaus JW. Definitions and Symbols. In: Payne JP, Severinghaus JW (eds). Pulse Oximetry. London: Springer, 1986: xxi.
6. Siggaard-Andersen O, Norgaard-Pedersen B, Rem J. Hemoglobin pigments. Spectrophotometric determinations of oxy-, carboxy-, met-, and sulfhemoglobin in capillary blood. Clin Chim Acta 1972; 42: 85.
7. Veyckemans F, Baele P, Guillaume JE, Willems E, Robert A, Clerbaux T. Hyperbilirubinemia does not interfere with hemoglobin saturation measured by pulse oximetry. Anesthesiology 1989; 70: 118.
8. Zander R, Vaupel P. Proposal for using a standardized terminology on oxygen transport to tissue. Adv Exp Med Biol 1985; 191: 965.
9. Zander R, Mertzlufft F (eds). The oxygen status of arterial blood. Basel: Karger, 1991.
10. Zijlstra WG, Oeseburg B. Definition and Notation of hemoglobin oxygen saturation. IEEE Trans Biomed Eng 1989; 36: 872.

NOMENCLATURE OF OXYGEN SATURATION

John W. Severinghaus

Professor Emeritus of Anesthesiology
1386HSE University of California Medical Center
San Francisco, CA 94143-0542

INTRODUCTION

This paper addresses a controversial question relating to the definition of oxygen saturation as O_2 content/O_2 capacity: Whether, O_2 capacity should include a) only oxyhemoglobin and deoxyhemoglobin, designated herein as O_2Hb + HHb, or b) total hemoglobin, tHb = O_2Hb + HHb + COHb + MetHb.

BACKGROUND

The introduction of multiwavelength oximeters permitted all four hemoglobin species to be quantified, either as fractions or percentages of the total, or in quantities (g/dl). Some of these instruments have defined "saturation" as O_2Hb/tHb. Others use "fractional saturation" when the denominator is tHb, and "functional saturation" or "HbO_2 Sat" when the denominator is O_2Hb + HHb. This nomenclature issue is to be addressed at this meeting in view of the imminent adoption of all-European standards by the European Community. This issue was recently reactivated by Zander and Mertzlufft[1] who proposed the term "partial saturation" for O_2Hb/[O_2Hb+HHb], and "saturation" for O_2Hb/tHb.

Four organizations have addressed this question, and may, I think, be said to have attained a concensus. The World Health Organization and the European Society for Clinical Respiratory Physiology held joint discussions over a four year period and published in 1978 a "working document" defining oxygen saturation as "the amount of oxygen combined with haemoglobin, expressed as a percentage of the oxygen binding capacity of that haemoglobin"[2]. The US National Committee on Clinical Laboratory Standards, NCCLS[3], the European Committee for Clinical and Laboratory Standards, ECCLS[4], and the International Federation of Clinical Chemistry, IFCC[5], and several groups of authors[6,7] have published equivalent definitions. These organizations and authors have agreed on the following: The term "oxygen saturation" and symbol S or s, expressed either as a fraction or percentage, shall be defined as O_2Hb/[O_2Hb+HHb]. When the denominator is total Hb, the resulting value shall be named "oxyhemoglobin fraction", "fraction of oxyhemoglobin", or if multiplied by 100, "oxyhemoglobin percentage". In order to accord with ISO terminology, Wimberley et al[7] suggest the following formal definitions and terminology:

$$\text{Oxygen saturation} = s_{O_2} = c_{O_2Hb}/(c_{HHb} + c_{O_2Hb}) \tag{1}$$

$$\text{Oxyhemoglobin fraction} = F_{O_2Hb} = c_{O_2Hb}/c_{tHb} \tag{2}$$

RATIONALE

The rationale supporting these decisions may be summarized as follows:

1) The term "saturation" was originally introduced in connection with analytic methods requiring extraction into vacuum of O_2 from blood, first as sampled and again after saturation of a portion with O_2 to determine the O_2 capacity*. These manometric methods are still regarded as the 'gold standard' for measurement of O_2 content of blood. A general principle in scientific nomenclature has been that terminology should reflect not only the data but the method with which it was originally associated. New methods in this concept require new terminology unless they are shown to result in the same value.

2) The term "saturation" recognises the fact that all HHb will be converted to O_2Hb at sufficiently high Po_2, i.e. 100% saturated. When S_aO_2 (arterial blood) is reported as less than 100%, the clinician understands that an increase of P_aO_2 for example by administration of a higher inspired O_2 concentration, can increase arterial blood O_2Hb content.

3) In the presence of dyshemoglobins, O_2 saturation calculated from blood gas electrode analyses of Po_2, pH and Pco_2 estimates $sO_2\%$ rather than $O_2Hb\%$[#].

4) Pulse oximeters estimate saturation, not oxyhemoglobin percentage, because they primarily detect deoxyhemoglobin, which strongly absorbs red light[8]. They cannot distinguish COHb from O_2Hb[†]. Their response in the presence of metHb is complex[†], and may be confusing[9].

Standards organizations have not fully addressed terminology. In a new review of over 500 publications on pulse oximetry in the last 3 years, I found the term S_pO_2 to have become nearly universal[10]. Modifiers are needed because neither pulse oximetry nor arterial blood gas analysis measure, but rather approximate or estimate, S_aO_2. Authors may need to distinguish S_aO_2 from S_pO_2 or $S_{abg}O_2$, for example when they measure or discuss both or all three. S_aO_2 may be appropriately used with either multiwavelength oximetry or direct (i.e. Van Slyke) O_2 content analysis.

CONCLUSIONS

To avoid the confusion of dual meaning of "saturation", considering the foregoing rationale, and in view of the actions taken by other standards organizations, I suggest that ISOTT find the nomenclature presented in equations 1 and 2 to be appropriate. In my opinion, ISOTT should suggest that either sO_2 or So_2 be an acceptable term.

Considering the multitude of terms used over the past several decades following introduction of the multi-wavelength blood oximeters, any standards proposed by ISOTT should also contain appropriate translation information to clarify meanings of terms such as 'O$_2$Hb SAT', 'fractional saturation', 'functional saturation', 'partial saturation' and 'true saturation', and the various symbols and styles, use of italics and case variants.

The multiwavelength oximeters do not completely eliminate uncertainty. They may not display HHb, sulfHb or other dyshemoglobins. In order to compute SO_2, one needs to determine HHb by subtraction from 100 of O_2Hb, MetHb and COHb, but it is not clear whether this result includes only HHb. ISOTT should point out this (small) uncertainty and request clarification from manufacturers.

* When saturation is done with air, a small unknown fraction of COHb is converted to O_2Hb. When saturation is done with a bubble of O_2, e.g. 1 part O_2 to 5 parts blood, the reduction of COHb will be less than 1 part in 200. A correction for dissolved O_2 is essential.

COHb shifts the O_2 dissociation curve left (to lower Po_2) especially at low saturation, such that $S_{abg}O_2$, calculated from a standard curve, will be too low. MetHb has little effect on the dissociation curve when expressed as % saturation vs Po_2.

† If O_2Hb = 75% and COHb = 15%, HHb = 10%, sO_2 is computed as $75/85$ = 88.2%, while pulse oximeters read saturation as approximately $(75+15)/100$ = 90%. For amounts between 0 and about 30%, MetHb reduces pulse oximeter reading by about half its actual amount. For example, 20% MetHb with 80% O_2Hb will read about 90% on pulse oximeters. As MetHb concentration increases further, S_pO_2 falls only to 85%.

REFERENCES

1. R. Zander, F. Mertzlufft, Oxygen parameters of blood: definitions and symbols, *Scand J Clin Lab Invest.* 50:177-185, (1990).

2. H. Matthys. "Clinical Respiratory Physiology: Abbreviations, Symbols, Units, Definitions." Dr. Karl Thomas GmbH, Biberach an der Riss, Germany, p66, (1978).

3. S. Ehrmeyer, R.W. Burnett, R.L. Chatburn et al. "Definitions of Quantities and Conventions Related to Blood pH and Gas Analysis" NCCLS Document C12-T2, (Tentative Standard), Villanova, Pa, USA, (1991).

4. A.H.J. Mass, G. Kokholm, R. Haeckel et al. "Guidelines for Multi-centre Evaluation of Analysers for the Measurement of Blood pH, pCO_2, and pO_2". ECCLS Document Number 1: ISSN 1011-6265, K. Jacobsen, University Hospital, Lund, Sweden, (1989).

5. O. Siggaard-Andersen, R.A. Durst, A.H.J. Maas, Physicochemical quantities and units in clinical chemistry. Approved IUPAC/IFCC recommendation (1984), *J Clin Chem Clin Biochem.* 25:369-391 (1987).

6. W.G. Zijlstra, B. Oeseburg, Definition and notation of hemoglobin oxygen saturation, *IEEE Trans Bio Med Eng.* 36:872 (1989).

7. P.D. Wimberley, O. Siggaard-Andersen, N. Fogh-Andersen, W.G. Zijlstra, J.W. Severinghaus, Haemoglobin oxygen saturation and related quantities; definitions, symbols and clinical use, *Scand J Clin Lab Invest.* 50: 455-459 (1990).

8. W.G. Zijlstra, A. Buursma, W.P. Meeuwsen-van der Roest, Absorbtion spectra of human fetal and adult oxyhemoglobin, de-oxyhemoglobin, carboxyhemoglobin and methemoglobin, *Clin Chem.* 37:1633-1638 (1991).

9. B. Oeseburg, Pulse oximetry in methaemoglobinaemia (Correspondence), *Anaesthesia* 45, 56, (1990).

10. J.W. Severinghaus, J.F. Kelleher, Recent developments in pulse oximetry, *Anesthesiology* 76: 1018-1038, (1992).

DEFINITION AND MEASUREMENT OF QUANTITIES PERTAINING TO OXYGEN IN BLOOD

B. Oeseburg[1], P. Rolfe[2], O. Siggaard Andersen[3], and W.G. Zijlstra[4]

[1]Dept. Physiology, Univ. Nijmegen, NL
[2]Dept. Biophysics, Univ. Keele, UK
[3]Dept. Clinical Chemistry, Herlev Hospital, Copenhagen, DK
[4]Professor Emeritus Physiology, Univ. Groningen, NL

INTRODUCTION

Since the introduction of more dedicated methods in blood gas analysis a lot of confusion started about definition and notation on oxygen related quantities in blood. The (US) National Committee for Clinical Laboratory Standards (NCCLS) has published a proposed guideline in which these problems are thoroughly discussed[18]. In the present paper a consistent set of definitions is given of the principal quantities pertaining to oxygen in blood in relation to the methods employed in the measurement of the quantities. Its core is the correct definition of oxygen saturation of hemoglobin as given in equations [3], [6], and [12a], which is in agreement with that given by NCCLS[19]. This system at least is consistent and the arguments are presented in this paper in a number of statements. The core of it is the correct definition on oxygen saturation of hemoglobin as given in and around equation [3].

STATEMENTS ON O_2 IN BLOOD

1. Molecular oxygen (O_2) in blood exists in two forms: that associated with hemoglobin and that dissolved in blood but not associated with any other substance. The substance concentration of total O_2 is defined as the sum of the substance concentrations of these two forms.

2. The substance concentration of total O_2 in blood (ctO_2) is given by

$$ctO_2 = cO_2(Hb) + cO_2 \qquad [1]$$

where $cO_2(Hb)$ and cO_2 are the substance concentrations of hemoglobin-bound O_2 and freely dissolved O_2, respectively. The commonly used unit is mmol/L.

Oxygen Transport to Tissue XV, Edited by P. Vaupel
et al., Plenum Press, New York, 1994

3. Substance concentration of total O_2 corresponds with the earlier designation O_2 content, which is usually expressed in mL(STPD)/dL or mL(STPD)/L.

4. Freely dissolved O_2 is given by

$$cO_2 = \alpha O_2 * pO_2 \qquad [2]$$

where pO_2 is the O_2 partial pressure and αO_2 is the concentrational solubility coefficient in blood. At 37°C $\alpha O2 = 0.01$ mmol/L* $kPa^{1,2}$.

5. The O_2 capacity of blood (BO_2) is defined as the maximum amount of O_2 that can be carried by the hemoglobin contained in one volume unit of blood. It is usually expressed in mL(STPD)/dL or mL(STPD)/L, but in some applications mmol/L is more practical.

6. The O_2 saturation of blood (sO_2) is defined as the actual amount of hemoglobin-bound O_2 per unit volume of blood divided by the O_2 capacity:

$$sO_2 = cO_2(Hb)/BO_2 = (ctO_2 - cO_2)/BO_2 \qquad [3]$$

7. Originally, sO_2 was determined by gasometric methods such as the manometric VanSlyke-Neill procedure[3]. The O_2 content of a blood specimen was measured before and after equilibration with air and sO_2 was calculated with equation [3].

8. The binding of O_2 by hemoglobin is reversible and depends primarily on pO_2. The sO_2 corresponding with a given pO_2 is determined by the O_2 affinity. The O_2 affinity is commonly described with the help of the O_2 dissociation curve (ODC), which is a graph of sO_2 vs. pO_2.

9. Many factors affect the O_2 affinity of blood and cause a change in the position and/or the shape of the ODC. As a simple measure of the actual O_2 affinity of a blood specimen the pO_2 corresponding with $sO_2 = 50$ % ($p50$) is used.

10. A decrease in pH, an increase in pCO_2 and a rise in temperature cause the O_2 affinity of blood to decrease and the ODC to shift to the right. The ODC at plasma-pH = 7.40, pCO_2 = 5.33 kPa and $T = 37$ °C is called the standard-ODC, the corresponding $p50$ is called standard-$p50$ ($p50$(stand.)). Its normal value is 3.55 $kPa^{4,5}$.

11. Several additional factors modulate the O_2 affinity of blood and, consequently, affect the standard-ODC and $p50$(stand.): 2,3-diphosphoglycerate concentration in the erythrocytes, difference in pH between plasma and erythrocytes, fetal hemoglobin, glycated hemoglobin, abnormal hemoglobins and dyshemoglobins.

12. Abnormal hemoglobins are hemoglobin species with genetically determined alterations in the globin moiety. There are many of them, but only a few have a significantly different O_2 affinity.

13. Dyshemoglobins (dysHb) are normal hemoglobins which have permanently or temporarily lost the capability of reversible O_2 binding at physiological pO_2[6]. Well-known dyshemoglobins are methemoglobin (MetHb; Hi), carboxyhemoglobin (COHb) and sulfhemoglobin (SulfHb; SHb). Only MetHb and COHb are frequently present in human blood[7].

14. The international reference method for hemoglobin in human blood[8] measures the total hemoglobin concentration ($ctHb$)[9]. Consequently, when BO_2 is calculated from $ctHb$, the dyshemoglobin concentration ($cdysHb$) has to be taken into account:

$$BO_2 = ctHb - cdysHb \qquad\qquad [4]$$

when B and c are expressed in mmol/L, or

$$BO_2 = \beta O_2 \, (ctHb - cdysHb) \qquad\qquad [5]$$

when B is expressed in mL/L and c in g/L; βO_2 is the volume of O_2 in mL(STPD) which can be bound by 1 g of hemoglobin.

15. Theoretically, $\beta O_2 = 22394/16114.5 = 1.39$ mL/g, where 22394 is the molecular volume of O_2 in mL(STPD) and 16114.5 is the quarter molecular mass of human HbA in g[10]. The experimental value of βO_2 has been found quite near the theoretical one[6].

16. The early one- and two-color photometric methods for the determination of sO_2 were calibrated against VanSlyke's method[11]. The usual spectrophotometric procedures are 2-λ methods analyzing the two-component system oxyhemoglobin/deoxyhemoglobin (O_2Hb/HHb).They donot measure the substance concentrations of the two hemoglobin species but only their ratio. For these methods the defining equation of sO_2 is usually written as

$$sO_2 = cO_2Hb/(cO_2Hb + cHHb) \qquad\qquad [6]$$

which is equivalent with [3]. By proper selection of the wavelengths, interference by other colored substances such as COHb, MetHb and indocyanine green can be minimized[9]. This also holds good for most pulse oximeters[12].

17. Multiwavelength spectrophotometric methods[13], and automated multiwavelength photometers for routine measurement of hemoglobin derivatives ("CO-oximeters"), such as the IL282[14] and 482, the Corning 2500 and 270, and the Radiometer OSM 3[15], actually determine the substance concentrations of the chosen hemoglobin derivatives. From the concentrations various other quantities are calculated. Usually only these derived quantities are displayed.

18. In the vast majority of cases it is sufficient to measure O_2Hb, HHb, COHb, and MetHb. From the substance concentrations of these hemoglobin species the following derived quantities can be calculated:

$$ctHb = cO_2Hb + cHHb + cCOHb + cMetHb \qquad\qquad [7]$$

$$FO_2Hb = cO_2Hb/ctHb \qquad\qquad [8]$$

$$FHHb = cHHb/ctHb \qquad\qquad [9]$$

$$FCOHb = cCOHb/ctHb \qquad\qquad [10]$$

$$FMetHb = cMetHb/ctHb \qquad\qquad [11]$$

$$sO_2 = cO_2Hb/(ctHb - cdysHb) \qquad\qquad [12a]$$

$$sO_2 \approx cO_2Hb/(ctHb - cCOHb - cMetHb) \qquad [12b]$$

$$cO_2(Hb) = FO_2Hb * ctHb = sO_2 * (ctHb - cdysHb) \qquad [13a]$$
when c is expressed in mmol/L

$$cO_2(Hb) = \beta O_2 * FO_2Hb * ctHb = \beta O_2 * sO_2 * (ctHb - cdysHb) \qquad [13b]$$
when $cO_2(Hb)$ is expressed in mL/L, and $ctHb$ and $cdysHb$ in g/L

Equation [12a] is equivalent with [6].

19. From [8] and [12a] it follows that when $cdysHb = 0$, $i.e$ when the blood does not contain any COHb and MetHb or any other dyshemoglobin, $sO_2 = FO_2Hb$. Because in healthy men and even in the majority of patients the blood actually contains little dyshemo-globin[6], the numerical difference between sO_2 and FO_2Hb is usually but slight. Yet the quantities should not be confused. Any discussion of the influence of dyshemoglobins on the oxygen affinity of hemoglobin is impossible when the distinction between sO_2 and FO_2Hb is lost.

20. Recently, the literature has been burdened with a futile discussion concerning which quantities are the most appropriate for being displayed by a CO-oximeter. The crucial quantity in the O_2 supply to the tissues is the end-capillary pO_2. This quantity is on the one hand determined by perfusion parameters and capillary architecture, and on the other hand by the O_2 transport properties of the blood and the arterial pO_2. About the latter a CO-oximeter can give a wealth of information: $ctHb$ is the principal determinant of the O_2 capacity, sO_2 represents pO_2, and knowledge of both **FCOHb** and **FMetHb** is desirable, because they similarly affect O_2 capacity and O_2 affinity, but need different therapeutic interventions. Therefore, since all four of them are available, all four should be displayed. This does not yield a complete picture of the O_2 transport capability of blood ($p50$ is still lacking), but for practical purposes it is usually enough.

21. Since FO_2Hb depends on pO_2 and $cdysHb$, $FO_2Hb > 95\%$ signals that pO_2 is high enough and that no appreciable amounts of COHb and MetHb are present. However, when FO_2Hb is too low, it does not convey much useful information anymore, because the decrease may be caused either by a fall in pO_2 or by an increase in $cdysHb$ or by both. Moreover, it should be stressed that FO_2Hb is **not** a measure of hemoglobin-bound O_2 in the blood (cf. equation [13a and b]).

22. Although reporting and interpretation may remain to a certain extent a matter of opinion, there can hardly be any disagreement about the necessity that it should be crystal-clear what appears on the display of a CO-oximeter and that users should understand how the quantities relevant to O_2 in blood are defined. The former is the responsibility of the manufacturer, the latter can easily be attained with the help of the literature[16,20].

23. The data processor of most automated blood gas analyzers contains an algorithm for calculating sO_2 from pO_2, pH, and pCO_2, which is based on the standard-ODC. For normal adult human blood this yields a fairly accurate estimate of sO_2. When, however, one or more additional determinants of the O_2 affinity are outside their normal range, the error in the calculated sO_2 may be considerable[9]. An appreciable difference between the calculated sO_2 and sO_2 as measured with a CO-oximeter points to a deviating O_2 affinity.

24. By using a blood gas analyzer in combination with a CO-oximeter[5], $p50$ can be estimated. The accuracy of such a determination of p50 is limited, but gross deviations in the O_2 affinity of blood can be reliably detected[21].

REFERENCES

1. Christoforides C, Hedley-White J. Effect of temperature and hemoglobin concentration on the solubility of O_2 in blood. J Appl Physiol 27, 592-59106, 1969.

2. Roughton FJW, Severinghaus JW. Accurate determination of O_2 dissociation curve of human blood above 98.7% saturation with data on O_2 solubility in unmodified human blood from 0 to 37 °C. J Appl Physiol 35, 861-869, 1973.

3. VanSlyke DD, Neill JM. Determination of gases in blood and other solutions by vacuum extraction and manometric measurement. J Biol Chem 61, 523-573, 1924.

4. Zwart A, Kwant G, Oeseburg B, Zijlstra WG. Oxygen dissociation curves for whole blood, recorded with an instrument that continously measures pO_2 and sO_2 independently at constant T, $pCO2$, and pH. Clin Chem 28, 1287-1292, 1982.

5. Wimberley PD, Burnett RW, Covington AK, Fogh-Andersen N, Maas AHJ, Müller-Plathe O, Siggaard-Andersen O, Zijlstra WG. Guidelines for routine measurement of blood hemoglobin oxygen affinity. Scand J Clin Lab Invest 50, suppl 203, 227-234, 1990.

6. Dijkhuizen P, Buursma A, Fongers TME, Gerding AM, Oeseburg B, Zijlstra WG. The oxygen binding capacity of human haemoglobin. Hüffner's factor redetermined. Pflügers Arch 369, 223-231, 1977.

7. Zwart A, van Kampen EJ, Zijlstra WG. Results of routine determination of clinically significant hemoglobin derivatives by multicomponent analysis. Clin Chem 32, 972--978, 1986.

8. International Committee for Standardization in Haematology. Recommendations for reference method for haemoglobinometry in human blood (ICSH standard 1986) and specifications for international haemiglobincyanide reference preparation (3rd edition). Clin lab Haemat 9, 73-79, 1987.

9. Van Kampen EJ, Zijlstra WG. Spectrophotometry of hemoglobin and hemoglobin derivatives. Adv Clin Chem 23, 199-257, 1983.

10. Braunitzer G, Gehring-Müller R, Hilschmann N, Hilse K, Hobom G, Rudolf V, Wittmann-Liebold B. Die Konstitution des normalen adulten Humanhämoglobins. Hoppe Seylers Z Physiol Chem 325, 283-288, 1961.

11. Brinkman R, Zijlstra WG. Determination and continuous registration of the percentage oxygen saturation in clinical condition. Arch Chir Neerl 1, 177-183, 1949.

12. Zijlstra WG, Buursma A, Meeuwsen-van der Roest WP. Absorption spectra of human fetal and adult oxyhemoglobin, de-oxyhemoglobin, carboxyhemoglobin, and methemoglobin. Clin Chem 37, 1633-1638, 1991.

13. Zwart A, Buursma A, Van Kampen EJ, Zijlstra WG. Multicomponent analysis of hemoglobin derivatives with a reversed-optics spectrophotometer. Clin Chem 30, 373-379, 1984.

14. Zwart A, Buursma A, Oeseburg B, Zijlstra WG. Determination of hemoglobin

derivatives with the IL 282 CO-oximeter as compared with a manual spectrophotometric five-wavelength method. Clin Chem 27, 1903-1907, 1981.

15. Zijlstra WG, Buursma A, Zwart A. Performance of an automated six-wavelength photometer (Radiometer OSM 3) for routine measurement of hemoglobin derivatives. Clin Chem 34, 149-152, 1988.

16. Zijlstra WG. Quantitative evaluation of the oxygen transport capability of human blood. Pflügers Arch 408, S9-S10, 1987.

17. Zijlstra WG, Oeseburg B. Definition and notation of hemoglobin oxygen saturation. IEEE Trans Biomed Eng 36, 872, 1989.

18. Moran RF, Clausen JL, Ehrmeyer S, Feil M, Van Kessel AL, Eichhorn JH. Oxygen content, hemoglobin oxygen saturation, and related quantities in blood: terminology, measurement, and reporting. NCCLS Document C25-P. Vol 10, No 2, 1990.

19. Ehrmeyer S, Burnett RW, Chatburn RL, Christiansen TF, Clausen JL, Cormier AD, Durst RA, Eichhorn JH, Fallon KD, Moran RG, Van Kessel AL. Definitions of quantities and conventions related to blood pH and gas analysis. NCCLS Document C12-T2. Vol 11, No 18, 1991.

20. Wimberley PD, Siggaard-Andersen O, Fogh-Andersen N, Zijlstra WG, Severinghaus JW. Haemoglobin oxygen saturation and related quantities: definitions, symbols and clinical use. Scand J Clin Lab Invest 50, 455-459, 1990.

21. Kwant G, Oeseburg B, Zijlstra WG. Reliability of the determination of whole-blood oxygen affinity by means of blood-gas analyzers and multiwavelength oximeters. Clin Chem 35, 773-777, 1989.

QUANTITIES AND UNITS IN GAS EXCHANGE PHYSIOLOGY

Jacob P. Zock

Department of Medical Physiology
University of Groningen
Bloemsingel 10, 9712 KZ Groningen, The Netherlands

INTRODUCTION

In 1971 Piiper *et al.* published a paper in which they discussed concepts and basic quantities in gas exchange physiology [1]. The goal of the paper was "an attempt to express basic concepts of gas transport in such a manner that, whatever the transport mechanism (convection and/or diffusion) and whatever the transport medium (gas, water or blood), the process can be presented in a general frame of reference with comparable units." The authors argued that it would be better to express amounts of substances in the unit "mol" instead of "liter" or "milliliter" as usual in respiratory physiology. This goal has still not been reached. A start seemed to be made when in the *Glossary on respiration and gas exchange* the "mmol" was given beside the "mL (STPD)" [1] to express the amount of oxygen in the definition of oxygen concentration but in the definitions of oxygen consumption, oxygen uptake, oxygen capacity, and the diffusing capacity of the lung, volumes of oxygen were used as a measure of the amount of substance [2].

Already in 1950, eleven renowned physiologists agreed upon a set of symbols to be used in respiratory physiology [3]. These symbols have played the role of a *de facto* standard in respiratory physiology for more than forty years. A disadvantage, already recognized by the authors, is the fact that there is abundant use of double subscripts, *i.e.* subscripts to subscripts, which makes it hard to use in typewriting and word processing. The symbols imply that an amount of gas is expressed as a volume.

In 1976, the editorial board of *Pflügers Archiv (European Journal of Physiology)* decided to recommend the use of the International System of Units (*SI*) in all papers to be published in the journal [4]. The *SI* is described in English *e.g.* in [5].

At its establishment the *European Coal and Steel Community* launched research programs concerning respiratory diseases. A part of one of the programs was the

---

[1]The capital "L" is a symbol admitted for the unit "liter". Its use, instead of "l", prevents confusion with the character "1".

harmonization and standardization of respiratory function tests. The results are given in a report published in 1983 [6]. The report contains an extensive list of symbols and units for quantities in respiratory physiology. The use of *SI* units is generally recommended (except for blood pressure).

The measurement and the presentation of blood gas and acid-base status has been standardized by the *International Federation of Clinical Chemistry* (IFCC) [7]. The standardization includes the terminology, the symbols and the units. The document is co-authored by the *International Union of Pure and Applied Chemistry* (IUPAC). The standards are, as far as applicable, in conformity with standards of physical chemistry agreed upon by the *International Union of Pure and Applied Physics* (IUPAP) [8]. Apart from the fact that in the IFCC recommendations time dependent quantities are lacking, the recommendations comply well with those of [6]. An overview regarding standards of hemoglobin oxygen saturation is given in [9, 10]. The IFCC standard of hemoglobin and related quantities in blood is now in the course of being adopted in the United States by the *National Committee on Clinical Laboratory Standards* [11, 12].

The development of transcutaneous measurement of oxygen in blood has given rise to a wealth of symbols to denote oxygen saturation measured with this technique [13]. The problem is that the outcome of transcutaneous measurement deviates from oxygen saturation determined with a reference method. In the special session on *Terminology and Definitions in Respiratory Physiology* at the 1992 meeting of the *International Society on Oxygen Transport to Tissue* (ISOTT) in Mainz (Germany) it was discussed whether clinical judgement would benefit from the introduction of new definitions and symbols to account for this. There was not much support and new symbols were considered superfluous [14]. Other subjects discussed concerned symbols and units used in oxygen exchange physiology and its clinical application. These symbols and terms are listed as well in [13].

In this paper it is argued that some terms and symbols used in oxygen exchange physiology should be more strictly defined. Symbols should clearly show what they stand for and they should comply as much as possible with accepted standards in related fields. The standards proposed and adopted in the fields of lung function testing and blood gas and acid-base measurement cover to a large extent the field of oxygen transport and may therefore be used as recommended standards in the ISOTT [6, 7]. Arguments in favor of the use of the "mol" as the unit to express the amount of substance in gas exchange physiology are repeated.

CONCEPTS, QUANTITIES AND SYMBOLS

Science consists of human activities aimed at maintaining and extending a logically coherent description of all observable phenomena. It cannot be separated from technology which consists of prescriptions, protocols and equations which if correctly applied by skilled people as techniques, give predictable and reproducible, observable effects. For communication of ideas among humans language is needed. Scientific language is a mixture of natural language – mainly English – and expressions and terminology specific for the various fields of science. Besides general conventions, fields in science have their own terminology and symbols. Although their use is inevitable, conventions generally agreed upon should be used as much as possible. This improves mutual understanding and enhances new developments which often occur between different fields. In equations the language of science is mathematics, at least for its grammar.

The idiom in the equations are the symbols for the various quantities. A consistent terminology is needed to describe quantities and the relations between them.

A physical quantity is a numerical value times a unit [8]. To get a coherent representation of observable phenomena a coherent system of units is necessary. A well chosen system of units minimizes the use of conversion coefficients or factors in equations which describe the relations between quantities. This is the most evident in large sets of equations interrelated by quantities they have in common.

Physiology as part of science is situated in between biology, chemistry, and physics. Medical practice is in part applied physiology. Only a small part of the descriptions in physiology are in the form of quantitative relations. In most cases equations are used separately or in connection with only a small number of other equations. and the necessity of a coherent set of quantities and units is not of much concern. In clinical medicine often only one or a few quantities are considered in decision making. Equations are not much favored in this respect and if necessary a dedicated apparatus contracts the quantitative information to a single value. As a result the many fields of medical physiology and medicine have their own, different symbols for the same quantity. Even in the same field symbols used for certain quantities may differ between authors. Readability would be much improved if a basic set of symbols would be agreed upon. Even more so, if - where applicable - these symbols are identical to those used in related fields for the same quantities.

Modeling reality has eventually be done in terms of observable quantities. However, models often contain quantities that cannot be determined directly as observable quantities but are idealizations, representing abstract ideas, concepts. Such a conceptual quantity used in ISOTT is the flowrate of oxygen from the environment to the tissues. The flowrate of oxygen is the result of many processes acting and interacting at different levels in series and in parallel. There is advantage in the use of one symbol for a conceptual quantity such as the flowrate of oxygen. This is similar to the use of one symbol for electric current in physics and electrical engineering. In agreement with the standards in clinical chemistry and respiratory physiology this symbol might be chosen $e.g.$ as $\dot{n}O_2$.

Einstein should have said that "the definition of a quantity is the way it is measured". This is a practical approach which leaves no room for doubt, but it also gives rise to problems. Conceptual quantities do not exist according to this statement. When a conceptual quantity is measured in two independent ways, this would mean two different quantities. However, comparison of these measured values would not make sense when we could not refer to the concept behind the quantities. Probably, the statement should not be understood that strictly. It stresses that one ought to be aware that the way quantities are obtained should be taken into consideration at the interpretation of results.

Well defined terms are important for the communication on and the correct use of concepts. The terms *oxygen supply* and *oxygen delivery* are often used as synonyms. The ambiguity in the every-day use of the terms *supply* and *delivery* might be prevented by strict definitions. The concept which contributes to the confusion is the steady state. A steady state is often implicitly assumed in reasonings on physiological experiments. Then the supply-side concept of delivered oxygen is automatically set equal to the demand-side concept of consumption. However, when considering non-steady state situations this is not correct most of the time. Part of the delivered oxygen is dissolved in the tissue and later used up. Low pO_2 in muscle tissue may be caused by the microcirculation being switched on and off. Oxygen is then temporarily stored as dissolved oxygen and in muscles bound to myoglobin. The delivery to the stores is intermittent. Temporarily, even a negative delivery may coexist with a positive supply if oxygen from the tissue is taken up by circulating blood. Over longer periods the time-averaged consumption will be virtually equal to the time-averaged delivery because the storage capacity of tissue for oxygen is limited.

Symbols for *oxygen supply* and *oxygen delivery* should be easy to understand and coherent with those used in related fields. With the symbol for *amount of oxygen per unit of time* mentioned they might be defined as follows.

OXYGEN SUPPLY is the amount of oxygen per unit of time brought to a tissue by the blood. This is mostly arterial blood: symbol $\dot{n}O_2(a)$, but oxygen supply may also be provided by the portal vein to the liver, $\dot{n}O_2(\text{portal vein})$, or the placental vein to the fetus, $\dot{n}O_2(\text{placental vein})$. For the indication of *arterial* and *mixed venous* the letters "a" and "$\bar{v}$" are used conform [3, 6, 7].

OXYGEN DELIVERY is the amount of oxygen per unit of time given off in a tissue. For most tissues or organs this is $\dot{n}O_2(a)$-$\dot{n}O_2(\bar{v})$. This may also be written as $\dot{n}O_2(a-\bar{v})$, but for the fetus this would mean $\dot{n}O_2(\text{umbilical vein - umbilical arteries})$ and for the liver $\dot{n}O_2(\text{hepatic artery + portal vein - hepatic veins})$.

AV DIFFERENCE. Confusion also may arise in the use of the term *arterio-venous difference*, because there are many differences. The problem may be resolved by the use of the symbol of the quantity concerned with the "Δ" prefixed to the symbol (*cf.* Table 1). Between brackets behind the synbol it can be indicated that the a-v difference is meant.

Table 1. Representation of av differences

Quantity	Example 1	Example 2
Oxygen pressure	$\Delta pO_2(a-v)$	$\Delta pO_2(av)$
Oxygen concentration	$\Delta cO_2(a-v)$	$\Delta cO_2(av)$
Oxygen saturation	$\Delta sO_2(a-v)$	$\Delta sO_2(av)$

UNITS

The use of a set of well chosen symbols is of little use if it does not have its complement in a well chosen set of coherent units. Such a set is the *SI*. In the *SI* the "mol" is the unit of amount of substance. The unit "mol" is unambiguous. Advantages of the use of the mol for the amount of substance in combination with symbols recommended for use in the representation of the results of pulmonary function tests and in clinical chemistry can be illustrated in equations of oxygen transport.

Equations concerning the gas phase can be best derived from the general ideal gas equation:

$$pX \cdot V = nX \cdot R \cdot T \tag{1}$$

Here, X stands for the gas considered, T is temperature in K (and not °K as in [15]) and $R = 8.3143$ joule/(mol·K). Differentiating the left and right hand side with respect to time leads to

$$pX \cdot \dot{V} = \dot{n}X \cdot R \cdot T \tag{2}$$

These equations in combination with knowledge of the partial pressure of water vapor can be used to derive the other gas equations of respiratory physiology, no matter what circumstances are present.

934

Alveolar ventilation and CO_2 given off:

$$\dot{V}_A = \frac{R \cdot T \cdot \dot{n}CO_2(E - I)}{1000 \cdot pCO_2(A)} \tag{3}$$

Here "E" stands for expired and "I" for inspired gas, and

$$\dot{n}CO_2(I - E) \equiv \dot{n}CO_2(I) - \dot{n}CO_2(E) \tag{4}$$

In the equation a factor 1000 has been introduced. It makes that $\dot{V}_A$ can be expressed in L/min, $\dot{n}CO_2$ in mmol/min and pCO_2 in kPa.

Ventilation and oxygen uptake:

$$\dot{n}O_2(I - E) \equiv \dot{n}O_2(I) - \dot{n}O_2(E) = \frac{1000}{R \cdot T} \cdot (pO_2 \cdot \dot{V}_I - pO_2 \cdot \dot{V}_E) \tag{5}$$

The right hand term can be converted into other expressions depending on the circumstances *e.g.* that given in [3].

Pulmonary transfer of oxygen:

$$\dot{n}O_2(A - a) = T_{L,O_2} \cdot (pO_2(A) - pO_2(a)) = T_{L,O_2} \cdot \Delta pO_2(A - a) \tag{6}$$

The symbol T_{L,O_2} for the transfer factor of oxygen and its unit mmol/(L · kPa) are both recommended in [6].

Transport of oxygen with blood, supply to the body:

$$\dot{n}O_2(\text{supply}) = \dot{Q}_{\text{pul}} \cdot [sO_2(a) \cdot (cHb(\text{tot}) - cHb(\text{dys})) + \alpha_{O_2} \cdot pO_2(a)] \tag{7}$$

Cardiac output is in L/min, cHb in mmol/L, sO_2 between 0 and 1, and the result $\dot{n}O_2$ in mmol/min.

Oxygen transport with the blood, delivered to the body:

$$\dot{n}O_2(\text{delivery}) = \dot{Q}_{\text{pul}} \cdot [(sO_2(a) - sO_2(\bar{v})) \cdot (cHb(\text{tot}) - cHb(\text{dys})) +$$
$$+ \alpha_{O_2} \cdot (pO_2(a) - pO_2(\bar{v}))] \tag{8}$$

If necessary in the equations it is simple to calculate the volume of a gas from the amount in mmol. For clinical applications where an accurate determination of the amount of oxygen is not present, it would be sufficient to take 25 mL as the equivalent of 1 mmol of gas at room temperature. In case an exact determination is required, a sophisticated measurement set-up is mostly already present which will be able to calculate the amount in mmol.

DISCUSSION AND CONCLUSION

A number of standards are already recommended or accepted covering a large part of gas exchange physiology [5, 6, 7, 11, 12]. For those quantities and symbols used in the ISOTT and not covered in these recommendations, terminology and symbols should be defined such as to get consistent with existing standards. The definitions should be formulated with utmost care because errors may be easily made. An example of a proposal which appears to be issued immaturely is [15]. In the paper some disturbing errors are present beside the one above-mentioned. The authors present 273.16 K as the zero point of the celsius temperature scale and the paper contains a table in which entries occur which do not belong to categories indicated in the caption. As papers like this may get the status of a *de facto* standard the errors they contain may get widespread. The paper mentioned may serve as a warning to the ISOTT that a recommendation for terminology and symbols should not too hastily be formulated. The decision at the session *Terminology and Definitions in Respiratory Physiology* at the ISOTT 1992 meeting to adopt the new symbol for delivered oxygen as "TO_2" should be reconsidered.

In the standards for clinical chemistry and for clinical respiratory physiology the "mol" is the accepted basic unit for the amount of substance. As this unit is independent of the circumstances it is well suited to be used in gas exchange physiology. The notion that "mL (STPD)" is better suited because it complies with real measurements is a fallacy. In both cases calculations are needed to eliminate the effects of temperature and water vapor pressure. The "mol" could therefore be recommended as the basic unit of amount substance to be used in oxygen exchange physiology as well.

In order to reach agreement on terminology, symbols and units for use in the ISOTT the possibility to install a working committee to prepare proposals on this issue might be considered. Proposals could be made available before the meeting. They may then be discussed in a special session at each meeting, like the one in Mainz, but without the need to reach instant agreement.

REFERENCES

1. J. Piiper, P. Dejours, P. Haab and H. Rahn, Concepts and basic quantities in gas exchange physiology, *Resp. Physiol.* 13: 292-304 (1971).
2. H. Bartels, P. Dejours, R.H. Kellog, J. Mead (Subcommitte for Respiration, International Union of Physiological Sciences), Glossary on respiration and gas exchange, *J. Appl. Physiol.* 34: 549-558 (1973).
3. J.R. Pappenheimer, Standardization of definitions and symbols in respiratory physiology, *Federation Proc.* 9: 602-605 (1950).
4. W.G. Zijlstra, Introduction to the use of the International System of Units (SI) in the papers to be published in Pflügers Archiv, *European Journal of Physiology. Pflügers Arch.* 368: 1-2 (1977).
5. D.T. Goldman and R.J. Bell (eds), "SI, The International System of Units," 4th edition, HMSO, London (1982).
   Tranlation of:
   Bureau de Poids et Mésures, "Le Système International d'Unités."
6. Ph.H. Quanjer (ed.), Standardized lung function testing, Report Working Party "Standardization of Lung Function Tests," European Community for Coal and Steel, Luxembourg, *Clin. Resp. Physiol. (Bull. Eur. de Physiopath. Resp.)*, suppl. 5, chap. 8 (1983).
7. O. Siggaard-Andersen, R.A. Durst, A.H.J. Maas (eds) (International Federation of Clinical Chemistry and International Union of Pure and Applied Chemistry), Approved recommendation (1984) on physico-chemical quantities and units in clinical chemistry, *J. Clin. Chem. Clin. Biochem.* 25: 369-391 (1987).
8. E.R. Cohen and P. Giacomo, "Symbols, Units, Nomenclature and Fundamental Constants in Physics (1987 Revision)," International Union of Pure and Applied Physics, SUNAMCO commission, *Document I.U.P.A.P.-25* (SUNAMCO 87-1) (1987).
9. W.G. Zijlstra and B. Oeseburg, Definition and notation of hemoglobin oxygen saturation, *IEEE Trans. Biomed. Eng.* 36: 872 (1989).

10. P.D. Wimberley, O. Siggaard-Andersen, N. Fogh-Andersen, W.G. Zijlstra and J.W. Severinghaus, Haemoglobin oxygen saturation and related quantities; definitions, symbols and clinical use, *Scand. J. Clin. Lab. Invest.* 50: 455-459 (1990).

11. R.F. Moran, J.L. Clausen, S. Ehrmeyer *et al.*, Oxygen content, hemoglobin oxygen "saturation," and related quantities in blood: terminology, measurement, and reporting, *National Committee on Clinical Laboratory Standards, Document* C25-P (Proposed Guideline) Vol. 10 number 2, ISSN 0273-3099 (1990).

12. S. Ehrmeyer, R.W. Burnett, R.L. Chatburn *et al.*, Definitions of quantities and conventions related to blood pH and gas analysis, *National Committee on Clinical Laboratory Standards, Document* C12-T2 (Tentative Standard) Vol. 11 number 18, ISSN 0273-3099 (1991).

13. R. Zander and F. Merzluft, Oxygen parameters of blood: definitions and symbols, *Scand. J. Clin. Lab. Invest.* 50, *Suppl.* 203: 177-185 (1990).

14. J.W. Severinghaus, Nomenclature of oxygen saturation, *This volume.*

15. J.B. Bassingthwaighte, F.P. Chinard, C. Crone *et al.*, Terminology for mass transport and exchange, *Am. J. Physiol.* 250 (*Heart Circ. Physiol.* 19): H539-H546 (1986).

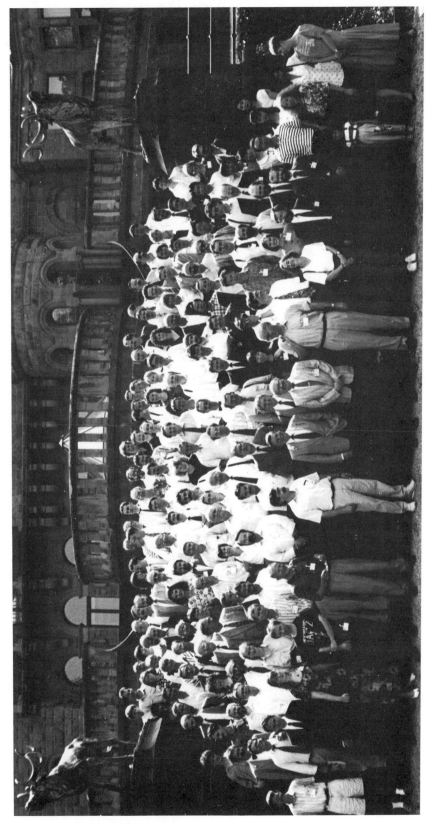

GROUP PHOTOGRAPH

AUTHOR INDEX

SUBJECT INDEX

Acetate hemodialysis, 139
Acid-base equilibria, modeling, 151
Acidosis, 133
   metabolic, 122
   non-respiratory, 140
   respiratory, 123
Adenosine, 260
Adenosine diphosphate, *see* ADP
Adenosine monophosphate, *see* AMP
Adenosine triphosphate, *see* ATP
ADP
   skeletal muscle, 400
   tumor, 396
Adult respiratory distress syndrome, 51, 55, 83,
         95, 113, 117, 741
Airway resistance, 67
Alveolar exudate, 90
AMP
   skeletal muscle, 400
   tumor, 396, 404
Anemia, 755
   organ blood flow, 377
   oxygen transport, 755
   tumor, 525
   tumor oxygenation, 521
Angiogenesis, brain hypoxia, 627
Angiotensin II, tumor blood flow, 423
Anion exchange
   catalytic cycle, 169
   electrodiffusion model, 174
   erythrocyte, 167, 169
Anion transport, ping-pong mechanism, 168, 174
Anion transporter, 168
Anoxia, myocardium, 255
Antioxidant enzymes, 59
Antioxidant vitamins, 191
Apnea, 126
   iatrogenic, 45
Arachidonic acid metabolites, 113
Arterial occlusive disease, 178, 731, 885
Artificial oxygen carriers, 197-240
Asphyxia, perinatal, 592
Astrup micromethod, 140, 145

Atelectasis, 90, 113
ATP
   skeletal muscle, 400
   tumor, 387, 396
Autoradiography, 388, 423
Autoregulation index, 320
Autoregulation, coronary blood flow, 317
Autoregulatory gain, 320

Basal metabolic rate, 764
Beer-Lambert Law, 861
Bicarbonate, 154
   hemodialysis, 139
   transport, 168
Bicarbonate-pH diagram, 157
Bioluminescence, 387
Bioreductive agents, 417, 498
Blood, oxygen status, 849
Blood exchange, isovolemic, 207
Blood flow, *see also* Perfusion
Blood flow
   brain, 576, 619
   gut, 238
   heart, 260, 299, 317-323, 904
   limb, 237
   lung, 7, 877
   microvascular, 853
   mismatch, 903
   oxygen transport, 755
   placenta, 149
   regional, 877
   skin, 425
   tumor, 367-373, 375-379, 403, 423, 501, 509,
      531
Blood gas equilibria, modeling, 151
Blood lamella method, 8
Blood volume, brain, 560, 619
Body plethysmography, 85
Bohr coefficient, 206
Bohr effect, 133
Brain, 559-658
   blood flow, 576, 619
   blood volume, 560, 619

Oxygen saturation
  arterial, 198
  definitions, 925-928
  fractional, 140, 145
  functional, 140, 145
  measurement, 925-928
  mixed venous, 198
  nomenclature, 921-923, 925-929
Oxygen solubility, 208, 236, 291
Oxygen solubility coefficient, blood, 926
Oxygen status, blood, 849
Oxygen store, intrapulmonary, 49
Oxygen supply
  brain, 34
  heart, 291
  placenta, 709
  skeletal muscle, 280
  volume substitution, 742
Oxygen tension
  distribution, 15, 901
  histograms, 567
  microvascular, 129
  transcutaneous, 731
Oxygen toxicity, 191
Oxygen transfer, maternal-fetal, 145
Oxygen transport, 747
  anemia, 755
  limitations, 747, 755
  modeling, 33, 893, 901
Oxygen transport rate, 209
Oxygen uptake, 208
  fetal, 149
  gut, 238
  limb, 237
  whole body, 237
Oxygen utilization, 236
Oxygenation
  apneic, 50
  arterial, 92
Oxygenation
  astrocytomas, 467
  benign breast tumors, 456
  brain, 559, 567, 579, 590, 603, 609
  brain metastases, 467, 474
  brain tumors, 465-469, 471-476
  breast cancer, 451, 459, 479, 485
  cervix cancer, 445
  gastric mucosa, 742
  heart, 275, 283, 293, 896
  hemodilution, 239
  human tumors, 445
  hyperbaric, 175, 181, 189
  intracellular, 563
  myocardium, 253-258
  rectal cancer, 459, 479
  recurrent tumors, 459, 479
  role of capillary flow, 280
  skeletal muscle, 276-279, 693, 896
  soft tissue sarcoma, 459, 479
  spheroids, 345, 351-356

Oxygenation (*cont'd*)
  subcutis, 503
  tumor, 395, 403, 445, 451, 459, 465, 471, 479,
      493, 501, 505, 509, 517, 531, 539
Oxystat
  cuvette, 849
  photometer, 850
  system, 849

Perflubron, 197, 215, 221, 228, 235
  carbon dioxide solubility, 198
  intratracheal administration, 51
  intravascular half-life, 199
  osmolality, 198
  oxygen extraction coefficient, 201
  oxygen solubility, 198
  particle sizes, 198
  physico-chemical properties, 52
Perfluorocarbons, 51, 215, 221, 227, 240
  biocompatibility, 227
  biodistribution, 229
  emulsion stability, 227
  excretion, 227, 229
  metabolism, 229
  molecular dowel, 227
  oxygen delivery, 197
  oxygen transport, 227
  retention time, 229
Perfusion, *see also* Blood flow
Perfusion
  limitations, 105
  placenta, 709
  skin, 694
Permeability coefficent, oxygen, 727
PET, *see* Positron emission tomography
pH, gastric mucosa, 742
pH electrode, 344
Phagocyte activity, 215, 221
Phase modulated spectroscopy, 807, 829
Phenylephrine, 413
Phosphorescence
  intensity, 540
  lifetime, 540
Phosphorescence imaging, tumor, 539-540
Phosphorescence quenching, 129, 539
  oxygen dependency, 545
Phosphorus-NMR spectroscopy, 531
Photodynamic therapy, 437
Photometry, time-resolved, 862
Photon diffusion, 27-28
Photon diffusion coefficient, 27
Photon diffusion waves, 29
Photon migration, Monte Carlo simulation, 24,
      816
Physical performance, 733
Ping-pong mechanism, anion transport, 168
Placenta
  blood flow, 149
  gas exchange, 149
  oxygen consumption, 709